Marine Biomaterials

Marine Biomaterials

Characterization, Isolation and Applications

Edited by
Se-Kwon Kim

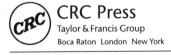

CRC Press
Taylor & Francis Group
Boca Raton London New York

CRC Press is an imprint of the
Taylor & Francis Group, an **informa** business

CRC Press
Taylor & Francis Group
6000 Broken Sound Parkway NW, Suite 300
Boca Raton, FL 33487-2742

© 2013 by Taylor & Francis Group, LLC
CRC Press is an imprint of Taylor & Francis Group, an Informa business

First issued in paperback 2017

No claim to original U.S. Government works
Version Date: 20121220

ISBN 13: 978-1-138-07638-9 (pbk)
ISBN 13: 978-1-4665-0564-3 (hbk)

Library of Congress Cataloging-in-Publication Data

Marine biomaterials : characterization, isolation, and applications / edited by Se-Kwon Kim.
    p. ; cm.
  Includes bibliographical references and index.
  ISBN 978-1-4665-0564-3 (alk. paper)
  I. Kim, Se-Kwon.
  [DNLM: 1. Biocompatible Materials--chemistry. 2. Biocompatible Materials--isolation & purification. 3. Aquatic Organisms--chemistry. 4. Aquatic Organisms--isolation & purification. 5. Biological Agents--therapeutic use. QT 37]

578.76--dc23   2012049633

Visit the Taylor & Francis Web site at
http://www.taylorandfrancis.com

and the CRC Press Web site at
http://www.crcpress.com

Contents

Part I Isolation and Characterization of Marine Biomaterials

Part II   Biological Activities of Marine Biomaterials

Part III Biomedical Applications of Marine Biomaterials

Part IV   Industrial Applications of Marine-Derived Biomaterials

Preface

Oceans not only consist of water but are also an abundant source of diverse biomaterials to mankind. Although marine biomaterial is an emerging area of research with significant applications, its usage is limited due to lack of research. To date, countable specific books are available for marine biomaterials as per my scientific knowledge. To bridge this gap and to provide a more comprehensive coverage of marine biomaterials, I decided to compile this literary work. This book presents the development of marine biomaterials and discusses various topics such as isolation and their characterization as well as applications from the preliminary research to clinical trials.

The focus of this book, *Marine Biomaterials: Characterization, Isolation and Applications,* is to provide an up-to-date coverage of marine biomaterials. The book has been divided into four major parts:

- Part I: Isolation and Characterization of Marine Biomaterials
  Marine biomaterials have a wide range of bioactivity, which can be utilized only once the isolation and characterization are accomplished in an appropriate manner. Part I covers the isolation and characterization of marine biomaterials (bioceramics, biopolymers, fatty acids, toxins and pigments, nanoparticles, and adhesive materials) and problems associated with them together with probable solutions for the same.

- Part II: Biological Activities of Marine Biomaterials
  Proper characterization ensures further use of the isolated/purified marine biomaterial in different applications. Part II deals mainly with biological applications of marine-derived biomaterials, for example, health benefits, potential biological activities of peptides, and biotoxins. In addition, antiviral activity, antidiabetic properties, and anticoagulant and anti-allergic effects of marine biomaterials have also been explored.

- Part III: Biomedical Application of Marine Biomaterials
  In recent days, significant development has been achieved with marine-derived bionanomaterials and nanocomposites in the area of biomedical applications (tissue engineering and drug delivery), and this is explored in Part III. Subsequently, several subsections deal with marine-derived chitosan and collagen usage in tissue engineering and scaffolding systems. The applicability of marine biomaterials in the drug delivery arena has also been discussed in light of the current available literature.

- Part IV: Industrial Application of Marine-Derived Biomaterials
  Last but not the least, the characterized material must reach the market, but for that it needs to be scaled up to the pilot plant level, which can be done only through industrialization. Part IV provides information about this important step of commercialization of marine biomaterials. This part includes the industrial application of marine polysaccharides and marine enzymes.

Various experts from around the globe (Europe, India, Asia-Pacific, Australia, Japan, Korea, and Vietnam) have contributed their knowledge and experience in the form of chapters in this book. I strongly believe that this book would provide sufficient knowledge about marine-derived biomaterials as it covers the key aspects of the majority of available marine biomaterials for biological and biomedical applications as well as presents techniques for future isolation of novel materials from the oceanic environment. The book covers a vast range of information available on isolation, characterization, as well as biological, biomedical, and industrial application of marine biomaterials, *all at one place*. It is essential reading for the novice and expert in the field of marine biomaterials, marine biotechnology, chemical sciences, natural products, materials science, pharmaceutical, nutraceuticals, and biomedical engineering sciences.

Prof. Se-Kwon Kim
Busan, South Korea

Acknowledgments

I would like to thank CRC Press, Taylor & Francis Group, for their encouragement and suggestions to get this wonderful compilation published. I would also like to extend my sincere gratitude to all the contributors for providing help, support, and advice to accomplish this task. Further, I would like to thank Dr. Jayachandran Venkatesan, who worked with me throughout the course of this book project. I strongly recommend this book for marine biomaterials researchers/students and hope that it helps to enhance their understanding in this field.

Editor

Professor Se-Kwon Kim, PhD, currently serves as a senior professor in the Department of Chemistry and the director of the Marine Bioprocess Research Center (MBPRC) at Pukyong National University in the Republic of Korea. He received his BSc, MSc, and PhD from the Pukyong National University and joined as a faculty member. He has previously served as a scientist in the University of Illinois, Urbana Champaign, Illinois (1988–1989), and was a visiting scientist at the Memorial University of Newfoundland in Canada (1999–2000).

Professor Se-Kwon Kim was president of the Korean Society of Chitin and Chitosan (1986–1990) and the Korean Society of Marine Biotechnology (2006–2007). He was also the chairman for the *7th Asia-Pacific Chitin and Chitosan Symposium*, which was held in South Korea in 2006. He is one of the board members of the International Society of Marine Biotechnology and the International Society for Nutraceuticals and Functional Foods. Moreover, he was the editor in chief of the *Korean Journal of Life Sciences* (1995–1997), the *Korean Journal of Fisheries Science and Technology* (2006–2007), and the *Korean Journal of Marine Bioscience and Biotechnology* (2006–present). His research has been credited with the best paper award from the American Oil Chemist's Society (AOCS) and the Korean Society of Fisheries Science and Technology in 2002.

Professor Se-Kwon Kim's major research interests are investigation and development of bioactive substances derived from marine organisms and their application in oriental medicine, nutraceuticals, and cosmeceuticals via marine bioprocessing and mass-production technologies. He has also conducted research on the development of bioactive materials from marine organisms for applications in oriental medicine, cosmeceuticals, and nutraceuticals. To date, he has authored over 500 research papers and holds 110 patents. In addition, he has written or edited more than 40 books.

Contributors

Snezana Agatonovic-Kustrin
School of Pharmacy and Applied Science
La Trobe University
Bendigo, Victoria, Australia

Abdul Bakrudeen Ali Ahmed
Faculty of Science
Institute of Biological Sciences
University of Kuala Lumpur
Kuala Lumpur, Malaysia

Toshihiro Akaike
Department of Biomolecular Engineering
Tokyo Institute of Technology
Yokohama, Japan

Muthuvel Arumugam
Faculty of Marine Sciences
Centre of Advanced Study in Marine
    Biology
Annamalai University
Chidambaram, India

R. Arun Kumar
Department of Biochemistry and
    Biotechnology
Annamalai University
Chidambaram, India

Thangavel Balasubramanian
Faculty of Marine Sciences
Centre of Advanced Study in Marine
    Biology
Annamalai University
Chidambaram, India

K.V. Bhaskara Rao
Environmental Biotechnology Division
School of Bio Sciences and Technology
VIT University
Vellore, India

A.N. Bedekar
Everest Biotech
Bangalore, India

Besim Ben-Nissan
Department of Chemistry
    and Forensic Science
University of Technology, Sydney
Broadway, New South Wales, Australia

Ira Bhatnagar
Marine Biochemistry Laboratory
Department of Chemistry
Pukyong National University
Busan, South Korea

and

Laboratory of Infectious Diseases
Centre for Cellular and Molecular Biology
Hyderabad, India

Subhasish Biswas
Department of Livestock Products
    Technology
West Bengal University of Animal
    and Fishery Sciences
Kolkata, India

Pablo R. Bonelli
Faculty of Exact and Natural Sciences
Department of Industry
University of Buenos Aires
and
National Council of Scientific and
    Technological Research
Buenos Aires, Argentina

Bruce F. Bowden
School of Pharmacy and Molecular
    Sciences
James Cook University
Douglas, Queensland, Australia

L. Brozova
Institute of Macromolecular Chemistry
Academy of Sciences of the Czech Republic
Prague, Czech Republic

Per Bruheim
Department of Biotechnology
Norwegian University of Science
    and Technology
Trondheim, Norway

Ana G. Cabado
Technological Centre for Seafood
    Preservation
National Association of Manufacturers of
    Canned Fish and Shellfish
Vigo, Spain

F. Carezzi
Centre of Nanoscience
Mavi Sud s.r.l
Aprilia, Italy

A. de Carlos
Faculty of Biology
Department of Biochemistry, Genetics and
    Immunology
University of Vigo
Vigo, Spain

Paula M.L. Castro
Biotechnology High School
Portuguese Catholic University
Porto, Portugal

Hyung Joon Cha
Department of Chemical Engineering
and
Marine BioMaterials Research Center
Pohang University of Science and
    Technology
Pohang, South Korea

María José Chapela
Technological Centre for Seafood
    Preservation
National Association of Manufacturers of
    Canned Fish and Shellfish
Vigo, Spain

Chong-Su Cho
Department of Agricultural Biotechnology
Institute for Agriculture
    and Life Sciences
Seoul National University
Seoul, South Korea

Myung-Haing Cho
Laboratory of Toxicology
College of Veterinary Medicine
Seoul National University
Seoul, South Korea

Yoo Seong Choi
Department of Chemical Engineering
Chungnam National University
Daejeon, South Korea

Yun-Jaie Choi
Department of Agricultural Biotechnology
Institute for Agriculture
    and Life Sciences
Seoul National University
Seoul, South Korea

Ana L. Cukierman
Faculty of Exact and Natural Sciences
Department of Industry
and
Faculty of Pharmacy and Biochemistry
Department of Pharmaceutical Technology
University of Buenos Aires
and
National Council of Scientific and
    Technological Research
Buenos Aires, Argentina

Uttam Datta
Department of Veterinary Gynaecology
    and Obstetrics
West Bengal University of Animal and
    Fishery Sciences
Kolkata, India

Keiichi Enomoto
School of Environmental Science and
    Engineering
Kochi University of Technology
Kami City, Japan

Tetsuya Furuike
Faculty of Chemistry, Materials and
    Bioengineering
Kansai University
Osaka, Japan

P. González
Department of Applied Physics
School of Industrial Engineering
University of Vigo
Vigo, Spain

David W. Green
Department of Chemistry and Forensic
    Science
University of Technology, Sydney
Broadway, New South Wales, Australia

Poul Erik Hansen
Department of Science, Systems
    and Models
Roskilde University
Roskilde, Denmark

Dong Soo Hwang
Ocean Science and Technology Institute
Pohang University of Science
    and Technology
Pohang, South Korea

R. Jayakumar
Amrita Centre for Nanosciences
    and Molecular Medicine
Amrita Institute of Medical Sciences
    and Research Centre
Kochi, India

Chidambaram Jayaseelan
Unit of Nanotechnology and Bioactive
    Natural Products
Post Graduate and Research Department
    of Zoology
C. Abdul Hakeem College
Vellore, India

Hu-Lin Jiang
Laboratory of Toxicology
College of Veterinary Medicine
Seoul National University
Seoul, South Korea

S.N. Joshi
Everest Biotech
Bangalore, India

Fatih Karadeniz
Department of Chemistry
Pukyong National University
Busan, South Korea

Mustafa Zafer Karagozlu
Department of Chemistry
Pukyong National University
Busan, South Korea

L. Karthik
Environmental Biotechnology Division
School of Bio Sciences and Technology
VIT University
Vellore, India

I. Kelnar
Institute of Macromolecular Chemistry
Academy of Sciences of the Czech
    Republic
Prague, Czech Republic

Christine Kettle
School of Pharmacy and Applied Science
La Trobe University
Bendigo, Victoria, Australia

Se-Kwon Kim
Department of Chemistry
and
Marine Bioprocess Research Center
Pukyong National University
Busan, South Korea

You-Kyoung Kim
Department of Agricultural Biotechnology
Institute for Agriculture
   and Life Sciences
Seoul National University
Seoul, South Korea

Arivarasan Vishnu Kirthi
Unit of Nanotechnology and Bioactive
   Natural Products
Post Graduate and Research Department of
   Zoology
C. Abdul Hakeem College
Vellore, India

L. Kobera
Institute of Macromolecular Chemistry
Academy of Sciences of the Czech
   Republic
Prague, Czech Republic

Gaurav Kumar
Environmental Biotechnology Division
School of Bio Sciences and Technology
VIT University
Vellore, India

Jorge Lago
Technological Centre for Seafood
   Preservation
National Association of Manufacturers of
   Canned Fish and Shellfish
Vigo, Spain

Ming Liu
Institute of Oceanology
Chinese Academy of Sciences
Qingdao, Shandong, People's Republic
   of China

M. López-Álvarez
Department of Applied Physics
School of Industrial Engineering
University of Vigo
Vigo, Spain

María C. Matulewicz
Faculty of Exact and Natural Sciences
Department of Organic Chemistry
University of Buenos Aires
and
National Council of Scientific and
   Technological Research
Buenos Aires, Argentina

Ambigapathi Moorthi
Department of Biotechnology
School of Bioengineering
SRM University
Chennai, India

P. Morganti
Department of Dermatology
University of Naples II
Naples, Italy

and

China Medical University
Shenyang, Liaoning, People's Republic of
   China

and

International Society of Cosmetics
   Dermatology
Rome, Italy

and

Centre of Nanoscience
Mavi Sud s.r.l,
Aprilia, Italy

David Morton
School of Pharmacy and Applied Science
La Trobe University
Bendigo, Victoria, Australia

Shantikumar V. Nair
Amrita Centre for Nanosciences and
   Molecular Medicine
Amrita Institute of Medical Sciences and
   Research Centre
Kochi, India

Samit Kumar Nandi
Department of Veterinary Surgery
   and Radiology
West Bengal University of Animal
   and Fishery Sciences
Kolkata, India

Ngo Dang Nghia
Institute of Biotechnology and
   Environment
Nha Trang University
Nha Trang, Vietnam

Dai-Hung Ngo
Department of Chemistry
Pukyong National University
Busan, South Korea

Dai-Nghiep Ngo
Faculty of Biology
Department of Biochemistry
University of Science
Vietnam National University
Ho Chi Minh City, Vietnam

Nitar Nwe
Dukkha Life Science Laboratory
Thanlyin, Myanmar

and

Food Engineering and Bioprocess
   Technology
Asian Institute of Technology
Bangkok, Thailand

and

Faculty of Chemistry, Materials and
   Bioengineering
Kansai University
Osaka, Japan

Alberto Otero
Technological Centre for Seafood
   Preservation
National Association of Manufacturers of
   Canned Fish and Shellfish
Vigo, Spain

Ramjee Pallela
Department of Chemistry
Institute of Biophysio Sensor
   Technology
Pusan National University
Busan, South Korea

and

International Centre for Genetic
   Engineering and Biotechnology
New Delhi, India

M. Palombo
Burn Center and Plastic Surgery
S. Eugenio Hospital
Rome, Italy

E. Pavlova
Institute of Macromolecular Chemistry
Academy of Sciences of the Czech
   Republic
Prague, Czech Republic

Clara Piccirillo
Biotechnology High School
Portuguese Catholic University
Porto, Portugal

Manuela M. Pintado
Biotechnology High School
Portuguese Catholic University
Porto, Portugal

Héctor J. Prado
Faculty of Exact and Natural Sciences
Department of Industry
and
Faculty of Pharmacy and Biochemistry
Department of Pharmaceutical
   Technology
University of Buenos Aires
and
National Council of Scientific and
   Technological Research
Buenos Aires, Argentina

Abdul Abdul Rahuman
Unit of Nanotechnology and Bioactive
  Natural Products
Post Graduate and Research Department of
  Zoology
C. Abdul Hakeem College
Vellore, India

R. Rajesh
Organic Chemistry Division
School of Advanced Sciences
VIT University
Vellore, India

Y. Dominic Ravichandran
Organic Chemistry Division
School of Advanced Sciences
VIT University
Vellore, India

Yuanfeng Ruan
Urological Department
Xuancheng Central Hospital
Xuancheng, Anhui, People's Republic of
  China

BoMi Ryu
Marine Bioprocess Research Center
Pukyong National University
Busan, South Korea

A. Malshani Samaraweera
Department of Animal Science
University of Peradeniya
Peradeniya, Sri Lanka

J.M. Sánchez
Faculty of Biology
Department of Plant Biology and Soil Science
University of Vigo
Vigo, Spain

Devarai Santhosh Kumar
Centre for Cellular and Molecular Biology
Council of Scientific and Industrial
  Research
Hyderabad, India

Sekaran Saravanan
Department of Biotechnology
School of Bioengineering
SRM University
Chennai, India

Nagarajan Selvamurugan
Department of Biotechnology
School of Bioengineering
SRM University
Chennai, India

Parimal C. Sen
Division of Molecular Medicine
Bose Institute
Kolkata, India

J. Serra
Department of Applied Physics
School of Industrial Engineering
University of Vigo
Vigo, Spain

Xiujuan Shi
School of Medicine
Shanghai Tenth People's Hospital
Tongji University
Yangpu, Shanghai, People's Republic of
  China

Yoon-Bo Shim
Department of Chemistry
Institute of Biophysio Sensor Technology
Pusan National University
Busan, South Korea

Bijay Singh
Department of Agricultural Biotechnology
Institute for Agriculture
  and Life Sciences
Seoul National University
Seoul, South Korea

Kota Sobha
Department of Biotechnology
RVR & JC College of Engineering
Guntur, India

Azamjon B. Soliev
School of Environmental Science
 and Engineering
Kochi University of Technology
Kami City, Japan

E. Song
Department of Ophthalmology First
 Affiliated Hospital
Jilin University
Changchun, Jilin, People's Republic of
 China

Na-Young Song
Tumor Microenvironment Global Core
 Research Center
Seoul National University
Seoul, South Korea

S. Sowmya
Amrita Centre for Nanosciences and
 Molecular Medicine
Amrita Institute of Medical Sciences and
 Research Centre
Kochi, India

M. Spirkova
Institute of Macromolecular Chemistry
Academy of Sciences of the Czech
 Republic
Prague, Czech Republic

Marit H. Stafsnes
Department of Biotechnology
Norwegian University of Science and
 Technology
Trondheim, Norway

P.N. Sudha
DKM College
Thiruvalluvar University
Vellore, India

Young-Joon Surh
Tumor Microenvironment Global Core
 Research Center
and
Department of Molecular Medicine and
 Biopharmaceutical Sciences
Graduate School of Convergence Sciences
 and Technology
and
Cancer Research Institute
Seoul National University
Seoul, South Korea

Quang Van Ta
Marine Biochemistry Laboratory
Department of Chemistry
Pukyong National University
Busan, South Korea

Rosna Mat Taha
Faculty of Science
Institute of Biological Sciences
University of Kuala Lumpur
Kuala Lumpur, Malaysia

Hiroshi Tamura
Faculty of Chemistry, Materials and
 Bioengineering
Kansai University
Osaka, Japan

G. Tishchenko
Institute of Macromolecular Chemistry
Academy of Sciences of the Czech
 Republic
Prague, Czech Republic

Mohita Trivedi
Department of Biotechnology
School of Bioengineering
SRM University
Chennai, India

Ioana M. Vasilescu
School of Pharmacy and Molecular
   Sciences
James Cook University
Douglas, Queensland, Australia

Jayachandran Venkatesan
Department of Chemistry
and
Marine Bioprocess Research Center
Pukyong National University
Busan, South Korea

Janak K. Vidanarachchi
Department of Animal Science
University of Peradeniya
Peradeniya, Sri Lanka

Juan M. Vieites
Technological Centre for Seafood
   Preservation
National Association of Manufacturers of
   Canned Fish and Shellfish
Vigo, Spain

Thanh-Sang Vo
Department of Chemistry
Pukyong National University
Busan, South Korea

Chen Zhang
School of Medicine
Shanghai Tenth People's Hospital
Tongji University
Yangpu, Shanghai, People's Republic of
   China

and

Marine Biochemistry Laboratory
Department of Chemistry
Pukyong National University
Busan, South Korea

Wei Zhang
Department of Science, Systems and
   Models
Roskilde University
Roskilde, Denmark

Part I

Isolation and Characterization of Marine Biomaterials

1

Introduction to Marine Biomaterials

Se-Kwon Kim and Jayachandran Venkatesan

CONTENTS

1.1 Introduction

The ocean not only consists of water but is also an abundant source of diverse biomaterials for mankind. Marine biomaterials are a new emerging area of research with significant applications. Recently, researchers have paid a considerable attention to marine-derived biomaterials for various applications. Due to vast diversity and biocompatibility marine-derived bioceramics, polysaccharides, enzymes, peptides, lipids, pigments, toxin, and algae-based products are widely used materials in biological and biomedical applications. The isolation, characterization, and application of marine biomaterials play an important role in developing the marine biotechnology industries. A recent advance in technologies helps to isolate bioactive materials from the marine source in an effective manner.

In the recent days, marine biomaterials have acquired a strong market position which, attracts various marine researchers and consumers as well. The global market for biomaterials is expected to reach from $25.6 billion in 2008 to $64.7 billion in 2015 with a compound annual growth rate of 15% from 2010 to 2015 (http://www.marketresearch.com/MarketsandMarkets-v3719/Global-Biomaterial-6294040/). The biomaterial market definitely holds a significant opportunity for innovators, but extensive research is required to develop new and improved products at competitive prices.

The main objective of the present book is to bring out the current trends in the marine biomaterials, especially with major implications of marine-originated biomaterials for biological and biomedical applications. The literature and information in this book promises to the concept of marine-derived biomaterials. In this context, our book chiefly deals with the latest approaches of isolating and characterizing the marine-derived materials and their biological and biomedical applications.

1.2 Biomaterials from Marine Origin

1.2.1 Biopolymers

Marine environment consists of several simple polymers to complicated polysaccharides such as chitin, chitosan, collagen, carrageenan, fucoidan, and alginate. These polymers are playing predominant role in biological and biomedical applications.

1.2.1.1 Chitin and Chitosan

Chitin is the second most abundant natural polymer after cellulose. Chitosan is produced from chitin, which is a natural polysaccharide found in crab, shrimp, lobster, coral, jellyfish, butterfly, ladybug, mushroom, and fungi (Figure 1.1). However, marine crustacean shells are widely used as primary sources for the production of chitosan (Madhavan

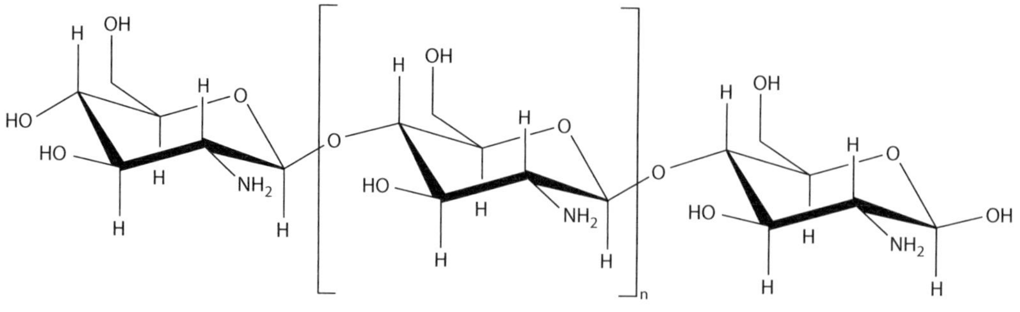

FIGURE 1.1
Structure of chitosan.

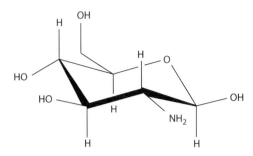

FIGURE 1.2
Structure of glucosamine.

and Nair, 1974; Shahidi and Abuzaytoun, 2005). Crab and shrimp are important marine species of great commercial importance in the tropical and subtropical waters of the Pacific, Atlantic, and Indian oceans. Processing the wastes of crab and shrimp has recently become a serious issue in coastal areas. Selective isolation of bioactive material from these wastes is the simplest way to decrease the pollution. It not only reduces the environmental pollution because of the disposal of these underutilized byproducts of crabs and shrimps but also increases the potential applications of chitosan. Moreover, the chemical hydrolysis and enzymatic methods, widely used for the isolation for chitosan from marine crustaceans shell, are quite inexpensive, and also glucosamine is produced from chitin and chitosan (Figure 1.2).

1.2.1.2 Collagen

Collagen is the most abundant protein in the vertebrates, and it acts as a structural matrix for organs such as bones, skin, muscle, and cartilage. Collagen from fish origin is also of the main source to mimic the same quality obtained from the other source and is used in numerous applications such as cosmeceuticals, nutraceuticals, pharmaceuticals, and functional food, and also widely used in biomedical area, especially bone-related diseases (Kim and Mendis, 2006).

Usually collagen from a bovine source carries a high risk of encephalopathy or transmissible spongiform encephalopathy. Thus, marine source is much important in this regard. There are several species that have been identified in the ocean to isolate collagen from marine sponge *Chondrosia reniformis Nardo* (Swatschek et al., 2002a); rhizostomous jellyfish (Nagai et al., 2000); fish waste materials, skin, bone, and fins (Nagai and Suzuki, 2000); jellyfish (Song et al., 2006); paper nautilus (Nagai and Suzuki, 2002); muscles and skins of marine animals (Sikorski and Borderias, 1994); cuttlefish (Nagai et al., 2001); squid skins (Kolodziejska et al., 1999); marine sponge (Garrone et al., 1975; Pallela et al., 2011a; Swatschek et al., 2002b); and *Sebastes mentella* (Kolodziejska et al., 1999).

1.2.1.3 Fucoidan

Fucoidan is a sulfated polysaccharide and is commonly found in marine species such as Hizikia fusiformis (Shiroma et al., 2003), mozuku, kombu, limu moui, bladderwrack, wakame, sea cucumber, and hijiki. The structure of fucoidan is shown in Figure 1.3. Fucoidan is used as an ingredient in dietary supplement products and is under development for many biological and biomedical activities (Aisa et al., 2005; Deux et al., 2002;

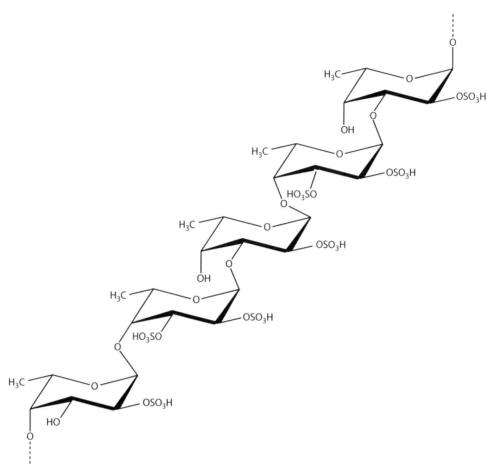

FIGURE 1.3
Structure of fucoidan.

Fitton, 2011; Irhimeh et al., 2007; Park et al., 2011). The marine-derived fucoidan has been checked for antitumor activity and immunological properties (Itoh et al., 1993), cosme-ceuticals (Fitton et al., 2007), anticoagulant (Colliec et al., 1991), and *Ascophyllum nodosum* (Marais and Joseleau, 2001).

Apart from the polymer discussed before, some other marine-derived polysaccharides are also isolated and characterized from several species. Among them, alginate (Figure 1.4), hyaluronan (Figure 1.5), chondroitin sulfate (Figure 1.6), and carrageenan (Figure 1.7) play a major role in the biological and biomedical products.

1.2.2 Bioceramics

1.2.2.1 Hydroxyapatite

Hydroxyapatite [HAp, $Ca_{10}(PO_4)_6(OH)_2$] is commonly prepared by a synthetic method with many advantages. In addition, several marine sources have been also used for the isolation of HAp with different kinds of methodologies such as the traditional thermal calcination method, the alkaline hydrolysis method, and the polymer-assisted method (Coelho et al.,

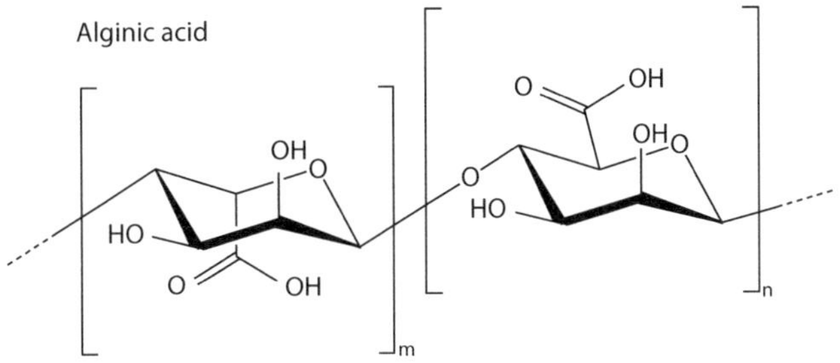

Alginic acid

FIGURE 1.4
Structure of alginic acid.

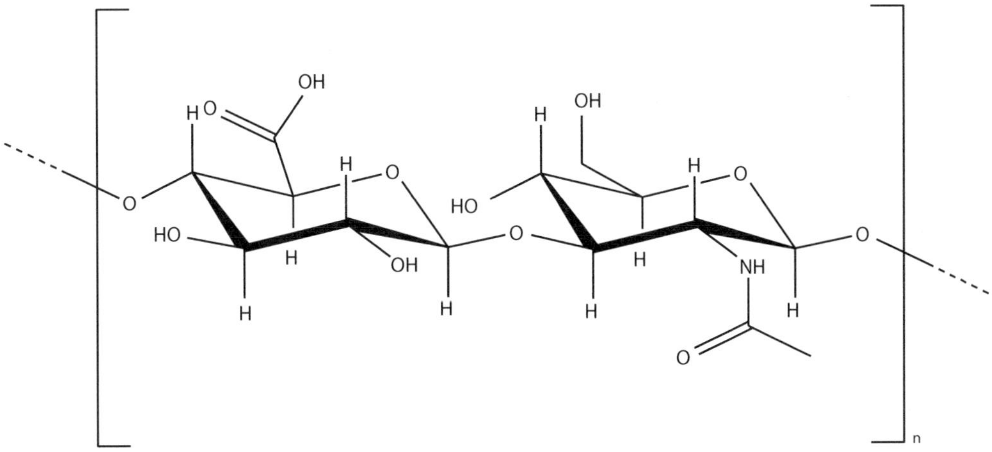

FIGURE 1.5
Structure of hyaluronan.

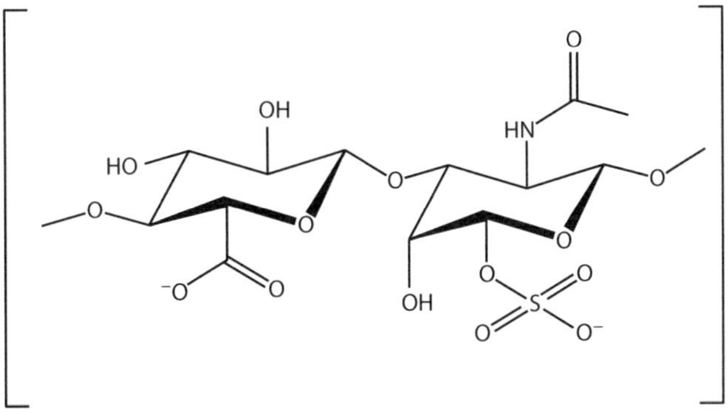

FIGURE 1.6
Structure of chondroitin sulfate.

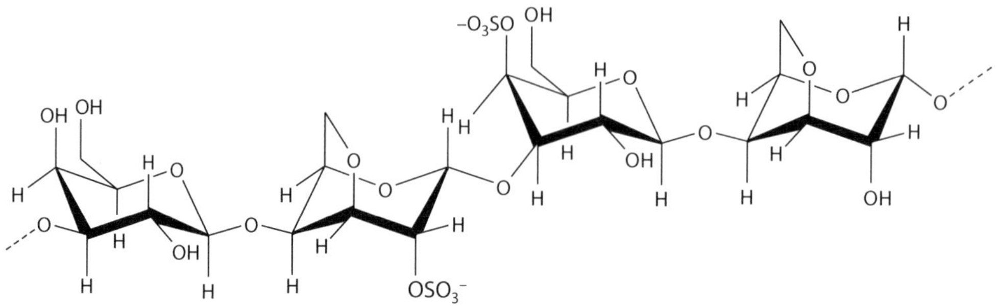

FIGURE 1.7
Structure of carrageenan.

2007; Ivankovic et al., 2009; Ozawa and Suzuki, 2002; Ozawa et al., 2003; Pallela et al., 2011c; Prabakaran and Rajeswari, 2006; Venkatesan and Kim, 2010b; Venkatesan et al., 2011b). HAp, especially in the form of nanocrystals, has been considered to play an important role in various bone-related applications (Best et al., 2008; Chesnutt et al., 2009; Palmer et al., 2008). HAp possesses significant biocompatibility in bone tissue, owing to its chemical composition that is similar to bone material (Sopyan et al., 2007).

1.2.3 Natural Products

Marine-derived natural compounds (derived from algae, fungi, bacteria, invertebrates, and fish) are promising candidates for various biological and biomedical applications. Thus, marine natural products have attracted the attention of biologists and chemists in the last several decades. To explain about marine-derived natural products in a detailed fashion, this book is not enough. From our lab, we have isolated several bioactive compounds from marine source and checked various biological and biomedical applications (Figure 1.8) (Heo et al., 2005; Li and Kim, 2011; Park et al., 2005; Wijesekara et al., 2010, 2011; Zhang and Kim, 2009). Marine-derived phlorotannins showed several biological properties similar to antioxidants (Li et al., 2009).

1.2.4 Fatty Acids

Fatty acid or omega-3 fatty acid is commercially prepared from microalgae (Viso and Marty, 1993). In addition, marine fish is also an important source for DHA (docosa-hexaenoic acids) and EPA (eicosapentaenoic acid). The structure of DHA is shown in Figure 1.9.

Marine fatty acids, particularly EPA and DHA, have been widely used for cancer treatment (Patterson et al., 2011; Terry et al., 2003) and cardiac disorders (Farzaneh-Far et al., 2010; Saravanan et al., 2010; Sekikawa et al., 2008) (Figure 1.10).

1.2.5 Marine Toxins

Marine biotoxins usually consist of organic compounds. The occurrence, isolation, and chemical characterization are the important processes to find out the bioactive compounds and are widely used for drug discovery for human diseases such as cancer. Marine toxins

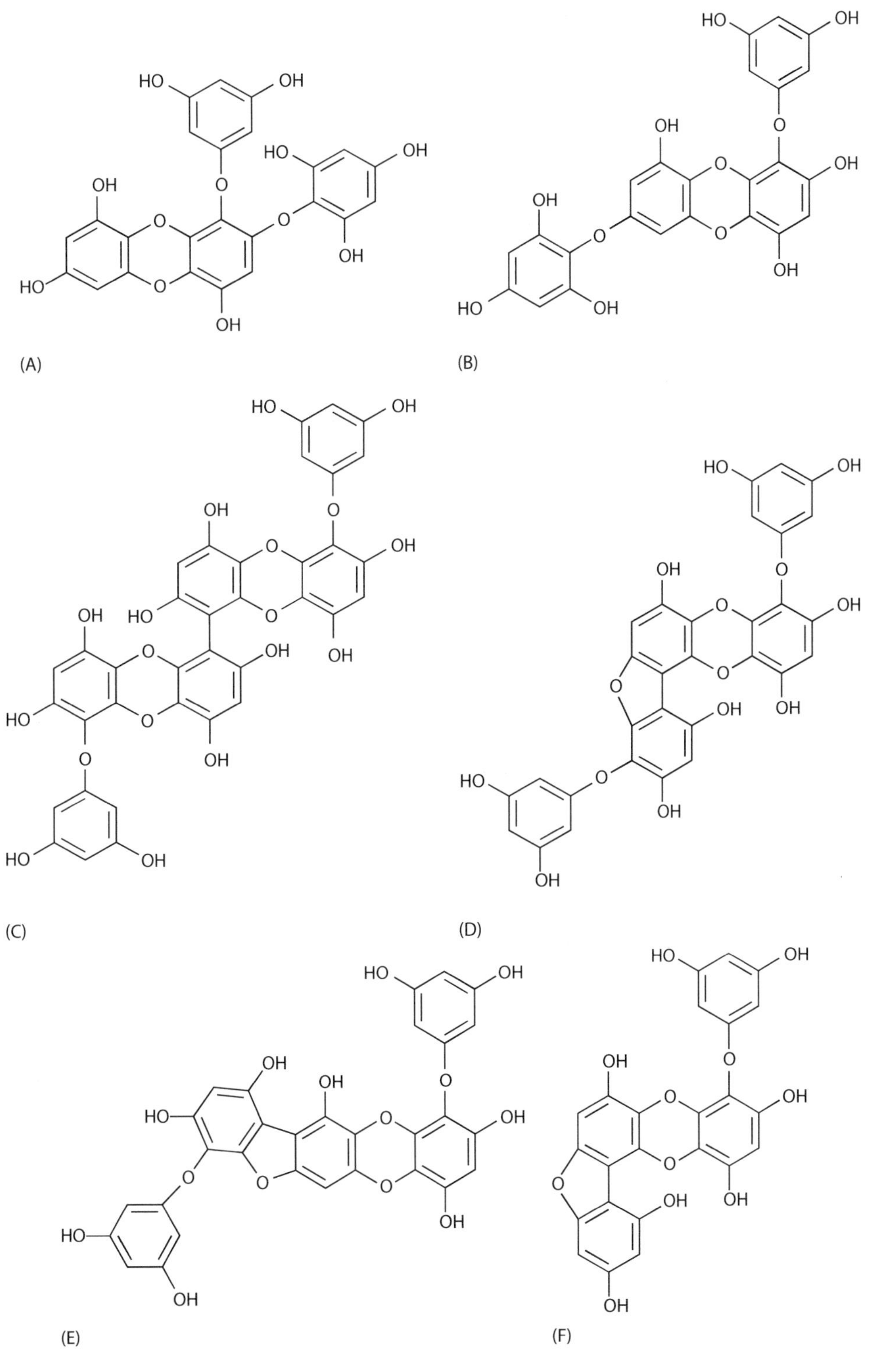

FIGURE 1.8
Marine-derived phlorotannins, (A) 2-phloroeckol, (B) 7-phloroeckol, (C) 6,6'-bieckol, (D) phlorofucofuroeckol-A, (E) phlorofucofuroeckol-B, and (F) fucofuroeckol-A.

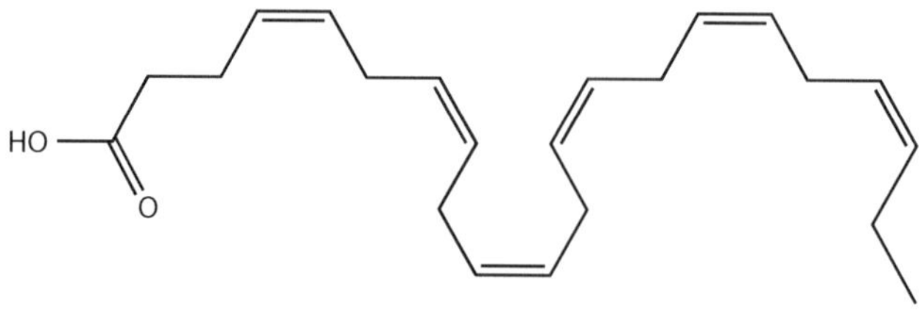

FIGURE 1.9
Structure of docosahexaenoic acid.

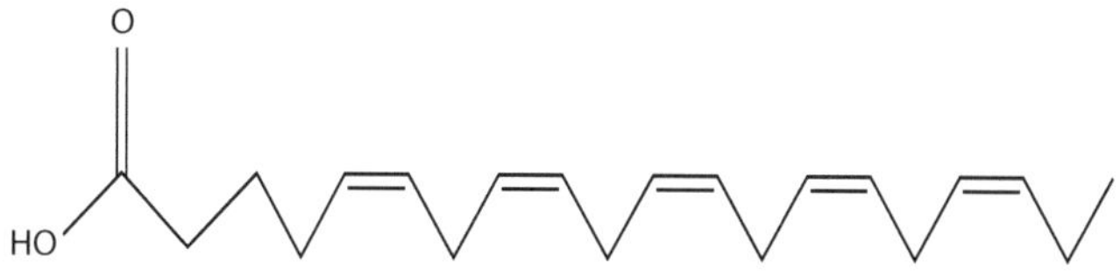

FIGURE 1.10
Structure of eicosapentaenoic acid.

have drawn scientist's attention due to their inordinately high biological and biomedical activity (Yasumoto and Murata, 1993). There are varieties of marine toxins, depending on their classification such as alkaloids, steroids, peptides, and proteins, and their functions are varied drastically in the biological activity. The important sources of marine biotoxins such as toxins, porifera, cnidarians, mollusk, echinoderms and vertebrates, sea snakes, and fishes (Fenical, 1993) have been discussed in this book. The production of toxins from marine animals is an important strategy that guarantees their survival in a highly competitive and challenging ecosystem.

1.2.6 Marine Pigments

Marine pigments are not only showing the color; they consist of diverse chemical components such as terpenoids and melanins, which are especially found in bacteria. The secondary metabolites from marine bacteria, especially colored ones, have diverse biological properties such as antibiotic and anticancer activities. Marine actinomycetes, marine pseudoalteromonas, and marine cyanobacteria are widely studied marine species. In this book, we have discussed marine pigments in detail.

1.2.7 Marine Nanoparticles

In the recent years, marine-derived nanoparticles play an important role in various biological and biomedical applications including cancer therapy, tissue engineering, drug delivery, catalysis, sensors, electronic materials, and wastewater treatment. Various nanoparticles (silver, titanium, and gold) have been isolated from marine sources and used for various applications including pharmaceutical, environmental, cosmeceutical, and drug delivery. Green approaches of nanoparticle synthesis have been discussed in this book using a rapid, single-step, and completely green biosynthetic method employing aqueous plant extracts, bacteria, and fungus.

1.3 Application

1.3.1 Biological Activity of Marine Biomaterials

1.3.1.1 Antioxidant and Anti-Inflammatory Activity

Reactive oxygen species (ROS) is generated in living organisms during human metabolic process, and it can be produced as hydrogen peroxide, superoxide, hydroxyl, and nitric oxide radical. The excess of ROS causes several diseases from cardiac problems to cancer. Hence, the reduction of ROS is the preliminary step for preventing various diseases.

Antioxidant activity of marine-derived biomaterials is playing a significant role in suppression of ROS. Recently, several papers have been published for antioxidant activity with marine biomaterials such as peptides, chitosan, and chitosan derivatives being discussed in the biological application part (Altiok et al., 2010; Knorr, 1982; Koryagin et al., 2006; Xie et al., 2001; Xing et al., 2005; Yen et al., 2007, 2008) and also sulfated polysaccharides, especially fucoidan and laminarn (Wang et al., 2009a,b; Xing et al., 2005).

1.3.1.2 Anticancer Activity

Some of the commercially available cancer drugs are derived from marine sources. Marine natural products are modeling materials for the synthetic chemist to prepare active molecules. Hence, marine-derived natural products, toxins, pigments, sulfated polysaccharides were also used as template for the designing the new anticancer potential drugs. Chitosan and its derivatives have been studied and discussed well in this book.

1.3.1.3 Anticoagulant Activity

Marine-derived sulfated polysaccharides, fucoidan, carrageenan, and heparin, have been widely used for anticoagulant activity, and it is explored well in this book.

1.3.1.4 Anti-HIV Activity

The inhibition of HIV-1 reverse transcriptase by chemical compounds is the primary role played by them to protect the host cell from HIV-1 infection. Numerous marine-derived substances such as phlorotannins, polysaccharides, and lectins have been isolated, and the activity was checked in vitro and also discussed in this book.

1.3.2 Biomedical Application of Marine Biomaterials

1.3.2.1 Tissue Engineering

Tissue engineering is an emerging field of research to prepare artificial materials for the treatment or replacement of infectious organs. Several synthetic and marine-derived materials have been widely used such as collagen, chitosan, hyaluronic acid, corals, algae (diatoms), and sponges (Allison and Grande-Allen, 2006; Clarke et al., 2011; DiMartino et al., 2005b; Kim et al., 2008; Nettles et al., 2002; Senni et al., 2011; Venkatesan and Kim, 2010a; Venkatesan et al., 2011a; Wang et al., 2003).

Marine-derived biomaterials are used for tissue engineering whether it is in the isolated form or the nature form. However, the marine-derived biomaterials should consist of pore distribution, pore adsorption, swelling studies, in vitro degradation, biomineralization, and biocompatibility for bone tissue engineering. Among the marine-derived biomaterials, chitosan is the widely used material until now. It can be used in different forms such as chitin nanofibers, chitosan nanocomposite with various bioactive materials, HAp, bioactive glass, silica nanoparticles, chitin nanoparticles, and chitin nanogel. Chitosan can be molded in any shape for the tissue engineering products (Ehrlich, 2010; Song et al., 2006).

Marine-derived collagen has been used in the scaffold preparation and for bone tissue engineering (Pallela et al., 2011b; Senaratne et al., 2006). The advantages and disadvantages of collagen materials in the usage of regenerative medicine and biomedical application have been explored well by other authors (Hayashi et al., 2012). Tissue-engineered vascular grafts composed of marine collagen and PLGA fibers using pulsatile perfusion bioreactors have been studied (Jeong et al., 2007).

Natural biopolymer composite materials are becoming increasingly important as scaffolds for bone tissue engineering. Next-generation biomaterials should combine bioactive and bioresorbable materials, which mimic the natural function of bone and activate in vivo mechanisms of tissue regeneration. Chitosan has been considerably employed as a scaffold in orthopedic and other biomedical applications due to its high biocompatibility, biodegradability, porous structure, suitability for cell ingrowth, and intrinsic antibacterial nature (DiMartino et al., 2005a; Muzzarelli, 2011; VandeVord et al., 2002). Chitosan-based composite biomaterials of low interconnected porosity for cell attachment and optimum mechanical strength need to be improved. Hence, instead of a single-component system that cannot assist and mimic all the properties of natural bones, an alternative multicomponent system has to be developed for bone repair and tissue engineering.

1.3.2.2 *Drug Delivery*

Drug delivery is the process to deliver the pharmaceutical compound into the specific place to avoid other side effects. Marine-derived polymers are biocompatible and also have surface characteristics and mechanical strength that are some vital features for a successful scaffold to be used as a drug delivery (Felt et al., 1998; Kim and Mendis, 2006; Olsen et al., 2003; Swatschek et al., 2002b).

1.3.3 Industrial Application of Marine Biomaterials

Biomaterials have potential for a range of industries, from engineering to pharmaceutical and cosmetic applications. Marine-derived polysaccharides are widely used in the areas such as biomedical, antimicrobial, agricultural, wastewater treatment, cosmetics, and paper technology industries (Kim and Mendis, 2006).

Carrageenan is used in food industry, pharmaceuticals, enzyme immobilization, cosmetic application, and wastewater treatment. Alginate and agar are also used in several industrialized areas such as food application, protein delivery, wound dressing, tissue engineering, nerve repair, paper, and adhesive industries.

1.4 Conclusion

Marine-derived biomaterials are abundant and biocompatible for mankind. However, marine biomaterials' field is a developing area; still several biomaterials should be isolated and characterized for several biological and biomedical applications.

Acknowledgment

This work was supported by a grant from Marine Bioprocess Research Centre of the Marine Bio 21 Center funded by the Ministry of Land, Transport and Maritime Affairs, Republic of Korea.

References

Aisa, Y., Miyakawa, Y., Nakazato, T., Shibata, H., Saito, K., Ikeda, Y., and Kizaki, M. (2005). Fucoidan induces apoptosis of human HS-Sultan cells accompanied by activation of caspase-3 and down-regulation of ERK Pathways. *American Journal of Hematology*, 78(1), 7–14.

Allison, D. D. and Grande-Allen, K. J. (2006). Review. Hyaluronan: A powerful tissue engineering tool. *Tissue Engineering*, 12(8), 2131–2140.

Altiok, D., Altiok, E., and Tihminlioglu, F. (2010). Physical, antibacterial and antioxidant properties of chitosan films incorporated with thyme oil for potential wound healing applications. *Journal of Materials Science: Materials in Medicine*, 21(7), 2227–2236.

Best, S. M., Porter, A. E., Thian, E. S., and Huang, J. (2008). Bioceramics: Past, present and for the future. *Journal of the European Ceramic Society*, 28(7), 1319–1327.

Chesnutt, B. M., Viano, A. M., Yuan, Y., Yang, Y., Guda, T., Appleford, M. R., Ong, J. L., Haggard, W. O., and Bumgardner, J. D. (2009). Design and characterization of a novel chitosan/nanocrystalline calcium phosphate composite scaffold for bone regeneration. *Journal of Biomedical Materials Research Part A*, 88A(2), 491–502.

Clarke, S., Walsh, P., Maggs, C., and Buchanan, F. (2011). Designs from the deep: Marine organisms for bone tissue engineering. *Biotechnology Advances*, 29(6), 610–617.

Coelho, T., Nogueira, E., Weinand, W., Lima, W., Steimacher, A., Medina, A., Baesso, M., and Bento, A. (2007). Thermal properties of natural nanostructured hydroxyapatite extracted from fish bone waste. *Journal of Applied Physics*, 101, 084701.

Colliec, S., Fischer, A., Tapon-Bretaudiere, J., Boisson, C., Durand, P., and Jozefonvicz, J. (1991). Anticoagulant properties of a fucoidan fraction. *Thrombosis Research*, 64(2), 143–154.

Deux, J.-F., Meddahi-Pellé, A., Le Blanche, A. F., Feldman, L. J., Colliec-Jouault, S., Brée, F., Boudghène, F., Michel, J.-B., and Letourneur, D. (2002). Low molecular weight fucoidan prevents neointimal hyperplasia in rabbit iliac artery in-stent restenosis model. *Arteriosclerosis, Thrombosis, and Vascular Biology*, 22(10), 1604–1609.

Di Martino, A., Sittinger, M., and Risbud, M. (2005). Chitosan: A versatile biopolymer for orthopaedic tissue-engineering. *Biomaterials*, 26(30), 5983–5990.

Ehrlich, H. (2010). *Biological Materials of Marine Origin*. Springer Verlag, New York.

Farzaneh-Far, R., Lin, J., Epel, E. S., Harris, W. S., Blackburn, E. H., and Whooley, M. A. (2010). Association of marine omega-3 fatty acid levels with telomeric aging in patients with coronary heart disease. *JAMA*, 303(3), 250–257.

Felt, O., Buri, P., and Gurny, R. (1998). Chitosan: A unique polysaccharide for drug delivery. *Drug Development and Industrial Pharmacy*, 24(11), 979–993.

Fenical, W. (1993). Chemical studies of marine bacteria: Developing a new resource. *Chemical Reviews*, 93(5), 1673–1683.

Fitton, J. H. (2011). Therapies from fucoidan; multifunctional marine polymers. *Marine Drugs*, 9(10), 1731–1760.

Fitton, J. H., Irhimeh, M., and Falk, N. (2007). Macroalgal fucoidan extracts: A new opportunity for marine cosmetics. *Cosmetics and Toiletries*, 122(8), 55.

Garrone, R., Huc, A., and Junqua, S. (1975). Fine structure and physicochemical studies on the collagen of the marine sponge *Chondrosia reniformis Nardo*. *Journal of Ultrastructure Research*, 52(2), 261–275.

Hayashi, Y., Yamada, S., Yanagi Guchi, K., Koyama, Z., and Ikeda, T. (2012). Chitosan and fish collagen as biomaterials for regenerative medicine. *Advances in Food and Nutrition Research, 65,* 107–120.

Heo, S. J., Park, P. J., Park, E. J., Kim, S. K., and Jeon, Y. J. (2005). Antioxidant activity of enzymatic extracts from a brown seaweed *Ecklonia cava* by electron spin resonance spectrometry and comet assay. *European Food Research and Technology, 221*(1), 41–47.

Irhimeh, M. R., Fitton, J. H., and Lowenthal, R. M. (2007). Fucoidan ingestion increases the expression of CXCR4 on human CD34+ cells. *Experimental Hematology, 35*(6), 989–994.

Itoh, H., Noda, H., Amano, H., Zhuaug, C., Mizuno, T., and Ito, H. (1993). Antitumor activity and immunological properties of marine algal polysaccharides, especially fucoidan, prepared from *Sargassum thunbergii* of Phaeophyceae. *Anticancer Research, 13*(6A), 2045.

Ivankovic, H., Gallego Ferrer, G., Tkalcec, E., Orlic, S., and Ivankovic, M. (2009). Preparation of highly porous hydroxyapatite from cuttlefish bone. *Journal of Materials Science: Materials in Medicine, 20*(5), 1039–1046.

Jeong, S., Kim, S. Y., Cho, S. K., Chong, M. S., Kim, K. S., Kim, H., Lee, S. B., and Lee, Y. M. (2007). Tissue-engineered vascular grafts composed of marine collagen and PLGA fibers using pulsatile perfusion bioreactors. *Biomaterials, 28*(6), 1115–1122.

Kim, S. K. and Mendis, E. (2006). Bioactive compounds from marine processing byproducts—A review. *Food Research International, 39*(4), 383–393.

Kim, I. Y., Seo, S. J., Moon, H. S., Yoo, M. K., Park, I. Y., Kim, B. C., and Cho, C. S. (2008). Chitosan and its derivatives for tissue engineering applications. *Biotechnology Advances, 26*(1), 1–21.

Knorr, D. (1982). Functional properties of chitin and chitosan. *Journal of Food Science, 47*(2), 593–595.

Kolodziejska, I., Sikorski, Z. E., and Niecikowska, C. (1999). Parameters affecting the isolation of collagen from squid (Illex argentinus) skins. *Food Chemistry, 66*(2), 153–157.

Koryagin, A., Erofeeva, E., Yakimovich, N., Aleksandrova, E., Smirnova, L., and Mal'kov, A. (2006). Analysis of antioxidant properties of chitosan and its oligomers. *Bulletin of Experimental Biology and Medicine, 142*(4), 461–463.

Li, Y. X. and Kim, S. K. (2011). Utilization of seaweed derived ingredients as potential antioxidants and functional ingredients in the food industry: An overview. *Food Science and Biotechnology, 20*(6), 1461–1466.

Li, Y., Qian, Z. J., Ryu, B. M., Lee, S. H., Kim, M. M., and Kim, S. K. (2009). Chemical components and its antioxidant properties in vitro: An edible marine brown alga, *Ecklonia cava. Bioorganic and Medicinal Chemistry, 17*(5), 1963–1973.

Madhavan, P. and Nair, K. (1974). Utilization of prawn waste: Isolation of chitin and its conversion to chitosan. *Fish Technology, 11*(1), 50–53.

Marais, M. F. and Joseleau, J. P. (2001). A fucoidan fraction from *Ascophyllum nodosum. Carbohydrate Research, 336*(2), 155–159.

Market Research.Com, http://www.marketresearch.com/MarketsandMarkets-v3719/Global-Biomaterial-6294040/, accessed on September 14, 2012.

Muzzarelli, R. A. A. (2011). Chitosan composites with inorganics, morphogenetic proteins and stem cells, for bone regeneration. *Carbohydrate Polymers, 83*(4), 1433–1445.

Nagai, T. and Suzuki, N. (2000). Isolation of collagen from fish waste material—Skin, bone and fins. *Food Chemistry, 68*(3), 277–281.

Nagai, T. and Suzuki, N. (2002). Preparation and partial characterization of collagen from paper nautilus (*Argonauta argo*, Linnaeus) outer skin. *Food Chemistry, 76*(2), 149–153.

Nagai, T., Worawattanamateekul, W., Suzuki, N., Nakamura, T., Ito, T., Fujiki, K., Nakao, M., and Yano, T. (2000). Isolation and characterization of collagen from rhizostomous jellyfish (*Rhopilema asamushi*). *Food Chemistry, 70*(2), 205–208.

Nagai, T., Yamashita, E., Taniguchi, K., Kanamori, N., and Suzuki, N. (2001). Isolation and characterisation of collagen from the outer skin waste material of cuttlefish (*Sepia lycidas*). *Food Chemistry, 72*(4), 425–429.

Nettles, D. L., Elder, S. H., and Gilbert, J. A. (2002). Potential use of chitosan as a cell scaffold material for cartilage tissue engineering. *Tissue Engineering, 8*(6), 1009–1016.

Olsen, D., Yang, C., Bodo, M., Chang, R., Leigh, S., Baez, J., Carmichael, D., Perälä, M., Hämäläinen, E. R., and Jarvinen, M. (2003). Recombinant collagen and gelatin for drug delivery. *Advanced Drug Delivery Reviews*, 55(12), 1547–1567.

Ozawa, M., Satake, K., and Suzuki, R. (2003). Removal of aqueous chromium by fish bone waste originated hydroxyapatite. *Journal of Materials Science Letters*, 22(7), 513–514.

Ozawa, M. and Suzuki, S. (2002). Microstructural development of natural hydroxyapatite originated from fish-bone waste through heat treatment. *Journal of the American Ceramic Society (USA)*, 85(5), 1315–1317.

Pallela, R., Bojja, S., and Janapala, V. R. (2011a). Biochemical and biophysical characterization of collagens of marine sponge, *Ircinia fusca* (Porifera: Demospongiae: Irciniidae). *International Journal of Biological Macromolecules*, 49(1), 85–92.

Pallela, R., Venkatesan, J., Janapala, V. R., and Kim, S. K. (2011b). Biophysicochemical evaluation of chitosan-hydroxyapatite-marine sponge collagen composite for bone tissue engineering. *Journal of Biomedical Materials Research: Part A*, 100, 486–495.

Pallela, R., Venkatesan, J., and Kim, S. K. (2011c). Polymer assisted isolation of hydroxyapatite from *Thunnus obesus* bone. *Ceramics International*, 37(8), 3489–3497.

Palmer, L. C., Newcomb, C. J., Kaltz, S. R., Spoerke, E. D., and Stupp, S. I. (2008). Biomimetic systems for hydroxyapatite mineralization inspired by bone and enamel. *Chemical Reviews*, 108(11), 4754–4783.

Park, P. J., Heo, S. J., Park, E. J., Kim, S. K., Byun, H. G., Jeon, B. T., and Jeon, Y. J. (2005). Reactive oxygen scavenging effect of enzymatic extracts from *Sargassum thunbergii*. *Journal of Agricultural and Food Chemistry*, 53(17), 6666–6672.

Park, M.-K., Jung, U., and Roh, C. (2011). Fucoidan from marine brown algae inhibits lipid accumulation. *Marine Drugs*, 9(8), 1359–1367.

Patterson, R. E., Flatt, S. W., Newman, V. A., Natarajan, L., Rock, C. L., Thomson, C. A., Caan, B. J., Parker, B. A., and Pierce, J. P. (2011). Marine fatty acid intake is associated with breast cancer prognosis. *The Journal of Nutrition*, 141(2), 201–206.

Prabakaran, K. and Rajeswari, S. (2006). Development of hydroxyapatite from natural fish bone through heat treatment. *Trends in Biomaterials Artificial Organs*, 20, 20–23.

Saravanan, P., Davidson, N. C., Schmidt, E. B., and Calder, P. C. (2010). Cardiovascular effects of marine omega-3 fatty acids. *The Lancet*, 376(9740), 540–550.

Sekikawa, A., Curb, J. D., Ueshima, H., El-Saed, A., Kadowaki, T., Abbott, R. D., Evans, R. W. et al. (2008). Marine-derived *n*-3 fatty acids and atherosclerosis in Japanese, Japanese-American, and white men: A cross-sectional study. *Journal of the American College of Cardiology*, 52(6), 417–424.

Senaratne, L., Park, P. J., and Kim, S. K. (2006). Isolation and characterization of collagen from brown backed toadfish (*Lagocephalus gloveri*) skin. *Bioresource Technology*, 97(2), 191–197.

Senni, K., Pereira, J., Gueniche, F., Delbarre-Ladrat, C., Sinquin, C., Ratiskol, J., Godeau, G., Fischer, A. M., Helley, D., and Colliec-Jouault, S. (2011). Marine polysaccharides: A source of bioactive molecules for cell therapy and tissue engineering. *Marine Drugs*, 9(9), 1664–1681.

Shahidi, F. and Abuzaytoun, R. (2005). Chitin, chitosan, and co-products: Chemistry, production, applications, and health effects. *Advances in Food and Nutrition Research*, 49, 93–135.

Shiroma, R., Uechi, S., Taira, T., Ishihara, M., Tawata, S., and Tako, M. (2003). Isolation and characterization of fucoidan from Hizikia fusiformis (Hijiki). *Journal of Applied Glycoscience*, 50(3), 361–366.

Sikorski, Z. E. and Borderias, J. A. (1994). *Collagen in the Muscles and Skins of Marine Animals*. Chapman and Hall, New York, pp. 58–70.

Song, E., Yeon Kim, S., Chun, T., Byun, H. J., and Lee, Y. M. (2006). Collagen scaffolds derived from a marine source and their biocompatibility. *Biomaterials*, 27(15), 2951–2961.

Sopyan, I., Mel, M., Ramesh, S., and Khalid, K. (2007). Porous hydroxyapatite for artificial bone applications. *Science and Technology of Advanced Materials*, 8(1–2), 116–123.

Swatschek, D., Schatton, W., Kellermann, J., Müller, W. E. G., and Kreuter, J. (2002a). Marine sponge collagen: Isolation, characterization and effects on the skin parameters surface-pH, moisture and sebum. *European Journal of Pharmaceutics and Biopharmaceutics*, 53(1), 107–113.

Swatschek, D., Schatton, W., Müller, W. E. G., and Kreuter, J. (2002b). Microparticles derived from marine sponge collagen (SCMPs): Preparation, characterization and suitability for dermal delivery of all-trans retinol. *European Journal of Pharmaceutics and Biopharmaceutics*, 54(2), 125–133.

Terry, P. D., Rohan, T. E., and Wolk, A. (2003). Intakes of fish and marine fatty acids and the risks of cancers of the breast and prostate and of other hormone-related cancers: A review of the epidemiologic evidence. *The American Journal of Clinical Nutrition*, 77(3), 532–543.

VandeVord, P. J., Matthew, H. W. T., DeSilva, S. P., Mayton, L., Wu, B., and Wooley, P. H. (2002). Evaluation of the biocompatibility of a chitosan scaffold in mice. *Journal of Biomedical Materials Research*, 59(3), 585–590.

Venkatesan, J. and Kim, S.-K. (2010a). Chitosan composites for bone tissue engineering—An overview. *Marine Drugs*, 8(8), 2252–2266.

Venkatesan, J. and Kim, S. K. (2010b). Effect of temperature on isolation and characterization of hydroxyapatite from tuna (*Thunnus obesus*) bone. *Materials*, 3(10), 4761–4772.

Venkatesan, J., Qian, Z. J., Ryu, B. M., Ashok Kumar, N., and Kim, S. K. (2011a). Preparation and characterization of carbon nanotube-grafted-chitosan-natural hydroxyapatite composite for bone tissue engineering. *Carbohydrate Polymers*, 83(2), 569–577.

Venkatesan, J., Qian, Z.-J., Ryu, B., Noel, V. T., and Kim, S.-K. (2011b). A comparative study of thermal calcination and an alkaline hydrolysis method in the isolation of hydroxyapatite from *Thunnus obesus* bone. *Biomedical Materials*, 6(3), 035003.

Viso, A.-C. and Marty, J.-C. (1993). Fatty acids from 28 marine microalgae. *Phytochemistry*, 34(6), 1521–1533.

Wang, J., Liu, L., Zhang, Q., Zhang, Z., Qi, H., and Li, P. (2009a). Synthesized oversulphated, acetylated and benzoylated derivatives of fucoidan extracted from *Laminaria japonica* and their potential antioxidant activity in vitro. *Food Chemistry*, 114(4), 1285–1290.

Wang, J., Wang, F., Zhang, Q., Zhang, Z., Shi, X., and Li, P. (2009b). Synthesized different derivatives of low molecular fucoidan extracted from *Laminaria japonica* and their potential antioxidant activity in vitro. *International Journal of Biological Macromolecules*, 44(5), 379–384.

Wang, L., Shelton, R., Cooper, P., Lawson, M., Triffitt, J., and Barralet, J. (2003). Evaluation of sodium alginate for bone marrow cell tissue engineering. *Biomaterials*, 24(20), 3475–3481.

Wijesekara, I., Pangestuti, R., and Kim, S. K. (2011). Biological activities and potential health benefits of sulfated polysaccharides derived from marine algae. *Carbohydrate Polymers*, 84(1), 14–21.

Wijesekara, I., Yoon, N. Y., and Kim, S. K. (2010). Phlorotannins from *Ecklonia cava* (Phaeophyceae): Biological activities and potential health benefits. *Biofactors*, 36(6), 408–414.

Xie, W., Xu, P., and Liu, Q. (2001). Antioxidant activity of water-soluble chitosan derivatives. *Bioorganic and Medicinal Chemistry Letters*, 11(13), 1699–1701.

Xing, R., Yu, H., Liu, S., Zhang, W., Zhang, Q., Li, Z., and Li, P. (2005). Antioxidant activity of differently regioselective chitosan sulfates in vitro. *Bioorganic and Medicinal Chemistry*, 13(4), 1387–1392.

Yasumoto, T. and Murata, M. (1993). Marine toxins. *Chemical Reviews*, 93(5), 1897–1909.

Yen, M. T., Tseng, Y. H., Li, R. C., and Mau, J. L. (2007). Antioxidant properties of fungal chitosan from shiitake stipes. *LWT-Food Science and Technology*, 40(2), 255–261.

Yen, M. T., Yang, J. H., and Mau, J. L. (2008). Antioxidant properties of chitosan from crab shells. *Carbohydrate Polymers*, 74(4), 840–844.

Zhang, C. and Kim, S. K. (2009). Matrix metalloproteinase inhibitors (MMPIs) from marine natural products: The current situation and future prospects. *Marine Drugs*, 7(2), 71–84.

2

Hydroxyapatite from Marine Fish Bone: Isolation and Characterization Techniques

Jayachandran Venkatesan and Se-Kwon Kim

CONTENTS

2.1 Introduction

Bone is a hierarchical structure and is made up of hydroxyapatite (HAp) and type I collagen as major portion. The average mineral content of bone tissue is species dependent and lies within the range of 50%–74% (Fratzl et al. 2004). HAp [$Ca_{10}(PO_4)_6(OH)_2$] is considered to play a vital role in various fields including the replacement of bone tissues (Tang et al. 2009), reconstruction of skull defects (Staffa et al. 2007), tissue engineering (Nair et al. 2008), artificial bone synthesis (Hirata et al. 2008; Venkatesan and Kim 2010a; Venkatesan et al. 2011a), biosensors (Salman et al. 2008), removal of heavy metals (Reichert and Binner 1996), and as a drug carrier (Kano et al. 1994). HAp can be derived either from a natural source or by a synthetic method. The production of HAp from natural sources is inexpensive and uncomplicated. The thermal calcination method is commonly used for the isolation of natural HAp.

Tuna (*Thunnus obesus*) is a fish species (length of 60 and 250 cm and weight 400 lb) of great commercial importance in the tropical and subtropical waters of the Pacific, Atlantic, and Indian oceans (Farley et al. 2006). Specifically, *Thunnus obesus* occupies 12% of the total amount of fish production in Korea (Production Database of Ministry of Maritime Affairs and Fisheries of Korea). The waste of *Thunnus obesus* has recently become a serious issue in coastal areas of Korea; one of the simplest ways to decrease pollution is the selective isolation of HAp from this waste.

Ozawa et al. (2003) have reported the removal of aqueous chromium by fish bone waste–originated HAp. HAp is the most stable calcium phosphate salt at normal temperatures and pH between 4 and 12. HAp derived from the powder processing method has a great potential as bone substitute owing to its excellent biocompatible and osteoconductive properties. In this chapter, we have discussed HAp isolation and characterization techniques (Venkatesan and Kim 2010; Pallela et al. 2011; Venkatesan et al. 2011b).

2.2 Methods in Hydroxyapatite Isolation

2.2.1 Synthetic Method

Chemicals such as $Ca(NO_3) \cdot 4H_2O$ and $(NH_4)_2 HPO_4$ have been widely used in synthesis of HAp. Several methods have been reported for the synthesis of HAp crystals, such as hydrothermal (Zhang et al. 2009), liquid membrane (Jarudilokkul et al. 2007), precipitation (Sarig and Kahana 2002), radio-frequency thermal plasma (Xu et al. 2004), ultrasonic precipitation (Cao et al. 2005), reverse microemulsion (Guo et al. 2005), sol–gel (Feng et al. 2005), and polymer-assisted method (Tseng et al. 2009).

2.2.2 Thermal Calcination Method

Raw bones were washed with hot water for 2 days to remove the traces of meat and skin. The washed bones were mixed with 1% sodium hydroxide (NaOH) and acetone to remove proteins, lipids, oils, and other organic impurities (the bone and sodium hydroxide solid/liquid ratio was 1:50). In the thermal calcination method, 2 g of bone was placed in a silica crucible and subjected to a temperature of 900°C in an electrical muffle furnace in the presence of air atmosphere (Venkatesan et al. 2011c).

By another researcher, the natural HAp was processed by calcining the bones at 900°C, for 8 h. Calcination for 8 h establishes the best conditions for achieving nanoparticles. They were then hand crushed inside an agate crucible prior to undergoing milling in a high-energy miller (Coelho et al. 2007).

2.2.3 Alkaline Hydrolysis Method

To hydrolyze collagen and other organic moieties, the alkaline hydrolysis method was followed. Grounded bones were treated with 2 M sodium hydroxide at 250°C for 5 h (solid/liquid ratio 1:30). 2 M sodium hydroxide was prepared with water as solvent. This procedure was repeated several times to ensure proper removal of organic moieties. The mixture was then filtered in a suction pump with continuous washing with water until the pH was neutral. The resultant product was dried in an oven at 100°C (Venkatesan et al. 2011b).

2.2.4 Subcritical Water Process

A cylindrical hydrothermal stainless steel autoclave with an internal diameter of 6 cm, external of 7.4 cm, and height of 15 cm has been used to isolate HAp from animal bones. The grounded bones were added to deionized water at a solid to liquid weight ratio of 1:40 and placed in an autoclave. The autoclave was tightly sealed and heated in a silicon oil bath at 275°C for 1 h. The obtained mixture was filtered; the solid product was washed with distilled water and dried at 80°C for 30 min (Barakat et al. 2008, 2009).

2.2.5 Polymer-Assisted Method

Grounded tuna fish bones were added to 1% NaOH solution to remove soluble impurities, stirred for 12 h, and dried at 100°C. The dried bones were mixed with 50% wt. amount of PEG $(-CH_2CH_2O-)_n - n = 6000$, PVA $(-CH_2CHOH-)_n - n = 1500$, and PEG-PPG-PEG $(C_3H_6O \cdot C_2H_4O)_n - n = 8400$ polymers and heated for 30 min at 250°C. The polymer and bone mixture was transferred into a silica crucible and calcined at 900°C for 5 h.

2.3 Hydroxyapatite Characterization Techniques

2.3.1 Thermal Gravimetric Analysis

Thermal gravimetric analysis (TGA) is a type of testing performed on the samples that determines changes in weight in relation to the temperature program in a controlled atmosphere such as nitrogen, helium, or in air. In most of the cases used in a nitrogen atmosphere, helium often provides the best baseline and air can sometimes improve the resolution. The TGA experiment depends on the environment consideration; thus, while performing the TGA experiments, avoid areas near heater or air conditioner ducts.

The TGA experiment is commonly employed to find out the level of inorganic and organic components in bone materials. Measurements are used primarily to determine the composition of materials and to predict their thermal stability at temperatures up to 1200°C. A DTG derivative weight loss curve can identify the point where weight loss is most apparent. The technique can characterize materials that exhibit weight loss or gain due to decomposition, oxidation, or dehydration. TGA can be used to determine the composition of a multicomponent system in the complex, thermal, and oxidative stability of materials, decomposition temperature, and moisture and volatiles content of the materials. About 10–20 mg of the samples was usually used for the TGA experiment in most of the applications, whereas 50–100 mg samples can be used for measuring the volatile compounds. Most of the TGA instruments have a baseline drift of ±0.025 mg, which is 0.25% of a 10 mg sample.

The raw marine fish bone of TGA and DTG has been found at 100.4°C and 365.6°C. The sample weight (4.76% and 30.02%) was significantly reduced based on the removal of water and organic moieties. The first derivative curve of the raw bone has shown a strong inflection at 365.6°C due to the collagen and other organic moieties (Figure 2.1).

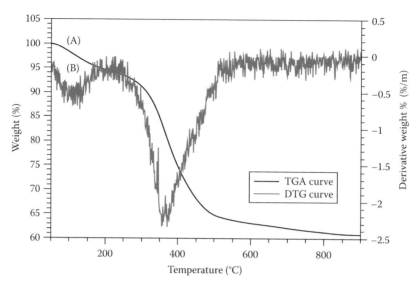

FIGURE 2.1
Thermal gravimetric and differential thermal gravimetric curves of fish bone.

The HAp obtained by thermal calcination and polymer-assisted thermal calcination method did not show any inflection at 365.6°C (figure not shown). This is confirmed by the absence of collagen and organic moieties in the derived HAp product. The small deflection point was observed in the first derivative peak of apatite derived by the alkaline hydrolysis method. This peak is due to the liberation of the high rich content of a carbonate group. Similar kind of weight loss had been observed in bovine bones by the alkaline hydrolysis method (Barakat et al. 2008).

2.3.2 Infrared Spectroscopy Analysis

Infrared spectroscopy deals with the infrared regions of the electromagnetic spectrum, which have longer wavelength and lower frequency than visible light. It can be used to identify and study chemicals. A common laboratory instrument used in this technique is the Fourier transform infrared (FT-IR) spectrometer. FT-IR is a promising tool to identify unknown substances and to determine the amount of components in a given sample. This test was performed to get authenticated information about the vibrational origin of the phosphate, carbonate, and amide groups and to confirm the production of HAp with no association of organic moieties. The raw fish bone contains an extracellular matrix mainly composed of HAp nanocrystals and collagen fibers.

The infrared region of the electromagnetic spectrum is divided into three regions:

1. Near infrared (14,000–4,000 cm^{-1})
2. Mid-infrared (4000–400 cm^{-1})
3. Far infrared (400–10 cm^{-1})

The near infrared region can excite overtone or harmonic vibration; mid-infrared is used to study the fundamental vibrations and associated rotational–vibrational structure.

HAp samples for the FT-IR analysis can be prepared in one of the following ways. Care is important to ensure that the film is not too thick; otherwise light cannot pass through it.

1. Crush the sample with an oily mulling agent in a marble or agate mortar, with a pestle. A thin film of the mull is smeared onto salt plates and measured.
2. Grind a quantity of the sample with a purified potassium bromide finely. This powder mixture is then pressed in a mechanical press to form a translucent pellet through which the beam of the spectrometer can pass.

In our laboratory, we have used FT-IR, PerkinElmer (United States), and spectrum GX spectrometers within the range of 400–4000 cm^{-1} and examined the stretching frequencies (vibrational origin) of HAp analysis.

The important stretching frequencies of HAp derived from fish bone are listed in Table 2.1 (Ducheyne et al. 1986; Pleshko et al. 1991; Rehman and Bonfield 1997; Joschek et al. 2000; Chen et al. 2002; Liu et al. 2002; Coelho et al. 2006; Prabakaran and Rajeswari 2006; Ooi et al. 2007; Boutinguiza et al. 2011).

TABLE 2.1

Important FT-IR Stretching Frequencies of HAp Derived with Thermal Calcination, Alkaline Hydrolysis, and Polymer-Assisted Thermal Calcination Methods

Methods	IR Absorption Bands (cm^{-1})	Description
Thermal calcination	1050, 1089	$v_3(PO_4^{3-})$
	962	$v_1(PO_4^{3-})$
	571	$v_4(PO_4^{3-})$
	1415, 1459	$v_3(CO_3^{2-})$
	634	Bending OH^-
Alkaline hydrolysis	1044, 1099	$v_3(PO_4^{3-})$
	963	$v_1(PO_4^{3-})$
	566	$v_4(PO_4^{3-})$
	1417, 1455	$v_3(CO_3^{2-})$
	875	$v_2(CO_3^{2-})$
	632	Bending OH^-
	3568	$v(OH)$
PEG-PPG-PEG with thermal calcination	1048, 1089	$v_3(PO_4^{3-})$
	961	$v_1(PO_4^{3-})$
	571	$v_4(PO_4^{3-})$
	1415, 1458	$v_3(CO_3^{2-})$
	634	Bending OH^-
	3571	$v(OH)$
PVA with thermal calcination	1048, 1089	$v_3(PO_4^{3-})$
	961	$v_1(PO_4^{3-})$
	571	$v_4(PO_4^{3-})$
	14,151,458	$v_3(CO_3^{2-})$
	634	Bending OH^-
	3571	$v(OH)$

2.3.3 X-Ray Diffraction Analysis

X-ray diffraction (XRD) analysis is a highly reliable technique to investigate the phase purity and crystallinity of compounds and also to determine the quantitative and qualitative aspects of solid compounds. The phase and the purity of the derived HAp crystals were confirmed with XRD analysis. XRD is a nondestructive technique and it can be used to identify crystalline phases and orientation, lattice parameters (10–4 Å), strain, grain size, epitaxy, phase composition, preferred orientation, and thermal expansion and to measure thickness of thin films and multilayers and atomic arrangements:

$$n\,\lambda = 2d\,\sin\theta$$

where
   d is the distance between atomic layers in a crystal
   λ is the wavelength of the incident x-ray beam
   n is an integer
   θ is the angle

Significance of peak shape, peak position, peak width, and peak intensity of HAp in XRD are important for the characterization of HAp. Thus, the XRD pattern obtained can be compared with known standards in the JCPDS file for the qualitative analysis.

In our laboratory, we used an x-ray diffractometer (PHILIPS X'Pert-MPD diffractometer, Netherlands) and Cu-Kα radiation of 1.5405 Å over a range of 5°–80° angle, step size 0.02, and scan speed 4°/min with 40 kV current and 30 mA voltage.

The intensity of the raw bone is usually found to be dispersed by x-ray radiation with a lowered intensity and wider peak. This may be due to the presence of an extracellular matrix and fibrous proteins. When subjected to calcination at higher temperatures, the subsequent peaks were highly intense and sharp, indicating the removal of organic portion (Glimcher 1959). The XRD results suggest that the HAp stability in the bone matrix was not disrupted when claimed in air up to 1000°C, as the chemical structure of HAp had not been affected and no other peak was obtained apart from HAp (Figure 2.2). It is well known that as the temperature increases, the intensity of the peak increases with a decrease in the peak width. The important high intensity peak of the x-ray spectrum of reference HAp by Joint Committee powder diffraction is shown in Table 2.2.

2.3.4 Field Emission Scanning Electron Microscopy

A field emission cathode in the electron gun of a scanning electron microscope provides narrower probing beams at low as well as high electron energy, resulting in improved spatial resolution. Field emission scanning electron microscopy (FE-SEM) produces clearer, less electrostatically distorted images with spatial resolution down to 1 1/2 nm. It is three to six times better than conventional SEM.

Sample preparation of FE-SEM analysis: first mount HAp particles on a mounting stub with double-sided carbon tape and blow off excess, unattached particles with compressed air. Attach the mounting stub to the mounting plate and gently screw it in place and measure with FE-SEM instruments. The surface morphology and crystal size of the derived HAp were studied using FE-SEM. Figure 2.3a through d show FE-SEM pictures of raw bone–derived HAp, by alkaline hydrolysis, thermal calcination, and polymer-assisted method, respectively.

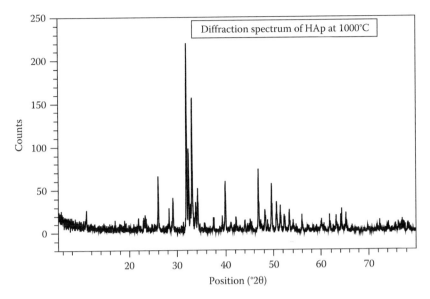

FIGURE 2.2
XRD spectrum of HAp at 1000°C derived from fish bone.

TABLE 2.2
XRD Data of Standard HAp JCPDS-090432—HAp

Crystallographic Plane (h k l)	Angle (θ)	d-Spacing (nm)	Intensity (%)
0 0 2	25.879	0.3440	40
2 1 1	31.774	0.2814	100
1 1 2	32.197	0.2778	60
3 0 0	32.902	0.2720	60
2 0 2	34.049	0.2631	25
3 1 0	39.819	0.2261	20
2 2 2	46.713	0.1943	30
2 1 3	49.469	0.1841	40
3 2 1	50.494	0.1806	20
0 0 4	53.145	0.1722	20

Microcrystals of HAp in the natural bone are very small, with a crystalline size of 5–10 nm, 10–15 nm wide, and more than a few micrometers long (Glimcher 1959; Ozawa and Suzuki 2002). The microstructures of raw *Thunnus obesus* bone appeared to be dense due to the presence of organic substances shown in Figure 2.3a. In Figure 2.3b and c, formation of microcrystals is clearly evident in the derived HAp at 900°C with dimensions 0.3–1.0 μm, whereas in the alkaline hydrolysis method, the size of the crystals is preserved <100 nm. It was conjectured from the surface morphology that the crystal size increases with respect to the temperature. The formation of these microstructures of derived HAp in the thermal process can be attributed to the tendency of particles to crystallize and agglomerate at high temperatures (Han et al. 2007; Barakat et al. 2009). HAp derived by

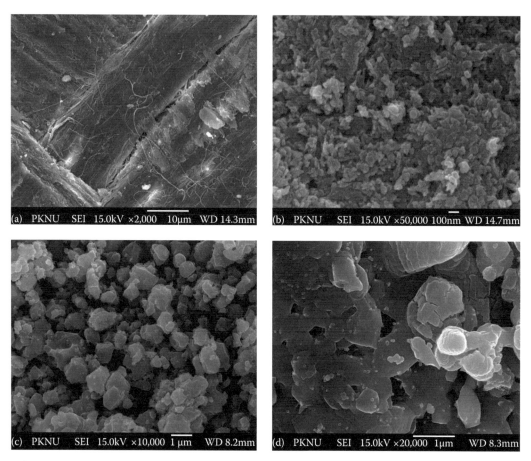

FIGURE 2.3
Scanning electron micrographs of (a) raw fish bone, HAp derived by (b) alkaline hydrolysis method, (c) thermal calcination method, and (d) polymer-assisted thermal calcination method.

the polymer-assisted thermal calcination method appears as a combination of nano- and microstructure arrangements (Figure 2.3d).

2.3.5 Electron Dispersive X-Ray Analysis

EDX is an analytical technique used for elemental analysis or chemical composition of a sample. According to the chemical formula of standard HAp, the Ca/P (calcium phosphorous) ratio is 1.67 (Koutsopoulos 2002). Based on the EDX signatures, the Ca/P weight ratio for derived HAp was calculated and was found to be 2.04, 1.94, and 1.99 at 600°C, 900°C, and 1200°C, respectively. The Ca/P ratios for the apatites obtained by alkaline hydrolysis and thermal calcination were 1.76 and 1.65, respectively, and the Ca/P weight ratio was 2.27 and 2.14, respectively.

2.3.6 Cytotoxicity Assay

The crystal size of HAp plays a major role in bone tissue engineering for nutrient supplementation and cell attachment. A highly porous and nanocrystal structure is a prerequisite to ensure that the biological environment is conductive for cell attachment, proliferation, tissue growth, and adequate nutrient flow. The cytotoxicity effects of derived HAp crystals at different temperatures were investigated by (3-(4,5-dimethylthiazol-2-yl)-2,5-diphenyltetrazolium bromide (MTT) assay.

The MTT assay method was used to find out the cytotoxicity of derived HAp. For this, osteoblastic cells are cultured in Dulbecco's Modified Eagle Medium (DMEM) supplemented with 5% fetal bovine serum, 2 mM glutamine, and 100 µg/mL penicillin–streptomycin and incubated at 37°C in a humidified atmosphere with 5% CO_2. The cells are grown at a concentration of 5×10^3 cells/well in a 96 well plate. After 24 h, cells were washed with fresh medium and treated with various concentrations of HAp crystals. After 24 h incubation, cells were rewashed with PBS; 2 mL of MTT (1 mg/mL) was added and further incubated for 4 h. Finally 2 mL of dimethyl sulfoxide (DMSO) was added to solubilize the formazan salt formed, and the amount of formazan salt was determined by measuring the optical density (OD) at 570 nm using a microplate reader. There are several contrary reports that have been published related to nanoparticle toxicity with cell experiment and several studies that explained that nanoparticles are toxic to cells (Liu et al. 2003).

2.4 Conclusion

This chapter shows the isolation of pure HAp from *fish* bone with different methodologies and characterization techniques. The emphasis was to isolate pure natural nano-HAp from tuna bone by employing alkaline hydrolysis and thermal calcination methods. Our work specifically signifies the potential use of thermally treated fish bone waste for the preparation of ceramics like HAp, which has a great potential as a viable and economical graft material in various biomedical and industrial applications. The HAp crystals obtained at different temperatures were found to be nontoxic, irrespective of the crystal size, suggesting their safe utility in bone tissue engineering.

Acknowledgment

This work was supported by a grant from Marine Bioprocess Research Centre of the Marine Bio 21 Center funded by the Ministry of Land, Transport and Maritime Affairs, Republic of Korea.

References

Barakat, N. A. M., K. A. Khalil, A. S. Faheem et al. 2008. Physiochemical characterizations of hydroxyapatite extracted from bovine bones by three different methods: Extraction of biologically desirable HAp. *Materials Science and Engineering: C* 28 (8):1381–1387.

Barakat, N. A. M., M. S. Khil, A. M. Omran, F. A. Sheikh, and H. Y. Kim. 2009. Extraction of pure natural hydroxyapatite from the bovine bones bio waste by three different methods. *Journal of Materials Processing Technology* 209 (7):3408–3415.

Boutinguiza, M., J. Pou, R. Comesaña, F. Lusquiños, A. de Carlos, and B. León. 2011. Biological hydroxyapatite obtained from fish bones. *Materials Science and Engineering: C* 32:478–486.

Cao, L.-Y., C.-B. Zhang, and J.-F. Huang. 2005. Synthesis of hydroxyapatite nanoparticles in ultrasonic precipitation. *Ceramics International* 31 (8):1041–1044.

Chen, F., Z. C. Wang, and C. J. Lin. 2002. Preparation and characterization of nano-sized hydroxyapatite particles and hydroxyapatite/chitosan nano-composite for use in biomedical materials. *Materials Letters* 57 (4):858–861.

Coelho, T. M., E. S. Nogueira, A. Steimacher et al. 2006. Characterization of natural nanostructured hydroxyapatite obtained from the bones of Brazilian river fish. *Journal of Applied Physics* 100:094312.

Coelho, T. M., E. S. Nogueira, W. R. Weinand et al. 2007. Thermal properties of natural nanostructured hydroxyapatite extracted from fish bone waste. *Journal of Applied Physics* 101:084701.

Ducheyne, P., W. Van Raemdonck, J. C. Heughebaert, and M. Heughebaert. 1986. Structural analysis of hydroxyapatite coatings on titanium. *Biomaterials* 7 (2):97–103.

Farley, J. H., N. P. Clear, B. Leroy, T. L. O. Davis, and G. Mcpherson. 2006. Age, growth and preliminary estimates of maturity of bigeye tuna, *Thunnus obesus*, in the Australian region. *Marine and Freshwater Research* 57 (7):713–724.

Feng, W., L. Mu-sen, L. Yu-peng, and Q. Yong-xin. 2005. A simple sol–gel technique for preparing hydroxyapatite nanopowders. *Materials Letters* 59 (8–9):916–919.

Fratzl, P., H. S. Gupta, E. P. Paschalis, and P. Roschger. 2004. Structure and mechanical quality of the collagen–mineral nano-composite in bone. *Journal of Materials Chemistry* 14 (14):2115–2123.

Glimcher, M. J. 1959. Molecular biology of mineralized tissues with particular reference to bone. *Reviews of Modern Physics* 31 (2):359.

Guo, G., Y. Sun, Z. Wang, and H. Guo. 2005. Preparation of hydroxyapatite nanoparticles by reverse microemulsion. *Ceramics International* 31 (6):869–872.

Han, Y., S. Li, X. Wang, L. Jia, and J. He. 2007. Preparation of hydroxyapatite rod-like crystals by protein precursor method. *Materials Research Bulletin* 42 (6):1169–1177.

Hirata, A., Y. Maruyama, K. Onishi, A. Hayashi, M. Saze, and E. Okada. 2008. A vascularized artificial bone graft using the periosteal flap and porous hydroxyapatite: Basic research and preliminary clinical application. *Wound Repair and Regeneration* 12 (1):A4.

Jarudilokkul, S., W. Tanthapanichakoon, and V. Boonamnuayvittaya. 2007. Synthesis of hydroxyapatite nanoparticles using an emulsion liquid membrane system. *Colloids and Surfaces A: Physicochemical and Engineering Aspects* 296 (1–3):149–153.

Joschek, S., B. Nies, R. Krotz, and A. Göpferich. 2000. Chemical and physicochemical characterization of porous hydroxyapatite ceramics made of natural bone. *Biomaterials* 21 (16):1645–1658.

Kano, S., A. Yamazaki, R. Otsuka, M. Ohgaki, M. Akao, and H. Aoki. 1994. Application of hydroxyapatite-sol as drug carrier. *Bio-Medical Materials and Engineering* 4 (4):283.

Koutsopoulos, S. 2002. Synthesis and characterization of hydroxyapatite crystals: A review study on the analytical methods. *Journal of Biomedical Materials Research* 62 (4):600–612.

Liu, Z. S., S. L. Tang, and Z. L. Ai. 2003. Effects of hydroxyapatite nanoparticles on proliferation and apoptosis of human hepatoma BEL-7402 cells. *World Journal of Gastroenterology* 9 (9):1968–1971.

Liu, D. M., Q. Yang, T. Troczynski, and W. J. Tseng. 2002. Structural evolution of sol–gel-derived hydroxyapatite. *Biomaterials* 23 (7):1679–1687.

Nair, M. B., S. Suresh Babu, H. K. Varma, and A. John. 2008. A triphasic ceramic-coated porous hydroxyapatite for tissue engineering application. *Acta Biomaterialia* 4 (1):173–181.

Ooi, C. Y., M. Hamdi, and S. Ramesh. 2007. Properties of hydroxyapatite produced by annealing of bovine bone. *Ceramics International* 33 (7):1171–1177.

Ozawa, M., K. Satake, and R. Suzuki. 2003. Removal of aqueous chromium by fish bone waste originated hydroxyapatite. *Journal of Materials Science Letters* 22 (7):513–514.

Ozawa, M. and S. Suzuki. 2002. Microstructural development of natural hydroxyapatite originated from fish-bone waste through heat treatment. *Journal of the American Ceramic Society (USA)* 85 (5):1315–1317.

Pallela, R., J. Venkatesan, and S. K. Kim. 2011. Polymer assisted isolation of hydroxyapatite from *Thunnus obesus* bone. *Ceramics International* 37 (8):3489–3497.

Pleshko, N., A. Boskey, and R. Mendelsohn. 1991. Novel infrared spectroscopic method for the determination of crystallinity of hydroxyapatite minerals. *Biophysical Journal* 60 (4):786–793.

Prabakaran, K. and S. Rajeswari. 2006. Development of hydroxyapatite from natural fish bone through heat treatment. *Trends in Biomaterials and Artificial Organs* 20:20–23.

Rehman, I. and W. Bonfield. 1997. Characterization of hydroxyapatite and carbonated apatite by photo acoustic FTIR spectroscopy. *Journal of Materials Science: Materials in Medicine* 8 (1):1–4.

Reichert, J. and J. G. P. Binner. 1996. An evaluation of hydroxyapatite-based filters for removal of heavy metal ions from aqueous solutions. *Journal of Materials Science* 31 (5):1231–1241.

Salman, S., S. Soundararajan, G. Safina, I. Satoh, and B. Danielsson. 2008. Hydroxyapatite as a novel reversible in situ adsorption matrix for enzyme thermistor-based FIA. *Talanta* 77 (2):490–493.

Sarig, S. and F. Kahana. 2002. Rapid formation of nanocrystalline apatite. *Journal of Crystal Growth* 237–239 (Part 1):55–59.

Staffa, G., A. Nataloni, C. Compagnone, and F. Servadei. 2007. Custom made cranioplasty prostheses in porous hydroxy-apatite using 3D design techniques: 7 years experience in 25 patients. *Acta Neurochirurgica* 149 (2):161–170.

Tang, P. F., G. Li, J. F. Wang, Q. J. Zheng, and Y. Wang. 2009. Development, characterization, and validation of porous carbonated hydroxyapatite bone cement. *Journal of Biomedical Materials Research. Part B, Applied Biomaterials* 90:886–893.

Tseng, Y.-H., C.-S. Kuo, Y.-Y. Li, and C.-P. Huang. 2009. Polymer-assisted synthesis of hydroxyapatite nanoparticle. *Materials Science and Engineering: C* 29 (3):819–822.

Venkatesan, J. and S. K. Kim. 2010a. Effect of temperature on isolation and characterization of hydroxyapatite from tuna (*Thunnus obesus*) bone. *Materials* 3 (10):4761–4772.

Venkatesan, J. and S.-K. Kim. 2010b. Chitosan composites for bone tissue engineering—An overview. *Marine Drugs* 8 (8):2252–2266.

Venkatesan, J., Z.-J. Qian, B. Ryu, N. A. Kumar, and S.-K. Kim. 2011a. Preparation and characterization of carbon nanotube-grafted-chitosan—Natural hydroxyapatite composite for bone tissue engineering. *Carbohydrate Polymers* 83:569–577.

Venkatesan, J., Z.-J. Qian, B. Ryu, V. T. Noel, and S.-K. Kim. 2011b. A comparative study of thermal calcination and an alkaline hydrolysis method in the isolation of hydroxyapatite from *Thunnus obesus* bone. *Biomedical Materials* 6 (3):035003.

Venkatesan, J., Z. J. Qian, B. M. Ryu, N. V. Thomas, and S. K. Kim. 2011c. A comparative study of thermal calcination and an alkaline hydrolysis method in the isolation of hydroxyapatite from *Thunnus obesus* bone. *Biomedical Materials* 6:035003.

Xu, J. L., K. A. Khor, Z. L. Dong, Y. W. Gu, R. Kumar, and P. Cheang. 2004. Preparation and characterization of nano-sized hydroxyapatite powders produced in a radio frequency (rf) thermal plasma. *Materials Science and Engineering A* 374 (1–2):101–108.

Zhang, H.-B., K.-C. Zhou, Z.-Y. Li, and S.-P. Huang. 2009. Plate-like hydroxyapatite nanoparticles synthesized by the hydrothermal method. *Journal of Physics and Chemistry of Solids* 70 (1):243–248.

3

Hydroxyapatite and Calcium Phosphates from Marine Sources: Extraction and Characterization

Clara Piccirillo, Manuela M. Pintado, and Paula M.L. Castro

CONTENTS

3.1 Hydroxyapatite and Calcium Phosphates: Properties and Applications as Biomaterials

Hydroxyapatite (HAp), $Ca_{10}(PO_4)_6(OH)_2$, is a chemical compound widely employed as a biomaterial, more specifically as a bone substitute (Dorozhkin, 2010). HAp is the main component of human and animal bones; it generally constitutes between 60 and 70 wt% of the bone, while the remaining part is collagen. The percentage of HAp in the bone can vary, if different animal species are considered; parameters such as the age of the animal can also affect this.

Using artificial HAp as a bone substitute is therefore the most obvious choice, as it replicates the mineral composition and the behavior of human bone. HAp is highly biocompatible and osteoconductive; in fact, it promotes the formation of new bone by favoring the growth of osteoblast cells.

HAp's biocompatibility and its effectiveness as a bone substitute material can depend on several factors; the ratio between calcium and phosphorus is particularly important. The stoichiometric ratio for HAp, and hence of human bones and teeth, is 1.67; therefore, in the material used as a bone substitute, the ratio should also be as close as possible to this value.

Another feature that can influence HAp biocompatibility is the possible presence of other elements as minor components in the HAp lattice. Magnesium, for instance, plays a key role, as it has an effect on HAp resorbability (Tomazic and Nancollas, 1975); the calcification of the bone itself and, therefore, its fragility can also be affected (Bigi et al., 1992). Chlorine and sodium, on the other hand, can have a positive influence on resorbability and osteoporosis, respectively (Kannan and Ferreira, 2006; Kannan et al., 2007a). Fluorine can also be important, as it can promote osteointegration (Cooper et al., 2006).

Surface characteristics, such as porosity, can also be a determining factor. Generally, a surface with high porosity favors cellular growth, as a greater area is available for osteoblast adhesion and migration (Tancred et al., 1998); this, in turn, facilitates the proliferation of the cells. Furthermore, the bonding between the bone and the HAp substitute material is more likely to take place on a porous surface.

In three-dimensional (3D) structures such as bone scaffolds, the dimension of the pores and their interconnectivity can also have an effect (Hutmacher et al., 2001). With well-interconnected pores, cells can easily reach all parts of the material, leading to a more complete osteointegration (Karageorgiu and Kaplan, 2005).

In some cases, however, a material with denser and more solid structure is necessary, exhibiting better mechanical properties; this is the case if HAp has to be used for the replacement of hard bones or for high load-bearing applications.

HAp is certainly the most used phosphate-based material for bone substitution, for all the characteristics described earlier. However, other phosphates are also employed as biomaterials (Dorozhkin, 2010). HAp is often used combined with tricalcium phosphate (TCP), $Ca_3(PO_4)_2$, in both its α and β forms. TCP generally has worse biocompatibility but a superior resorbability; therefore, a combination of the two materials can be used— a biphasic calcium phosphate (BCP). Studies on BCP materials are reported in literature (Gauthier et al., 1999; Peña and Vallet-Regi, 2003; Dorozhkin, 2012); their formation is favored when the atomic ratio between calcium and phosphorus is lower than 1.67 and closer to 1.5 (stoichiometric values for HAp and TCP, respectively) (Kannan et al. 2006). Several BCP products with both α and β forms are commercially available.

Fluorapatite (FAp), $Ca_{10}(PO_4)_6F_2$, on the other hand, has also been considered, particularly for dental materials (Rodriguez-Lorenzo, 2003). Due to its lower solubility, FAp is more stable in slightly acidic physiological environments; at the same time, however, its biocompatibility is comparable to that of HAp (Dhert et al., 1993). Furthermore, it can show antibacterial behavior toward both gram-positive and gram-negative strains (Ge et al., 2010).

3.2 Hydroxyapatite/Calcium Phosphates of Natural Origin

The majority of HAp and calcium phosphate materials used today are synthetic; several methods have been used to prepare HAp, TCP, and BCP materials in the form of powders, cements, thin films, or scaffolds. A review of all these methods is beyond the scope of this work; therefore, this topic will not be considered further.

In parallel to this, a series of process have been developed to prepare HAp from natural sources. In the next sections, a detailed description will be given of HAp and/or calcium phosphate biomaterials prepared using marine sources as starting materials.

The sources considered will be fish bones, fish scales, corals, cuttlefish, other shellfish, and finally marine algae.

3.2.1 Hydroxyapatite/Calcium Phosphates from Fish Bones

Producing HAp from sources like fish bones presents several advantages. Fish bones are a by-product of the fishing industry; in recent years, increasing amounts of these by-products have been generated. Their treatment poses a serious challenge for society, due to the associated potential environmental and safety issues. In the last decade, the extraction of valuable compounds from food by-products has been increasingly encouraged and developed (AWARENET, 2002). Therefore, the use of fish bones for HAp extraction fits this trend, and it could be of great benefit to both society and the environment.

Another issue to be considered is the availability of phosphorus necessary for the production of synthetic HAp. Phosphorus is not a scarce element on Earth. Despite this, however, recent reports have shown that if consumed at the current rate, world reserves will be depleted in about 50 years (Gilbert, 2009). This is because phosphorus is used in fertilizer production, and so there is an increasing demand, due to the growth of both the global population and economy. Hence, the development of alternative methods which do not require the addition of new phosphorus but, on the contrary, employ phosphorus naturally present in by-products is particularly valuable.

Considering the characteristics of the material, HAp of natural origin can actually be an improvement compared to synthetic ones. In fact, in animal bones, several elements are present as minor components (Grynpas et al., 1993), including the elements described in Section 3.2.1 (i.e., sodium, magnesium), which can have beneficial effects on HAp properties and its performance as biomaterial. In HAp extracted from fish bones, therefore, it is not necessary to add these elements, as they are already present in the lattice structure.

The use of animal bones to extract HAp is a process which was already performed for bovine and pig bones. Such studies are reported in literature (Barakat et al., 2008; Janus et al., 2008; Figueiredo et al., 2010); furthermore, HAp products from bovine origin are commercially available (Tadic and Epple, 2004; Dorozhkin, 2010). Examples of these products are Endobon®, Cerabon®, and PepGen P-15®.

Considering fish bones, at present, no HAp commercial product is available; several investigations, however, have been reported in literature.

The simplest process to extract HAp from animal bones is by thermal treatment. As mentioned in Section 3.2.1, HAp is the main component of bone, the remaining part being organic molecules such as collagen; therefore, a calcination process at high temperatures can remove the organic fraction, leaving only the HAp as the mineral component.

This procedure was employed by Ozawa on the bones of Japanese sea bream (Ozawa and Suzuki, 2002). Annealing was performed for temperatures up to 1300°C, with the weight loss monitored by thermogravimetric analysis. Three main weight losses were observed, between 30°C–250°C, 250°C–380°C, and 380°C–525°C; the first corresponded to the removal of the water from the bone lattice, while the second and the third to the elimination of organic matter. X-ray diffraction (XRD) analysis confirmed that the material was single-phase HAp; for the sample annealed at the 1300°C, however, some β-TCP was also detected. Ozawa observed a decrease of both surface area and pore volume with increasing annealing temperatures.

Several investigations were performed by Buitinguiza and coworkers. They extracted HAp using thermal processes from the bones of swordfish (*Xiphia gladius*) and tuna (*Thunnus thynnus*); annealing was performed at 600°C and 900°C (Buitinguiza et al., 2012). XRD analysis showed that samples annealed at 600°C from both fishes consisted of HAp only, but at higher temperatures, β-TCP was observed, in a concentration of about 13 wt%. These results were surprising considering that the Ca/P ratio was 1.82, i.e., not lower than the stoichiometric HAp value. For the samples annealed at 600°C, carbonate ions were detected by IR spectroscopy; these are normally associated with carbonate-substituted HAp (CHAp). In this case, the carbonate substitutes the phosphate ion, according to the formula $(Ca_{10-x/2}(PO_4)_{6-x}(CO_3)_x(OH)_2)$; this is referred to as B-type CHAp (El Feki et al., 1999). This feature is particularly important as both human bones and teeth contain CHAp. In samples annealed at 900°C, these ions are not present anymore, due to the complete removal of the organic species. BCPs obtained from both fishes showed no cytotoxicity (i.e., comparable to commercial products); therefore, they could be employed to fabricate bone substitute materials.

In another study published by the same authors, a two-step process was carried out to prepare HAp in the form of nanoparticles. Firstly, HAp was extracted from swordfish bones (*Xiphia gladius*) with a standard thermal treatment; subsequently, the material was treated with an appropriate laser source, to obtain HAp nanoparticles (Buitinguiza et al., 2009). Two laser sources were used: an Nd:YAG laser, applying pulses of power, and Ytterbium doped fiber laser, applying continuous power. HAp powder obtained from the calcination of the bones was dissolved in deionized water and irradiated; this caused the fragmentation of the powder into nanoparticles as small as 10 nm. The shape of the particles, however, was not always regular, and nanorods were also observed by microscopy. Furthermore, the composition of the material changed during the process, from single-phase HAp prior to the irradiation to BCP after (β-TCP was detected).

Further experiments were performed using a CO_2 laser source (Buitinguiza et al., 2011). In this case, HAp powder obtained by bone calcination was pressed into a cylindrical pellet and placed in deionized water. This target was then irradiated with the laser (ablation process). This led to the formation of nanoparticles with a spherical shape and an average diameter of 24.8 nm; Figure 3.1 shows the majority of nanoparticles have a diameter smaller than 38 nm, with a narrow distribution (sd = 8.7). In this case, however, a conversion into either β-TCP or whitlockite, $(Ca,Mg)_3(PO_4)_2$, was observed.

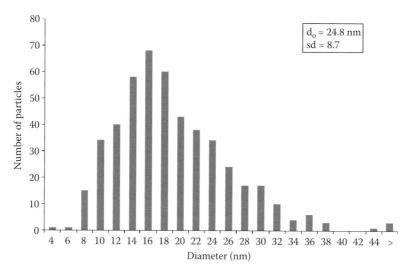

FIGURE 3.1
Diameter of nanoparticles produced by pulse CO_2 laser ablation in deionized water. (From Boutinguiza, M. et al., *Appl. Surf. Sci.*, 257, 5195, 2011. With permission.)

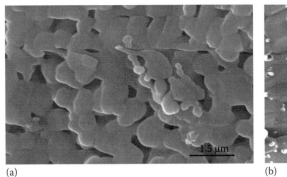
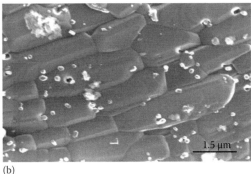

(a)   (b)

FIGURE 3.2
SEM images of HAp obtained by codfish bones with treatment in (a) $CaCl_2$ and (b) $CaAc_2$ solution and subsequent annealing at 1000°C.

Extraction of HAp and other phosphate compounds from Atlantic codfish (*Gadus morhua*) bones was also reported (Piccirillo et al., submitted). In this study, bones were annealed at temperatures between 600°C and 1200°C. XRD analyses showed that single-phase HAp was obtained only for the sample treated at 600°C. For the other annealing temperatures, a biphasic material HAp:β-TCP was detected; this was due to the Ca/P ratio being lower than 1.67. The proportions of the two phases changed, depending on the temperature used.

Moreover, the composition of the material was modified by treating the bones in a solution of an appropriate salt prior to the annealing process. The use of Ca-containing salts ($CaCl_2$ or $CaAc_2$) increased the Ca/P ratio; this led to the formation of single-phase HAp. Figure 3.2 shows SEM micrographies of HAp obtained from (a) $CaCl_2$ and (b) $CaAc_2$; it can be seen how the treatment in different solutions affects the surface morphology; this in turn can affect the properties of the biomaterial. Using a F-containing salt such as NaF, either a F-doped HAp or a completely substituted FAp was obtained. This last result was particularly interesting, considering the importance of FAp-based compounds described in Section 3.2.1. Furthermore, the concentration of minor elements such as sodium could be changed. These changes in the composition were possible due to the HAp structure and its excellent properties as an ion exchanger (Nzihou and Sharrock, 2010); the ion exchange process was especially effective due to the porous nature of the bones. This work showed that fish bones could be used not just to extract HAp but also to obtain HAp with a particular composition, tailored to specific applications.

3.2.2 Hydroxyapatite/Calcium Phosphates from Fish Scales

Fish scales are also by-products in the fish industry; therefore, all the environmental issues considered in Section 3.2.3 for the bones are valid for the scales as well. The main components of fish scales are collagen and HAp (Holá et al., 2011). A detailed study of the structure and morphology of the scales of sea bream (*Pagrus major*) was reported by Ikoma et al. (2003); XRD analyses confirmed the presence of HAp.

Despite being a potential source for HAp extraction, in literature not many studies are published on this topic, as the majority of investigations reported focused on the extraction and characterization of the collagen (Chen et al., 2010; Pati et al., 2010).

Mondal et al. (2010) reported on the extraction of HAp from the scales of *Labeo rohita* fish. Prior to the annealing, the scales were soaked in an acid solution (HCl), and then in an alkaline one (NaOH). Subsequently, the scales were annealed at different temperatures, between 600°C and 1400°C, and XRD analyses showed the effect of the annealing temperature on the sample phase composition. For temperatures up to 800°C, only HAp was detected; in the temperature range 1000°C–1200°C, however, some β-TCP was observed. At 1400°C, on the other hand, a dehydrated form of calcium phosphate—tetra calcium phosphate (TTCP), $Ca_4(PO_4)_2O$—was observed.

The extraction of HAp from the scales of tilapia (*Oreochromis sp.*) was studied by Huang (Huang et al., 2011). The extraction was performed by an enzymatic method, using protease and subsequently flavourzyme. The products were successively annealed at 800°C; XRD patterns showed that samples were single-phase HAp. To test the suitability of these materials as bone substitutes, cell promotion and differentiation were tested, using MG63 osteoblast-like cells. The results showed an activity comparable to that of commercial HAp samples.

This last study confirms the potential use of fish scales as a HAp source; this is surely a topic which deserves more investigation and further development.

3.2.3 Hydroxyapatite/Calcium Phosphates Derived from Corals

Corals have also been widely employed to manufacture HAp and/or other phosphate materials. The main advantage of the use of these marine species is their characteristic morphology. In fact, they have a 3D skeleton structure, very porous and with high levels of interconnectivity; as described in Section 3.2.1, this is an essential parameter for the efficacy of HAp as biomaterial.

In contrast to fish bones or scales, however, the main component of corals is not HAp or any other phosphate compounds but calcium carbonate, normally in the form of calcite. It is, therefore, necessary to convert the carbonate into phosphate, with the use of appropriate reagents/phosphate sources. It is important, however, to carefully choose the reaction conditions, to preserve the natural interconnected porous structure of the starting material.

The conversion of corals into HAp was first reported by Roy (Roy and Linnehan, 1973); the reaction was performed using hydrothermal synthesis at high temperature and pressure—103 MPa and 270°C, respectively (Roy and Linnehan, 1973). As a phosphate source, they used diammonium phosphate, according to the reaction

$$10CaCO_3 + 6(NH_4)_2 HPO_4 + 2H_2O \rightarrow Ca_{10}(PO_4)_6 (OH)_2 + 6(NH_4)_2 CO_3 + 4H_2CO_3$$

This process has been widely employed; today, several HAp-based commercial products, prepared using this reaction, are present in the market; examples are ProOsten® and Interpore200® made from *Goniopora* species (Dorozkhin, 2010). These materials are widely used for many different applications; several studies were performed to assess their effectiveness as bone substitutes (White and Shors, 1986, and references therein).

Following this first synthesis, other processes were successively developed. The main aims were either to use different corals as starting materials or to perform the reaction in less drastic conditions, i.e., at lower pressure and temperature.

Indian corals (*Goniopora* species) were successfully converted into HAp, as reported by Sivakuram et al. (1996). A hydrothermal process was used; coral powder was first preheated at high temperatures, to remove all the organics, and subsequently reacted with diammonium phosphate in a pressurized vessel. Some processing parameters were changed to determine the possible effect on the characteristics of the produced material; varying the preheating temperatures and the phosphate concentration seemed to particularly affect the crystalline structure.

The same researchers later used *Goniopora* coral species as starting material to prepare FAp (Sivakuram and Manjubala, 2001). Two methods were used for this synthesis: in the first one, hydrofluoric acid was added to the reaction vessel containing the coral powder and the phosphate. In the second, HAp was prepared as described earlier, and then, it was reacted with sodium fluoride (10% mol) at 900°C. These results were very important, as they showed how coral-derived HAp could be modified into different products. Moreover, a composite of both HAp and FAp with zirconia was also prepared; this was achieved by adding appropriate amounts of zirconia either into the hydrothermal reaction vessel (with the phosphate and hydrofluoric acid) or to the reaction mixture (with the sodium fluoride). Zirconia has very good mechanical properties; its use with HAp to make composites, therefore, could give materials with better mechanical performance. When zirconia was used, however, β-TCP was also detected; this indicates that HAp conversion into β-TCP was favored by the zirconia presence.

Further research on coral-derived HAp was performed by Ben-Nissan et al. (2004); they developed a two-stage process using *Porites sp.* corals. The corals were firstly converted into HAp with a hydrothermal process; subsequently, a HAp nano-coating was applied on the surface of this material, using the sol-gel technique. In this second step, salts such as calcium ethoxide, calcium acetate monohydrate, and diethyl hydrogen phosphonate were employed in the sol. The preparation and the aging of the sol was a critical point in the overall process; an aging of 72 h was essential to obtain single-phase HAp, with no other phases present (i.e., CaO). A substantial improvement in the mechanical properties was observed in the material prepared with this method, in comparison to the standard coral-line HAp obtained with simple hydrothermal process. The value of the biaxial strength was, in fact, almost double.

3.2.4 Hydroxyapatite/Calcium Phosphates from Cuttlefish Bones

Despite the very good performance shown by coral-derived materials, in recent years, different HAp sources have been considered. One reason is that the use of corals in big quantities may affect the ecology and equilibrium of their marine environments; some coral species, for instance, have been classified as endangered and, therefore, can be harvested only in very limited amounts and in specific periods (CITES). Furthermore, corals are not available everywhere in the world but only in some areas. There is, therefore, a need to find alternative sources, from unendangered species and/or species available worldwide.

Cuttlefish bones were one of the possibilities considered. Like coral, they have a carbonate-based porous interconnected structure, which would favor cellular growth and the osteointegration. Furthermore, they are available in many more locations in comparison to corals. As with fish bones (Section 3.2.3), cuttlefish bones also contain other elements as minor components, which can improve biocompatibility.

The use of cuttlefish bones was described in several papers; Rocha and his coworkers, for instance, used the bones of *Sepia officinalis* (Rocha et al., 2005a,b, 2006). The conversion reaction was performed at 200°C and 15 atm, using either diammonium phosphate or ammonium diphosphate as a source of phosphorus; several reaction times (between 1 and 72 h) were tested to study the kinetics of the reaction. Both XRD and IR data showed complete conversion into HAp after 9 h. IR spectroscopy confirmed the presence of carbonate in the HAp lattice, substituting both the hydroxyl and the phosphate ions, according to the

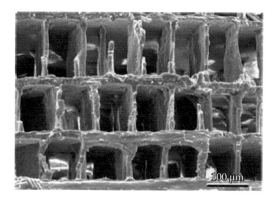

FIGURE 3.3
SEM image of HAp scaffold derived from *Sepia officinalis* annealed at 1250°C. (From Rocha, J.H.G. et al., *Bone*, 37, 850, 2005a.)

formula $Ca_{10}[(PO_4)_{6-x}(CO_3)_x][(OH)_{2-y}(CO_3)_y]$. This dicarbonated HAp is known as AB-type CHAp (Lafon et al., 2008). SEM microscopy confirmed that the original scaffold structure was maintained unaltered during the synthesis. Some selected samples were also annealed at higher temperatures (up to 1250°C), to improve the crystallinity of the material; also in this case, however, the interconnected structure was preserved (see Figure 3.3). Indeed, tests on cellular growth confirmed the biocompatibility of these materials.

Further work in this field was reported by the same research group; they also studied the synthesis of fluorine-substituted HAp, using the same starting material (bones from *Sepia officinalis*). To achieve this, they performed a similar reaction, using ammonium fluoride as a reactant together with the diammonium phosphate. Depending on the amount of fluoride employed, they obtained either F-substituted HAp or FAp (Kannan et al., 2007b); these are very interesting results, considering the importance of both these compounds (Section 3.2.1). Similarly to what was observed for the unsubstituted HAp, neither the hydrothermal synthesis nor the annealing affected the porous structure. The reaction kinetics, however, were different, as a longer time (12 h) was necessary to obtain the complete conversion of the carbonate into phosphates. Annealing at 1200°C caused the formation of some β-TCP in the material; this observation makes the material even more interesting, considering the good properties of the biphasic compound HAp:β-TCP.

Similar investigations on the use of cuttlefish bones were reported by Ivankovic et al. (2009). In their research, the bones from a Mediterranean cuttlefish (*Sepia officinalis* L.) were used; the hydrothermal synthesis was carried out with ammonium biphosphate at 200°C for different periods of time (between 1 and 48 h). Changes in the lattice structure (unit cell parameters and atomic coordinates) were monitored for the different reaction times due to the different degree of carbonate substitution. In a second series of experiments, a kinetic study of the reaction was performed (Ivankovic et al., 2010); this was performed by changing the reaction temperatures to values between 140°C and 220°C. In this way, the rate constant and the activation energy for this process were calculated.

Further work on cuttlefish bones was published by Sarin et al. (2011); the synthesis of BCP compounds, with different proportions of HAp and β-TCP, was studied in detail. Bones from cuttlefish from the Yellow Sea were treated in solutions containing variable amounts of phosphoric acid (between 12 and 20 wt%); after the treatment, a two-phase annealing process was performed on the bone first at 800°C, to eliminate the organic fraction, and then at 1200°C–1300°C, to improve the crystallinity. XRD results showed that the proportion of β-TCP in the material increased with increasing phosphoric acid concentration in solution. This method is important, as it allows the synthesis of BCP with different HAp proportions, which can be tailored to specific applications. Furthermore, the original porous structure of the cuttlefish bones was maintained, guaranteeing good biocompatibility and osteointegration.

3.2.5 Hydroxyapatite from Seashells

Similarly to fish bones and scales, seashells are also a by-product of the fishing industry; there is, therefore, interest in their reuse, to obtain valuable compounds. Different kinds of seashells have been used to prepare biological HAp.

The use of oysters, for instance, was reported by Lemos et al. (2006), employing the shells from *Mytilus galloprovincialis* and *Ostrea edulis*. As the main component of oysters is calcium carbonate, a hydrothermal process similar to that used for cuttlefish bones (described earlier) was employed (Rocha et al., 2005a). In this case, however, different reaction conditions were also tried—a different phosphate salt (potassium biphosphate) and a peptizing agent (tetraethyl ammonium hydroxide) were added together with the diammonium phosphate. This was done to avoid by-product formation. Moreover, the shells were ball milled prior to the reaction, to obtain nanoparticles as a starting material. Results showed the formation of CHAp, AB type, in the form of nanoparticles with average dimensions of 100 nm.

Oyster shells from *Crassostrea angulata* were employed in the study reported by Yang et al. (2011); similarly to Lemos, the hydrothermal synthesis was carried out with diammonium phosphate. The material obtained from this reaction, however, was not single-phase HAp but a BCP composite, with β-TCP present; this was due to a Ca/P ratio smaller than 1.67. This composite was then used to make 3D scaffolds, using polyvinyl alcohol and polyurethane, following a procedure already reported in literature (Teixeira et al., 2009) and depicted in Figure 3.4. The biocompatibility tests showed that the scaffolds prepared with oyster-derived BCP have comparable, or better, properties than those prepared with synthetic HAp.

Oyster shells, more exactly from *Crassostrea gigas*, were also used by Wu et al. (2011); the approach they used, however, was different, as they did not use hydrothermal synthesis but ball milling. First, the shells were milled to obtain a very fine powder; then they were mixed, by milling, with calcium phosphate compounds (either calcium pyrophosphate, $Ca_2P_2O_7$, or dicalcium phosphate dihydrate, $CaHPO_4 \cdot 2H_2O$ (DCPD)), making very homogenous mixtures. Subsequently, the mixtures were annealed at high temperatures.

The conversion of the carbonate into HAp, favored by the high temperatures, took place according to the reactions

$$6CaHPO_4 \cdot 2H_2O + 4CaCO_3 \rightarrow Ca_{10}(PO_4)_6(OH)_2 + 14H_2O + 4CO_2$$

$$3Ca_2P_2O_7 + 4CaCO_3 + xH_2O \rightarrow Ca_{10}(PO_4)_6(OH)_2 + (x-1)H_2O + 4CO_2$$

Several milling times (between 1 and 8 h) and different annealing temperatures (900°C, 1000°C, and 1100°C) were tested. Results showed a complete disappearance of the carbonate present in the starting material when $Ca_2P_2O_7$ was used; however, β-TCP was

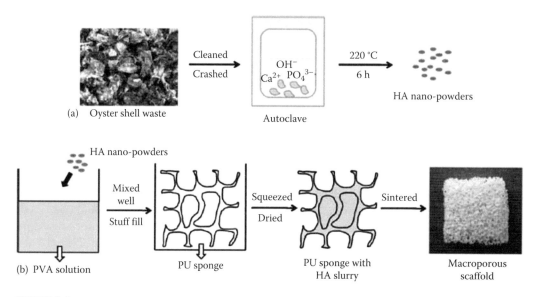

FIGURE 3.4
Schematic process: (a) hydrothermal conversion of the oyster shells to HAp nano-powders (b) fabrication of macroporous scaffolds. (From Yang, Y. et al., *Chem. Eng. J.*, 173, 837, 2011. With permission.)

also formed along with HAp, in different proportions depending on the experimental conditions. With DCPD, on the other hand, a complete conversion into single-phase HAp was observed.

The conversion of nacre (also known as mother-of-pearl) into HAp was also published. Gastropod (red abalone) nacre was used by Zaremba et al. (1998); a hydrothermal process was employed to obtain HAp. A comparison with other natural carbonate-based species (i.e., crab shell, lobster shell, coral) was performed, to better understand the reaction mechanisms and, consequently, the characteristics of the product. Results suggested that the complete conversion into HAp took place via a dissolution–recrystallization mechanism and not via a topotactic ion exchange. This mechanism was not observed for the other species tested; therefore, it could have been induced by the characteristic lamellar structure of the nacre used.

Clams were also used for conversion into HAp. Zhang and Vecchio (2006) described the use of the shells from *Tridacna gigas* (giant clam) and from *Strombus gigas* (conch). HAp was obtained by the hydrothermal process, by reacting with diammonium phosphate at temperatures between 180°C and 200°C. Several reaction times were tested—between 2 and 20 days—to see how this affected the conversion yield and the properties of the prepared material. As the shells had a compact dense structure, the formed HAp also had these characteristics; this is a very important aspect to consider for high load-bearing applications (see Section 3.2.1). Measurements of their mechanical properties indeed showed that the values of the fracture stress were comparable to those of human bones.

More studies were performed by the same research group on these HAp materials (Vecchio et al., 2007). Further to the mechanical properties, they also tested their biocompatibility and osteoconductivity with in vivo tests on rats; results showed that shell-derived HAp implants promoted bone growth, without causing fibrosis or any other problems.

Further to oysters, nacre, and clams, mussels were also employed to prepare HAp. Jones reported on the use of New Zealand mussels (Jones et al., 2011); the reaction to obtain HAp was performed using monopotassium phosphate at room temperature, in a nitrogen atmosphere. A conversion to HAp of about 95% was observed. Successive annealing treatments were performed to improve the crystallinity of the material.

3.2.6 Hydroxyapatite and Calcium Phosphates Derived from Algae

Algae have also been employed as a source of natural HAp or other calcium phosphate materials. Coralline algae, or red algae (sometimes called red seaweed), were the ones used for this application; this is because they contain calcium carbonate in their structure, more exactly in their thallus. Similar to that described for corals and cuttlefish (see Sections 3.2.5 and 3.2.6), they have a porous structure which makes them very suitable as bone filler material. Moreover, they are a renewable source, as they can be replanted in an appropriate environment very easily. Also in this case, hydrothermal syntheses were performed to convert the calcium carbonate into HAp, trying to maintain the 3D skeleton structure.

A high-pressure hydrothermal synthesis is used in the production of Algipore®. Algipore is produced and commercialized by DENTSPLY Friadent (Germany); in the U.S. market, however, it is referred to as algisorb (Osseus Technology).

Corallina officinalis and *Amphiroa ephedra* algae are employed to prepare Algipore; the hydrothermal conversion is performed for the reaction of the calcium carbonate with ammonium phosphate at 700°C. Tadic (Tadic and Epple, 2004) compared several HAp-based products of natural origin, including Algipore. From these analyses, it could be seen that Algipore showed a lower level of crystallinity; in its IR spectrum, on the other hand, the presence of residual carbonate and water in its structure could be observed. Indeed, its thermogravimetric curve confirmed these data, indicating residual concentrations of water and carbonate of 0.3 and 2.3 wt%, respectively (Tadic and Epple, 2004). In the SEM micrography, a porous structure could be observed, with grains smaller than 1 µm.

Subsequently, using the same algae, the hydrothermal process was modified by Spassova et al. (2007), to obtain either single-phase HAp or a HAp:β-TCP BCP material. These modifications were introduced considering the importance and the wider applications of BCP compounds, described in Section 3.2.1.

The formation of β-TCP was controlled with the addition of Mg^{2+} to the phosphate solution; in fact, this ion acts as a catalyst for the formation of this phosphate phase. Varying the amount of Mg^{2+}, it was possible to vary the percentage of β-TCP formed in the biphasic material, up to a value of 95% wt. XRD patterns confirmed the nature of the two different phases; in some cases, residues of carbonate (calcite) were also detected. For both single-phase and biphasic materials the channel-like structure of the algae was maintained; comparing the different materials, however, some differences could be observed due to the changes in composition. Single-phase HAp was the material which retained more of the original structure of the algae; in both cases, however, channels with an average diameter of about 10 µm could be observed. When β-TCP was formed, on the contrary, the average dimension of the channel was smaller (5–6 µm); this difference is due to the dimensions of the β-TCP grains, much larger than the HAp ones. This made the channel walls thicker and, consequently, their diameter smaller; the effect was more enhanced for the samples with a higher β-TCP content. This effect can be seen in Figure 3.5, where the SEM images of single-phase HAp and BCP materials are shown (a and b, respectively).

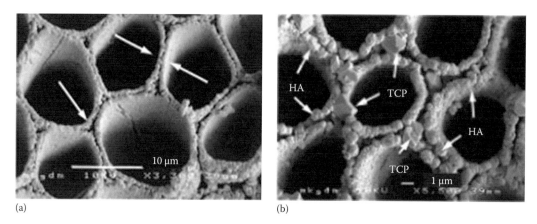

(a)   (b)

FIGURE 3.5
Cross-section SEM images of (a) single-phase HAp (b) BCP HAp:βTCP composite. (From Spassova, E. et al., *Mat.-wiss.u Werkstofftech*, 38(12), 1027, 2007.)

A low-pressure process using *Corallina officinalis* was reported by Oliveira et al. (2007); in this work, a combination of thermal and chemical treatments were used to achieve a conversion into HAp without losing the algae skeleton structure. The first step is a calcination at 400°C for 6 h, to remove most of the organic matter present in the algae, without decomposing the carbonate and/or losing the algae structure. Successively, the algae were soaked in an ammonium phosphate solution for 28 days; this allowed the conversion of the carbonate into HAp. The conversion, however, was not complete, as peaks belonging to the carbonate were still detected in both IR spectra and XRD patterns of the final phosphate-based material.

Walsh and coworkers also developed a low-pressure process for *Corallina officinalis* (Walsh et al., 2008). The principle is the same as that described by Oliveira (see earlier details), as a preliminary thermal treatment is then followed by a chemical reaction. There were differences, however, in the experimental conditions employed during the process. The first difference was the calcination, as it was performed at a higher temperature (650°C–700°C) and for a longer period (12 h); a very slow ramp was used (0.5°C/min) to avoid the decomposition of the skeleton of the algae. Subsequently, the reaction with the ammonium phosphate was performed at 100°C for 12 h. A complete conversion into HAp was observed. The 3D algae structure was maintained; the average channel size, however, was slightly bigger—10.72 μm for the HAp versus 10.01 μm for the algae starting material. The size distribution was also bigger, as the standard deviation increased to 1.99 from 1.27 μm.

The same research group successively performed a more detailed study of this process, focused on the first step—the annealing of the algae (Walsh et al., 2010). They showed how the annealing conditions—both the annealing temperature and the heating ramp—remarkably affect the characteristics of the final HAp-based material. Their investigation showed that a temperature of 600°C–650°C, a ramp of 2°C/min and an annealing time of 12 h obtained the material with the best morphology. Figure 3.6 shows the difference in morphology for samples annealed with different temperature ramps.

The low-pressure process described earlier was also employed using a different algae as a starting material, *Phymatolithon calcareum* (Kusmanto et al., 2008). Similarly to what was reported for *Corallina officinalis*, a conversion into HAp was observed, maintaining

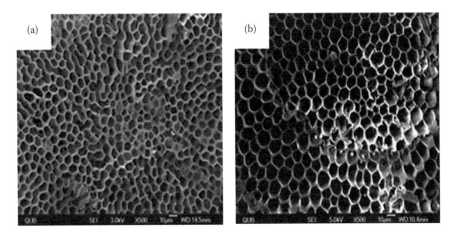

FIGURE 3.6
SEM images of algae annealed at 600°C for 12 h, temperature ramp: (a) 2°C/min (b) 10°C/min. (From Walsh, P.J. et al., *J. Mater. Sci. Mater. Med.*, 21, 2281, 2010. With permission.)

a high level of porosity. The material also showed good biocompatibility. Subsequently, the HAp so produced was mixed with a polymer (polycaprolactone, PCL) to manufacture scaffolds. Such scaffolds showed improved mechanical properties, without losing their characteristic porous structure.

3.3 Conclusions

HAp and other calcium phosphate–based materials were successfully produced from different sources of marine origin, such as fish bones and scales, corals, cuttlefish bones, seashells, and algae. In some cases, i.e., fish bones, the major component was already HAp; therefore, the focus was on the optimization of the extraction process. In other cases, i.e., corals, the starting material was a carbonate-based compound; hence, a reaction to convert it into phosphates was necessary.

Corals and algae-derived products are already commercially available; this is not yet the cases for the materials prepared from other sources. The work described here, however, confirms the potentials of all these compounds. Indeed the performances of the materials—biocompatibility and cellular growth—obtained from all different sources were comparable, if not better, of other HAp or phosphate compounds prepared with other methods.

Considering these results, further developments are expected in the future.

Acknowledgments

This work was financially supported by iCOD (Inovadora Tecnologias para a Valorização de Subproductos do Processamento do Bacalhau, funded by FTC, contract QREN AdI I|466). The authors thank Dr. R. Pullar for the help with the English language.

References

AWARENET. 2002. Handbook for the prevention and minimization of waste and valorisation of by-products in European agro-food industries. Agro-food waste minimization and reduction network (AWARENET). Growth Programme, European Commission, Bruxelles, Belgium.

Barakat, N.A.M., Khalil, K.A., Sheikh, F.A., Omran, A.M., Gaihre, B., Khil, S.M., and Kim, H.Y. 2008. Physiochemical characterization of hydroxyapatite extracted from bovine bones by three different methods: Extraction of biologically desirable HAp. *Materials Science and Engineering C*, 28:1381–1387.

Ben-Nissan, B., Milev, A., and Vago, R. 2004. Morphology of sol-gel derived nano-coated coralline hydroxyapatite. *Biomaterials*, 25:4971–4975.

Bigi, A., Foresti, E., Gregoriani, R., Ripamonti, A., Roveri, N., and Shah, J.S. 1992. The role of magnesium in the structure of biological apatites. *Calcified Tissue International*, 50:439–444.

Boutinguiza, M., Lusquiños, F., Riveiro, R., Comesaña, R., and Pou, J. 2009. Hydroxylapatite nanoparticles obtained by fiber laser-induced fracture. *Applied Surface Science*, 255:5382–5385.

Boutinguiza, M., Pou, J., Comesaña, R., Lusquiños, F., de Carlos, A., and León, B. 2012. Biological hydroxyapatite obtained from fish bones. *Materials Science and Engineering C*, 32:478–486.

Boutinguiza, M., Pou, J., Lusquiños, F., Comesaña, R., and Riveiro, R. 2011. Laser-assisted production of tricalcium phosphate nanoparticles from biological and synthetic hydroxyapatite in aqueous medium. *Applied Surface Science*, 257:5195–5199.

Chen, S., Hirota, N., Okuda, M., Takeguchi, M., Kobayashi, H., Hangata, N., and Ikoma, T. 2010. Microstructure and rheological properties of *tilapia* fish scales collagen hydrogels with aligned fibrils fabricated under magnetic fields. *Acta Biomaterialia*, 7(2):644–652.

CISPE—Convention on International Trade in Endangered Species of Wild Fauna and Flora. Appendices I, II and III, valid from September 25, 2012. http://www.cites.org/eng/app/appendices.php, accessed November 2012.

Cooper, L.F., Zhou, Y., Takebe, J., Guo, J., Abron, A., Holmén, A., and Ellingsen, J.E. 2006. Fluoride modification effects on osteoblast behaviour and bone formation at TiO_2 grit-blasted c.p. titanium endosseous implants. *Biomaterials*, 27:926–936.

Dhert, W.J.A., Klein, C.P.A.T., Jansen, J.A., Van der Velde, E.A., Vriesde, R.C., Rozing, P.M., and De Groot, K. 1993. A histological and histomorphometrical investigation of fluoroapatite, magnesium whitlockite, and hydroxylapatite plasma-sprayed coatings in goats. *Journal Biomedical Materials Research*, 27:127–138.

Dorozhkin, S.V. 2010. Bioceramics of calcium orthophosphates. *Biomaterials*, 31:1465–1485.

Dorozhkin, S.V. 2012. Biphasic, triphasic and multiphasic calcium orthophosphates. *Acta Biomaterialia*, 8(3):963–977.

El Feki, H.E., Savariault, J.M., and Bensalah, A. 1999. Structure refinements by the Rietveld method of partially substituted hydroxyapatite $Ca_9Na_{0.5}(PO_4)_{4.5}(CO_3)_{1.5}(OH)_2$. *Journal Alloys and Compounds*, 287:114–120.

Figueiredo, M., Fernando, A., Martins, G., Freitas, J., Judas, F., and Figueiredo, H., 2010. Effect of the calcination temperature on the composition and microstructure of hydroxyapatite derived from human and animal bone. *Ceramics International*, 36:2383–2393.

Gauthier, O., Bouler, J.M., Weiss, P., Bosco, J., Daculsi G., and Aguado, E. 1999. Kinetic study of bone ingrowth and ceramic resorption associated with the implantation of different injectable calcium-phosphate bone substitutes. *Journal Biomedical Materials Research*, 47:28–35.

Ge, X., Leng, Y., Bao, C., Xu, S.L., Wang, R., and Ren, F. 2010. Antibacterial coatings of fluorinated hydroapatite for percutaneous implants. *Journal Biomedical Materials Research A*, 95(2):588–599.

Gilbert, N. 2009. The disappearing nutrient. *Nature*, 461:716–718.

Grynpas, M.D., Hancock, R.G.V., Greenwood, C., Turnquist, J., and Kessler, M.J. 1993. The effects of diet, age and sex on the mineral content of primate bones. *Calcification Tissue International*, 52:399–405.

Holá, M., Kalvoda, J., Nováková, H., Skoda, R., and Kanicky, V. 2011. Possibility of LA-ICP-MS technique for the spatial elemental analysis of recent fish scales: Line scan vs. Depth profiling. *Applied Surface Science*, 257(6):1932–1940.

Huang, Y.C., Hsiao, P.C., and Chai, H.J. 2011. Hydroxyapatite extracted from fish scale: Effects on MG63 osteoblast-like cells. *Ceramics International*, 37:1825–1831.

Hutmacher, D.W., Schantz, T., Zien, I., Ng, K.W., Teoh, S.H., and Tan, K.C. 2001. Mechanical properties and cell cultural response of polycaprolactone scaffolds designed and fabricated via fused deposition modeling. *Journal Biomedical Materials Research*, 55:203–216.

Ikoma, T., Kobayashi, H., Tanaka, J., Walsh, D., and Mann, S. 2003. Microstructure, mechanical and biomimetic properties of fish scales from *Pagrus major*. *Journal of Structural Biology*, 142:327–333.

Ivankovic, H., Gallego-Ferrer, G., Tkalced, E., Orlic, S., and Ivankovic, M. 2009. Preparation of highly porous hydroxyapatite from cuttlefish bones. *Journal Materials Science: Materials in Medicine*, 20:1039–1046.

Ivankovic, H., Tkalced, E., Orlic, S., Gallego-Ferrer, G., and Schauperl, Z. 2010. Hydroxyapatite formation from cuttlefish bones: Kinetics. *Journal Materials Science: Materials in Medicine*, 21:2711–2722.

Janus, A.M., Faryna, M., Haberko, K., Rakowska, A., and Panz, T. 2008. Chemical and microstructural characterization of natural hydroxyapatite derived from pig bones. *Microchimica Acta*, 161:349–353.

Jones, M.I., Barakat, H., and Patterson, D.A. 2011. Production of hydroxyapatite from waste mussel shells. *IOP Conference Series: Materials Science and Engineering*, 18:192002.

Kannan, S. and Ferreira, J.M.F. 2006. Synthesis and thermal stability of hydroxyapatite-b-tricalcium phosphate composites with cosubstituted sodium, magnesium and fluorine. *Chemistry of Materials*, 18:198–203.

Kannan, S., Rebelo, A., Lemosa, A.F., Barba, A., and Ferreira, J.M.F. 2007a. Synthesis and mechanical behaviour of chloroapatite and chloroapatite/β-TCP composites. *Journal European Ceramic Society*, 27:2287–2294.

Kannan, S., Rocha, J.H.G., Agathopoulos, S., and Ferreira, J.M.F. 2007b. Fluorine-substituted hydroxyapatite scaffolds hydrothermally grown from aragonitic cuttlefish bones. *Acta Biomaterialia*, 3:243–249.

Karageorgiu, V. and Kaplan, D. 2005. Porosity of 3D biomaterial scaffolds and osteogenesis. *Biomaterials*, 26(27):5474–5491.

Kusmanto, F., Walker, G., Gan, Q., Walsh, P., Buchnan, F., Dickson, G., McCaigue, M., Maggs, C., and Dring, M. 2008. Development of composite tissue scaffolds containing naturally sourced microporous hydroxyapatite. *Chemical Engineering Journal*, 139:398–407.

Lafon, P., Champion, E., and Bernache-Assollant, D. 2008. Processing of AB-type carbonated hydroxyapatite $Ca_{10-x}(PO_4)_{6-x}(CO_3)_x(OH)_{2-x-2y}(CO_3)_y$ ceramics with controlled composition. *Journal European Ceramic Society*, 28(1):139–147.

Lemos, A.F., Rocha, J.H.G., Quaresma, S.S.F., Kannan, S., Oktar, F.N., Agathopoulos, S., and Ferreira, J.M.F. 2006. Hydroxyapatite nano-powders produced hydrothermally from nacreous material. *Journal European Ceramic Society*, 26:3639–3646.

Mondal, S., Mahata, S., Kundu, D., and Mondal, B. 2010. Processing of natural resourced hydroxyapatite ceramics from fish scales. *Advances in Applied Ceramics*, 109:234–239.

Nzihou, A. and Sharrock, P. 2010. Role of phosphate in the remediation and reuse of heavy metal polluted wastes and sites. *Waste and Biomass Valorization*, 1:163–174.

Oliveira, J.M., Grech, J.M.R., Leonor, I.B., Mano, J.F.M., and Reis, R.L. 2007. Calcium-phosphate derived from mineralized algae for bone tissue engineering applications. *Materials Letters*, 61:3495–3499.

Osseus Technology. Algisorb brochure. http://www.osseoustech.com/pdf/algisorb/algisorb-Brochure-2008.pdf, accessed April 2012.

Ozawa, M. and Suzuki, S. 2002. Microstructural developments of hydroxyapatite originated from fish bones waste though heat treatment. *Journal American Ceramic Society*, 85(5):1315–1317.

Pati, C., Adhikari, B., and Dhara, S. 2010. Isolation and characterization of fish scales collagen of higher thermal stability. *Bioresource Technology*, 101(10):3737–3742.

Peña, J. and Vallet-Regí, M., 2003. Hydroxyapatite, tricalcium phosphate and biphasic materials prepared by a liquid mix technique. *Journal European Ceramic Society*, 23:1687–1696.

Piccirillo, C., Silva, M.F., Pular, R.C., Braga da Cruz, I., Jorge, R., Pintado, M.M.E., and Castro, P.M.L. 2013. Extraction and characterization of apatites and tricalcium phosphates-based materials from cod fish bones. *Materials Science and Engineering C*, 33:103–110.

Rocha, J.H.G., Lemos, A.F., Agathopoulos, Kannan, S., Valério, P., and Ferreira, J.M.F. 2006. Hydrothermal growth of hydroxyapatite scaffolds from aragonitic cuttlefish bones. *Journal Biomedical Materials Research A*, 77(1):160–168.

Rocha, J.H.G., Lemos, A.F., Agathopoulos, S., Valério, P., Kannan, S., Oktar, F.N., and Ferreira, J.M.F. 2005a. Scaffolds for bone restoration from cuttlefish. *Bone*, 37:850–857.

Rocha, J.H.G., Lemos, A.F., Kannan, S., Agathopoulos, S., and Ferreira, J.M.F. 2005b. Hydroxyapatite scaffolds hydrothermally grown from aragonitic cuttlefish bones. *Journal Materials Chemistry*, 15:5007–5011.

Rodrigues-Lorenzo, L.M., Hart, J.N., and Gross, K.A. 2003. Influence of fluorine in the synthesis of hydroxyapatite. Synthesis of solid solutions of hydroxy-fluorapatite. *Biomaterials*, 24:3777–3785.

Roy, D.M. and Linnehan, S.K. 1973. Hydroxyapatite formed from coral skeleton carbonate by hydrothermal exchange. *Nature*, 247:220–222.

Sarin, P., Lee, S.J., Apostolov, Z.D., and Kriven, W.M. 2011. Porous biphasic calcium phosphate scaffolds from cuttlefish bone. *Journal of American Ceramic Society*, 94(8):2362–2370.

Spassova, E., Gintenreiter, S., Halwax, E., Moser, D., Schopper, C., and Ewers, R. 2007. Chemistry, ultrastructure and porosity of monophasic and biphasic bone forming materials derived from marine algae. *Mat.-wiss.u Werkstofftech*, 38(12):1027–1034.

Sivakuram, M., Kumart Sampath, T.S., Shantha, K.L., and Panduranga Rao, K. 1996. Development of hydroxyapatite derived from Indian coral. *Biomaterials*, 17:1709–1714.

Sivakuram, M. and Manjubala, I. 2001. Preparation of hydroxyapatite/fluoroapatite-zirconia composited using Indian corals for biomedical applications. *Materials Letters*, 50:199–205.

Tadic, D. and Epple, M. 2004. A thorough physicochemical characterisation of 14 calcium phosphate-based bone substitution materials in comparison to natural bone. *Biomaterials*, 25:987–994.

Tancred, D.C., McCormack, B.A., and Carr, A.J. 1998. A synthetic bone implant macroscopically identical to cancellous bone. *Biomaterials*, 19:2303–2311.

Teixeira, S., Rodriguez, M.A., Peña, P., De Aza, A.H., Ferraz, M.P., and Monteiro, F.J. 2009. Physical characterization of hydroxyapatite porous scaffolds for tissue engineering. *Materials Science and Engineering C*, 29:1510–1514.

Tomazic, B. and Nancollas, T.M. 1975. Growth of calcium phosphate on hydroxyapatite crystals: The effect of magnesium. *Archives of Oral Biology*, 20:803–808.

Vecchio, K.S., Zhang, X., Massie, J.B., Wang, M., and Kim, C.W. 2007. Conversion of bulk seashells to biocompatible hydroxyapatite for bone implants. *Acta Biomaterialia*, 3:910–918.

Walsh, P.J., Buchnan, F.J., Dring, M., Maggs, C., Bell, S., and Walker, G.M. 2008. Low-pressure synthesis and characterisation of hydroxyapatite derived from mineralise red algae. *Chemical Engineering Journal*, 137:173–179.

Walsh, P.J., Walker, G.M., Maggs, C.A., and Buchnan, F.J. 2010. Thermal preparation of highly porous calcium phosphate bone filler derived from marine algae. *Journal Materials Science: Materials in Medicine*, 21:2281–2286.

White, E. and Shors, E.C. 1986. Biomaterial aspects of Interpore-200 porous hydroxyapatite. *Dental Clinics of North America*, 30:49–67.

Wu, S.C., Hsu, H.C., Wu, Y.N., and Ho, W.F. 2011. Hydroxyapatite synthetized from oyster shell powders by ball milling and heat treatment. *Materials Characterization*, 62:1180–1187.

Yang, Y., Yao, Q., Pu, X., Hou, Z., and Zhang, Q. 2011. Biphasic calcium phosphate macroporous scaffolds derived from oyster shells for bone tissue engineering. *Chemical Engineering Journal*, 173:837–845.

Zaremba, C.M., Morse, D.E., Mann, S., Hansma, P.K., and Stucky, G.D. 1998. Aragonite-hydroxyapatite conversion in gastropod (abalone) nacre. *Chemistry of Materials*, 10:3813–3824.

Zhang, X. and Vecchio, K.S. 2006. Creation of dense hydroxyapatite (synthetic bone) by hydrothermal conversion of seashells. *Materials Science and Engineering C*, 26:1445–1450.

4

Isolation and Characterization of Chitin and Chitosan as Potential Biomaterials

Nitar Nwe, Tetsuya Furuike, and Hiroshi Tamura

CONTENTS

4.1 Introduction

Natural biopolymers such as gelatin, agar, agarose, alginate, carrageen, chitin, and chitosan can be produced from marine materials (e.g., gelatin is obtained from fish skin, pork skin, cattle bones, etc; alginates are obtained from seaweed; chitin and chitosan are obtained from shells of shrimps, crabs, and lobsters and bone plates of squids, crayfishes, krill, and cuttlefishes). Among them, chitin and chitosan have been used in various products such as antioxidative agents, bone-healing agent, cholesterol reduction agent, dental enamel de-remineralization, edible film, flocculating agent, growth stimulating agent for plant, hemostatic agent, immune stimulating agent, immobilization of cell, and juice clarification (Nwe et al. 2011).

Commercially, chitins and chitosans are produced from biowastes obtained from aquatic organisms, in which the physicochemical characteristics of chitosan are batch-to-batch variability due to seasonality of raw materials, freshness of the shell, quality of shell, species present, climate and distance of the shell supply, variability in raw materials, and difficulties in process control (Ashford et al. 1977 cited in White et al. 1979, Ornum 1992). To solve these problems, several excellent research contributions on the production of chitin and chitosan from different sources and on the properties and applications of chitin and chitosan have been made by scientists from all over the world for about 200 years. The success of the applications of chitin and chitosan depends on the properties of chitin and chitosan. All chitins and chitosans are not applicable in all sectors. For example, the application of chitosan as antibacterial agent or plant growth stimulator requires low-molecular-weight (LMW) chitosan. All chitosans do not support to make those applications successfully. Up to now, the terms "chitin" and "chitosan" are used for all products of chitin and chitosan. There is a need to develop a nomenclature system to represent each type of chitin and chitosan product. We already proposed to develop a nomenclature system for chitin and chitosan (Nwe et al. 2011). To development a systematic nomenclature system for chitin and chitosan, there is a need to establish international official standard methods to determine the degree of deacetylation (DD) and molecular weight of chitin and chitosan. Up to now, international official standard methods to determine physicochemical properties of chitin and chitosan have not been determined yet.

This article presents the production processes of chitin and chitosan from marine biowaste. Moreover, various forms of chitin and chitosan are presented based on solubility properties of chitin and chitosan. In addition, methods for determination of DD and molecular weight of chitin and chitosan are presented to propose a standard method to determine DD and molecular weight of chitin and chitosan that needs to develop a systematic nomenclature system to present each type of chitin and chitosan.

4.2 Production of Chitin and Chitosan from Marine Materials

In South East Asia, most shrimps and crabs are produced in aquaculture by both natural and high popular breeding techniques. The production of shrimp and crab meat for transport and export to prepare various seafood products results into massive amounts of shells of shrimps and crabs as biowaste (Figure 4.1). This waste has been used as fertilizer, feed for ducks and chickens, and others. Nowadays, this waste is used to produce chitin and chitosan in commercial scale. The production of chitin and chitosan from marine crustacean sources has been reported using several experimental conditions in laboratory scale.

4.2.1 Production of Chitin and Chitosan

The procedure for the production of chitin from shells of shrimps and crabs, and bone plates of squids includes demineralization and deproteination process, and then, chitosan is produced by deacetylation of chitin (Figure 4.2). The different quality of chitosan from these sources was obtained by treatment of chitin with concentrated NaOH at different conditions (Tables 4.1 and 4.2).

The demineralization of shrimp waste is completed within 15 min using 0.25 M HCl at room temperature (Roberts 2008 cited in Nwe et al. 2011). High DD (80%–100% DD)

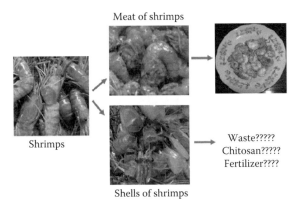

Meat of shrimps

Shrimps

Shells of shrimps

Waste?????
Chitosan?????
Fertilizer????

FIGURE 4.1
Shells of shrimps obtained from seafood processing.

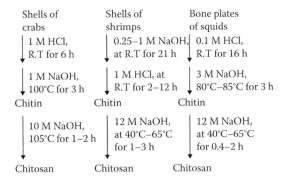

Shells of crabs → 1 M HCl, R.T for 6 h → 1 M NaOH, 100°C for 3 h → **Chitin** → 10 M NaOH, 105°C for 1–2 h → **Chitosan**

Shells of shrimps → 0.25–1 M NaOH, at R.T for 21 h → 1 M HCl, at R.T for 2–12 h → **Chitin** → 12 M NaOH, at 40°C–65°C for 1–3 h → **Chitosan**

Bone plates of squids → 0.1 M HCl, R.T for 16 h → 3 M NaOH, 80°C–85°C for 3 h → **Chitin** → 12 M NaOH, at 40°C–65°C for 0.4–2 h → **Chitosan**

FIGURE 4.2
Production of chitosan from shells of crabs and shrimps and bone plates of squids. (From Yen, M. et al., *Carbohydr. Polym.*, 75, 15, 2009; Lertsutthiwong, P. et al., *J. Metals, Mater., Miner.*, 12, 11, 2002; Methacanon, P. et al., *Carbohydr. Polym.*, 52, 119, 2003.)

of chitosan could be obtained by treatment of chitin from squid pens with 10–15 M NaOH at 80°C–100°C for 1–2 h (Table 4.1). The resultant chitosan has medium molecular weight. However, chitosans with medium molecular weight, 810 kDa, and various DD have been produced by treatment of chitin from shells of shrimps with 12.5 M NaOH under different treatment conditions (Table 4.2), in which Lertsutthiwong et al. (2002) reported that the DD and molecular weight of chitosan produced from shells of shrimps depend on the conditions of extraction process, including the concentration of NaOH and HCl, the soaking time and the sequence of treatments for deproteination, decalcification, and deacetylation. The scale-up shrimp chitin deacetylation was carried out with strong alkaline under ambient temperature for 3 days; the DD was 75.10%. The higher DD of chitosan with 90% was obtained by second treatment with strong alkaline (Chinadit et al. 1998 cited in Nwe et al. 2011). The molecular weight of native chitin is usually larger than one million while commercial chitosan products fall between 100,000 and 1,200,000 (Muzzarelli 1973 cited in Nwe et al. 2011).

Moreover, the production of chitin and chitosan by chemical process has a lot of problems such as environmental pollution, inconsistent molecular weight, and degree of acetylation. To solve these problems, fermentation processes have been studied to produce chitin and

TABLE 4.1

Condition for Deacetylation of Squid Chitin and Degree of
N-Deacetylation of Squid Chitosan Obtained under Various
Conditions (1 g of Chitin Was Treated with 10 mL of NaOH Solution)

NaOH Concentration (%)	Temperature (°C)	Time (min)	%DD (Average)[a]
40	40	120	43.3
40	60	120	68
40	80	120	84
40	100	120	88.7
60	40	120	27.5
60	60	120	70.7
60	80	45	84.2
60	80	60	90.2
60	80	120	94.7
60	100	30	94.0
60	100	60	97.3

Source: Methacanon, P. et al., *Carbohydr. Polym.,* 52, 119, 2003.
[a] The DD was measured using ^{13}C CP/MAS NMR spectra.

TABLE 4.2

Conditions Used for Preparation of Chitosan from Shells of Shrimps

NaOH Concentration (M)	Deacetylation Conditions			DD of Chitosan[a]
	Temperature (°C)	Time (h)	Times of Deacetylation	
12.5	40	24	1	75
12.5	65	20	1	87
12.5	65	20	2	96

Source: Trung, T.S. et al., *Bioresour. Technol.,* 97, 659, 2006.
[a] The DD was measured according to Tan et al. (1996).

chitosan from shells of shrimps and crabs and bone plates of squids (Nwe et al. 2011). The enzymatic deacetylation of various chitin preparations has been investigated using the fungal chitin deacetylase (CDA) isolated from *Rhizopus oryzae* growth in solid-state and submerged fermentation medium (Aye et al. 2006). The results showed that natural crystalline chitin is a very poor substrate for the enzyme.

4.2.2 Production of Low-Molecular-Weight Chitosan and Chitooligosaccharides

In agriculture and medical applications, LMW chitosans and chitooligosaccharide (CTS-O) are more effective than high-molecular-weight (HMW) chitosan (Nwe et al. 2011). The LMW chitosan and CTS-O have been produced from the HMW chitosan by physical method such as treatment with γ-ray irradiation and with microwave irradiation; chemical method such as treatment with dilute and concentrated HCl, with $NaNO_2$, with H_2O_2, with HNO_2, and with phosphoric acid; mechanical method such as treatment with sonication; and enzymatic method such as treatment with cellulose, with lysozyme, with chitinase, with chitosanase, with lipase, with hyaluronidase, with papain, with pectinase, with pepsin, with protease, and with hemicellulase (Nwe et al. 2011). Although the different protocols for the production of LMW chitosan and CTS-O have been published, acid and enzymatic depolymerization of chitosan is most frequently used.

4.2.2.1 Depolymerization of Chitosan with Chemical Method

The chitosan with desired molecular weight can be obtained by varying the mixing days in deacetylation–degradation or sodium nitrite in oxidative degradation (Luyen 1994) and controlling the ratio of nitrite to chitosan (Thomas and Philip 2000). Kasaai et al. (2001) reported that the fragmentation with HCl at 65°C and oxidation with $NaNO_2$ at room temperature was more effective than the fragmentation with H_2O_2 at room temperature. The HNO_2 attacks the amino group of glucosamine units and cleavages the glycosidic linkage of the D-A and D-D which are known by determining the identity and the relative amounts of new nonreducing ends of depolymerized chitosans (Vårum et al. 1996a cited in Vårum et al. 2001). Thomas and Philip (2000) pointed out that sodium nitrite must be carefully removed from the LMW chitosan to use safely in medical application. Among the chemicals used, HCl is widely used for the production of LMW chitosan and CTS-O. The O-glycosidic linkages (depolymerization) and the N-acetyl linkages (de-N-acetylation) in the chitosan polymers are hydrolyzed during treatment with dilute and concentrated HCl (Vårum et al. 2001). The rate of hydrolysis of the glycosidic linkages was equal to that of N-acetyl linkage in dilute acid, in which the glycosidic linkages were hydrolyzed more than 10 times faster than the N-acetyl linkage in concentrated HCl (Vårum et al. 2001).

4.2.2.2 Depolymerization of Chitosan with Enzymatic Method

Kasaai et al. (2001) reported that papain and wheat bran lipase were most effective for the depolymerization of chitosan as compared to other enzymes (pectinase, lysozyme, *Candida rugosa* lipase, and hyaluronidase). Chang et al. (1998) reported that the degradation of chitosan to an average molecular weight of 30,000 Da, as observed during treatment with crude pepsin, was performed by the chitosanase present in the enzyme preparation and not by the proteolytic enzyme itself. The conditions for depolymerization of chitin and chitosan using some enzymes are shown in Table 4.3.

4.2.2.3 Depolymerization of Chitosan by γ-Ray Irradiation

Depolymerization of chitosan (powder or solution form) has been carried out under different dosages of γ-ray irradiation (Table 4.4). Rate of degradation of chitosan powder in dried form by γ-ray irradiation was lower than that of hydrated form of chitosan.

4.3 Physicochemical Properties of Chitin and Chitosan

4.3.1 Solubility Properties of Chitin and Chitosan

Chitin is a copolymer of N-acetyl-D-glucosamine and D-glucosamine units linked with β-(1–4) glycosidic bond; here, N-acetyl-D-glucosamine units are predominant in that polymer chain. Crystalline form of chitin occurs in nature as α-, β-, and γ-chitin (Rudall 1963 cited in Nwe and Stevens 2008). α-Chitin can be obtained from shells of

TABLE 4.3

Enzymatic Depolymerization of Chitin and Chitosan Using Various Enzymes and Conditions

Enzyme	Chitin/Chitosan	Treatment Conditions			Results
		pH	Temp (°C)	Time (h)	
Pepsin[a]	Amorphous chitin (100 mg/20 mg enzyme)	5.4	44	24	71.5% of chitobiose, 19% of GlcNAc and 9.5% chitotriose
Neutral protease[b]	Chitosan (92% DD)	5.4	50	—	The DD of the main hydrolysis products decreased compared with the initial chitosan. The degree of polymerization of chito-oligomers was mainly from 3 to 8
Hemicellulase[c]	Chitosan (2.5%)	5.5	50	1–4	The enzymatic hydrolysis was endo-action and mainly occurred in a random fashion. The total degree of acetylation of chitosan did not change after degradation

[a] Ilankovan et al. (2006).
[b] Li et al. (2005).
[c] Qin et al. (2003).

TABLE 4.4

Effect of Radiation Dose and Form of Chitosan on the Depolymerization of Chitosan by γ-Ray Irradiation

Radiation Doses (kGy)	Form of Chitosan	MW of Sample after Radiation (kDa)	Remarks
0[a]	Powder	577	The DD of chitosan samples before and after irradiation showed a negligible effect on the exposure of γ-ray radiation under the doses of 10–100 kGy
10[a]	Powder	458	
25[a]	Powder	242	
50[a]	Powder	159	
100[a]	Powder	106	
0[b]	Powder	~740	"The molecular weight of chitosan decreased remarkably with increasing radiation dose and tapers off at 200 kGy and above"
100[b]	Powder	~100	
200[b]	Powder	~70	
0[c]	Powder	369	Chitosan in powder form (3 g chitosan powder was hydrated by mixing with 3 mL of distilled water) and chitosan in solution form (chitosan powder, 1 g was dissolved in 100 mL of 0.35 M acetic acid at room temperature) were irradiated under γ-ray for degradation of their polymer chains
100[c]	Powder	10	
90[c]	Solution	0.9	

[a] Zainol et al. (2009).
[b] Hai et al. (2003).
[c] Nwe et al. (2010).

crabs and shrimps and from cell walls of fungi, and β-chitin can be isolated from the bone plates of squids and cuttlefishes (Lopez-Romero and Ruiz-Herrera 1986, Stevens 1996 cited in Nwe and Stevens 2008). In α-chitin, the chains run in antiparallel fashion bound by strong hydrogen bounding. In β-chitin, the chains run in parallel and are connected by weak intermolecular forces. The γ-chitin is a mixed form of α- and β-chitin

(Rudall 1963 cited in Nwe and Stevens 2008). The deacetylated form of chitin is chitosan. In the deacetylation process of chitin, the aligned structure of chitin molecules has no influence on removal of protein, calcium phosphate, and amide groups from crab tendon chitin through a strong treatment in 50% NaOH at 100°C (Itoh et al. 2003 cited in Nwe et al. 2011). This means the aligned structure of chitosan molecules is similar to that of chitin molecules.

Solubility properties of chitin and chitosan are highly dependent on the number of free amino groups in the molecules. Chitin possesses a low content of amino groups. Therefore, most chitins are not soluble and do not swell in common solvents; however, very partially deacetylated chitin (degree of acetylation [DA] 25%) and β-chitin can be swollen in water (Hein et al. 2007, Kurita 2001 cited in Nwe and Stevens 2008). Chitins dissolve in concentrated acids (HCl, H_2SO_4, formic, acetic, dichloroacetic, and trichloroacetic acid), in (dimethylformamide)-N_2O_4 mixtures, in hexafluoro-2-propanol, in hexafluoroacetone, in dimethylacetamide-LiCl, in N-methyl pyrrolidone-LiCl, and in $CaCl_2.2H_2O$-methanol (Kurita 2001, Roberts 1992 cited in Nwe and Stevens 2008, Tamura et al. 2006). Conditions to dissolve chitin in some solvents are presented in Table 4.5. Chitosan is soluble in dilute inorganic acids, HCl, HBr, HI, HNO_3, and $HClO_4$; in concentrated H_2SO_4; in organic acids, citric, formic, lactic, acetic, and pyruvic acid; in tetrahydrofuran; in ethyl acetate; and in 1,2-dichloroethane, but it is insoluble in benzoic acid, in cinnamic acid, and in oxalic acid (Nwe et al. 2010a cited in Nwe et al. 2011, Roberts 1992). CTS-O is soluble in water and in solutions at acid and alkaline pH. It has low viscosity.

TABLE 4.5

Solubility Properties of Chitin in Different Solvents

Solvents	Conditions for Solubility	Remarks
8% (w/v) NaOH/4% (w/v) Urea[a]	4 g chitin in 200 g solvent, −20°C for 36 h	Homogeneous and transparent solution at −20°C and transform it to gel when temperature increases
Dimethylacetamide-5% LiCl[b,c]	0.3–1.5 g chitin in 100 mL of solvent at room temperature for 48 h	Clear and transparent chitin solution was obtained. Undissolved materials remained
N-methyl pyrrolidone-5% LiCl[c]	0.3–1.5 g chitin in 100 mL of solvent at room temperature for 48 h	Clear and transparent chitin solution was obtained. Undissolved materials remained
$CaCl_2 \cdot 2H_2O$-methanol[d]	1–2 g of chitin powder in 100 mL of Ca solvent (1.25% for β-chitin and 2% for α-chitin)	The properties of chitin solution depend on degree of N-acetylation, molecular weight of chitin, concentration of $CaCl_2$, and number of water molecules composed in $CaCl_2$
85% phosphoric acid[e]	—	Chitin could recover from solution by adding 6 M NaOH to pH 8.0
37% HCl acid[e]	—	Chitin could recover from solution by adding 6 M NaOH to pH 8.0

[a] Hu et al. (2007).
[b] Yusof et al. (2004).
[c] Yilmaz and Bengisu (2003).
[d] Tamura et al. (2006).
[e] Ilankovan et al. (2006).

Under acidic pH, the amino groups in the chitosan molecule become protonated and the polymers dissolve in polar solvents. In the neutral and alkaline pH, chitosan molecules lose their positive charge and precipitate. These properties can be exploited to prepare chitosan matrices in various forms: powder, capsule, hydrogels, macro- and microfiber, nano-fiber, membrane, macro- and micro-beads, and scaffolds (Nwe et al. 2011).

4.3.1.1 Preparation of Chitin and Chitosan Hydrogel

Preparation of chitin hydrogel: Chitin hydrogels have been prepared using different solvents and using different methods. In 2004, Yusof et al. reported to prepare chitin hydrogel using DMAc–5%LiCl as solvent. Briefly, chitin flake, 0.5 g, was dissolved in 100 mL of DMAc–5%LiCl at 10°C, and the solution was filtered through glass wool. The chitin solution, 155 mL, was cast into a deep mold, and the mold was covered with aluminum foil, which has pinholes. After that, the mold was incubated in a fume hood at 25°C–27°C for 24 h. In 2006, Tamura et al. investigated a method to prepare chitin hydrogel using saturated $CaCl_2.2H_2O$ in methanol as solvent to dissolve chitin. Briefly, a large amount of distilled water (around 20 L) was added to 1 L of chitin solution with vigorous stirring and then filtered to collect the chitin precipitate, followed by extensive dialysis against distilled water to remove the calcium ions and methanol. The chitin content in the hydrogel was about 3%–6% (w/v). For the preparation of anhydrous chitin gel, a large amount of methanol or isopropanol was added to the chitin solution in order to precipitate chitin. The chitin precipitate was loaded into a glass column, and then, methanol was passed through to the column to remove calcium ions in the chitin gel. Moreover, Tamura et al. (2006) prepared β-chitin using distilled water as solvent. Briefly, 10 g of β-chitin powder was suspended in 20 mL of distilled water and subjected to a high-speed mechanical agitation in a Waring blender for 30 s at room temperature. The procedure was repeated several times by the stepwise addition of distilled water until a homogeneous gel was formed. The chitin content was adjusted by centrifugation to 3%–6% (w/v).

4.3.1.2 Preparation of Chitin and Chitosan Membrane

4.3.1.2.1 Preparation of Chitin Membranes

Yusof et al. (2004) used chitin gel, obtained by dissolving chitin in DMAc–5%LiCl for 24 h, to cast the chitin film. Briefly, chitin gel was placed between two sheets of filter paper. Two glass plates were next placed, one on either side of the filter paper, to form a "sandwich" where the chitin gel was in the middle. The glass plates were held together by paper clamps at room temperature, and the gel assembly was next heated at 50°C in an oven for 12 h to remove residual solvent. The obtained film was subsequently soaked in 95% ethanol, and the cold-press procedure was repeated and maintained for 48 h to give dry and free DMAc. The chitin film is transparent and colorless. In 2006, Tamura et al. prepared chitin membrane using distilled water as chitin solvent. Chitin gel was suspended in water (approximately 0.1% w/v) and then filtered through a saranmeshed filter to remove the water. The resulting chitin thread was pressed dry between filter papers at room temperature for 20 h.

4.3.1.2.2 Preparation of Chitosan Membrane

Solvent casting method was used mostly to prepare membranes of chitosan (Figure 4.3). Chitosan solution was prepared by dissolving 0.2 g of each type of chitosan powder in

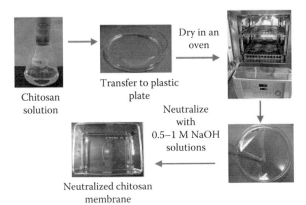

FIGURE 4.3
Preparation of chitosan membrane.

20 mL of 0.35 M acetic acid at 25°C, 150 rpm for 48 h. After homogeneous solution was obtained, each chitosan solution was transferred to plastic cultivation dishes (diameter 99 mm) and dried at 45°C in an oven. The dried membrane was neutralized in 0.5 M NaOH solution and then washed with distilled water up to neutral pH. Finally, the neutralized membrane was placed between two filter papers and dried at room temperature.

4.3.1.3 Preparation of Chitosan Scaffolds

Nwe et al. (2009) used freeze-dried method to prepare chitosan scaffold (Figure 4.4). Chitosan powder (1 g) was dissolved in 0.35 M acetic acid (100 mL), which is a common solvent to dissolve all chitosans, at room temperature for 1–2 days until the solutions became viscous, transparent, and homogeneous. Each chitosan solution (8 mL) was transferred to a cultivation dish (diameter 35 mm) and frozen at −20°C and then freeze-dried.

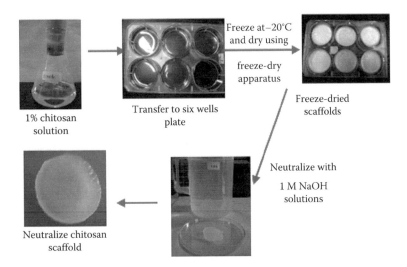

FIGURE 4.4
Preparation of chitosan scaffold.

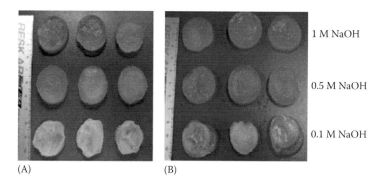

FIGURE 4.5
Morphology of crab chitosan scaffolds after neutralization with 1, 0.5, and 0.1 M NaOH in distilled water (A) and in 70% ethanol (B). (From Nwe, N. et al., *Materials*, 2, 374, 2009.)

After freeze-drying, the acetate molecules are in solid form in the scaffold cavities, as ions bound to the cationic amine groups in the chitosan. To remove acetate ions from scaffold cavities, chitosan scaffold was neutralized in 10 mL of 0.01, 0.1, 0.5, and 1 M NaOH dissolved in distilled water or 70% ethanol (Figure 4.5) to determine the right NaOH concentration for the neutralization of chitosan scaffolds. It was observed that scaffolds completely dissolved in 0.01 M NaOH in distilled water or in 70% ethanol solution during 5 h. The aggregation of scaffold cavities could be observed in scaffold neutralized in 0.1 M NaOH in distilled water or in 70% ethanol solution. Porous chitosan scaffolds could be obtained using 0.5 and 1 M NaOH in distilled water or in 70% ethanol solution as neutralized media. The best neutralization medium is 1 M NaOH dissolved in distilled water or 70% ethanol. Here, air bubbles trapped inside the scaffolds were observed in the freeze-dried scaffolds when the scaffolds were stored for 1–2 weeks and then neutralized with 1 M NaOH. The reason might be the moisture in the air will bind to acetate ions and amino groups on the surface of the scaffold. As a consequence, the surface tension of the scaffold will decrease, and trapped air remains trapped for a long time during neutralization. Therefore, immediately, freeze-dried chitosan scaffolds were neutralized with 10 mL of 1 M NaOH solution in order to prevent air trapping inside the scaffold during neutralization. After neutralization, scaffold was thoroughly washed with double distilled water up to neutral pH.

4.3.1.4 Preparation of Chitin Beads

Yilmaz and Bengisu (2003) prepared chitin beads using chitin solution of 0.3%–1.0% in either DMAc/LiCl or NMP/LiCl. The chitin solution was slowly dropped into the nonsolvent (i.e., ethanol or acetone) with the help of 3 mL plastic transfer pipette and the solution formed beads instantaneously. Beads were left in the nonsolvent for 24 h to allow solvent exchange, and the nonsolvent was replaced every 12 h. After 48 h, the beads were filtered and dried under vacuum at 40°C to constant weight.

4.3.1.5 Preparation of Chitosan Fibers

In 2004, Tamura et al. reported a method for preparation of chitosan fibers (Figure 4.6). Chitosan solution (7%–10% w/v) was prepared using 10% aqueous acetic acid under vigorous agitation. The solution was filtered to remove insoluble materials from

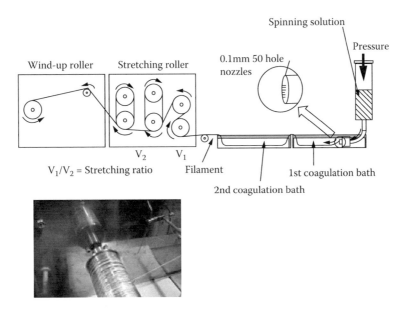

FIGURE 4.6
Preparation of chitosan fiber.

chitosan sample. The viscous solution was placed in a column and stand for overnight at room temperature to remove air bubbles. The column outlet pipe was connected with stainless steel nozzle (3 cm of diameter) with 0.1 mmφ × 50 holes. Calcium chloride saturated aqueous methanol (or ethanol) (water: methanol, 1:1 v/v) was prepared and followed by cooling down the viscous solution for first coagulation bath (Figure 4.6). Second coagulation bath was composed of 50% aqueous methanol or ethanol depending on the composition of first coagulation bath. The rate of first wind up roller was 6.3 m/min under the pressure of 0.6–0.8 kg/cm² applying stainless steel nozzle (3 cm of diameter) with 0.1 mmφ × 50 holes. The stretching was performed under wet state at the ratio of 1.0–1.2. Chitosan filament on cassette was treated immediately with NaOH solution. After the treatment, chitosan filament on cassette was washed with distilled water and finally dried in air.

4.3.2 Determination of Degree of Deacetylation and Degree of Acetylation

Many techniques have been developed for the determination of DA of chitin and chitosan. Among them liquid-state NMR spectroscopic method, first derivative UV spectrophotometric method, high-performance liquid chromatographic (HPLC) method, acid–base titration method, and UV spectrophotometry with phosphoric acid as solvent (PUV) method are valid for perfectly soluble materials. For the elemental analysis, sample must be absolutely pure from residual proteins. "The X-ray diffraction (XRD), differential scanning calorimetry (DSC), and Fourier transform infrared spectroscopy (FTIR) (KBr pellet) methods showed poor accuracy with the samples of diverse preparations and sources" (Hein et al. 2008 cited in Nwe et al. 2011).

FTIR methods are suitable for all chitosan samples (i.e., low- to high-DA chitosan samples); however, these methods depend on their calculation methods, sample forms, patterns of glucosamine, and *N*-acetyl glucosamine (GlcNAc) in chitosan molecules (Van de

Velde and Kiekens 2004 cited in Nwe et al. 2011). The PUV, solid-state cross-polarization magic angle spinning carbon-13 nuclear magnetic resonance (^{13}C CP/MAS NMR), and acid hydrolysis–HPLC method showed the best methods to determine DA of chitin and chitosan; moreover, these methods are suitable for determination of acetyl content over the whole range of chitin and chitosan (Hein et al. 2008 cited in Nwe et al. 2011).

4.3.2.1 Potentiometric Determination of Degree of Deacetylation

Qin et al. (2003) used potentiometric titration method to determine DD of chitosan. The chitosan solution (1.5%) was prepared by dissolving chitosan in 0.1 M HCl acid. The solution was titrated with a 0.1 M NaOH solution, and a curve with two inflection points was obtained. The difference of the volumes of these two points corresponded to the acid consumed for the protonation of amine groups and allows the determination of degree of deacetylation (DDA) of the chitosan. The titration was performed with a pH meter.

4.3.2.2 First Derivative UV Spectrophotometry Method

First derivative UV spectrophotometry method was described by Muzzarelli and Rocchetti (1985), and in later years, this method was modified by Tan et al. (1998). Nwe and Stevens (2002) used this method to determine DD. The first derivative spectra were obtained from the Unicam spectrophotometry at a bandwidth of 0.2 nm, a scanning speed of 30 nm/min (Figure 4.7). The zero crossing point (ZCP) was obtained by overlapping the first derivative spectra of 0.0100, 0.0200, and 0.0300 M of acetic acid solution at 202.4 nm. GlcNAc (Sigma, USA) solution of 0.005, 0.01, 0.02, 0.03, 0.04, and 0.05 mg/mL in 0.01 M acetic acid solution was prepared, and their first derivative spectra were obtained. The vertical distance was measured from the ZCP to the GlcNAc absorbance at 202.4 nm. A linear calibration curve was obtained by plotting the first derivative absorbance value versus GlcNAc concentration (Figure 4.8). Dried-chitosan sample 0.01 g (weight to the accuracy of 0.0001 g) was dissolved in 10 mL of 0.1 M acetic acid solution and topped up to 100 mL distilled water. Three

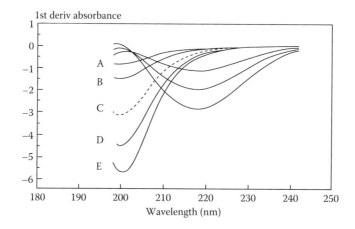

FIGURE 4.7
Acetic acid zero crossing point by overlapping the first derivative spectra of 0.01, 0.02, and 0.03 M of acetic acid and first derivative spectra of NAcGlu solutions (A) 0.005 mg/ml NAcGlu, (B) 0.01 mg/ml NAcGlu, (C) 0.02 mg/ml NAcGlu, (D) 0.03 mg/ml NAcGlu, and (E) 0.04 mg/ml NAcGlu.

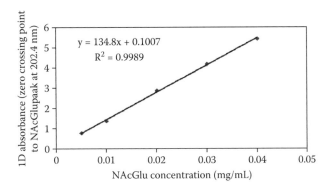

FIGURE 4.8
Standard curve for the determination of DD of chitosan sample by 1DUV spectrophotometry method.

replicates were prepared for each sample. The absorbance values of the first derivative spectra of chitosan samples were measured. The concentration of GlcNAc was determined by using the calibration curve. After that the DD of fungal chitosan was determined by the formula

$$DD = \left[100 - \left\{A/(W - 204A)/161 + A)\right\}\right] \times 100$$

where
   A is the amount of GlcNAc determined/204
   W is the mass of chitosan sample used
   204 is the molecular weight of N-acetyl D-glucosamine
   161 is the molecular weight of D-glucosamine

4.4 Determination of Molecular Weight of Chitosan

For the determination of molecular weight of chitosan, gel permeation chromatographic (GPC), light-scattering and viscosity method are widely used. Chitosans produced using aquatic crustaceans under heterogeneous conditions and using fungal mycelia contain a population of chitosan molecules with varying molecular weight. Most research used the GPC method to determine the distribution of molecular weights of chitosan molecules in the sample.

Weight-average molecular weight (Mw), number-average molecular weight (Mn), and molecular weight dispersion (Mw/Mn) of sample were measured by GPC. The GPC system consists of the Waters Ultrahydrogel™ columns 500, 1000, and 2000 (packing materials, hydroxylated polymethacrylate–based gel; column length, 300 mm; internal diameter, 7.8 mm), pump and detector (differential refractometer) (Figure 4.9A). The solvent was prepared by dissolving 43.38 g of 2.5 M CH_3COONa and 31.57 g of 6.6 M glacial acetic acid in a 1 L volumetric flask and topped up with ultrapure water. The solvent was filtered through 0.45 µm cellulose acetate filter before use (Figure 4.9B).

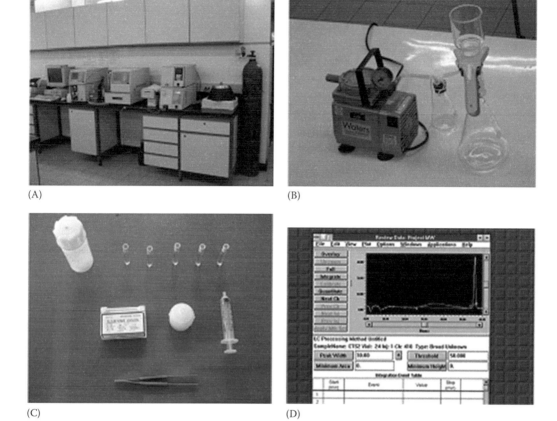

(A)   (B)

(C)   (D)

FIGURE 4.9
Determination of molecular weight of chitosan by gel permeation chromatography method. (A) GPC apparatus, (B) solvent filtration apparatus, (C) items required for filtration of chitosan samples, and (D) graph of chitosan sample.

The flow rate was 0.6 mL/min, and He gas was used for degas at 15 mL/min. Dextran standard solutions of 0.2% were prepared for the molecular weight of 9,900, 17,900, 35,600, 74,300, and 170,000, and 0.1% solutions were prepared for the molecular weight of 230,000, 535,000, and 2,000,000 in the sodium acetate buffer. The standard solutions were filtered through 0.45 μm cellulose acetate filter and put into the vial. The vials were arranged in the autosampler vial tray for sample injection (100 μL) into the pump. The temperature of the column and detector were set at 55°C and 40°C, respectively. The flow rate of the solvent was 0.6 mL/min, and the sample running time is 60 min/sample. A calibration curve was obtained by plotting the retention time versus log of molecular weight of the standards. The chitosan sample (0.03 g) was dissolved in 22.5 mL of 0.266 M acetic acid at 100 rpm, 25°C for 12 h. After chitosan was dissolved in acetic acid, 7.5 mL of 0.4 M sodium acetate solution was added and shaken at 100 rpm, 25°C for 12 h. The chitosan sample was filtered, and samples were placed to the test vial (Figure 4.9C). After that test vial was placed in the tray of auto injector, molecular weight of chitosan sample was determined using calibration curve (Figure 4.9D).

References

Aye, K. N., Karuppuswamy, R., Ahamed, T., and Stevens, W. F. 2006. Peripheral enzymatic deacetylation of chitin and reprecipitated chitin particles. *Bioresource Technology* 97: 577–582.

Chang, C. T., Liao, Y. M., and Li, S. J. 1998. Preparation of low molecular weight chitosan and chito-oligosaccharides by the enzymatic hydrolysis of chitosan. In *Advances in Chitin Science, Proceedings of the 3rd Asia Pacific Symposium*, eds. R. H. Chen and H. C. Chen, Keelung, Taiwan, pp. 233–238.

Hai, L., Diep, T. B., Nagasawa, N., Yoshii, F., and Kume, T. 2003. Radiation depolymerization of chitosan to prepare oligomers. *Nuclear Instruments and Methods in Physics Research B* 208: 466–470.

Hu, X., Du, Y., Tang, Y., Wang, Q., Feng, T., Yang, J., and Kennedy, J. F. 2007. Solubility and property of chitin in NaOH/urea aqueous solution. *Carbohydrate Polymers* 70: 451–458.

Ilankovan, P., Hein, S., Ng, C. H., Trung, T. S., and Stevens, W. F. 2006. Production of N-acetyl chitobiose from various chitin substrates using commercial enzymes. *Carbohydrate Polymers* 63: 245–250.

Kasaai, M. R., Malaekeh, M., Charlet, G., and Arul, J. 2001. Depolymerization of chitosan. In *Chitin and Chitosan, Chitin and Chitosan in Life Science*, eds. T. Uragami, K. Kurita, and T. Fukamizo, Yamaguchi, Japan, pp. 28–35.

Lertsutthiwong, P., How, N. C., Chandrkrachang, S., and Stevens, W. F. 2002. Effect of chemical treatment on the characteristics of shrimp chitosan. *Journal of Metals, Materials and Minerals* 12: 11–18.

Li, J., Du, Y., Yang, J., Feng, T., Li, A., and Chen, P. 2005. Preparation and characterization of low molecular weight chitosan and chito-oligomers by a commercial enzyme. *Polymer Degradation and Stability* 87: 441–448.

Luyen, D. V. 1994. Partially hydrolyzed chitosan. In *Asia-Pacific Chitin and Chitosan Symposium*, Bangi, Malaysia.

Methacanon, P., Prasitsilp, M., Pothsree, T., and Pattaraarchachai, J. 2003. Heterogeneous N- deacetylation of squid chitin in alkaline solution. *Carbohydrate Polymers* 52: 119–123.

Muzzarelli, R. A. A. and Rocchetti, R. 1985. Determination of the degree of acetylation of chitosans by first derivative ultraviolet spectrophotometry. *Carbohydrate Polymers* 5: 461–472.

Nwe, N., Furuike, T., and Tamura, H. 2009. The mechanical and biological properties of chitosan scaffolds for tissue regeneration templates are significantly enhanced by chitosan from *Gongronella butleri*. *Materials* 2: 374–398.

Nwe, N., Furuike, T., and Tamura, H. 2010. Production of low molecular weight chitosan and chito-oligosaccharides: Gamma-ray irradiation, acid hydrolysis and enzymatic hydrolysis method. *Chitin and Chitosan Research* 16: 238.

Nwe, N., Furuike, T., and Tamura, H. 2011. Chitosan from aquatic and terrestrial organisms and microorganisms: Production, properties and applications. In *Biodegradable Materials: Production, Properties and Applications*, eds. B. M. Johnson and Z. E. Berkel, pp. 29–50. Nova Science publishers, New York.

Nwe, N., and Stevens, W. F. 2002. Production of fungal chitosan by solid substrate fermentation followed by enzymatic extraction. *Biotechnology Letters* 24:131–134.

Nwe, N. and Stevens, W. F. 2008. Production of chitin and chitosan and their applications in the medical and biological sector. In *Recent Research in Biomedical Aspects of Chitin and Chitosan*, ed. H. Tamura, pp. 161–176, Research Signpost, India.

Ornum, J. 1992. Shrimp waste must it be wasted. *Infofish International* 6: 48–52.

Qin, C., Du, Y., Zong, L., Zeng, F., Liu, Y., and Zhou, B. 2003. Effect of hemicellulase on the molecular weight and structure of chitosan. *Polymer Degradation and Stability* 80: 435–441.

Tamura, H., Nagahama, H., and Tokura, S. 2006. Preparation of chitin hydrogel under mild conditions. *Cellulose* 13: 357–364.

Tamura, H., Tsuruta, Y., Itoyama, K., Worakitkanchanakul, W., Rujiravanit, R., and Tokura, S. 2004. Preparation of chitosan filament applying new coagulation system. *Carbohydrate Polymers* 56: 205–211.

Tan, S. C., Khor, E., Tan, T. K., and Wong, S. M. 1998. The degree of deacetylation of chitosan: Advocating the first derivative UV-spectrophotometry method of determination. *Talanta* 45: 713–719.

Thomas, P. and Philip, B. 2000. Production of partially degraded chitosan with desire molecular weight. In *Advance in Chitin Science, Proceedings of the 3rd International Conference of the European Chitin Society*, eds. M.G. Peter, A. Domard, and R. A. A. Muzzarelli, University of Potsdam, Potsdam, Germany, pp. 63–67.

Trung, T. S., Thein-Han, W. W., Qui, N. T., Ng, C. H., and Stevens, W. F. 2006. Functional characteristics of shrimp chitosan and its membranes as affected by the degree of deacetylation. *Bioresource Technology* 97: 659–663.

Vårum, K. M., Ottøy, M. H., and Smidsrød, O. 2001. Acid hydrolysis of chitosans. *Carbohydrate Polymers* 46: 89–98.

White, S. A., Farina, P. R., and Fulton, I. 1979. Production and isolation of chitosan from *Mucor rouxii*. *Applied Environmental Microbiology* 38: 323–328.

Yen, M., Yang, J., and Mau, J. 2009. Physicochemical characterization of chitin and chitosan from crab shells. *Carbohydrate Polymers* 75: 15–21.

Yilmaz, E. and Bengisu, M. 2003. Preparation and characterization of physical gels and beads from chitin solutions. *Carbohydrate Polymers* 54: 479–488.

Yusof, N. L. B. M., Lim, L. Y., and Khor, E. 2004. Flexible chitin films: Structural studies. *Carbohydrate Research* 339: 2701–2711.

Zainol, I., Akil, H. M., and Mastor, A. 2009. Effect of γ-irradiation on the physical and mechanical properties of chitosan powder. *Materials Science and Engineering C* 29: 292–297.

5

Structure Elucidation and Biological Effects of Carrageenans from Red Algae

Wei Zhang, Ming Liu, and Poul Erik Hansen

CONTENTS

5.1 Introduction

Marine polysaccharides from algae have wide applications in food, cosmetic, and pharmaceutical industry, due to their excellent thickening, stabilizing, and gel-forming property (Imeson 2000; van de Velde and De Ruiter 2002). Besides the applications in traditional industry, marine polysaccharides have a great potential to become a major resource of biomass for producing biofuel (Bringezu et al. 2009; Huesemann et al. 2010).

Carrageenans are a family of linear sulfated galactans extracted from certain species of red algae (Rhodophyta). The yearly global production of carrageenans is 45,000 tons, of which 70% is used in food industry and the rest used in cosmetic, pharmaceutical industry, etc. (Campo et al. 2009). Carrageenan has a repeating disaccharides unit of β-ᴅ-galactose and α-ᴅ-galactose or α-ᴅ-3,6-anhydrogalactose (Figure 5.1). Depending on different content of half-ester sulfate, carrageenans can be divided into ι-carrageenan, κ-carrageenan, etc. (Knutsen et al. 1994).

Carrageenan polysaccharides undergo conformational transition from random coils to ordered double helical structure under proper conditions (decreasing temperature or increasing salt concentration, etc.). The branched polymer chains could further develop into a macromolecular network through cross-linking of the double helices, thus form gel or aggregates.

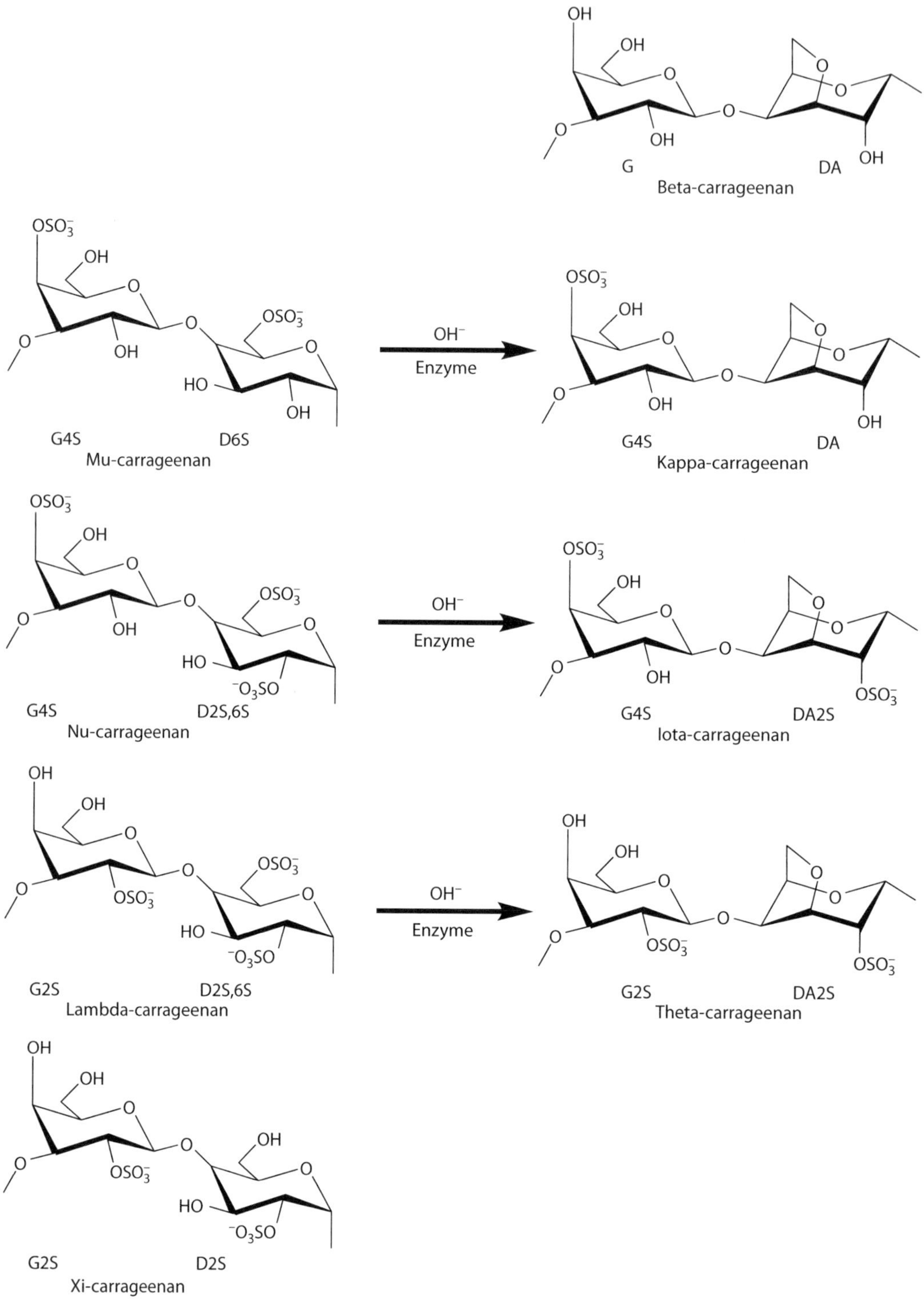

FIGURE 5.1
Structures of carrageenans. The names beta, kappa, iota, lambda, mu, nu, theta, and xi are often used instead of the Greek symbols β, κ, ι, λ, μ, ν, τ, and ξ.

The carrageenan double helix structure was solved by x-ray fiber diffraction (Anderson et al. 1969; Arnott et al. 1974; Millane et al. 1988; Cairns et al. 1991). ι-Carrageenan has a parallel half-staggered double helix structure with a pitch of 2.6 nm (Anderson et al. 1969; Arnott et al. 1974). κ-Carrageenan has a parallel double helix with a pitch of 2.5 nm, but the two chains are offset by a 28° rotation and a 0.1 nm translation from the half-staggered arrangement (Millane et al. 1988). Although the difference in ordered helical structure of κ-and ι-carrageenan is very small, there is a significant difference in the nonelectrostatic free energy changes of the coil–helix transition between κ- and ι-carrageenan (Nilsson et al. 1989). κ-Carrageenan has a strong tendency of gel formation, but ι-carrageenan has a very weak tendency of gel formation. κ-Carrageenan has a pronounced ion specificity of certain cations and anions on its conformational transition and gel formation (Rochas and Rinaudo 1980). In contrast, the ion specificity is not observed for ι-carrageenan (Piculell et al. 1987, 1989, 1990). The marked difference in their physical–chemical property between κ- and ι-carrageenan demonstrates the importance in clarifying their structure–function relationship.

Several carrageenase enzyme structures by x-ray diffraction were published in recent years, disclosing the molecular mechanism of enzyme and carrageenan/ions interaction (Michel et al. 2001a,b, 2003). The electrostatic interaction seems to be one of the dominant forces in the carrageenan binding to enzyme (Michel et al. 2003).

In the past decades, nuclear magnetic resonance (NMR) technique has developed rapidly to become one of the main experimental methods to study structure and dynamics of biomolecules. In contrast to x-ray diffraction, NMR could study structure and dynamics of biomolecules in aqueous solution, which is very similar to the physiological condition of the living organisms. In the following sections, we will review the updated biological NMR spectroscopy and its application to carrageenan studies.

5.2 NMR Methodology

The first experimental observation of NMR was made between 1945 and 1946, by Bloch and Purcell (Bloch et al. 1946; Purcell et al. 1946). The discovery of NMR chemical shift greatly broadened its application in chemistry (Knight 1949; Arnold et al. 1951). In the 1960s, the concept of Fourier transform spectroscopy and hence two-dimensional NMR spectroscopy was introduced by Ernst et al. (Ernst and Anderson 1966), which revolutionized the NMR methodology of biological molecules. A systematic NMR method for assignment and structure determination of proteins and nucleic acids was developed by Wüthrich in the 1980s (Wüthrich 1986). The isotope labeling of recombinant proteins and nucleic acids fostered a new wave of NMR development in the 1990s (Bax 1994; Gardner and Kay 1998). Many 3D and 4D ^{1}H, ^{13}C, ^{15}N triple resonance spectra were designed, which greatly simplified the NMR assignment of proteins and nucleic acids (Bax 1994; Clore and Gronenborn 1998; Wider and Wüthrich 1999). The methodology development of NMR was also accompanied by technological development of NMR spectrometer, with the development of high-field and ultrahigh-field superconducting magnet, advancement in computer and electronic technology, etc.

While great progress has been made in NMR studies of proteins and nucleic acids in the past several decades, the NMR application to polysaccharides and oligosaccharides is still very limited. The limiting factor is the difficulty in synthesizing polysaccharides and oligosaccharides, hence their isotope labeling (Duus et al. 2000). Therefore, the ^{1}H, ^{13}C, ^{15}N triple resonance NMR spectroscopy, which has been successfully applied to studies of proteins and nucleic acids, could not be generally applied to studies of polysaccharides and oligosaccharides. The NMR study of polysaccharides and oligosaccharides mostly relies on the conventional proton homonuclear 2D spectra (COSY, NOESY, ROESY, TOCSY, etc.) and 2D heteronuclear spectra (^{1}H, ^{13}C-HSQC, HMQC, HMBC, etc.) of natural abundance samples (Duus et al. 2000).

The limitation in applying modern NMR spectroscopy to polysaccharide and oligosaccharides could be partially offset by a careful selection of 2D NMR experiments and experimental parameters. A total NMR assignment of oligosaccharides up to 30–40 sugar residues has been achieved in the past (du Penhoat et al. 1999).

Natural abundance ^{13}C edited 3D experiment was also reported for oligosaccharides, if there was enough quantity of the sample (Vuister et al. 1989; Homans 1992; Homans and Rutherford 1992).

Besides the most commonly used nuclei like ^{1}H, ^{13}C, and ^{15}N in NMR studies of biological molecules, other nuclei were also deployed to extract structural information of biomolecules, e.g., ion NMR (Lindman and Forsen 1976).

5.3 Carrageenan Structural Studies by NMR

NMR is widely used in characterization of components and their chemical structures of carrageenan samples (Knutsen and Grasdalen 1992; Ueda et al. 2001, 2004; Yu et al. 2002). There are several reviews in NMR of carrageenan covering this issue (van de Velde et al. 2002; van de Velde and De Ruiter 2008; Jiao et al. 2011). The ^{1}H and ^{13}C chemical shifts of different saccharide units of carrageenan are assigned based on corresponding monosaccharide and oligosaccharide derivatives (Knutsen and Grasdalen 1992; Ueda et al. 2001; Yu et al. 2002). Examples of 1D ^{1}H NMR spectra of κ-, ι-, and λ-carrageenans are given in the review by Campo et al. (2009) and by van de Velde et al. (2002). Examples of 1D ^{13}C NMR spectra are likewise given in the latter. In addition to these reviews, van de Velde et al. (van de Velde et al. 2004) revised the NMR chemical shifts for a series of carrageenans. This is clearly important. The data of Abad et al. (2011) are clearly different from those of van de Velde (2004) although DSS is used as internal standard in both cases (Table 5.1). From Table 5.2, the effects of the sugar unit not being central ones can be seen.

In addition to ^{1}H chemical shifts of non-exchangeable protons, OH proton chemical shifts can also be obtained in non-protic solvents such as Me_2SO-d_6. The OH chemical shifts of κ-carrageenan show temperature variation (Bosco et al. 2005) in the temperature range 303–358 K. For OGS2, an increase in temperature results in a decrease of the chemical shift difference between the OH signal and the water signal, whereas the opposite is true for the OH protons ODA2 and OGS6. This means that the latter are involved in well-defined hydrogen bonds in which the OH group is hydrogen donors. Very interestingly, the hydrogen bonds are defined as intramolecular ones and possibly have an SO_4^- group as acceptor. The use of these effects is usually referred to as XH temperature coefficients (Sosnicki and Hansen 2004).

While most of these NMR studies of carrageenan are focused on characterization of chemical structures of saccharides, very few of them have studied spatial structures of carrageenan polysaccharides and their oligosaccharide derivatives. Since the physical–chemical

TABLE 5.1

^{13}C Chemical Shifts of DA and GS Units of Carrageenans

Carbon	van de Velde[a]	Zhang[b]	Abad[c]
GA	104.70	104.77	101.87
C-1			
C-2	71.72	71.71	69.81
C-3	80.98	80.44	78.51
C-4	76.25	76.03	74.12
C-5	77.00	77.08	75.18
C-6	63.49	63.71	61.68
DA	97.34	96.97	96.08
C-1			
C-2	72.11	71.94	70.01
C-3	81.41	81.50	79.60
C-4	80.54	80.70	78.87
C-5	79.07	78.96	77.08
C-6	71.72	71.74	70.01

[a] van de Velde et al. (2004).
[b] Zhang et al. (2010).
[c] Abad et al. (2011).

property of different carrageenan varies significantly from each other, it is of great importance to study their spatial structure to find structure–function relationship.

Studies of carrageenan structures are done on both natural products and oligomers. The oligomers can be obtained by mild hydrolysis (Zhang et al. 2010). Also irradiation can be used to obtain oligomers (Abad et al. 2011). Irradiations at 100 kGy as well as 2 kGy are used to obtain different degrees of depolymerization and subsequently different molecular weights of the oligomers. Slightly different results are obtained by irradiation of solid (100 kGy) or 1% aq. solutions (2 kGy). In the first instance, more of a fraction with molecular weight below 3 kDa is obtained.

A general NMR methodology for de novo primary structure assignment and spatial structure characterization of carrageenan oligosaccharides has been developed by Zhang et al. (2010). There are two types of 2D NMR spectroscopy applied to carrageenan studies: the through-bond correlation spectroscopy and through-space correlation spectroscopy. The through-bond correlation spectroscopy includes DQF-COSY, TOCSY and ^1H–^{13}C HMQC, HMBC. The through-space correlation spectroscopy includes NOESY and ROESY.

The individual sugar spin systems in carrageenan samples are identified by the through-bond correlation spectroscopy. The homonuclear ^1H–^1H three-bond and two-bond correlations in the same sugar spin system could be identified in DQF-COSY. The homonuclear ^1H–^1H long-range correlations through the magnetization relaying mechanism could be identified in TOCSY. The ^{13}C resonances could be assigned in ^1H–^{13}C HMQC, HMBC, based on the assignment of the ^1H resonances. The assignment of the ^1H resonances could be further confirmed in ^1H–^{13}C HMQC, HMBC.

The important glycosidic linkage information between the different sugar spin systems is identified by the through-space correlation spectroscopy, together with ^1H–^{13}C HMBC. Hence, the sequential connectivity of the oligosaccharides is also identified.

TABLE 5.2

^{1}H and ^{13}C-NMR Chemical Shifts (in ppm) Data of Carr-A, B, and C[a]

Compound	Spin System	Nucleus	1	2	3	4	5	6a	6b
Carr-A	S1	^{1}H	5.310	3.910	4.167	4.893	4.182	3.793	3.720
		^{13}C	94.72	69.61	77.50	77.24	72.46	63.86	
	S2	^{1}H	5.113	4.136	4.517	4.591	4.635	4.224	4.053
		^{13}C	97.05	71.94	81.52	80.61	78.93	71.69	
	S3	^{1}H	5.095	4.136	4.517	4.591	4.635	4.224	4.053
		^{13}C	96.92	71.93	81.52	80.61	78.93	71.69	
	S4	^{1}H	4.646	3.588	3.972	4.833	3.768	3.768	
		^{13}C	98.87	72.97	80.61	76.21	76.98	63.78	
	S5	^{1}H	4.610	3.503	3.798	4.670	3.862	3.798	3.786
		^{13}C	104.95	73.36	74.39	79.18	77.24	63.59	
Carr-B	S1	^{1}H	5.314	3.914	4.168	4.891	4.180	3.798	
		^{13}C	94.70	69.57	77.53	77.20	72.45	63.62	
	S2	^{1}H	5.111	4.136	4.522	4.598	4.642	4.218	4.056
		^{13}C	96.99	71.94	81.50	80.70	78.96	71.74	
	S3	^{1}H	5.098	4.136	4.522	4.598	4.642	4.218	4.056
		^{13}C	96.97	71.94	81.50	80.70	78.96	71.74	
	S4	^{1}H	4.645	3.589	3.972	4.834	3.770	3.760	
		^{13}C	98.91	72.92	80.62	76.14	76.91	63.69	
	S5	^{1}H	4.612	3.509	3.800	4.673	3.863	3.780	
		^{13}C	105.21	73.37	74.34	79.21	77.24	63.71	
	S6	^{1}H	4.653	3.596	4.005	4.855	3.813	3.780	
		^{13}C	104.77	71.71	80.44	76.03	77.08	63.71	
Carr-C	S1	^{1}H	5.312	3.907	4.167	4.892	4.179	3.784	3.725
		^{13}C	94.69	69.58	77.48	77.22	72.43	63.88	
	S2	^{1}H	5.108	4.128	4.519	4.596	4.641	4.219	4.050
		^{13}C	96.89	71.91	81.49	80.71	78.90	71.65	
	S3	^{1}H	5.097	4.128	4.519	4.596	4.641	4.219	4.050
		^{13}C	96.89	71.91	81.49	80.71	78.90	71.65	
	S4	^{1}H	4.643	3.594	3.990	4.832	3.766	3.789–3.745	
		^{13}C	98.84	71.65	80.45	76.05	76.83	63.75	
	S5	^{1}H	4.61	3.503	3.789	4.670	3.862	3.789–3.745	
		^{13}C	105.05	73.33	74.36	79.16	77.22	63.48	
	S6	^{1}H	4.658	3.610	4.014	4.852	3.815	3.801	
		^{13}C	104.79	71.65	80.45	76.05	77.09	63.49	

Source: Zhang, W. et al., *J. Psychol.*, 46, 831, 2010.

[a] For a definition of carr-A, B, and C as well as spin systems S, see Figure 5.6.

The through-space correlation spectroscopy (NOESY and ROESY) reveals conformational information of the carrageenan molecules.

The NMR methodology has been successfully applied to study a series of κ-carrageenan oligosaccharides (Zhang et al. 2010).

The sugar spin systems are initially identified in the anomeric region of the ^{1}H–^{13}C HMQC spectrum (Figure 5.2). DQF-COSY, TOCSY, HMQC, and HMBC spectra are used in the analysis of these spin systems. The proton connectivities in these spin systems are

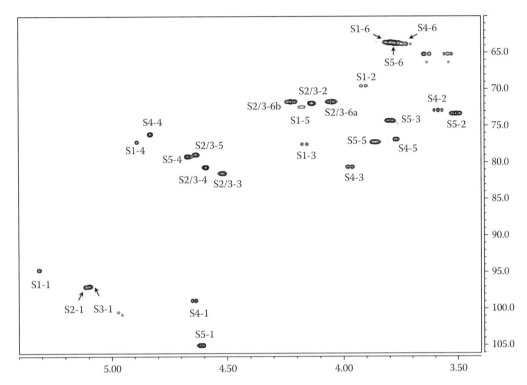

FIGURE 5.2
^{1}H-^{13}C HMQC spectrum of carr-A. The cross-peaks were labeled by their respective spin systems and resonance positions, e.g., S1-1 was the resonance peak at position 1 of the spin system S1. (From Zhang, W. et al., *J. Psychol.*, 46, 831, 2010. With permission.)

shown in the DQF-COSY (Figure 5.3) and the TOCSY spectrum (Figure 5.4). With the identification of the ^{1}H resonances, the ^{13}C signals in these spin systems could be assigned from the HMQC (Figure 5.2) and HMBC (Figure 5.5) spectra. The ^{1}H and ^{13}C chemical shifts are listed in Table 5.2.

The three-bond ^{1}H–^{1}H coupling constants and intraresidue NOEs greatly help to identify the sugar types and conformations of the spin systems. In S1, $^3J_{H1-H2} \sim 3.9$ Hz, $^3J_{H2-H3} \sim 9.7$ Hz, $^3J_{H3-H4} \sim 3.9$ Hz, and $^3J_{H4-H5}$ is very small; in S4 and S5, $^3J_{H1-H2} \sim 7.8$ Hz, $^3J_{H2-H3} \sim 9.7$ Hz, $^3J_{H3-H4} \sim 3.9$ Hz, and $^3J_{H4-H5}$ is very small. Based on the coupling constants, it is deduced that S1 is an α-D-Gal-based unit and S4 and S5 are β-D-Gal-based units. The observed intraresidue NOE contacts for S4 and S5 (Table 5.3) are consistent with the chair conformation of β-D-Gal indicated in Figure 5.6. It is difficult to confirm the conformation of α-D-Gal for S1 by intraresidue NOEs, due to the proton signal degeneracies and weak signals.

For S2 and S3, not all the coupling constants could be observed. However, $^3J_{H1-H2} \sim 3.0$ Hz and $^1J_{C,H} \sim 167$ Hz, indicating an α-configuration of S2 and S3; the long-range H6-C3 and H3-C6 correlations in HMBC (Figure 5.5) indicate the existence of a 3,6-oxo-bridge. Due to the oxo-bridge between position 3 and position 6 in S2 and S3, $^3J_{H3,H4}$ gets smaller, H3 and H4 only giving a weak cross-peak in TOCSY, and no correlations in DQF-COSY. The NOE signals from H6b at 4.035 ppm to H5 and from H6a at 4.224 ppm to H1 in both S2 and S3 are observed, revealing the chair conformation of S2 and S3 (Figure 5.6).

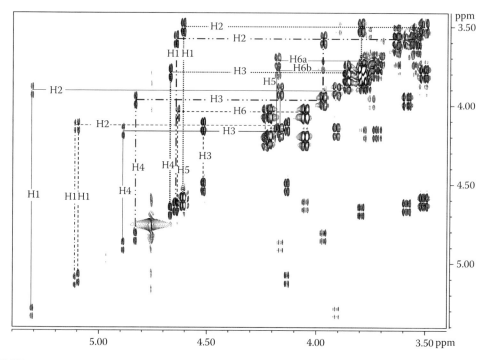

FIGURE 5.3
DQF-COSY spectrum of carr-A. (From Zhang, W. et al., *J. Psychol.*, 46, 831, 2010. With permission.)

All the sugar spin systems including their chemical structures and conformations could be assigned and identified for carr-A, mainly based on the through-bond connectivities, coupling constants, and intraresidue NOEs in various 2D-NMR spectra.

Long-range correlation HMBC spectra supplemented by NOESY/ROESY data are used to identify the sequential connectivity of these spin systems. The determined sequences are shown in Figure 5.6. The positions of the glycosidic linkages are assigned by the long-range ^1H, ^{13}C couplings in HMBC (Figure 5.5).

In conclusion, de novo primary structure (sugar residue type and sequence connectivity) determination is achieved for the studied samples. Semiquantitative conformational information of the oligosaccharides is also obtained. It is concluded that the carrageenan oligosaccharides adopted an ordered helical structure.

In general, the earlier mentioned NMR methodology could be applied to any other oligosaccharides, as long as a millimolar concentration of the pure oligosaccharides sample in aqueous solution could be obtained. Another limitation of the NMR methodology is the molecular weight of the studied oligosaccharides. The oligosaccharides are generally rigid molecules; therefore, the oligosaccharides with a large number of sugar residues would tumble slowly in solution, causing broadened weak NMR signals.

Bosco et al. (2005) investigated κ-carrageenan with a molecular weight of $\sim 3 \times 10^5$ D. In this large molecule, spin diffusion plays a major role. A series of NOE, ROESY, and TROSY experiments confirmed that a NOE effect could be seen between DA1 and GS1 and between DA1 and GS5. These effects were determined to be intramolecular, so no evidence for a double chain was found. Considering the difficulty in achieving a sufficient number of parameters to define the structure of carbohydrates including carrageenans, molecular

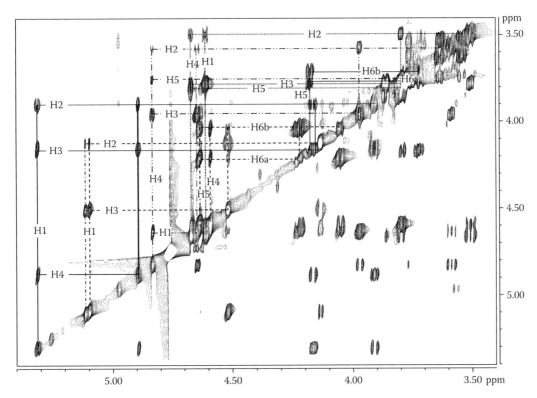

FIGURE 5.4
TOCSY spectrum of carr-A, with a spin lock time of 150 ms. (From Zhang, W. et al., *J. Psychol.*, 46, 831, 2010. With permission.)

modeling has been used extensively. Bosco et al. (2005) used molecular mechanics calculations to prepare Ramachandran-like conformational energy maps using the CVFF force field. In this case, it was to explore the possible θ and χ angle space (θ and χ angle as defined in Figure 5.7).

One important area for the application of NMR methodology is to study interactions between carrageenan oligosaccharides and proteins/enzymes, clarifying the molecular mechanism of their interactions. Such application is especially important for studying the pharmaceutical effects of carrageenans and biofuel productions from carrageenans.

Ion NMR is a very useful method for detecting specific interactions between ions (cations/anions) and carrageenans (Lindman and Forsen 1976; Grasdalen and Smidsrød 1981a,b; Smidsrød and Grasdalen 1984). Nuclei, such as ^{133}Cs, ^{14}N, and ^{127}I, are used for this kind of study (Grasdalen and Smidsrød 1981a,b; Zhang et al. 1991, 1992; Zhang and Furo 1993). Ion NMR discloses specific ion binding to κ-carrageenan helical conformers but not to coil conformers. The ion binding constant and intrinsic ion NMR chemical shift at the binding site can be extracted from the NMR data (Zhang et al. 1991, 1992).

Derivatives of κ-carrageenan have also been investigated. The O-succinyl derivative of κ-carrageenan is analyzed and ^1H and ^{13}C chemical shifts assigned (Jiang et al. 2005). In addition, pyruvate derivatives may be found in carrageenans (Cáceres et al. 2000). A polysaccharide rich in pyruvylated β-carrageenan is prepared by solvolytic desulfation and a full assignment achieved. In addition, the structure is investigated by 2D NMR (Falshaw et al. 2003).

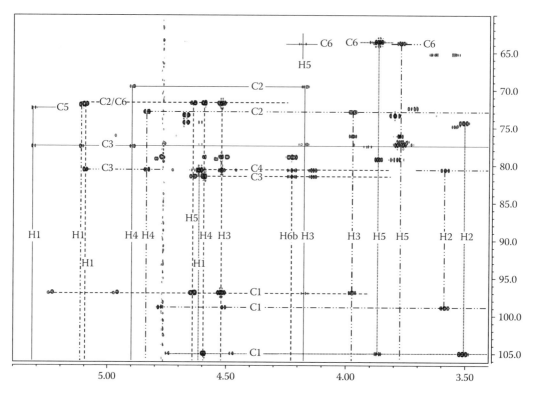

FIGURE 5.5
¹H-¹³C HMBC spectrum of carr-A. The resonances from individual spin systems were labeled by the curve (S1), (S2), (S3), (S4), and (S5), respectively. (From Zhang, W. et al., *J. Psychol.*, 46, 831, 2010. With permission.)

TABLE 5.3

Intraresidue NOEs Detected in ROESY Spectrum of Carr-A[a]

Spin System	S1	S2	S3	S4	S5
NOE's	H2–H3	H1–H2	H1–H2	H3–H4	H1–H3
	H3–H4	H1–H6a	H1–H6a	H3–H5	H1–H5
		H2–H3	H2–H3	H4–H5	H3–H4
		H5–H6b	H5–H6b		H4–H5
		H6a–H6b	H6a–H6b		

Source: Zhang, W. et al., *J. Psychol.*, 46, 831, 2010.
[a] NOE relations for carr-B and carr-C are similar to those given for carr-A.

In order to carry out a comprehensive study of carrageenan conformational change and hence gel formation, a model system of carrageenan oligosaccharides, which forms double helical conformation under the proper condition, should be searched. With the availability of such a model system, the ion binding site to carrageenan helices could be identified. The structural basis of other factors affecting the carrageenan conformational transition could also be well studied.

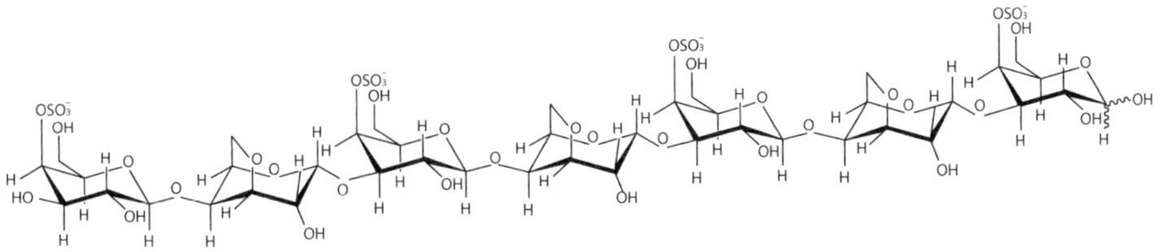

Compound	G4S$_{nre}$	DA	G4S$_{int}$	DA	G4S$_{int}$	DA	G4S$_{re}$
Carr-A	S5					S2	S1α
	S5					S3	S4β
Carr-B	S5			S3	S6	S2	S1α
	S5			S3	S6	S3	S4β
Carr-C	S5	S3	S6	S3	S6	S2	S1α
	S5	S3	S6	S3	S6	S3	S4β

FIGURE 5.6
Spin system and sequences of carr-A, carr-B, and carr-C. (From Zhang, W. et al., *J. Psychol.*, 46, 831, 2010. With permission.)

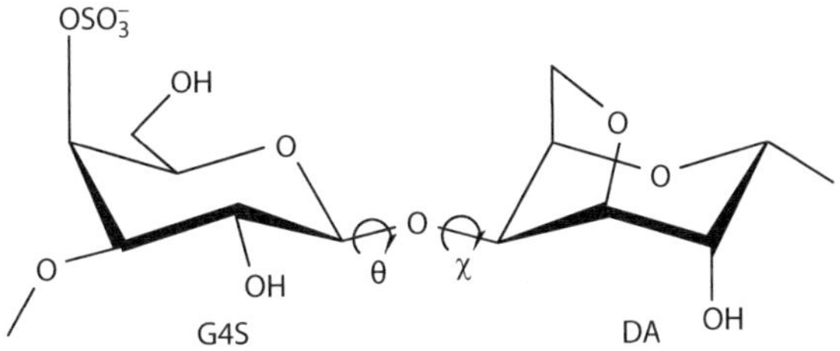

FIGURE 5.7
θ and χ angles.

5.4 Pharmacology and Biological Activities of Carrageenan

5.4.1 Antitumor and Immunomodulation Activities

λ-Carrageenans from *Chondrus ocellatus* (650, 240, 140, 15, 9.3 kDa) show both antitumor and immunomodulation activities in vivo. However, these λ-carrageenan samples do not show cytotoxicity against S180 and H22 tumor cells directly in vitro but enhances the nature killer cell activities and lymphocyte proliferation. These results suggest that the antitumor activities of λ-carrageenan are not due to their cytotoxicity but due to their immunomodulation of immune system, samples with molecular weight 15 and 9.3 kDa has the highest activities (Zhou et al. 2004). And these λ-carrageenan samples could increase the antitumor activity of 5-Fu and renew the immune function of treated mice decreased by 5-Fu (Zhou et al. 2006). κ-Carrageenan (MW:1726) could markedly inhibit Sarcoma 180 tumor in mouse without obvious cytotoxicity in vitro. The immunological regulation, especially the phagocytosis ratio and phagocytosis index of macrophage, is observed, further supporting that this immunomodulation contributed to the antitumor activities of carrageenan (Haijin et al. 2003).

In vitro lymphocyte activation induced by carrageenan was investigated and the results found that carrageenan could activate B cells and induce the production of polyclonal antibody (Ishizaka et al. 1980). Carrageenan also stimulates macrophages to release immunostimulatory agent interleukin 1 (IL-1) (Nicklin and Miller 1989). These immunomodulatory activities, effects on the cytokine production, were reported to have a relationship with the basic polysaccharide structure; monosaccharide composition, number, and position; and distribution of sulfate groups along the galactan chain (Yermak et al. 2012).

The antitumor activities of carrageenan may also have a relationship with the growth factor–binding activity of carrageenan. For example, τ-carrageenan may act as antagonists of heparin-binding growth factors and exert antitumor activity either by inhibiting growth factor–induced proliferation of tumor cells or indirectly by inhibiting angiogenesis (Hoffman et al. 1995). Oligo-λ-carrageenans could bind to bFGF and inhibit bFGF-induced cell proliferation, and oligo-λ-carrageenans (dp2–8) were the most potent bFGF antagonists. These oligo-λ-carrageenans and oligo-κ-carrageenans (dp9–17) also showed high inhibitory effect against heparanase activity, and these bFGF binding and heparanase inhibition activities of carrageenan oligosaccharides are closely related to the molecular weight, carbohydrate structure, and content and linking position of sulfur groups (Chen et al. 2011). Another study showed that the affinity of κ-carrageenan to aFGF is higher than λ-carrageenan and ι-carrageenan (Belford et al. 1993).

λ-, ι-, and κ-carrageenans could bind to the granulocyte colony-stimulating factor (G-CSF) and inhibited G-CSF-induced growth of NFS-60 cells, but κ-carrageenan oligosaccharide could not. λ-Carrageenan could also induce the maturation of the cells, but ι- and κ-carrageenans could not. This research suggested that G-CSF-carrageenan bindings and their activities in the growth and differentiation of NFS-60 cells were dependent on carrageenans sulfate contents and chain lengths (Liang et al. 2006).

5.4.2 Antiviral Properties

Carrageenan possesses antiviral properties in vitro by inhibiting the replication of hepatitis A viruses. Carrageenans isolated from the red seaweed *Gigartina skottsbergii* inhibits herpes simplex virus type 1 (HSV-1) and type 2 (HSV-2) infection of murine astrocytes (Carlucci et al. 1999). Carrageenans extracted from cystocarpic and tetrasporic *Stenogramme interrupta* with the major component of α-carrageenan and minor components of pyruvated carrageenan also interfere the replication cycle of HSV (Cáceres et al. 2000). Another study also showed that the inhibitory effect on the in vitro replication of HSV-1 and HSV-2 was related to the electric charge, the polymeric backbone, the carbohydrate moieties, and the degree of polymerization (Marchetti et al. 1995), and the amount of α-D-galactose 2,6-disulfate residues in the carrageenans was directly correlated to the antiviral activity (Carlucci et al. 1997).

Carrageenan is an extremely potent infection inhibitor of a broad range of genital human papillomaviruses (HPVs), and there are indications that carrageenan-based sexual lubricant gels may offer protection against HPV transmission, by preventing the binding of HPV virions to cells (Buck et al. 2006). Carrageenan contained in some vaginal lubricants might serve as an effective topical HPV microbicide (Roberts et al. 2007). ι-, λ-, and κ-carrageenans showed a potent inhibitory effect on the replication of hepatitis A virus (HAV) (Girond et al. 1991). λ-Carrageenan type IV blocked feline herpes virus (FHV)-1 adsorption in the plaque assay and shortened the time period in which infected cats had positive virus isolation from the conjunctiva but did not alter the clinical course of FHV-1 conjunctivitis in cats (Stiles et al. 2008).

5.4.3 Anticoagulant Activity

Oversulfated κ-carrageenan was found to show dual properties of inhibiting coagulation and also significantly enhancing the in vitro activation of glutamic plasminogen (Glu-Plg) and tissue plasminogen activator (t-PA) (Opoku et al. 2006). λ- and κ-/ι-Carrageenans possess higher anticoagulant activity than κ-/β-carrageenan, and the monosaccharide composition of polysaccharides and number, position, and distribution of sulfate groups along galactan chain play an important role in the anticoagulant activity (Yermak et al. 2012). Structure and activity relationship of a sulfated galactan from the red alga *Gelidium crinale* has showed that the sulfation pattern and the nature of the saccharide chain play an important role in the anticoagulant activity (Pereira et al. 2005).

5.4.4 Induction of Experimental Inflammation

Carrageenan could induce inflammation in the rat paw, which is extensively used as a classical model of edema formation and hyperalgesia in the development of nonsteroidal anti-inflammatory drugs and selective COX1–2 inhibitors (Morris 2003; Guay et al. 2004).

5.4.5 Antioxidant Activity

Carrageenan oligosaccharides and their derivatives exhibited significant antioxidant activities both in vitro and in a cell system (Yuan et al. 2005, 2006). Different sulfated carrageenans showed antioxidant properties activity and stimulate catalytic activity of SOD (Sokolova et al. 2011).

5.4.6 Blood Cholesterol and Lipid-Lowering and Hypoglycemic Effects

Carrageenan in the diet may result in reduced blood cholesterol and lipid levels in human subjects (Panlasigui et al. 2003), and the hypoglycemic effect of carrageenan may be potential in the prevention and treatment of metabolic conditions such as diabetes (Dumelod et al. 1999).

5.4.7 Effects on Plant Growth

The effects of κ-carrageenan oligomers as plant growth promoters are investigated. The biological activity depends on the number of sulfate groups and the molecular size. The optimum activity was found for MWs below 10 kDa. NMR investigations also showed that no change in the composition had occurred as a consequence of the radiation used to produce the oligomers (Abad et al. 2011).

5.5 Conclusions

From the many biological studies of carrageenans, a common feature seems to be that the more sulfate groups, the more pronounced the biological effects are. Also the size of the molecules plays a role. The recent study of plant growth promotion (Abad et al. 2011) points toward a molecular weight below 10 kDa as the most efficient. What is still lacking is a better insight into structure. The NMR foundations are clearly laid, but more work needs to be done in this direction. However, studies of smaller oligomers seem very relevant as these may also be the biologically most active. As the high NMR instruments are becoming increasingly more sensitive, 1D techniques can probably help solve some of these problems. Deuterium isotope effects on ^{13}C chemical shift (the OH group exchanged partially with deuterium) can be measured in carbohydrates. Measurements in Me_2SO-d_6 were pioneered by Davies (Hansen 1983, 1988; Christofides et al. 1986), and recently, progress has been made in mixed solvents (Coxon 2005) and an example of a monosulfated D-galactose is also available (Archibald 1981). The deuterium isotope effects on ^{13}C chemical shifts can tell us about inter- and intramolecular hydrogen bonding. ^{13}C–^{1}H coupling constants are indirectly used in HMBC spectra, but values are not easily determined this way. Measurements of long-range ^{13}C–^{1}H couplings can be very useful and are used extensively in carbohydrates (Hansen 1981; Duus et al. 2000); combined with measurements of ^{13}C–^{13}C coupling constants, they can tell about the θ and χ angles (Figure 5.7).

References

Abad, L.V., Saiki, S., Nagasawa, N., Kudo, H., Katsumura, Y., and De La Rosa, A.M. 2011. NMR analysis of fractionated irradiated κ-carrageenan oligomers as plant growth promotors. *Radphyschem* 80: 977–982.

Anderson, N.S., Campbell, J.W., Harding, M.M., Rees, D.A., and Samuel, J.W.B. 1969. X-ray diffraction studies of polysaccharide sulphates: Double helix models for κ- and ι-carrageenans. *J. Mol. Biol.* 45: 85–88.

Archbald, P.J., Fenn, M.D., and Roy, A.B. 1981. ^{13}C NMR studies of D-glucose and D-galactose monosulphates. *Carbohydr. Res.* 93: 177–190.

Arnold, J.T., Dharmatti, S.S., and Packard, M.E. 1951. Chemical effects on nuclear induction signals from organic compounds. *J. Chem. Phys.* 19: 507–510.

Arnott, S., Scott, W.E., Rees, D.A., and McNab, C.G.A. 1974. ι-Carrageenan: Molecular structure and packing of polysaccharide double helices in oriented fibres of divalent cation salts. *J. Mol. Biol.* 90: 253–256.

Bax, A. 1994. Multidimensional nuclear-magnetic resonance methods for protein studies. *Curr. Opin. Struct. Biol.* 4: 738–744.

Belford, D.A., Hendry, I.A., and Parish, C.R. 1993. Investigation of the ability of several naturally occurring and synthetic polyanions to bind to and potentiate the biological activity of acidic fibroblast growth factor. *J. Cell Physiol.* 157: 184–189.

Bloch, F., Hansen, W.W., and Packard, M. 1946. Nuclear induction. *Phys. Rev.* 69: 127.

Bosco, M., Segre, A., Miertus, S., Cesàro, A., and Paoletti, S. 2005. The disordered conformation of kappa-carrageenan in solution as determined by NMR experiments and molecular modeling. *Carbohydr. Res.* 340: 943–958.

Bringezu, S., Schütz, H., O'Brien, M., Kauppi, L., Howarth, R.W., and McNeely, J. 2009. *Towards Sustainable Production and Use of Resources: Assessing Biofuels*, United Nations Environment Programme.

Buck, C.B., Thompson, C.D., Roberts, J.N., Müller, M., Lowy, D.R., and Schiller, J.T. 2006. Carrageenan is a potent inhibitor of papillomavirus infection. *PLoS Pathog.* 2: e69.

Cáceres, P.J., Carlucci, M.J., Damonte, E.B., Matsuhiro, B., and Zúñiga, E.A. 2000. Carrageenans from Chilean samples of *Stenogramme interrupta* (Phyllophoraceae): Structural analysis and biological activity. *Phytochemistry* 53: 81–86.

Cairns, P., Atkins, E.D.T., Miles, M.J., and Morris, V.J. 1991. Molecular transforms of kappa carrageenan and furcellaran from mixed gel systems. *Int. J. Biol. Macromol.* 13: 65–68.

Campo, V.L., Kawano, D.F., da Silva D.B., and Carvalho, I. 2009. Carrageenans: Biological properties, chemical modifications and structural analysis—A review. *Carbohydr. Polymer.* 77: 167–180.

Carlucci, M.J., Pujol, C.A., Ciancia, M. et al. 1997. Antiherpetic and anticoagulant properties of carrageenans from the red seaweed *Gigartina skottsbergii* and their cyclized derivatives: Correlation between structure and biological activity. *Int. J. Biol. Macromol.* 20: 97–105.

Carlucci, M.J., Scolaro, L.A., and Damonte, E.B. 1999. Inhibitory action of natural carrageenans on Herpes simplex virus infection of mouse astrocytes. *Chemotherapy* 45: 429–436.

Chen, H.-M., Gao, Y., and Yan, X.-J. 2011. Carrageenan oligosaccharides inhibit growth-factor binding and heparanase activity. *Acta Pharmaceutica Sinica* 46: 280–284.

Christofides, J.C., Davies, D.B., Marin, J.A., and Rathborne, E.B. 1986. Intramolecular hydrogen bonding in 1'-sucrose derivatives determined by SIMPLE ^{1}H NMR spectroscopy. *J. Am. Chem. Soc.* 108: 5738.

Clore, G.M. and Gronenborn, A.M. 1998. Determining the structures of large proteins and protein complexes by NMR. *Trends Biotechnol.* 16: 22–34.

Coxon, B.C. 2005. Deuterium isotope effects in carbohydrates revisited. Cryoprobe studies of the anomerization and NH to DD deuterium isotope induced ^{13}C NMR chemical shifts of acetamidodeoxy and aminodeoxy sugars. *Carbohydr. Res.* 340: 1714–1721.

Dumelod, B.D., Ramirez, R.P., Tiangson, C.L., Barrios, E.B., and Panlasigui, L.N. 1999. Carbohydrate availability of arroz caldo with lambda-carrageenan. *Int. J. Food Sci. Nutr.* 50: 283–289.

duPenhoat, C.H., Gey, C., Pellerin, P., and Perez, S. 1999. An NMR solution study of the mega-oligosaccharide, rhamnogalacturonan II. *J. Biomol. NMR* 14: 253–271.

Duus, J.O., Gotfredsen, C.H., and Bock, K. 2000. Carbohydrate structural determination by NMR spectroscopy: Modern methods and limitations. *Chem. Rev.* 100: 4589–4614.

Ernst, R.R. and Anderson, W.A. 1966. Application of Fourier transform spectroscopy to magnetic resonance. *Rev. Sci. Instrum.* 37: 93–102.

Falshaw, R., Furneaux, R.H., and Wong, H. 2003. Analysis of pyruvylated b-carrageen by 2D NMR spectroscopy and reductive partial hydrolysis. *Carbohydr. Res.* 338: 1403–1414.

Gardner, K.H. and Kay, L.E. 1998. The use of ^{2}H, ^{13}C, ^{15}N multidimensional NMR to study the structure and dynamics of proteins. *A. Rev. Biophys. Biomol. Struct.* 27: 357–406.

Girond, S., Crance, J.M., Van Cuyck-Gandre, H., Renaudet, J., and Deloince, R. 1991. Antiviral activity of carrageenan on hepatitis A virus replication in cell culture. *Res. Virol.* 142: 261–270.

Grasdalen, H. and Smidsrød, O. 1981a. ^{133}Cs NMR in the sol-gel states of aqueous carrageenan. Selective site binding of cesium and potassium ions in κ-carrageenan gels. *Macromolecules* 14: 229–231.

Grasdalen, H. and Smidsrød, O. 1981b. Iodide-specific formation of κ-carrageenan single helices. ^{127}I NMR spectroscopic evidence for selective site binding of iodide anions in the ordered conformation. *Macromolecules* 14: 1842–1845.

Guay, J., Bateman, K., Gordon, R., Mancini, J., and Riendeau, D. 2004. Carrageenan-induced paw edema in rat elicits a predominant prostaglandin E2 (PGE2) response in the central nervous system associated with the induction of microsomal PGE2 synthase-1. *J. Biol. Chem.* 279: 24866–24872.

Haijin, M., Xiaolu, J., and Huashi, G. 2003. A κ-carrageenan derived oligosaccharide prepared by enzymatic degradation containing anti-tumor activity. *J. Appl. Phycol.* 15: 297–303.

Hansen, P.E. 1981. Carbon-hydrogen coupling constants, a review. *Prog. NMR Spectrosc.* 14: 175–296.

Hansen, P.E. 1983. Isotope effects on nuclear shielding, a review. *Annu. Rep. NMR Spectrosc.* 15: 106–231.

Hansen, P.E. 1988. Isotope effects in nuclear shielding. *Prog. NMR Spectrosc.* 20: 207–255.

Hoffman, R., Burns, W.W., and Paper, D.H. 1995. Selective inhibition of cell proliferation and DNA synthesis by the polysulphated carbohydrate ι-carrageenan. *Cancer Chemother. Pharmacol.* 36: 325–334.

Homans, S.W. 1992. Homonuclear three-dimensional NMR methods for the complete assignment of proton NMR spectra of oligosaccharides-application to Galβ1–4(Fucα1–3)GlcNAcβ1–3Galβ1–4Glc. *Glycobiology* 2: 153–159.

Homans, S.W. and Rutherford, T.J. 1992. Reducing the overlap problem in the proton NMR spectra of oligosaccharides by application of pseudo-four-dimensional homonuclear HOHAHA-HOHAHA-COSY. *Glycobiology* 2: 293–298.

Huesemann, M., Roesjadi, G., Benemann, J., and Metting, F.B. 2010. Biofuels from microalgae and seaweeds. In *Biomass to Biofuels: Strategies for Global Industries*, eds. A. Vertés, N. Qureshi, H.P. Blaschek, and H. Yukawa, pp. 165–184. John Wiley & Sons, Hoboken, NJ.

Imeson, A.P. 2000. Carrageenan. In *Handbook of Hydrocolloids*, eds. G.O. Philips and P.A. Williams, pp. 87–102. Woodhead Publishing Limited, Cambridge, U.K.

Ishizaka, S., Hasuma, T., Otani, S., and Morisawa, S. 1980. Lymphocyte activation by purified carrageenan. *J. Immunol.* 125: 2232–2235.

Jiang, Y.-P., Guo, X.-K., and Tian, X.-F. 2005. Synthesis and NMR structural analysis of O-succinyl derivative of low-molecular weight k-carrageenan. *Carohydr. Polymer.* 61: 399–406.

Jiao, G., Yu, G., Zhang, J., and Ewart, H.S. 2011. Chemical structures and bioactivities of sulfated polysaccharides from marine algae. *Mar. Drugs* 9: 196–223.

Knight, W.D. 1949. Nuclear magnetic resonance shift in metals. *Phys. Rev.* 76: 1259.

Knutsen, S.H. and Grasdalen, H. 1992. The use of neocarrabiose oligosaccharides with different length and sulphate substitution as model compounds for ^{1}H-NMR spectroscopy. *Carbohydr. Res.* 229: 233–244.

Knutsen, S.H., Myladobodski, D.E., Larsen, B., and Usov, A.I. 1994. A modified system of nomenclature for red algal galactans. *Botanica Marina* 37: 163–169.

Liang, A., Zhou, X., Wang, Q., Liu, X., Liu, X., Du, Y., Wang, K., and Lin, B. 2006. Structural features in carrageenan that interact with a heparin-binding hematopoietic growth factor and modulate its biological activity. *J. Chromatogr. B* 843: 114–119.

Lindman, B. and Forsen, S. 1976. *Chlorine, Bromine and Iodine NMR. Physico-Chemical and Biological Applications.* Springer-Verlag, Berlin, Germany.

Marchetti, M., Pisani, S., Pietropaolo, V., Seganti, L., Nicoletti, R., and Orsi, N. 1995. Inhibition of herpes simplex virus infection by negatively charged and neutral carbohydrate polymers. *J. Chemother.* 7: 90–96.

Michel, G., Chantalat, L., and Kloareg, B. 2001a. The iota-carrageenase of *Alteromonas fortis*. A beta-helix fold-containing enzyme for the degradation of a highly polyanionic polysaccharide. *J. Biol. Chem.* 276: 40202–40209.

Michel, G., Chantalat, L., and Kloareg, B. 2001b. The kappa-carrageenase of *P. carrageenovora* features a tunnel-shaped active site: A novel insight in the evolution of clan-B glycoside hydrolases. *Structure* 9: 513–525.

Michel, G., Helbert, W., Kahn, R., Dideberg, O., and Kloareg, B. 2003. The structural bases of the processive degradation of iota-carrageenan, a main cell wall polysaccharide of red algae. *J. Mol. Biol.* 334: 421–433.

Millane, R.P., Chandrasekaran, R., Arnott, S., and Dea, I.C.M. 1988. The molecular structure of kappa-carrageenan and comparison with iota-carrageenan. *Carbohydr. Res.* 182: 1–17.

Morris, C.J. 2003. Carrageenan-induced paw edema in the rat and mouse. In *Inflammation Protocols. Methods in Molecular Biology*, eds. P.G. Winyard and D.A. Willoughby, vol. 225, pp. 115–121. Humana Press, Totowa, NJ.

Nicklin, S. and Miller, K. 1989. Intestinal uptake and immunological effects of carrageenan—Current concepts. *Food Addit. Contam.* 6: 425–436.

Nilsson, S., Piculell, L., and Joensson, B. 1989. Helix-coil transitions of ionic polysaccharides analyzed within the Poisson-Boltzmann cell model. 1. Effects of polyion concentration and counterion valency. *Macromolecules* 22: 2367–2375.

Opoku, G., Qiu, X., and Doctor, V. 2006. Effect of oversulfation on the chemical and biological properties of kappa carrageenan. *Carbohydr. Polym.* 65: 134–138.

Panlasigui, L.N., Baello, O.Q., Dimatangal, J.M., and Dumelod, B.D. 2003. Blood cholesterol and lipid-lowering effects of carrageenan on human volunteers. *Asia Pac. J. Clin. Nutr.* 12: 209–214.

Pereira, M.G., Benevides, N.M.B., Melo, M.R.S., Valente, A.P., Melo, F.R., and Mourão, P.A.S. 2005. Structure and anticoagulant activity of a sulfated galactan from the red alga, *Gelidium crinale*. Is there a specific structural requirement for the anticoagulant action? *Carbohydr. Res.* 340: 2015–2023.

Picullel, L., Håkansson, C., and Nilsson, S. 1987. Cation specificity of the order—Disorder transition in iota carrageenan: Effects of kappa carrageenan impurities. *Int. J. Biol. Macromol.* 9: 297–301.

Picullel, L., Nilsson, S., and Ström, P. 1989. On the specificity of the binding of cations to carrageenans: Counterion N.M.R. spectroscopy in mixed carrageenan systems. *Carbohydr. Res.* 188: 121–135.

Picullel, L. and Rochas, C. 1990. $^{87}Rb^+$ spin relaxation in enzymatically purified and in untreated iota-carrageenan. *Carbohydr. Res.* 208: 127–138.

Purcell, E.M., Torrey, H.C., and Pound, C.V. 1946. Resonance absorption by nuclear magnetic moments in a solid. *Phys. Rev.* 69: 37–38.

Roberts, J.N., Buck, C.B., Thompson, C.D., Kines, R., Bernardo, M., Choyke, P.L., Lowy, D.R., and Schiller, J.T. 2007. Genital transmission of HPV in a mouse model is potentiated by nonoxynol-9 and inhibited by carrageenan. *Nat. Med.* 13: 857–861.

Rochas, C. and Rinaudo, M. 1980. Activity coefficients of counterions and conformation in kappa-carrageenan systems. *Biopolymers* 19: 1675–1687.

Smidsrød, O. and Grasdalen, H. 1984. Conformations of κ-carrageenan in solution. *Hydrobiologia* 116/117: 178–186.

Sokolova, E., Barabanova, A., Homenko, V., Solov'eva, T., Bogdanovich, R., and Yermak, I. 2011. In vitro and ex vivo studies of antioxidant activity of carrageenans, sulfated polysaccharides from red algae. *Bull. Exp. Biol. Med.* 150: 426–428.

Sosnicki, J.G. and Hansen, P.E. 2004. Temperature coefficients of NH chemical shifts of thioamides in relation to structure. *J. Mol. Struct.* 700: 91–103.

Stiles, J., Guptill-Yoran, L., Moore, G.E., and Pogranichniy, R.M. 2008. Effects of λ-carrageenan on in vitro replication of feline herpesvirus and on experimentally induced herpetic conjunctivitis in cats. *Invest. Ophthalmol. Vis. Sci.* 49: 1496–1501.

Ueda, K., Saiki, M., and Brady, J.W. 2001. Molecular dynamics simulation and NMR study of aqueous neocarrabiose 4-sulfate, a building block of κ-carrageenan. *J. Phys. Chem. B* 105: 8629–8638.

Ueda, K., Ueda, T., Sato, T., Nakayama, H., and Brady, J.W. 2004. The conformational free-energy map for solvated neocarrabiose. *Carbohydr. Res.* 339: 1953–1960.

van de Velde, F. and De Ruiter, G.A. 2002. Carrageenan. In *Biopolymers (vol. 6) Polysaccharide II Polysaccharides from Eukaryotes*, eds. A. Steinbüchel, S. DeBaets, and E.J. VanDamme, pp. 245–274. Wiley-VCH, Weinheim, Germany.

van de Velde, F. and De Ruiter, G.A. 2008. *Biopolymers*, pp. 254–256. Wiley-VCH-Verlag, Weinheim, Germany.

van de Velde, F., Knutsen, S.H., Rollema, H.S., and Cerezo, A.S. 2002. ^1H and ^{13}C high resolution NMR spectroscopy of carrageenans: Application in research and industry. *Trends Food Sci. Technol.* 13: 73–92.

van de Velde, F., Pereira, L., and Rollema, H.S. 2004. The revised NMR chemical shift data of carrageenans. *Carbohydr. Res.* 339: 2309–2313.

Vuister, G.W., De Waard, P., Boelens, R., Vliegenthart, J.F.G., and Kaptein, R. 1989. The use of three-dimensional NMR in structural studies of oligosaccharides. *J. Am. Chem. Soc.* 111: 772–774.

Wider, G. and Wüthrich, K. 1999. NMR spectroscopy of large molecules and multimolecular assemblies in solution. *Curr. Opin. Struct. Biol.* 9: 594–601.

Wüthrich, K. 1986. *NMR of Proteins and Nucleic Acids.* Wiley, New York.

Yermak, I.M., Barabanova, A.O., Aminin, D.L., Davydova, V.N., Sokolova, E.V., Solov'eva, T.F., Kim, Y.H., and Shin, K.S. 2012. Effects of structural peculiarities of carrageenans on their immunomodulatory and anticoagulant activities. *Carbohydr. Polym.* 87: 713–720.

Yu, G., Guan, H., Ioanoviciu, A.S. et al. 2002. Structural studies on kappa-carrageenan derived oligosaccharides. *Carbohydr. Res.* 337: 433–440.

Yuan, H., Song, J., Zhang, W., Li, X., Li, N., and Gao, X. 2006. Antioxidant activity and cytoprotective effect of κ-carrageenan oligosaccharides and their different derivatives. *Bioorg. Med. Chem. Lett.* 16: 1329–1334.

Yuan, H., Zhang, W., Li, X., Lü, X., Li, N., Gao, X., and Song, J. 2005. Preparation and in vitro antioxidant activity of κ-carrageenan oligosaccharides and their oversulfated, acetylated, and phosphorylated derivatives. *Carbohydr. Res.* 340: 685–692.

Zhang, W. and Furo, I. 1993. [127]I-NMR studies of anion binding to κ-carrageenan. *Biopolymers* 33: 1709–1714.

Zhang, W., Liu, M., Hansen, P.E., Yu, G., Yang, B., and Zhao, X. 2010. Sequence and structure analysis of κ-carrageenan-derived oligosaccharides by two-dimensional nuclear magnetic resonance. *J. Psychol.* 46: 831–838.

Zhang, W., Piculell, L., and Nilsson, S. 1991. Salt dependence and ion specificity of the coil-helix transition of Furcellaran. *Biopolymer* 31: 1727–1736.

Zhang, W., Piculell, L., and Nilsson, S. 1992. Effects of specific anion binding on the helix-coil transition of lower charged carrageenans. NMR data and conformational equilibria analyzed within the Poisson-Boltzmann cell model. *Macromolecules* 25: 6165–6172.

Zhou, G., Sheng, W., Yao, W., and Wang, C. 2006. Effect of low molecular λ-carrageenan from *Chondrus ocellatus* on antitumor H-22 activity of 5-Fu. *Pharmacol. Res.* 53: 129–134.

Zhou, G., Sun, Y., Xin, H., Zhang, Y., Li, Z., and Xu, Z. 2004. In vivo antitumor and immunomodulation activities of different molecular weight lambda-carrageenans from *Chondrus ocellatus*. *Pharmacol. Res.* 50: 47–53.

6

Study of Marine-Derived Fatty Acids and Their Therapeutic Importance

Parimal C. Sen

CONTENTS

6.1 Introduction

The Bay of Bengal is the largest bay in the world. It is bordered predominantly by Sri Lanka and India to the west, Bangladesh to the north, and Myanmar to the east. It comprises an area of about 2,172,000 km². The coastal area of the Bay of Bengal has a large number of marine organisms more specifically fish containing high level of polyunsaturated fatty acids (PUFAs) particularly n-3 (omega 3) series with potential therapeutic importance. During the last 30 years of extensive studies on PUFAs of n-3 series, the major components of marine lipids have been found to modulate blood lipid profiles in a number of chronic diseases and other pathophysiological disorders like diabetes, arthritis, cataract development of eye, kidney defects, atherosclerosis, heart attack, depression, cancer, and ulcerative colitis neoplasm (Simopoulos 1991). Recent report suggests important beneficial effects of EPA-/DHA-enriched PUFA in combating a number of diseases (http://www. umms.org 2009) and nutritional importance of n-3 fatty acids (http://www.articlebase. com/health-articles/omega-3-fish-oil-epaand-dha-explained-4011.html). Further study in recent times indicates the therapeutic effects on cardiovascular disease (Pei-Chen et al. 2009) and depression (Jazayeri et al. 2008). The essential fatty acids, namely, EPA, 20:5 n-3 and DHA, 22:6 n-3, are required to be provided as dietary supplements (Rose 1997) since human body is incapable of de novo synthesis of these fatty acids. Major marine lipid components are essential constituents of mammalian cell membranes (Hazra et al. 2003), which act as triene prostaglandin (PG) precursors. Dietary intake of these fatty acids is effective in lowering plasma concentration of triacylglycerol (TG) (Sanders et al. 1981).

Metabolic experiments in humans and rats led to suggest a decrease in the production of very low–density lipoproteins (VLDL) and chylomicrons by liver and intestine, respectively (Harris 1989; Harris and Muzio 1993; Nestle et al. 1982), and in improving insulin sensitivity (Andersen et al. 2008). The mechanism for this effect has been evaluated in cell cultures (Nossen et al. 1986; Wong et al. 1985), and the results indicated that decreased TG synthesis is a major cause for the reduced secretion of VLDL TG (Rustan et al. 1998). TG is known to be an essential constituent of cell membranes. Further, phospholipids, which occur in three different forms, namely, alkylacyl, alkenylacyl, and diacyl forms, are rich in marine PUFA and excellent substrates for PG biosynthesis.

A large number of marine fishes are available in the coastal area of Bay of Bengal (along the West Bengal belt); however, they are yet to be investigated in the context of its lipid content and the EPA and DHA level therein. EPA and DHA are called as essential fatty acids or n-3 PUFAs (Pereira et al. 2004) of n-3 series. Although there is no doubt about the beneficial effects of EPA and DHA, indeed they might even be considered essential to be one of the basic nutritional components of daily nutrition. However, their efficacy is dependent upon the ratio of n-6: n-3 and the condition being treated. It has been established that only lower ratios between 2.5:1 and 5:1 (n-6:n-3) are beneficial; a daily intake of 2.5:1 has been proven to act beneficially in case of colorectal cancer, 2.3:1 on rheumatoid arthritis, and 5:1 on asthma (Simopoulos 2008). It has been reported with strong evidence that intake of adequate level of EPA and DHA (main components of most fish oil) is effective against cardiovascular disease, rheumatoid arthritis, macular degeneration, etc. The minimum recommended daily dose of EPA+DHA intake is 500 mg. Report suggested that both children (age group 8–14) and elderly ones are likely to be deficient in EPA+DHA (Fratesi et al. 2009; Madden et al. 2009).

In the western countries particularly in the United States health authorities are suggesting for consumption of fish at least two to three times per week specifically those who are suffering from some diseases as mentioned earlier. However, there is a point of caution that a large many fish are now heavily contaminated with highly toxic compound particularly mercury, with profound toxic effects on cardiovascular and nervous system. This is even more alarming to pregnant women and infants (Ginsberg and Toal 2009). Attempt was also made to find a relation between seafood-based n-3 PUFAs and plant-based n-3 PUFAs. It has been found that when intake of seafood-based n-3 PUFAs is low, plant-based n-3 PUFAs was effective in reducing chronic heart disease risk. Therefore, it was suggested that plant source PUFAs are equally important (Mozaffarian et al. 2005). Because of the unsaturated nature (multiple double bonds) of PUFAs, they are prone to oxidation which makes them rancid and potential initiators of chain reactions which can lead to oxidation of fat and cholesterol molecules in the body. This so-called lipid peroxidation reaction is believed to be implicated in atherosclerosis, cancer, and inflammation (Eritsland 2000). However, most studies confirmed that DHA benefits nervous system functions, cardiovascular health. In one study, men who took DHA supplements for 6–12 weeks were found to decrease the concentrations of several inflammatory markers in their blood by approximately 20% (Farzaneh-Far et al. 2010). Heart disease patients with higher intakes of DHA and EPA have been reported to survive longer. A new study found that higher intake of DHA was associated with slower rates of telomere shortening, which is a basic DNA-level marker of aging (Farzaneh-Far et al. 2010). A study with over 14,000 men and women showed that vegans with no intake of dietary EPA or DHA still had very high levels of plasma DHA and EPA, suggesting that conversion of linolenic acid and shorter carbon chain n-3 fatty acids is very efficient. Male vegans had only slightly lower levels of DHA than female subjects and only slightly lower levels than fish eaters (195 compared to 240). EPA levels were found to be higher in male vegans than in meat-eating and fish-eating

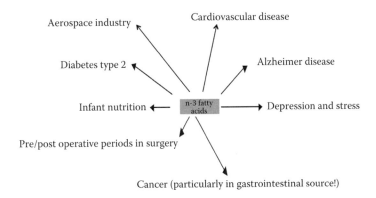

FIGURE 6.1
Application of EPA-/DHA-enriched PUFAs.

males (Welch et al. 2010), vegetarians, and vegans and the precursor-to-product ratio of α-linolenic acid to long-chain n-3 PUFAs (Welch et al. 2010).

Marine fatty acids, particularly the long-chain EPA and DHA, have been shown to inhibit the proliferation of breast and prostate cancer cell lines in vitro and to reduce the risk and progression of these tumors in experimental animals. However, whether a high consumption of marine PUFAs can reduce the risk of these cancers or other hormone-dependent cancers in human populations is not quite clear. Most of the studies failed to draw a correlation between fish consumption or marine fatty acid intake and the risk of hormone-related cancers (Terry et al. 2003).

Long-chain n-3 fatty acids, EPA (20:5n-3), and DHA (22:6n-3) are associated with decreased triglyceride levels in hypertriglyceridemic patients and lowered the risk of developing coronary heart disease (CHD). Dietary trans-fatty acids on the other hand are associated with increased LDL cholesterol levels. Therefore, a diet low in saturated and trans-fatty acids, with sufficient amounts of monounsaturated and PUFAs, particularly long-chain n-3 fatty acids, would be recommended to reduce the risk of developing CHD. It has been demonstrated by Zainal et al. (2009) that isolated in presence of EPA and DHA, chondrocytes reduce catabolic gene expression profiles. They have also shown that in a cartilage explant model, PUFAs are translated into reduction in tissue degradation. The n-3 PUFAs, particularly EPA, have been found to be of therapeutic potential for the treatment of inflammatory joint diseases such as osteoarthritis (Angus et al. 2010; Lichtenstein 2003). Further to the earlier mentioned beneficial effect, the application of n-3 PUFA has been described by Gogus and Smith (2010) in their recent review. The report suggests various useful effects of PUFs (Figure 6.1).

6.2 Isolation and Preparation of EPA- and DHA-Enriched Polyunsaturated Fatty Acids

6.2.1 Extraction of Total Lipids from Marine Fish

Flesh is to be separated from fins and bones and pooled separately and finely minced in a blender. Total lipids could be extracted with methanol and chloroform according to the method of Bligh and Dyer (1959). The solvent containing lipids is to be removed by flash rotavapor and weighted to obtain the quantity of lipid per gm of tissue. 2,6 Ditertiary butyl-p-cresol at a concentration of 10 µg/mL is suggested to be used as an antioxidant. The antioxidants at this concentration do not have any visible side effect. The lipid may be redissolved in a minimum volume of $CHCl_3$ and stored under nitrogen at –20°C.

6.2.2 Separation of Phospholipids by Preparative Thin Layer Chromatography

Polar and nonpolar lipids extracted from different fishes can be separated by preparative thin layer chromatography (TLC) (20 cm × 20 cm) after developing in a solvent system—acetone: diethyl ether (3:1, vol/vol). Plates after air-drying in a stream of nitrogen flow following each sample spots are visualized by molybdenum blue reagent; polar lipids appear at the lower portion of TLC could be scrapped off. Mostly, phospholipids present in this silica scrap can be extracted three times with solvent system, $CHCl_3:CH_3OH:H_2O$ (2:1:0.5, v/v/v). The combined extracts may be dried by rotavapor.

6.2.3 Analysis of Fatty Acids Composition in Different Marine Fishes

Fatty acid compositions are to be determined after methylation with H_2SO_4/methanol according to Christie (1982). The FAME can be quantified by gas chromatography using a flame-ionization detector and 10% DEGS polar column (30 m × 0.25 mm × 0.25 µm). Analyses are preferably carried out with a programmed oven temperature rise of 1°C/min from 160°C to 200°C. Nitrogen is used as carrier gas with a flow rate 40 mL/min. Fatty acids are identified by comparing their retention times of their separation with respect to appropriate standards. When proper standards are not available, unknown one can be identified from logarithmic plot.

6.2.4 Large-Scale Preparation of EPA-/DHA-Enriched Fraction

Lipid can be extracted in large quantity at 10°C as stated earlier from lotte fish (however, same approach is applicable to other fishes also) (reason explained later) since it is found to be rich in EPA/DHA. Total phospholipids are saponified, and free fatty acid was released by acidification with 4(N) H_2SO_4. This should be dried overnight on anhydrous Na_2SO_4 and converted into methyl esters by standard method with methanol in 1% concentrated H_2SO_4. Dried fatty acid methyl esters (FAME) are dissolved in methanol. EPA-/DHA-enriched PUFA fraction is prepared by urea fractionation method according to Ghosh et al. (1975).

Fatty acids can be separated with increasing concentration of urea based on unsaturation, and at the final stage, EPA and DHA were collected together. From 1 g of total fatty acid mixture about 200 mg EPA/DHA is obtained with about 75%–80% enrichment. It takes about three days to complete one cycle of purification. The composition of fatty acids at each step is monitored with gas chromatography and modified till the desired enriched product (~80% EPA-/DHA-enriched PUFA) is obtained. The sample should be stored under nitrogen at –20°C. EPA-/DHA-enriched PUFA fraction so prepared could be used in any subsequent study.

6.2.5 EPA-/DHA-Enriched PUFA Preparation for Cell Culture

PUFAs are highly unstable and undergo lipid peroxidation in the air, forming free radicals such as peroxyl and alkoxyl radicals which are very toxic on cell. So it is required to minimize the oxidation of PUFA using an antioxidant as described earlier. Similarly, they are usually not soluble in aqueous medium. Therefore, to study their biological response, these are usually emulsified with protein such as bovine serum albumin (1 mg/mL) (Zhang et al. 1990). PUFAs were dissolved in $CHCl_3{:}CH_3OH$ (2:1, vol/vol); the required amount was taken in a sterile vial and evaporated to dryness completely in the absence of oxygen. To the vial containing the dried PUFA, Dulbecco's Modified Eagle's Medium (DMEM) containing 10% heat-inactivated fetal bovine serum (FBS) was added to make the final desired concentration and the mixture was sonicated under nitrogen in a water bath sonicator for use in subsequent experiments. As mentioned before, marine fishes are abundant in the coastal area of Bay of Bengal (West Bengal, India). Recently, seven of them have been studied in detail with respect to their lipid content in the context of EPA and DHA contribution (Bera et al. 2010). Vangan fish (*Mugil tade*) was found to contain the highest percentage of total lipid (~15%) and lotte fish (*Harpadon nehereus*) the lowest (~2.5%); however, phospholipids content was found to be highest in lotte (~68%) fish. Percentage of PUFAs in lotte fish is higher (about 53%) than other fishes. When the quantity of EPA/DHA per gram of total lipid was calculated, not much difference was found between lotte and pomfret. Phospholipid content was found to be quite high in the lotte fish, hence easy to separate phospholipid from the total mixture; therefore, we have selected this particular fish in our study for large-scale preparation of EPA- and DHA-enriched PUFA (more than 50%). All fish samples though contained different types of saturated and unsaturated fatty acids along with EPA/DHA acids.

The marine fishes available in any geographical location are to be considered important and valuable when their oil has an appreciable content of such EPA/DHA. In our study, we have found that a local marine fish called lotte (*Harpadon nehereus*) contains highest level of EPA and DHA in its oil among seven species of marine fishes analyzed from the coastal area of Bay of Bengal. The fish is consumed primarily by local people; however, there is always a gap between the volume of its catch in the season and consumption of fresh fish during that period; therefore, it is required to be preserved as a dried fish for the off-season time. There are plenty of reports of having high level of EPA/DHA in different marine fishes particularly in murrells (Sen et al. 1976) and sardine (Gamez-Meza et al. 1999); however, their content is found to vary from season to season and from place to place. It was also reported by Khalid et al. (1968) that PUFA content in 13 species of marine fish varied widely. The cholesterol content in the oil of lotte fish is found to be quite low. Therefore, its consumption would be beneficial along with high content of (n-3) PUFA (Bera et al. 2010). In a study from our laboratory, we have found that EPA and DHA act as protective agent against mercury poisoning studied in cell culture (LLC-PK1 pig kidney cell line) as well as in animal model (rat kidney). It is found to be highly preventive against diabetes (Bera et al. 2010).

Mercuric chloride is a known human and animal nephrotoxicant. The uptake of mercury shows that kidney accumulates the highest level of mercury compared to brain and liver causing a dose-dependent induction of kidney damage, thereby causing an increase in leakage of mercury through the kidney (Emanuelli et al. 1996; Hussain et al. 1999). It is well established that mercuric chloride damages kidney and rectal region of renal tubules. Brown et al. (1998) have shown that the composition of dietary PUFA modifies glomerular thermodynamics in normal rats and affects the chronic course of renal disease in partially nephrectonized rats and that dietary supplementation prevented deterioration of the glomerular filtration rate and preserved renal structure. The dietary lipids derived from coconut oil, soya oil, or cod-liver oil have been reported to reduce the whole body retention of mercury in mice significantly (Hojbjerg et al. 1992). Findings of our laboratory have shown that damage of the kidney by mercuric chloride can be restricted by intake of food supplemented with EPA/DHA. In cell culture study, EPA- and DHA-enriched PUFA were found to be highly protective against cell damage mainly through the mediation of resistance by changing the mitochondrial membrane potential. So PUFAs with EPA-/DHA-enriched preparation are extremely useful in protecting the mercury-induced renal failure (Bera et al. 2010).

The study from our laboratory for the first time has shown that intake of EPA and DHA prepared from lotte fish oil lowers glucose level from ~375 to ~175 mg/dL in experimentally induced (with streptozotocin, STZ) diabetic rat. It was reported that patients with diabetes mellitus are at increased risk of developing CHD, and the potential effect of fish oil in reducing this risk is likely to be useful to these patients (Toft et al. 1995; Vessby et al. 1992). The sugar level of the diabetic rat was found to be quite high and was considered to be hyperglycemic when treated with STZ. Mild glycemic condition was found by Henquin et al. (1994) when sugar level was about 200 mg/dL, whereas Bonner-Weir et al. (1981) reported that during hyperglycemic condition, sugar level went up to around 350 mg/mL on STZ-induced diabetes in rat. In our animal model study, we have clearly demonstrated the lowering of the blood glucose with the desired amount PUFA having high content of EPA/DHA. It has been also reported that fish oil does not have any adverse effects on glucose or insulin metabolism in diabetic patients; on the other hand, it was reported to lower the TG levels effectively (Friedberg et al. 1998).

PUFAs may cause oxidative stress in biological systems as they undergo lipid peroxidation; however, in in vivo experiments when PUFAs are incorporated as dietary supplement, lipid peroxidation has been proposed to be restricted by the presence of multiple antioxidants in food and the physiological system. Oxidative stress in diabetes coexists with reduced antioxidant status, and in STZ-induced diabetic rat, pancreatic beta cell damage is reversed by antioxidant treatment. The marine fish EPA/DHA is highly effective as antioxidant, by reverting the damaged pancreatic beta cell to normal, suggesting enhancement of protective antioxidant status.

The fish oil with enriched EPA/DHA lipid fraction would improve glycemic condition and diabetes as well (Arulselvan and Subrmanian 2007). It has been reported that hilsa fish oil which contains high level of EPA and DHA acts as antioxidative defense of STZ-induced diabetes in rats (Mahmud et al. 2004). Thus beneficial activity of EPA-/DHA-enriched PUFA from lotte fish led us to believe that use of selective amount may produce the effective results in health care. EPA-/DHA-enriched PUFA is found to be quite effective in reversing the diabetes in rat when induced with STZ. In one study from author's laboratory, a protein of 70 kDa molecular weight isolated from goat spermatozoa has been reported to have dual functions: inhibition of Na,K-ATPase on the one hand and arylsulfatase (ASA) activity on the other. The enzyme activity is found to be affected during diabetes induced by STZ. EPA- and DHA-enriched PUFA treatment reversed the condition (Dhara et al. 2012). The changes in tissue morphology and ASA activity have been monitored during the diabetes recovery following treatment with PUFA. The use of PUFA as beneficiary vehicle for the changes in metabolic diseases toward its recovery as well as control factor (preventive) is well documented (http://www.articlebase.com/health-articles/omega-3-fish-oil-epaand-dha-explained-4011.html). Carvalho et al. (2003) have reported the increase in ASA activity of cytosolic fraction of STZ-induced diabetes. We have shown that the enzyme activity of the individual organ of such diabetic rats increased (in average, 40%–50%) when compared with the respective tissues of normal animal. Interestingly, such increase in ASA activity due to diabetes can be reversed and returned close to almost normal level by DHA- and EPA-enriched PUFA treatment (Dhara et al. 2012).

The mean body weight in STZ-induced diabetic rat was found to be decreased compared to control one as documented previously (Brozoska et al. 2003; Puranik et al. 2007) which is in consistent with our study (Bera et al. 2010). In our study, the body weight of STZ-induced animals is found to be regained considerably after several weeks of EPA-/DHA-enriched PUFA treatment (Bera et al. 2010). Western blot analysis with anti-p70 antibody shows that cytosolic fraction exhibits significant intensity with highest level observed in diabetic rats. This is probably due to the higher expression of ASA A activity during STZ-induced diabetes. Mahmood et al. (2000) have reported that ASAs A and B were affected during STZ-induced diabetes and starvation in rats. The intensity of band in different organs is reduced to almost the control subject when diabetic rat was treated with PUFA. The result thus clearly suggests that PUFA antagonizes the STZ effect, suggesting that the treatment indeed recovers the damage caused due to artificially induced diabetes. The increase in the expression of ASA, a cytosolic enzyme, is very interesting which corroborates the increase of this enzyme activity during diabetes induction.

The scanning electron microscopic analyses of brain, liver, and kidney of control, diabetic-induced, and PUFA-treated rat showed some external morphological changes during induction of diabetes, which indicates some abnormalities in the normal physiology of these organs, possibly due to cell damage caused during diabetes. Significant changes in external morphology were seen in brain and liver segments when analyzed with SEM. PUFA treatment reversed most of the effect (Dhara et al. 2012). The morphological changes were examined by further experiment with hematoxylin- and eosin-stained section of control, STZ-induced diabetic, and PUFA-treated rat organs (brain, liver, and kidney), i.e., by histological studies. Histological examination of the rat organs revealed change in internal morphology. In the diabetic rat, the liver size becomes larger and, on PUFA treatment, becomes normal. Some abnormalities were observed in case of kidney during diabetes induction also. However, in most of the cases, EPA-/DHA-enriched PUFA treatment of the diabetic subject led to the reversal of the changes (Dhara et al. 2012). Kim et al. (2006) also observed morphological and other biochemical changes in different organs during diabetes induced by STZ.

6.3 Conclusion

Based on the previous discussion, it may be suggested that the PUFAs, namely, DHA- and EPA-enriched lipid, have been found to be effective in curing different diseases. Therefore, these types of PUFA treatment could be highly beneficial in protecting human health from damage caused due to various diseases.

Acknowledgments

Author is thankful to the Department of Biotechnology, Government of India, and Bose Institute for the financial support.

References

Andersen, G., K. Harnack, H.F. Erbersdobler, and V. Somoza. 2008. Dietary eicosapentaenoic acid and docosahexaenoic acid are more effective than alpha-linolenic acid in improving insulin sensitivity in rats. *Annals of Nutrition and Metabolism* 52: 250–256.

Angus, K.T., E.J. Wann, E.J. Blaine, A.T. Michael-Titus, and M.M. Knight. 2010. Eicosapentaenoic acid and docosahexaenoic acid reduce interleukin-1β-mediated cartilage degradation. *Arthritis Research Therapy* 12: R207. doi:10.1186/ar3183.

Arulselvan, P. and S.P. Subrmanian. 2007. Beneficial effects of *Murraya koenigii* leaves on anti-oxidant defence system and ultra structural changes of pancreatic beta cell in experimental diabetes in rats. *Chemico-Biological Interactions* 165: 155–164.

Bera, R., T.K. Dhara, R. Bhadra, G.C. Majumder, and P.C. Sen. 2010. Eicosapentaenoic and docosahexaenoic acids enriched polyunsaturated fatty acids from the coastal marine fish of Bay of Bengal and their therapeutic value. *Indian Journal of Experimental Biology* 48: 1194–1203.

Bligh, E.G. and W.J. Dyer. 1959. A rapid method of total lipid extraction and purification. *Canadian Journal of Biochemistry and Physiology* 37: 911–917.

Bonner-Weir, S., D.F. Trent, R. Honey, and G.C. Weir. 1981. Responses of neonatal rat islets to streptozotocin: Limited B- cell regeneration and hyperglycemia. *Diabetes* 30:64–69.

Brown, S.A., C.A. Brown, W.A. Crowell, J.A. Barsanti, T. Allen, C. Cowell, and D.R. Finco. 1998. Beneficial effects of chronic administration of dietary omega-3 polyunsaturated fatty acids in digs with renal insufficiency. *Journal of Laboratory and Clinical Medicine* 131: 447–455.

Brozoska, M.M., J. Moniuszko-Jakoniuk, B. Pilat-Marcinkiewicz, and B. Sawicki. 2003. Liver and kidney function and histology in parts exposed to cadmium and ethanol. *Alcohol and Alcoholism* 38: 2–10.

de Carvalho, E.N., N.A.S. de Carvalho, and L.M. Ferreira. 2003. Experimental model of induction of diabetes mellitus in rats. *Acta Cirurgica Brasileira* 8: 60–64.

Christie, W. W. 1982. *Lipid Analysis*, 2nd edn., Pergamon Press, Oxford, U.K.

Dhara, T.K., R. Bera, R. Bhadra, and P.C. Sen. 2012. Arylsulphatase and ultrastructural changes in different organs of rat during streptozotocin induced diabetes and the effect of polyunsaturated fatty acids. *Journal of Pharmaceutical and Biomedical Sciences* 16(3): 1–8.

Emanuelli, T., J.B. Rocha, M.E. Pereira, L.O. Porciuncula, V.M. Morsch, A.F. Martins, and D.O. Souza. 1996. Effect of mercuric chloride intoxication and dimercaprol treatment on delta-aminolevulinate dehydratase from brain, liver and kidney of adult mice. *Pharmacology and Toxicology* 79: 136–143.

Eritsland, J. 2000. Safety considerations of polyunsaturated fatty acids. *American Journal of Clinical Nutrition* 71: 197S–201S.

Farzaneh-Far, R., J. Lin, E.S. Epel, W.S. Harris, E.H. Blackburn, and M.A. Whooley. 2010. Association of marine omega-3, fatty acid levels with telomeric aging in patients with coronary heart disease. *Journal of American Medical Association* 303: 250–257.

Fratesi, J.A., R.C. Hogg, G.S. Young-Newton, A.C. Patterson, P. Charkhzarin, B.K. Thomas, M.T. Sharratt, and K.D. Stark. 2009. Direct quantitation of omega-3 fatty acid intake of Canadian residents of a long-term care facility. *Applied Physiology, Nutrition and Metabolism* 34: 1–9.

Friedberg, C.E., M.J. Jansen, R.J. Heine, and D.E. Grobbee. 1998. Fish oil and glycemic control in diabetes. A meta-analysis. *Diabetes Care* 21: 494–500.

Gamez-Meza, N., L. Higuera-Ciapara, A.M. Calderon, C.L. de La Barca, J. Vazquez- Moreno, J. Noriega- Rodriguez, and O. Angulo-Guerrero. 1999. Seasonal variation in the fatty acid composition and quality of sardine oil from *Sardinops sagax caeruleus* of the Gulf of California. *Lipids* 34: 639–642.

Ghosh, A., A. Ghosh, M. Haque, and J. Dutta. 1975. Fatty acids of boal fish oil by urea fractionation and gas-liquid chromatography. *Journal of Food Science and Agriculture* 27: 159–167.

Ginsberg, G.L. and B.F. Toal. 2009. Quantitative approach for incorporating methyl mercury risks and omega-3 fatty acid benefits in developing species-specific fish consumption advice. *Environmental Health Perspectives* 117: 267–275.

Gogus, U. and C. Smith. 2010. Current application of omega-3 PUFA. *International Journal of Food Science and Technology* 45: 417–436.

Harris, W.S. 1989. Fish oils and plasma lipid and lipoprotein metabolism in humans: A critical review. *Journal of Lipid Research* 30: 785–807.

Harris, W.S. and F. Muzio. 1993. Fish oil reduces postprandial triglyceride concentrations without accelerating lipid-emulsion removal rates. *American Journal of Clinical Nutrition* 58: 68–74.

Hazra, A.K., S. Ghosh, S. Banerjee, and B. Mukherjee. 2003. The multifaceted fish oil. *Science and Culture* 69: 319–322.

Henquin, J.C., F. Carton, L.N. Ongemba, and D.J. Becker. 1994. Improvement of mild hypoinsulinae-mic diabetes in the rat by low non-toxic doses of vanadate. *Journal of Endocrinology* 142: 555–561.

Hojbjerg, S., J.B. Nielsen, and O. Adersen. 1992. Effects of dietary lipids on whole-body retention and organ distribution of organic and inorganic mercury in mice. *Food Chemistry and Toxicology* 30: 703–708.

http://www.articlebase.com/health-articles/omega-3-fish-oil-epaand-dha-explained-4011.html

http://www.umms.org, 2009.

Hussain, S., A. Atkinson, S.J. Thompson, and A.T. Khan. 1999. Accumulation of mercury and its effect on antioxidant enzymes in brain, liver and kidneys of mice. *Journal of Environmental Science and Health B* 34: 645–660.

Jazayeri, S., M. Tehrani-Doost, S.A. Keshavarz, M. Hosseini, A. Djazavery, H. Amini, M. Jalali, and M. Peet. 2008. Comparison of therapeutic effects of omega-3 fatty acid, eicosapentaenoic acid and fluoxetine separately and in combination, in major depressive disorder. *Australian and New Zealand Journal of Psychiatry* 42: 192–198.

Khalid, Q., A.S. Mirza, and A.H. Khan. 1968. The fatty acid composition of edible marine fish oils. *Journal of American Oil Chemists' Society* 45: 247–249.

Kim, N.N., M. Stankovi, T.T. Cushman, I. Goldstein, R. Munarriz, and A.M. Traish. 2006. Streptozotocin-induced diabetes in the rat is associated with changes in vaginal hemodynam-ics, morphology and biochemical markers. *BMC Physiology* 6: 4–11.

Lichtenstein, A.H. 2003. Dietary fat and cardiovascular disease risk: Quantity or quality? *Journal of Women's Health (Larchmt)* 12: 109–114.

Madden, S.M.M., C.F. Garrioch, and B.J. Holub. 2009. Direct diet quantification indicates low intakes of n-3 fatty acids in children 4 to 8 years old. *Journal of Nutrition* 139: 528–532.

Mahmood, V., J.-P., Mansoureh, J. Shahrzad, and R. Mojgan. 2000. Hepatic arylsulfatases A and B activities in streptozotocin-induced diabetic rats. *Archives of Iranian Medicine* 4: 3–6.

Mahmud, D., A. Hossain, S. Hossain, A. Hanna, L. Ali, and M. Hashimoto. 2004. Effects of Hilsa fish oil on the atherogenic lipid profile and glycemic status of streptozotocin-treated type 1 diabetic. *Clinical and Experimental Pharmacology and Physiology* 31: 76–81.

Mozaffarian, D., A. Ascherio, F.B. Hu, M.J. Stampfer, W.C. Willett, D.S. Siscovick, and E.D. Rinm. 2005. Interplay between different polyunsaturated fatty acids and risk of coronary heart dis-ease in men. *Circulation* 111: 157–164.

Nestle, P.J., W.E. Connor, M.E. Reardon, S. Connor, S.H. Wong, and R. Boston. 1982. Suppression by diets rich in fish oil of very low density lipoprotein production in man. *Journal of Clinical Investigation* 74: 82–89.

Nossen, J.O., A.C. Rustan, S.H. Gloppestad, S. Mabakken, and C.A. Drevon. 1986. Eicosapentaenoic acid inhibits synthesis and secretion of triacylglycerols by cultured rat hepatocytes. *Biochimica Biophysica Acta* 879: 56–62.

Pei-Chen, J.C., C. Yi-Ting, and S. Kuan-Pin. 2009. Omega-3 polyunsaturated fatty acids (n-3 PUFAs) in cardiovascular diseases (CVDs) and depression: The missing link? *Cardiovascular Psychology and Neurology* 725316 (PMCID: PMC2791235).

Pereira, S.L., A.E. Leonard, Y.S. Huang, L.T. Chuang, and P. Mukerji. 2004. Identification of two novel microalgal enzymes is involved in the conversion of the omega-3 fatty acids, eicosapentaenoic acid to docosahexaenoic acid. *Biochemical Journal* 384: 357–366.

Puranik, K.N., K.F. Kammar, and S. Devi. 2007. Modulation of morphology and some gluconeo-genic enzymes activity by *Tinospora cordifolia* (Willd.) in diabetic rat kidney. *Biomedical Research* 18: 179–183.

Rose, D.P. 1997. Effects of dietary fatty acids on breast and prostate cancers: Evidence from in vitro experiments and animal studies. *American Journal of Clinical Nutrition* 66 (suppl): 1513S–1522S.

Rustan, A.C., J.O Nossen, E.N. Christiansen, and C.A. Drevon. 1998. Eicosapentaenoic acid reduces hepatic synthesis and secretion of triacylglycerol by decreasing the activity of acyl-CoA: 1.2-diacylglycerol acyltransferase. *Journal of Lipid Research* 29: 1417–1426.

Sanders, T.A.B., M. Vickers, and A.P. Haines. 1981. Effect on blood lipids and haemostasis of a supplement of cod liver oil, rich in EPA and DHA, in healthy young men. *Clinical Science* 61: 317–324.

Sen, P.C., A. Ghosh, and J. Datta. 1976. Fatty acids of lipids of murrells. *Journal of Food Science and Agriculture* 27: 811–818.

Simopoulos, A.P. 1991. Omega-3 fatty acids in health and disease and in growth and development. *American Journal of Clinical Nutrition* 54: 438–463.

Simopoulos, A.P. 2008. The importance of the omega-6 and omega-3 fatty acid ration in cardiovascular disease and other chronic diseases. *Experimental Biology and Medicine* 233: 674–688.

Terry, P.D., T.E. Rohan, and A. Wolk. 2003. Intakes of fish and marine fatty acids and the risks of cancers of the breast and prostate and of other hormone-related cancers: A review of the epidemiologic evidence. *American Journal of Clinical Nutrition* 77: 532–543.

Toft, I., K.H. Bønaa, O.L.E.C. Ingebretsen, A. Nordøy, and J. Jenssen. 1995. Effects of ω-3 polyunsaturated fatty acids on glucose homeostasis and blood pressure in essential hypertension: A randomized, controlled trial. *Annals of Internal Medicine* 123: 911–918.

Vessby, B., B. Karlstrom, M. Boberg, H. Lithell, and C. Berne. 1992. Polyunsaturated fatty acid may impair blood glucose control in type 2 diabetic patients. *Diabetes and Medicine* 9: 126–132.

Welch, A.A., A.A. Shakya-Srestha, M.A.H. Lentjes, N.J. Wareham, and K.-T. Khaw. 2010. Dietary intake and status of n–3 polyunsaturated fatty acids in a population of fish-eating and non-fish-eating meat-eaters, vegetarians, and vegans and the precursor-product ratio of α-linolenic acid to long-chain n–3 polyunsaturated fatty acids: results from the EPIC-Norfolk cohort. *American Journal of Clinical Nutrition* 92: 1040–1051.

Wong, S.H., M. Reardon, and I.J. Nestle. 1985. Reduced triglyceride formation from long- chain polyenoic fatty acids in rat hepatocytes. *Metabolism* 34: 900–905.

Zainal, Z., A.J. Longman, S. Hurst, K. Duggan, B. Caterson, C.E. Hughes, and J.L. Harwood. 2009. Relative efficacies of omega-3 polyunsaturated fatty acids in reducing expression of key proteins in a model system for studying osteoarthritis. *Osteoarthritis Cartilage* 17: 896–905.

Zhang, H., N.N. Desai, J.M. Murphey, and S. Spiegel. 1990. Sphingosine stimulates cellular proliferation via a protein kinase C-independent pathway. *Journal of Biological Chemistry* 265: 21309–21316.

7

Marine Toxins for Natural Products Drug Discovery

Muthuvel Arumugam, Thangavel Balasubramanian, and Se-Kwon Kim

CONTENTS

7.1 Introduction

The production of toxins from marine animals is an important strategy that guarantees their survival in a highly competitive and challenging ecosystem. These animals produce an enormous number of metabolites, whose combinations result in a great variety of chemical structures and complex molecules, as alkaloids, steroids, peptides, and proteins with chemical and pharmacological properties that are entirely different from the terrestrial animal venoms (Russel 1971). Further, the biological properties of the venoms of terrestrial animals such as snakes, spider, and scorpions have been extensively investigated. The venomous invertebrates have developed, through their adaptive evolution, a huge number of toxins having, in each case, a single scaffold. They have evolved highly refined specificity and selectivity in targeting different types of ion channels and receptors (Kordis and Gubensek 2000). However, less research has been undertaken on marine creatures; this is due to the difficulties of obtaining and storing the venom extract and their extreme liability. The marine toxins are inevitable source of novel compounds due to the diversity of marine organisms and their competitive living habitat. These strategies have produced many valuable drugs and are likely continue to produce lead molecules for chemotherapeutic in future. Invertebrate venoms have attracted considerable interest as a potential source of bioactive compounds, especially neurotoxins and cardiotoxins. These molecules have proved to be extremely useful tools for the understanding of synaptic transmission events, ion channel blockers, and they have contributed to the design of novel drugs for the various medicinal purposes (Mortai et al. 2007).

7.2 Marine Invertebrates Toxin

7.2.1 Toxins from Porifera

Phylum Porifera consist of 5000 or more species of sponges and are known to be toxic to human or to contain substances toxic to other animals. The glass-like spicules may provoke traumatic injuries in humans, and these animals can release a material into their environment that is toxic to fishes and other marine animals. So far, more than 75 substances have been isolated from the poriferans. Most of the sponges consist of biogenic amines that have been reported from *Haliclona viridis* and *Toxadocia violacea*, which are of relatively high molecular weight and appear to be of interest as potential cytoxan and neurotropic agents. However, the instability of these substances in aqueous solutions would suggest a rather limited use. Most of the sponge extracts consist of sulfated polysaccharide that is responsible for aggregation activity upon removal of the carbohydrate fraction such as glycoprotein responsible for aggregation activity that contains sulfate residues. However, the presence of nonspecific cytotoxic molecules in sponges that are capable of producing the aggregation phenomena that has been observed and the indications that the aggregation process may be nonspecific, requiring either metabolic function or formation of protoplasmic continuity to accomplish true redifferentiation, lend little support to this speculation. The unusual metabolites of sponges have, in this case, led out one of the ways in which marine products of potential interest may stimulate the idea for synthetic products of medicinal value. At the outset, the arabinose nucleosides (*Ara-A and Ara-C*) exist in nature, and the impetus for experimental work came to see how similar synthetic compounds might affect other cellular systems. Although cytosine arabinoside is not a constituent of marine organism, it is clear that the research on marine organisms led to the production of a potentially useful drug. A sesquiterpenoid hydroquinone with a rearranged drimane skeleton (avarol) was first isolated from the marine sponge *Dysidea avara*, which shows potent antiviral activity (Rosa et al. 1976; Sarma and Chattopadhyay 1982). Manzamine A was isolated from *Haliclona sp.* as an antitumor compound in Okinawa waters near Japan (Figure 7.1) (Sakai et al. 1986).

7.2.2 Toxins from Cnidarians

The phylum Cnidaria or Coelenterata is mainly composed of the hydroids, jellyfish, sea anemones, and corals, of which there are approximately 9000 species (Figures 7.2 and 7.3). Of these, about 90 have been implicated in significant injuries to man through their potent toxins. The toxin/toxic molecules that have been isolated from cnidarians

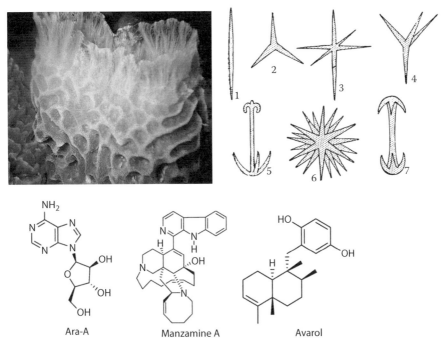

FIGURE 7.1
The typical marine sponge and their spicule patterns. (From Rocha, J. et al., *Mar. Drugs*, 9, 1860, 2011.)

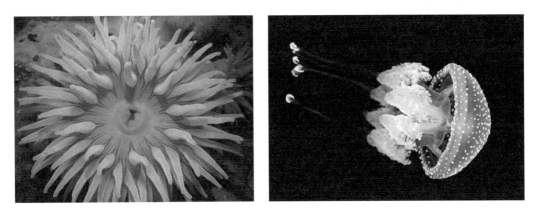

FIGURE 7.2
The sea anemone and jellyfishes. (Courtesy of Bryan McCloskey.)

include homarine, trigonelline, anemonine, sterols (*asterolaurin A*), waxed, triglycerides, and phospholipids; basic proteins capable of disrupting membrane structure and
function; thalasin; "cyanea principle," a histamine releaser; elastases, DNase, and histamine; collagenase; alkaline protease; anticholinesterases; and muscarine toxins, i.e.,
substances that inhibit the binding of ligands. Most of the coelenterates show very good
antimicrobial activity and cytotoxic effects. Most significant antibiotic compounds,

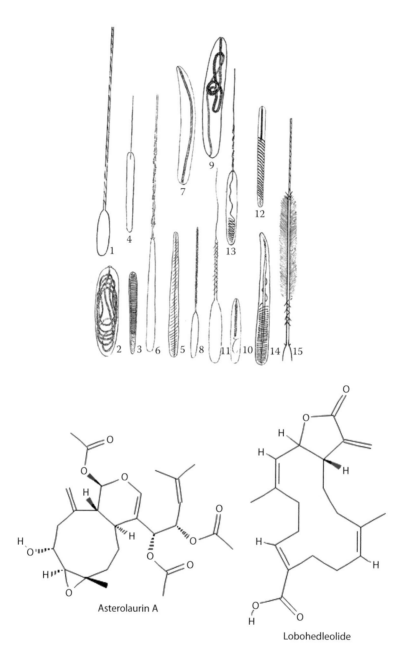

FIGURE 7.3
The nematocysts of sea anemones.

viz., terpenes and terpenoids, have been isolated from cnidarians and appear to act as defensive agents against other sessile organisms. The terpenoids are believed to originate in symbiotic zooxanthellae. The presence of low molecular weight substances (lobohedleolide) of cnidarians would appear to offer no new pharmacological agents of interest in medicine. The macromolecular toxins, which exhibit strong actions on the heart and appear to inhibit nerve activity through mechanisms of alteration of ionic permeability in many animal species, appear to possess some biomedical potential. However, since the materials appear to be highly toxic and antigenic in nature, their direct use will probably be rather limited and their most important biomedical value may be in elucidation of important physiological mechanisms. Over 3000 marine natural products have been described from this phylum alone, mostly in the last decade (Rocha et al. 2011).

7.2.3 Toxins from Mollusk

Phylum Mollusca shows extensive species diversity and their by-products have received much attention from the beginning of the twentieth century. Among the mollusk, most have pronounced pharmacological activities or other properties useful in the biomedical arena. Of the 80,000 or so molluskan species, about 85 poison man either upon ingestion or by way of venom apparatus. They consist of different bioactive molecules, viz., neuromuscular and CNS drugs, which contains amines and peptides; tetramine; murexine or urocanylcholine; photodynamic, antibacterial (*paolin I*) and antiviral (*paolin II*) substances; antitumor and growth-inhibiting factors; biologically active amines such as tyramine, histamine, serotonin, and lotoxin; a glycoprotein; eledoisin, a peptide; hypotensive agents; and heterocyclic aromatic bromo compounds known as aplysin and aplysinol with hypotensive and cardioactive properties.

Marine cone snails have developed many distinct types of venom that contain biologically active peptides as part of an envenomation survival strategy for feeding and defense. These peptides, known as conopeptides, have been optimized through evolution to target-specific ion channels and receptors with very high affinities and selectivities. Side effects of currently available therapies often arise from their lack of selectivity between pharmacologically relevant targets and targets that have a similar structure but different function. Some of the most intriguing marine natural products are those derived from marine snails of the genus *Conus*.

Cone snails are typically found on, or near, coral reefs in tropical waters throughout the world. As part of defensive and feeding strategy, these unique mollusks have a complex venom delivered through a specialized radular tooth that serves both as a harpoon and as a disposable hypodermic needle to immobilize their prey. In *Conus* snails, the toxins are unusually small peptides, the majority being in the range of 12–30 amino acids (Olivera 1997; Olivera et al. 1999). Conotoxins are smaller than polypeptide toxins used by other venomous animals and represent exceptionally small channel-blocking ligands. Conotoxins are invariably highly constrained conformational and exhibit one of three characteristic arrangements of cysteine residues, the two-, three-, or four-loop frameworks (Olivera 1997). All of the substances isolated from gastropods appear to have an effect on the neuromuscular tissues of animals. Murexine has a neuromuscular blocking action about one-fifth that of succinylcholine and, like succinylcholine, exerts this effect by a depolarizing action on the end plate region. Prialt®, the first drug, enters into the market for potent analgesic that consists of ziconotide (Figure 7.4D) from *C. magus*. Further, *murexine* has also been proposed as an alternative to succinylcholine as muscle relaxant in clinical use, but its nicotinic properties and greater instability seem to contraindicate this.

In the case of cephalopods, the cephalotoxin exhibits a number of interesting pharmacological activities on smooth muscle and cardiovascular system, which parallel to a fair

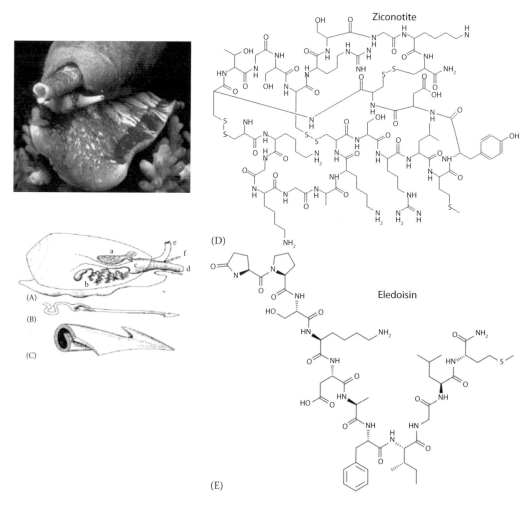

FIGURE 7.4
A cone shell's venom apparatus. (A) Anatomical organization of the venom apparatus and organs involved. (B) Venom harpoon during application. (C) Close-up illustration of a single venom harpoon. (D) Structure of ziconotide. (E) Structure of eledoisin. a, harpoon sac; b, venom gland; c, pharynx; d, proboscis; e, sipho; f, eyestalks. (From Frings, S. and Grammig, D., Conotoxine-MuskelgiftederKegelschnecken.)

extent the actions of eledoisin. However, the thermolability and potential antigenic properties of this substance would indicate a limited biomedical potential. Eledoisin has been found to be effective in clinical trials, and this peptide and other synthetic substances would seem to have potential in treatment of human cardiovascular disease. In addition, extracts of the squid *Loligo* sp. contain substances that have antivirus and antitumor activity in vivo (Figure 7.4).

7.2.4 Toxins from Echinoderms

The echinoderms are generally considered to be harmless. However, there is an exception to every rule. Of these 6000 species, the crown-of-thorns starfishes of the genus Acanthaster

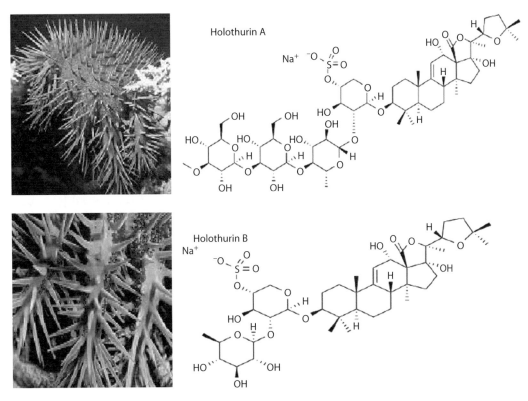

FIGURE 7.5
The sea urchin (*Acanthaster planci*) and their spine patterns.

are the only ones with long venomous spines that can cause painful and sometimes debilitating wounds by the secretion of highly poisonous steroid glycoside. The starfish has a glandular tissue embedded in calcite that secretes a toxin; the sea urchins have pedicellaria venom apparatus usually between their spines, while the sea cucumbers contain their toxin in specialized tubules that can be eviscerated. Sea urchin consists of sharp, needlelike spines containing a slightly toxic substance that greatly increases the pain. Some tropical sea urchins, most notably the fire urchins and flower urchins, have highly toxic venom with special delivery systems (Figure 7.5).

Apart from these, several saponin-type compounds have been isolated from the echinoderms, and these include *asterosaponin A & B* and toxin saponins, some of which show sperm immobilizing properties and induction of egg and sperm shedding effects. A toxic protein is having acetylcholine-like nerve-blocking activity, and a mixture of steroidal glycosides (*holothurin A & B*) having hemolytic, cytotoxic, neuromuscular, and antitumor activities have also been identified (Chanley et al. 1959; Kitagawa 1979). Possible "invertebrate insulin" in the sea star *Pisaster ochraceus* has also been reported (Wilson and Falkmer 1965). The toxins isolated from sea cucumbers appear to have interesting pharmacological potential as both neuromuscular drugs and cancer chemotherapeutic agents.

7.3 Marine Vertebrates Toxin

7.3.1 Toxins from Sea Snakes

The sea snakes are the most venomous reptilian group in the world. They are encountered around the coast that includes reefs, estuaries, rivers, and sea. Sea snake venoms are 2–10 times more potent toxin than the terrestrial snakes like king cobra, although they tend to deliver much less venom. However, they are rarely aggressive or menacing due to their laziness. The sea snake venoms consist of potent neurotoxin (Tu 1988; Acott and Williamson 1996). The sea snake venom which commonly act as a potent neurotoxin (Tu 1988; Acott and Williamson 1996) also contains several other factors like anticoagu-lant and anticancer agents (Mora et al. 2005; Tang et al. 2005) of thermostable nature. Typical short and long neurotoxin was identified from snake venoms such as Eb from *Laticauda semifasciata* (a) and toxins B and C from *Astrotia stokesii* (b) (Figure 7.6) (Tamiya and Yagi 2011).

Some toxic phospholipases A$_2$ from snake venoms act prefunctionally to reduce acetylcholine release, while others have additional myotoxic effects that are pronounced in vivo (Chang 1985). LcPLA-II had little action on the direct muscle stimulation induced by depolarization with K$^+$ and did not produce contractures. Hence, LcPLA-II probably acts to block neuromuscular transmission by occupying the acetylcholine-binding site and

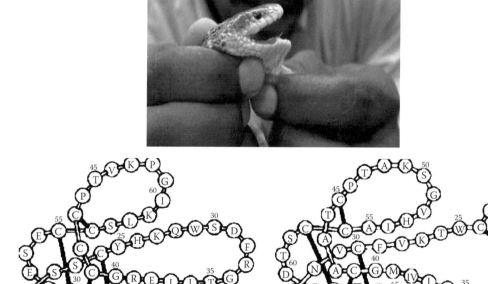

FIGURE 7.6
The milking of sea snake. Amino acid sequence of neurotoxins identified from sea snakes (A) *Laticauda semifas-ciata* and (B) *Astrotia stokesii*. (From Yang, R.S. et al., *Toxicon*, 45, 661, 2005; Mora, R. et al., *Toxicon*, 45, 651, 2005.)

not by uncoupling or blocking receptor ion channels (Andreasen and Mc Namee 1977; Harvey and Tamiya 1980).

7.3.2 Toxins from Fishes

In aquatic environment, large numbers of venomous and poisonous animals were found. Of these, more than 200 species of marine fish, including stingrays, scorpion fish, zebra fish, stonefish, weever fish, toadfish, stargazers, and some species of shark, ratfish, catfish, surgeonfish, and blenny, are known or suspected to be venomous (Russel 1996). The vast majorities of these fish are nonmigratory, are slow moving, and tend to live in shallow waters in protected habitats (Maretic 1988). It has been suggested that this tendency toward inactivity is linked to the evolution of venom apparatus (Cameron and Endean 1973). Stonustoxin (SNTX) is a multifunctional lethal protein isolated from venom elaborated by the stonefish, *Synanceia horrida*, which consists of two subunits with respective molecular masses of 71 and 79 kDa (Ghadessy et al. 1996). In addition, tetrodotoxin (TTX) is a potent marine neurotoxin, named after the order of fish from which it is most commonly associated, the Tetraodontiformes or the Tetraodon puffer fishes (Figure 7.7) (Mosher 1986).

The production of toxins by aquatic animals is an important strategy that guarantees its survival in a highly competitive ecosystem such as marine habitat that shows attack and defense behavior that includes the production of substances expressing repellent, paralytic, or other biological actions. In this way, these animals tend to defend themselves or their territories by producing a significant number of metabolites, which in combination result in a great variety of chemical structures and complex molecules such as alkaloids, steroids, peptides, and proteins with chemical and pharmacological properties, different from those in venoms of terrestrial animals (Russel 1971). These toxins present a wide array of biological activities (cytolytic, neurotoxic, cardiotoxic, neuromuscular, edematogenic, and hemolytic) and a high molecular mass of about 150 kDa (Poh et al. 1991; Chhatwal and Dreyer 1992; Garnier et al. 1995; Colassante et al. 1996; Hahn and O'Connor 2000). Therefore, marine toxins are still representing sources of pharmacological compounds that may be useful as research tools or lead compounds for drugs, and as such their pharmacological actions have been the focus of recent works (Table 7.1).

7.4 Concluding Remarks

The marine environment undoubtedly holds an enormous source for providing potential new molecules for the development of drug discovery. Especially toxins from marine vertebrates and invertebrates have broad applications because of their origin and complex nature. The revealed molecules derived from the marine venom are offering us a great opportunity to evaluate not only totally new chemical classes of natural products but also novel and potentially relevant target of human diseases. Among the venomous marine animals, *Conus* contributes more number of lead molecules in terms of venomous peptides. At the outset, the world's oceans will play an important part in the future to control the global infectious diseases. Although substantial progress has been made in identifying novel drug leads from the marine resources, great effort is still needed to commercial application.

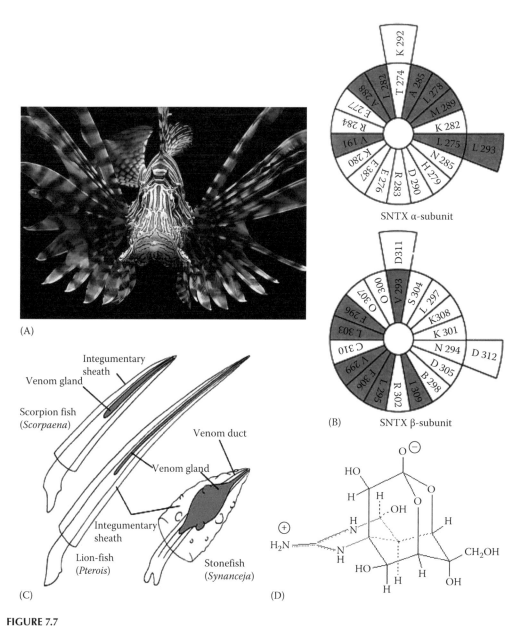

FIGURE 7.7
(A) The venomous lion-fish. (B) The α and β subunit of SNTX from the venom of stonefish. (C) The venomous spine of stonefish, scorpion fish, and lion-fish. (D) The structure of TTX from puffer fish. (From Ghadessy, F.J. et al., *J. Biol. Chem.*, 271, 25575, 1996.)

TABLE 7.1

List of Compounds from Marine Invertebrates and Vertebrates

S. No	Sources	Toxin/Chemistry	Chemical Compound	Activity	Reference
	Porifera				
1.	*Aaptos* sp.	Alkaloid	4-Methylaaptamine	Antiviral	Coutinho et al. (2002)
2.	*Acanthella* sp.	Diterpenoid	Kalihinol A	Antimalarial	Miyaoka et al. (1998)
3.	*Acanthodendrilla* sp.	Sterol	Acanthosterols	Antifungal	Tsukamoto et al. (1998)
4.	*Amphimedon viridis*	Cytotoxic and neurotoxic	Halitoxin	Hemolytic, antimitotic, cytotoxic, and neurotoxic activities	Marisa Rangel et al. (2001)
5.	*Aplysina aerophoba*	Alkaloid toxin	Aeroplysinin I	Cytotoxic	Koulman et al. (1996)
6.	*Arenosclera brasiliensis*		Arenosclerins A–C Haliclonacyclamine E	Cytotoxic and antimicrobial	Torres et al. (2002)
7.	*Callyspongia truncata*	Polyketide	Callystatin A	Antitumor	Kobayashi et al. (1997)
8.	*Cymbastela hooperi*	Pyrrol	Oroidin	Antimalarial	Konig et al. (1996)
9.	*Dysidea avara*	Sesquiterpenoid hydroquinone	Avarol	Antiviral	Minale et al. (1974)
10.	*Halicortex* sp.	Bromoindole alkaloid	Dragmacidin F	Antiviral	Cutignano et al. (2000)
11.	*Haliclona* sp.	Alkaloid	Manzamine A	Antitumor	Sakai et al. (1986)
12.	*Hamigera tarangaensis*	Phenolic macrolides	Hamigeran B	Antiviral	Muller et al. (2000)
13.	*Hyrtios erecta*	Macrolide	Spongistatin	Antifungal	Pettit et al. (1998)
14.	*Mycale* sp.	Nucleosides	Mycalamide A Mycalamide B	Antiviral	Perry et al. (1988)
15.	*Plakinastrella* sp.	Alkylphenol	Elenic acid	Antitumor	Juagdan et al. (1995)
16.	*Reniera sarai*	Cytolytic, cytotoxic	3-Alkylpyridinium polymers	Anti-AChE activity	Sepcic et al. (1997)
17.	*Reniera sarai*		3-Alkylpyridines and related pyridinium salts	Antifouling activity	Chelossi et al. (2006)
18.	*Sidonops microspinosa*	Cyclic depsipeptide	Microspinosamide	Anti-HIV	Rashid et al. (2001)
19.	*Theonella mirabilis and Theonella swinhoei*	Cytotoxic cyclic depsipeptides	Papuamides A, B, C, and D	Anti-HIV	Ford et al. (1951)
20.	*Tethya crypta*	Nucleosides	Vidarabine or Ara-A	Antiviral	Bergmann and Feeney (1951)

(continued)

TABLE 7.1 (continued)

List of Compounds from Marine Invertebrates and Vertebrates

S. No		Sources	Toxin/Chemistry	Chemical Compound	Activity	Reference
21.	Cnidarians	*Bunodosoma caissarum* / sea anemone	Neurotoxic	BcIV	Paralyzing peptides	Oliveira et al. (2006)
22.		*Heteractis crispa* / sea anemone	Polypeptide inhibitor of vanilloid receptor 1	TRPV1	Analgesic compound	Andreev et al. (2008)
23.		Sea whip	Diterpene	Pseudopterosin N	Anti-inflammatory	Ata et al. (2003)
24.		*Veretillum malayense* / sea pen	Diterpenes	Malayenolides A–D		Fu et al. (1999)
25.	Mollusks	*Conus radiates*	Neurotoxin	Conantokin-R	Anticonvulsant	Mortari et al. (2007)
26.		*Conus lynceus*	Neurotoxin	Conantokin-L	Anticonvulsant	Mortari et al. (2007)
27.		*Conus geographus*	Neurotoxin	Conantokin-G	Anticonvulsant	Mortari et al. (2007)
28.		*Dolabella auricularia* / sea hare	Peptide	Dolabellanin B2	Antibacterial	Iijima et al. (2003)
29.		*Dolabella auricularia* / sea hare		Dolastatin	Antineoplastic	Pettit et al. (1989)
30.		*Dolabella auricularia* / sea hare		Dolastatin-10	Anticancer	Yamada et al. (2000)
31.		*Elysia rufescens*	Polypeptide	Kahalalide A and F	Antituberculosis	Hamann et al. (1996)
32.		*Kelletia kelletii*	Tetra esterase	Kelletinins I and II	Antibacterial	Tymiak and Rinehart (1983)
33.	Echinoderms	*Certonardoa semiregularis* / starfish	Saponins	Certonardosides A–J	Antiviral	Wang et al. (2004)
34.		*Dermasterias imbricate* / starfish	Cytotoxic metabolite	Imbricatine		Burgoyne et al. (1991)
35.		*Psolus patagonicus* / sea cucumber	Triterpene glycoside	Patagonicoside A	Antifungal	Murray et al. (2001)
36.		Sea cucumber	Polysaccharide	Fucosylated chondroitin sulfate	Anticoagulant	Zancan and Mourao (2004)
37.		Sea cucumber	Triterpenoid glycoside	Holothurin B	Antifungal	Kumar et al. (2007)

No.	Group	Species	Component	Activity	Toxin	Reference
38.	Fishes	*Notesthes robusta*		Algesic substance	Nocitoxin	Hahn and O'Connor (2000)
39.		*Plotosus canius*	Lethal protein	Neuromuscular blocking	Toxin-PC	Auddy and Gomes (1996)
40.		*Potamotrygon gr. orbignyi*		Novel vasoconstrictor peptide	Orpotrin	Conceicao et al. (2006)
41.		*Pterios volitans*	Venom	Antitumor, hepatoprotective, antimetastatic effects		Sri Balasubashini et al. (2006)
42.		*Synanceja horrida*	Lethal factor	Endothelium-dependent vasodilation	SNTX	Ghadessy et al. (1996)
43.		*Synanceja trachynis*	Neurosecretory protein	Endothelium-independent contraction	Trachynilysin	Colasante et al. (1996)
44.		*Synanceja verrucosa*	Cytolytic factor	Cardiotoxicity	Verrucotoxin	Garnier et al. (1995)
45.		*Thalassophryne nattereri*	Proteins	Kininogenase activity	Natterins	Magalhães et al. (2005)
46.		*Trachinus draco*		Hemorrhagic activity	Dracotoxin	Chhatwal and Dreyer (1992)
47.		*Trachinus vipera*		Lethal activity	Trachinine	Perriere et al. (1998)
48.		Puffer fishes	Neurotoxin		TTX	Mosher (1986)
49.	Sea snakes	*Astrotia stokesii*	Two long-chain neurotoxic proteins with amidated C-termini	Lethal protein	Neurotoxins	Maeda and Tamiya (1978)
50.		*Enhydrina schistosa*	Neurotoxins	Lethal effect	Schistosa 4 Schistosa 5	Geh and Toh (1978)
51.		*Enhydrina schistosa*	Neurotoxic components	Irreversibly blocked neuromuscular transmission	Enhydrotoxins a, b, and c	Gawade and Gaitonde (1982)
52.		*Hydrophis cyanocinctus*	Venom	Toxicity	Phospholipases A2	Ali et al. (1999)
53.		*Hydrophis spiralis*	Venom	Antitumor activity		Karthikeyan et al. (2007)
54.		*Laticauda colubrina* *Laticauda laticaudata*	Neurotoxic protein	Attacks the postsynaptic membrane, competing with acetylcholine	Laticotoxin A	Sato et al. (1969)
55.		*Laticauda semifasciata*	Neurotoxins	Blocking respiration	Erabutoxins a and b	Tamiya and Yagi (2011)
56.		*Laticauda semifasciata*	Neurotoxins	Neurotoxic activity	Erabutoxin c	Tamiya and Abe (1972)
57.		*Laticauda semifasciata*	Neurotoxicity	Reversible neurotoxin	Laticauda semifasciata III	Maeda and Tamiya (1974)

Acknowledgments

The authors are thankful to the authorities of Annamalai University, Tamil Nadu, India, and the Ministry of Earth Sciences (MoES) through the "Drugs from the Sea Programme" for the financial support and encouragements.

References

Acott, C. and J. Williamson. 1996. Sea snake. In: *Venomous and Poisonous Marine Animals: A Medical and Biological Handbook*. Eds. Williamson, J.A., Fenner, P.J., Burnett, J.W., and Rifkin, J.F., University of New South Wales Press, Kensington, New South Wales, Australia, pp. 396–402.

Ali, S.A., J.M. Alam, S. Stoeva, J. Schütz, A. Abbasi, Z.H. Zaidi, and W. Voelter. 1999. Sea snake *Hydrophis cyanocinctus* venom. I. Purification, characterization and N-terminal sequence of two phospholipases A2. *Toxicon* 37: 1505–1520.

Andreasen, T.J. and M.G. McNamee. 1977. Phospholipase A, inhibition of acetylcholine receptor functions in *Torpedo californica* membrane vesicles. *Biochemical and Biophysical Research Communications* 79: 958–965.

Andreev, Y.A., S.A. Kozlov, S.G. Koshelev, E.A. Ivanova, M.M. Monastyrnaya, E.P. Kozlovskaya, and E.V. Grishin. 2008. Analgesic compound from sea anemone *Heteractis crispa* is the first polypeptide inhibitor of vanilloid receptor 1 [TRPV1]. *Journal of Biological Chemistry* 283: 23914–23921.

Ata, A., R.G. Kerr, C.E. Moya, and R.S. Jacobs. 2003. Identification of anti-inflammatory diterpenes from the marine gorgonian *Pseudopterogorgia elisabethae*. *Tetrahedron* 59: 4215–4222.

Auddy, B. and A. Gomes. 1996. Indian catfish [*Plotosus canius*, Hamilton] venom. Occurrence of lethal protein toxin [toxin-PC]. *Advances in Experimental Medicine and Biology* 391: 225–229.

Bergmann, W. and R.J. Feeney. 1951. Contributions to the study of marine products XXXII. The nucleosides of sponges. *Journal of Organic Chemistry* 16: 981–987.

Burgoyne, D., S. Miao, C. Pathirana, and R.J. Andersen. 1991. The structure and partial synthesis of imbricatine, a benzyltetrahydroisoquinoline alkaloid from the starfish *Dermasterias imbricata*. *Canadian Journal of Chemistry* 69: 20–26.

Cameron, A.M. and R. Endean. 1973. Epidermal secretions and the evolution of venom glands in fishes. *Toxicon* 11: 401–406.

Chang, C.C. 1985. Neurotoxin with phospholipase A2 activity in sea snake venom. *Proceedings of National Science Council–Republic of China. Part B: Basic Sciences* 9: 126–142.

Chanley, J.D., R. Ledeen, J. Wax, R.F. Nigrelli, and S. Harry. 1959. Holothurin. I. Isolation, properties, and sugar components of Holothurin A. *Journal of the American Chemical Society* 81: 5180–5183.

Chelossi, E., E. Mancini, K. Sepcic, T. Turk, and M. Faimali. 2006. Comparative antibacterial activity of polymeric 3-alkylpyridinium salts isolated from the Mediterranean sponge *Reniera sarai* and their synthetic analogues. *Biomolecular Engineering* 23: 317–323.

Chhatwal, I. and F. Dreyer. 1992. Isolation and characterization of dracotoxin from the venom of the greater weever fish *Trachinus draco*. *Toxicon* 30: 87–93.

Colassante, C., F.A. Meunier, A.S. Kreger, and J. Molgo. 1996. Selective depletion of clear synaptic vesicles and enhanced quantal transmitter release at frog motor nerve endings produced by Trachynilysin, a protein toxin isolated from stonefish [*Synanceia trachynis*] venom. *European Journal of Neuroscience* 8: 2149–2156.

Conceicao, K., K. Konno, R.L. Melo, E.E. Marques, A.C. Hiruma-Lima, C. Lima, M. Richardson, D.C. Pimenta, and M. Lopes-Ferreira. 2006. Orpotrin: A novel vasoconstrictor peptide from the venom of the Brazilian Stingray *Potamotrygon gr. orbignyi*. *Peptides* 27: 3039–3046.

Coutinho, A.F., B. Chanas, T.M.L. Souza, I.C.P.P. Frugrulhetti, and R.A. de Epifanio. 2002. Anti HSV-1 alkaloids from a feeding deterrent marine sponge of the genus *Aaptos*. *Heterocycles* 57: 1265–1272.

Cutignano, A., G. Bifulco, I. Bruno, A. Casapullo, L. Gomez-Paloma, and R. Riccio. 2000. Dragmacidin F: A new antiviral bromoindole alkaloid from the Mediterranean sponge *Halicortex sp.* *Tetrahedron* 56: 3743–3748.

Ford, P., K. Gustafson, T. McKee, N. Shigematsu, L. Maurizi, L. Pannell, D. Williams, E. de Silva, P. Lassota, and T. Allen. 1951. Papuamides A–D, HIV-inhibitory and cytotoxic depsipeptides from the sponges *Theonella mirabilis* and *Theonella swinhoei* collected in Papua New Guinea. *Journal of the American Chemical Society* 121: 5899–5909.

Fu, X., F.J. Schmitz, and G.C. Williams. 1999. Malayenolides A-D, novel diterpenes from the Indonesian sea pen *Veretillum*. *Journal of Natural Products* 62: 584–586.

Garnier, P., F. Goudey-Perrière, P. Breton, C. Dewulf, F. Petek, and C. Perrière. 1995. Enzymatic properties of the stonefish [*Synanceia verrucosa* Bloch and Schneider, 1801] venom and purification of a lethal, hypotensive and cytolytic factor. *Toxicon* 33: 143–155.

Gawade, S.P. and B.B. Gaitonde. 1982. Isolation and characterisation of toxic components from the venom of the common Indian sea snake [*Enhydrina schistosa*]. *Toxicon* 20: 797–801.

Geh, S.L. and H.T. Toh. 1978. Ultra structural changes in skeletal muscle caused by a phospholipase A_2 fraction isolated from the venom of a sea snake, *Enhydrina schistosa*. *Toxicon* 16: 633–643.

Ghadessy, F.J., D. Chen, R.M. Kini, M.C.M. Chung, K. Jeyaseelan, H.E. Khoo, and R. Yuen. 1996. Stonustoxin is a novel lethal factor from stonefish [*Synanceja horrida*] venom cDNA cloning and characterization. *Journal of Biological Chemistry* 271: 25575–25581.

Hahn, S.T. and J.M. O'Connor. 2000. An investigation of the biological activity of bullrout [*Notesthes robusta*] venom. *Toxicon* 38: 79–89.

Hamann, M.T., P.J. Scheuer, and M. Kelly-Borges. 1996. Kahalalides: Bioactive peptides from marine mollusk *Elysia rufescens* and its algal diet *Bryopsis sp.* *Journal of Organic Chemistry* 61: 6594–6660.

Harvey, A.L. and N. Tamiya. 1980. Role of phospholipase A activity in the neuromuscular paralysis produced by some components isolated from the venom of the seasnake, *Laticauda semifasciata*. *Toxicon* 18: 65–69.

Iijima, R., J. Kisugi, and M. Yamazaki. 2003. A novel antimicrobial peptide from the sea hare *Dolabella auricularia*. *Development of Comparative Immunology* 27: 305–311.

Juagdan, E.G., R.S. Kalindindi, P.J. Scheuer, and M. Kelly-Borges. 1995. Elenic acid, an inhibitor of Topoisomerase II, from a sponge, *Plakinastrella sp.* *Tetrahedron Letters* 36: 2905–2908.

Karthikeyan, R., S. Kathigayan, M. SriBalasubasini, S. Vijayalakshmi, S.T. Somasundaram, and T. Balasubramanian. 2007. Antitumour effect of snake venom [*Hydrophis spiralis*] on Ehrlich Ascites Carcinoma bearing mice. *International Journal of Cancer Research* 3: 167–173.

Kitagawa, I. 1979. Structure of Holothurin A, a biologically active triterpene-oligoglycoside from the sea cucumber *Holothuria leucospilota* brandt. *Tetrahedron Letters* 20: 1419.

Kobayashi, M., K. Higuchi, N. Murakami, H. Tajima, and S. Aoki. 1997. Callystatin A, a potent cytotoxic polyketide from the marine sponge, *Callyspongia truncata*. *Tetrahedron Letters* 38: 2859–2862.

Konig, G.M., A.D. Wright, and C.K. Angerhofer. 1996. Novel potent antimalarial diterpene isocyanates, isothiocyanates, and isonitriles from the tropical marine sponge *Cymbastela hooperi*. *Journal of Organic Chemistry* 61: 3259–3267.

Kordis, D. and F. Gubensek. 2000. Horizontal transfer of non-LTR retrotransposons in vertebrates. In: *Transposable Elements and Genome Evolution*, Georgia Genetics Review, vol. 1. Ed. MacDonald, J.F., Kluwer, Dordrecht, the Netherlands, pp. 121–128.

Koulman, A., P. Proksch, R. Ebel, A.C. Beekman, W. VanUden, A.W. Konings, J.A. Pedersen, N. Pras, and H.J. Woerdenbag. 1996. Cytotoxicity and mode of action of aeroplysinin-1 and a related dienone from the sponge *Aplysina aerophoba*. *Journal of Natural Products* 59: 591–594.

Kumar, R., A.K. Chaturvedi, P.K. Shukla, and V. Lakshmi. 2007. Antifungal activity in triterpene glycosides from the sea cucumber *Actinopyga lecanora*. *Bioorganic and Medicinal Chemistry Letters* 17: 4387–4391.

Maeda, N. and N. Tamiya. 1974. The primary structure of the toxin *Laticauda semifasciata* III, a weak and reversibly acting neurotoxin from the venom of a sea snake, *Laticauda semifasciata*. *Biochemical Journal* 141: 389400.

Maeda, N. and N. Tamiya. 1978. Three neurotoxins from the venom of a sea snake *Astrotia stokesii*, including two long-chain neurotoxic proteins with amidated C-termini. *Biochemical Journal* 175: 507–517.

Magalhães, G.S., M. Lopes-Ferreira, I.L.M. Junqueira-de-Azevedo, P.J. Spencer, M.S. Araújo, F.C.V. Portaro, L. Ma et al. 2005. Natterins, a new class of proteins with kininogenase activity characterized from *Thalassophryne nattereri* fish venom. *Biochimie* 87: 687–699.

Maretic, Z. 1988. Fish venoms. In: *Handbook of Natural Toxins: Marine Toxins and Venoms*. Ed. Tu, A.T., Marcel Dekker, New York, pp. 445–477.

Minale, L., R. Riccio, and G. Sodano. 1974. Avarol a novel sesquiterpenoid hydroquinone with a rearranged drimane skeleton from the sponge. *Tetrahedron Letters* 15: 3401–3404.

Miyaoka, H., M. Shimomura, H. Kimura, Y. Yamada, H.S. Kim, and Y. Wataya. 1998. Antimalarial activity of kalahinol A and new relative diterpenoids from the Okinawan sponge, *Acanthella sp. Tetrahedron* 54: 13467–13474.

Mora, R., B. Valverde, C. Diaz, B. Lomonte, and J.M. Gutierrez. 2005. A Lys49 phospholipase A2 homologue from *Bothrops asper* snake venom induces proliferation, apoptosis and necrosis in a lymphoblastoid cell line. *Toxicon* 45: 651–660.

Mortari, M.R., A.O.S. Cunha, L.B. Ferreira, and W.F.D. Santos. 2007. Neurotoxins from invertebrates as anticonvulsants: From basic research to therapeutic application. *Pharmacology & Therapeutics* 114: 171–183.

Mosher, H.S. 1986. Tetrodotoxin, saxitoxin and the molecular biology of the sodium channel. *Annals of the New York Academy of Sciences* 479: 1–448.

Muller, W., M. Bohm, R. Batel, S. De Rosa, G. Tommonaro, I. Muller, and H. Schroder. 2000. Application of cell culture for the production of bioactive compounds from sponges: Synthesis of avarol by primmorphs from *Dysidea avara. Journal of Natural Products* 63: 1077–1081.

Murray, A.P., C. Munian, A.M. Seldes, and M.S. Maier. 2001. Patagonicoside A: A novel antifungal disulfated triterpene glycoside from the sea cucumber *Psolus patagonicu. Tetrahedron* 57: 9563–9568.

Oliveira, J.S., A.J. Zaharenko, W.A. Ferreira Jr, K. Konn, C.S. Shida, M. Richardson, A.D. Lúcio, P.S.L. Beirão, and J.S. de Freitas. 2006. BcIV, a new paralyzing peptide obtained from the venom of the sea anemone *Bunodosoma caissarum*. A comparison with the Na+ channel toxin BcIII. *Biochimica et Biophysica Acta* 1764: 1592–1600.

Olivera, B.M. 1997. *Conus* venom peptides, receptor and ion channel targets and drug design: 50 million years of neuropharmacology. *Molecular Biology of Cell* 8: 2101–2109.

Olivera, B.M., C. Walker, G.E. Cartier, D. Hooper, R. Santos, M. Watkin, P. Bandyopadhyay, and D.R. Hillyard. 1999. Specification of cone snails and interspecific hyperdivergence of their venom peptides. Potential evolutionary significance of introns. *Annals of the New York Academy of Sciences* 870: 223–237.

Perriere, C., G. Le Gall, J.M. Grosclaude, P. Garnier, C. Dewulf, and F. Goudey-Perriere. 1998. Storage influence on stonefish venom components activity. *Toxicon* 36: 1313–1314.

Perry, N., J. Blunt, M. Munro, and L. Pannell. 1988. Mycalamide A, an antiviral compound from a New Zealand sponge of the genus Mycale. *Journal of the American Chemical Society* 110: 4850–4851.

Pettit, R.K., S.C. McAllister, G.R. Pettit, C.L. Herald, J.M. Johnson, and Z.A. Cichacz. 1998. A broad-spectrum antifungal from the marine sponge *Hyrtios erecta. International Journal of Antimicrobial Agents* 9: 147–152.

Pettit, G.R., F. Singh, P. Hogan, L. Williams., C.L. Herald, D.D. Burbett, and P.J. Clewlow. 1989. The absolute configuration and synthesis of natural [-]-dolostatin 10. *Journal of the American Chemical Society* 70: 5463–5465.

Poh, C.H., R. Yuen, H.E. Khoo, M.C.D. Chung, M.C.E. Gwee, and P. Gopalakrishnakone. 1991. Purification and partial characterization of Stonustoxin [lethal factor] from *Synanceja horrida* venom. *Comparative Biochemistry and Physiology* 99: 793–798.

Rangel, M., B. de Sanctis, J.S. de Freitas, J.M. Polatto, A.C. Granato, R.G.S. Berlinck, and E. Hajdu. 2001. Cytotoxic and neurotoxic activities in extracts of marine sponges [Porifera] from Southeastern Brazilian coast. *Journal of Experimental Marine Biology and Ecology* 262: 31–40.

Rashid, M., K. Gustafson, L. Cartner, N. Shigematsu, L. Pannell, and M. Boyd. 2001. Microspinosamide, a new HIV-inhibitory cyclic depsipeptide from the marine sponge *Sidonops microspinosa*. *Journal of Natural Products* 64: 117–121.

Rocha, J., L. Peixe, N.C.M. Gomes, and R. Calado. 2011. Review: Cnidarians as a source of new marine bioactive compounds—An overview of the last decade and future steps for bioprospecting. *Marine Drugs* 9: 1860–1886.

Rosa, S., L. Minale, R. Riccio, and G. Sodano. 1976. The absolute configuration of avarol, a rearranged sesquiterpenoid hydroquinone from a marine sponge. *Journal of the Chemical Society, Perkin Transactions* 1: 1408–1414.

Russell, F.E. 1971. *Poisonous Marine Animals*, TFH Publications, New York.

Russell, F.E. 1996. Toxic effects of animals toxins. In: *Casarett and Doull's Toxicology—The Basic Science of Poisons*. Ed. Klaasen, C.D., McGraw-Hill, New York, pp. 801–839.

Sakai, R., T. Higa, C.W. Jefford, G. Bernardinelli, and A. Manzamine. 1986. A novel antitumor alkaloid from a sponge. *Journal of the American Chemical Society* 108: 6404–6405.

Sarma, A. and P. Chattopadhyay. 1982. Synthetic studies of trans-clerodane diterpenoids and congeners: Stereocontrolled total synthesis of [±]-avarol. *Journal of Organic Chemistry* 47: 1727–1731.

Sato, S., H. Yoshida, H. Abe, and N. Tamiya. 1969. Properties and biosynthesis of a neurotoxic protein of the venoms of sea snakes *Laticauda laticaudata* and *Laticauda colubrine*. *Biochemistry Journal* 115: 85.

Sepcic, K., U. Batista, J. Vacelet, P. Macek, and T. Turk. 1997. Biological activities of aqueous extracts from marine sponges and cytotoxic effects of 3-alkylpyridinium polymers from *Reniera sarai*. *Comparative Biochemistry and Physiology* 117C: 47–53.

Sri Balasubashini, M., S. Karthigayan, S.T. Somasundaram, T. Balasubramanian, V. Viswanathan, P. Raveendrand, and V.P. Menona. 2006. Fish venom [*Pterios volitans*] peptide reduces tumor burden and ameliorates oxidative stress in Ehrlich's ascites carcinoma xenografted mice. *Bioorganic and Medicinal Chemistry Letters* 16: 6219–6225.

Tamiya, N. and H. Abe. 1972. The isolation, properties and amino acid sequence of Erabutoxin c, a minor neurotoxic component of the venom of a sea snake *Laticauda semifasciata*. *Biochemistry Journal* 130: 547–555.

Tamiya, N. and T. Yagi. 2011. Studies on sea snake venom. *Proceedings of the Japanese Academy-Series B: Physical and Biological Sciences* 87: 41–52.

Torres, Y.R., G.S. Roberto, B. Gislene, G.F. Nascimento, S.C. Fortier, C. Pessoa, and M.O. de Moraes. 2002. Antibacterial activity against resistant bacteria and cytotoxicity of four alkaloid toxins isolated from the marine sponge *Arenosclera brasiliensis*. *Toxicon* 40: 885–891.

Tsukamoto, S., S. Matsunaga, N. Fusetani, and R.W.M. Van Soest. 1998. Acanthosterol sulfates A-J: Ten new antifungal steroidal sulfates from a marine sponge *Acanthodendrilla sp. Journal of Natural Products* 61: 1374–1378.

Tu, A.T. 1988. Pharmacology of sea snake venoms. In: *Poisonous and Venomous Marine Animals of the World*. Ed. Halstead, B.W., Darwin Press, Princeton, NJ, pp. 235–258.

Tymiak, A.A. and K.L. Rinehart Jr. 1983. Structures of Kelletinins I and II, antibacterial metabolites of the marine mollusk *Kelletia kelletii*. *Journal of the American Chemical Society* 105: 7396.

Wang, W., J. Hong, C.O. Lee, K.S. Im, J.S. Choi, and J.H. Jung. 2004. Cytotoxic sterols and saponins from the starfish *Certonardoa semiregularis*. *Journal of Natural Products* 67: 584–591.

Wilson, S. and S. Falkmer. 1965. Starfish insulin. *Canadian Journal of Biochemistry* 43: 1615–1624.

Yamada, K., M. Okija, H. Kigoshi, and K. Suenaga. 2000. Cytotoxic substances from Opisthobranch mollusks. In *Drugs from the Sea*. Ed. Fusetani, N., Karger, Basel, Switzerland, pp. 59–73.

Yang, R.S., C.H. Tang, W.J. Chuang, T.H. Huang, H.C. Peng, T.F. Huang, and W.M. Fu. 2005. Inhibition of tumor formation by snake venom disintegrin. *Toxicon* 45: 661–669.

Zancan, P. and P.A. Mourao. 2004. Venous and arterial thrombosis in rat models: Dissociation of the antithrombotic effects of glycosaminoglycans. *Blood Coagulation & Fibrinolysis* 15: 45–54.

8

Conotoxins: A Source of Biomaterial for Pharmacology and Neuroscience

Ngo Dang Nghia

CONTENTS

8.1 Introduction

Cone snails are widely distributed marine mollusks of the family Conidae of about 500–700 species (Olivera and Teichert 2007) and a half of species living in the Indo-Pacific region (Figure 8.1) (Rockel et al. 1995). These snails have a highly evolved apparatus for hunting prey. This venom system consists of a venom bulb connected to a long duct that opens into the pharynx. The role of the bulb is still unclear, while the venom is produced and matures in the venom duct. The size of the venom bulb and the length of the venom duct are different from species to species. For injecting venom into the prey, the *Conus* snails develop teeth inside the radular sac composed of two parts, the long arm where the teeth develop and the short arm where the teeth are ready to use. Upon contact with prey, a tooth is forcibly launched into the victim through the long proboscis and the venom is injected through the channel inside the hollow tooth (Marshall et al. 2002, Terlau and Olivera 2004). In a single attack, the cone snail can launch a few teeth. This property of prey capture of cone snails may be unique at the very high level of evolution (Figure 8.2).

Depending on the kind of the prey, *Conus* snails belong to one of three categories: fish (piscivorous species), mollusks (molluscivorous species), and worms (vermivorous species). The estimated number of *Conus* as well as the number of peptides in every species has

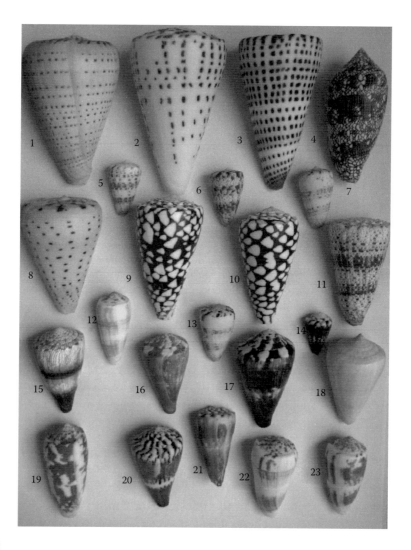

FIGURE 8.1
Shells of some cone snails collected in Vietnam. 1,8: *Conus betulinus*; 2: *Conus leopardus*; 3: *Conus litteratus*; 4: *Conus textile*; 5: *Conus tessulatus*; 6,7,13: *Conus caracteristicus*; 9: *Conus bandanus*; 10: *Conus marmoreus*; 11: *Conus imperialis*; 12: *Conus terebra*; 14: *Conus lividus*; 15: *Conus miles*; 16: *Conus vexillum*; 17: *Conus* sp.; 18: *Conus quercinus*; 19: *Conus striatus*; 20: *Conus capitaneus*; 21: *Conus distans*; and 22,23: *Conus magus*.

changed continuously. The earlier data estimated 500 species with the peptides ranging from 50 to 100 in every species, and in consequence the total peptides are about 50,000. Now with the *Conus* species of 500–700 producing from 1000 to 1900 different bioactive peptides (Davis et al. 2009), the total quantity of peptides from *Conus* snail is remarkable over the estimation given earlier (Olivera and Teichert 2007) and becomes a huge resource of biomaterial for study in neuroscience and pharmacology (Lew et al. 1997, Olivera 1997, Lewis 2009). However, the number of peptides isolated and identified so far is very small with 1180 mature peptides (Kaas et al. 2012).

The conotoxins are classified according to three schemes: gene superfamilies, cysteine frameworks, and pharmacological families.

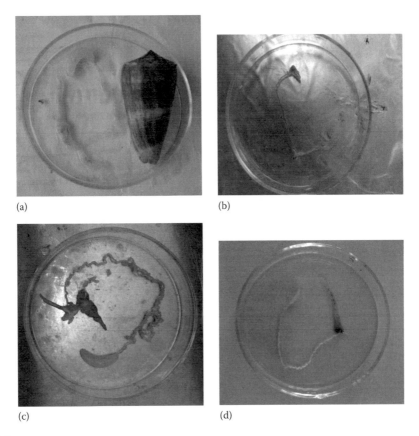

(a) (b)

(c) (d)

FIGURE 8.2
Venom apparatus of cone snails in Vietnam. (a) *Conus magus*; (b) *Conus miles*; (c) *Conus imperialis*; and (d) *Conus terebra*.

In biochemistry, the *Conus* venoms are peptides divided into two categories: disulfide-rich conotoxins and peptides that lack multiple disulfide cross-links. The specific feature of conotoxins is based on the framework of amino acid cysteine and characterized by the number of cysteines, the number and the distribution of pairs of cysteine, the distance in terms of the number of different amino acids (from 0 to 6) between two cysteines, and the number and the position of the connectivity of disulfide. So far, there are 22 different frameworks reported (Table 8.1) (Kaas et al. 2010, 2012).

In molecular genetic aspects, the conopeptides are expressed as protein precursor by epithelial cells lining the venom ducts of cone snails. They are distributed into 16 gene superfamilies A, D, I1, I2, I3, J, L, M, O1, O2, O3, P, S, T, V, and Y based on the sequence similarity of their ER signal sequences. The conopeptide precursor consists of four regions: an ER signal sequence region, an N-terminal proregion, the mature peptide region, and the C-terminal proregion. In the maturation process, the ER signal and the N- and C-terminal proregions are cleavaged via proteolytic processing; some amino acids in the mature region can be posttranslationally modified, form the disulfide bonds, and finally fold into their active 3D configuration (Olivera 2002). The sequence length of mature peptides currently reported is of 8–86 amino acids with an average of 26 residues and standard deviation of 10 residues (Kaas et al. 2010).

TABLE 8.1

Cysteine Framework of Conotoxins

Framework	Cysteine Pattern	Number of Cysteine
I	CC–C–C	4
II	CCC–C–C–C	6
III	CC–C–C–CC	6
IV	CC–C–C–C–C	6
V	CC–CC	4
VI/VII	C–C–CC–C–C	6
VIII	C–C–C–C–C–C–C–C–C–C	10
IX	C–C–C–C–C–C	6
X	CC–C.[PO]C	4
XI	C–C–CC–CC–C–C	8
XII	C–C–C–C–CC–C–C	8
XIII	C–C–C–CC–C–C–C	8
XIV	C–C–C–C	4
XV	C–C–CC–C–C–C–C	8
XVI	C–C–CC	4
XVII	C–C–CC–C–CC–C	8
XVIII	C–C–CC–CC	6
XIX	C–C–C–CCC–C–C–C–C	10
XX	C–CC–C–CC–C–C–C–C	10
XXI	CC–C–C–C–CC–C–C–C	10
XXII	C–C–C–C–C–C–C–C	8

Source: Kaas, Q. et al., *Nucleic Acids Res.,* 40, D325, 2012.

When examining the targets of conotoxins, they are classified into different pharmacological families based on the receptors and the physiological activity. These families are α (alpha), γ (gamma), δ (delta), ε (epsilon), ι (iota), κ (kappa), μ (mu), ρ (rho), σ (sigma), χ (chi), and ω (omega) (Table 8.2) (Kaas et al. 2010).

The standard toxin name consists of three parts, in which the first one is one or two letters indicating the *Conus* species, followed by a Roman number indicating the cysteine framework category and the last part is the uppercase letter denoting the order of discovery. For example, EVIA is the first conotoxin (A) with cysteine framework VI extracted from *Conus ermineus* (E).

The huge quantity, the diversity in structures, and their bioactivities in targeting the receptors in the neuron system make conotoxins a very valuable source of biomaterial for study in neuroscience, physiological activities, and pharmacology.

8.2 Conotoxins as Tools in Neuroscience

8.2.1 Conopeptides Targeted to Voltage-Gated Ion Channels

The voltage-gated ion channels are the membrane proteins activated by a change in the transmembrane potential. They permit the selective permeability through the cell membrane of monovalent cations such as K^+, Na^+, Ca^{2+}, and Cl^-. The most important physiological

TABLE 8.2

Conotoxin Pharmacological Families Corresponding to Membrane Receptor Family, the Number of Wild-Type Conotoxins Identified and the Gene Superfamily

Pharmacological Families	Membrane Receptor Family	Mature Conotoxins	Gene Superfamily
α (alpha)	Nicotinic acetylcholine receptor (nAChR)	55	A, D, L, M, S
χ (chi)	Neuronal noradrenaline transporter	4	T
	Voltage-gated Na channels		
δ (delta)	Presynaptic Ca channels or G	18	O1
ε (epsilon)	protein couple	1	T
	Neuronal pacemaker cation current		
γ (gamma)	Voltage-gated Na channels	4	O1, O2
	Voltage-gated K channels		
ι (iota)	Voltage-gated Na channels	2	I1, M
κ (kappa)	Voltage-gated Ca channels	8	A, I2, J, M, O1
μ (mu)	Alpha 1-adrenoceptors	23	M, O1, T
ω (omega)	Serotonin-gated ion channels	31	O1
ρ (rho)		1	A
σ (sigma)		1	S

Source: Kaas, Q. et al., *Toxicon*, 55, 1491, 2010.

role of these channels is the generation, shaping, and transduction of the electrical signals of the cell. These proteins have specific structures with a pore that opens or close with the change in electrical potential. Although every channel from different cell types seems to have similar functional properties, there are much many distinct genes for each type of voltage-gated ion channels. For example, 10 human Na^+ channel genes and more than 80 K^+ channel genes are currently known (Terlau and Olivera 2004). The genes within the same type of ion channel produce proteins that differ in their structure, function, and distribution in specific tissues.

Voltage-gated Ca^{2+} channels serve many different actions in neurons such as controlling the shape of potentials and generating action potentials in the same way as sodium channels, but the most important function is the release of neurotransmitters at synapses. There are six groups of calcium channels classified according to their electrophysiological and pharmacological properties, termed L, N, P, Q, T, and R types. With many functions charged to calcium channels, drugs that block these channels can be used to treat a wide range of diseases, from heart problems to anxiety disorders.

The Na channels play a key role in controlling neuronal excitability, initiation, and transmission of action potentials along nerves. According to the susceptibility to block by the tetrodotoxin, TTX, sodium channels are divided into TTX-sensitive and TTX-insensitive classes. These channels have nine homologous α subunit subtypes Na_v 1.1–1.9 (Goldin et al. 2000). The sodium channels relate to clinical states such as pain, stroke, and epilepsy.

K channels play a key role not only in repolarization phase of action potentials but also in setting the resting membrane potentials and bursting activity. With more than 80 genes related to K channels, it is clear that these channels are responsible for the large range of purposes in different cell types.

μ-Conotoxins were originally isolated from *Conus geographus*, the fish-hunting cone snail. This toxin in M-superfamily is composed of 22–25 amino acids with six cysteine residues in the class III framework. μ-Conotoxin is so far the only polypeptide that blocks sodium currents by acting at site I of the Na channel. The *Conus* species collected to isolate μ-conotoxins are *C. geographus*, *Conus purpurascens*, and *Conus stercusmuscarum* according to μ-GIIIA, μ-GIIIA, μ-PIIIA, and μ-SIIIA peptides (Jacob and McDougal 2010).

μO-conotoxins and δ-conotoxins are unusually hydrophobic peptides belonging to the O-superfamily. Although μO-conotoxins inhibit Na channel conductance like μ-conotoxin but do not interact in site I (Terlau et al. 1996). μO-MrVIA and μO-MrVIB are isolated from the venom of *Conus marmoreus*, a snail-hunting species with the disulfide bonding pattern closer to ω-conotoxins than μ-conotoxins. μO-MrVIA blocks Na$_v$1.2 and both TTX-sensitive and TTX-insensitive Na channels (Daly et al. 2004).

δ-Conotoxin inhibits the fast inactivation of Na currents, an important mechanism to achieve proper shape and duration of action potentials. The effects of δ-conotoxin depend largely on the system being investigated. The "King Kong" peptide, δ-TxVIA, isolated from *Conus textile* (Garrett et al. 2005), could prolong the Na current in molluskan neuronal membranes, while δ-PVIA, isolated from *C. purpurascens*, can elicit excitatory symptoms in mice and fish but is inactive in mollusks even at doses 100-fold higher (Shon et al. 1995, 1998).

The conotoxins that target K channels reported so far are κ-conotoxin PVIIA, κM-RIIIK, and κA-SIVA isolated from *C. purpurascens*, *Conus radiatus*, and *Conus striatus*. The κ-PVIIA is the key venom component that immobilizes the fish prey quickly. Combining with the δ-conotoxin PVIA, κ-PVIIA causes the hyperexcitation of the victim, leading to instant titanic paralysis (Terlau and Olivera 2004).

Conotoxins that target Ca channels attract more attention and are intensively applied in neuroscience. These peptides, termed ω-conotoxins, are isolated mainly from the venom of fish-hunting snails. The ω-MVIIA identified from *Conus magus* inhibits selectively N-type calcium channel Ca$_v$2.2, while ω-MVIIC preferentially targets P/Q channels Ca$_v$2.1. It is proved that the tyrosine residue in both peptides is responsible for binding to Ca$_v$2.1 and Ca$_v$2.2 channels (Kim et al. 1994). One of the ω-conotoxins, MVIIA from *C. magus*, has been approved by FDA and has become the drug for treatment of intractable pain under generic name ziconotide and commercial name Prialt by the developer Elan Pharmaceuticals (Olivera 2000).

8.2.2 Conopeptides Targeted to Ligand-Gated Ion Channels

Ligand-gated ion channels are the transmembrane ion channels activated in response to the binding of a ligand, usually a transmitter. One major group of these channels, all belonging to the same gene superfamily, are those sensitive to acetylcholine, serotonin, GABA, or glycine. The other gene superfamily of ligand-gated ion channels is glutamate receptors that are subdivided into N-methyl-D-aspartate (NMDA) and non-NMDA (AMPA) receptors. The third family is ATP receptors.

Conotoxins are targeted to three different families of ligand-gated ion channels. Most of conopeptides target nicotinic acetylcholine receptors. Among them, α-conotoxins are widely distributed and highly subtype-selective nicotinic antagonists. Based on this property, α-conotoxins are valuable in discriminating between closely related neuronal nicotinic acetylcholine receptor isoforms (Nicke et al. 2003, 2004, Terlau and Olivera 2004).

8.3 Conotoxins as the Template for Designing New Drugs in Pharmacology

8.3.1 Pain Treatment

Pain is a form of somatic sensation that occurs in response to actual or potential tissue damage. The sensation of pain is initiated by noxious chemicals or extreme temperature or pressure that activate a variety of protein in nociceptors, the terminals of specific peripheral nerve fibers, resulting in depolarization and generation of the action potentials. The signals from peripheral nociceptors, by the release of neurotransmitters, activate receptors on spinal dorsal horn neurons that transfer through several pathways to the brainstem, thalamus, and ultimately to the cerebral cortex.

Pain states are separated into two categories: acute and chronic. Acute pain is an alert signal to the body for avoiding the dangerous situation for survival. Chronic pain is the result of a dysfunctional reorganization of the pain system, often long time after injury has healed. Chronic pain can be found in many diseases or disorders such as back pain, cancer pain, complex regional pain syndrome, diabetic neuropathy, HIV/AIDS neuropathy, etc. The need of effective treatment strategies for chronic pain is now still remained because of low efficacy or undesirable side effects of the current treatments.

Conotoxins reveal high selectivity for pain targets, avoiding side effects like drug addiction to opioids. The peptides having analgesic properties are MVIIA (Prialt), CVID (AM336), contulakin-G (CGX-1160), MrIA (Xen-2174), conantokin-G (CGX-1007), Vc1.1 (ACV-1), and MrVIB (CGX-1002). Among them, only Prialt has been approved and others are under development or are being explored (Alonso et al. 2003, Layer and McIntosh 2006).

8.3.2 Treatment of Stroke

Stroke is one of the leading causes of death or disability, including impairment of cognition and function. The ischemic stroke initiates from occlusion of blood current in vessels of brain. This is the result of atherosclerotic plaque formation in brain vessels or blood clots in coronary arteries of the heart. The occlusion of blood vessel results in the lack of oxygen and glucose, depletion of brain ATP, and loss of ability to maintain and restore ionic gradients in neurons. The concentration of calcium rises to toxic levels. Neurons in the core of the infarcted region swell and burst. The region of neuronal damage and cell death will expand over time.

The conotoxin that inhibits the Ca channels and NMDARs can be used for treatment of stroke. ω-Conotoxins and conantokins inhibit Ca_v channels and NMDARs, respectively. The experiment of using Prialt in rats has a positive result. The intravenous infusion of MVIIA reduced the cortical volume of infarction and extracellular glutamate. This drug has performed the phase I of clinical trail (human pharmacology) in healthy volunteers (McGuire et al. 1997).

8.3.3 Neuromuscular Block

The neuromuscular junction is the synapse of the axon terminal of a motor neuron that initiates the action potential across the muscle's surface causing the contraction of muscle. In vertebrates, acetylcholine is used to transmit the signal through the neuromuscular junction. When blocking the neuromuscular transmission, the muscle function can be lost relatively or completely.

Neuromuscular-blocking drugs block neuromuscular transmission at the neuromuscular junction by acting presynaptically via the inhibition of action of acetylcholine. These drugs are used in surgery to provide muscle relaxation to facilitate positive pressure ventilation during and after anesthesia and to facilitate tracheal intubation. One of the neuromuscular-blocking drugs being chosen to facilitate the tracheal intubation is succinylcholine. However, this drug has side effects such as fasciculation, postoperative muscle pain, hyperkalemia, vagally mediated bradycardia, and histamine-induced hypotension and anaphylaxis (Layer and McIntosh 2006).

Each nAChR is composed of five subunits and every subunit contains four transmembrane domains. In neuronal and sensory mammalian tissues, 11 nAChR subunits, $\alpha 2$–$\alpha 7$, $\alpha 9$, $\alpha 10$, and $\beta 2$–$\beta 4$, have been found. The different subunit compositions provide the nAChRs different structures and show the diversity in pharmacological and physiological properties of the channel. Different neuronal nAChR subtypes have been known to be involved in learning, antinociception, nicotine addiction, and neurological disorders such as Parkinson's and Alzheimer's disease.

Among peptides isolated from cone snails, the α-conotoxin class provides a powerful tool for going further in structure and function of neuronal nicotinic acetylcholine receptor subtypes (Ellison et al. 2003, Nicke et al. 2004). The $\alpha 3/5$-conotoxins such as GI, MI, and SI display distinct binding site selectivity (Hann et al. 1994). Based on their properties in selective binding and competitive blocking, the $\alpha 3/5$-conotoxins show high potential in becoming the new neuromuscular-blocking drugs.

8.3.4 Cardioprotection

When the blood circulation in a coronary artery is blocked by the thrombosis, it causes lack of blood supply to a part of the heart, and in severe situation, acute myocardial infarction occurs. The treatment for this disease is to limit the size of the infarction through thrombolytic drugs or by surgery. Many drugs have been developed for this purpose but not perfectly as they do not reduce the size of the infarct region if the ischemia has initiated before the drugs are given. Another side effect is hypotension (Layer and McIntosh 2006).

The κ-PVIIA, a conopeptide isolated from *C. purpurascens*, has shown activity in reducing the infarct size in models of acute myocardial infarction in animals such as rabbits, rats, and dogs. The cardioprotection of κ-PVIIA was sustained even when the reperfusion lasted for 72 h (Zhang et al. 2003, Lubbers et al. 2005). It is important that κ-PVIIA is effective just before the time of reperfusion. Although the mechanism of cardioprotection produced by this peptide is still unclear, based on the result of studies, it has shown ability in coronary artery thrombolytic therapy.

8.4 Conclusion

The small peptides isolated from marine cone snails surprise the scientists by their diversity but very high selectivity in targeting specific sites of the neuronal system. They become precise tools for further studies in neuroscience, and with the relative ease of synthesis, they open a wide horizon for designing new drugs for treatment of many severe diseases in a wide range from pain to heart stroke. Perhaps in nature, it is hard to find a similar case like this. With more than hundred thousand distinct peptides but only a very small part, less than 0.1%, of them having been characterized and developed, this valuable resource of the marine biomaterials requires much efforts and long time to achieve the knowledge of whole entity.

References

Alonso, D., Z. Khalil, N. Satkunanathan, B.G. Livett. 2003. Drugs from the sea: Conotoxins as drug leads for neuropathic pain and other neurological conditions. *Mini Rev. Med. Chem.* 3: 785–787.

Daly, N.L., J.A. Ekberg, L. Thomas, D.J. Adams, R.J. Lewis, D.J. Craik. 2004. Structures of μO-conotoxins from *Conus marmoreus*: Inhibitors of tetrodotoxin (TTX)-sensitive and TTX-resistant sodium channels in mammalian sensory neurons. *J. Biol. Chem.* 279: 25774–25782.

Davis, J., A. Jones, R.J. Lewis. 2009. Remarkable inter- and intra-species complexity of conotoxins revealed by LC/MS. *Peptides* 30: 1222–1227.

Ellison, M., J.M. McIntosh, B.M. Olivera. 2003. α-Conotoxins ImI and ImII. *J. Biol. Chem.* 278: 757–764.

Garrett, J.E., O. Buczek, M. Watkins, B.M. Olivera, G. Bulaj. 2005. Biochemical and gene expression analyses of conotoxins in *Conus textile* venom ducts. *Biochem. Biophys. Res. Commun.* 328: 362–367.

Goldin, A.L., R.L. Barchi, J.H. Caldwell, F. Hofmann, J.C. Howe Hunter et al. 2000. Nomenclature of voltage-gated sodium channels. *Neuron* 28: 365–368.

Hann, R.M., O.R. Pagan, V.A. Eterovic. 1994. The alpha-conotoxins GI and MI distinguish between the nicotinic acetylcholine receptor agonist sites while SI does not. *Biochemistry* 33: 14058–14063.

Jacob, R.B., O.M. McDougal. 2010. The M-superfamily of conotoxin: A review. *Cell Mol. Life Sci.* 67: 17–27.

Kaas, Q., J.C. Westermann, D.J. Craik. 2010. Conopeptide characterization and classifications: An analysis using ConoServer. *Toxicon* 55: 1491–1509.

Kaas, Q., R. Yu, A.H. Jin, S. Dutertre, D. Craik. 2012. Conoserver: Updated content, knowledge, and discovery tools in the conopeptide data base. *Nucleic Acids Res.* 40: D325–D330.

Kim, J.I., M. Takahashi, A. Ogura, T. Kohno, Y. Kudo, K. Sato. 1994. Hydroxyl group of Tyr$^+$ is essential for the activity of ω-conotoxin GVIA, a peptide toxin for N-type calcium channel. *J. Biol. Chem.* 273: 23876–23878.

Layer, R.T., J.M. McIntosh. 2006. Conotoxins: Therapeutic potential and application. *Mar. Drugs* 4: 119–142.

Lew, M.J., J.P. Flinn, P.K. Pallaghy, R. Murphy, S.L. Whorlow et al. 1997. Structure-function relationships of ω-conotoxin GVIA. Synthesis, structure, calcium channel binding, and functional assay of alanine-substituted analogues. *J. Biol. Chem.* 272: 12014–12023.

Lewis, R.J. 2009. Conotoxins: Molecular and therapeutic targets. In *Marine Toxins as Research Tools*, eds. N. Fusetani, W. Kem. Springer-Verlag, Berlin, Germany.

Lubbers, N.L., T.J. Campbell, J.S. Polakowski, G. Bulaj, R.T. Layer et al. 2005. Postischemic administration of CGX-1051, a peptide from cone snail venom, reduces infarct size in both rat and dog models of myocardial ischemia and reperfusion. *J. Cardiovasc. Pharmacol.* 46: 141–146.

Marshall, J., W.P. Kelley, S.S. Rubakhin, J.P. Bingham, J.V. Sweedler, W.F. Gilly. 2002. Anatomical correlates of venom production in *Conus californicus*. *Biol. Bull.* 203: 27–41.

McGuire, D., S. Bowersox, J.D. Fellman, R.R. Luther. 1997. Sympatholysis after neuron-specific, N-type, voltage-sensitive calcium channel blockage: First demonstration of N-channel function in humans. *J. Cardiovasc. Pharmacol.* 30: 400–403.

Nicke, A., M.L. Loughnan, E.L. Millard, P.F. Alewood, D.J. Adams et al. 2003. Isolation, structure, and activity of GID, a novel alpha 4/7-conotoxin with an extended N-terminal sequence. *J. Biol. Chem.* 278: 3137–3144.

Nicke, A., S. Wonnacott, R.J. Lewis. 2004. α-Conotoxins as tools for the elucidation of structure and function of neuronal nicotinic acetylcholine receptor subtypes. *Eur. J. Biochem.* 271: 2305–2319.

Olivera, B.M. 1997. *Conus* venom peptides, receptor and ion channel targets and drugs design: 50 million years of neuropharmacology (EE Just Lecture). *Mol. Biol. Cell* 8: 2101–2109.

Olivera, B.M. 2000. ω-Conotoxins MVIIA: From marine snail venom to analgesic drug. In *Drugs from the Sea*, ed. N. Fusetani. Karger, Basel, Switzerland, pp. 75–85.

Olivera, B.M. 2002. *Conus* venom peptides: Reflections from the biology of clades and species. *Annu. Rev. Ecol. Syst.* 33: 25–47.

Olivera, B.M., R.W. Teichert. 2007. Diversity of the neurotoxic *Conus* peptides. *Mol. Interven.* 7: 251–260.

Rockel, D., W. Korn, A.J. Kohn. 1995. *Manual of the Living Conidae*. Verlag Christa Hemmen, Weisbaden, Germany, 517pp.

Shon, K., M.M. Grilley, M. Marsh, D. Yoshikami, A.R. Hall et al. 1995. Purification, characterization and cloning of the lockjaw peptide from *Conus purpurascens* venom. *Biochemistry* 34: 4913–4918.

Shon, K., M. Stocker, H. Terlau, W. Stuhmer, R. Jacobsen et al. 1998. k-Conotoxin PVIIA: A peptide inhibiting the *Shaker* K$^+$ channel. *J. Biol. Chem.* 273: 33–38.

Terlau, H., B.M. Olivera. 2004. *Conus* venoms: A rich source of novel ion channel-targeted peptides. *Physiol. Rev.* 84: 41–68.

Terlau, H., M. Stocker, K.J. Shon, J.M. McIntosh, B.M. Olivera. 1996. Mo-conotoxin MrVIA inhibits mammalian channels but not through site J. *J. Neurosci.* 76: 1423–1429.

Zhang, S.J., X.M. Yang, G.S. Liu, M.V. Cohen, K. Pemberton, J.M. Downey. 2003. CGX-1051, a peptide from *Conus* snail venom, attenuates infarction in rabbit hearts when administered at reperfusion. *J. Cardiovasc. Pharmacol.* 42: 764–771.

9

Pigmented Marine Heterotrophic Bacteria: Occurrence, Diversity, and Characterization of Pigmentation

Marit H. Stafsnes and Per Bruheim

CONTENTS

9.1 Introduction

The oceans, which cover approximately 70% of the earth's surface (Fenical 1993), contain a variety of species, many of which have no terrestrial counterparts. The high organic matter confined in the oceans may be considered favorable for the evolution and growth of life in general. One of the pioneers of marine microbiology, Claude Zobell, began his work in delineating the vast numbers and diversity of marine bacteria in the 1930s, and his classic book *Marine Microbiology* was published in 1946 (ZoBell 1946). Microbiologically, the oceans are massively complex and consist of a diverse assemblage of microbial life forms, which occur in environments of extreme variations in pressure, salinity, and temperature. Hence, the concentration of the microbial population varies significantly, and a typical mL of seawater contains 10^6 microorganisms, ranging from 10^3 to 10^7 (Jensen and Fenical 1996; Chin et al. 2006; Valentine 2007).

The diversity of marine environments has exerted a driving force on microbial evolution and selection leading to new adaptive strategies and the synthesis of new metabolites. In the early 1960s, researchers started to explore the microbial diversity as a source of potentially useful unique bioactive compounds. Many of these compounds are produced by the microorganisms without an apparent function in the growth and development of the microbial cells and are referred to as secondary metabolites. Thus, marine microorganisms offer the potential for the production of metabolites of potential interest for commercial exploration (Jensen and Fenical 1996; Valentine 2007). As a result, more than 10,000 marine microbial metabolites have been isolated and characterized over the past five decades (Chin et al. 2006).

Although several studies have been carried out to characterize the marine microbial life in general in ocean sites and in different coastal areas, few studies have been performed with the scope of identifying the total diversity of marine heterotrophic bacteria (MHB) (Du et al. 2006). One of the first comprehensive studies on MHB describes the isolation of 500 *actinomycete* strains and antibiotics (quinones) produced by these (Okazaki et al. 1975). Besides being a source for valuable natural dyes, pigmentation in MHB is often linked to other potentially interesting properties such as antioxidant effects, antibacterial, or anticancer properties. With more efficient sampling and identification of bioactive metabolites, the ocean offers a promising potential for isolating novel molecules with beneficial effect for the human health (Dufosse 2006). A summary of the diversity of MHB and their pigment production will be presented in this chapter. This comprises an overview of reported pigments and their functionality and a general guide of how to characterize the pigments.

9.2 Occurrence and Diversity of Pigmented Heterotrophic Bacteria in Marine Ecosystems

An enormous bacterial diversity is found in the oceans, and it is generally acknowledged that the bacteria are one major agent shaping the organic composition of the oceans (Amon et al. 2001). Bacteria maintain a broad array of genetic, metabolic, and physiological capabilities that allow for a high degree of adaptability and metabolic diversification into numerous environmental niches and habitats. Thus, bacteria are important contributors of the biological transformation in various nutrient cycles (e.g., carbon, nitrogen, and sulfur cycles). Also, the marine ecosystems are presumed more heterogeneous than the soil ecosystems at the bacterial level (Tringe et al. 2004), and almost all the currently described bacterial phyla are represented in the ocean, while only about half have terrestrial members (Ray 1988). The other prokaryotic domain, *Archaea*, has been well known for its presence in extreme habitats, and recent studies indicate that *Archaea* in general might also be a significant contributor to the marine pelagic picoplankton biomass, though especially below the euphotic zone (Karner et al. 2001; Valentine 2007).

Certain bacterial species and even genera have until now only been found in marine environments, for example, the *Roseobacter* clade or the genus *Pseudoalteromonas*. They would therefore, by definition, be true marine bacteria. But the definition is not always that unambiguous as many genera are found in both marine and terrestrial habitats. This is frequently observed even at the species level and it could simply be that the marine isolates are originating from terrestrial habitats. Seawater and/or sodium requirements are unequivocal physiological characteristics of indigenous marine bacteria. The generally accepted definition of marine bacteria is "microorganisms which were isolated from the marine habitat and which are functionally reproductive under typical marine conditions" (Jensen et al. 1996). It is obvious that this description may also include terrestrial contaminants if they tolerate the 3.4% salt concentration of the oceans. Therefore many choose to call them "isolates from a marine habitat" (Laatsch 2006), and this broader definition is used throughout this chapter without further discussion if the genus/species is a true marine one. The number of bacteria isolated from the ocean territories continues to increase each year. The World Register of Marine species (WoRMS) currently contains 3684 marine bacterial species (Appeltans et al. 2012), and the genome sequence of 182 marine bacterial species has been published through the *CAMERA* portal (Sun et al. 2011).

9.2.1 Assessment of Diversity and Identification of Marine Bacteria

Distribution of bacteria depends on changes in water temperature, salinity, and other physicochemical parameters (Alavandi 1990; Das et al. 2006). Generally, only a small fraction of the bacteria present in natural samples multiply in laboratory media, that is, are able to form colony-forming units (CFU). It is assumed that 0.1%–1% of marine bacteria are culturable (Amann et al. 1995; Pedrós-Alió 2006b), but culture-independent methods like microautoradiography, direct viable count technique, or flow cytometry have revealed that up to 50%, and in some cases even 90%, of the bacterial cells may be metabolically active (Gerdts and Luedke 2006). Bacteria adapted to higher nutrient values in their natural habitat are more likely to survive and proliferate in artificial nutrient compositions in the laboratory. Therefore, in general, the percentage of culturable heterotrophic bacteria is less in nutrient-poor waters and higher in nutrient-rich waters (Porter et al. 2004). Marine free-living bacteria are regarded facultatively oligotrophs (require low-nutrient media to grow), but the definition is somewhat controversial (Schut et al. 1997). The number of total bacterial cell counts also varies in the water column, with highest number in the sea surface microlayer and decreasing downward, probably as a consequence of gradients in nutrient availability and composition (Bruns et al. 2002; Du et al. 2006). However, it is difficult to compare different studies as the results are highly dependent upon isolation and incubation condition. Artificial nutrient compositions are obviously lacking the full range of environmental requirements for marine bacteria (Roszak and Colwell 1987), and it is a common experience that bacterial cultures are rapidly losing their metabolic capabilities under laboratory conditions if they are too often subcultured (Laatsch 2006). This phenomenon has also been observed with pigmentation; selected pigmented colonies might no longer be pigmented after several rounds of subculturing (Jones 1946). Also, during the original sampling and screening procedure, the agar plates may have harbored co-cultured microorganisms that potentially mutually benefit each other (Mearns-Spragg et al. 1998). Thus, new media components and incubation conditions are continuously being developed and introduced with the scope of increasing the cultivation efficiency and expression of secondary metabolites (Fry 1990; Bruns et al. 2002).

The diversity of marine samples has increased by one or two orders of magnitude per year and was previously recognized from conventional cultivation but later with molecular approaches (Pedrós-Alió 2006a). The 16S ribosomal RNA gene is used as it is highly conserved between different species of *Bacteria* and *Archaea*. Many 16S rRNA sequences have been found that do not belong to any known cultured species and is thus a proof for the unculturability and diversity in the ocean (Lee et al. 2011). Thus, for example, latitudinal patterns in the distribution of the bacterial genera that form the diversity have been found by cloning and sequencing large clone libraries from different oceans (Venter et al. 2004; Kennedy et al. 2008). Even a 16S rRNA community analysis can be biased and underreport uncultivable bacteria as the rare genera not necessarily will be hybridized with universal PCR primers and thereby remain undetected. Furthermore, the presence of DNA from phages and higher organisms in the community could also contaminate the samples and introduce noise in the analysis. The genes encoding small subunit rRNA also reflect the evolutionary relationship of microorganisms and are used to group and identify microorganisms (Woese et al. 1990). Lately, a high-throughput technology, the PhyloChip, has become available to assess microbial profiles. This microarray-based technology uses genetic probes and covers over 32,000 taxa. The chip was, for example, used to characterize the deep-sea microbial flora after the Deepwater Horizon oil blowout in 2010 (Hazen et al. 2010).

As cloning and sequencing of 16S RNA genes are laborious and costly for analyzing a large number of samples, genetic fingerprinting techniques enabling higher throughput have been developed. Polymerase chain reaction–denaturing gradient gel electrophoresis (PCR-DGGE) fingerprinting is the most common tool used for monitoring variations in microbial genetic diversity, providing a minimum estimate of the richness of predominant community members (Schäfer and Muyzer 2001).

Fluorescence in situ hybridization (FISH) with rRNA-targeted probes is a staining technique that allows phylogenetic identification of bacteria in mixed assemblages without prior cultivation (Pernthaler et al. 2002). While some bacterial genera have been found dominant by using traditional cultivation methods, FISH data have revealed that they are in fact minor component of the total bacterioplankton (Du et al. 2006). Clearly, there can be, and not unexpectedly, discrepancies between cultivation-dependent and cultivation-independent microbial community analyses.

Another promising technique for identifying marine bacteria is chemotaxonomy—the identification of bacteria by protein markers. Matrix-assisted laser desorption ionization–time of flight mass spectrometry (MALDI-ToF MS) is a powerful tool for such identification (Lay 2000). By making a customized database of MALDI-ToF metabolic fingerprints of previously characterized bacteria by their 16S rDNA sequences, rapid identification was achieved (Salaün et al. 2010), and the diversity of bacteria in marine sponges has been described by application of MALDI-ToF MS (Dieckmann et al. 2005). The method can even allow the analysis of complex bacterial mixtures (Wahl et al. 2002; Liu et al. 2007). The present commercial databases are not sufficiently comprehensive and positive identification based solely on MALDI-ToF MS of most marine bacterial isolates cannot be expected. However, it is likely that identification will become more accurate in the future due to technological advancements and extension of databases with spectra from new bacterial species (Lay 2000). Not only whole-cell proteome but also secreted secondary metabolites representing the secretome can be analyzed with the MALDI-ToF technique (Vater et al. 2002; Hindré et al. 2003). Thus, this method can be applied for rapid screening of unexplored microorganisms in different habitats in order to identify novel bioactive compounds available for industrial exploitation. Wietz et al. also showed that the profiling of small molecules can be used for species discrimination (Wietz et al. 2010).

For the reasons mentioned earlier, it is impossible to determine diversity indices and species diversity of heterotrophic bacteria accurately in most communities using either cultivation or molecular approaches. The right order of magnitude of species diversity is not known. The low estimates (10^4) are close to the number of currently described species (3.7×10^3) (Pommier et al. 2005) and high estimates vary between 10^6 and 10^9 (Pedrós-Alió 2006).

9.2.2 Pigmented Heterotrophic Bacteria

It is impossible to give a general number of the abundance of pigmented heterotrophic bacteria (PHB) to total MHB due to the enormous diversity of marine bacteria. This will definitively vary with sampling site, seasonal variation, etc., and several studies of the pigmentation of heterotrophic bacteria indicate a great variety in percentage pigmentation ranging from 10% to almost 70% of the total CFU (Zobell and Feltham 1934; ZoBell 1946; Hermansson et al. 1987; Du et al. 2006; Cetina et al. 2010). Older publication in general gives a higher number. However, this could just express that earlier used isolation methods favored pigmented strains or that they were selectively chosen as "unique" isolates, and therefore there would be a higher percentage of pigmented bacteria in the collection. Pigment synthesis is also dependent on light, pH, temperature, and various media constituents (Buck 1974). The pigmented bacteria display almost all the colors of the rainbow including light or dark tinges and unusual colors like black, white, brown, golden, silver, and fluorescent green, yellow, or blue. In general, the pigmented bacteria cannot be constringed to specific bacterial genera and often not even to the species level. Therefore the total diversity of heterotrophic bacteria will be discussed and representative pigmented isolates will be enlightened in this section. Table 9.1 gives an overview of pigmented marine isolated mainly based on studies with the aim of describing their diversity. As specific species can express several pigmented metabolites they might exhibit various colors depending on the relative production of each pigment. Therefore the reported colors and pigment groups have to be viewed in light of the isolation and cultivation conditions.

Marine bacteria have different ways of living, either free-living (referred to as pelagic or planktonic), attached to biotic and abiotic surfaces/particles, or in internal space of invertebrate. Particularly in the latter case, they are likely to benefit from a symbiotic relationship. What was earlier considered pigment-producing coral, fish, sea grass, sponges, mollusks, and tunicates might in reality be produced by their attached bacteria (Okazaki et al. 1975), and the study of symbiotic marine microorganisms is a rapidly growing field (Bhatnagar and Kim 2010). Several studies have been carried out to characterize heterotrophic bacteria in ocean sites and in different coastal areas of temperate, tropical, and polar zones, but it would be an impossible task to describe the total diversity of MHB in the oceans unless their habitat is defined, and this depends in particular on whether they are pelagic or surface attached although the most abundant genera are ubiquitously present (DeLong et al. 1993). In general the abundance and diversity is influenced by their availability or lack of nutrients and surrounding stress including predators.

TABLE 9.1

Overview of Identified Marine PHB from Recent Studies (2002–2011)

Marine Isolate[a]	Color	Main Pigment[b]	Habitat	Reference
Algibacter lectus	Yellow		Surface	Agogué et al. (2005)
Altererythrobacter ishigakiensis	Orange-red	Astaxanthin	Sediment	Matsumoto et al. (2011)
Alteromonas sp.			Seaweeds, invertebrates, surface, subsurface	Zheng et al. (2005); Du et al. (2006)
Arthrobacter agilis	Dark rose-red	Carotenoid	Antarctic	Dieser et al. (2010)
Arthrobacter nicotianae	Yellow		Biofilm	Lee et al. (2003)
Bacillus licheniformis	Red	Diadinoxanthin	Sea grass	Nugraheni et al. (2010)
Bacillus sp.	Species specific		Seaweed, invertebrates, biofilm	Lee et al. (2003); Zheng et al. (2005); Du et al. (2006)
Bacillus horikoshii	Orange		Surface, subsurface	Agogué et al. (2005)
Blastococcus aggregates	Pink		Surface, subsurface	Agogué et al. (2005)
Brevibacterium epidermidis	Yellow		Biofilm	Lee et al. (2003)
Brevundimonas sp.	Orange	C40-carotenoid	Surface, subsurface	Agogué et al. (2005); Misawa (2011)
Cellulophaga lytica	Orange		Surface, subsurface	Agogué et al. (2005)
Cytophaga laterculla	Brown, yellow		Subsurface	Lee et al. (2003); Agogué et al. (2005)
Cytophaga sp.	Yellow-orange		Pelagic	Das et al. (2007)
Deleya sp.			Surface, subsurface	Du et al. (2006)
Dietzia sp.	Orange		Surface, subsurface	Agogué et al. (2005); Du et al. (2006)
Enterobacter sakazakii	Orange		Surface, subsurface	Agogué et al. (2005)
Erythrobacter citreus	Brown		Surface, subsurface	Agogué et al. (2005)
Erythrobacter litoralis	Red		Surface	Agogué et al. (2005)
Erythrobacter sp.	Yellow	Nostoxanthin glucoside	Surface, subsurface	Agogué et al. (2005); Du et al. (2006); Stafsnes et al. (2010)
Exiguobacterium sp.	Yellow-orange		Pelagic	Agogué et al. (2005); Das et al. (2006); Du et al. (2006)
Flavobacterium sp.	Orange, yellow	Xeaxanthin	Antarctic, pelagic, seaweed, invertebrates	Zheng (2005); Das et al. (2007); Dieser et al. (2010)
Flexibacter sp.	Yellow-orange		Pelagic	Agogué et al. (2005); Das et al. (2007)
Halomonas sp.			Surface, subsurface	Du et al. (2006)
Hongiella sp.	Pink		Surface, subsurface	Agogué et al. (2005)
Hyphomonas johnsonii	Orange		Subsurface	Agogué et al. (2005)
Kocuria sp.	Yellow		Surface, subsurface	Du et al. (2006)

TABLE 9.1 (continued)

Overview of Identified Marine PHB from Recent Studies (2002–2011)

Marine Isolate[a]	Color	Main Pigment[b]	Habitat	Reference
Leeuwenhoekiella sp.	Yellow	Zeaxanthin	Surface	Stafsnes et al. (2010)
Leeuwenhoekiella blandensis	Yellow	Zeaxanthin	Pelagic	Pedrós-Alió (2006)
Maribacter sedimenticola	Yellow		Surface	Agogué et al. (2005)
Marinomonas sp.			Surface, subsurface	Du et al. (2006)
Microbacterium maritypicum	Light yellow		Pelagic	Williams et al. (2007)
Micrococcus luteus	Yellow	Sarcinaxanthin	Surface	Goodwin (1980); Stafsnes et al. (2010)
Micrococcus sp.			Surface, subsurface	Du et al. (2006)
Muricauda ruestringensis	Brown		Pelagic	Agogué et al. (2005)
Muricauda sp.	Yellow		Cyanobacteria	Hube et al. (2009)
Nocardioides jensenii	Yellow		Pelagic	Agogué et al. (2005)
Paracoccus sp.	Yellow, red	C40-carotenoid	Surface, subsurface	Das et al. (2006); Du et al. (2006); Misawa (2011)
Paracoccus carotinifaciens	Orange		Biofilm	Lee et al. (2003)
Paracoccus aminovorans	Orange		Subsurface	Agogué et al. (2005)
Planococcus sp.	Orange	C30-type carotenoid acid	Surface, subsurface	Agogué et al. (2005); Du et al. (2006); Misawa (2011)
Polaribacter sp.	Orange	β-carotene, zeaxanthin	Pelagic	Pedrós-Alió (2006)
Porphyrobacter sp.	Red		Cyanobacteria	Hube et al. (2009)
Pseudoalteromonas luteoviolacea	Purple	Violacein	Pelagic	Lee et al. (2003); Vynne et al. (2011)
Pseudoalteromonas maricoloris	Yellow	Bromoalterochromides	Sponges	Lee et al. (2003); Speitling et al. (2007)
Pseudoalteromonas phenolica	Brown		Pelagic	Lee et al. (2003); Isnansetyo and Kamei (2009)
Pseudoalteromonas piscicida	Yellow	Xanthophyll	Green algae, biofilm	Lee et al. (2003); Radjasa et al. (2009)
Pseudoalteromonas rubra	Red	Prodiginines	Pelagic	Lee et al. (2003); Soliev et al. (2011)
Pseudoalteromonas sp.	Yellow	Bromoalterochromide	Biofilm	Du et al. (2006); Tebben et al. (2011); Vynne et al. (2011)
Pseudoalteromonas sp.	Yellow		Seawater, sediment	Cetina et al. (2010)
Pseudoalteromonas tunicata	Green, purple, yellow	Tambjamine, violacein	Algae	Egan et al. (2002); Matz et al. (2004); Franks et al. (2005)

(continued)

TABLE 9.1 (continued)

Overview of Identified Marine PHB from Recent Studies (2002–2011)

Marine Isolate[a]	Color	Main Pigment[b]	Habitat	Reference
Pseudomonas aeruginosa	Blue-green, yellow, brown	Phenazines, melanin	Mangrove, pelagic	Lee et al. (2003); Nosanchuk and Casadevall (2003); Saha et al. (2008)
Pseudomonas jessenii	Black		Subsurface	Agogué et al. (2005)
Pseudomonas pseudoalcaligenes	Brown		Surface	Agogué et al. (2005)
Pseudomonas putida			Surface, subsurface	Du et al. (2006)
Pseudonocardia sp.	Yellow	Phenozostatin D	Marine sediment	Maskey et al. (2003); Teasdale et al. (2009)
Rhodobacter sp.	Pink		Aggregates with cyanobacteria	Hube et al. (2009)
Rhodococcus sp.	Orange-red-pink		Surface, subsurface	Du et al. (2006)
Roseobacter sp.	Bright colors, pink, red		Cyanobacteria, subsurface	Agogué et al. (2005); Du et al. (2006); Hube et al. (2009)
Rubritalea squalenifaciens	Red	Acyl glyco-carotenoic acids	Sponge	Shindo et al. (2007); Misawa (2011)
Ruegeria atlantica sp.	Pink		Surface	Du et al. (2006)
Salinibacter sp.	Red		Saltern pound	Agogué et al. (2005); Soliev et al. (2011)
Saprospira grandis	Red	Saproxanthin	Seashore	Lewin (1997)
Shewanella sp.	Brown, yellow		Subsurface	Lee et al. (2003); Agogué et al. (2005); Du et al. (2006)
Sphingomonas echinoides	Yellow	Nostoxanthin	Antarctic	Bowman (2007); Dieser et al. (2010)
Sphingomonas bakryungensis	Yellow	Nostoxanthin	Surface	Stafsnes et al. (2010)
Staphylococcus warnerii	Yellow		Pelagic	Agogué et al. (2005)
Tenacibaculum mesophilum	Yellow, orange		Biofilm	Lee et al. (2003); Agogué et al. (2005)
Tsukamurella paurometabola	Orange		Biofilm	Lee et al. (2003)
Vibrio sp.		Phenazine	Surface associated	Du et al. (2006)
Vibrio sp.	Red	Prodigiosin	Estuarine waters	Du et al. (2006); Boric et al. (2011)
Zooshikella rubidus	Red	Prodigiosin, cycloprodigiosin	Sediment	Lee et al. (2011)

[a] Closest match based on 16S rRNA sequences.
[b] Most studies focused on the diversity of PHB and not on the identification of the pigment; therefore in most cases the main pigment is not identified.

Marine bacteria must be able to survive and grow in the water environment with low nutrition, high salinity, low and high temperature, and high pressure. Zobell estimated the Gram-negative groups to comprise 90% of the heterotrophic bacteria, of which the majority of the isolates belong to the genera *Pseudomonas*, *Vibrio*, and *Flavobacterium* and thereby believed to be the most abundant (ZoBell 1946). The high abundance of Gram-negative bacteria is consistent with the postulation that their outer membrane structure is evolutionarily adapted to aquatic environmental factors (Soliev et al. 2011).

The presence of Gram-positive bacteria as indigenous members of marine bacterial communities ubiquitously distributed (Jensen and Fenical 1995) has been revealed by establishment of clone libraries (Stevens et al. 2007) or by hybridization with 16S rRNA genus-specific probes (Bruns et al. 2003). Jensen and Fenical isolated nearly 500 Gram-positive strains, which accounted for 12%–31% of the CFU obtained from samples taken from seawater, sediments, algal surfaces, and invertebrates (Jensen and Fenical 1995). An obligate requirement of seawater for growth was demonstrated by 82% of the strains, which is an important proof for characterizing them as originating from marine environments. *Rhodococcus marinonascens* (Helmke and Weyland 1984), *Dietzia maris* (Rainey et al. 1995), and *Microbacterium maritypicum* (Takeuchi and Hatano 1998) *are examples of marine* Gram-positive bacteria that have been characterized in detail. The Gram-positive *Aeromicrobium marinum* has been demonstrated to be an abundant member of the pelagic bacterial community in the German Wadden Sea representing about 1% of the total bacterial population (Bruns et al. 2003). The presence of *Bacillus* in diverse marine environments may indicate that this genus is an important component of the marine microbial community. *Bacillus* species are usually colorless, but several studies report pigmented marine *Bacillus* strains (see Table 9.1). Also members of the Actinobacteria have been found to account for a significant portion of the total bacteria (4%–7%), and these were distinctly different from that in the freshwater system (Stevens et al. 2007). The Actinobacteria are more abundant in terrestrial systems and the abundance in marine habitats has been proven to decrease with increasing distance from land. Many terrestrial Streptomycetes have a high degree of salt tolerance and together this supports the "wash-in" hypothesis of Gram-positive bacteria (Okazaki and Okami 1976; Goodfellow and Haynes 1984).

Das et al. (2007) proposed a simplified scheme for identifying marine bacteria based on fast and easy biochemical tests starting with identifying the Gram type. They proposed that pigmented nonmotile Gram-negative bacteria comprise the genera *Flexibacter*, *Flavobacterium*, and *Cytophaga*, whereas the nonpigmented isolates belonged to *Photobacter*, *Enterobacter*, *Aeromonas*, *Acinetobacter*, *Moraxella*, *and Pseudomonas*. Furthermore, it has been observed that motility is a frequent property of marine bacterial isolates and that some genera identified in this study were *Enterobacteriaceae*, *Alcaligenes*, *Pseudomonas*, *Alteromonas*, *Photobacterium*, *Vibrio*, *Aeromonas*, *Bacillus*, *Corynebacterium*, *Streptococcus*, *Arthrobacter*, *Micrococcus*, and *Staphylococcus* (Baumann et al. 1972). Thus, major and well-known heterotrophic bacterial genera have been isolated from marine habitats.

In 2006, Du et al. conducted a systematic investigation of PHB based on axenic cultures of their MHB culture collection with isolates from the Chinese coastal and shelf waters and the Pacific Ocean (Du et al. 2006). They described both the abundance of PHB and the ratio of PHB to CFU as it decreased along trophic gradients from coastal to oceanic waters, with the highest values of 10^4 cell/mL PHB and 40%. The 247 characterized isolates covering 25 genera of six phylogenetic classes exhibited various colors, for example, golden, yellow, red, pink, and orange. They showed that PHB have a broad genetic diversity and are widely distributed in the marine environment. PHB predominated in the euphotic zone in terms of vertical distribution and showed a close association with light. The ratio of PHB to CFU in the surface layer was nearly twice that in subsurface layers in turbid estuaries, while it differed little between surface and subsurface water in the clear eastern tropical North Pacific Ocean. Nair and Simidu focused on marine bacteria with antibacterial activity and reported more than 700 strains from various habitats. They obtained 37 producer strains, whereof 30% were pigmented (Nair and Simidu 1987). The highest percentage of strains showing antibacterial activity was observed in phytoplankton isolates, and the minimum was observed in those obtained from sponges. A more recent and comprehensive study of sea sediment and sea samples from 30 m depth from the East China Sea collected in total 30,000 strains (Lu et al. 2011). In this study, they presented 395 isolated strains belonging to 33 different genera, of which 100 strains possess various biological activities based on different large-scale screening models (antibacterial, cytotoxicity, and antioxidant activities).

The γ-proteobacteria genus *Pseudoalteromonas* are present globally in marine waters where they constitute between 0.5% and 6% of the total bacterial biomass (Wietz et al. 2010). They are heterotrophic aerobes and non-fermentative and the cells are motile by one or more polar flagella. The genus can be divided relatively distinctly into pigmented and nonpigmented species clades, and the pigmented species are often producers of bioactive secondary metabolites (Egan et al. 2002). Pigmented strains appeared to be more frequent in coastal areas, whereas the nonpigmented strains are associated with open waters. Pigmented species show greater sequence divergence and are concentrated within the other two major clades making up the genus (Bowman 2007). Bioactive *Pseudoalteromonas* are primarily originating from biotic or abiotic surfaces in contrast to planktonic strains (Holmström and Kjelleberg 1999); their association with higher organisms suggests an ecological role in which some bioactive species might play an active part in host defense against pathogens and fouling organisms (Holmström et al. 1996; Egan et al. 2008). Vynne et al. (2011) concluded that the pigmented antibacterial *Pseudoalteromonas* have a niche specificity, and sampling from marine biofilm environments is a strategy for isolating novel marine bacteria that produce antibacterial compounds. The bacterium *Pseudoalteromonas tunicata* is a successful competitor on marine surfaces owing primarily to its ability to produce a number of inhibitory molecules. As such, *P. tunicata* has become a model organism for the studies of surface colonization and eukaryotic host–bacteria interactions (Egan et al. 2008; Thomas et al. 2008). Furthermore, the isolation and structural similarity of an isolated secondary metabolite to the yellow pigment tambjamine isolated from sponges and bryozoans suggests that these compounds may be of bacterial origin and related to the presence of *Pseudoalteromonas* (Franks et al. 2005).

Pigmented bacteria, especially orange and yellow, have been found to dominate on green and red algae, but not in the bacterial population of the brown algae, which were similar to pelagic bacteria (Shiba and Taga 1980). Most of the pigmented bacteria were identified as belonging to the *Flavobacterium-Cytophaga* group, and a low number of *Vibrio* were identified on the green algae. A beneficial relationship was suggested between the green algae and the pigmented bacteria. Chan reported that the bacterial numbers attached to the algae *Ascophyllum nodosum* and *Polysiphonia lanosa* were 100–10,000 times higher than those in the seawater (Chan and McManus 1969). The dominant bacteria were *Vibrio* and *Flavobacter*, while the other identified isolates were members of the genera *Escherichia*, *Pseudomonas*, *Sarcina*, *Staphylococcus*, and *Achromobacter* (*Alcaligenes*) as well as a pink yeast (*Rhodotorula*). Hube et al. reported heterotrophic bacteria in association with cyanobacteria (Hube et al. 2009). Of a total of 30 isolates, eight strains were pigmented. They described three pigmented strains belonging to the genera *Porphyrobacter, Roseobacter,* and *Muricauda.* They all associated with cyanobacteria but were not dependent on them for survival. Members of the *Roseobacter* clade is reported to dominate among marine phytoplankton-associated bacteria and is exclusively marine or hypersaline (Brinkhoff et al. 2008; Slightom and Buchan 2009; Newton et al. 2010). The genus *Muricauda* was described in 2001 by Bruns et al. and belongs to the *Bacteroidetes* group (Bruns et al. 2001). The genus comprises four species that are known to be marine, yellow pigmented, and obligate or facultatively aerobic. In sum, the present cases highlight the potential use of green algae-associated bacteria as a sustainable source of marine pigments as well as marine antimicrobial compounds. Also bacterial symbionts of sea grass are considered a rich group of pigment-producing bacteria (Nugraheni et al. 2010).

In general, pigmented bacteria are described using culture-dependent techniques, but genetic approaches for the detection of secondary metabolite pathways might be applied. As an example, Mavrodi et al. designed a universal primer system able to study a wide range of bacterial groups including actinomycetes and pseudomonades, in order to detect genes of phenazine production in unidentified new isolates without prior performance of a phylogenetic classification (Mavrodi et al. 2006).

9.3 Pigments Produced by Marine Heterotrophic Bacteria and Their Physiological Role

Why do heterotrophic bacteria produce pigments? In heterotrophic bacteria, pigment formation is associated with morphological characteristics (Weber and de Bont 1996), pathogenesis (Lewis and Corpe 1964), protection, and survival (Courington and Goodwin 1955; Gauthier 1969; Nair and Simidu 1987; Agogué et al. 2005). Pigments are considered secondary metabolites implying that they are not strictly needed for growth, but one must assume that they have some kind of inherent activity. The secondary metabolites, in general, may be evolved in nature as some kind of response to the effects of the environment, including living (e.g., competition, symbiosis) and physical environments. The microbial secondary metabolites represent a kind of chemical interface between microbes and the rest of the living world. In many cases, these activities have not yet been discovered or fully elucidated. However, since some heterotrophic bacteria are prioritizing valuable nutrients to pigment synthesis, there clearly must be an ecological beneficial role. It might also be that the observable color is not directly relevant for the bioactive functionality of the colored compound: It is just colored due to the evolved chemical structure, which is contrary to pigmentation in light absorption processes of photosynthetic organisms where color reflects absorption of visible lights. MHB produce a wide variety of pigments of which many have antioxidant, antibiotic, anticancer, or immunosuppressive activities. The main physiological properties and characteristics of the major pigment groups identified in MHB will be presented in the following sections of this chapter.

9.3.1 Physiological Role

The physiological properties clearly vary between different pigment groups as these will have different physicochemical properties and have been developed for various purposes. But, on the general basis, one important physiological role of pigments in heterotrophic bacteria is, as it is for photosynthetic organisms, related to protection of light exposure. MHB have to be able to adapt to excessive sunlight and survive under harmful UV irradiation (Margalith 1992). UV-A radiation (320–400 nm) is catalyzing the intracellular formation of chemical intermediates such as reactive oxygen species (ROS). Many pigments have been shown to confer resistance to ROS as they are able to absorb excess energy from ROS (Agogué et al. 2005; Liu and Nizet 2009). Generally, a much higher pigmented fraction of MHB has been found in the sea surface microlayer relative to the subsurface. Hermansson et al. reported nearly 80% pigmented bacteria in the surface versus 15% from the other and less UV-exposed sampling sites (Hermansson et al. 1987). The higher proportion of pigmented isolates at the surface may reflect a physiological response for protection against the intense solar radiation at the interface. The high frequency of pigment production in isolates from ice cores (Zhang et al. 2008), glaciers (Christner et al. 2000; Miteva et al. 2004), or various marine surface waters (Agogué et al. 2005) further supports that pigmentation plays a role in adaptation to these highly UV-exposed sites as well as to cold environments (Dieser et al. 2010). Dieser et al. (2010) linked the carotenoid pigmentation in Antarctic heterotrophic bacteria to their strategy to withstand environmental stresses; they found that after 2 h of solar radiation exposure, 61% of the pigmented organisms survived versus 0.01% for the nonpigmented isolates. However, the literature is not solely consistent and unambiguous. Agogue et al. (2005) drew the opposite conclusion; pigmented strains are not more resistant to solar radiation than nonpigmented bacteria. They isolated similar percentages (43%–48%) of pigmented strains from the surface microlayer, underlying waters, and both layers. The majority of pigmented strains (53%) had a medium resistance, but pigmented strains had a smaller relative contribution (10%) to the highly resistant class than nonpigmented strains (33%). Among the sensitive and weakly resistant strains, pigmented and nonpigmented strains were equally distributed. That different reports reach different conclusions is not directly surprising and there could be many reasons for that, for example, focus on different pigments groups with various light-protecting properties, season variation, sampling from different sites and habitats, and different cultivation conditions in the laboratories performing the microbial testing.

Some antibiotic producers are pigmented per se, but the color can also be due to another secondary metabolite produced by the same host. *Streptomyces coelicolor*, a well-known secondary metabolite producer, harbors more than 20 secondary metabolite gene clusters in its genome (Bentley et al. 2002). Of those few antibiotics that are usually produced by *S. coelicolor*, some are colored (actinorhodin and undecylprodigiosin) while others are not (calcium-dependent antibiotic). Thus, studies based on colony inspection and/or crude extracts should be separated from studies on purified compounds. Several studies on *Pseudoalteromonas tunicata* and other PHB revealed close association between bioactivity and pigmentation (Lichstein and van de Sand 1945; Hermansson et al. 1987; Holmström et al. 1996; Egan et al. 2002; Vynne et al. 2011). Nair and Simidu tested a total of 726 strains for antibacterial activity (Nair and Simidu 1987). Thirty percent of the 54 bioactive-producing isolates were pigmented. Cetina et al. observed that only 15% of the pigmented strains exhibited antibacterial activity, but did not investigate how many of the nonpigmented strains had antibacterial activity (Cetina et al. 2010). Vynne et al. (2011) extracted the pigment of antimicrobial strains and tested their inhibitory effect against *Vibrio anguillarum* and found that they had no inhibitory effect. Hence the pigments, in general, should not be linked to the antibacterial activity before tested as purified compound and preferentially with complete structure being elucidated. Holmström et al. found pigmented surface-associated bacteria that were effective in the inhibition of the settlement of various fouling invertebrates and algae (Holmström et al. 2002). Based on subsequent analyses, they found that pigmented *Pseudoalteromonas* species possess a broad range of bioactivity associated with the secretion of extracellular compounds, which is in agreement with studies by Bowman (Bowman 2007). The correlation between pigmentation and inhibitory activity was also reported in an earlier study by Holmström (Holmström et al. 1996). Twenty-two out of the twenty-four dark pigmented bacterial strains that were tested against the settlement of two fouling organisms showed inhibition. Given that the production of pigment(s) is dependent on the specific nutrients that are available, it may be speculated that the host organisms induce the bacterially mediated protection against biofouling by altering the release of compounds utilized by the surface-associated bacteria.

Furthermore, a correlation between pigmentation and increased metal tolerance has been forwarded. The pigments might function as complexation agents and Hermansson et al. (1987) observed increased resistance to mercury among pigmented strains tested. Other studies support these findings (Nair et al. 1992). The higher incidence of pigmentation, mercury, and drug resistance and, possibly, plasmids in bacteria of the surface microlayers than in the subsurface microflora suggests that the interface bacteria display a range of characteristics in response to the selective pressures that operate in this habitat.

In general, if one is to affiliate some general roles of the pigments for MHB, one can conclude that pigments are produced to provide an adaption to environmental conditions and provide defense against predators (Bhatnagar and Kim 2010).

9.3.2 Pigment Groups

9.3.2.1 Carotenoids

Carotenoids are a large group of pigments found in bacteria, fungi, plants, and animals. They are responsible for most natural red, orange, and yellow coloration in many biological systems. Approximately 750 natural carotenoids have so far been found (Britton et al. 2004). Although best known as auxiliary components of the photosynthetic light-harvesting apparatus, many carotenoids are also produced by non-photosynthetic heterotrophic bacteria and fungi (Krinsky 1998; Klassen and Foght 2008). Thus, they are generally regarded as the dominant group of pigments in MHB.

Carotenoids are divided in two groups, carotenes and xanthophylls, where the latter are carotenoids containing –OH groups. Most carotenoids have a C_{40} skeleton made from isoprenoid precursors, but many C_{30} and C_{50} carotenoids have also been identified. Different structural end groups (e.g., cyclization, glycosylation, acetylation) give further variation. More on the diversity of carotenoid can be found in the book series *Carotenoids: Handbook* (Britton et al. 2004). Carotenoids absorb light most efficiently in the 400–500 nm range. Most carotenoids have absorption spectrum that does not appear as a single band but shows three more or less distinct peaks. This is known as the vibrational fine structure. It is seen to various extents with different carotenoids and provides an important diagnostic element. By examining the spectral fine structure, it should be possible to deduce the probable chromophore of an unknown carotenoid. Conjugated ketocarotenoids give in general no fine spectrum, thus only one λ max peak (e.g., astaxanthin, cantaxanthin).

Certain microorganisms produce carotenoids with structural characteristics very different from those commonly found in foods, such as a higher number of carbon atoms, of conjugated double bounds and of hydroxyl groups, which all contribute to their great antioxidant capacity (Osawa et al. 2010). The carotenoids produced by marine bacteria do not differ significantly from terrestrial bacteria, the main characteristics being a comparative lack of carotenes, synthesis of xanthophyll compounds, and inability to synthesize lutein (Courington and Goodwin 1955). Many bacteria that have been isolated from marine environments can synthesize a variety of carotenoid pigments. Acetylenic carotenoids appear to be restricted to aquatic, including marine, environments (Liaaen-Jensen 1991). For example, acyclic C_{30}-type carotenoic acids were identified in some marine bacteria such as *Planococcus maritimus* and *Rubritalea squalenifaciens* (Misawa 2011). C_{50}-carotenoids are frequently found in halophile bacteria and are found to play a role in both membrane stabilization and protection against oxidizing agents; thus these compounds are essential for the survival of such extremophile microorganisms (Mandelli et al. 2011). The commercial interesting carotenoid astaxanthin has been found to be produced in several marine bacteria, for example, *Paracoccus haeundaensis*, *Altererythrobacter ishigakiensis*, and *Agrobacterium arantiacum* (Yokoyama et al. 1995; Lee et al. 2004; Matsumoto et al. 2011).

The antioxidant properties of carotenoids are dependent on their chemical structure, including aspects such as the number of conjugated double bounds, type of structural end groups, and oxygen-containing substituents (Britton 1995; Albrecht et al. 2000). The carotenoids are efficient scavengers of reactive nitrogen species; ROS, especially of singlet oxygen species; and nonbiological radicals (Chew and Park 2004; Liu and Nizet 2009).

9.3.2.2 Phenazine Compounds

Phenazines are crystalline tricyclic compounds that constitute a large group of nitrogen-containing heterocyclic compounds. The color of phenazines ranges from yellow to orange (Gerber 1969a). Presently, biosynthesis of phenazines is only known in bacteria, and it seems to be frequently distributed among a diverse range of bacteria. Many phenazine-producing bacteria are commonly found associated with host organisms. Today, more than 100 natural and biologically active (antibacterial, antifungal, antiviral, antitumor) phenazines, synthesized mainly by *Pseudomonas* and *Streptomyces* species, are known (Schneemann et al. 2011). Different marine *Streptomyces* spp. are known for production of various phenazine structures (Pusecker et al. 1997); in contrast the only known phenazine-producing *Pseudomonas* species isolated from marine habitats is *Pseudomonas aeruginosa* (Angell et al. 2006; Isnansetyo and Kamei 2009). Most studies on the production and biosynthetic pathways of the various phenazine pigments have been conducted with representatives of the fluorescent *Pseudomonas* genus, in particular with *P. aeruginosa*, which produces the blue pigment pyocyanin. Other marine phenazine producers can be found in the genera *Brevibacterium*, *Bacillus* and *Pelagibacter* (Choi et al. 2010), *Micromonospora*, *Kiloniella*, and *Pseudovibrio* (Schneemann et al. 2011). Phenazines have been used as chemical backbone for semisynthetic derivatization, and over 6000 compounds that contain phenazine as a central moiety have been described (Laursen and Nielsen 2004).

Bacteria often produce a wide range of phenazine compounds and they are believed to play multiple roles and contribute to the ecological fitness of the producing bacterium. Phenazines serve as electron shuttles altering electron flow patterns, modify cellular redox states, act as cell signals that regulate patterns of gene expression, contribute to biofilm formation, and enhance bacterial survival (Pierson and Pierson 2010).

9.3.2.3 Prodiginines

Prodigiosin synthesis in different bacteria was described already in 1964 (Lewis and Corpe 1964), while the first isolation of the pigment was reported in 1975 (Gerber 1975). This was isolated from the ubiquitous bacterium *Serratia marcescens*, but later several other prodigiosin producers have been identified: actinomycetes (*Streptomyces coelicolor* and *Streptomyces variegatus*) and specific marine bacteria, *Hahella chejuensis*, *Pseudoalteromonas denitrificans*, *Zooshikella rubidus*, various *Vibrio* species (Lee et al. 2011), and *Alteromonas denitrificans* (Enger et al. 1987). Prodigiosin has a strong absorption maximum at 535 nm and a shoulder at about 510 nm and is member of the pigment group prodiginines, which share a common pyrrolyldipyrromethene core structure (Gerber 1969b). Several other compounds belonging to the prodiginines have been identified (e.g., magnesidins and marineosins) (Olano et al. 2009). Prodiginines have a wide variety of biological properties, including antibacterial, antifungal, antimalarial, antibiotic, immunosuppressive, and anticancer activities (Boric et al. 2011). Prodiginines are known as potent algicidal components, as for *Hahella chejuensis*, suggesting that the extracellular algicidal compounds might be used as a biological control agent in natural seawaters. Completely purified prodigiosin was found to have a significant algicidal activity against *Cochlodinium polykrikoides* even at low concentrations as 10.3 mg/L (10 ppb) (Kim 2008). Boric et al. showed the UV-protective abilities of prodigiosin for the first time as they compared prodigiosin-producing and nonproducing *Vibrio* strains. Pigmented cells survived high UV exposure (324 J/m^2) around 1000-fold more successfully compared to the nonpigmented mutant cells (Boric et al. 2011).

9.3.2.4 Tambjamines

Tambjamines are yellow alkaloids that have been isolated from marine bacteria and invertebrates including bryozoans, nudibranchs, and ascidians. Most evidence points to bacteria, colonizing the surface of higher organisms, as the source of these compounds when isolated from invertebrate samples (Bowman 2007). A member of the tambjamine pigment has been isolated from the marine bacteria *Pseudoalteromonas tunicata* (Franks et al. 2005). A common structural feature is a 2,2′-bipyrrole ring system containing an enamine moiety at the C_2 position of the pyrrole ring and an adjacent methoxy group at C_3 that may contain a bromine atom. The enamine nitrogen is normally substituted with a two to four carbon-saturated alkyl chain. Other members of this class, which include tri- and tetrapyrrole compounds, possess a range of biological activities including antimicrobial, antitumor, and immunosuppressive activities (Kojiri et al. 1993; Franks et al. 2005). Tambjamines possess antifungal, antimicrobial, antitumorigenic, immunosuppressive, anti-proliferation, and ichthyodeterrent activities and are likely produced as natural defensive compounds against predators (Blackman and Li 1994).

9.3.2.5 Melanins

Melanins are polyphenolic pigments synthesized by different organisms through all the phylogenetic scale, from bacteria to mammals. Melanins are a diverse group of pigments derived from the hydroxylation, oxidation, and polymerization of phenolic compounds. Several studies and reviews are available on the genetics, synthesis, properties, roles, and biomedical aspects of melanins in human and higher animals, but less is known about microbial melanins, and less still about melanins in marine microorganisms (Nosanchuk and Casadevall 2003). Several types of melanins have been described: eumelanins (black or brown), phaeomelanins (yellow–red), allomelanins, and pyomelanins (Liu and Nizet 2009). *Vibrio cholerae*, *Shewanella colwelliana*, and *Alteromonas nigrifaciens* were some of the first marine bacterial strains reported to produce melanin or melaninlike pigments (Soliev et al. 2011). *Cellulophaga tyrosinoxydans* was reported to produce a yellow pigment suggested being a pheomelanin. Production of pyomelanin has been reported in many species of bacteria, like *P. aeruginosa*, *Hyphomonas* sp., *Shewanella colwelliana*, some of which consist of both pelagic and surface-attached pathogenic strains (Plonka and Grabacka 2006). *Streptomyces* strains isolated from marine environments share the characteristics of being able to synthesize melanins (Vasanthabharathi et al. 2011). Another important melanin-synthesizing bacterium is *Marinomonas mediterranea*, which is able to produce black eumelanin (Plonka and Grabacka 2006).

Melanins are reported to protect the producing organisms against several stress conditions such as high temperatures, starvation, or hyperosmotic media (Coyne and Al-Harthi 1992). Melanins can serve as energy transducers, bind diverse drugs and chemicals, and affect cellular integrity (Plonka and Grabacka 2006; Sanchez-Amat et al. 2010). The ability of certain microbes to produce melanin has been linked with virulence and pathogenicity for their respective animal or plant hosts (Nosanchuk and Casadevall 2003; Valeru et al. 2009). It has also been attributed a role in UV protection, to be able to chelate metal ions, to function as a physiological redox buffer, to provide structural rigidity to cell walls, and to help to store water and ions (Huang et al. 2011).

9.3.2.6 Violacein

The members of this pigment group are indole derivatives and represent a wide range of colors: light violet, dark violet, almost black, and blue with a variety of biological activities. It has predominantly been isolated from bacteria of the genus *Chromobacterium* and *Janthinobacterium* that inhabit the soil and water of tropical and subtropical areas, but Hakvåg et al. (2009) report a violacein-producing *Collimonas* sp. isolated from the neuston layer of the Norwegian Trondheimsfjord. Despite that the *Collimonas* bacteria were isolated from marine samples, the isolates showed inhibited (or no) growth on seawater-containing media. Violacein has earlier been found in bacteria isolated from marine environment, and this might suggest that the *Collimonas* are growing as biofilm in the tidal zone of brackish water or in soils/freshwater and had been washed out into the sea not long before sampling. Several strains of violacein-producing *Pseudoalteromonas luteoviolacea* were isolated from Kinko Bay in Japan (Kobayashi et al. 2007). It has also been isolated from the surface of a marine sponge (Yada et al. 2008).

Violacein has been demonstrated to possess strong antioxidant properties, and it can protect lipid membranes from peroxidation caused by hydroxyl radicals. Violacein has potent antimicrobial activity against many bacteria and protozoa. Hence, secretion of this pigment might protect against protozoal predation (Matz et al. 2004) and promote survival of *C. violaceum* in the environment (Liu and Nizet 2009). Due to its very low aqueous solubility, violacein probably protects against predation rather than acts as a true antibiotic, and it has been shown to induce cell death in grazing organisms (Matz et al. 2004).

9.3.2.7 Other Pigments

Xanthomonadines are a unique class of carotenoid-like pigments produced by members of the phytopathogenic genus *Xanthomonas* (Starr et al. 1977). These pigments are brominated, aryl-polyene, yellow, water-insoluble pigments that are associated exclusively with the outer membrane of the bacterial cell wall. The absorption spectra of xanthomonadines look like a typical carotenoid absorption specter with three maximums (425, 440, 480 nm) and is therefore not easily distinguished by HPLC-DAD but also requires the mass spectrometric analysis. Gauthier reported isolation of *Xanthomonas* in marine habitats (Gauthier 1969). Also Stafsnes et al. (2010) identified a yellow *Xanthomonas* sp. from the marine environment, but the pigments produced were not identified. So xanthomonadines have not been positively identified in true marine bacteria yet. A possible correlation of xanthomonadine production and UV protection in bacteriahas been investigated, but no positive correlation was found (Poplawsky et al. 2000).

Flexirubin-type pigments are yellow to orange pigments consisting of a ω-phenyloctaenic acid chromophore esterified with resorcinol carrying two hydrocarbon chains. Their chemical structures are characterized by non-isoprenoid ω-phenyl-substituted polyene carboxylic acids (Reichenbach et al. 1974). This basic chemical structure may be modified by variation of the length and branching of the hydrocarbon chains on the resorcinol and by the introduction of additional substituents on the omega-phenyl ring, specifically methyl and chlorine; actually, for all pigment species, chlorinated counterparts are found in every flexirubin-producing organism. In this way, a large variety of different flexirubin-type pigments arise, and one single strain may synthesize more than 25 different compounds. They are so far only found in bacteria belonging to *Cytophagales* and in true *Flavobacteria* (Reichenbach et al. 1980; Achenbach et al. 1981; Reichenbach 2006). However, not all *Cytophagales* contain flexirubin-type pigments, and even closely related species, and perhaps even strains of the same species, may differ in that respect (Reichenbach 2006). The presence of flexirubin in *Flavobacteria* from soil and freshwater samples is nearly regarded as a taxonomic marker, but marine isolate usually does not produce these pigments (Reichenbach et al. 1980). The yellow pigmentation of marine isolates is mostly attributed to carotenoids (zeaxanthin) (Reichenbach 2006). However, the simple flexirubin test developed by Fautz and Reichenbach (1980) continues to be performed when characterizing marine pigments from the *Flavobacteriaceae* family (Brettar et al. 2004; Nedashkovskaya et al. 2005; Oh et al. 2009; Choi et al. 2011). The marine bacterium *Cytophaga uliginosa* (Bowman 2000) and members of the genus *Zobellia* (Nedashkovskaya et al. 2004) were positive for flexirubin. In contrast to carotenoid production is the synthesis of the flexirubins, light independent but dependent on nutrient conditions as high phosphate content and a low pH appeared to reduce pigment synthesis (Reichenbach et al. 1974). Flexirubin has been proven to be located in the outer membrane of *Flexibacter*, and the concentration was found to be about 10 times as high as the phospholipid content in the outer membrane of ordinary Gram-negative bacteria. Thus it is unlikely that flexirubin functions as photoprotective compound or is involved in the respiratory chain. Their presence and high concentration in the outer membrane suggests that they may have a structural function (Irschik and Reichenbach 1978).

Quinones are yellow to red compounds with an aromatic ring structure that exhibit antiviral, anti-infective, antimicrobial, insecticidal, and anticancer activities (Margalith 1992). *Streptomycetes* spp. are especially frequent producers of biologically highly active quinones. The yellow 2-methyl-pyrimidine-5-carboxamide has been isolated from another unidentified marine bacterium (Laatsch 2006). When faced with a perceived enemy, some *Roseobacter* strains synthesize the quinine compound indigoidine, a blue compound that acts as an antibacterial agent, preventing the other bacterium from growing and potentially outcompeting *Roseobacter*. Indigoidine could be one of the reasons that some *Roseobacter* strains are so adept at colonization. Kobayashi purified a new violet pigment derived from *Shewanella violacea* DSS12, which was identified as 5,5'-didodecylamino-4,4'-dihydroxy-3,3'-diazodiphenoquinone-(2,2'), containing the same chromophore as indigoidine known as microbial blue pigment (Kobayashi et al. 2007).

Bromoalterochromide A and B are pigments produced by an epibiotic bacterial strain *Pseudoalteromonas maricaloris* KMM 636T, isolated from the Great Barrier Reef sponge *Fascaplysinopsis reticulata* (Speitling et al. 2007; Vynne et al. 2011). The UV/Vis spectrum of the pigments was unusual, showing only an absorption maximum at λ_{max} 395 nm with a tailing into the visible region. They showed moderate cytotoxicity to the eggs of the sea urchin *Strongylocentrotus intermedius*. Pigments were not produced in liquid cultures in the laboratory, only on agar plates. *Pseudomonas aurantiaca, Pseudoalteromonas prydzensis, Pseudoalteromonas rubra*, and *Pseudoalteromonas flavipulchra* are other species of the *Pseudoalteromonas* genus that have been identified as bromoalterochromide producers (Vynne 2011).

Glaukothalin is a deep blue pigment isolated from two pelagic *Rheinheimera* strains isolated from the German Wadden Sea and from Øresund, Denmark (Grossart et al. 2009). The molecule is highly symmetrically and consists of two heterocyclic halves to which aliphatic side chains are attached. The UV spectrum of glaukothalin exhibits characteristic absorption maxima at 636 nm, and antibacterial cytotoxic activities have been linked to this molecule.

Tetrabromopyrrole was identified in four bacterial *Pseudoalteromonas* strains as responsible for inducing larval metamorphosis (Tebben et al. 2011). The yellow pigment has also been found to be antibacterial acting on a group of bacteria, including the producing organism (Andersen et al. 1974).

In conclusion, many pigments have already been characterized, some uniquely produced by MHB but many also by other organisms. It is very likely that more members and even new pigment groups will be discovered during the search for bioactive compounds in marine bacteria as improvement in extraction and purification methods as well as analytical instrumentation permits the efficient isolation of minor agents in the fermentation broth and the efficient elucidation of new chemical structures.

9.4 Isolation and Identification of Pigments

One advantage with heterotrophic bacteria is their ease of cultivation. There is no seasonal harvest and biomass production can easily be scaled up for purification, structure elucidation, and bioactivity testing purposes. However, care must be taken when designing medium and incubation conditions as pigmentation is heavily dependent upon growth conditions. It can therefore be advisable to run preliminary experimentation to establish optimal pigment production by varying temperature, richness/poorness of medium, osmolarity, light exposure conditions, etc. Initial stages in isolation of PHB usually are conducted on solid medium, which makes it possible to visually evaluate the pigment production. It is also easy to observe on solid medium if the pigment is retained inside the cells or is excreted and diffused out into the agar, thereby making it possible for an early decision if this could be a pigment with potential interesting properties. However, production of biomass for purification of pigment is most conveniently carried out in liquid culture, which easily can be scaled up to tens of liters in benchtop bioreactors. A standard growth medium can be easily designed to support cell densities up to 50 g dry weight per liter, implying that total biomass yields of hundreds of grams to kilogram are possible to obtain in a routine microbiology laboratory. If the fresh culture is not going to be used immediately, it is recommended to separate cells and supernatant by centrifugation and store them separately below −20°C, preferentially −80°C, or alternatively remove the water by lyophilization. The lyophilizated samples should also be stored cold and in darkness.

9.4.1 Extraction

The first step in isolating pigments is the extraction step. As a general precaution it is advisable to work under conditions with minimized exposure to oxygen, light, heat, and acidic/alkaline conditions since the pigments can be unstable, especially after extracted from the biomass. Pigmentation greatly eases isolation as it makes monitoring of the purification process possible, and it is easy to follow the partition of the pigment during liquid–liquid extraction. Also, potential degradation is immediately observed during loss or change in color. Excreted pigments are most easily concentrated through lyophilization of culture supernatant and preferentially reconstituted in organic solvents to hinder resolution of proteins and other polymers. The extraction step should be regarded also as an initial fractionation step as this can make the following purification steps simpler. Water-soluble pigments are readily amenable to further purification steps, but they can form strong complexes, for example, with metal ions, and thereby complicate further isolation steps as seen for the actinorhodins (Bystrykh et al. 1996). Adding chelators to the extraction solvent might help dissolve strong complexes. Usually extraction of bacterial biomass is executed with an appropriate organic solvent as methanol, acetone, dichloromethane, and chloroform, depending on the hydrophobicity of the pigment. An enzymatic treatment step to weaken the bacterial cell wall, especially Gram-positive bacteria, might be necessary in order to release the majority of pigments. Physical methods as ultrasound, French press, and bead homogenizer are also alternatives. DMSO is a frequently used extraction solvent and it has strong extraction capacities for a large number of compounds. It is therefore very popular in bioprospecting projects where the physicochemical properties of potential novel bioactive and pigmented compounds are unknown. However, due to its overall dissolving properties, the DMSO extracts will contain many contaminants that complicate the further isolation steps. DMSO has a high boiling point and it is therefore not easy to remove during concentrating steps (i.e., lyophilization, high-temperature vacuum drying) either. This property can also be detrimental on the ionization during LC-MS analysis (see next paragraph), and it is therefore advised to try other more volatile organic solvents as methanol and dichloromethane first.

9.4.2 High-Throughput Screening

Bioprospecting is frequently connected to high-throughput screening as a large number of isolates must be evaluated for identification of a potential novel lead. Many lead compounds are already described and use of resources to rediscover these are just waste of time and money. Therefore, technology to screen a large number of isolates is employed. Fast LC-MS is probably the most prominent tool for such a task as it is possible to screen a large number of samples, and it should be possible to rank and make a priority list of extracts containing potential interesting leads (Stafsnes et al. 2010). Especially the latest instrumental developments in ultrahigh-pressure liquid chromatography (UPLC) with increased resolution capacities make it possible to establish robust analysis down to and below 5 min, even including column regeneration when employing gradient elution. Therefore it should be possible to screen 50–100 isolates per day on a single instrument. This initial characterization step could also be connected to a fraction collection by splitting the eluent between the MS inlet and a fraction collector. Since MS detection is very sensitive, it is possible to split over 95% to the fraction collector. A fraction collection step is not necessary for pigment screening only, but if bioactivity testing is wanted, then parallel MS detection and fraction collection saves time. The LC-MS analysis of a pigmented extract must be optimized for the particular pigment group of interest. The reason is that many choices on both LC conditions and MS conditions must be made. The preferred choice of LC column stationary phase is reverse phase, but then the pigment structure must carry some nonpolar substructures that enable retainment on a reverse-phase column. Hydrophilic interaction chromatography (HILIC) is an alternative for highly charged and polar pigments (Jandera 2008; Cubbon et al. 2010). It is getting increasing attention in the metabolomics field, but it is not considered as robust as reverse phase, and it might not therefore be suitable, at least for high-throughput screening purposes. The usual mobile-phase constituents are water, methanol, acetonitrile, and dichloromethane (HILIC even though it is derivative of normal-phase chromatography works with water and acetonitrile gradients and can therefore be used to analyze highly charged and hydrophilic metabolites), and only volatile salts must be used as salt can have detrimental effect on the ionization, for example, ammonium hydroxide and acetic acid are preferentially used to adjust the pH of the mobile phase. High pH is used to ease negative ionization and, contrary, low pH for positive ionization. There are in particular two ionization sources of choice for LC-MS pigment analysis, that is, electrospray (ESI) and atmospheric pressure chemical ionization (APCI). ESI is considered the standard choice and should be tested first. APCI is a stronger ionization method and is used when ESI initially fails. For pigment identification, the diode array detection (DAD) is also a powerful instrumentation that supplies complimentary information to MS detection. The DAD is included in the LC-MS instrument between the LC column and the MS detector and before any flow splitting if fraction collection is performed. Actually, during LC-DAD-MS analysis of pigmented extracts, it is the DAD chromatogram that is inspected first, and this guides the evaluation of the MS chromatogram. This is exemplified in the following case that shows a 20 min reverse-phase LC-DAD-MS analysis of a methanol extract for a bacterial isolate in our culture collection of marine PHB, which is dominated by carotenoid-producing bacteria (Stafsnes et al. 2010). LC-MS analysis of carotenoids is usually performed with reverse-phase chromatography in conjunction with positive APCI (Rivera 2012). Xanthophylls are readily ionized by ESI, but the non-oxygenated carotenes need the stronger APCI source.

9.4.3 Worked Example to Characterize a PHB Extract by LC-MS

This example is taken from an analysis of a bacterial isolate from the Norwegian coastline, and it was assumed that the pigments belonged mainly to the carotenoid group (Stafsnes et al. 2010). The upper panel in Figure 9.1 shows the isoplot of the diode array chromatogram, and four major peaks are easily identified. The corresponding UV/Vis scan is shown in the lower panel of Figure 9.1. All four scans resemble strongly carotenoid absorption spectra with having three peak profiles. Many carotenoids have a one peak profile also, among them astaxanthin, and conclusion about chemical group cannot be drawn based on UV/Vis spectra only. The absorption properties are determined by the polyene structure of the carbon backbone, and other chemical groups have also polyene substructures, for example, macrolide antibiotics produced by polyketide synthases. There are extensive literature resources of physicochemical properties of carotenoids available, and they can be accessed for verification/hypothesis purposes (Britton et al. 2004; Roy et al. 2011). However, UV/Vis data are usually obtained in pure solvents, while the gradient elution in an LC-MS run might lead to λ_{max} that slightly deviates from literature data depending on mobile-phase composition at time of DAD recording. The total ion chromatogram (TIC) indicates the abundance of ionizable analytes, and there is clearly more compounds

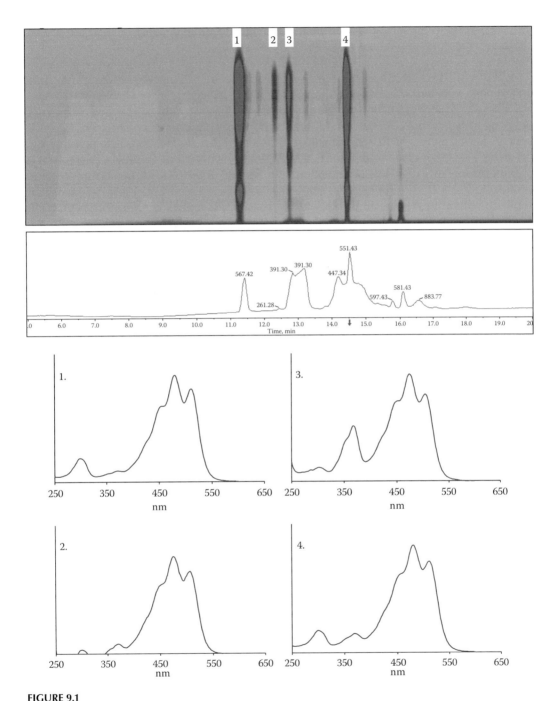

FIGURE 9.1
The results from an LC-DAD-MS analysis of a methanol extract of a MHB. The upper panel displays the DAD isoplot and the four most abundant pigments are numbered. The next panel shows the corresponding TIC from the ToF MS analysis. The lowest panel shows the UV/Vis spectra from the four pigments.

present in the extract than those that also exhibit UV/Vis absorption properties. Anyway, the DAD isoplot guides the interpretation of the TIC and assignment of potential masses (i.e., m/z) to the pigments. This can be a challenging task and usually there are several choices in the mass spectrum. This MS analysis is therefore preferentially performed on high mass accuracy and high-resolution MS detectors of time of flight (Tof), orbitrap, or FT-ICR types. The current analysis was performed on a Tof MS that enables routinely mass assignment with better accuracies than 3 ppm. This is sufficient for carotenoid analysis as a limited number of brutto formulas are probable. The MS analysis for peak 1 revealed only one potential mass (m/z 567.4198) that could correspond to a carotenoid of C_{40} backbone. A search on this brutto formula ($C_{40}H_{54}O_2$, accurate mass search is also possible, e.g., by using a ±5 ppm error window) in the Dictionary of Natural Products (http://www.chemnetbase.com/) reported 24 carotenoid hits. Several of the hits originate from the same carotenoid but with different stereochemistry. Peak 2 is interesting as the m/z 569.4337 ion show up with almost same abundance as the 567.4202. The peak is minor but is probably originating from two co-eluting carotenoids. Peak 3 could solely be associated with m/z 567 ion again. The increased absorption around 300 nm in the UV/Vis spectra of peak 3 gives an indication that this is the *cis* isomer of peak 1. The cis isomer could very likely be introduced during sample processing steps and therefore not be present in situ. Peak 4 can be associated with a carotenoid brutto formula with one less oxygen atom. It might be that this carotenoid is a precursor in the biosynthetic pathway to the carotenoid detected in peak 1 or it could be a branch off. Nevertheless, this example shows the resolving power of the LC-MS analysis and that much relevant information can be obtained in a fast and straightforward manner. Thus, this shows how far one obtains with LC-DAD-MS analysis and that the next step involves purification and NMR. Therefore, as indicated in Table 9.2, a number of different carotenoids with the same brutto formula have been identified, and the next step would be to purify enough (at least 10–50 mg is needed) for complete structural elucidation with NMR, circular dichroism, and other analytical techniques needed for stereochemical determination. For such applications there exist good commercial solutions for scaling up analytical LC conditions to preparative conditions. A 5 cm ID preparative column operating at 70–100 mL/min has capacity to load over 100 mg of compound, implying that enough material could be purified in a few run. However, subsequent purification employing other purification strategies might be needed, as non-UV-absorbing contaminants (e.g., lipids) quite often co-elute in such 1D LC fractionation. This is also seen in the TIC in Figure 9.1 as there clearly are analytes eluting at other time points than the four carotenoids.

TABLE 9.2

The Most Likely Masses That Can Be Correlated to the Pigments, Their Potential Brutto Formula, and Number of Hits in the Dictionary of Natural Products Database When Constraining the Search to Carotenoids

Compound	Measured Mass	Potential Brutto Formula	Accurate Mass	(M + H)⁺	ppm Error	#Hits in DNP
1	567.4198	$C_{40}H_{54}O_2$	566.4123	567.4196	0.3	24
2	567.4202	$C_{40}H_{54}O_2$	566.4123	567.4196	1.0	24
	569.4337	$C_{40}H_{56}O_2$	568.4280	569.4337	−2.8	61
3	567.4192	$C_{40}H_{54}O_2$	566.4123	567.4196	−0.8	24
4	551.4250	$C_{40}H_{54}O$	550.4175	551.4247	0.5	19

9.5 Concluding Remarks

Clearly, MHB make their contribution to coloring the Earth, especially along the yellow–orange–red color scale. The diversity in pigment structures and distribution among bacterial species is huge. Pigmented bacteria are especially present in the upper surface layer of the oceans. The physiological role of the pigmentation vary among the pigment groups, and even though they are not directly needed for cell growth, as cell material building blocks or functioning in energy generation, there must be an ecological beneficial role of maintaining and expressing the pigment-synthesizing potential. Pigments can have desirable bioactive properties, and culture collections of MHB are valuable sources for identifying and exploiting this potential.

Acknowledgment

This study was supported by a grant from the Norwegian Research Council.

References

Achenbach, H., W. Kohl, A. Böttger-Vetter, and H. Reichenbach. 1981. Untersuchungen an stoffwech-selprodukten von mikroorganismen,-XXII: Untersuchung der pigmente aus flavobacterium spec. stamm C12. *Tetrahedron* 37(3): 559–563.

Agogué, H., F. Joux, I. Obernosterer, and P. Lebaron. 2005. Resistance of marine bacterioneuston to solar radiation. *Appl. Environ. Microbiol.* 71(9): 5282–5289.

Alavandi, S. V. 1990. Relationship between heterotrophic bacteria and suspended particulate matter in the Arabian sea (Cochin). *Indian J. Mar. Sci.* 30: 89–92.

Albrecht, M., S. Takaichi, S. Steiger, Z.-Y. Wang, and G. Sandmann. 2000. Novel hydroxycarotenoids with improved antioxidative properties produced by gene combination in *Escherichia coli. Nat. Biotechnol.* 18(8): 843–846.

Amann, R., W. Ludwig, and K. H. Scheifer. 1995. Phylogenetic identification and in situ detection of individual microbial cells without cultivation. *Microbiol. Rev.* 59(1): 143–169.

Amon, R. M. W., H.-P. Fitznar, and R. Benner. 2001. Linkages among the bioreactivity, chemical composition, and diagenetic state of marine dissolved organic matter. *Limnol. Oceanogr.* 46(2): 287–297.

Andersen, R. J., M. S. Wolfe, and D. J. Faulkner. 1974. Autotoxic antibiotic production by a marine *Chromobacterium. Mar. Biol.* 27(4): 281–285.

Angell, S., B. J. Bench, H. Williams, and C. M. H. Watanabe. 2006. Pyocyanin isolated from a marine microbial population: Synergistic production between two distinct bacterial species and mode of action. *Chem. Biol.* 13(12): 1349–1359.

Appeltans, W., P. Bouchet, G. A. Boxshall et al. 2012. World register of marine species. http://www.marinespecies.org (accessed January 26, 2012).

Baumann, L., P. Baumann, M. Mandel, and R. D. Allen. 1972. Taxonomy of aerobic marine eubacteria. *J. Bacteriol.* 110(1): 402–429.

Bentley, S. D., K. F. Chater, A. M. Cerdemp-Tarraga et al. 2002. Complete genome sequence of the model actinomycete *Streptomyces coelicolor* A3(2). *Nature* 417(6885): 141–147.

Bhatnagar, I. and S. K. Kim. 2010. Immense essence of excellence: Marine microbial bioactive compounds. *Mar. Drugs* 8(10): 2673–2701.

Blackman, A. and C. Li. 1994. New tambjamine alkaloids from the marine bryozoan *Bugula dentata*. *Aust. J. Chem.* 47(8): 1625–1629.

Boric, M., T. Danevcic, and D. Stopar. 2011. Prodigiosin from *Vibrio* sp DSM 14379: A new UV-protective pigment. *Microbiol. Ecol.* 62(3): 528–536.

Bowman, J. P. 2000. Description of *Cellulophaga algicola* sp. nov., isolated from the surfaces of Antarctic algae, and reclassification of *Cytophaga uliginosa* (ZoBell and Upham 1944) Reichenbach 1989 as *Cellulophaga uliginosa* comb. nov. *Int. J. Syst. Evol. Microbiol.* 50(5): 1861–1868.

Bowman, J. P. 2007. Bioactive compound synthetic capacity and ecological significance of marine bacterial genus *Pseudoalteromonas*. *Mar. Drugs* 5(4): 220–241.

Brettar, I., R. Christen, and M. G. Höfle. 2004. *Belliella baltica* gen. nov., sp. nov., a novel marine bacterium of the Cytophaga–Flavobacterium–Bacteroides group isolated from surface water of the central Baltic Sea. *Int. J. Syst. Evol. Microbiol.* 54(1): 65–70.

Brinkhoff, T., H.-A. Giebel, and M. Simon. 2008. Diversity, ecology, and genomics of the *Roseobacter clade*: A short overview. *Arch. Microbiol.* 189(6): 531–539.

Britton, G. 1995. Structure and properties of carotenoids in relation to function. *FASEB J.* 9: 1551–1558.

Britton, G., S. Liaaen-Jensen, and H. Pfander. 2004. *Carotenoids—Handbook*. Birkhäuser Verlag, Basel, Switzerland.

Bruns, A., H. Cypionka, and J. Overmann. 2002. Cyclic AMP and acyl homoserine lactones increase the cultivation efficiency of heterotrophic bacteria from the Central Baltic Sea. *Appl. Environ. Microbiol.* 68(8): 3978–3987.

Bruns, A., H. Philipp, H. Cypionka, and T. Brinkhoff. 2003. *Aeromicrobium marinum* sp. nov., an abundant pelagic bacterium isolated from the German Wadden Sea. *Int. J. Syst. Evol. Microbiol.* 53(6): 1917–1923.

Bruns, A., M. Rohde, and L. Berthe-Corti. 2001. *Muricauda ruestringensis* gen. nov., sp. nov., a facultatively anaerobic, appendaged bacterium from German North Sea intertidal sediment. *Int. J. Syst. Evol. Microbiol.* 51(6): 1997–2006.

Buck, J. D. 1974. Effects of medium composition on the recovery of bacteria from sea water. *J. Exp. Mar. Biol. Ecol.* 15(1): 25–34.

Bystrykh, L. V., M. A. FernandezMoreno, J. K. Herrema, F. Malpartida, D. A. Hopwood, and L. Dijkhuizen. 1996. Production of actinorhodin-related 'blue pigments' by *Streptomyces coelicolor* A3(2). *J. Bacteriol.* 178(8): 2238–2244.

Cetina, A., A. Matos, G. Garma, H. Barba, R. Vázquez, A. Zepeda-Rodríguez, D. Jay, V. Monteón, and R. López-A. 2010. Antimicrobial activity of marine bacteria isolated from Gulf of Mexico. *Rev. Peru. Biol.* 17(2): 231–236.

Chan, E. C. S. and E. A. McManus. 1969. Distribution, characterization, and nutrition of marine microorganisms from the algae *Polysiphonia lanosa* and *Ascophyllum nodosum. Can. J. Microbiol.* 15(5): 409–420.

Chew, B. P. and J. S. Park. 2004. Carotenoid action on the immune response. *J. Nutr.* 134(1): 257S–261S.

Chin, Y.-W., M. J. Balunas, H. B. Chai, and A. D. Kinghorn. 2006. Drug discovery from natural sources. *AAPS J.* 8(2): E239–E253.

Choi, E. J., H. C. Kwon, J. Ham, and H. O. Yang. 2010. ChemInform abstract: 6-Hydroxymethyl-1-phenazine-carboxamide and 1,6-Phenazinedimethanol from a marine bacterium, *Brevibacterium* sp. KMD 003, associated with marine purple vase sponge. *ChemInform* 41(14): 1349–1359.

Choi, A., H.-M. Oh, S.-J. Yang, and J.-C. Cho. 2011. *Kordia periserrulae* sp. nov., isolated from a marine polychaete *Periserrula leucophryna*, and emended description of the genus *Kordia*. *Int. J. Syst. Evol. Microbiol.* 61(4): 864–869.

Christner, B. C., E. Mosley-Thompson, and L. G. Thompson. 2000. Recovery and identification of viable bacteria immured in glacial ice. *Icarus* 144(2): 479–485.

Courington, D. P. and T. W. Goodwin. 1955. A survey of pigments of a number of chromogenic marine bacteria, with special reference to the carotenoids. *J. Bacteriol.* 70(5): 568–571.

Coyne, V. E. and L. Al-Harthi. 1992. Induction of melanin biosynthesis in *Vibrio cholerae. Appl. Environ. Microbiol.* 58(9): 2861–2865.

Cubbon, S., C. Antonio, J. Wilson, and J. Thomas-Oates. 2010. Metabolomic applications of HILIC-LC-MS. *Mass Spectrom. Rev.* 29(5): 671–684.

Das, S., P. S. Lyla, and S. A. Khan. 2006. Marine microbial diversity and ecology: Importance and future perspectives. *Curr. Sci.* 90(10): 1325–1335.

Das, S., P. S. Lyla, and S. A. Khan. 2007. A simple scheme for the identification of marine heterotrophic bacteria. *Thalassas* 23(2): 17–21.

DeLong, E. F., D. G. Franks, and A. L. Alldredge. 1993. Phylogenetic diversity of aggregate-attached vs. free-living marine bacterial assemblages. *Limnol. Oceanogr.* 38(5): 924–934.

Dieckmann, R., I. Graeber, I. Kaesler, U. Szewzyk, and H. von Döhren. 2005. Rapid screening and dereplication of bacterial isolates from marine sponges of the sula ridge by intact-cell-MALDI-TOF mass spectrometry (ICM-MS). *Appl. Microbiol. Biotechnol.* 67: 539–548.

Dieser, M., M. Greenwood, and C. M. Foreman. 2010. Carotenoid pigmentation in Antarctic heterotrophic bacteria as a strategy to withstand environmental stresses. *Arct. Antarct. Alp. Res.* 42(4): 396–405.

Du, H. L., N. Z. Jiao, Y. H. Hu, and Y. H. Zeng. 2006. Diversity and distribution of pigmented heterotrophic bacteria in marine environments. *FEMS Microbiol. Ecol.* 57(1): 92–105.

Dufosse, L. 2006. Microbial production of food grade pigments. *Food Technol. Biotechnol.* 44(3): 313–321.

Egan, S., S. James, C. Holmström, and S. Kjelleberg. 2002. Correlation between pigmentation and antifouling compounds produced by *Pseudoalteromonas tunicata. Environ. Microbiol.* 4(8): 433–442.

Egan, S., T. Thomas, and S. Kjelleberg. 2008. Unlocking the diversity and biotechnological potential of marine surface associated microbial communities. *Curr. Opin. Microbiol.* 11(3): 219–225.

Enger, Ø., H. Nygaard, M. Solberg, G. Schei, J. Nielsen, and I. Dundas. 1987. Characterization of *Alteromonas denitrijicans* sp. nov. *Int. J. Syst. Bacteriol.* 37(4): 416–421.

Fautz, E. and H. Reichenbach. 1980. A simple test for flexirubin-type pigments. *FEMS Microbiol. Lett.* 8(2): 87–91.

Fenical, W. 1993. Chemical studies of marine bacteria: Developing a new resource. *Chem. Rev.* 93(5): 1673–1683.

Franks, A., P. Haywood, C. Holmstöm, S. Egan, S. Kjelleberg, and N. Kumar. 2005. Isolation and structure elucidation of a novel yellow pigment from the marine bacterium *Pseudoalteromonas tunicata. Molecules* 10(10): 1286–1291.

Fry, J. C. 1990. Direct methods and biomass estimation. *Methods Microbiol.* 22(C): 41–85.

Gauthier, M. J. 1969. Substances antibacteriennes produits par les bacteries marines. I, étude systématique de l'activité antagoniste de souches bactériennes marines, vis-á-vis de germes telluri ques aerobios. *Rev. Int. Ocean. Méd.* 15–16: 41–61.

Gerber, N. N. 1969a. New microbial phenazines. *J. Heterocycl. Chem.* 6(3): 297–300.

Gerber, N. N. 1969b. Prodigiosin-like pigments from *Actinomadura (Nocardia) pelletieri* and *Actinomadura madurae. Appl. Microbiol.* 18(1): 1–3.

Gerber, N. N. 1975. Prodigiosin-like pigments. *Crit. Rev. Microbiol.* 3(4): 469–485.

Gerdts, G. and G. Luedke. 2006. FISH and chips: Marine bacterial communities analyzed by flow cytometry based on microfluidics. *J. Microbiol. Methods* 64(2): 232–240.

Goodfellow, M. and J. A. Haynes. 1984. Actinomycetes in marine sediments. In *Biological, Biochemical and Biomedical Aspects of Actinomycetes.* Eds. L. Oritz-Oritz, L. F. Bojalil, and V. Yakoleff. Academic Press, London, U.K.

Goodwin, T. W. 1980. *The Biochemistry of the Carotenoids.* Chapman & Hall, Ltd, London, U.K.

Grossart, H.-P., M. Thorwest, I. Plitzko, T. Brinkhoff, M. Simon, and A. Zeeck. 2009. Production of a blue pigment (Glaukothalin) by marine *Rheinheimera* spp. *Int. J. Microbiol.* 2009: 1–7.

Hakvåg, S., E. Fjærvik, G. Klinkenberg, S. E. F. Borgos, K. D. Josefsen, T. E. Ellingsen, and S. B. Zotchev. 2009. Violacein-producing *Collimonas* sp. from the sea surface microlayer of costal waters in Trøndelag, Norway. *Mar. Drugs* 7: 576–588.

Hazen, T. C., E. A. Dubinsky, T. Z. DeSantis et al. 2010. Deep-sea oil plume enriches indigenous oil-degrading bacteria. *Science* 330(6001): 204–208.

Helmke, E. and H. Weyland. 1984. *Rhodococcus marinonascens* sp. nov., an actinomycete from the sea. *Int. J. Syst. Bacteriol.* 34(2): 127–138.

Hermansson, M., G. W. Jones, and S. Kjelleberg. 1987. Frequency of antibiotic and heavy metal resistance, pigmentation, and plasmids in bacteria of the marine air-water interface. *Appl. Environ. Microbiol.* 53(10): 2338–2342.

Hindré, T., S. Didelot, J.-P. Le Pennec, D. Haras, A. Dufour, and K. Vallée-Réhel. 2003. Bacteriocin detection from whole bacteria by matrix-assisted laser desorption ionization-time of flight mass spectrometry. *Appl. Environ. Microbiol.* 69(2): 1051–1058.

Holmström, C., S. Egan, A. Franks, S. McCloy, and S. Kjelleberg. 2002. Antifouling activities expressed by marine surface associated *Pseudoalteromonas* species. *FEMS Microbiol. Ecol.* 41(1): 47–58.

Holmström, C., S. James, S. Egan, and S. Kjelleberg. 1996. Inhibition of common fouling organisms by marine bacterial isolates ith special reference to the role of pigmented bacteria. *Biofouling* 10(1–3): 251–259.

Holmström, C. and S. Kjelleberg. 1999. Marine *Pseudoalteromonas* species are associated with higher organisms and produce biologically active extracellular agents. *FEMS Microbiol. Ecol.* 30(4): 285–293.

Huang, S., Y. Pan, D. Gan, X. Ouyang, S. Tang, S. Ekunwe, and H. Wang. 2011. Antioxidant activities and UV-protective properties of melanin from the berry of *Cinnamomum burmannii* and *Osmanthus fragrans*. *Med. Chem. Res.* 20(4): 475–481.

Hube, A. E., B. Heyduck-Söller, and U. Fischer. 2009. Phylogenetic classification of heterotrophic bacteria associated with filamentous marine cyanobacteria in culture. *Syst. Appl. Microbiol.* 32(4): 256–265.

Irschik, H. and H. Reichenbach. 1978. Intracellular location of flexirubins in *Flexibacter elegans* (cytophagales). *Biochim. Biophys. Acta (BBA)—Biomembr.* 510(1): 1–10.

Isnansetyo, A. and Y. Kamei. 2009. Bioactive substances produced by marine isolates of *Pseudomonas*. *J. Ind. Microbiol. Biotechnol.* 36(10): 1239–1248.

Jandera, P. 2008. Stationary phases for hydrophilic interaction chromatography, their characterization and implementation into multidimensional chromatography concepts. *J. Sep. Sci.* 31(9): 1421–1437.

Jensen, P. R. and W. Fenical. 1995. The relative abundance and seawater requirements of gram-positive bacteria in near-shore tropical marine samples. *Microbiol. Ecol.* 29(3): 249–257.

Jensen, P. R. and W. Fenical. 1996. Marine bacterial diversity as a resource for novel microbial products. *J. Ind. Microbiol. Biotechnol.* 17(5–6): 346–351.

Jones, K. L. 1946. Further notes on variation in certain *Saprophytic actinomycetes*. *J. Bacteriol.* 51(2): 211–216.

Karner, M. B., E. F. DeLong, and D. M. Karl. 2001. Archaeal dominance in the mesopelagic zone of the Pacific Ocean. *Nature* 409(6819): 507–510.

Kennedy, J., J. Marchesi, and A. Dubson. 2008. Marine metagenomics: Strategies for the discovery of novel enzymes with biotechnologcal applications from marine environments. *Microb. Cell Fact.* 7(1): 27.

Kim, D., J. Kim, J. H. Yim, S. K. Kwon, C. H. Lee, and H. K. Lee. 2008. Red to red—The marine bacterium *Hahella chejuensis* and its product prodigiosin for mitigation of harmful algal blooms. *J. Microbiol. Biotechnol.* 18(10): 1621–1629.

Klassen, J. L. and J. M. Foght. 2008. Differences in carotenoid composition among hymenobacter and related strains support a tree-like model of carotenoid evolution. *Appl. Environ. Microbiol.* 74(7): 2016–2022.

Kobayashi, H., Y. Nogi, and K. Horikoshi. 2007. New violet 3,3'-bipyridyl pigment purified from deep-sea microorganism *Shewanella violacea* DSS12. *Extremophiles* 11(2): 245–250.

Kojiri, K., S. Nakajima, H. Suzuki, A. Okura, and H. Suda. 1993. A new antitumor substance, BE-18591, produced by a streptomycete. 1. Fermentation, isolation, physico-chemical and biological properties. *J. Antibiot.* 46(12): 1799–1803.

Krinsky, N. I. 1998. The antioxidant and biological properties of the carotenoids. *Ann. NY Acad. Sci.* 854(1): 443–447.

Laatsch, H. 2006. Marine bacterial metabolites. In *Frontiers in Marine Biotechnology.* Eds. P. Proksch and W. E. G. Müller. Horizon Bioscience, Norfolk, U.K.

Laursen, J. B. and J. Nielsen. 2004. Phenazine natural products: Biosynthesis, synthetic analogues, and biological activity. *Chem. Rev.* 104(3): 1663.

Lay, Jr. J. O. 2000. MALDI-TOF mass spectrometry and bacterial taxonomy. *TrAC Trends Anal. Chem.* 19(8): 507–516.

Lee, J. H., Y.-S. Kim, T.-J. Choi, W. J. Lee, and Y. T. Kim. 2004. *Paracoccus haeundaensis* sp. nov., a gram-negative, halophilic, astaxanthin-producing bacterium. *Int. J. Syst. Evol. Microbiol.* 54(5): 1699–1702.

Lee, J. S., Y.-S. Kim, S. Park, J. Kim, S.-J. Kang, M.-H. Lee, S. Ruy, J. M. Choi, T.-K. Oh, and J.-H. Yoon. 2011. Exceptional production of both prodigiosin and cycloprodigiosin as major metabolic constituents by a novel marine bacterium, *Zooshikella rubidus* S1–1. *Appl. Environ. Microbiol.* 77(14): 4967–4973.

Lee, Y. K., K.-K. Kwon, K. H. Cho, H. W. Kim, J. H. Park, and H. K. Lee. 2003. Culture and identification of bacteria from marine biofilms. *J. Microbiol.* 41(3): 183–188.

Lewin, R. A. 1997. *Saprospira grandis*: A flexibacterium that can catch bacterial prey by "Ixotrophy." *Microbiol. Ecol.* 34(3): 232–236.

Lewis, S. M. and W. A. Corpe. 1964. Prodigiosin-producing bacteria from marine sources. *Appl. Microbiol. Biotechnol.* 12(1): 13–17.

Liaaen-Jensen, S. 1991. Marine carotenoids: Recent progress. *Pure Appl. Chem.* 63(1): 1–12.

Lichstein, H. C. and V. F. van de Sand. 1945. Violacein, an antibiotic pigment produced by *Chromobacterium violaceum. J. Infect. Dis.* 76: 47–51.

Liu, H., Z. Du, J. Wand, and R. Yang. 2007. Universal sample preparation method for characterization of bacteria by matrix-assisted laser desorption ionization-time of flight mass spectrometry. *Appl. Environ. Microbiol.* 73(6): 1899–1907.

Liu, G. Y. and V. Nizet. 2009. Color me bad: Microbial pigments as virulence factors. *Trends Microbiol.* 17(9): 406–413.

Lu, X., X. Liu, C. Long, G. Wang, Y. Gao, J. Liu, and B. Jiao. 2011. A preliminary study of the microbial resources and their biological activities of the East China Sea. *Evid.-Based Complement. Alternat. Med.* 2011: 1–8.

Mandelli, F., V. Miranda, E. Rodrigues, and A. Mercadante. 2011. Identification of carotenoids with high antioxidant capacity produced by extremophile microorganisms. *World J. Microbiol. Biotechnol.* 28(4): 1781–1790.

Margalith, P. Z. 1992. *Pigment Microbiology.* Chapman & Hall, London, U.K.

Maskey, R., I. Kock, E. Helmke, and H. Laatsch. 2003. Isolation and structure determination of phenazostatin D, a new phenazine from a marine actinomycete isolate *Pseudonocardia* sp. B6273. *Zeitschrift fur Naturforschung Section b-a J. Chem. Sci.* 58: 692–694.

Matsumoto, M., D. Iwama, A. Arakaki, A. Tanaka, T. Tanaka, H. Miyashita, and T. Matsunaga. 2011. *Altererythrobacter ishigakiensis* sp. nov., an astaxanthin-producing bacterium isolated from marine sediments. *Int. J. Syst. Evol. Microbiol.* 61(12): 2956–2961.

Matz, C., P. Deines, J. Boenigt, H. Arndt, L. Eberl, S. Kjelleberg, and K. Jürgens. 2004. Impact of violacein-producing bacteria on survival and feeding of bacterivorous nanoflagellates. *Appl. Environ. Microbiol.* 70(3): 1593–1599.

Mavrodi, D. V., W. Blankenfeldt, and L. S. Thomashow. 2006. Phenazine compounds in fluorescent *Pseudomonas* spp. biosynthesis and regulation. *Annu. Rev. Phytopathol.* 44: 417–445.

Mearns-Spragg, A., M. Bregu, K. G. Boyd, and J. G. Burgess. 1998. Cross-species induction and enhancement of antimicrobial activity produced by epibiotic bacteria from marine algae and invertebrates, after exposure to terrestrial bacteria. *Lett. Appl. Microbiol.* 27(3): 142–146.

Misawa, N. 2011. Carotenoid β-ring hydroxylase and ketolase from marine bacteria-promiscuous enzymes for synthesizing functional xanthophylls. *Mar. Drugs* 9(5): 757–771.

Miteva, V. I., P. P. Sheridan, and J. E. Brenchley. 2004. Phylogenetic and physiological diversity of micro-organisms isolated from a deep greenland glacier ice core. *Appl. Environ. Microbiol.* 70(1): 202–213.

Nair, S., D. Chandramohan, and P. A. L. Bharathi. 1992. Differential sensitivity of pigmented and non-pigmented marine bacteria to metals and antibiotics. *Water Res.* 26(4): 431–434.

Nair, S. and U. Simidu. 1987. Distribution and significance of heterotrophic marine-bacteria with antibacterial activity. *Appl. Environ. Microbiol.* 53(12): 2957–2962.

Nedashkovskaya, O., S. Kim, A. Lysenko, N. Kalinovskaya, V. Mikhailov, I. Kim, and K. Bae. 2005. *Polaribacter butkevichii* sp. nov., a novel marine mesophilic bacterium of the family flavobacteriaceae. *Curr. Microbiol.* 51(6): 408–412.

Nedashkovskaya, O. I., M. Suzuki, M. Vancanneyt, I. Cleenwerck, A. M. Lysenko, V. V. Mikhailov, and J. Swings. 2004. *Zobellia amurskyensis* sp. nov., *Zobellia laminariae* sp. nov. and *Zobellia russellii* sp. nov., novel marine bacteria of the family Flavobacteriaceae. *Int. J. Syst. Evol. Microbiol.* 54(5): 1643–1648.

Newton, R. J., L. E. Griffin, K. M. Bowles et al. 2010. Genome characteristics of a generalist marine bacterial lineage. *ISME J.* 4(6): 784–798.

Nosanchuk, J. D. and A. Casadevall. 2003. The contribution of melanin to microbial pathogenesis. *Cell. Microbiol.* 5(4): 203–223.

Nugraheni, S. A., M. M. Khoeri, L. Kusmita, Y. Widyastuti, and O. K. Radjasa. 2010. Characterization of carotenoid pigments from bacterial symbionts of seagrass *Thalassia hemprichii*. *J. Coastal Dev.* 14(1): 51–60.

Oh, H.-M., K. Lee, and J.-C. Cho. 2009. *Lewinella antarctica* sp. nov., a marine bacterium isolated from Antarctic seawater. *Int. J. Syst. Evol. Microbiol.* 59(1): 65–68.

Okazaki, T., T. Kitahara, and Y. Okami. 1975. Studies on marine microorganisms. IV. A new antibiotic SS-228 Y produced by Chainia isolated from shallow sea mud. *J. Antibiot.* 28(3): 176–184.

Okazaki, T. and Y. Okami. 1976. Studies on actinomycetes isolated from shallow sea and their antibiotic substances. In *Actinomycetes, the Boundary Microorganisms*. Ed. T. Ari. Toppan, Tokyo, Japan.

Olano, C., C. Méndez, and J. Salas. 2009. Antitumor compounds from marine actinomycetes. *Mar. Drugs* 7(2): 210–248.

Osawa, A., Y. Ishii, N. Sasamura, M. Morita, H. Kasai, T. Maoka, and K. Shindo. 2010. Characterization and antioxidative activities of rare C(50) carotenoids-sarcinaxanthin, sarcinaxanthin mono-glucoside, and sarcinaxanthin diglucoside-obtained from *Micrococcus yunnanensis*. *J. Oleo. Sci.* 59(12): 653–659.

Pedrós-Alió, C. 2006a. Genomics and marine microbial ecology. *Int. Microbiol.* 3: 191–197.

Pedrós-Alió, C. 2006b. Marine microbial diversity: Can it be determined? *Trends Microbiol.* 14(6): 257–263.

Pernthaler, A., J. Pernthaler, and R. Amann. 2002. Fluorescence in situ hybridization and catalyzed reporter deposition for the identification of marine bacteria. *Appl. Environ. Microbiol.* 68(6): 3094–3101.

Pierson, L. and E. Pierson. 2010. Metabolism and function of phenazines in bacteria: Impacts on the behavior of bacteria in the environment and biotechnological processes. *Appl. Microbiol. Biotechnol.* 86(6): 1659–1670.

Plonka, P. M. and M. Grabacka. 2006. Melanin synthesis in microorganisms—Biotechnological and medical aspects. *Acta Biochim. Pol.* 53(3): 429–443.

Pommier, T., J. Pinhassi, and Å. Hagström. 2005. Biogeographic analysis of ribosomal RNA clusters from marine bacterioplankton. *Aquat. Microb. Ecol.* 41(1): 79–89.

Poplawsky, A. R., S. C. Urban, and W. Chun. 2000. Biological role of xanthomonadin pigments in *Xanthomonas campestris* pv. campestris. *Appl. Environ. Microbiol.* 66(12): 5123–5127.

Porter, J., S. A. Morris, and R. W. Pickup. 2004. Effect of trophic status on the culturability and activity of bacteria from a range of lakes in the English Lake District. *Appl. Environ. Microbiol.* 70(4): 2072–2078.

Pusecker, K., H. Laatsch, E. Helmke, and H. Weyland. 1997. Dihydrophencomycin methyl ester, a new phenazine derivative from a marine *Streptomycete*. *J. Antibiot. (Tokyo)*. 50(6): 479–483.

Radjasa, O. K., L. Limantara, and A. Sabdono. 2009. Antibacterial activity of a pigment producing bacterium associated with *Halimeda* sp. from Land-locked marine lake Kakaban, Indonesia. *J. Coastal Dev.* 12(2): 100–104.

Rainey, F. A., S. Klatte, R. M. Kroppenstedt, and E. Stackebrandt. 1995. Dietzia, new genus including *Dietzia maris* comb. nov., formerly *Rhodococcus maris. Int. J. Syst. Bacteriol.* 45(1): 32–36.

Ray, G. C. 1988. Ecological diversity in coastal zones and oceans. In *Biodiversity.* Ed. E. O. Wilson. National Academy Press, Washington, DC.

Reichenbach, H. 2006. The order cytophagales. In *The Prokaryotes.* Eds. M. Dworkin, S. Falkow, E. Rosenberg, K.-H. Schleifer, and E. Stackebrandt. Springer, New York, pp. 549–590.

Reichenbach, H., H. Kleinig, and H. Achenbach. 1974. The pigments of *Flexibacter elegans*: Novel and chemosystematically useful compounds. *Arch. Microbiol.* 101(1): 131–144.

Reichenbach, H., W. Kohl, A. Böttger-Vetter, and H. Achenbach. 1980. Flexirubin-type pigments in flavobacterium. *Arch. Microbiol.* 126(3): 291–293.

Rivera, S. M. and R. Canela-Garayoa. 2012. Analytical tools for the analysis of carotenoids in diverse materials. *J. Chromatogr. A* 1224: 1–10.

Roszak, D. B. and R. R. Colwell. 1987. Survival strategies of bacteria in the natural environment. *Microbiol. Rev.* 51(3): 365–379.

Roy, S., C. A. Llewellyn, E. S. Egeland, and G. Johnson. 2011. *Phytoplankton Pigments.* Cambridge University Press, Cambridge, U.K.

Saha, S., R. Thavasi, and S. Jayalakshmi. 2008. Phenazine pigments from *Pseudomonas aeruginosa* and their application as antibacterial agent and food colourants. *Res. J. Microbiol.* 3: 122–128.

Salaün, S., N. Kervarec, P. Potin, D. Haras, M. Piotto, and S. La Barre. 2010. Whole-cell spectroscopy is a convenient tool to assist molecular identification of cultivatable marine bacteria and to investigate their adaptive metabolism. *Talanta* 80(5): 1758–1770.

Sanchez-Amat, A., F. Solano, and P. Lucas-Elio. 2010. Finding new enzymes from bacterial physiology: A successful approach illustrated by the detection of novel oxidases in marinomonas mediterranea. *Mar. Drugs* 8(3): 519–541.

Schäfer, H. and G. Muyzer. 2001. Denaturing gradient gel electrophoresis in marine microbial ecology. In *Methods in Microbiology.* Ed. H. P. John. Academic Press, London, U.K.

Schneemann, I., J. Wiese, A. L. Kunz, and J. F. Imhoff. 2011. Genetic approach for the fast discovery of phenazine producing bacteria. *Mar. Drugs* 9(5): 772–789.

Schut, F. R., A. Prins, and J. C. Gottschal. 1997. Oligotrophy and pelagic marine bacteria: Facts and fiction. *Aquat. Microb. Ecol.* 12: 177–202.

Shiba, T. and N. Taga. 1980. Heterotrophic bacteria attached to seaweeds. *J. Exp. Mar. Biol. Ecol.* 47(3): 251–258.

Shindo, K., K. Mikami, E. Tamesada, S. Takaichi, K. Adachi, N. Misawa, and T. Maoka. 2007. Diapolycopenedioic acid xylosyl ester, a novel glyco-C30-carotenoic acid produced by a new marine bacterium *Rubritalea squalenifaciens. Tetrahedron Lett.* 48(15): 2725–2727.

Slightom, R. N. and A. Buchan. 2009. Surface colonization by marine roseobacters: Integrating genotype and phenotype. *Appl. Environ. Microbiol.* 75(19): 6027–6037.

Soliev, A. B., K. Hosokawa, and K. Enamoto. 2011. Bioactive pigments from marine bacteria: Applications and physiological roles. *Evid.-Based Complement. Alternat. Med.* 2011: 1–17.

Speitling, M., O. F. Smetanina, O. F. Kuznetsova, and H. Laatsch. 2007. Bromoalterochromides A and A', unprecedented chromopeptides from a marine *Pseudoalteromonas maricaloris* strain KMM 636T. *J. Antibiot.* 60(1): 36–42.

Stafsnes, M., K. Josefsen, G. Kildahl-Andersen, S. Valla, T. Ellingsen, and P. Bruheim. 2010. Isolation and characterization of marine pigmented bacteria from Norwegian coastal waters and screening for carotenoids with UVA-blue light absorbing properties. *J. Microbiol.* 48(1): 16–23.

Starr, M. P., C. L. Jenkins, L. B. Bussey, and A. G. Andrewes. 1977. Chemotaxonomic significance of the xanthomonadins, novel brominated aryl-polyene pigments produced by bacteria of the genus *Xanthomonas. Arch. Microbiol.* 113(1): 1–9.

Stevens, H., Brinkhoff, T., Rink, B., Vollmers, J., and Simon, M. 2007. Diversity and abundance of gram-positive bacteria in a tidal flat ecosystem. *Environ. Microb.* 9(7): 1810–1822.

Sun, S., J. Chen, W. Li et al. 2011. Community cyberinfrastructure for advanced microbial ecology research and analysis: The CAMERA resource. http://camera.calit2.net/ (accessed February 12, 2012).

Takeuchi, M. and K. Hatano. 1998. Proposal of six new species in the genus *Microbacterium* and transfer of *Flavobacterium marinotypicum* ZoBell and Upham to the genus *Microbacterium* as *Microbacterium maritypicum* comb. nov. *Int. J. Syst. Bacteriol.* 48(3): 973–982.

Teasdale, M. E., J. Liu, J. Wallace, F. Akhlaghi, and D. C. Rowley. 2009. Secondary metabolites produced by the marine bacterium *Halobacillus salinus* that inhibit quorum sensing-controlled phenotypes in gram-negative bacteria. *Appl. Environ. Microbiol.* 75(3): 567–572.

Tebben, J., D. M. Tapiolas, C. A. Motti, D. Abrego, A. P. Negri, L. L. Blackall, P. D. Steinberg, and T. Harder. 2011. Induction of larval metamorphosis of the coral acropora millepora by tetrabromopyrrole isolated from a *Pseudoalteromonas bacterium. PLoS ONE* 6(4): e19082.

Thomas, T., F. F. Evans, D. Schleheck et al. 2008. Analysis of the *Pseudoalteromonas tunicata* genome reveals properties of a surface-associated life style in the marine environment. *PLoS ONE* 3(9): 1–11.

Tringe, S. G., C. von Mering, A. Kobayashi et al. 2004. Comparative metagenomics of microbial communities. *Escholarship* (December): 1–46. http://www.escholarship.org/uc/item/7bd0j5b0

Valentine, D. L. 2007. Adaptations to energy stress dictate the ecology and evolution of the archaea. *Nat. Rev. Microbiol.* 5: 316–323.

Valeru, S. P., P. K. Rompikuntal, T. Ishikawa, K. Vaitkevicius, Å. Sjöling, N. Dolganov, J. Zhu, G. Schoolnik, and S. N. Wai. 2009. Role of melanin pigment in expression of *Vibrio cholerae* virulence factors. *Infect. Immun.* 77(3): 935–942.

Vasanthabharathi, V., R. Lakshminarayanan, and S. Jayalakshmi. 2011. Melanin production from marine *Streptomyces. African J. Biotechnol.* 10(54): 11224–11234.

Vater, J., B. Kablitz, C. Wilde, F. Peter, N. Mehta, and S. S. Cameotra. 2002. Matrix-assisted laser desorption ionization-time of flight mass spectrometry of lipopeptide biosurfactants in whole cells and culture filtrates of *Bacillus subtilis* C-1 isolated from petroleum sludge. *Appl. Environ. Microbiol.* 68(12): 6210–6219.

Venter, J. C., K. Remington, J. F. Heidelberg et al. 2004. Environmental genome shotgun sequencing of the Sargasso Sea. *Science* 304(5667): 66–74.

Vynne, N., M. Månsson, K. Nielsen, and L. Gram. 2011. Bioactivity, chemical profiling, and 16S rRNA-based phylogeny of *Pseudoalteromonas* strains collected on a global research cruise. *Mar. Biotechnol.* 13(6): 1062–1073.

Wahl, K. L., S. C. Wunschel, K. H. Jarman, N. C. Valentine, C. E. Petersen, M. T. Kingsley, K. A. Zartolas, and A. J. Seanz. 2002. Analysis of microbial mixtures by matrix-assisted laser desorption/ionization time-of-flight mass spectrometry. *Anal. Chem.* 74(24): 6191–6199.

Weber, F. J. and J. A. de Bont. 1996. Adaptation mechanisms of microorganisms to the toxic effects of organic solvents on membranes. *Biochim. Biophys. Acta* 1286(3): 225–245.

Wietz, M., M. Mansson, C. H. Gotfredsen, T. O. Larsen, and L. Gram. 2010. Antibacterial compounds from marine vibrionaceae isolated on a global expedition. *Mar. Drugs* 8(12): 2946–2960.

Williams, P., S. Eichstadt, T. Kokjohn, and E. Martin. 2007. Effects of ultraviolet radiation on the gram-positive marine bacterium *Microbacterium maritypicum. Curr. Microbiol.* 55(1): 1–7.

Woese, C. R., O. Kandler, and M. L Wheelis. 1990. Towards a natural system of organisms: Proposal for the domains archaea, bacteria, and eucarya. *Proc. Natl Acad. Sci. USA* 87(12): 4576–4579.

Yada, S., Y. Wang, Y. Zou et al. 2008. Isolation and characterization of two groups of novel marine bacteria producing violacein. *Mar. Biotechnol.* 10(2): 128–132.

Yokoyama, A., K. Adachi, and Y. Shizuri. 1995. New carotenoid glucosides, astaxanthin glucoside and adonixanthin glucoside, isolated from the astaxanthin-producing marine bacterium, *Agrobacterium aurantiacum. J. Nat. Prod.* 58(12): 1929–1933.

Zhang, X. F., T. D. Yao, L. D. Tian, S. J. Xu, and L. Z. An. 2008. Phylogenetic and physiological diversity of bacteria isolated from puruogangri ice core. *Microbiol. Ecol.* 55: 476–488.

Zheng, L., X. Han, H. Chen, W. Lin, and X. Yan. 2005. Marine bacteria associated with marine macroorganisms: The potential antimicrobial resources. *Culture* 55: 119–124.

ZoBell, C. E. 1946. *Marine Microbiology: A Monograph on Hydrobacteriology.* Chronica Botanica Company, Waltham, MA.

Zobell, C. E. and C. B. Feltham. 1934. Preliminary studies on the distribution and characteristics of marine bacteria. *Bull. Scripps Imst. Oceanogr., Tech. Ser.* 3: 279–296.

10

Antitumor Pigments from Marine Bacteria

Azamjon B. Soliev and Keiichi Enomoto

CONTENTS

10.1 Introduction

Transformation of normal cells to malignant cells is known to occur as a result of mutagenesis, which has as a consequence the uncontrollable and abnormal multiplication of these cells within the body. Chemotherapy, the use of biologically active chemical compounds to interrupt and stop the growth of cancer cells, remains one of the most effective ways to cure cancer. However, the lack of effective chemotherapeutic drugs that can completely annihilate cancer cells remains an unsolved problem for modern science. Finding those desirable bioactive compounds has become a challenging task for researchers facing the limited efficacy of drugs used in clinical practice. Another challenge for the treatment of cancer is the ability of cancer cells to develop chemoresistance against drugs. Therefore, highly effective chemical compounds that can selectively eliminate tumor cells while not affecting normal cells are still in urgent demand. The newly designed drugs should preferably have selective inhibitory effects toward molecules that initiate anti-apoptotic mechanisms, while inducing pro-apoptotic proteins (Almond and Cohen 2002).

Historically, nature was the main source of the medicines used to treat the various illnesses that humans suffered from. This remains the case even now, as researchers still gather valuable materials from the diverse ecosystems of our planet, including the marine environment. The advents of modern technology that enable us to go much deeper into the ocean have facilitated the exploration of untouched environments. As a result, the oceans, which cover more than half of the surface of the Earth, have proven to be rich in bioresources. The study of the vast marine ecosystem has tremendously expanded in the last two decades, resulting in the development of new fields specializing on marine-based biology, biochemistry, and biotechnology. Consequently, the active metabolites obtained from the sea that are used to treat human diseases have taken the name of *marine drugs*. This term is becoming more popular as the number of bio-active compounds from marine sources, including invertebrates and microorganisms, increases. It is estimated that more than 50% of the 100 isolates obtained from marine sources are potentially useful bioactive substances (Jha and Zi-rong 2004). Most of these compounds have either antibiotic or cytotoxic activities. Thus, in the period between 1998 and 2008, 592 marine compounds with cytotoxic activity were reported to have entered the stage of preclinical investigation. During this period, other 666 chemicals demonstrated antibiotic activities including antibacterial, antifungal, antihelmintic, antiprotozoal, and antiviral activities, as well as anticoagulant, anti-inflammatory, and antiplatelet effects, which have impact on the cardiovascular, endocrine, immune, and nervous systems (Mayer 2011). Among these active metabolites, the compounds from marine bacteria are of special interest.

Although it is difficult to isolate and harvest marine bacteria (Soliev et al. 2011), they are preferred over eukaryotes because of their higher productivity and because it is easier to optimize their culturing conditions. Consequently, marine bacteria represent a rich source of bioactive compounds compared to other organisms. In fact, a continuously increasing number of bacteria isolated from the sea have demonstrated potential value as a research tool for biochemical, biotechnological, and clinical research. Microbial metabolites, especially colored ones, are attracting scientific interest (Soliev et al. 2011). Until now, thousands of biologically active bacterial metabolites have been isolated from marine *Streptomyces*, *Pseudomonas*, *Pseudoalteromonas*, *Bacillus*, *Vibrio*, and *Cytophaga* found in seawater, sediments, algae, and marine invertebrates. These toxic secondary metabolites not only play an important role in bacterial life as a defense against predators and/or for survival against harsh environmental conditions (Soliev et al. 2011) but also show different biological activities against various human illnesses including cancer. While most of these compounds are reported to have potential antibiotic activities, a number of them also show cytotoxic effects (Li 2009). The chemical spectrum of antitumor compounds derived from marine bacteria is wide, including indolocarbazoles, polyketides, alkaloids, isoprenoids (terpenoids), and even peptides (Table 10.1).

Despite thousands of bioactive metabolites having been isolated from marine bacteria, this chapter focuses only on colored compounds that have demonstrated either in vitro or in vivo apoptotic effects against cancer cells. Table 10.1 summarizes some of the bioactive antitumor pigments isolated from marine bacteria. The listed compounds do not show equal effects to all kinds of tumor cells, but they are rather selective to particular types of cells, showing cell type–specific action. This may be the reason why the bioactivity of the compounds is expressed in different half effective concentrations such as IC_{50} (IC_{70}), GI_{50}, TGI_{50}, LC_{50}, LD_{50}, EC_{50}, ED, GIC, and MIC (Table 10.1). At present, the true bioactivity of some compounds regarding selectivity and sensitivity toward cancer cells is unknown. For this reason, finding these values through further research will be necessary to be able to select suitable tumor cell lines that are more sensitive to the compounds of interest, as a prerequisite for drug development. Although the cytotoxic compounds discussed later belong to a specific bacterial family, it is well known that one specific compound can be produced by many different species of bacteria, regardless if they are from terrestrial or marine origin. This indicates that the same or similar gene clusters responsible for the production of specific biomolecules may exist in many different species of bacteria, probably as product of the horizontal transfer of gene clusters among them.

Antitumor Pigments from Marine Bacteria

151

TABLE 10.1

Antitumor Pigments Isolated from Marine Bacteria

No	Compound	Appearance	Structural Class	Source	Active Against (Cell Lines)	Effective Dose	Reference
Actinomycetes							
1.	Actinofuranones A and B	Yellow oils	Polyketide	*Streptomyces* sp. CNQ766	Mouse splenocyte T cells and macrophages	IC_{50}: 20 μg/mL	Cho et al. (2006)
2.	Ammosamides A and B	Blue and red solids	Pyrroloiminoquinone	*Streptomyces* sp. CNR-698	HCT-116 (colorectal carcinoma), HeLa	IC_{50}: 0.02–1 μM	Hughes et al. (2009)
3.	Arcyriaflavin A	Orange crystal	Indolocarbazole	Marine actinomycete $Z_2$039-2	K562 (leukemia)	IC_{50}: 100 μM	Liu et al. (2007)
4.	Butenolides	Yellow syrup	Butenolide	*Streptoverticillium luteoverticillatum*	K562; P388 (leukemia)	IC_{50}: 8.73, 6.29, 1.05 μmol/mL; 0.34, 0.19, 0.18 μmol/mL	Li et al. (2006)
5.	Chandrananimycins A–C	Orange solid	Phenoxazinone	*Actinomadura* sp. M048	CCL HT29 (colon carcinoma), MEXF 514L (melanoma), and others	IC_{70}: <1.4 μg/mL	Maskey et al. (2003)
6.	Chartreusin	Yellow solid	Polyketide	*Streptomyces* sp. QD518	L1210 (leukemia), B16 (melanoma)	NM	Wu et al. (2006); McGovren et al. (1977)
7.	Chinikomycin A	Yellowish-brown solid	Polyketide	*Streptomyces* sp. M045	MAXF 401NL (mammary cancer), RXF 944L (renal cancer), and others	IC_{50}: 2.41, 4.02 μg/mL	Li et al. (2005)

(continued)

TABLE 10.1 (continued)

Antitumor Pigments Isolated from Marine Bacteria

No	Compound	Appearance	Structural Class	Source	Active Against (Cell Lines)	Effective Dose	Reference
8.	Chinikomycin B	Red solid	Polyketide	*Streptomyces* sp. M045	MAXF 401NL	IC_{50}: 3.04 μg/mL	Li et al. (2005)
9.	Chlorinated dihydroquinones	Pale yellow crystals	Terpenoid dihydroquinones	*Streptomyces* sp. CNQ-525	HCT-116	IC_{50}: 0.97–2.40 μg/mL	Soria-Mercado et al. (2005)
10.	Daryamides A–C	Yellow powder	Polyketide	*Streptomyces* sp. CNQ-085	HCT-116	IC_{50}: 3.15–10.03 μg/mL	Asolkar et al. (2006)
11.	Gutingimycin	Yellow	Polyketide	*Streptomyces* sp. B8652	NM	IC_{70}: 3.4 μg/mL	Maskey et al. (2004b)
12.	IB-00208	Orange	Polyketide	*Actinomadura* sp. BL-42-PO13-046	P-388, A-549 (lung carcinoma), HT-29 (colon cancer), SK-MEL-28 (melanoma)	MIC: 1 nM	Malet-Cascón et al. (2003)
13.	Iodinin	Violet solid	Phenazine	*Actinomadura* sp. *M048*	MAXF 401NL, RXF 944L, and others	IC_{50}: 3.6 μg/mL	Maskey et al. (2003)
14.	Questiomycin A	Orange solid	Phenoxazinone	*Actinomadura* sp. M048	CCL HT29, MEXF 514L, and others	IC_{70}: <1.4 μg/mL	Maskey et al. (2003)
15.	K252c	Yellow crystal	Indolocarbazole	Marine actinomycete Z_2039-2	K562	IC_{50}: 10 μM	Liu et al. (2007)
16.	Lajollamycin	Yellow solid	Mixed polyketide/non-ribosomal peptide	*Streptomyces nodosus* (NPS007994)	B16-F10 (melanoma)	EC_{50}: 9.6 μM	Manam et al. (2005)
17.	Lomaiviticins A and B	Amorphous red powder	Diazobenzofluorene glycosides	*Micromonospora lomaivitiensis*	A panel of cancer cells	IC_{50}: 0.01–98 ng/mL	He et al. (2001)
18.	Lucentamycins A and B	Yellow oil	Peptides	*Nocardiopsis lucentensis* (CNR-712)	HCT-116	IC_{50}: 0.20, 11 μM	Cho et al. (2007)

No.	Name	Appearance	Type	Source	Cell lines	Activity	References
19.	Manumycin A	Yellow solid	Polyketide	*Streptomyces* sp. M045	L-1210	IC_{50}: 3.1 µg/mL	Li et al. (2005); Sattler et al. (1998)
20.	Marinomycins A–D	Yellow powder	Polyketide	Marine actinomycete *Marinispora* CNQ-140	NCI's 60 cancer cell line panel	LC_{50}: 0.2–2.7 µM	Kwon et al. (2006)
21.	Marmycin A	Red crystalline solid	Polyketide	*Streptomyces* sp.	HCT-116; 12 other cancer cells	IC_{50}: 0.06 µM; 0.022 µM	Martin et al. (2007)
22.	Marmycin B	Pink crystalline solid	Polyketide	*Streptomyces* sp.	HCT-116; 12 other cancer cells	IC_{50}: 1.09 µM; 3.5 µM	Martin et al. (2007)
23.	N-carboxamido-staurosporine	Yellow solid	Indolocarbazole	*Streptomyces* sp. QD518	37 cancer cells	IC_{50}: 0.016 µg/mL; IC_{70}: 0.17 µg/mL	Wu et al. (2006)
24.	Parimycin	Orange solid	Polyketide	*Streptomyces* sp. B8652	GXF 251L (gastric cancer), H460 (lung cancer), and others	IC_{70}: 0.9–6.7 µg/mL	Maskey et al. (2002)
25.	Piericidins C7 and C8	Yellow	Polyketide	*Streptomyces* sp. YM14-060	Rat glial cells; mouse Neuro-2a cells (neuroblastoma)	IC_{50}: 1.5, 0.45 nM; 0.83, 0.21 nM	Hayakawa et al. (2007)
26.	Resistoflavine	Yellow solid	Polyketide	*Streptomyces chibaensis* AUBN$_1$/7	HMO2 (gastric adenocarcinoma) HePG2 (hepatic carcinoma)	GI_{50}: 0.007 µg/mL; TGI: 0.009 µg/mL; LC_{50}: 0.013 µg/mL GI_{50}: 0.010 µg/mL; TGI: 0.013 µg/mL; LC_{50}: 0.016 µg/mL	Gorajana et al. (2007)
27.	Resistomycin	Yellow solid	Polyketide	*Streptomyces* sp. B8005, *Streptomyces* sp. B4842	MCF-7 (breast cancer), UACC-62 (melanoma), and others	>50 ng/mL	Kock et al. (2005); Lee et al. (1993)

(continued)

TABLE 10.1 (continued)

Antitumor Pigments Isolated from Marine Bacteria

No	Compound	Structural Class	Appearance	Source	Active Against (Cell Lines)	Effective Dose	Reference
28.	SS-228 Y	Polyketide	Yellowish-brown powder	*Chainia* sp. SS-228	Ehrlich ascites tumor cells	LD_{50}: 1.56–6.25 mg/kg	Okazaki et al. (1975)
29.	Streptochlorin	Indole	Yellow crystalline solid	*Streptomyces* sp. 04DH110	U937 (leukemia)	IC_{50}: 10–12 µg/mL	Park et al. (2008); Shin et al. (2008)
30.	Tetracenomycin D	Polyketide	Yellow-orange solid	*Streptomyces* sp. B8005	L1210	IC_{50}: 22.1 µM	Kock et al. (2005); Martin et al. (2002)
31.	Thiocoraline	Cyclic thiodepsipeptide	Pale yellow crystalline	*Micromonospora* sp. L-13-ACM2-092	P388, A549, HT-29, MEL-28 (melanoma)	IC_{50}: 0.002–0.01 µg/mL	Romero et al. (1997); Baz et al. (1997)
32.	Trioxacarcins A–D	Polyketide	Yellow solid	*Streptomyces* sp. B8652	HT-29, MEXF 514L, and others	IC_{70}: 0.001–2.161 µg/mL	Maskey et al. (2004a)
33.	1-Hydroxy-1-norresistomycin	Polyketide	Pale yellow solid	*Streptomyces chibaensis* AUBN$_1$/7	HMO2, HePG2	GI_{50}: 0.009 µg/mL; TGI_{50}: 0.012 µg/mL; LC_{50}: 0.015 µg/mL; GI_{50}: 0.014 µg/mL; TGI_{50}: 0.018 µg/mL; LC_{50}: 0.021 µg/mL	Gorajana et al. (2005)
34.	1,6-Phenazinediol	Phenazine	Yellow solid	*Actinomadura* sp. M048	LXFA 629L, LXFL 529L, (lung carcinoma), and others	IC_{50}: 3.2 µg/mL	Maskey et al. (2003)
Pseudoalteromonas							
35.	Cycloprodigiosin	Pyrrole alkaloid	Red solid	*Pseudoalteromonas denitrificans*	Six liver cancer cell lines	IC_{50}: 276–592 nmol/L	Yamamoto et al. (1999)
36.	Prodigiosin	Pyrrole alkaloid	Red solid	*Streptomyces, Pseudomonas, Pseudoalteromonas, Actinomadura* sp.	Standard 60 human tumor cell line panel	GIC_{50}: 0.014 µM; LC_{50}: 2.1 µM	Pandey et al. (2009)

No.	Name	Color/form	Type	Source	Cell line/cancer	Activity	Reference
37.	Tambjamines	Yellow oil	Alkaloid	*Pseudoalteromonas tunicata*	HL60 (leukemia), MDA-MB435 (breast carcinoma), HCT-8 (colorectal carcinoma), and others	IC_{50}: 0.23–3.42 µg/mL	Franks et al. (2005); Pinkerton et al. (2010)
38.	Violacein	Purple solid	Indolocarbazole	*Pseudoalteromonas tunicata* *Pseudoalteromonas* sp. 520P1 *Collimonas* CT	U937, K562, and others	IC_{50}: 0.5–1 µM	Ferreira et al. (2004); Kodach et al. (2006)
39.	9H-pyrido[3,4-b] indole (Norharman)	Light yellow crystalline	β-Carboline alkaloid	*Pseudoalteromonas piscicida*	HeLa, BGC-823 (stomach cancer)	IC_{50}: 5 µg/mL	Zheng et al. (2006)
Cyanobacteria							
40.	Curacin D	Pale yellow oil	Lipid	*Lyngbya majuscula*	MCF-7	IC_{50}: 0.34 µM	Marquez et al. (1998)
41.	Hectochlorin	Pale yellow solid	Lipopeptide	*Lyngbya majuscula*	60 cancer cell lines	GI_{50}: 5.1 µM	Marquez et al. (2002)
42.	Homodolastatin 16	Pale yellow oil	Cyclic depsipeptide	*Lyngbya majuscula*	WHCO1 and WHCO6 (esophageal cancer); ME180 (cervical cancer)	IC_{50}: 4.3 and 10.1 µg/mL; 8.3 µg/mL	Davies-Coleman et al. (2003)
43.	Jamaicamides A, B and C	Pale yellow oils	Mixed polyketide–peptide	*Lyngbya majuscula*	NCL-H460 (lung cancer) and Neuro-2a	LC_{50}: 15 µM	Edwards et al. (2004)
44.	Lyngbyabellin B	Pale yellow oil	Cyclic depsipeptide	*Lyngbya majuscula*	KB (epidermal carcinoma)	IC_{50}: 0.1 µM	Milligan et al. (2000)
45.	Phycocyanin	Light blue	Phycobiliprotein	*Spirulina platensis*	K562, Hep3B (hepatoma)	IC_{50}: 50 µM	Subhashini et al. (2004)

(*continued*)

TABLE 10.1 (continued)

Antitumor Pigments Isolated from Marine Bacteria

No	Compound	Appearance	Structural Class	Source	Active Against (Cell Lines)	Effective Dose	Reference
Other bacteria							
46.	Alteramide A	Yellow powder	Alkaloid	*Alteromonas* sp.	P388, L1210, KB	IC_{50}: 0.1, 1.7, 5.0 μg/mL	Shigemori et al. (1992)
47.	Heptylprodigiosin	Red solid	Pyrrole alkaloid	*Pseudovibrio denitrificans* Z143-1	L5178Y (lymphoma)	IC_{50}: 0.677 μM	Bojo et al. (2010)
48.	PG-L-1	Red solid	Prodigiosin-like Pyrrole alkaloid	γ-Proteobacterium MS-02-063	U937, CHO, HeLa, and others	ED_{50}: 70–150 ng/mL	Nakashima et al. (2005b)
49.	Unknown phenazine derivatives	Yellow needles	Phenazine	*Bacillus* sp.	P388; K562	IC_{50}: <50 μM; 74, 87 μM	Li et al. (2007)

NM—not mentioned.

10.2 Cytotoxic Pigments from Marine Actinomycetes

When referring to pigmented cytotoxic compounds isolated from aquatic flora, marine *Pseudoalteromonas*, cyanobacteria, and especially *Streptomyces* stand out as they are the most important sources of these active metabolites. Terrestrial *Streptomyces* sp., first described by Waksman and Henrici (1943), has proved to be the richest source of compounds with biological activities among bacterial species. Nearly 75% of the active metabolites isolated from *Streptomyces* have antibiotic and antitumor activities (Miyadoh 1993). In a survey of active metabolites isolated from microorganisms, published in *The Journal of Antibiotics* between 1984 and 1993, Miyadoh (1993) reported that actinomycetes are the most important sources of bioactive compounds, with a total of 93% of all antitumor antibiotics having been isolated from this group of bacteria. Despite the lack of reports, marine-derived counterparts have also demonstrated to be significant sources of active metabolites, both quantitatively and qualitatively. The number of active metabolites isolated from marine strains of actinomycetes is increasing considerably. In fact, it has been discovered that the aquatic species of actinomycetes produce not only the same compounds as their terrestrial counterparts (Fiedler et al. 2005) but also other types of compounds with unique structures and pharmacological activities. The search for new antitumor antibiotics from marine bacteria has led to the discovery of a wide range of pigmented cytotoxic compounds with different potency and selectivity, obtained from marine *Streptomyces* species found in different marine environments (Table 10.1). Varying not only in their appearance but also in their chemical structures, these toxic compounds induce apoptosis in different ways, acting through various yet not fully understood pathways. These may include extrinsic pathways, through death receptor signaling, and intrinsic ones that involve multiple other intracellular signaling pathways. An example of this is streptochlorin, a yellowish crystalline solid isolated from marine *Streptomyces* sp. 04DH110 (Figure 10.1 and Table 10.1, No.29) (Shin et al. 2007). This compound was reported to activate caspases, upregulate the pro-apoptotic Bax and FasL, decrease the mitochondrial membrane potential, and increase the degradation of poly-(ADP-ribose) polymerase(PARP) and phospholipase C-γ1 proteins while inhibiting the action of the anti-apoptotic Bcl-2 protein toward U937 leukemia cells (Park et al. 2008). Other examples are the blue- and red-colored ammosamides A and B isolated from the *Streptomyces* strain CNR-698 (Figure 10.1 and Table 10.1, No.2), which were reported to have pronounced selectivity against various cancer cell lines, with IC_{50} values ranging from 20 nM to 1 μM. In vitro cytotoxicity assay of both compounds against HCT-116 (HeLa) colon carcinoma cells produced an IC_{50} value of 320 nM. A preliminary investigation of their molecular mechanisms of action, carried out by converting them to highly conjugated fluorescent molecules, revealed that these compounds act on proteins of the myosin family, which are responsible for numerous cell processes, including cell cycle regulation, cytokinesis, and cell migration (Hughes et al. 2009).

There are dozens of other compounds isolated from marine actinomycetes whose anticancer activity mechanisms have yet to be determined (Table 10.1). It is interesting to note that the yellow-colored *N*-carboxamido-staurosporine isolated from marine *Streptomyces* sp. QD518 has a more potent anticancer activity than its colorless analogs *N*-formyl-staurosporine and sesquiterpene (Figure 10.1 and Table 10.1, No.23). Exhibiting a mean IC_{50} value of 0.016 μg/mL and a mean IC_{70} value of 0.17 μg/mL, this compound showed high tumor selectivity against 37 cancer cell lines from bladder, central nervous system, colon, gastric, head and neck, lung, mammary, ovarian, pancreatic, prostate, renal, skin, pleural mesothelium, and uterine cancers (Wu et al. 2006). However, the mechanism of action of this compound remains elusive.

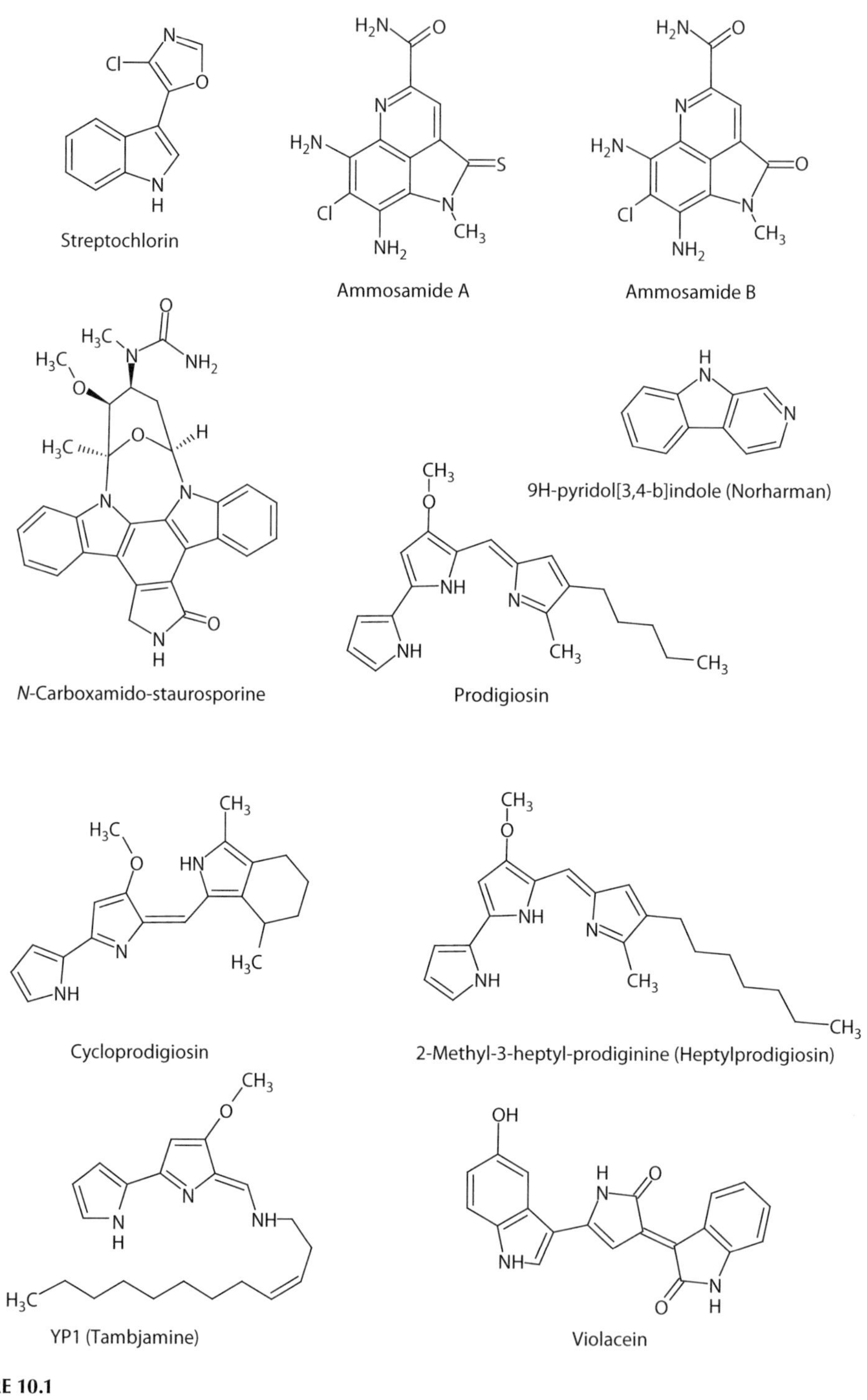

FIGURE 10.1
Representative antitumor pigments from marine bacteria.

10.3 Cytotoxic Pigments from Marine *Pseudoalteromonas*

The genus *Pseudoalteromonas*, solely belonging to a marine type of bacteria, has two kinds of species: pigmented and nonpigmented. According to some reports, the pigmented species are more effective than the nonpigmented species in terms of producing more potent biologically active compounds (Vynne et al. 2011). Holmström et al. reported that the pigmented species were more effective against biofouling than their nonpigmented counterparts (Holmström et al. 1996, 1998). The pigmented strains seem to produce much stronger toxic secondary metabolites with a wide range of bioactivities, an essential requirement for drug development. Among these compounds, the ones with antitumor activities attract special interest. These compounds are discussed later and are also listed in Table 10.1.

9H-pyrido[3,4-b]indole (norharman), a light yellow-colored compound isolated from *Pseudoalteromonas piscicida*, has been reported to have apoptotic effects (Figure 10.1 and Table 10.1, No.39). Although the exact molecular mechanisms of action are still elusive, the reported effects involved chromatin condensation and DNA degradation, which are characteristic of apoptosis (Zheng et al. 2006).

The red-colored prodigiosins take an important place, as research on their cytotoxicity has increased considerably since the last decade due to their immense clinical relevance. The strikingly red-colored prodiginines were first isolated from the terrestrial *Serratia marcescens*, previously known as *Bacillus prodigiosus* (Gerber 1975a), from which their name derives (Gerber 1969). Sharing a common pyrrolyldipyrromethene core skeleton, prodigiosin was the first prodiginine having its chemical structure elucidated (Figure 10.1 and Table 10.1, No.36) (Rapoport and Holden 1962). Due to their wide range of biological properties, such as antibiotic, immunosuppressive, and anticancer activities (Montaner and Pérez-Tomás 2003; Williamson et al. 2007), prodiginines have become an attractive research tool. These compounds gained fame especially for their immunosuppressive and prominent antitumor activities. Prodiginines were reported to have anticancer activity against nearly 60 human cancer cell lines with little or no effect on normal cells (Williamson et al. 2007; Pandey et al. 2009). In fact, these compounds were proved to induce apoptosis even in drug-resistant tumor cells, thus being able to overcome one of the main problems in chemotherapy. Synthetic prodiginine derivatives such as PNU156804 and GX15-070 have already entered clinical trials to develop immunosuppressive and anticancer drugs, respectively (Williamson et al. 2007). Although advanced studies have been conducted on these compounds to determine their molecular mechanisms of cytotoxicity, information regarding the way they induce apoptosis remains elusive because of their extremely wide cellular targets (Figure 10.2). Despite the lack of information regarding the cytotoxicity mechanisms of prodiginines, four main possible pathways leading to apoptosis of cancer cells have been proposed: (1) regulation of intracellular pH by proton pumping ATPases (Sato et al. 1998), (2) arrest of cell cycle at different levels of G- or S-stages by inhibition of protein activities promoting cell differentiation and proliferation (Montaner and Pérez-Tomás 2003; Pérez-Tomás and Montaner 2003; Montaner et al. 2005), (3) copper (II)-mediated DNA fragmentation (Pérez-Tomás et al. 2003), and (4) regulation of signal transduction pathway molecules (Ramoneda and Pérez-Tomás 2002; Fürstner et al. 2004).

Prodigiosin has also demonstrated antimetastatic activity against 95-D human lung carcinoma and B16BL6 mouse melanoma cells by inhibiting their migration and invasion, both in vitro and in vivo. The action of prodigiosin is dose dependent, reaching 50%

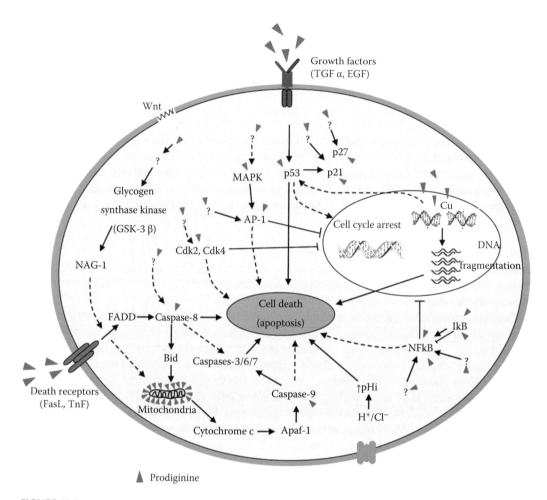

FIGURE 10.2
Possible cellular targets of prodiginines leading to apoptosis. The figure shows intrinsic (mitochondrial) and extrinsic pathways that participate in the apoptotic process by prodiginines. These two pathways, comprising four main mechanisms, are suggested to induce apoptosis by prodiginines in the following ways: (1) regulation of intracellular pH by proton pumping ATPases, (2) arrest of cell cycle at different levels of G- or S-stages by inhibition of protein activities promoting cell differentiation and proliferation, (3) copper (II)-mediated DNA fragmentation, and (4) regulation of signal transduction pathway molecules.

metastasis inhibition of 95-D cells at 4.66 μM for 12 h (Zhang et al. 2005). These findings indicate that prodigiosin-like compounds are potential chemotherapeutic drug candidates against cancer.

Previously, prodiginines were known to be produced exclusively by *Serratia* and *Streptomyces* living in the soil (Wasserman et al. 1966a,b; Gerber 1975b; Gerber and Lechevalier 1976; Tsao et al. 1985), but now there are plenty of reports on prodiginines isolated from marine *Streptomyces* (Laatsch et al. 1991), *Pseudomonas* (Gandhi et al. 1976), and others (Lewis and Corpe 1964). *Pseudoalteromonas* in particular seems to be a rich source of these active metabolites (Gauthier 1976a; Gerber and Gauthier 1979; Enger et al. 1987; Sawabe et al. 1998; Yamamoto et al. 1999; Fehér et al. 2008).

Marine-derived cycloprodigiosin was first isolated from *Pseudoalteromonas rubra* (Gerber and Gauthier 1979) and was later found to be produced by *Pseudoalteromonas denitrificans* too (Figure 10.1 and Table 10.1, No.35). Cycloprodigiosin demonstrated strong in vitro and in vivo apoptotic effects on liver cancer cell lines including Huh-7, HCC-M, HCC-T (human hepatocellular carcinoma), HepG2 (human hepatoblastoma), dRLh-84, and H-35 (rat hepatocellular carcinoma) (Yamamoto et al. 1999). This compound has also antimalarial (Kim et al. 1999) and immunosuppressive activities (Kawauchi et al. 1997). Suppressed cellular proliferation as a result of apoptosis was suggested to be due to the decrease of intracellular pH, caused by the uncoupling effect of cycloprodigiosin on proton transport by V-ATPase. The anti-apoptotic NF-κB protein activity responsible for DNA transcription was also reported to be suppressed by cycloprodigiosin (Kamata et al. 2001). Undecylprodigiosin was also found to suppress the proliferation of human lymphocytes by blocking the cell cycle at G1 phase, which was attributed to the inhibition of the phosphorylation of the retinoblastoma protein and the inhibition of the induction of cyclin A, cyclin E, cyclin-dependent kinase-2, and cyclin-dependent kinase-4 (Songia et al. 1997). However, undecylprodigiosin has no effect on the proliferation of different leukemia cell lines. Heptylprodigiosin, isolated from a marine α-proteobacterium, was reported to have in vitro cytotoxic activity against L5178Y mouse lymphocytes in addition to its antimalarial activity against *Plasmodium falciparum* 3D7 (Figure 10.1 and Table 10.1, No.47) (Lazaro et al. 2002). This compound displayed synergistic effect with another cytotoxic compound, adociaquinone B, isolated from the marine sponge *Xestospongia* sp., against MCF-7 breast cancer cells (Bojo et al. 2010). A 3:1 ratio of adociaquinone B: heptylprodigiosin was the most effective, resulting in the greatest reduction of the IC_{50} values of the individual compounds, thus reducing the possible toxicity against normal cells.

Prodigiosin-like pigments were also reported to be produced by marine *Vibrio* (D'Aoust and Kushner 1972; Shieh et al. 2003), *Hahella* (Lee et al. 2001; Nakashima et al. 2005a; Kim et al. 2007), *Zooshikella* (Yi et al. 2003), and actinomycetes (Laatsch et al. 1991) isolated from different aquatic fauna. The biological activities of these pigments have been studied using different methods.

The prodigiosin-like pigment PG-L-1, isolated from the bacterial strain MS-02-063 belonging to γ-proteobacterium, was reported to have a strong cytotoxic effect against MDCK, CHO, HeLa, Vero, XC, and PtK_1 cells (Nakashima et al. 2005b). PG-L-1 also induced apoptosis of U937 cells, accompanied by the increase of intracellular pH, activation of p38 MAP kinase, inhibition of O^{2-} generation, and DNA fragmentation. The apoptosis mechanisms of PG-L-1 may be attributed to the increase of intracellular pH and the activation of p38 MAP kinase (Nakashima et al. 2005b). The bacterial strain 1020R, which is closely related to the prodigiosin-producing bacterium *Pseudoalteromonas rubra*, was previously isolated from the Pacific Ocean by our research group (Wang et al. 2012). This strain produces seven similar prodigiosin compounds, the structures of four of which were successfully elucidated using physicochemical methods such as NMR and LC-MS. The compounds were identified as 2-methyl-3-butyl-prodiginine, 2-methyl-3-pentyl-prodiginine (prodigiosin), 2-methyl-3-hexyl-prodiginine, and 2-methyl-3-heptyl-prodiginine. They differ from each other only in the length of the alkyl chain attached to the C-3 position of the C-ring. Investigation of their biological activity revealed that all of these compounds have cytotoxic effects against U937, K562, and HL60 leukemia cancer cells. Structure activity relationship (SAR) studies found 2-methyl-3-pentyl-prodiginine (prodigiosin) to be the most potent cytotoxic compound against all the tested cancer cell lines, based on cell survival rates evaluated by the MTS assay. Investigations of the molecular mechanisms of action of these compounds have revealed that they induce DNA fragmentation and caspase-3 activation characteristic to apoptosis. Recently, we found that protein phosphatases actively involved in the signal transduction pathway regulating cell functions, namely, protein tyrosine phosphatase 1B and protein phosphatase 2A, served as the target molecules of these compounds in vitro (Soliev and Enomoto 2011). Unlike protein phosphatases, protein kinases do not seem to be the direct targets of prodigiosins. Tests conducted by our research group found that the activities of protein tyrosine kinase (Src kinase), CaM kinase, PKA, and PKC were not significantly inhibited, indicating the selective action of prodigiosins toward phosphatases. SAR investigations revealed that the inhibitory activity of these compounds toward protein phosphatases decreases when the length of the alkyl chain in the C-3 position of the C-ring increases. Thus, 2-methyl-3-butyl-prodiginine was the most potent inhibitor among this group of compounds against protein phosphatases. These data suggest that the chemical structures of the compounds determine the affinity to enzymes they can bind to and consequently inhibit. Fürstner et al. (2004) also reported the inhibition of protein tyrosine phosphatase by synthetic prodigiosin-related compounds and proposed the use of these compounds in the treatment of cancer.

Biologically active components of the marine *Pseudoalteromonas tunicata* have been identified as alkaloid tambjamines, the chemical structures of which are partly similar to prodiginines (Figure 10.1 and Table 10.1, No.37) (Franks et al. 2005). Screening of the biological activities of some tambjamines against certain human cancer cell lines has revealed that they possess moderate antitumor activity compared to the doxorubicin control (Pinkerton et al. 2010).

Another pigment that has prominent biological properties, including anticancer activity, is a purple-colored violacein (Figure 10.1 and Table 10.1, No.38). This compound is a well-known indole derivative also known as 3-(1,2-dihydro-5-(5-hydroxy-1H-indol-3-yl)-2-oxo-3H-pyrrol-3-ilydene)-1,3-dihydro-2H-indol-2-one. It is produced by *Chromobacterium violaceum*, an opportunist pathogenic bacterium inhabiting the soil and water of tropical and subtropical areas (Leifson 1956; Sneath 1956; Rettori and Durán 1998). However, Hamilton and Austin (1967) were among the first researchers who reported violacein from marine bacteria, followed by Gauthier (Gauthier et al. 1975; Gauthier 1976b) and others (Novick and Tyler 1985; Yang et al. 2007; Yada et al. 2008; Hakvåg et al. 2009).

Violacein is reported to have a wide range of biological properties, including antibacterial, antiprotozoal, antiparasitic, antifungal, and antiviral activities, as well as cytotoxic activity against cancer cells (Durán et al. 2007). Some reports highlighted the defensive role of violacein in bacteria (Matz et al. 2004). Despite unique antibiotic properties, the anticancer activity of violacein has attracted special attention, and many studies have been recently conducted to understand its apoptotic mechanisms.

Investigations on the molecular mechanisms of cytotoxicity of violacein isolated from *Chromobacterium violaceum* revealed the activation of caspase-8 and p38 MAP kinase, as well as the transcription of NF-κB target genes in HL60 leukemia cells (Ferreira et al. 2004). The IC_{50} value of violacein against HL60 cells was determined to be 700 nM. In addition to activation of the TNF receptor, upregulation of the expression of p21 protein, activation of caspase-3, phosphatidylserine exposure, fragmentation of poly (ADP-ribose) polymerase (PARP), decrease of c-jun expression, and downregulation of the inhibitor of apoptosis protein 1 (IAP1), all leading to facilitate the apoptosis process, were also observed (Ferreira et al. 2004). In another study by the same research group, violacein-induced apoptosis of four colon cancer cell lines was associated with cell cycle blockage at the G1 phase, upregulating the levels of p53, p27, and p21 proteins and decreasing the expression of cyclin D1 (Kodach et al. 2006). However, the main cause of apoptosis was attributed to the inhibition of Akt (PKB) phosphorylation, which changed the levels of the proteins mentioned earlier, with subsequent activation of the apoptotic pathway and downregulation of NF-κB signaling. This signaling pathway in colon cancer cells was suggested to be more sensitive to 5-fluorouracil (5-FU), a potent chemotherapeutic agent, in a synergistic fashion with violacein. The elevated levels of the pro-apoptotic BAD protein were thought to be promoted by the activation of caspase-3, in addition to the activation of caspase-8 and caspase-9, and the decreased level of FADD was suggested to be indicative of the exclusion of the extrinsic apoptotic pathway (Kodach et al. 2006).

Our research group has also been investigating the molecular mechanisms of cytotoxicity of violacein isolated from the marine bacterial strain 520P1 belonging to *Pseudoalteromonas* (Yada et al. 2008; Zhang and Enomoto 2011), to contribute to a better understanding of the possible apoptotic pathways in cancer cells. Preliminary results obtained using U937, K562, and HL60 leukemia cell lines showed potent cytotoxic activity, with IC_{50} values of 0.5–1 μM, confirming the data previously reported in the literature (Ferreira et al. 2004). The stimuli leading to apoptosis, including caspase-3 activation, chromatin condensation, and DNA fragmentation, were experimentally confirmed (Hosokawa and Enomoto 2010). In contrast to the red-colored prodiginines, which inhibit protein phosphatases, violacein showed higher affinity for protein kinases than for phosphatases (Hosokawa et al. 2010). In the experiment with the catalytic subunits of protein kinases A and C, violacein dose-dependently inhibited their enzymatic activities with IC_{50} values of 6 and 2 μM, respectively. However, the pigment's effect toward protein kinases A and C seems to be selective, as it failed to inhibit other kinase family enzymes like Ca^{2+}/calmodulin-dependent protein kinase and protein tyrosine (Src) kinase. Subsequent experiments with enzymes of the PKC subfamily, consisting of classical (α, βI, βII, γ), novel (δ, ε, θ, η), and atypical (ζ, μ, τ, ι), revealed that the classical-type enzymes are the most sensitive to the pigment's effect. The results obtained suggest the involvement of PKC and its downstream pathway in the cytotoxic action of violacein against tumor cells, because phorbol myristate acetate (PMA), a strong activator of PKC enzyme added to the culture medium of HL60 cells, prevented pigment-induced DNA fragmentation. However, further research is needed to reveal the direct target molecule(s) of violacein in tumor cells.

10.4 Cytotoxic Pigments from Marine Cyanobacteria

Marine cyanobacteria, previously known as blue–green algae, are also productive microorganisms that have been known for their ability to produce a wide variety of unique secondary metabolites. Although more than 300 structurally diverse biomolecules have been obtained from marine cyanobacteria, they are especially famous for the production of lipopeptides and depsipeptides (Tan 2007), most of which are biologically active. A number of these bioactive compounds have demonstrated anticancer activity, with different potency against various cancer cell lines (Table 10.1). It should be noted that many well-known potent antitumor compounds (e.g., dolastatin), previously believed to originate from marine invertebrate species such as sea hares and mollusks, have recently be found to actually originate from marine cyanobacteria living in symbiosis with those species.

Phycocyanin, a pigment produced by the cyanobacterium *Spirulina platensis* (Boussiba and Richmond 1980), belongs to the light-harvesting phycobiliprotein family and is used as a fluorescent agent in immunoassay analysis (Kronick 1986). Phycocyanin has a characteristic light blue color, absorbs orange and red light near 620 nm, and emits fluorescence at about 650 nm. Being an accessory pigment that works in conjunction with chlorophyll *a*, it is also a well-known natural food colorant. In addition to its anti-oxidative and anti-inflammatory effects, phycocyanin was also found to have cytotoxicity against cancer cells, the molecular mechanisms of which displayed characteristic features of apoptosis, such as cell shrinkage, membrane blebbing, and nuclear condensation followed by mitochondrial cytochrome *c* release, PARP cleavage, and downregulation of the anti-apoptotic Bcl-2 protein (Table 10.1, No.45) (Subhashini et al. 2004).

Nevertheless, not only pigmented compounds show bioactivities. There are also a number of nonpigmented, highly potent cyanobacterial active metabolites with antitumor activity against various cancer cell lines, isolated from different species, representing potential candidates for future drug development. It is expected that more compounds with interesting biological activities will be discovered in the future, since this family of bacteria remains virtually uninvestigated. Therefore, researchers specializing in chemistry, biology, pharmacology, and medicine have a challenging task to accomplish in the study of bioactive compounds from marine microorganisms.

10.5 Concluding Remarks

Marine bacteria play a very important role among aquatic fauna and flora. Symbiosis of bacteria with marine invertebrates and other higher eukaryotes seems to be beneficial for both hosts and their symbionts in mutualistic and commensalistic associations. Bacteria provide survival and defensive tools to their hosts by producing various toxic compounds. On the other hand, the hosts may provide a nutrient-rich, biologically favorable place for bacteria to live, although more research is needed to clarify their role in the symbiosis. The discovery of symbiotic bacteria meant the reevaluation of the previous knowledge on compounds isolated from marine sources. It was found that many biologically active chemical compounds thought to originate from marine invertebrates were actually produced by symbiotic bacteria.

Today, thousands of bioactive compounds with anticancer activities have been isolated from the marine environment, dozens of which are in preclinical or clinical test trials. However, the biotechnological production in large scale of biologically active compounds from marine multicellular organisms has limitations in terms of culturing conditions, because they are generally found at very low concentrations. This is an important point as it may influence the cost of chemotherapeutic drugs being commercialized. Some experts warn that the actual prices of these drugs are much higher than originally expected. Hence, anticancer drugs like oxaliplatin and irinotecan, which have been recently developed and approved by the European Medicines Evaluation Agency and the U.S. Food and Drug Administration, can often cost more than $10,000 for a course of treatment, yet their effectiveness is not substantially higher than that of the conventional drugs (Garattini and Bertele 2002). This price may double or even triple if combinatorial chemotherapy is used. There are many reasons why the prices of these drugs are high, with long-term funding of R&D by pharmaceutical companies being the costliest. However, one of the main reasons for the high prices is the source from which the bioactive compounds are isolated. As mentioned earlier, some bioactive metabolites are found in very low amounts, and in addition, they are often isolated from rare organisms. For example, more than half a ton of sea squirt is needed to obtain 1 g of ET743, an extremely potent chemotherapeutic drug being commercialized as Yondelis™. Many rare dogfish sharks (*Squalus acanthias*) are needed to obtain the necessary amount of squalamine lactate, a novel antiangiogenic aminosteroid that by 2003 was in phase II clinical trials for ovarian and non–small cell lung cancer (Haefner 2003). The rarity of the compounds makes the isolation procedure much more complicated, eventually affecting the cost of the product. To circumvent this, chemical synthesis of the compounds has been carried out. However, due to their structural complexity, total synthesis of some natural anticancer compounds has faced extreme difficulties, as in the case of bryostatin-1, a potent antineoplastic drug (Keck et al. 2011).

Unlike the situation with higher organisms, harvesting natural products from microorganisms including bacteria seems less costly, and their culturing conditions could be easily optimized, making it possible to obtain higher amounts of the required compounds. Thus, the optimization of the culture media led to a 40-fold increase in the production of the red-pigmented prodigiosin and at least a 23-fold increase in the production of undecylprodigiosin from *S. marcescens* (Giri et al. 2004; Wei and Chen 2005; Wei et al. 2005).

Despite the large number of cytotoxic antibiotics isolated from marine bacteria, it is difficult to name one that has become a commercially available drug. Most of the isolated anticancer compounds that attracted the enthusiasm of researchers have failed in clinical trials, due to their life threatening side effects toward normal functioning cells. Some scientists hold the opinion that these failures might have been caused by the lack of research, which prevented getting crucial information about the properties of the compounds (Arif et al. 2004). However, this problem is not exclusive of marine bacteria, as the same situation has happened with bioactive compounds isolated from marine invertebrates, although a few of them have already been commercialized (Thakur et al. 2005). Nevertheless, we must be optimistic and take into account that the research on marine bacteria is still in its infancy. According to some calculations, the number of marine microorganisms can exceed 10^9 organisms/mL (Fenical and Jensen 2006). Therefore, there is no doubt that in the future novel species of marine bacteria, producing bioactive chemicals with unique biological properties will be discovered. Among the biomolecules found, there might be compounds with potent anticancer activities that will cure patients in advanced illness stage like miraculous drugs. Nature created both illnesses and the medicines to treat them. The cure for cancer may also lay hidden in nature. Our task is to find it and make it available to patients. And who knows, this cure may be found in the oceans!

References

Almond, J. B. and G. M. Cohen. 2002. The proteasome: A novel target for cancer chemotherapy. *Leukemia* 16 (4):433–443.

Arif, J. M., A. A. Al-Hazzani, M. Kunhi, and F. Al-Khodairy. 2004. Novel marine compounds: Anticancer or genotoxic? *J. Biomed. Biotechnol.* 2004 (2):93–98.

Asolkar, R. N., P. R. Jensen, C. A. Kauffman, and W. Fenical. 2006. Daryamides A-C, weakly cytotoxic polyketides from a marine-derived actinomycete of the genus *Streptomyces* strain CNQ-085. *J. Nat. Prod.* 69 (12):1756–1759.

Baz, J. P., L. M. Canedo, and J. L. F. Puentes. 1997. Thiocoraline, a novel depsipeptide with antitumor activity produced by a marine *Micromonospora* II. Physico-chemical properties and structure determination. *J. Antibiot.* 50 (9):738–741.

Bojo, Z. P., C. D. Deano, S. D. Jacinto, and G. P. Concepcion. 2010. Synergistic in vitro cytotoxicity of adociaquinone B and heptylprodigiosin against MCF-7 breast cancer cell line. *Philipp. Sci. Lett.* 3 (2):48–58.

Boussiba, S. and A. E. Richmond. 1980. C-phycocyanin as a storage protein in the blue-green alga *Spirulina platensis*. *Arch. Microbiol.* 125 (1–2):143–147.

Cho, J. Y., H. C. Kwon, P. G. Williams, C. A. Kauffman, P. R. Jensen, and W. Fenical. 2006. Actinofuranones A and B, polyketides from a marine-derived bacterium related to the genus *Streptomyces* (Actinomycetales). *J. Nat. Prod.* 69 (3):425–428.

Cho, J. Y., P. G. Williams, H. C. Kwon, P. R. Jensen, and W. Fenical. 2007. Lucentamycins A-D, cytotoxic peptides from the marine-derived actinomycete *Nocardiopsis lucentensis*. *J. Nat. Prod.* 70 (8):1321–1328.

D'Aoust, J. Y. and D. J. Kushner. 1972. *Vibrio psychroerythrus* sp. n.: Classification of the psychrophilic marine bacterium, NRC 1004. *J. Bacteriol.* 111 (2):340–342.

Davies-Coleman, M. T., T. M. Dzeha, C. A. Gray et al. 2003. Isolation of homodolastatin 16, a new cyclic depsipeptide from a Kenyan collection of *Lyngbya majuscula*. *J. Nat. Prod.* 66 (5):712–715.

Durán, N., G. Z. Justo, C. V. Ferreira, P. S. Melo, L. Cordi, and D. Martins. 2007. Violacein: Properties and biological activities. *Biotechnol. Appl. Biochem.* 48 (Pt 3):127–133.

Edwards, D. J., B. L. Marquez, L. M. Nogle et al. 2004. Structure and biosynthesis of the jamaicamides, new mixed polyketide-peptide neurotoxins from the marine cyanobacterium *Lyngbya majuscula*. *Chem. Biol.* 11 (6):817–833.

Enger, Ø., H. Nygaard, M. Solberg, G. Schei, J. Nielsen, and I. Dundas. 1987. Characterization of *Alteromonas denitrificans* sp. nov. *Int. J. Syst. Bacteriol.* 37 (4):416–421.

Fehér, D., R. S. Barlow, P. S. Lorenzo, and T. K. Hemscheidt. 2008. A 2-substituted prodiginine, 2-(p-hydroxybenzyl)prodigiosin, from *Pseudoalteromonas rubra*. *J. Nat. Prod.* 71 (11):1970–1972.

Fenical, W. and P. R. Jensen. 2006. Developing a new resource for drug discovery: Marine actinomycete bacteria. *Nat. Chem. Biol.* 2 (12):666–673.

Ferreira, C. V., C. L. Bos, H. H. Versteeg, G. Z. Justo, N. Durán, and M. P. Peppelenbosch. 2004. Molecular mechanism of violacein-mediated human leukemia cell death. *Blood* 104 (5):1459–1464.

Fiedler, H. P., C. Bruntner, A. T. Bull et al. 2005. Marine actinomycetes as a source of novel secondary metabolites. *Antonie van Leeuwenhoek* 87 (1):37–42.

Franks, A., P. Haywood, C. Holmström, S. Egan, S. Kjelleberg, and N. Kumar. 2005. Isolation and structure elucidation of a novel yellow pigment from the marine bacterium *Pseudoalteromonas tunicata*. *Molecules* 10 (10):1286–1291.

Fürstner, A., K. Reinecke, H. Prinz, and H. Waldmann. 2004. The core structure of roseophilin and the prodigiosin alkaloids define a new class of protein tyrosine phosphatase inhibitors. *ChemBioChem* 5 (11):1575–1579.

Gandhi, N. M., J. R. Patell, J. Gandhi, N. J. De Souza, and H. Kohl. 1976. Prodigiosin metabolites of a marine *Pseudomonas* species. *Mar. Biol.* 34 (3):223–227.

Garattini, S. and V. Bertele. 2002. Efficacy, safety, and cost of new anticancer drugs. *Br. Med. J.* 325 (7358):269–271.

Gauthier, M. J. 1976a. *Alteromonas rubra* sp. nov., a new marine antibiotic producing bacterium. *Int. J. Syst. Bacteriol.* 26 (4):459–466.

Gauthier, M. J. 1976b. Morphological, physiological, and biochemical characteristics of some violet-pigmented bacteria isolated from seawater. *Can. J. Microbiol.* 22 (2):138–149.

Gauthier, M. J., J. M. Shewan, D. M. Gibson, and J. V. Lee. 1975. Taxonomic position and seasonal variations in marine neritic environment of some gram-negative antibiotic-producing bacteria. *J. Gen. Microbiol.* 87 (2):211–218.

Gerber, N. N. 1969. Prodigiosin-like pigments from *Actinomadura (Nocardia) pelletieri* and *Actinomadura madurae*. *Appl. Microbiol.* 18 (1):1–3.

Gerber, N. N. 1975a. Prodigiosin-like pigments. *CRC Crit. Rev. Microbiol.* 3 (4):469–485.

Gerber, N. N. 1975b. A new prodiginine (prodigiosin-like) pigment from *Streptomyces*. Antimalarial activity of several prodiginines. *J. Antibiot.* 28 (3):194–199.

Gerber, N. N. and M. J. Gauthier. 1979. New prodigiosin-like pigment from *Alteromonas rubra. Appl. Environ. Microbiol.* 37 (6):1176–1179.

Gerber, N. N. and M. P. Lechevalier. 1976. Prodiginine (prodigiosin-like) pigments from *Streptomyces* and other aerobic actinomycetes. *Can. J. Microbiol.* 22 (5):658–667.

Giri, A. V., N. Anandkumar, G. Muthukumaran, and G. Pennathur. 2004. A novel medium for the enhanced cell growth and production of prodigiosin from *Serratia marcescens* isolated from soil. *BMC Microbiol.* 4 (11):1–10.

Gorajana, A., B. V. V. S. N. Kurada, S. Peela, P. Jangam, S. Vinjamuri, E. Poluri, and A. Zeeck. 2005. 1-Hydroxy-1-norresistomycin, a new cytotoxic compound from a marine actinomycete, *Streptomyces chibaensis* AUBN$_1$/7. *J. Antibiot.* 58 (8):526–529.

Gorajana, A., M. Venkatesan, S. Vinjamuri et al. 2007. Resistoflavine, cytotoxic compound from a marine actinomycete, *Streptomyces chibaensis* AUBN$_1$/7. *Microbiol. Res.* 162 (4):322–327.

Haefner, B. 2003. Drugs from the deep: Marine natural products as drug candidates. *Drug Discov. Today* 8 (12):536–544.

Hakvåg, S., E. Fjærvik, G. Klinkenberg et al. 2009. Violacein producing *Collimonas* sp. from the sea surface microlayer of coastal waters in Trøndelag, Norway. *Mar. Drugs* 7 (4):576–588.

Hamilton, R. D. and K. E. Austin. 1967. Physiological and cultural characteristics of *Chromobacterium marinum* sp. n. *Antonie van Leeuwenhoek* 33 (3):257–264.

Hayakawa, Y., S. Shirasaki, S. Shiba, T. Kawasaki, Y. Matsuo, K. Adachi, and Y. Shizuri. 2007. Piericidins C7 and C8, new cytotoxic antibiotics produced by a marine *Streptomyces* sp. *J. Antibiot.* 60 (3):196–200.

He, H., W. D. Ding, V. S. Bernan et al. 2001. Lomaiviticins A and B, potent antitumor antibiotics from *Micromonospora lomaivitiensis. J. Am. Chem. Soc.* 123 (22):5362–5363.

Holmström, C., S. James, S. Egan, and S. Kjelleberg. 1996. Inhibition of common fouling organisms by marine bacterial isolates with special reference to the role of pigmented bacteria. *Biofouling* 10 (1–3):251–259.

Holmström, C., S. James, B. A. Neilan, D. C. White, and S. Kjelleberg. 1998. *Pseudoalteromonas tunicata* sp. nov., a bacterium that produces antifouling agents. *Int. J. Syst. Bacteriol.* 48 (4):1205–1212.

Hosokawa, K. and K. Enomoto. 2010. Molecular mechanisms of cytotoxicity by prodigiosin and violacein pigments from marine bacteria. Paper presented at the *Annual Meeting of the Japanese Pharmacological Society*, Osaka, Japan. *J. Pharmacol. Sci.* 112 (Suppl.):172.

Hosokawa, K., A. B. Soliev, A. Kajihara, and K. Enomoto. 2010. Inhibition of protein kinases by an anti-tumor pigment violacein. Paper presented at the *Annual Meeting of the Japanese Biochemical Society*, Kobe, Japan, 4P-0397.

Hughes, C. C., J. B. MacMillan, S. P. Gaudêncio, P. R. Jensen, and W. Fenical. 2009. The ammosamides: Structures of cell cycle modulators from a marine-derived *Streptomyces* species. *Angew. Chem. Int. Ed. Engl.* 48 (4):725–727.

Jha, R. K. and X. Zi-rong. 2004. Biomedical compounds from marine organisms. *Mar. Drugs* 2 (3):123–146.

Kamata, K., S. Okamoto, S. Oka, H. Kamata, H. Yagisawa, and H. Hirata. 2001. Cycloprodigiosin hydrochloride suppresses tumor necrosis factor (TNF) α-induced transcriptional activation by NF-κB. *FEBS Lett.* 507 (1):74–80.

Kawauchi, K., K. Shibutani, H. Yagisawa et al. 1997. A possible immunosuppressant, cycloprodigiosin hydrochloride, obtained from *Pseudoalteromonas denitrificans. Biochem. Biophys. Res. Commun.* 237 (3):543–547.

Keck, G. E., Y. B. Poudel, T. J. Cummins, A. Rudra, and J. A. Covel. 2011. Total synthesis of bryostatin 1. *J. Am. Chem. Soc.* 133 (4):744–747.

Kim, H. S., M. Hayashi, Y. Shibata et al. 1999. Cycloprodigiosin hydrochloride obtained from *Pseudoalteromonas denitrificans* is a potent antimalarial agent. *Biol. Pharm. Bull.* 22 (5):532–534.

Kim, D., J. S. Lee, Y. K. Park et al. 2007. Biosynthesis of antibiotic prodiginines in the marine bacterium *Hahella chejuensis* KCTC 2396. *J. Appl. Microbiol.* 102 (4):937–944.

Kock, I., R. P. Maskey, M. A. Biabani, E. Helmke, and H. Laatsch. 2005. 1-Hydroxy-1-norresistomycin and resistoflavin methyl ether: New antibiotics from marine-derived *Streptomycetes*. *J. Antibiot.* 58 (8):530–534.

Kodach, L. L., C. L. Bos, N. Durán, M. P. Peppelenbosch, C. V. Ferreira, and J. C. H. Hardwick. 2006. Violacein synergistically increases 5-fluorouracil cytotoxicity, induces apoptosis and inhibits Akt-mediated signal transduction in human colorectal cancer cells. *Carcinogenesis* 27 (3):508–516.

Kronick, M. N. 1986. The use of phycobiliproteins as fluorescent labels in immunoassay. *J. Immunol. Methods* 92 (1):1–13.

Kwon, H. C., C. A. Kauffman, P. R. Jensen, and W. Fenical. 2006. Marinomycins A-D, antitumor-antibiotics of a new structure class from a marine actinomycete of the recently discovered genus "*Marinispora*." *J. Am. Chem. Soc.* 128 (5):1622–1632.

Laatsch, H., M. Kellner, and H. Weyland. 1991. Butyl-*meta*-cycloheptylprodiginine—A revision of the structure of the former *ortho*-isomer. *J. Antibiot.* 44 (2):187–191.

Lazaro, J. E., J. Nitcheu, R. Z. Predicala et al. 2002. Heptyl prodigiosin, a bacterial metabolite, is anti-malarial in vivo and nonmutagenic in vitro. *J. Nat. Toxins* 11 (4):367–377.

Lee, H. K., J. Chun, E. Y. Moon et al. 2001. *Hahella chejuensis* gen. nov., sp. nov., an extracellular-polysaccharide-producing marine bacterium. *Int. J. Syst. Evol. Microbiol.* 51 (2):661–666.

Lee, S. W., S. E. Kim, Y. H. Kim et al. 1993. Antitumoral compound, MCS-202, an effector on prolifera-tion and morphology of human breast tumor cell line, MCF-7. *Kor. J. Appl. Microbiol. Biotechnol.* 21 (6):594–599.

Leifson, E. 1956. Morphological and physiological characteristics of the genus *Chromobacterium*. *J. Bacteriol.* 71 (4):393–400.

Lewis, S. M. and W. A. Corpe. 1964. Prodigiosin-producing bacteria from marine sources. *Appl. Microbiol.* 12 (1):13–17.

Li, Z. 2009. Advances in marine microbial symbionts in the China Sea and related pharmaceutical metabolites. *Mar. Drugs* 7 (2):113–129.

Li, F., R. P. Maskey, S. Qin et al. 2005. Chinikomycins A and B: Isolation, structure elucidation, and biological activity of novel antibiotics from a marine *Streptomyces* sp. isolate M045. *J. Nat. Prod.* 68 (3):349–353.

Li, D., F. Wang, X. Xiao, X. Zeng, Q. Q. Gu, and W. M. Zhu. 2007. A new cytotoxic phenazine deriva-tive from a deep sea bacterium *Bacillus* sp. *Arch. Pharm. Res.* 30 (5):552–555.

Li, D. H., T. J. Zhu, H. B. Liu, Y. C. Fang, Q. Q. Gu, and W. M. Zhu. 2006. Four butenolides are novel cytotoxic compounds isolated from the marine-derived bacterium, *Streptoverticillium luteoverti-cillatum* 11014. *Arch. Pharm. Res.* 29 (8):624–626.

Liu, R., T. Zhu, D. Li, J. Gu, W. Xia, Y. Fang, H. Liu, W. Zhu, and Q. Gu. 2007. Two indolocarbazole alkaloids with apoptosis activity from a marine-derived actinomycete Z2039–2. *Arch. Pharm. Res.* 30 (3):270–274.

Malet-Cascón, L., F. Romero, F. Espliego-Vázquez, D. Grávalos, and J. L. Fernández-Puentes. 2003. IB-00208, a new cytotoxic polycyclic xanthone produced by a marine-derived *Actinomadura* I. Isolation of the strain, taxonomy and biological activities. *J. Antibiot.* 56 (3):219–225.

Manam, R. R., S. Teisan, D. J. White et al. 2005. Lajollamycin, a nitro-tetraene spiro-β-lactone-γ-lactam antibiotic from the marine actinomycete *Streptomyces nodosus*. *J. Nat. Prod.* 68 (2):240–243.

Marquez, B., P. Verder-Pinard, E. Hamel, and W. H. Gerwick. 1998. Curacin D, an antimitotic agent from the marine cyanobacterium *Lyngbya majuscula*. *Phytochemistry* 49 (8):2387–2389.

Marquez, B. L., K. S. Watts, A. Yokochi et al. 2002. Structure and absolute stereochemistry of hecto-chlorin, a potent stimulator of actin assembly. *J. Nat. Prod.* 65 (6):866–871.

Martin, P., S. Rodier, M. Mondon et al. 2002. Synthesis and cytotoxic activity of tetracenomycin D and of saintopin analogues. *Bioorg. Med. Chem.* 10 (2):253–260.

Martin, G. D. A., L. T. Tan, P. R. Jensen et al. 2007. Marmycins A and B, cytotoxic pentacyclic C-glycosides from a marine sediment-derived actinomycete related to the genus *Streptomyces*. *J. Nat. Prod.* 70 (9):1406–1409.

Maskey, R. P., E. Helmke, H. H. Feibig, and H. Laatsch. 2002. Parimycin: Isolation and structure elucidation of a novel cytotoxic 2,3-dihydroquinizarin analogue of γ-indomycinone from a marine *Streptomycete* isolate. *J. Antibiot.* 55 (12):1031–1035.

Maskey, R. P., E. Helmke, O. Kayser et al. 2004a. Anti-cancer and antibacterial trioxacarcins with high anti-malaria activity from a marine *Streptomycete* and their absolute stereochemistry. *J. Antibiot.* 57 (12):771–779.

Maskey, R. P., F. C. Li, S. Qin, H. H. Fiebig, and H. Laatsch. 2003. Chandrananimycins A–C: Production of novel anticancer antibiotics from a marine *Actinomadura* sp. isolate M048 by variation of medium composition and growth conditions. *J. Antibiot.* 56 (7):622–629.

Maskey, R. P., M. Sevvana, I. Usón, E. Helmke, and H. Laatsch. 2004b. Gutingimycin: A highly complex metabolite from a marine streptomycete. *Angew. Chem. Int. Ed. Engl.* 43 (10):1281–1283.

Matz, C., P. Deines, J. Boenigk, H. Arndt, L. Eberl, S. Kjelleberg, and K. Jürgens. 2004. Impact of violacein-producing bacteria on survival and feeding of bacterivorous nanoflagellates. *Appl. Environ. Microbiol.* 70 (3):1593–1599.

Mayer, A. M. S. 2011. Marine pharmaceuticals: The preclinical pipeline in the World Wide. http://marinepharmacology.midwestern.edu/preclinPipeline.htm (accessed January 31, 2012).

McGovren, J. P., G. L. Neil, S. L. Crampton, M. I. Robinson, and J. D. Douros. 1977. Antitumor activity and preliminary drug disposition studies on chartreusin (NSC 5159). *Cancer Res.* 37 (6):1666–1672.

Milligan, K. E., B. L. Marquez, R. T. Williamson, and W. H. Gerwick. 2000. Lyngbyabellin B, a toxic and antifungal secondary metabolite from the marine cyanobacterium *Lyngbya majuscula*. *J. Nat. Prod.* 63 (10):1440–1443.

Miyadoh, S. 1993. Research on antibiotic screening in Japan over the last decade: A producing microorganisms approach. *Actinomycetologica* 7 (2):100–106.

Montaner, B., W. Castillo-Ávila, M. Martinell, R. Öllinger, J. Aymami, E. Giralt, and R. Pérez-Tomás. 2005. DNA interaction and dual topoisomerase I and II inhibition properties of the anti-tumor drug prodigiosin. *Toxicol. Sci.* 85 (2):870–879.

Montaner, B. and R. Pérez-Tomás. 2003. The prodigiosins: A new family of anticancer drugs. *Curr. Cancer Drug Targets* 3 (1):57–65.

Nakashima, T., M. Kurachi, Y. Kato, K. Yamaguchi, and T. Oda. 2005a. Characterization of bacterium isolated from the sediment at coastal area of Omura bay in Japan and several biological activities of pigment produced by this isolate. *Microbiol. Immunol.* 49 (5):407–415.

Nakashima, T., T. Tamura, M. Kurachi, K. Yamaguchi, and T. Oda. 2005b. Apoptosis-mediated cytotoxicity of prodigiosin-like red pigment produced by γ-proteobacterium and its multiple bioactivities. *Biol. Pharm. Bull.* 28 (12):2289–2295.

Novick, N. J. and M. E. Tyler. 1985. Isolation and characterization of *Alteromonas luteoviolacea* strains with sheathed flagella. *Int. J. Syst. Bacteriol.* 35 (1):111–113.

Okazaki, T., T. Kitahara, and Y. Okami. 1975. Studies on marine microorganisms. IV. A new antibiotic SS-228 Y produced by *Chainia* isolated from shallow sea mud. *J. Antibiot.* 28 (3):176–184.

Pandey, R., R. Chander, and K. B. Sainis. 2009. Prodigiosins as anti cancer agents: Living up to their name. *Curr. Pharm. Des.* 15 (7):732–741.

Park, C., H. J. Shin, G. Y. Kim et al. 2008. Induction of apoptosis by streptochlorin isolated from *Streptomyces* sp. in human leukemic U937 cells. *Toxicol. In Vitro* 22 (6):1573–1581.

Pérez-Tomás, R. and B. Montaner. 2003. Effects of the proapoptotic drug prodigiosin on cell cycle-related proteins in Jurkat T cells. *Histol. Histopathol.* 18 (2):379–385.

Pérez-Tomás, R., B. Montaner, E. Llagostera, and V. Soto-Cerrato. 2003. The prodigiosins, proapoptotic drugs with anticancer properties. *Biochem. Pharmacol.* 66 (8):1447–1452.

Pinkerton, D. M., M. G. Banwell, M. J. Garson et al. 2010. Antimicrobial and cytotoxic activities of synthetically derived tambjamines C and E–J, BE-18591, and a related alkaloid from the marine bacterium *Pseudoalteromonas tunicata*. *Chem. Biodivers.* 7 (5):1311–1324.

Ramoneda, B. M. and R. Pérez-Tomás. 2002. Activation of protein kinase C for protection of cells against apoptosis induced by the immunosuppressor prodigiosin. *Biochem. Pharmacol.* 63 (3):463–469.

Rapoport, H. and K. G. Holden. 1962. The synthesis of prodigiosin. *J. Am. Chem. Soc.* 84 (4):635–642.

Rettori, D. and N. Durán. 1998. Production, extraction and purification of violacein: An antibiotic pigment produced by *Chromobacterium violaceum. World J. Microbiol. Biotechnol.* 14 (5):685–688.

Romero, F., F. Espliego, J. P. Baz et al. 1997. Thiocoraline, a new depsipeptide with antitumor activity produced by a marine *Micromonospora* I. Taxonomy, fermentation, isolation, and biological activities. *J. Antibiot.* 50 (9):734–737.

Sato, T., H. Konno, Y. Tanaka et al. 1998. Prodigiosins as a new group of H^+/Cl^- symporters that uncouple proton translocators. *J. Biol. Chem.* 273 (34):21455–21462.

Sattler, I., R. Thiericke, and A. Zeeck. 1998. The manumycin-group metabolites. *Nat. Prod. Rep.* 15 (3):221–240.

Sawabe, T., H. Makino, M. Tatsumi et al. 1998. *Pseudoalteromonas bacteriolytica* sp. nov., a marine bacterium that is the causative agent of red spot disease of *Laminaria japonica. Int. J. Syst. Bacteriol.* 48 (3):769–774.

Shieh, W. Y., Y. W. Chen, S. M. Chaw, and H. H. Chiu. 2003. *Vibrio ruber* sp. nov., a red, facultatively anaerobic, marine bacterium isolated from sea water. *Int. J. Syst. Evol. Microbiol.* 53 (2):479–484.

Shigemori, H., M. A. Bae, K. Yazawa, T. Sasaki, and J. Kobayashi. 1992. Alteramide A, a new tetracyclic alkaloid from a bacterium *Alteromonas* sp. associated with the marine sponge *Halichondria okadai. J. Org. Chem.* 57 (15):4317–4320.

Shin, H. J., H. S. Jeong, H. S. Lee, S. K. Park, H. M. Kim, and H. J. Kwon. 2007. Isolation and structure determination of streptochlorin, an antiproliferative agent from a marine-derived *Streptomyces* sp. 04DH110. *J. Microbiol. Biotechnol.* 17 (8):1403–1406.

Shin, D. Y., H. J. Shin, G. Y. Kim et al. 2008. Streptochlorin isolated from *Streptomyces* sp. induces apoptosis in human hepatocarcinoma cells through a reactive oxygen species-mediated mitochondrial pathway. *J. Microbiol. Biotechnol.* 18 (11):1862–1867.

Sneath, P. H. A. 1956. Conservation of the generic name *Chromobacterium* and designation of type species and type strains. *Int. Bull. Bacteriol. Nomencl. Taxon.* 6 (2):65–91.

Soliev, A. B. and K. Enomoto. 2011. Molecular mechanisms of cytotoxicity by prodigiosin and violacein pigments from marine bacteria. Paper presented at the *Annual Meeting of the Japanese Biochemical Society*, Kyoto, Japan. 4T15a-17.

Soliev, A. B., K. Hosokawa, and K. Enomoto. 2011. Bioactive pigments from marine bacteria: Applications and physiological roles. *Evid. Based Complement. Alternat. Med.* Vol. 2011, Article ID 670349, 17 pages, doi:10.1155/2011/670349.

Songia, S., A. Mortellaro, S. Taverna et al. 1997. Characterization of the new immunosuppressive drug undecylprodigiosin in human lymphocytes: Retinoblastoma protein, cyclin-dependent kinase-2, and cyclin-dependent kinase-4 as molecular targets. *J. Immunol.* 158 (8):3987–3995.

Soria-Mercado, I. E., A. Prieto-Davo, P. R. Jensen, and W. Fenical. 2005. Antibiotic terpenoid chlorodihydroquinones from a new marine actinomycete. *J. Nat. Prod.* 68 (6):904–910.

Subhashini, J., S. V. Mahipal, M. C. Reddy, R. M. Mallikarjuna, A. Rachamallu, and P. Reddanna. 2004. Molecular mechanisms in c-phycocyanin induced apoptosis in human chronic myeloid leukemia cell line-K562. *Biochem. Pharmacol.* 68 (3):453–462.

Tan, L. T. 2007. Bioactive natural products from marine cyanobacteria for drug discovery. *Phytochemistry* 68 (7):954–979.

Thakur, N. L., A. N. Thakur, and W. E. G. Müller. 2005. Marine natural products in drug discovery. *Nat. Prod. Rad.* 4 (6):471–478.

Tsao, S. W., B. A. M. Rudd, X. G. He, C. J. Chang, and H. G. Floss. 1985. Identification of a red pigment from *Streptomyces coelicolor* A3(2) as a mixture of prodigiosin derivatives. *J. Antibiot.* 38 (1):128–131.

Vynne, N., M. Månsson, K. F. Nielsen, and L. Gram. 2011. Bioactivity, chemical profiling, and 16S rRNA-based phylogeny of *Pseudoalteromonas* strains collected on a global research cruise. *Mar. Biotechnol.* 13 (6):1062–1073.

Waksman, S. A. and A. T. Henrici. 1943. The nomenclature and classification of the actinomycetes. *J. Bacteriol.* 46 (4):337–341.

Wang, Y., A. Nakajima, K. Hosokawa et al. 2012. Cytotoxic prodigiosin family pigments from *Pseudoalteromonas* sp. 1020R isolated from the Pacific coast of Japan. *Biosci. Biotechnol. Biochem.* 76 (6):1229–1232.

Wasserman, H. H., G. C. Rodgers, and D. D. Keith. 1966a. The structure and synthesis of undecylprodigiosin. A prodigiosin analogue from *Streptomyces*. *Chem. Commun.* 22:825–826.

Wasserman, H. H., G. C. Rodgers, and D. D. Keith. 1966b. Metacycloprodigiosin, a tripyrrole pigment from *Streptomyces longisporus ruber*. *J. Am. Chem. Soc.* 91 (5):1263–1264.

Wei, Y. H. and W. C. Chen. 2005. Enhanced production of prodigiosin-like pigment from *Serratia marcescens* SMΔR by medium improvement and oil-supplementation strategies. *J. Biosci. Bioeng.* 99 (6):616–622.

Wei, Y. H., W. J. Yu, and W. C. Chen. 2005. Enhanced undecylprodigiosin production from *Serratia marcescens* SS-1 by medium formulation and amino-acid supplementation. *J. Biosci. Bioeng.* 100 (4):466–471.

Williamson, N. R., P. C. Fineran, T. Gristwood, S. R. Chawrai, F. J. Leeper, and G. P. C. Salmond. 2007. Anticancer and immunosuppressive properties of bacterial prodiginines. *Future Microbiol.* 2 (6):605–618.

Wu, S. J., S. Fotso, F. Li et al. 2006. *N*-carboxamido-staurosporine and selina-4(14),7(11)-diene- 8,9-diol, new metabolites from a marine *Streptomyces* sp. *J. Antibiot.* 59 (6):331–337.

Yada, S., Y. Wang, Y. Zou et al. 2008. Isolation and characterization of two groups of novel marine bacteria producing violacein. *Mar. Biotechnol.* 10 (2):128–132.

Yamamoto, C., H. Takemoto, K. Kuno et al. 1999. Cycloprodigiosin hydrochloride, a new H^+/Cl^- symporter, induces apoptosis in human and rat hepatocellular cancer cell lines in vitro and inhibits the growth of hepatocellular carcinoma xenografts in nude mice. *Hepatology* 30 (4):894–902.

Yang, L. H., H. Xiong, O. O. Lee, S. H. Qi, and P. Y. Qian. 2007. Effect of agitation on violacein production in *Pseudoalteromonas luteoviolacea* isolated from a marine sponge. *Lett. Appl. Microbiol.* 44 (6):625–630.

Yi, H., Y. H. Chang, H. W. Oh, K. S. Bae, and J. Chun. 2003. *Zooshikella ganghwensis* gen. nov., sp. nov., isolated from tidal flat sediments. *Int. J. Syst. Evol. Microbiol.* 53 (4):1013–1018.

Zhang, X. and K. Enomoto. 2011. Characterization of a gene cluster and its putative promoter region for violacein biosynthesis in *Pseudoalteromonas* sp. 520P1. *Appl. Microbiol. Biotechnol.* 90 (6):1963–1971.

Zhang, J., Y. Shen, J. Liu, and D. Wei. 2005. Antimetastatic effect of prodigiosin through inhibition of tumor invasion. *Biochem. Pharmacol.* 69 (3):407–414.

Zheng, L., X. Yan, X. Han et al. 2006. Identification of norharman as the cytotoxic compound produced by the sponge (*Hymeniacidon perleve*)-associated marine bacterium *Pseudoalteromonas piscicida* and its apoptotic effect on cancer cells. *Biotechnol. Appl. Biochem.* 44 (3):135–142.

11

Structural Characteristics of Bioactive Marine Natural Products

Snezana Agatonovic-Kustrin, David Morton, and Christine Kettle

CONTENTS

11.1 Introduction

The marine environment, with its enormous wealth of biological and chemical diversity, is unique in terms of the specific composition in both organic and inorganic substances present. Sessile marine invertebrates such as sponges, bryozoans, and tunicates, which mostly lack morphological defense structures, are producing a wide range of secondary metabolites, some of which provide a chemical defense function to the organism. These compounds have diverse and unusual structures which generally differ greatly to terrestrial natural products, with their exact function within the organism not always known. Due to their structural novelty, intricate carbon skeletons, and the ease at which the human body accepts these molecules with minimal manipulation, marine natural products are an important source of compounds that have had a crucial role in identifying novel chemical entities with useful drug properties (Cragg et al. 2006).

However, compounds from marine organisms were rarely used in medicine until relatively recently. Before the development of reliable deepwater scuba-diving technology, the collection of marine organisms was limited to those available in more shallow water using standard skin diving equipment (Fenical 2006). Effective methods of isolation of compounds from these organisms have provided many potent compounds in pure form. Advancement in instrumentation methods such as nuclear magnetic resonance (NMR), mass spectrometric (MS) techniques, and x-ray diffraction (XRD) has helped to determine their often complex and stereochemical structures. In recent years, a significant number of novel metabolites with potent pharmacological properties have been discovered from a number of marine organisms.

Interest in natural products as sources of novel drugs has fallen in recent decades, due to high-throughput combinatorial chemistry approaches (Newman and Cragg 2007) becoming more popular. Unfortunately, these approaches have not been all that successful in the development of new pharmaceuticals, so there is now a revival of interest in natural product drug discovery (Newman et al. 2003). The search for new biomedicals from marine organisms has resulted in the isolation of around 10,000 metabolites (Fusetani 2000), many of which have been found to possess pharmacodynamic properties. This includes antibiotic, antifungal, toxic, cytotoxic, neurotoxic, antimitotic, antiviral, antineoplastic, and cardiovascular activities. In more recent years, a number of compounds derived from marine sources have shown to be pharmacodynamically active for AIDS, immunosuppression, anti-inflammation, Alzheimer's disease, aging processes, and some tropical diseases (Kelecom 1999).

Research into the pharmacological properties of marine natural products has led to the discovery of many potently active agents considered worthy of clinical application:

a. Anti-inflammatory and analgesic effects of Egyptian Red Sea sponge extracts (Fakhr et al. 2006)

b. Angiogenic effects either by disabling the agents that activate and promote cell growth or by directly blocking the growing blood vessel cells of fucoidans on endothelial cells (Matsubara et al. 2005), antiangiogenic and antimicrobial activity of sponge-associated bacterial extracts (Thakur et al. 2005)

c. Antioxidative and anti-inflammatory effects of phlorotannin-containing extracts with potential for treating osteoarthritis from the brown alga *Ecklonia cava* (Shin et al. 2006)

d. Immunostimulating activity in vivo of a novel sulfated exopolysaccharide derived from a red-tide microalga *Gyrodinium impudicum* (Yim et al. 2005)

e. Anti-infective or antimicrobial (from Red Sea corals) (Kelman et al. 2006), broad-spectrum antibacterial (from *Marinomonas mediterranea*) (Lucas-Elio et al. 2005), antifungal activity (from red algae *Chondria armata*) (Al-Fadhli et al. 2006), antiviral activity (from *Stoechospermum marginatum*, marine sponges, *Bacillus licheniformis*, and *Arthrospira*) (Adhikari et al. 2006, Arena et al. 2006, Rechter et al. 2006, da Silva et al. 2006), and anti-HIV-1 (from marine worm *Chaetopterus variopedatus*) (Wang et al. 2006)

f. Potent anticoagulant activity of a sulfated polysaccharide from the brown alga *Ecklonia cava* (Athukorala et al. 2006)

Two antiviral drugs, cytosine arabinoside (Ara-C) and adenine arabinoside (Ara-A), which are synthetic analogues of sponge metabolites, were approved by the Food and Drug Administration (FDA) in 1969 and 1980, respectively (Sneader 2005). The first marine natural product to become commercially available as a drug for pain relief was ω-conotoxin MVIIA (ziconotide), a peptide that was isolated from a cone snail in 1987 and approved for use by the FDA in 2004 (Chaplan et al. 2010). In 2007, the marine natural product trabectedin, which was isolated from a tunicate in 1987, was approved by the European Medicines Agency for the treatment of soft-tissue sarcoma, and it is currently in clinical trials for breast, prostate, and pediatric cancers (Gennigens and Jerusalem 2011). Many other marine natural products have been, or currently are, also in clinical trials. Didemnin B was the first defined marine natural product to enter clinical trials as a potential anticancer drug (Taylor et al. 1992) to treat adenocarcinoma, advanced epithelial ovarian cancer (Cain et al. 1992), and metastatic breast cancer (Montgomery and Zukoshi 1985). Although didemnin B was never carried into phase III trials, the activity focused on developing the compound as a potential cancer treatment which helped pave the way for the rest of the marine-derived products that followed it into the development pipeline (Newman and Cragg 2004a). Bryostatin 1 (Mutter and Wills 2000), a macrolactone isolated from the marine bryozoan, *Bugula neritina*, is a potent modulator of protein kinase C activity and is currently under investigation as an anticancer agent and a memory-enhancing agent

(Gschwend et al. 2000). Structurally related γ-lactams salinosporamide A, omuralide, and lactacystin, isolated from microbacteria, inhibit proteasome activity and have been used as lead compounds for the development of anticancer agents (Hogan and Corey 2005).

11.2 Natural Products

Natural products are organic molecules derived from plants, animals, or microorganisms. They are generally complex molecules often with multiple chiral centers that have specific biological function(s) within the organism from which they are derived (Young 1999, Cordell 2000). For instance, they may provide a chemical defense function for the organism (da Rocha et al. 2001). Because of these properties compared to molecules obtained using combinatorial synthesis, they now represent the starting point for most of the anti-infective and anticancer drugs on the market today.

Recent progress in drug discovery from natural product sources has resulted in numerous therapeutic agents developed to treat cancer, resistant bacteria and viruses, and immunosuppressive disorders. The opportunity to discover new species and, therefore, new types of natural product molecules has increased through the application of new tools to explore the marine environment. Recent advances in understanding the genetics of secondary metabolites in marine actinomycete bacteria and new screening technologies have led to the discovery of several new drug candidates.

Living systems produce a vast and diverse range of organic compounds, small molecules that can be classified as either primary or secondary metabolites. Primary metabolites are substances widely distributed in nature, occurring in one form or another in virtually all organisms. The primary metabolites, such as phytosterols, vitamins, purine nucleotides, amino acids, and organic acids, are necessary to sustain the life of the living system, and they perform metabolic roles that are usually evident. Secondary metabolites are not involved in the normal growth and development of an organism and therefore are not essential for survival, but are beneficial to the survival of the organism and provide a survival advantage. They often have an ecological role for the producing organisms such as defense against predators, competition for space, roles in reproduction, and antimicrobial activity (Coll 1992, Paul 1992, Sammarco and Coll 1992, Pawlik 1993, Hay 1996). Plant and microorganisms being devoid of motility and an immune system have developed alternative defense strategies, involving the huge variety of secondary metabolites as tools to overcome stress constraints enabling them to adapt to the changing environment and survive. Their functions, many of which remain unknown, are being elucidated with increasing frequency. Marine organisms generally live in symbiotic association. Sessile marine organisms, that is, seaweeds, corals, and other benthic organisms, face constant challenges on coral reefs. Fish may take more than 150,000 bites per square meter on the ocean floor every day, removing nearly 100% of daily productivity (Carpenter 1986). Sessile marine organisms also fight for space on limited reef substrates (McClintock and Baker 2001), and microbial pathogens can devastate susceptible species (Harvell et al. 1999).

The multitude of enemies faced by marine organisms creates substantial selection pressure for the evolution of mechanisms to improve survival in the face of these challenges.

Many sessile invertebrates such as sponges, corals, and tunicates feed by filtering seawater. Since seawater contains high concentrations of bacteria, these organisms produce antibiotics to defend themselves from potentially harmful microorganisms. This production of antibacterial compounds provides a chemical defense for sponges and antibiotics for humans. Natural products released into the water are rapidly diluted and therefore need to be highly potent to have any effect (Mayer et al. 2000, Proksch et al. 2002). Furthermore, in the case of encrusting sponges growing together, the sponge that will survive is the one that will produce the most effective chemical to kill the rapidly dividing cells of the neighboring sponges. This ability of a chemical to kill rapidly dividing cells is the foundation for the chemotherapy treatment. Chemotherapy works by interfering with the cancer cell's ability to grow. Anticancer drugs often act by killing the rapidly dividing cells of a tumor but generally do not harm normal healthy cells.

In general, secondary metabolites have been found to be medicinally more important than primary metabolites. Marine organisms, sponges, corals, microorganisms, etc., have provided natural products chemists with a rich source of unusual and diverse secondary metabolites. Many of these compounds have potent pharmacological activities, including antitumor, antifungal, antiviral, and antibacterial properties, some of which are currently in preclinical or clinical trials (Newman and Cragg 2004b). They are biosynthetically derived from primary metabolites but are more limited in distribution and are strain specific.

11.3 Origin of Bioactive Marine Metabolites

The importance of terrestrial microorganisms, bacteria and fungi, as sources of valuable bioactive metabolites is well-established, and some of the most important medicines in use today (penicillins, cyclosporin A, adriamycine, etc.) are obtained from terrestrial microorganisms. Similarly, it seems that marine microorganisms are the true producers of a number of secondary marine metabolites.

The marine environment is a vast and largely unexplored source of natural products with wide chemical and pharmacological diversity. Marine habitats provide unique conditions for microbial growth and secondary metabolite expression that are not found in terrestrial ecosystems. The coevolution of many marine macroorganisms, particularly invertebrate animals with microbes, has often led to the development of very close associations or symbiotic relationships between the host organism and a specific microbe. For instance, in sponges, there are a number of natural products present that are not produced by the sponge itself but by symbiotic bacteria growing inside the sponge. As the microbial world displays the greatest biodiversity, it has the potential to be the most important source of natural products that can be utilized to generate novel compounds with therapeutic activity.

It has been estimated that at best only about 1% of the world's microbes can be cultured with the technology currently being used. As a result, the DNA from these microbes is now being isolated and inserted into cultivatable organisms in the hope that the host organism will express the foreign DNA and produce novel compounds that otherwise would be unobtainable (Brady et al. 2001).

There are a number of general structural characteristics observed in the isolated bioactive molecules being discovered in marine microorganisms. Nitrogenated and acetate-derived products constitute the main principal classes (56%) of metabolites, 30% are acetate-derived metabolites, and around 13% are terpenoids. This distribution is very different from the distribution observed for marine invertebrates where the main classes of metabolites belong to the terpenoids (Kelecom 1999). However, natural products obtained from marine invertebrates and those from marine microorganisms (e.g., microalgae, cyanobacteria, heterotrophic bacteria, and fungi) generally show many structural similarities, suggesting that microorganisms living in their invertebrate hosts (e.g., tunicates, sponges, and soft corals) could be the actual producers of these secondary metabolites (Leusch et al. 2002, König et al. 2006). This was confirmed when cell populations within the marine sponge *Theonella swinhoei* were separated by differential centrifugation and the fractions obtained were chemically analyzed (Bewley et al. 1996). The peptide theopalauamide was localized in filamentous heterotrophic bacteria and the cytotoxic macrolide swinholide A in heterotrophic unicellular bacteria, suggesting a possible biosynthetic origin of some of these secondary metabolites.

Ascidians of the family Didemnidae are found to be in obligate symbiosis with the unicellular cyanobacterium *Prochloron* spp. (Donia et al. 2006). Numerous biologically active cyclic peptides have been isolated from the didemnin ascidians, including members of the patellamide and lissoclinamide families (Degnan et al. 1989). Recently, the *pat* gene cluster for patellamide biosynthesis was described, demonstrating that the symbiotic bacterium *Prochloron* spp. is responsible for patellamide production (Schmidt et al. 2005). Numerous structurally similar peptides and depsipeptides were isolated from both free-living cyanobacteria and sponges. The cyclic peptide leucamide A was isolated as the biologically active constituent of an organic extract of the sponge *Leucetta microraphis* (Kehraus et al. 2002). Scanning electron micrographs of *L. microraphis* revealed the presence of microbial symbionts, including cyanobacteria, in the sponge tissue. Leucamide A closely resembles the cyanobacterial peptides tenuecyclamide A (Banker and Carmeli 1988), dendroamide A (Ogino et al. 1996), nostocyclamide (Todorova et al. 1995), and the venturamides (A and B) (Linington et al. 2007), which also contain methyloxazole and thiazole rings. Pseudodysidenin, dysidenamide, nordysidenin, and barbamide are trichlorinated lipopeptides isolated from Panamanian and Curaçao strains of cyanobacteria *Lyngbya majuscula* (Orjala and Gerwick 1996, Jimenez and Scheuer 2001). Similar compounds (e.g., dysidenin and barbaleucamides A and B) were isolated from specimens of the sponge *Dysidea herbacea* (Kazlauskas et al. 1977, Harrigan et al. 2001).

11.4 Classes of Natural Products

Most natural products can be classified as terpenoids, polyketides, alkaloids, or nitrogen-containing compounds and nonribosomal peptides based on how they are biosynthesized. Terpenes include primary and secondary metabolites, all biosynthesized from the five carbon isoprene building units (Ruzicka 1953). Structural modification of these isoprene units leads a massively diverse range of derivatives with a wide array of chemical structures and biological properties. While higher plants' terpenoids were already studied and ethnopharmacologically rationalized centuries ago, those from their marine counterparts were not explored until the first half of the twentieth century. Some natural products have a mixed biosynthetic origin, where different parts of the molecule are synthesized by different biochemical pathways. Common examples of this are mixed polyketide–nonribosomal peptides and meroterpenoids, which are terpenoids with a nonterpenoid portion.

Natural products can be divided according to whether they act inside the organism or outside the organism. Endometabolites are substances exercising their biological function(s) within the organism itself (e.g., oxylipins, hormones, and phytoalexins), whereas exometabolites are released into the environment by the organism (e.g., toxins, antibiotics, and different signaling compounds). It is useful to note that in general there are many more exometabolites produced than endometabolites by marine organisms. As expected, the chemical structure of secondary metabolites varies greatly and includes steroids, terpenoids, alkaloids, polyketides, phenolic metabolites, some carbohydrates, lipids, and peptides. Often, secondary metabolites are classified on the basis of their biological function(s), for example, as hormones, antibiotics, toxins, and pheromones. Chemically the bioactive metabolites of marine flora include brominated phenols, oxygen heterocyclics, nitrogen heterocyclics, sulfur nitrogen heterocyclics, sterols, terpenoids, polysaccharides, peptides, and proteins (Faulkner 1991).

11.5 Marine Natural Products with Antitumor Properties

Some of the most effective cancer treatments to date are natural products or compounds derived from natural products. Over the past two decades, marine organisms including sponges (Hickford et al. 2009), sponge–microbe symbiotic association (Thomas et al. 2010), gorgonian (Rodriguez and Martinez 1993), actinomycetes (Olano et al. 2009), and soft coral (Hassan et al. 2010) have been widely explored for potential anticancer agents. Several dozen marine metabolites have been found to be extremely toxic against tumor cells. Many of these metabolites can be classified into fundamentally new structural classes of antitumor agents, therefore providing potential new sources for many new lead antitumor drug candidates. Before these substances were discovered, all of the natural products used in chemotherapy could be classified into only four to five structural types. However, marine natural products are difficult to access and sometimes impossible to harvest in sufficient quantities from the marine organisms. Marine organisms that produce these compounds are usually rare and are scattered around the oceans which makes them hard to collect in sufficient numbers. There is potential for growing and harvesting these organisms in order to be able to collect these secondary metabolites in sufficient quantities for use. However, current aquaculture methods do not enable these organisms to be grown successfully. Furthermore, a laboratory synthesis of these metabolites is not yet economically possible, due to the complexity of their structures and abundance of asymmetric centers. It is important to note that with compounds that showed antitumor activity, although these compounds are highly toxic against tumor cells, they do not always demonstrate good anticancer activity in vivo, and some of them cause side effects which exclude their clinical application.

Promising anticancer clinical candidates like salinosporamide A and bryostatin show the incredible importance of drug leads derived from marine organisms. Polyketide salinosporamide A (Figure 11.1) is a highly bioactive β-lactone, cytotoxic proteasome inhibitor isolated from the salt-tolerant marine bacterium *Salinispora tropica* (Feling et al. 2003). Salinosporamide A inhibits p26 proteosomes (Lopez-Macia et al. 2001) by covalently modifying the active site threonine residues of the 20S proteasome. It is currently in several phase I clinical trials for the treatment of drug-resistant multiple myelomas and three other types of cancers (Ahn et al. 2007, Molinski et al. 2009).

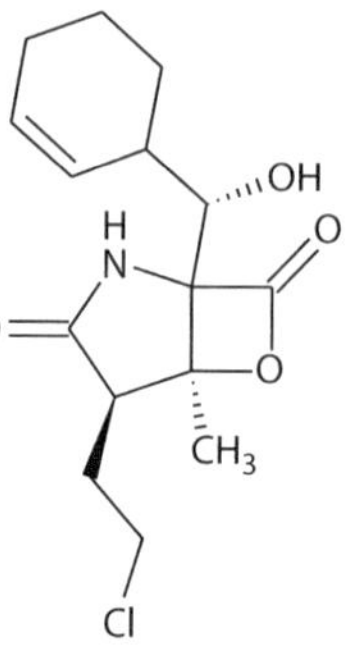

FIGURE 11.1
Salinosporamide A.

11.5.1 Bryostatins

The bryostatins are complex, rare natural products produced by a bacterial symbiont (Davidson et al. 2001, Lopanik et al. 2004), the marine bryozoan *B. neritina*, a fouling organism that grows in thick colonies on pier pilings and docks in oceans around the world (Pettit et al. 1970). The structure of the primary active constituent from extracts of this marine organism, bryostatin 1 (Figure 11.2), was elucidated with the help of x-ray analysis in 1982 (Pettit et al. 1982). Since then, 19 additional bryostatins have been described. The bryostatins are a family of 26-membered ring macrocyclic lactones consisting of three highly substituted tetrahydropyran rings with varying ester functionality on two of these rings. They belong to a diverse class of complex products called polyketides. Bryostatin 1 was first isolated from the bryozoan sponge *B. neritina* in 1981 by Pettit et al. (1982), and since then, 19 other bryostatin macrolides have been discovered, differing in their functionality at the C-7 and C-20 oxygens, as well as the complexity of the C-ring (formed by the C19–C23 chain). Bryostatin has 11 asymmetric centers, and it is very unlikely that it

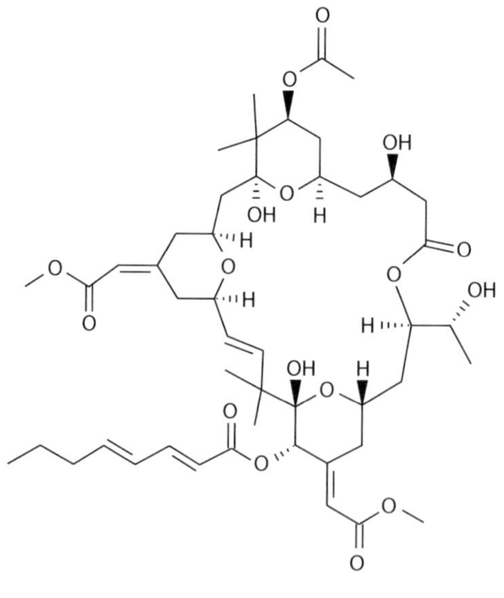

FIGURE 11.2
Bryostatin 1.

could be obtained with a sufficient yield by organic synthesis. Its content in the bryozoan extract is insignificant (0.00001%), but scientists have managed to obtain 18 g of bryostatin for clinical and preclinical testing from 10,000 gal of bryozoan collected. This substance has been determined to be a modulator of protein kinase C, a stimulator of the immune system, and an inductor of cell differentiation. It intensifies the antitumor action of some drugs but causes myalgias as a side effect. Bryostatin 1 shows affinity for protein kinase C isozymes and, through this pathway, has been shown to exhibit anticancer properties, reverse multidrug resistance, stimulate the immune system, and treat several central nervous system diseases, such as Alzheimer's disease and depression.

Bryostatin 1 possesses a remarkable spectrum of biological activities relevant to cancer therapy including modulation of apoptotic function (Wall et al. 1999), reversal of multidrug resistance (Elgie et al. 1998, Spitaler et al. 1998), and stimulation of the immune system (Oz et al. 2000). Studies have shown that bryostatin 1 can enhance the clinical efficacy of known oncolytics in several cases (Dowlati et al. 2003, Ajani et al. 2006, Barr et al. 2009). Additionally, bryostatins provide a starting point for the conception and design of novel immunotherapeutic approaches to cancer treatment (Shaha et al. 2009). The required clinical dose of bryostatin is extremely low, and only approximately 1 mg is needed for an 8 week clinical treatment cycle. It was also found that bryostatin 1 enhances learning and extends memory in animal models (Sun and Alkon 2005, Kuzirian et al. 2006), due to its ability to induce synaptogenesis (Hongpaisan and Alkon 2007). Thus, it could serve as a first-in-class clinical lead for the treatment of Alzheimer's disease (Etcheberrigaray et al. 2004) and other neurodegenerative disorders (Sun and Alkon 2006). Bryostatin also exhibits neuroprotective capabilities in animal models of cerebral ischemia, indicating its potential use for minimizing the destructive neurological effects of stroke (Sun et al. 2009). Of special recent significance, bryostatin, not unlike prostratin (Wender et al. 2008), has been found to activate latent HIV reservoirs, providing a potential strategy for the eradication of HIV (Mehla et al. 2010).

11.5.2 Ecteinascidins

The investigation of tropical marine ecosystems has resulted in the isolation and subsequent clinical development of two anticancer agents, trabectedin, also known as ecteinascidin 743 (ET-743; Etrabectedin), and aplidin (Figure 11.3). Ecteinascidin is a family of tetrahydroisoquinoline alkaloids derived from the Caribbean sea squirt (Ascidia) *Ecteinascidia turbinate* (Rinehart et al. 1990, Wright et al. 1990), a colony-forming tunicate that grows in the coastal platform of several temperate seas and is a common component of the intertidal/subtidal mangrove prop root community. Ecteinascidin 743 (Figure 11.3) has recently emerged as the first active drug (Yondelis) developed against sarcoma in the last two decades, with promising results especially against soft-tissue sarcoma and Ewing's sarcoma (ES). Yondelis was approved in European Union countries for treatment of soft-tissue sarcoma in 2007. Although the structure of the ecteinascidin 743 was elucidated in 1990 (Rinehart et al. 1990), the high antitumor activity of extract of *Ecteinascidia turbinata* has been known since 1969. The natural scarcity of ecteinascidins (1 mg of ET-743 per 1 kg of tunicate) prevented their isolation and structure elucidation for nearly 20 years. The initial in vitro cytotoxicity and relative high stability of ecteinascidin 743 prompted further investigation of its utility as an anticancer drug (van Kestren et al. 2003). The low toxic concentration of ET-743 ($IC_{50}=0.5$ ng/mL) against the tumor cells L-1210 demonstrated a high antitumor activity against different types of mouse cancer. ET-743 is currently in several phase II (prostate cancer and osteosarcoma) and phase III (metastatic

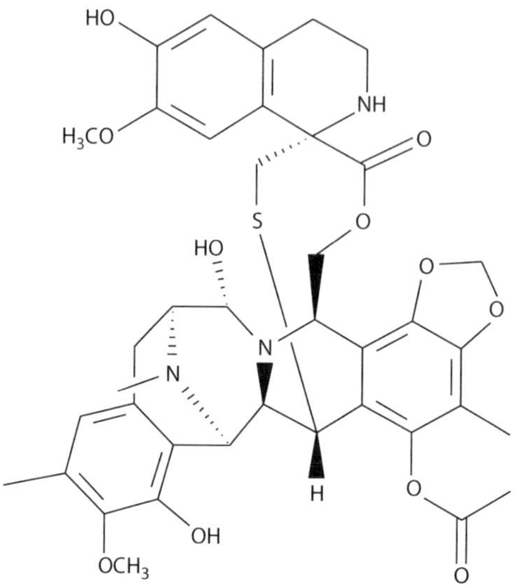

FIGURE 11.3
Ecteinascidin 743.

breast cancer and ovarian cancer) clinical trials alone and in combination with other drugs (http://www.clinicaltrials.gov). In addition, ET-743 was granted orphan drug status from the European Commission (EC) and the U.S. FDA for soft-tissue sarcomas and ovarian cancer and received authorization for commercialization from the EC for advanced soft-tissue sarcoma.

There were a number of issues in obtaining sufficient quantities of ET-743 for clinical use. Complete laboratory synthesis of ET-743 could not provide a sufficient amount of material for bioassay (Corey et al. 1996), while ascidian cultivation did not produce sufficient quantities due to the wide variation in the content of ecteinascidins obtained from these organisms. Finally, after much work, scientists managed to synthesize this alkaloid from the antibiotic cyanosafracin B which is able to be produced in good yield from the terrestrial bacterium *Pseudomonas fluorescens* (Cuevas et al. 2000).

The mechanism of biological action of ecteinascidin 743 on tumor cells is related to its ability to penetrate the DNA's minor groove and to alkylate guanine residues, thereby inducing a curvature in the DNA helix toward the major groove (Pommier et al. 1996, Zewail-Foote and Hurley 1999). This mode of action is different from other agents currently being used in cancer chemotherapy. Moreover, ecteinascidin 743 causes programmed death (apoptosis) of tumor cells and intensifies the antitumor action of some well-known drugs (doxorubicin, paclitaxel [Taxol], etc.). In spite of the fact that ecteinascidin 743 was approved only for the treatment of soft-tissue sarcoma, it showed good results in the course of clinical testing for the treatment of other types of malignant tumors.

Several highly active depsipeptides from ascidians, including didemnin B from *Trididemnum solidum* (Rinehart et al. 1981), were intensely studied for many years as potential antitumor drugs. Nevertheless, the clinical investigations of didemnin B (Figure 11.4) were discontinued due to significant neuromuscular toxicity and insufficient effectiveness for patients in terminal stages of cancer. Its analogue, aplidin (dehydrodidemnin B), exhibited marked anticancer properties, outperforming the related compound didemnin B by a factor of 6. Aplidin was discovered in the Mediterranean ascidian (tunicate) *Aplidium albicans*

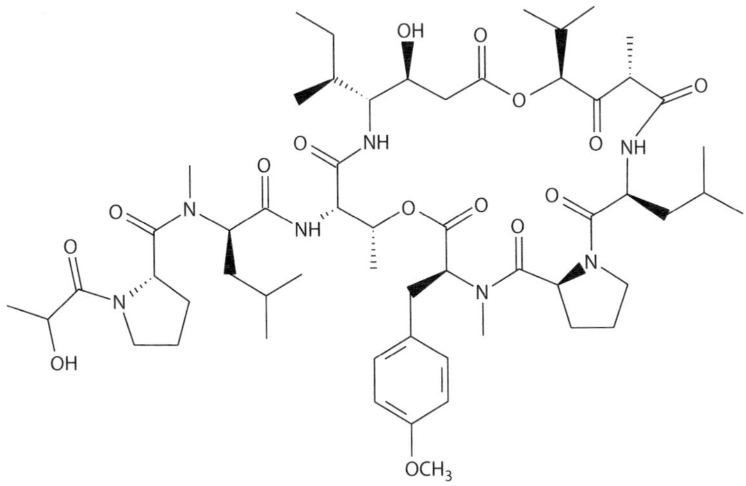

FIGURE 11.4
Didemnin B.

and has been developed as an antineoplastic agent. Aplidin differs chemically from didemnin B and the other didemnins only in the structure of its side chain. This fact, along with its small size and relatively simple structure, has allowed researchers to achieve total synthesis of didemnin analogues. The replacing of some amino acids nonessential for bioactivity with covalent bonds has increased resistance to enzymatic degradation and prolonged the biological lifetime of the molecule. Analogues more active than any of the original natural didemnins have also been produced in this manner. Aplidin initiates oxidative stress which results in apoptosis in tumor cells (Gajate et al. 2003). Aplidin is also an inhibitor of angiogenesis and disturbs the blood supply to tumors. In spite of the fact that aplidin is at the second stage of clinical testing as a drug for myeloma treatment, a good method to produce it has not yet been developed, because neither the technology for the corresponding ascidian cultivation nor an appropriate synthesis for the production of sufficient amounts of this substance has been achieved (Pommier et al. 1996).

11.5.3 Dolastatins

Dolastatins, a group of peptides isolated from the Indian Ocean sea hare *Dolabella auricularia* (Pettit et al. 1987, 1989a,b) (sea slug or snail), have been shown to have remarkable anticancer properties. They bind to tubulin subunits and inhibit tubulin-dependent GTP hydrolysis in vitro (Bai et al. 1990). In vivo, these actions inhibit the assembly of new microtubules, induce the depolymerization of existing microtubules, and inhibit cell cycle progression in mitosis (Bai et al. 1992, Beckwith et al. 1993). However, due to the extremely small abundance of the active dolastatin 10 (Figure 11.5) present in these organisms, the structure elucidation of dolastatin 10 took nearly 15 years to complete. In order to obtain the first milligram of dolastatin 10, an enormous amount of the rare mollusk was required (about 2 tons). Dolastatin 10 was found to be a linear pentapeptide with a unique structure comprising five units, an essential amino acid valine, and four previously unknown amino acids: *N,N*-dimethylvaline, dolaisoleucine, dolaproine, and dolaphenine (Pettit et al. 1987). A few years later, researchers carried out a total synthesis of that peptide,

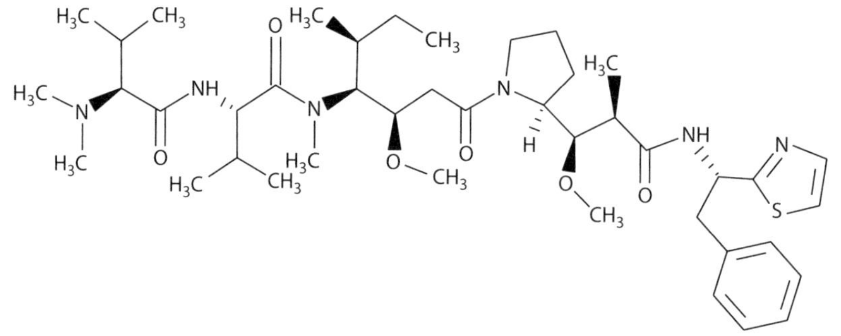

FIGURE 11.5
Dolastatin 10.

which confirmed the structure suggested and established its absolute stereochemistry (Pettit et al. 1989).

It was suggested the source of the dolastatin 10 in sea hares was the result of a diet of cyanobacteria which contained the bioactive secondary metabolite (Harrigan et al. 1998). This was subsequently confirmed by direct isolation of dolastatin 10 from field collections of the marine cyanobacterium *Symploca* sp. (Luesch et al. 2001).

Dolastatin 10 is extremely toxic against tumor cells. At the time of its discovery, it was the most potent antiproliferative agent known with an IC_{50} of 4.6×10^{-5} µg/mL against P388 leukemia cells (Pettit et al. 1987). Subsequently, dolastatin 10 was shown to be a potent noncompetitive inhibitor of vinca alkaloid binding to tubulin ($Ki = 1.4$ µmol/L) and strongly affected microtubule assembly and tubulin-dependent guanosine triphosphate hydrolysis (Bai et al. 1990). Further work revealed that dolastatin 10 binds to the rhizoxin/maytansine binding site (Jordan et al. 1998) (adjacent to vinca alkaloid site) as well as to the exchangeable guanosine triphosphate site on tubulin, causing cell cycle arrest in metaphase (Bai et al. 1992). However, clinical testing of dolastatin 10 was discontinued due to its high antitumor activity not being confirmed at the first and second stages of clinical evaluation (Pitot et al. 1999, Vaishampayan et al. 2000, Hoffman et al. 2003). Attempts to create a dolastatin-based antitumor drug were not abandoned, and dolastatin 10 was used as an excellent lead for structure–activity relationship (SAR) studies and synthetic drug design, ultimately leading to the development of the tetrapeptide analogue TZT-1027 (Figure 11.6).

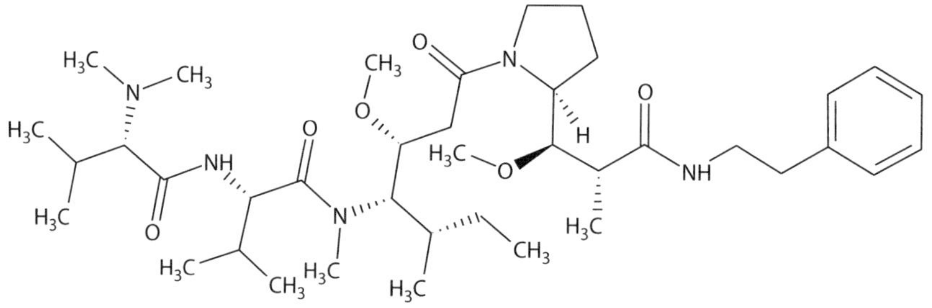

FIGURE 11.6
TZT-1027.

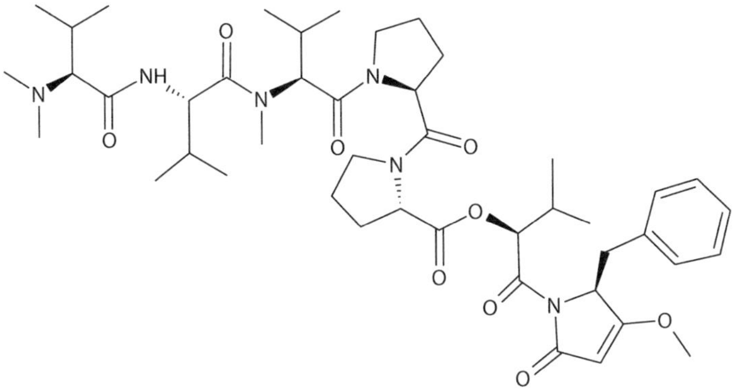

FIGURE 11.7
Dolastatin 15.

TZT-1027 (soblidotin, auristatin PE) was designed with the goal of maintaining potent antitumor activity while reducing the toxicity of the parent compound (Miyazaki et al. 1995). The structure of TZT-1027 differs from dolastatin 10 only in the absence of the thiazole ring from the original dolaphenine residue, resulting in a terminal phenyl-ethanamine moiety. Just like dolastatin 10, it is a strong inhibitor of tubulin polymer-ization, stops the division of cancer cells in very low concentrations, and reduces blood supply to tumors (inhibits angiogenesis) (Watanabe et al. 2007). TZT-1027 is a mitotic spindle poison that interacts with tubulin in the same domain as the vinca alkaloid binding region.

Dolastatin 15 (Figure 11.7) was also isolated from extracts of the Indian Ocean sea hare *D. auricularia* in trace amounts, also strongly implicating a cyanobacterial source for this metabolite (Gerwick et al. 2001). It is a linear depsipeptide sequence composed of seven amino acid or hydroxyl acid residues. In initial bioassays with the P388 lym-phocytic leukemia cell line, dolastatin 15 displayed an $ED_{50} = 2.4 \times 10^{-3}$ µg/mL (Pettit et al. 1989). In contrast to dolastatin 10, dolastatin 15 binds directly to the *vinca* domain of tubulin (Cruz-Monserrate et al. 2003). Obstacles to further clinical evaluation of dol-astatin 15 include molecular complexity, low yield from chemical synthesis, and poor water solubility. However, these impediments have prompted the development of vari-ous synthetic analogue compounds with enhanced chemical properties (e.g., cematodin and synthadotin).

In 1995, cematodin (LU-103793) was synthesized as a water-soluble and water-stabilized analogue of dolastatin 15 with a terminal benzylamine moiety in place of the original dolapyrrolidone. Cematodin retains the high in vitro cytotoxicity of the parent compound ($IC_{50} = 0.1$ µmol/L), disrupts tubulin polymerization ($IC_{50} = 7.0$ µmol/L), and induces depo-lymerization of preassembled microtubules. Cell cycle arrest occurs at the G2/M phase transition (de Arruda et al. 1995). Recently, cematodin underwent six phase I clinical trials with dose-limiting toxicity, including cardiac toxicity, hypertension, and acute myocardial infarction. Overall, neutropenia was the most common dose-limiting effect observed in phase I testing (Villalona-Calero et al. 1998, Amador et al. 2003). Unfortunately, phase II evaluations with malignant melanoma, metastatic breast cancer, and non-small cell lung cancer have produced no objective results to date (Smyth et al. 2001, Kerbrat et al. 2003, Marks et al. 2003). Therefore, current clinical evaluation of LU-103793 has been discontinued (Newman and Cragg 2004b).

ILX-651 (synthadotin) is an orally active third-generation synthetic dolastatin 15 analogue possessing a terminal *tert*-butyl moiety (vs. the original dolapyrrolidone). Synthadotin (ILX-651) is a pentapeptide with a unique mechanism of action that potentially differs from that of microtubule stabilizers (taxanes and epothilones) and tubulin inhibitors (vinca alkaloids and dolastatins), and it is postulated that it inhibits microtubule nucleation. The drug has been chemically modified to provide improved pharmacological properties and has a better potential therapeutic window over previous generations of dolastatins. Although ILX-651 is known to be an inhibitor of tubulin assembly, further refinements on its mechanism of action have been reported recently (Ray et al. 2007, Bai et al. 2009) where the "active version" is probably the pentapeptide produced by hydrolysis of the C-terminal amide bond.

Tubulin is a well-established target for anticancer agents. Although available antitubulin agents, including the taxanes and *vinca* alkaloids, are highly effective in cancer therapy, their clinical usefulness is limited by intrinsic or acquired resistance and systemic toxicity (Kavallaris et al. 2001). Thus, it is important to develop new agents that target the tubulin/microtubule system with efficacy against resistant tumors and also have an improved side effect profile. However, initial clinical evaluation of dolastatin 10 and cemadotin, a synthetic analogue of dolastatin 15, showed disappointing results (Hoffman et al. 2003, Kerbrat et al. 2003, Marks et al. 2003) possibly due, in part, to poor cellular uptake. In addition, cemadotin is rapidly converted to a metabolite with dose-limiting cardiovascular toxicities, including hypertension, angina, and myocardial infarction, that limited its therapeutic efficacy (Figure 11.8) (Mross et al. 1996, Wolff et al. 1996, Villalona-Calero et al. 1998).

To address these problems, a new generation of dolastatins, represented by tasidotin, has been created. These dolastatins offer several advantages over most other antitubulins. Tasidotin is a pentapeptide (*N,N*-dimethyl-L-valyl-L-valyl-*N*-methyl-L-valyl-L-prolyl-L-proline-*tert*-butylamide hydrochloride), chemically modified to improve the pharmacological properties of cemadotin, resulting in a more metabolically stable compound. Tasidotin induces a prolonged lag phase in microtubule assembly at concentrations of 25–40 µmol/L (16–26 µg/mL) followed by recovery with microtubule assembly returning to normal levels (Stephenson et al. 2004). These effects are in contrast to those seen with other antitubulins, such as podophyllotoxin and vinblastine (Wilson et al. 1999, Jordan 2002, Okouneva et al. 2003, Bunker et al. 2004, Jordan and Wilson 2004), which produce cell cycle arrest in the G2 and M cell cycle phases. At concentrations ≥50 µmol/L (32 µg/mL), tasidotin inhibits the extent of microtubule assembly, which is also an atypical finding for antitubulins. Finally, in addition to its potentially enhanced therapeutic window, tasidotin is bioavailable when administered orally (Figure 11.9) (Hopper et al. 2003).

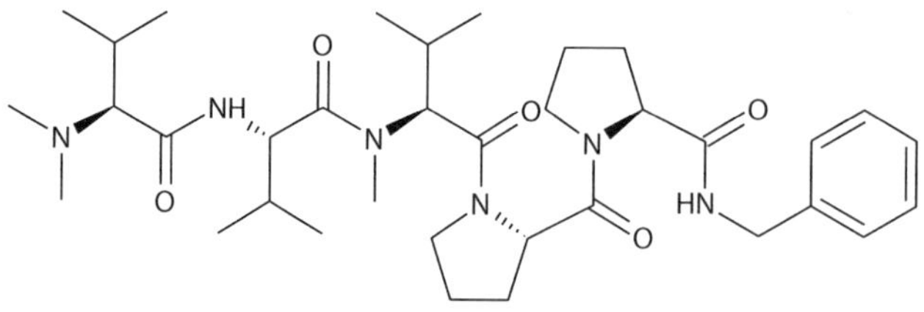

FIGURE 11.8
Cemadotin.

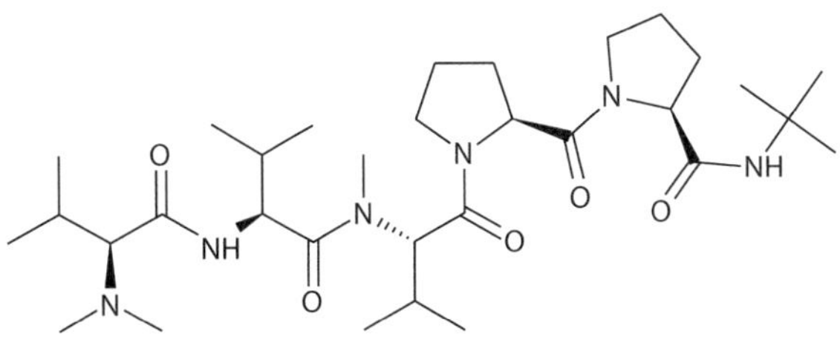

FIGURE 11.9
Tasidotin.

11.5.4 Hemiasterlin

Hemiasterlin (Figure 11.10) is an antimitotic tripeptide that was extracted for the first time from the deepwater sponge *Hemiastrella minor* by Kashman and his coworkers in 1986 (Talpir et al. 1994). Initial screening showed that it was highly cytotoxic with an IC_{50} value of ~0.01 µg/mL against the P388 leukemia cell line (Talpir et al. 1994). In 1995, the related isomers hemiasterlins A and B (Figure 11.10), isolated by Andersen and coworkers from sponges of the genus *Auletta* and *Cymbastela* in 1995 (Coleman et al. 1995), were found to be even more potent. All hemiasterlins showed cytotoxicity in the nanomolar range (concentrations ~1 × 10^{-9} M) against a variety of cultured human and murine cell lines. In 1996, an x-ray crystal structure analysis of the hemiasterlin methyl ester confirmed the linear structure of hemiasterlin and its unusual constituent amino acids (Coleman et al. 1995, 1996). A fourth analogue, hemiasterlin C (Figure 11.10), was described in 1999 (Gamble et al. 1999). Its synthetic analogue HTI-286, with a phenyl substituent instead of *N*-methylindole, appeared to be more active and, in nanomolecular concentrations, inhibited cell division by disrupting the polymerization of the monomeric units of tubulin (Niu et al. 2004). In preclinical testing, it showed good activity against tumors resistant to paclitaxel, one of the best antitumor drugs used currently. However, the clinical testing did not confirm that it was active in the case of patients in terminal stages of cancer. Recently, scientists demonstrated the antitumor action of this drug on androgen-dependent tumors, which has inspired renewed interest in further clinical studies of HTI-286 (Hadaschik et al. 2008).

Extensive SAR studies demonstrated that the simpler synthetic analogue of hemiasterlin, HTI-286 (Figure 11.11), with a phenyl substituent replacing the *N*-methyltryptophan, is more potent than hemiasterlin (Coleman et al. 1996). An analogue of HTI-286 with a

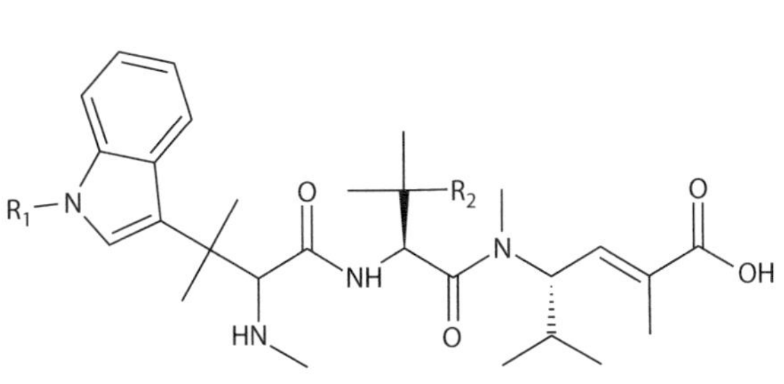

FIGURE 11.10
Hemiasterlin (R_1 = CH_3, R_2 = CH_3); hemiasterlin A (R_1 = H, R_2 = CH_3); hemiasterlin B (R_1 = H, R_2 = H); hemiasterlin C (R_1 = CH_3, R_2 = H).

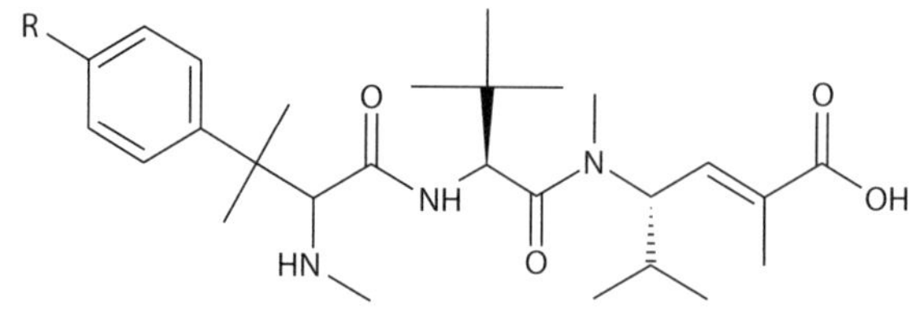

FIGURE 11.11
HTI-286 (R = H); HTI-286 analogue (R = OCH$_3$).

para-methoxyl substituent on the benzene ring was even more potent (Gamble et al. 1999). Other structural elements, including the gem β,β-dimethyl group and the *N*-methyl on the first amino acid residue (N terminus), the isopropyl and an double bond in the homolo-gated γ-amino acid (C terminus), including a terminal carboxylic acid or methyl ester, were essential for activity.

The aryl side chain on the *N* terminus could be replaced synthetically by alkyl groups (e.g., *tert*-butyl) while still retaining potent activity (Nieman et al. 2003, Niu et al. 2004, Yamashita et al. 2004, Zask et al. 2004a,b). The binding of hemiasterlin and HTI-286 to β-tubulin takes place at the vinca peptide site, near the α/β interface (Nunes et al. 2005), in a ratio of one to one (Lo et al. 2004).

11.5.5 Discodermolide

The difficulty of developing drugs from marine sources has limited development in this area for a long time. Because the ocean is a much more demanding environment in which to sample and harvest enough quantities of rare natural compounds, and since due to their complexity they are generally difficult to synthesize, obtaining these compounds in sufficient quantities for use has often been an issue. For example, the chemically versatile marine sponges, the source of many potential therapeutic compounds such as discoder-molide and hemiasterlin, are primitive metazoans that live almost exclusively in marine habitats. Discodermolide (Figure 11.12) was isolated from the rare deepwater sponge *Discodermia dissoluta* at depths of up to 300 m using a submarine. Sponges and their micro-bial fauna are mostly unculturable, and the natural products that they produce must be extracted and purified from specimens collected by hand using scuba diving or some-times with the aid of submersibles equipped with robotic arms. Both of these techniques are expensive endeavors that are unwieldy and foreign to the modern pharmaceutical industry. Nevertheless, interest in the remarkable properties of marine natural products

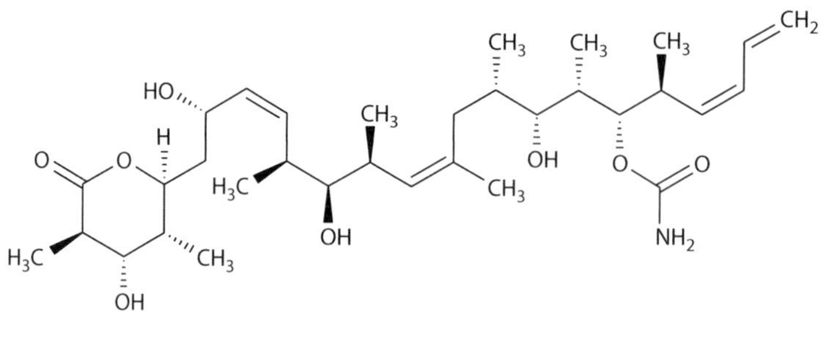

FIGURE 11.12
(+)-Discodermolide.

has remained high enough so that inspired innovative solutions to the supply problem have been proposed on a case-by-case basis, ranging from aquaculture of marine invertebrates to semisynthesis of the natural products under investigation (Mendola 2000).

The structure of the naturally occurring isomer (+)-discodermolide was first elucidated by analysis of NMR and MS data, with its relative stereochemistry determined using x-ray crystal structure analysis (Gunasekera et al. 1990, 1991). The isomer (–)-discodermolide, while not naturally occurring, has since been synthesized in the laboratory (Nerenberg et al. 1993). (–)-Discodermolide is not as potent as (+)-discodermolide, arresting the cell cycle in vitro, at much higher concentrations (72–135 nM) when compared with the naturally occurring (+) enantiomer (3–80 nM). It has also been found that their mechanism of action is quite different with (+)-discodermolide blocking the cell cycle at the G2/M phase and (–)-discodermolide blocking the cell cycle at the S phase (Hung et al. 1994).

(+)-Discodermolide has also been synthesized in the laboratory (Harried et al. 2003). Due to the exceedingly limited natural supply of (+)-discodermolide, much work has been undertaken to develop more efficient methods to synthesize the compound, resulting in several inventive multistep, scaled-up processes for total syntheses of the isomer (Paterson and Lyothier 2004, Paterson et al. 2005). This enabled Novartis to obtain sufficient material for phase I clinical trials (Mickel et al. 2004a–e). The outcome of these trials was that (+)-discodermolide showed no neuropathy or neutropenia and demonstrated mild-to-moderate toxicity from 0.6 to 19.2 mg/m². The pharmacokinetics of (+)-discodermolide were shown to be nonlinear with recycling of (+)-discodermolide between tissues and the circulatory system (Mita et al. 2004). At present, Novartis has discontinued phase I trials with (+)-discodermolide, owing to lack of efficacy and toxicity problems. However, it may possibly still prove useful in the future as a therapeutic agent when used in combination with other antitumor drugs (Molinski et al. 2009).

11.5.6 Cryptophycins

The cryptophycins (Figure 11.13) are a unique family of 16-membered macrolide antimitotic agents isolated from the cyanobacteria *Nostoc* sp. The name cryptophycin is due to its extremely potent activity against filamentous fungi of the genus *Cryptococcus* (Cole et al. 1992). Cryptophycin-1 is a cyclic depsipeptide, and it is the major cytotoxic metabolite isolated from two blue-green algae, *Nostoc* sp. Moore and coworkers (Schwartz et al. 1990, Trimurtulu et al. 1994, Subbaraju et al. 1997) isolated 26 closely related natural products from the strain GSV 224 with cryptophycin-1 being the major isolate. Originally

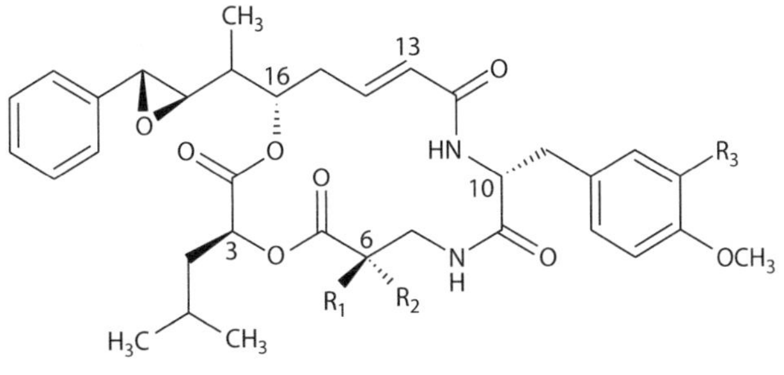

FIGURE 11.13
Cryptophycin-1 ($R_1 = CH_3$, $R_2 = H$, $R_3 = Cl$); cryptophycin-24 ($R_1 = H$, $R_2 = H$, $R_3 = H$); cryptophycin-52 ($R_1 = CH_3$, $R_2 = H$, $R_3 = Cl$).

cryptophycin was investigated as an antifungal agent. However, preliminary investigations indicated that it was too toxic for human use and development of the compound for this purpose was not pursued. At the same time, a structurally related cytotoxic compound, initially named arenastatin, was isolated from the Okinawan marine sponge *Dysidea arenaria* (Kobayashi et al. 1994c). It was found that arenastatin A was identical to cryptophycin-24, and it has been postulated that cryptophycin's presence in the Okinawan marine sponge was due to the presence of a cyanobacterial symbiont. Cryptophycin-1 has shown potent broad-spectrum antitumor activity in both preclinical in vitro and in vivo models, with IC_{50} values in the pM range (Kobayashi et al. 1994a,b). It is a potent inhibitor of tubulin polymerization and strongly binds to tubulin and disrupts microtubule assembly. It is important to note that there is reduced susceptibility of the cryptophycins to P-glycoprotein-mediated multiple drug resistance when compared to the antitumor agents vinblastine, colchicine, and paclitaxel (Smith et al. 1994).

SAR studies have indicated that most modifications of the cryptophycin structure result in a dramatic decrease in activity. In vitro studies have shown the least detrimental change appeared to be the removal of the C6 methyl substituent. However, in vivo studies show removal of the C6 methyl substituent results in a significant loss in activity (marginal to negative) likely due to an increase in hydrolytic susceptibility of the C5 ester (Golakoti et al. 1995). The instability of this bond was firstly examined during the initial isolation of the cryptophycins when methanol extracts produced several methanolysis products (Trimurtulu et al. 1994).

11.5.7 Halichondrins

In 1986, Uemura and Hirata isolated eight minor metabolites, polyether macrolides, called halichondrins from *Halichondria okadai* (Hirata and Uemura 1986), a widely distributed sponge in the Pacific coast of Japan. Those compounds were strong inhibitors of tumor cell development (IC_{50} 10^{-9} M), bound to tubulin on the same site as the vinca peptides applied in clinical treatment, and were selected for further investigation of their antitumor properties. An initial attempt to determine the structure of halichondrin B (Figure 11.14), the most effective antitumor substance among those, failed due to its relatively large molecular weight ($M = 1110$) and then the absence of any heavy atoms such as bromine or iodine

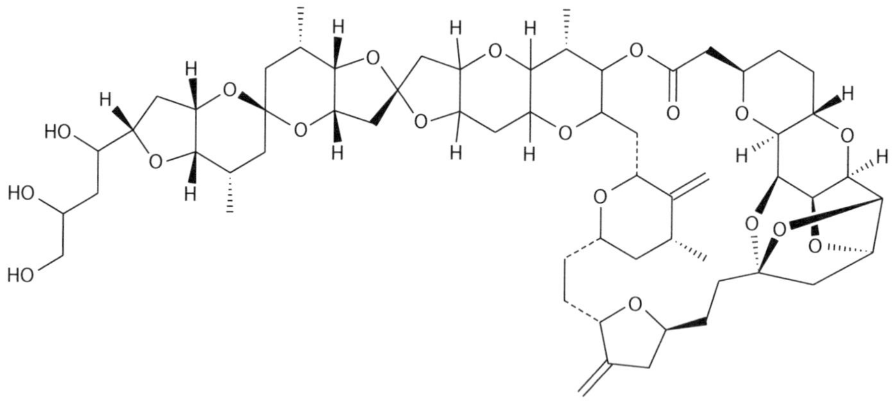

FIGURE 11.14
Halichondrin B.

atoms. Hence, structural elucidation of norhalichondrin A, the major component of this series, has been done (Uemura et al. 1985). The length of a molecule of halichondrins, 30–35 Å, corresponds to half of the lipid bilayer of biomembrane. Structural variations of this series depend on a lipophilic and hydrophilic part of a long molecule, which are assigned to the tricyclo system and the terminal moiety. It is very important for antitumor activity that the tricyclo ring is relatively lipophilic and then the terminal moiety contains two or three hydroxyls but not a carboxylate.

The important features of these molecules are (1) a long, straight carbon chain such as (2) the first naturally found 2,6,9-trioxatricyclo[3.3.2] decane system; (3) a polyether macrolide; (4) two spirosystems, involving a 1,6-dioxaspiro[4.4]nonane system; (5) two boat-shaped pyranose rings; and (6) two *cis*-fused pyranose rings.

However, it was rather difficult to produce halichondrins in sufficient amount. Halichondrin B has a staggering 32 stereocenters, meaning that there are 2^{32} (more than 4 billion) possible isomers of the molecule. Due to a complex structure, the total synthesis of halichondrin B developed in 1992 (Aicher et al. 1992) consisted of 90 stages and could not solve that problem. Almost at the same time, New Zealand scientists discovered a new source of halichondrins, the deepwater sponge *Lissodendoryx* n. sp.1. A ton of that sponge was obtained by dredging. Moreover, plantations of *Lissodendoryx* were created in shallow waters in New Zealand, though the content of the target agents was much lower in the cultivated tube than in the wild one (Munro et al. 1990). After putting it into clinical development in the early 1990s, NCI funded the collection of 1 ton of the host sponge, which is found in deep water off the coast of New Zealand. That boiled down to a mere 300 mg of product, not nearly enough to further develop the drug.

Those efforts made it possible to obtain 310 mg of halichondrin B and to begin clinical testing in 2002. Then, Japanese scientists, in collaboration with the Eisai Company, found out that a much simpler derivative of halichondrin, eribulin mesylate, shows the same biological activity. This activity is retained in structurally simplified macrocyclic ketone analogues (Towle et al. 2001), and the development candidate, eribulin mesylate, retains the promising biological properties of the natural product as well as favorable pharmaceutical attributes including water solubility and chemical stability (Yu 2005). Like the widely used taxane and vinca alkaloid chemotherapeutics, eribulin (Figure 11.15) and halichondrin B are tubulin-targeted agents. However, eribulin and halichondrin B inhibit microtubule

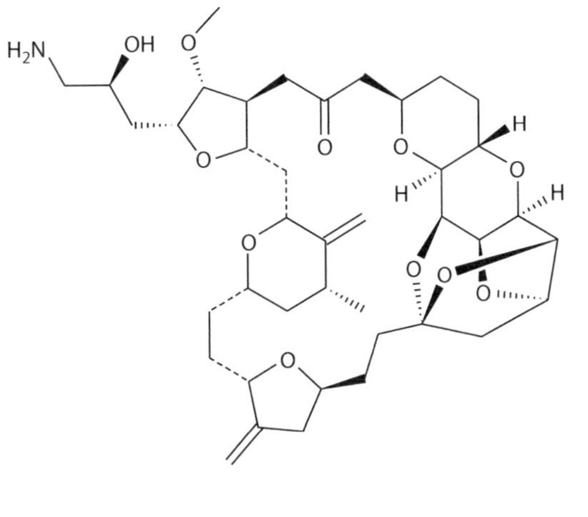

FIGURE 11.15
Eribulin.

dynamics through a unique mechanism distinct from those of the taxanes and vincas (Jordan et al. 2005, Okouneva et al. 2008). Against cancer cells, eribulin exerts potent and irreversible antimitotic effects, leading to cell death by apoptosis (Kuznetsov et al. 2004).

Currently, eribulin mesylate is in the third stage of clinical testing as a potential drug for the treatment of breast cancer (Molinski et al. 2009). Moreover, it is being tested for the treatment of prostate cancer and sarcoma. Eribulin, previously known as E7389, is a structurally simplified synthetic analogue of halichondrin B, a fully synthetic polyether macrocyclic ketone. On November 15, 2010, the FDA granted approval for eribulin mesylate (Halaven™ Injection) for the treatment of patients with metastatic breast cancer (Huyck et al. 2011).

11.5.8 Squalamine

Squalamine is a sulfated aminosterol, water-soluble cationic steroid, originally isolated in 1993 (Moore et al. 1993) from the tissues of the spiny dogfish shark *Squalus acanthias* and later identified within the circulating white blood cells of the sea lamprey (*Petromyzon marinus*) (Yun and Li 2007). When it was discovered in 1993, the compound was reported to exhibit broad-spectrum antibiotic activity.

Squalamine 1 (Figure 11.16) possesses a steroid skeleton with a *trans*-AB ring junction, a cholestane-related sulfated side chain and a flexible polyamino-hydrophilic spermidine group linked to the hydrophobic unit at the C-3 position (Wehrli et al. 1993). Squalamine has numerous therapeutic properties, including antimicrobial and antiangiogenic properties (Brunel et al. 2005, Salmi and Brunel 2007). It was found to have pharmacological activity in endothelial cells, inhibiting several growth factor-dependent processes (such as angiogenesis, migration, and proliferation) both in vitro and in vivo (Sills et al. 1998).

This water-soluble cationic steroid displays a range of antibacterial properties including effective bactericidal activity and the ability to permeabilize the outer membranes of Gram-negative bacteria sensitizing them to hydrophobic antibiotics that ineffectively traverse the outer membrane. Squalamine acts by disrupting the outer membranes of Gram-negative bacteria by a detergent-like mechanism of action and by depolarizing the bacterial membranes of Gram-positive bacteria (Alhanout et al. 2010). Squalamine carries a net positive charge by virtue of its polyamine spermidine moiety and exhibits a high affinity for anionic phospholipids (Selinsky et al. 1998, Yeung et al. 2008) in the cell membrane and neutralizes the negative charge of the surface to which it binds. Squalamine enters cells and causes displacement of proteins that are associated through electrostatic interactions

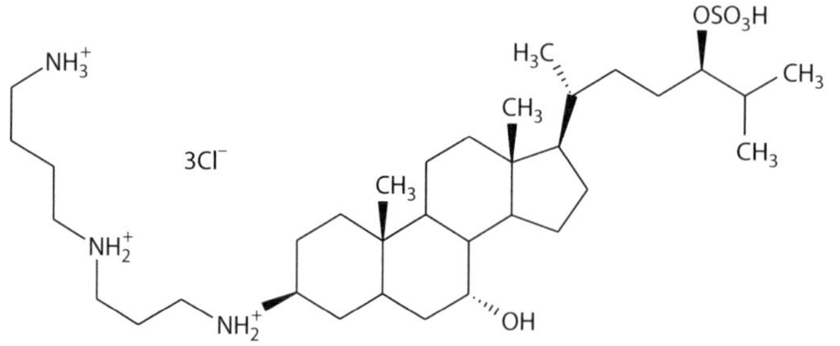

FIGURE 11.16
Squalamine 1.

with the inner face of the cytoplasmic membrane (Yeung et al. 2008). Surprisingly, this disruption of electrostatic potential can occur without obvious structural damage to the cell membrane as measured by changes in permeability (Sumioka et al. 2010). After it has gained entry into a cell, squalamine subsequently exits over the course of hours, which has been shown by its pharmacokinetic properties in numerous mammalian species, including humans (Bhargava et al. 2001, Hao et al. 2003). The ability of squalamine to alter the electrostatic charge is so strong that it causes displacement of membrane-anchored proteins, suggesting that squalamine might have, as a consequence, antiviral properties (Zasloff et al. 2011).

11.5.9 Kahalalide

Kahalalide F (Figure 11.17) is a cyclic depsipeptide that was first isolated in 1993 by Hamann and Scheuer from a marine mollusk, *Elysia rufescens*, and from the algae that the mollusk feeds on, *Bryopsis pennata* (Hamann and Scheuer 1993). In fact, it is the algae *Bryopsis* spp. that actually produces kahalalide F. The mollusk accumulates this biologically active substance and is present at a concentration 5000 times higher than that found in the algae. It has also been reported in another mollusk, *Elysia grandifolia* (Ashour et al. 2006, Tilvi and Naik 2007). It acts as a chemical protective agent against predators and belongs to a group of depsipeptides known as the kahalalides.

Kahalalide F shows in vitro activity against prostate and colon cancer cells and, to a lesser extent, antiviral, antifungal, and bactericide activity (Hamann et al. 1996). It also induces oncosis and has a 5- to 40-fold greater effect on cancer cells than healthy cells (Garcia-Rocha et al. 1996, Janmaat et al. 2005, Rademaker-Lakhai et al. 2005). Its mechanism of action involves severely compromising the integrity of crucial organelles such as mitochondria, endoplasmic reticulum, and lysosomes while leaving the nuclear structure of the cell intact. The effects of kahalalide F indicate that the osmotic balance of the cell may be altered, possibly as a result of cellular membrane damage. Thus, it appears that kahalalide F does not induce apoptosis which is the main mechanism by which tumor cells are killed by anticancer drugs or radiotherapy. Moreover, it is found

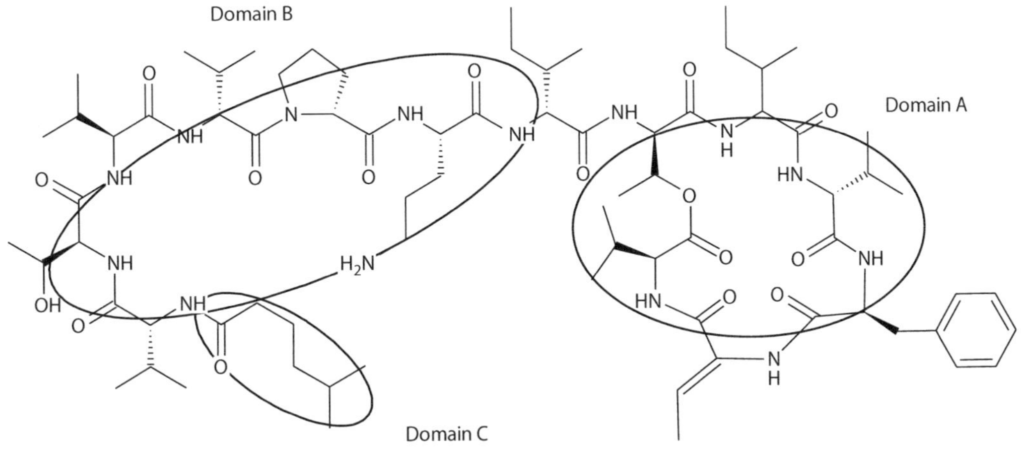

FIGURE 11.17
Kahalalide F.

that the mechanism of action of kahalalide F is caspase independent and not affected by DNA expression.

In order to identify new kahalalide F analogues with improved pharmacological properties, the role of each residue on the biological activity of this compound was investigated by developing a SAR. In order to understand the importance of the different parts of the molecule, kahalalide F structure was divided into three domains: domain A includes the macrocycle, domain B contains the peptide tail, and domain C is the N-terminal aliphatic acid (Jiménez et al. 2008).

It was shown that kahalalide F has a more defined structure than expected. This is not surprising in cyclic domain A, but surprisingly, it also occurs in domain B, which a priori is much more flexible. Kahalalide F is highly sensitive to stereotopical changes, namely, those changes that affect chirality at the R-carbon of the residue. It is not sensitive to side chain substitutions in almost every residue, the electronic density of the substituting chain being more relevant than its volume. For almost every side chain, it was possible to find a distinct side chain that could preserve or even improve the activity.

11.5.10 Bengamides

Bengamides (Figure 11.18) are a family of compounds first isolated by Crews and coworkers in 1986 (Quinoa et al. 1986), from an abundant, fingerlike, orange sponge (*Japsis* sp.), collected from around the Fiji islands and reported to be biotoxic to eukaryotic cells, nematodes, and bacteria.

They have a unique molecular structure and differ only in the lactam moiety, while a polyhydroxylated C10 side chain is the common feature. The first examples of bengamides were bengamides A and B, which are dodecanoyl-substituted on the caprolactam ring. They have shown a broad array of biological activities that include antitumor, antibiotic, and anthelmintic properties (Groweiss et al. 1999).

Because of their striking and attractive antitumor properties, these molecules have been the focus of much work to prepare them synthetically (Broka and Ehrler 1991, Kinder et al. 2001a, Fonseca and Seoane 2005, Sarabia and Sanchez-Ruiz 2005) and to test their biological (Thale et al. 2001, Kim et al. 2004) activity.

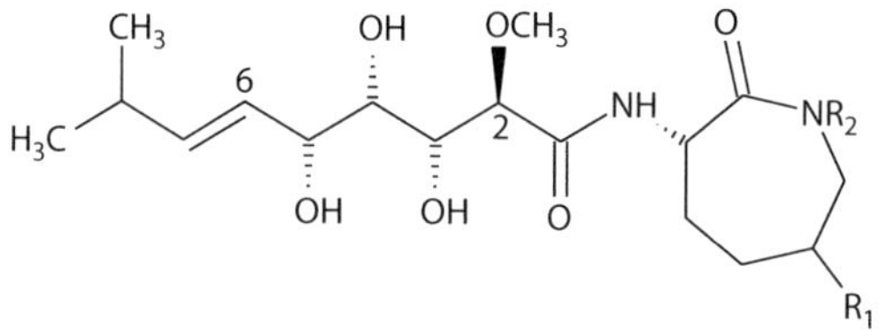

Bengamide	R_1	R_2
A		H
B	$OCO(CH_2)_{12}CH_3$	CH_3
C	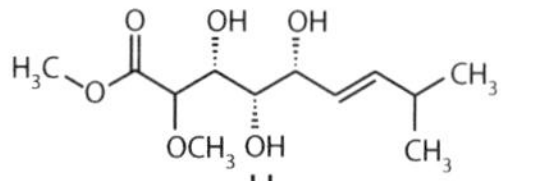	H
D		CH_3
E	H	H
F	H	CH_3

FIGURE 11.18
Bengamides.

Although bengamide B was a potent lead structure (Faulkner 2000), its limited availability from natural sources, the complexity of its synthesis, and its relatively poor solubility prevented further development of the compound as a therapeutic agent. Therefore, a synthetic chemistry program was initiated to develop analogues of bengamide B with enhanced solubility and ease of synthesis. Like its natural congeners, LAF389 (Xu et al. 2003), the synthetic bengamide analogue is a general inhibitor of cell proliferation that was developed as an anticancer agent and has been used in a clinical trial. LAF389 was selected from a number of analogues because of its equivalent activity in vitro against a broad panel of human tumor cell lines and its improved activity in human tumor xenograft models (Kinder et al. 2001b). However, the poor pharmacokinetic properties and unclear side effects of LAF389, which appeared early in the trial, have prevented its further development.

11.6 Marine Natural Products as Anti-Infective Agents

Although much progress has been made in the treatment of infectious diseases, they are still a significant public health issue and are the second leading cause of death and disability-adjusted life years throughout the world. The World Health Organization Report (2000) (The World Health Report 2000) indicated that the major problems and lethal infectious diseases are acute lower respiratory tract infections, HIV/AIDS, diarrheal diseases, tuberculosis, and malaria. Most of the antibiotics in clinical use today have been developed from compounds isolated from bacteria and fungi (Peláez 2006), with the majority isolated from soil-derived actinomycetes of the genus *Streptomyces*. However, due to continuous evolution of antibiotic-resistant microbial pathogens, there is a need for the development of new and effective antimicrobial compounds. The consequent decrease in discoveries of new antimicrobial compounds from terrestrial microbial sources, and the development of antibiotic-resistant clinical pathogens such as *Mycobacterium tuberculosis*, *Enterococcus*, *Pseudomonas* sp., *Streptococcus pneumoniae*, and *Staphylococcus aureus*, has led to an increased interest in natural marine products as a potential source for new effective antibiotics.

The search for new antimicrobials has in recent years been increasingly directed to unexploited marine environments (Sheridan 2006). In particular, marine microorganisms have become an important source of investigation in the search for novel antibiotics. Since the 1960s, many novel pharmaceutical compounds produced by a diverse range of marine bacteria have been reported in the literature. The biodiversity of marine organisms reflects the chemodiversity of compounds isolated from the marine environment. Most streptomycetes and other filamentous actinomycetes possess numerous gene clusters for the biosynthesis of secondary metabolites (Omura et al. 2001, Bentley et al. 2002), and genome sequence studies have shown that large portions of their genomes are devoted to secondary metabolite biosynthesis. Therefore, the marine environment provides a huge source of diverse secondary metabolites, many of which may turn out to be potent anti-infective agents. In addition, structural modification of existing marine compounds also provides a source of new chemical entities and may increase the potency of these compounds.

Bacteria and other microorganisms are ubiquitous in the marine environment. They are taxonomically diverse and biologically active and colonize all marine habitats, from the deep oceans to the shallowest estuaries (Rheinheimer 1992), as well as coral reefs (Ducklow 1990). Corals and sponges are frequently colonized by bacteria. The surface of these ben-thic invertebrates is covered by a mucus layer, which is colonized by bacteria, allowing for the establishment of a bacterial community that can be characteristic of a particular coral species (Rohwer et al. 2002). However, corals and sponges need the ability to regulate the bacteria they encounter and to resist/control microbial colonization and the invasion of potential pathogens in order to remain healthy and viable. One method of combating microbial attack is to use a chemical defense mechanism which involves producing potent antiviral and antibacterial compounds to combat any opportunistic infectious organisms. Marine invertebrates have also been found to be producers of antifungal as well as anti-bacterial agents (Molinski 2004).

In addition, marine microorganisms also offer tremendous potential in producing new antimicrobial and antifungal agents (Bernan et al. 2004, Kasanah and Hamann 2004). There are many potential advantages in the investigation of biologically active molecules from marine microorganisms compared to other natural product sources. These are the following:

a. Diversity of microorganisms may yield diversity in the production of secondary metabolites.

b. The production and diversity of microbial metabolites can be regulated by modi-fication of culture conditions.

c. Most bioactive compounds are produced by a specific strain rather than a taxonom-ically defined species of microorganisms. Therefore, new bioactive compounds can be obtained by the cultivation of isolated strains without prior taxonomic classification.

d. Only a small amount of plant and/or animal tissue is required to cultivate marine microorganisms so it protects macroorganisms from oversampling.

e. Preservation of natural habitats since once microbes are cultured and preserved, recollection is not required.

f. Culturable marine microorganisms will provide an adequate supply of bioactive compounds required for scientific and economic development.

g. Microorganisms are more readily manipulated than macroorganisms.

11.6.1 Manzamine Alkaloids

Due to their unique structural properties and potent biological activities, marine alkaloids extracted from sponges have become an increasingly important focus of research since the late 1990s in terms of natural product synthesis and pharmaceutical research. However, one particular class of alkaloid that has received considerable attention for their chemistry and pharmacology is the manzamines (Figure 11.19). They are a group of marine-derived alkaloids, found exclusively in sponges, and are characterized by a complex heterocyclic ring system attached to a β-carboline moiety. The first manzamine (manzamine A) was isolated from a Japanese *Haliclona* sponge in 1986, and its structure, including absolute configuration, was established by XRD (Sakai et al. 1986). It consists of a complicated 5-, 6-, 7-, 8-, and 13-membered heterocyclic ring system coupled to a β-carboline. The piperidine and cyclohexene ring systems adopt chair and boat conformations, respectively, and are bridged by an eight-carbon chain creating a 13-membered macrocycle. The conformation of the eight-membered ring is in an envelope boat, with a mirror plane passing through

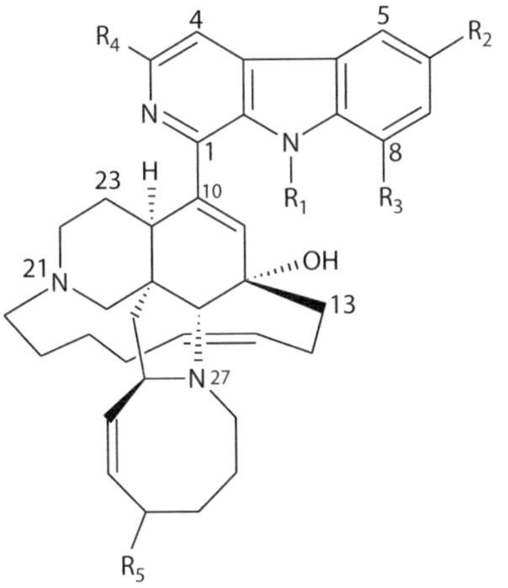

FIGURE 11.19
Manzamine alkaloids: manzamine A (R1 – R5 = H), 8-hydroxymanzamine A (R1, R2, R4, R5 = H, R3 = OH), manzamine F (R1, R2, R4 = H, R3 = OH, R5 = O).

C-32 and C-28. The chloride ion is held by hydrogen bonding with two NH and one OH groups. The positive charge on the pyrrolidinium nitrogen atom was indicated by the longer than usual bond lengths of the attached α-carbon atoms (Sakai et al. 1986).

Since the discovery of manzamine A, more than 80 manzamine and manzamine-related alkaloids have been isolated from more than 16 different species, belonging to five families and two orders of marine sponges distributed throughout the world (Edrada et al. 1996). These sponges have been collected from oceans around Okinawa, the Philippines, Indonesia, Italy, South Africa and Papua New Guinea, and the Red Sea (Crews et al. 1994, Bourguet-Kondracki et al. 1996, Guo et al. 1998, Koren-Goldshlager et al. 1998, Hu et al. 2003). The wide distribution of manzamine alkaloids in taxonomically unrelated sponges strongly implies that microorganism(s) present as symbionts in these sponges may play a critical role in the biosynthesis of these compounds and be the real producer of these alkaloids (Kobayashi et al. 1994c, Tsuda and Kobayashi 1997, Hu et al. 2003, Peng et al. 2008).

Although many manzamines have been isolated and their biological activities evaluated, little is known about the SAR necessary for the potent biological activity observed with these alkaloids. The bioactivity of manzamine alkaloids is impressive and diverse. They are cytotoxic against a number of bacteria and fungi (Ichiba et al. 1988, Longley et al. 1993, Peng et al. 2008); display anti-inflammatory (Mayer et al. 2005), antineuroinflammatory (Yousaf et al. 2004), insecticidal (Edrada et al. 1996, El Sayed et al. 1997), antimicrobial (Nakamura et al. 1987a, El Sayed et al. 2001, Rao et al. 2003), and antiparasitic properties; and show the greatest potential as agents for the treatment of malaria (Ang et al. 2000) and *Mycobacterium tuberculosis* (Yousaf et al. 2002, Rao et al. 2003, 2004). Manzamine A shows antimicrobial activity against *S. aureus* and methicillin-resistant *S. aureus* (Yousaf et al. 2002, 2004) with IC_{50} values of 0.5 and 0.7 μg/mL, respectively (Kondo et al. 1992).

SAR studies were carried out by chemical modification of manzamine A, 8-hydroxymanzamine A, manzamine F, and ircinal, isolated from the sponge *Acanthostrongylophora* (Peng et al. 2010). The derived analogues were evaluated for antimalarial, antimicrobial, and antineuroinflammatory activities, and they exhibited potent and improved in vitro antineuroinflammatory, antimicrobial, and antimalarial activity.

Although further investigations are required to completely understand the SAR for this class of compounds, the greatest potential for the manzamine alkaloids appears to be against malaria and neuroinflammation. This dual action may make it possible to treat both the infection and the symptoms of malaria with a single drug. Manzamine A was shown to permeate across the blood–brain barrier (BBB) (Peng et al. 2010), which means the potent antineuroinflammatory activity of the manzamines could provide great benefit for the prevention and treatment of cerebral infections (e.g., *Cryptococcus* and *Plasmodium*).

Presently, the most effective and *widely* used antimalarial drugs are those derived from quinine and artemisinin (natural products from terrestrial plants). Peng and coworkers showed there is significant potential both from in vitro and in vivo data that there is significant potential for the use of manzamine A and 8-hydroxymanzamine analogues in the treatment of malaria as they *show improved antimalarial activity over chloroquine and artemisinin in animal models*. Although toxicity has been seen in high doses and daily dosing schedules of manzamines, they show promise as the potentially effective novel class of antimalarial drugs from manzamines by optimization of both structure and drug administration. Note that small changes in the manzamine structure can significantly affect its toxicity. For instance, there is significantly reduced toxicity of 8-hydroxymanzamine A compared to manzamine A in intraperitoneal administration to mice (Peng et al. 2010). This suggests that investigation of the properties of manzamine analogues may result in an optimized candidate with suitably potent antimalarial activity with a better therapeutic window.

11.7 Anti-Infective Agents from Marine Actinomycetes

The majority of natural antibiotics in use today were originally found in soil-borne actinomycetes. For over half a century, the cultivation of terrestrial actinomycetes has yielded structurally diverse secondary metabolites with remarkable biological activities (Newman and Cragg 2007). Studies of these chemically prolific bacteria have been expanded from traditional soil habitats to include strains obtained from marine samples. The exploitation of marine actinomycetes is only at the beginning, but it has already proved to be very a promising source of novel antibiotic compounds (Donia and Hamann 2003, Bull et al. 2005, Fenical and Jensen 2006). Comparisons of 16S rRNA sequence data have shown that deep-ocean sediments harbor new actinomycete taxa, some of which are fully restricted to life in the sea (Maldonado et al. 2005). Moreover, phylogenetic analyses based on sequences of 16S rRNA have provided evidence that marine actinomycetes are distinct from their terrestrial counterparts (Mincer et al. 2002). Rare actinomycetes have become more important as sources for the discovery of novel compounds from undescribed species (Tanaka and Omura 1993), and there are several less exploited genera of rare actinomycetes that will likely be particularly important for the discovery of new drug leads including *Actinomadura, Actinoplanes, Amycolatopsis, Dactylosporangium, Kibdelosporangium, Microbiospora, Micromonospora, Planobiospora, Streptosporangium,* and *Planomonospora*. Rare actinomycetes are also present in the marine environment as exemplified by the isolation of new genus *Salinospora* from marine sediment and the sponge *Pseudoceratina clavata*. Several important antibiotics on the market are derived from rare actinomycetes (Berdy 2005). Cultivation of these strains in the laboratory has yielded many structurally unique metabolites of

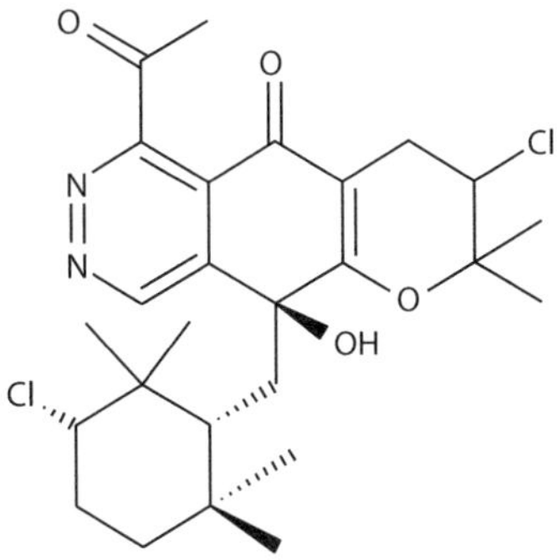

FIGURE 11.20
Azamerone.

considerable biological interest (Hughes et al. 2009). Thus, it is not surprising that a number of novel secondary metabolites have been isolated from these taxonomically unique populations of marine-derived actinomycetes (Feling et al. 2003) (http://www.ncbi.nlm. nih.gov/pubmed/15726290). Certain strains of these marine-derived actinomycetes produce chlorine-containing meroterpenoids, compounds of mixed polyketide–terpenoid origins (Simpson 1987) of the napyradiomycin class, which are highly unusual for actinomycetes (Jensen and Fenical 2005, Soria-Mercado et al. 2005). These compounds possess significant antibacterial and cancer cell cytotoxic activities in in vitro bioassays. These studies lead to the isolation of azamerone (Cho et al. 2006) (Figure 11.20), the first natural product with a phthalazinone ring that was isolated by the Fenical-Jensen lab from the marine sediment-derived bacterium *Streptomyces* sp. CNQ-766. Azamerone is composed of a unique chloropyranophthalazinone core with a 3-chloro-6-hydroxy-2,2,6-trimethylcyclohexylmethyl side chain.

Until the phthalazinone meroterpenoid azamerone was isolated from the marine sediment-derived *Streptomyces* sp. CNQ-766 (Winter et al. 2009), pyridazomycin was the only known natural product containing a pyridazine ring, and it was speculated that the pyridazine ring moiety in azamerone was also derived from the cyclization of amino acid residues. However, identification of coproduced chlorinated dihydroquinones and diazo meroterpenoids suggested that azamerone is biosynthetically linked to the nitrogenated compounds and that its phthalazinone core may be derived from a naphthoquinone precursor. These data suggest that azamerone is biosynthetically linked to the napyradiomycin family of natural products.

11.8 Lipoxazolidinones

A number of structurally less complex natural products with activity against methicillin-resistant *S. aureus* (MRSA) and vancomycin-resistant *Escherichia coli* (VRE) have also been isolated from cultures of marine bacteria since 2000. A new class of 2-alkylidene-5-alkyl-4-oxazolidinone, with a unique antibiotic pharmacophore, was isolated from a marine actinomycete strain NPS8920 (Macherla et al. 2007, Michelle et al. 2008), which is a member of the new genus *Marinispora*. A series of three compounds in this class,

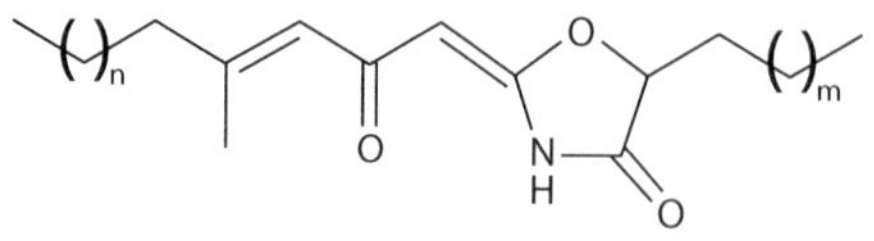

FIGURE 11.21
Lipoxazolidinone A: $x = 5$, $y = 2$; lipoxazolidinone B: $x = 5$, $y = 3$; lipoxazolidinone C: $x = 4$, $y = 2$.

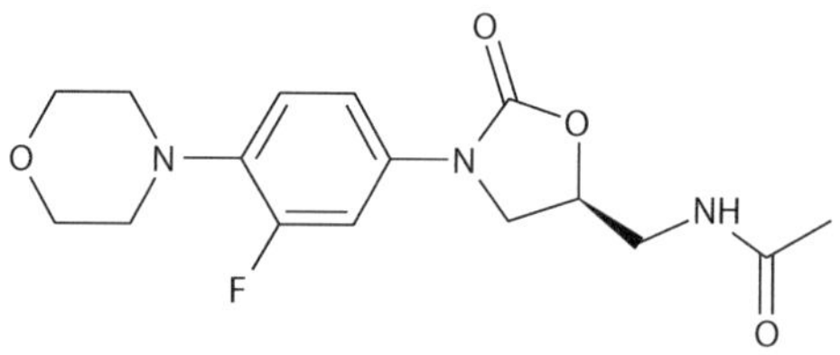

FIGURE 11.22
Linezolid.

lipoxazolidinones A, B, and C (Figure 11.21), were isolated and showed broad-spectrum antimicrobial activity similar to that of the commercial antibiotic linezolid (Figure 11.22), a 2-oxazolidinone. Lipoxazolidinone A was found to possess good potency (1–2 µg/mL) against drug-resistant pathogens MRSA and VRE. Hydrolysis of the amide bond of the 4-oxazolidinone ring of lipoxazolidinone A results in the loss of antibacterial activity. The 2-alkylidene-4-oxazolidinone represents a new antibiotic pharmacophore and is the first molecule of this type to be found in nature.

11.9 Marinopyrroles

Cultivation of the marine actinomycete *Streptomyces* strain CNQ-418 in a seawater-based medium resulted in the isolation of marinopyrroles A and B (Hughes et al. 2008), which are densely halogenated, axially chiral natural products consisting of two sali-cyloyl substituents on a 1,3'-bipyrrole core (an uncommon N,C2-linked bispyrrole structure) (Figure 11.23). The unusual biaryl bond, surrounded by four ortho substitu-ents, establishes an axis of chirality that further distinguishes these interesting natu-ral products. X-ray analysis of marinopyrrole B showed that the natural product exists as an atropo-enantiomer with the M-configuration. Though configurationally stable at room temperature, M-(–)-marinopyrrole A can be racemized at elevated tempera-tures to yield the nonnatural P-(+)-atropo-enantiomer. Marinopyrroles possess potent antibiotic activities against MRSA. Optimization of culture conditions has resulted in the isolation of further members (C–F) of the marinopyrrole series (Hughes et al. 2010) (Figure 11.23). All of the marinopyrroles were isolated as single M-configured atropo-enantiomers and thus were configurationally stable at room temperature, except for marinopyrrole F, which was isolated as a racemic mixture. Like marinopyrroles A and B, marinopyrrole C exhibited potent activity against MRSA and moderate activity against HCT-116 cells.

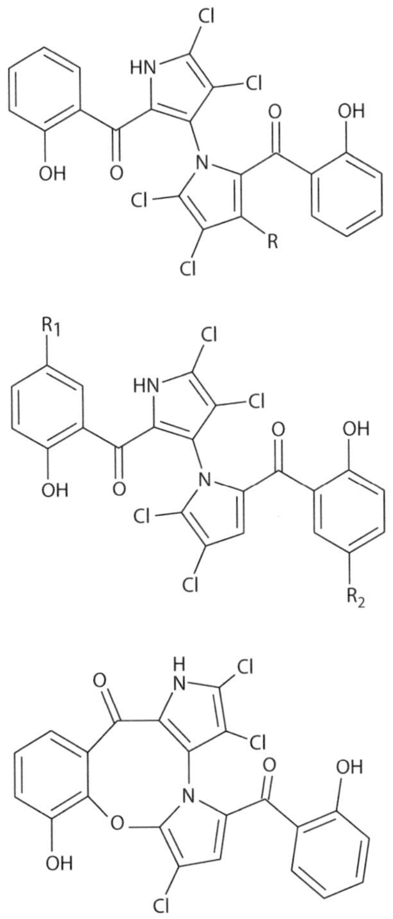

(–) A : R = H

(–) B : R = Br

(–) C : R_1 = Cl, R_2 = H

(–) D : R_1 = Cl, R_2 = H

(–) E : R_1 = Cl, R_2 = H

(±) F

FIGURE 11.23
Marinopyrrole A–F.

11.10 Thiopeptide Antibiotics

The first thiopeptide antibiotic, micrococcin, was isolated in 1948. Since then, around 80 different thiopeptide antibiotics have been discovered. However, up until recently, they have not received much interest as therapeutic agents. Structurally, they are quite complex and consist of a peptide macrocyclic structure which is comprised of a number of heteratomic rings (mainly thiazoles, oxazoles, indoles, and a six-membered tri- or tetrasubstituted nitrogen ring) and dehydroamino acids. They are divided into five classes (*a–e*) according to the oxidation state of the tri- or tetrasubstituted nitrogen ring (Bagley et al. 2005). Most of them function by inhibiting protein synthesis in bacteria. Generally, they show little activity against Gram-negative bacteria but are highly active against Gram-positive bacteria, and a number are active against MRSA. Thiopeptide antibiotics thiostrepton and micrococcin have also been found to inhibit protein synthesis in the malaria virus *Plasmodium falciparum* (McConkey et al. 1997, Rogers et al. 1998).

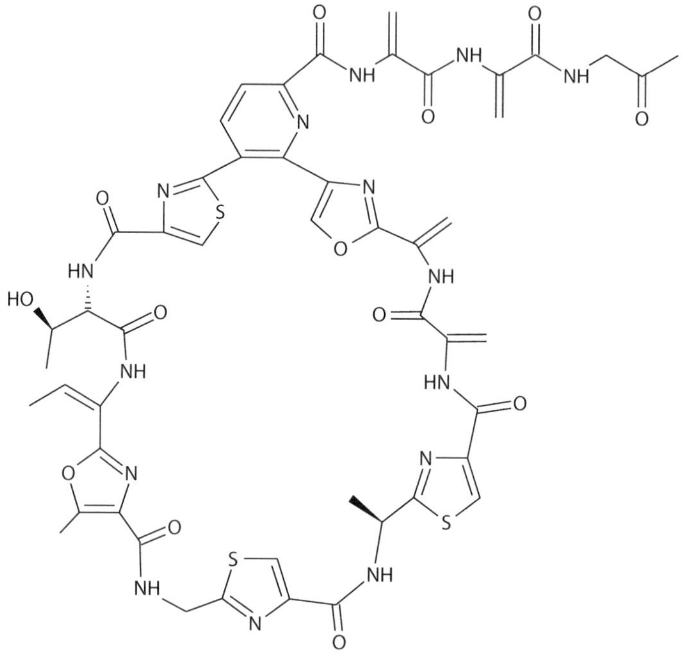

FIGURE 11.24
Thiopeptide antibiotic TP-1161.

Most of them have been isolated from terrestrial actinomycetes (genus *Streptomyces*); however, more recent work has focused on isolating them from bacteria found in the marine environment. Engelhardt and coworkers (Engelhardt et al. 2010) recently isolated a new (series *d*) thiopeptide antibiotic (TP-1161) (Figure 11.24) from a marine *Nocardiopsis* sp. that was found to be active against a number of Gram-positive bacterial strains but inactive to the Gram-negative bacterial strains tested. Other thiopeptides include YM-266183 and YM-266184 produced by *Bacillus cereus* isolated from the marine sponge *Halichondria japonica* (Nagai et al. 2003).

11.11 Marine *Micromonospora* spp. as a Source for Novel Antibiotics

Micromonospora (family *Micromonosporaceae*) is one of the rare genera of actinomycetes which are a minor component of soil actinomycetes, but are found to be significantly more abundant in the marine environment. This genus is well known for their biosynthesis of two important classes of antibiotics: gentamicins and rifamycins. They are Gram-positive, spore-forming, generally aerobic, form branched mycelium and occur as saprotrophic forms in both soil and water. Although the genus *Micromonospora* has long been recognized as a significant source of secondary metabolites, it is only recently that the importance of *Micromonospora* species on plant growth and development has been acknowledged. *Micromonospora* species produce many of the best-known antibiotics and are best known for synthesizing antibiotics, especially aminoglycoside antibiotics (gentamicin and netamicin)

(Bérdy 2005), anthracycline antibiotics, anthraquinones, lupinacidins A and B, with anti-tumor activity (Igarashi et al. 2007), vitamin B12 (Wagman et al. 1969), and antifungal compounds (Nolan and Cross 1988, Ismet et al. 2004). Marine *Micromonospora* species have recently been reviewed with respect to their broad distribution and their potential for use as probiotics (Das et al. 2008). The compounds isolated from marine *Micromonospora* spp. are diverse with activity as antibiotics or anticancer leads (Kwok et al. 2008). Several new generations of antibiotics derived from *Micromonospora* are under development. The antibiotics have potent activity that may help solve emergent problems in antibiotic resistance due to their spectrum and/or novel mechanisms of action.

11.12 Everninomicins: A Novel Class of Complex Oligosaccharide Antibiotics

Everninomicins are produced by *Micromonospora carbonaceae* and are found to be highly active against Gram-positive bacteria including MRSA and VRE (Jones and Barrett 1995). SCH27899 (Ziracin®, Schering-Plough Corporation) is a novel everninomicin derivative which made it through to phase II and phase III clinical trials, but was withdrawn in March 2000 after safety concerns arose from patients using the drug. Ziracin is a protein synthesis inhibitor with unique binding to ribosomal protein L16 (Terakubo et al. 2001), and this was the reason there was susceptibility of multidrug-resistant bacterial pathogens to the everninomicin family of compounds. SCH27899 (Figure 11.25) consists of eight saccharides and two highly substituted aromatic ester moieties. SCH27899 contains two ortho ester linkages, a nitro sugar, a methylene dioxy group, two aromatic ester residues, and 35 centers of asymmetries. The saccharide hydroxyl groups were one area for modification that would alter the hydrogen bonding properties of the molecules and, in some cases, water solubility, which consequently may affect their pharmacokinetic properties. Extensive SAR studies indicated that they are structurally quite diverse (in terms of size, polarity, and charge), while amino acid modifications yielded similar activities, suggesting that the nitro group in SCH27899 could be modified without loss of biological activity (Ganguly et al. 1999).

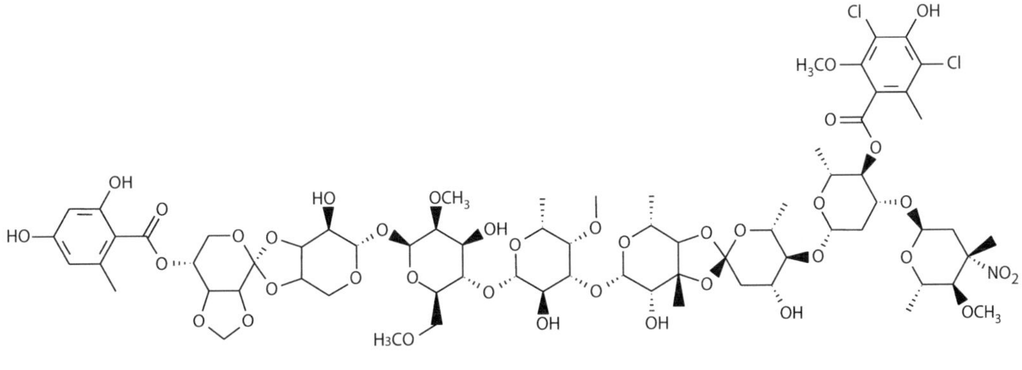

FIGURE 11.25
Everninomicin SCH27899.

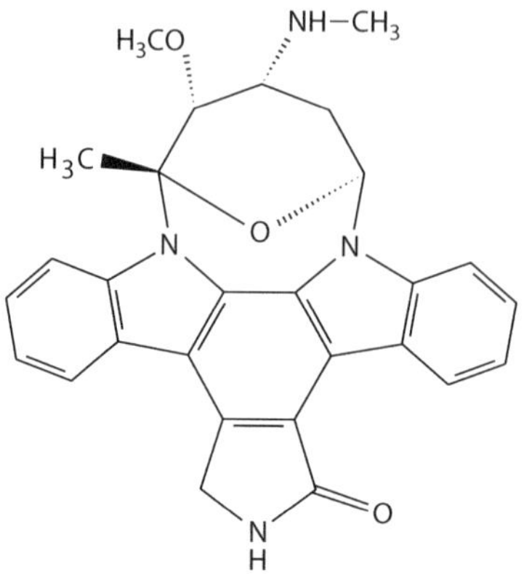

FIGURE 11.26
SB-219383.

Aminoacyl-tRNA synthetases (ARS) are novel targets in drug discovery of antibiotics. The enzymes perform a crucial role in protein biosynthesis, catalyzing the attachment of an amino acid onto its cognate tRNA. Selective inhibition of bacterial isoleucyl-tRNA synthetase gives rise to potent antibacterial activity (Walker et al. 1993) and provides a promising platform on which to develop novel antibiotics that show no cross-resistance (Kim et al. 2003). A novel natural product, SB-219383 (Figure 11.26), isolated from *Micromonospora* NCIMB 40684 is a potent, selective inhibitor of bacterial tyrosyl-tRNA synthetase. However, it exhibits weak antibacterial activity due to its high polarity preventing penetration through the bacterial cell wall (Houge-Frydrych et al. 2000, Stefanska et al. 2000).

11.13 Staurosporine

Staurosporine was first isolated in 1977 from the bacterium *Streptomyces staurosporeus* by Omura and coworkers while searching for new alkaloids in actinomycetes (Omura et al. 1977). Structurally, staurosporine can be divided into two distinct parts: the nonsugar indolocarbazole aglycon part and the carbohydrate portion of the molecule (Figure 11.27) (Furusaki et al. 1978). The aglycon part is itself a natural product, commonly referred to as staurosporinone or K-252c, and it constitutes a major structural unit of many of the indolocarbazole natural products (Sapi and Massiot 1995). SAR suggested that the presence of the carbohydrate moiety (sugar part) is important for the biological activity, that is, recognition by these cellular targets, as is the planar six-ring scaffold. It was the first of a number of alkaloids to be isolated with this type of chemical structure. Since 1977, more than 60 natural products incorporating the indolo[2,3-*a*]pyrrolo[3,4-*c*]carbazole have been reported (Gribble and Berthel 1993). Due to the novel structures and wide range of activities of its members, this group of alkaloids has attracted the interest of many researchers. Staurosporine was discovered to have a number of biological activities including smooth muscle relaxation, antifungal activity, antiplatelet aggregation, and antitumor activity (Omura et al. 1995). *It is interesting to note that* staurosporine possesses inhibitory activity against fungi and yeast but has no significant effect on bacteria. It has been found to be one

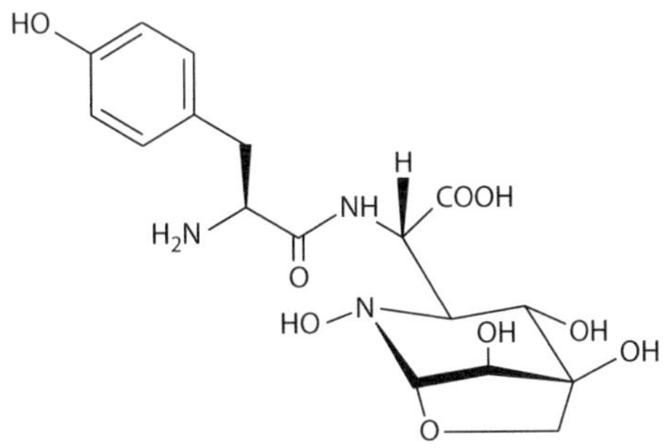

FIGURE 11.27
Staurosporine.

of the strongest known cell-permeable inhibitors of protein kinases, with IC_{50} values in the 1–20 nM range (Tamaoki et al. 1986), and is often used to study the involvement of protein kinases in signal transduction pathways.

11.14 Abyssomicins

Abyssomicins B, C, and D (Figure 11.28) are natural polycyclic polyketide antibiotics recently isolated from the Japanese sea actinomycete *Verrucosispora* strain which is a rare actinomycete genus belonging to the family *Micromonosporaceae* (Riedlinger et al. 2004). Among these three polycyclic polyketide compounds, only abyssomicin C possesses potent activity against Gram-positive bacteria, including MRSA and vancomycin-resistant *S. aureus* (VRSA) strains. Abyssomicin C inhibits the inhibitors of the *p*-aminobenzoic acid (PABA) pathway in the folic acid biosynthesis at an earlier stage than the well-known synthetic sulfa drugs (Bister et al. 2004). The atropisomer of abyssomicin C (atrop-abyssomicin C) is the main metabolite produced by *Verrucosispora* and was found to be 25% more active than abyssomicin C (Keller et al. 2007). Since abyssomicin D, lacking the enone unit present in abyssomicin C, is biologically inactive, the reactive enone functionality of abyssomicin C is thought to be crucial for the observed biological activity. Abyssomicin C and its analogues (Rath et al. 2005) present promising lead structures for the development of new antibacterial agents for use against drug-resistant pathogens.

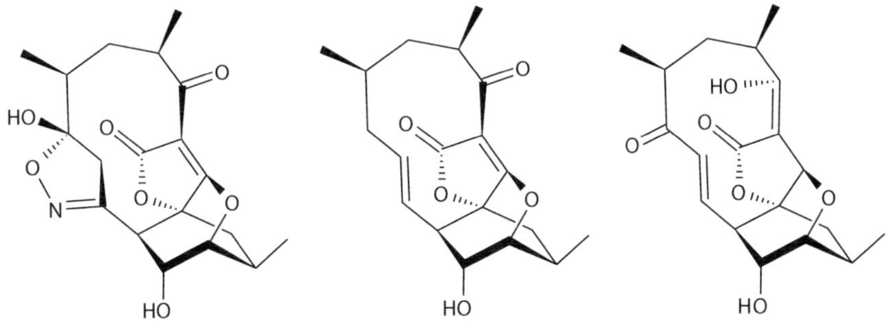

FIGURE 11.28
Abyssomicin B–D.

11.15 Diazepinomicin (ECO-4601)

Azoprenylated (N-prenylated) secondary metabolites (anthranilic acid derivatives, diaz-epinones, and indole, and xanthine alkaloids) have been recognized in recent years as interesting secondary metabolites with promising biological activities. Many of the iso-lated prenylazo secondary metabolites and their semisynthetic derivatives are shown to exert valuable in vitro and in vivo anticancer, anti-inflammatory, antibacterial, antiviral, and antifungal effects.

Diazepinomicin, also known as ECO-4601, is a secondary metabolite produced by a *Micromonospora strain* (Charan et al. 2004) that possesses antibacterial, anti-inflammatory, and antitumor activity. It has atypical tricyclic dibenzodiazepinone nucleus linked to farne-syl side chain (Figure 11.29). The dibenzodiazepinone nucleus is extremely rare among natural products, and the biogenetic origin of this moiety is of great interest (McAlpine et al. 2008). The first isolation of diazepinomicin was by an antibacterial activity-guided fractionation from the fermentation broth of *Micromonospora* sp., strain DPJ12, obtained from the Japanese ascidian *Didemnum proliferatum* collected from Shishijima island and is closely related to *Micromonospora chalcea* (Charan et al. 2004). It possesses antibacterial, anti-inflammatory, and antitumor activity. It has a broad spectrum of in vitro cytotoxic-ity and has demonstrated in vivo activity against glioma, breast, and prostate cancer in mouse models. The preclinical development of ECO-4601 as an anticancer agent has been completed (Lam 2006).

11.15.1 Tetrocarcins

Tetrocarcins constitute a growing class of spirotetronic acids with activities against some Gram-positive bacteria (e.g., *Bacillus subtilis*). In 1980, Tomita and Tamaoki reported the isolation of a novel antibiotic complex from actinomycete strain DO-11 isolated from a soil sample collected in Sendai-shi, Miyagi, Japan, which displayed antibacterial and antitumor activity (Morimoto et al. 1982). The complex was isolated and separated into three components designated as tetrocarcins A, B, and C. Tetrocarcins A, B, and C dis-played moderate activity against *S. aureus* and strong activity against *B. subtilis*, while no activity was observed against the Gram-negative bacteria tested (Tomita et al. 1980). Tetrocarcin A (Figure 11.30) showed activity against cells of sarcoma 180, P388 leukemia, and B16 melanoma (Nakashima et al. 2000). The generic name, tetrocarcin, was proposed due to the unique structure of the aglycone that consists of a derivative of tetronic acid. Tetrocarcins A, B, and C contain the novel polycyclic aglycone tetronolide that is common to all tetrocarcins.

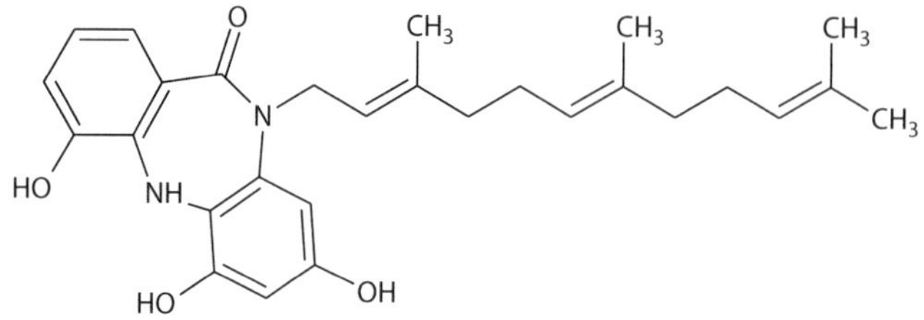

FIGURE 11.29
Diazepinomicin (ECO-4601).

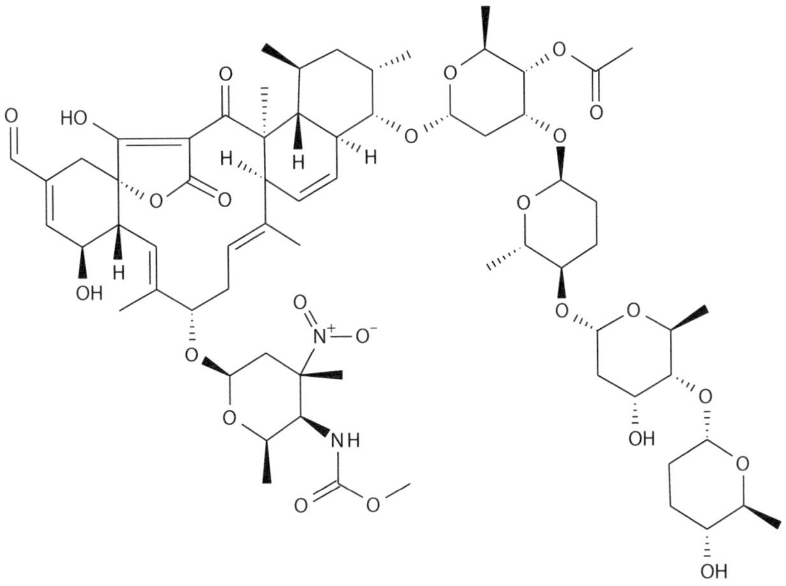

FIGURE 11.30
Tetrocarcin A.

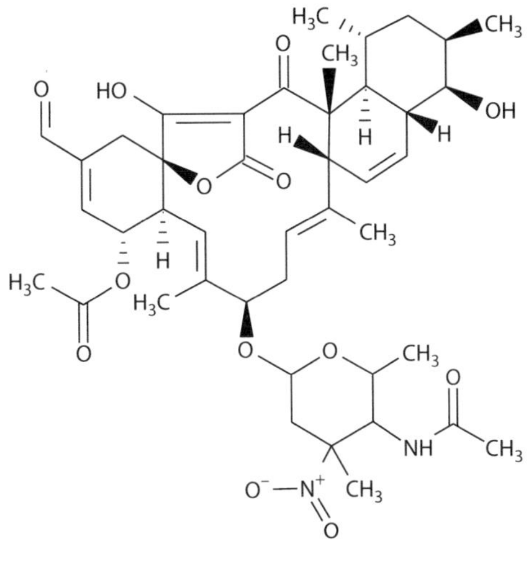

FIGURE 11.31
Tetronolide.

Tetronolide (Figure 11.31) has a unique structural feature of a 14-membered macrolide in which a spirotetronic acid constitutes the lactone group. The same structure, with differing functional groups and the location of the double bond on the cyclohexene ring, is found with kijanolide (Figure 11.32), the aglycone of kijanimicin (Mallams et al. 1981), which was reported shortly afterward by the Schering-Plough group.

Tetrocarcin analogues aristotatins A and B, along with tetrocarcin A, were isolated from *Micromonospora* sp. from seawater collected in Toyama Bay, Japan (Furumai et al. 2000), in 2000. Aristotatins have an iso-butanoyldigitoxose unit instead of acetyldigitoxose

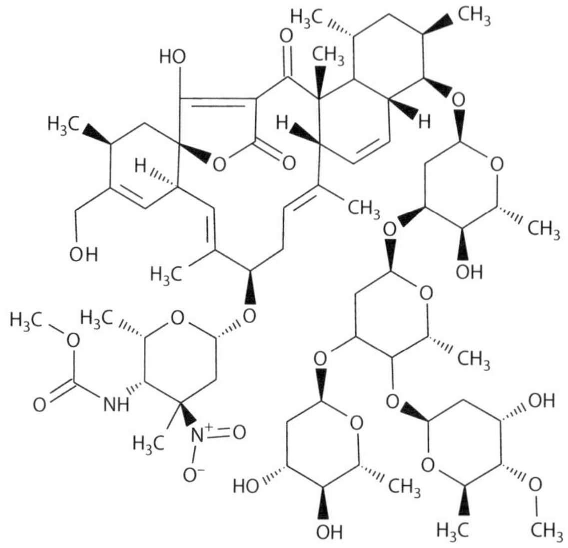

FIGURE 11.32
Kijanimicin.

(Igarashi et al. 2000). They showed potent in vitro activity against Gram-positive bacteria and tumors on some solid tumor cell lines but displayed no activity against Gram-negative bacteria and yeast. Their cytotoxic activity was tested on a human myeloid leukemia U937 cell line with an IC_{50} of 0.4 μg/mL for aristotatin A and 4.0 μg/mL for aristotatin B. Aristotatin A inhibits neuritogenesis of NGF-stimulated P12 cells at less than 1 μM, by inhibiting tubulin polymerization, while tetrocarcin A inhibits the antiapoptotic function of Bcl-2 (Figure 11.33) (Furumai et al. 2000).

11.16 Marine Natural Products as Anti-Inflammatory Agents

During the past few decades, intensive collaborative research in the area of chronic and acute inflammatory diseases has resulted in the better understanding of the pathophysiology of these diseases. However, due to the multitude of cellular-derived inflammatory mediators, treatment is still an unresolved problem. These mediators include prostaglandins (PGs), leukotrienes (LTs), nitric oxide (NO), tumor necrosis factor-α (TNF-α), and cytokines of the interleukin (IL) families.

Phospholipase A_2 is an enzyme involved in the pathogenesis of variety of inflammatory diseases. It catalyzes the hydrolysis of membrane phospholipids releasing fatty acids such as arachidonic acid and is the rate-limiting step in the production of eicosanoid mediators of inflammation. Arachidonic acid provides the substrate for proinflammatory mediators such as LTs, PGs, and thromboxanes, collectively known as the eicosanoids (Potts and Faulkner 1992). As a result, phospholipase A_2 inhibitors have been considered as potential targets for the development of anti-inflammatory drugs (Giannini et al. 2001). It has been reported that some unsaturated aldehyde sesterterpenoids show anti-inflammatory properties via phospholipase A_2 inhibition.

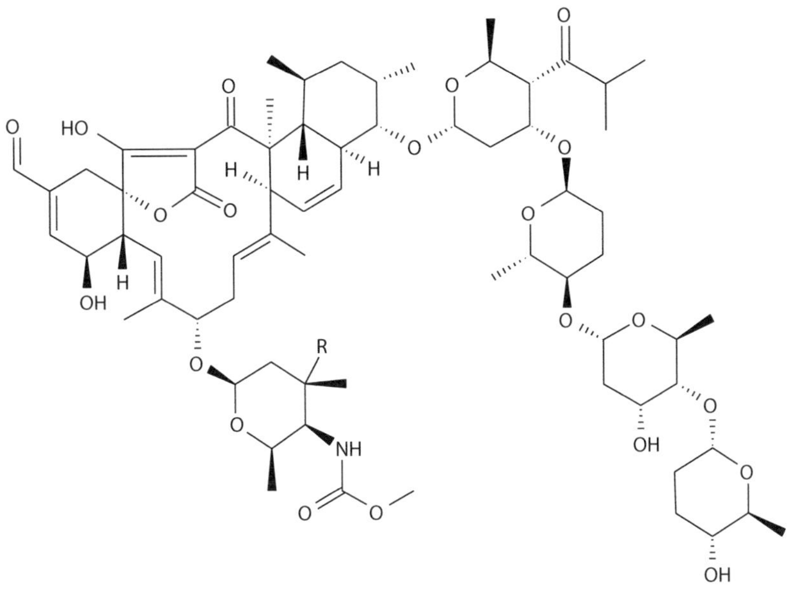

FIGURE 11.33
Aristotatin A (R = NO$_2$) and aristotatin B (R = NH$_2$).

Marine organisms and microorganisms have provided a large proportion of the anti-inflammatory and natural antioxidant products over the last years, and marine organisms, especially sponges, have proved to be a rich source of aldehyde sesterterpenoid. The inhibitory profile of most molecules of marine origin shows a high degree of selectivity (both in vivo and in vitro) against secretory enzymes (sPLA2) compared to cystolic (cPLA2). The sesterterpenes are the smallest class of terpenoid compounds and consist of alcohol, aldehyde, and ketone derivatives of terpene hydrocarbons.

Phospholipase A$_2$ activity has been reported in several marine organisms, including hard and soft corals, jellyfish, starfish, sea anemones, soft corals, and marine snails (Nevalainen et al. 2004, Zarai et al. 2010). Thus, it is not surprising that marine organisms have developed potent phospholipase A$_2$ inhibitors, which may be used as chemical defenses in their natural environment. Marine phospholipase A$_2$ inhibitors reported to date are primarily terpenoids isolated from sponges, nudibranchs, and algae with some of the earliest examples of these sesterterpenoids including manoalide and scalaradial.

In the last few years, several investigations appeared in the literature that deal with the identification of the molecular mechanism of sPLA2 inactivation by marine natural products that bear diverse pharmacophoric groups such as γ-hydroxybutenolide, quinone, or dialdehyde moieties (Soriente et al. 1999).

11.16.1 γ-Hydroxybutenolide Sesterterpenoids

Manoalide is the first anti-inflammatory agent of marine origin isolated in 1980 from the Indo-Pacific sponge *Luffariella variabilis* (Potts et al. 1992). It was found to irreversibly inhibit the release of arachidonic acid from membrane phosphor by the enzyme PLA2 (Soriente et al. 1999, Pommier et al. 2003), resulting in inhibition of the formation of proinflammatory mediators such as LTs and PGs (Reynolds et al. 1988, Glaser et al. 1989). The chemical basis of manoalide's inhibitory activity is the formation of a Schiff base between the mano-alide hemiacetals and lysine residue of the PLA2 protein, which prevents the enzyme from binding to the membranes.

Subsequently, many other related molecules have been isolated, such as secomanoalide, luffariellolide, luffariellins, luffolide, the cacospongionolides, and the petrosaspongiolides M-R (De Silva et al. 1981, Albizati et al. 1987, Kernan et al. 1987, De Rosa et al. 1994, Kernan et al. 1989, Randazzo et al. 1998), all of which are irreversible inhibitors of PLA2.

Manoalide is the parent compound of a series of marine sponge metabolites belong-ing to the sesterterpene class, a γ-hydroxybutenolide sesterterpenoid, the first sub-stance ever observed to selectively inhibit phospholipase A_2. Although this compound ultimately failed as a drug, its use as a model for designing inhibitors of this important enzyme will have lasting effect in medicinal research. Although this natural product was originally reported by Scheuer's group as an antibiotic with antibacterial activity against Gram-positive bacteria (*S. aureus* and *B. subtilis*) (De Silva and Scheuer 1980, 1981), later work revealed that manoalide possesses potent analgesic and anti-inflammatory properties. Manoalide was further investigated and found to be a potent inhibitor of phospholipase A_2 (Lombardo and Dennis 1985, Glaser and Jacobs 1986, 1987, Glaser et al. 1989, Jacobson et al. 1990). Manoalide had reached phase II clinical trials as a topical antipsoriatic. Its development was, however, discontinued due to formulation problems, as sufficient quantities of the compound would not pass through the skin using the formulations developed for the trials (Newman and Cragg 2004b). It was, however, developed as a biochemical standard probe for phospholipase A_2 inhibition (Gross and Konig 2006).

A series of isomers or derivatives of manoalide have been isolated from the same sponge species or the sponges of the same genus, namely, secomanoalide, (*E*)-neomanoalide, and (*Z*)-neomanoalide (De Silva and Scheuer 1981). All three compounds, as well as the par-ent compound, displayed antibacterial activity against Gram-positive bacteria (*S. aureus* and *B. subtilis*) but were inactive against *E. coli*, *Pseudomonas aeruginosa*, and *Candida albi-cans*. Manoalide and its isomer secomanoalide (Figure 11.34) possess the same trimeth-ylcyclohexenyl and γ-hydroxybutenolide moieties and antibiotic activity (De Silva and Scheurer 1981).

In some specimens of *L. variabilis*, manoalide and secomanoalide are replaced, either totally or partially, by luffariellin A and luffariellin B, respectively (Figure 11.35). Luffariellins A and B have the same γ-hydroxybutenolide group as manoalide but a differ-ent structure in the other parts while having the same anti-inflammatory activity (Kernan et al. 1987). Luffariellins are all characterized by the 1-isoproprenyl-2-methylcyclopentane ring system replacing the trimethylcyclohexenyl moiety in other manoalide analogues. Despite this discrepancy in chemical structure, luffariellins A and B retain identical

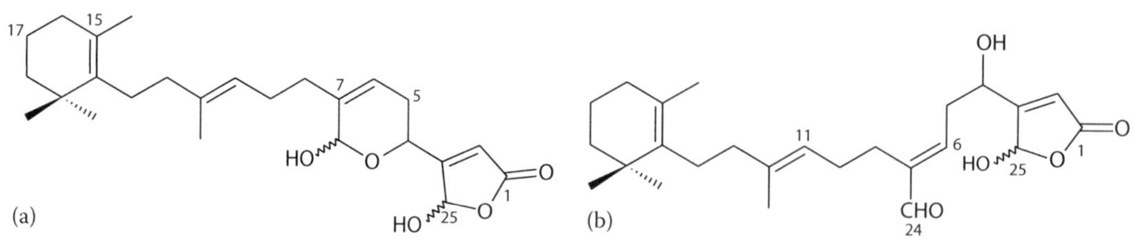

FIGURE 11.34
Manoalide (a), secomanoalide (b).

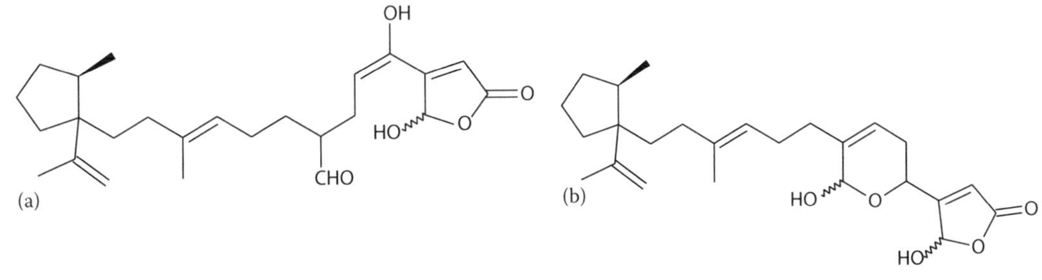

FIGURE 11.35
Luffariellin A (a) and luffariellin B (b).

functional groups as those present in manoalide and secomanoalide, respectively, and show similar anti-inflammatory properties (Kernan et al. 1987).

Although manoalide could be obtained in good yield from natural sources and has also been synthesized (Shigeo et al. 1985), the search for other anti-inflammatory agents, especially those with reversible phospholipase inhibition, has continued. The sponge *L. variabilis* has shown to contain other bioactive compounds, luffariellolides, structurally related to manoalide and with similar biological properties. Luffariellolide is a sesterterpenoid analogue of secomanoalide, which was first reported from a Palauan sponge *Luffariella* sp. (Albizati et al. 1987). Structurally, luffariellolide differed in having C-24 as methyl group instead of aldehyde functionality, and it was obtained as the (Z) isomer as well.

Since manoalide inhibits phospholipase A_2 irreversibly (Glaser and Jacobs 1986), SAR analysis was performed on natural analogues and chemical derivatives of manoalide to rationalize the contributions of the various functional groups incorporated in the structure, such as the γ-hydroxybutenolide, α-hydroxydihydropyran, and trimethylcyclohexenyl ring systems, to the efficacy in the phospholipase A_2 inhibition process (Glaser et al. 1989, Potts et al. 1992, Soriente et al. 1999). These studies indicated that (1) the existence of the hemiacetal in the α-hydroxydihydropyran ring is crucial for irreversible binding, (2) the γ-hydroxybutenolide ring is involved in the initial interaction with phospholipase A_2, and (3) the hydrophobic nature of the trimethylcyclohexenyl ring system allows nonbonded interactions with the enzyme that enhances the potency of these analogues.

The closed ring form of manoalide is the predominant molecular moiety that accounts for the selective and potent inhibition of phospholipase A_2. Recent studies (Dal Piaz et al. 2002) have clarified the fine details of the molecular mechanism of PLA2 inactivation, reaching the unexpected conclusion that the γ-hydroxybutenolide moiety alone undergoes a PLA2 nucleophilic attack.

Luffariellolide is a slightly less potent phospholipase A_2 inhibitor than manoalide. However, it is a more preferable anti-inflammatory agent for potential pharmacological investigation (Albizati et al. 1987) since it is a partially reversible inhibitor.

11.16.2 Scalarane Sesterterpenoids and 1.4-Dialdehyde Marine Terpenoids

Scalarane sesterterpenoids are bioactive natural products isolated exclusively from sponges and shell-less mollusks (marine snails that have no shell or nudibranchs) and are believed to be capable of sequestering the scalarane-based metabolites (Figure 11.36) from the sponges on which they feed. Most of these compounds play a key role as eco-physiological mediators (chemical defense) and are of interest for potential applications

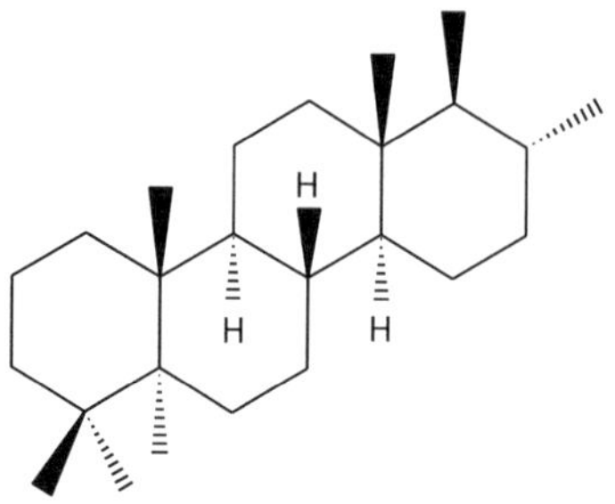

FIGURE 11.36
Scalarane skeleton.

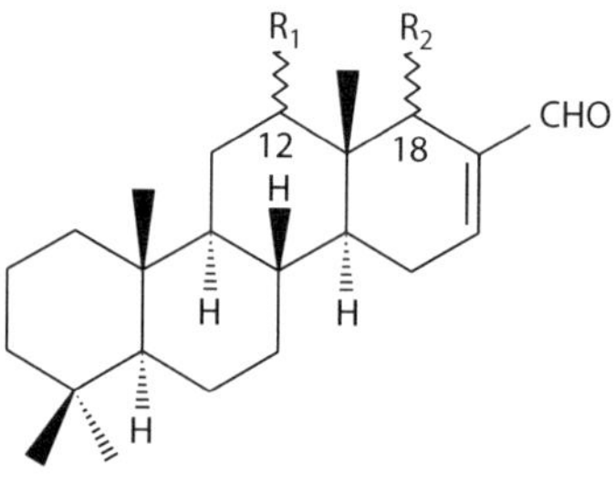

FIGURE 11.37
Scalaradial and related metabolites. Scalaradial: $R_1 = $ OAc; $R_2 = $ CHO. Related metabolites: $R_1 = $ OAc, OH, H, $= $ O; $R_2 = CH_2OH$, CHO.

as therapeutic agents. In addition, scalarane sesterterpenoids are considered to represent useful chemotaxonomic markers within sponges.

Scalaranes are well-known PLA2 inhibitors among sponge sesterterpenes. They have a characteristic carbon skeleton and are named after scalaradial, a 1,4-dialdehyde marine terpenoid, isolated from *Cacospongia mollior* in 1974 (Cimino et al. 1974, Puliti et al. 1990, Potts et al. 1992).

Scalaradial (Figure 11.37) is a sesterterpene molecule featuring a tetracyclic *trans*-anti-*trans*-anti-*trans* cyclohexane-perhydrophenanthrene skeleton and D-ring containing a 1,4-dialdehyde functionality (Puliti et al. 1995). The presence of an α,β-unsaturated aldehyde is somehow reminiscent of structural elements seen in the open chain form of manoalide.

Since several marine terpenoids contain at least one reactive aldehyde group, such as manoalide and its congeners, and possess anti-inflammatory activities that are mediated by the covalent inactivation of secretory phospholipase A_2, scalaradial has been considered to be an irreversible covalent inhibitor of phospholipase A. The 1,4-dialdehyde moiety was expected to play a crucial role in eliciting the scalaradial biological activity, because it is prone to attack by nitrogen nucleophiles. However, analysis of the molecular-level interaction between scalaradial and phospholipase A has disclosed an unexpected and complex reaction profile. On the basis of all the experimental data and in silico calculations, it was proposed that the key step of the inhibition process is the noncovalent anchoring of scalaradial into the enzyme active site, which is guided by strong hydrophobic contacts and the chelation of the catalytic calcium ion. Thus, even though the covalent interaction of scalaradial with the phospholipase A Lys85 (less than 3%) is a remarkable example of a specific small-molecule–protein binding, it should be considered to be a side reaction and irrelevant in terms of enzymatic inhibition.

Presently, the most convincing hypothesis is that, upon binding to phospholipase A, scalaradial is able to reversibly form a covalent species that actively contributes to the inhibition process. Either this kind of intermediate or, more likely, scalaradial itself may proceed along the reaction pathway described earlier to afford the final pyrrole-containing adduct which is now believed to have characterized. The chemical nature of this additional elusive intermediate is still unclear, even if the chemical reactivity revealed by the present model study seems to rule out any kind of scalaradial adduct with a nitrogenous nucleophile. The possibility of an important role played by oxygen (Ser, Thr, or Tyr) and/ or sulfur (Cys) nucleophiles needs to be investigated and presently can be neither excluded nor confirmed.

11.16.3 Sesquiterpenes (Quinone-Containing Sesterterpenoids)

The recently discovered sesquiterpene, having a phenolic or quinoid moiety, constitutes a fascinating family of natural products with a wide range of remarkable biological properties, including cytotoxic, antimicrobial, antiviral, and anti-inflammatory activities. Hence, they are valuable targets in medicinal chemistry and synthesis (Capon 1995, Popov et al. 1999, Lucas et al. 2003). These intriguing compounds are most commonly found in marine sponges of the genus *Dysidea* (family Dysideidae), some of them have been reported from brown algae, and at least three compounds were described from the fungus (Kondracki and Guyot 1989, Alvi et al. 1992, de Guzman et al. 1998, Giannini et al. 2000, Salmoun et al. 2000).

The first is the hydroquinone avarol (Figure 11.38a), originally isolated from the sponge *Dysidea avara*, and its quinone isomer avarone (Figure 11.38b) (Minale et al. 1974). Bolinaquinone (Figure 11.38c), a hydroxyquinone sesquiterpene, was isolated from a *Dysidea* sp. collected in the Philippines (de Guzman et al. 1998). Subsequently, bolinaquinone has also been isolated from a species of *Dysidea* (Giannini et al. 2001) along with dysidotronic acid (Figure 11.38d) (Giannini et al. 2000), dysidenones A (Figure 11.38e) and B (Figure 11.38f), and dysidine (Figure 11.38g). All of these metabolites possess anti-inflammatory activity against secretory PLA2 enzymes.

Most sesquiterpene quinines/quinoles have a sesquiterpene decalin-type unit of bicyclic normal drimane skeleton, or a rearranged drimane skeleton (Kazlauskas et al. 1978, Kobayashi et al. 1989), coupled to a quinoid system, to quinone, or to hydroquinone (quinol) (Figure 11.39).

The sesquiterpene quinones share a common drimane rearranged *cis*- or *trans*-decalin ring varying at the relative position of the double bond at the C-4 carbon and/or the stereochemical configuration about C-5. The C-9 position is substituted with a variably hydroxylated or heteroatom-substituted benzoquinone side chain. Given the interesting and diverse medicinal activities of this class of compounds, this chemical structure has been intensively studied (Ling et al. 2002). Aoki et al. recently reported a SAR study of 10 sesquiterpene quinone/hydroquinones and found that the quinone and amine groups are essential for activity (low μM) but that the configuration at C-5 is not important (Aoki et al. 2004).

SAR analyses indicate that a hydroxyquinone functionality with a short hydroxide/alkoxide side chain at C-20 will potentiate pyruvate orthophosphate dikinase (PPDK) activity (herbicides), while an aminoquinone with a larger substituent at C-20 is tolerated for PLA2 inhibitory activity (Figure 11.38g).

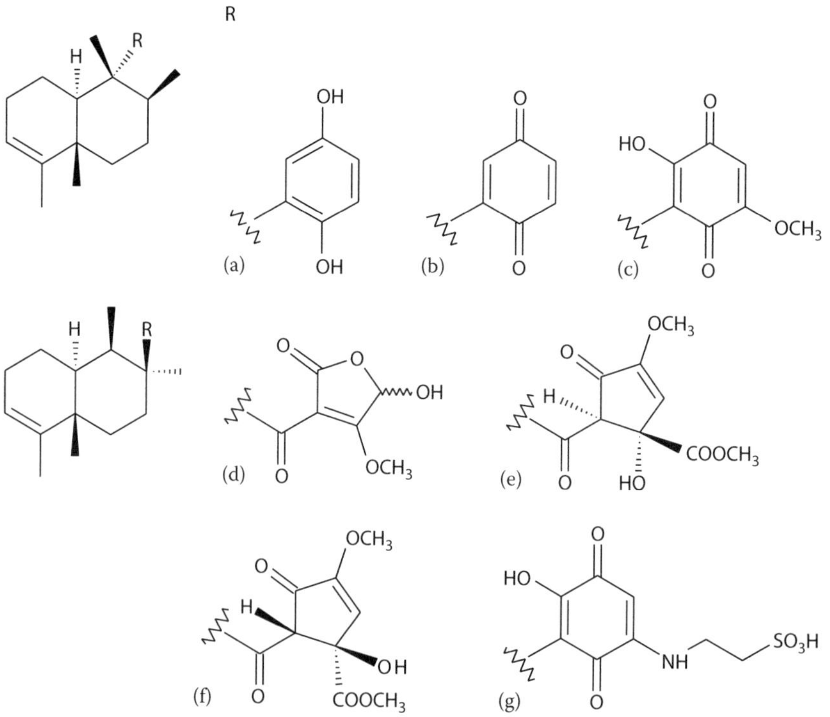

FIGURE 11.38
Sesquiterpenes: (a) the hydroquinone avarol, (b) the quinone isomer avarone, (c) bolinaquinone; (d) dysidotronic acid, (e) dysidenone A, (f) dysidenone B, and (g) dysidine.

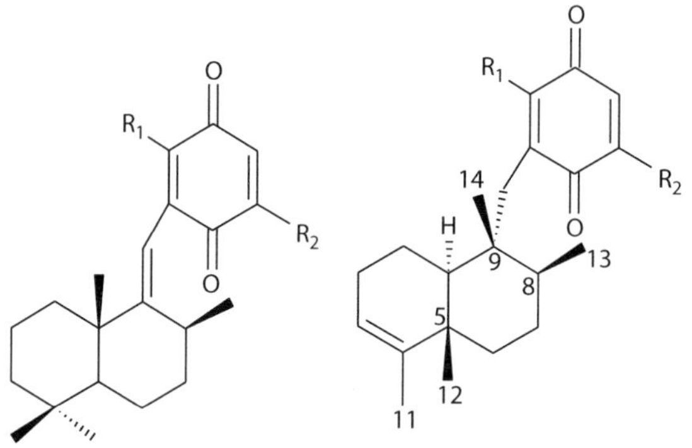

FIGURE 11.39
Drimane skeleton coupled to a quinoid system.

PLA2 inhibitory activity of sesquiterpene quinones/hydroquinones relies on the presence of a hydroxyquinone structure with a large side chain at C-20 and also amine substitution at C-20. Substitution at C-20 plays a significant role in PLA2 inhibitory activity and can be improved through synthetic modification of the drimane rearranged decalin ring and the quinone scaffold, especially the size of the C-20 nitrogen substituent. The C-9 position at which the quinone group is attached to the decalin ring may also be a useful site for synthetic modification (Motti et al. 2007).

Avarol, avarone, boliquinone, and other quinone and quinole products have been shown to be PLA2 inhibitors with typical selective profile against secretory enzymes. Avarol was able to inhibit human recombinant synovial phospholipase A_2 activity with an IC_{50} ¼ 158 mM, while the quinone derivative avarone failed to show inhibitory activity (Ferrandiz et al. 1994). Bolinaquinone, sharing a hydroxyl-p-quinone moiety connected to a *trans*-decalin terpene unit in a rearranged drimane skeleton, is one of the most active metabolites with a selective profile against secretory PLA2's (Giannini et al. 2001).

Bolinaquinone (Figure 11.38c), a sesquiterpenoid recently isolated from a *Dysidea* sp. sponge (Giannini et al. 2001), exhibits activity against the human colon tumor cell line, mild inhibition of *B. subtilis*, and remarkable anti-inflammatory activity (Kobayashi et al. 1989, 1992, de Guzman et al. 1998, Soriente et al. 1999). Bolinaquinone has a characteristic in vitro inhibitory profile against different secretory PLA2 without any effect on cytosolic PLA2. Its potency was higher than that of the reference inhibitor manoalide. In addition, bolinaquinone is chemically very close to other molecules, such as avarol and avarone (Ferrandiz et al. 1994), which have been reported as potent anti-inflammatory agents. Notably, bolinaquinone, sharing with avarol and avarone a very similar sesquiterpenoid substructure moiety, differs in the benzenoid part attached to the sesquiterpene moiety. In this regard, bolinaquinone simultaneously contains in its structure the hydroquinone system present in avarol together with the quinone system of avarone and contributes to some of its pharmacological properties.

11.16.4 Pseudopterosin

The pseudopterosins represent a class of structurally diverse amphilectane-type (Figure 11.40) diterpene glycosides isolated from the Caribbean soft coral species called a sea whip gorgonian octocoral *Pseudopterogorgia elisabethae* (Look et al. 1986a). The structurally related seco-pseudopterosins A–D belong to the serrulatane class of diterpenes and were initially isolated from *Pseudopterogorgia kallos* (Look and Fenical 1987).

The pseudopterosins (Figure 11.41) and seco-pseudopterosins (Figure 11.42) are anti-inflammatory agents, with a novel spectrum of activity when compared to existing topical anti-inflammatory agents. Recent studies have indicated that the release of eicosanoids is blocked without interrupting biosynthesis, usually involving versatile modes of action (Fenical 1987). They function as superior anti-inflammatory and analgesic agents when compared to the commercial drug indomethacin (Look et al. 1986b, Look and Fenical 1987, Potts and Faulner 1992, Mayer et al. 1998, Ata et al. 2003). Furthermore, these compounds appear to inhibit eicosanoid biosynthesis by inhibiting PLA2, 5-lipoxygenase (5-LO), and

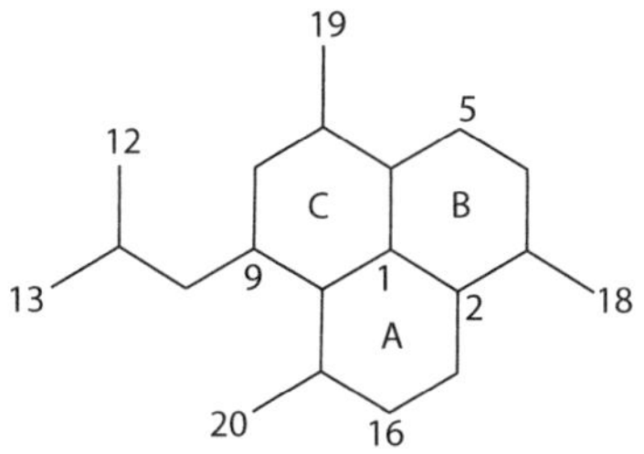

FIGURE 11.40
Amphilectane skeleton.

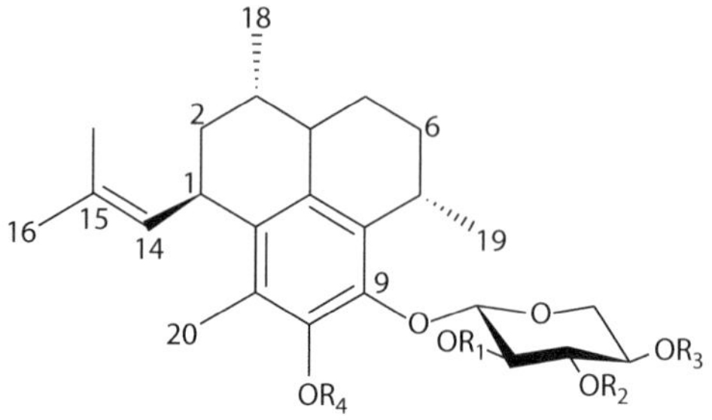

FIGURE 11.41
Pseudopterosins. Pseudopterosin A ($R_1 = R_2 = R_3 = R_4 = H$); B ($R_1 = Ac$, $R_2 = R_3 = R_4 = H$); C ($R_2 = Ac$, $R_1 = R_3 = R_4 = H$) and D ($R_3 = Ac$, $R_1 = R_2 = R_4 = H$).

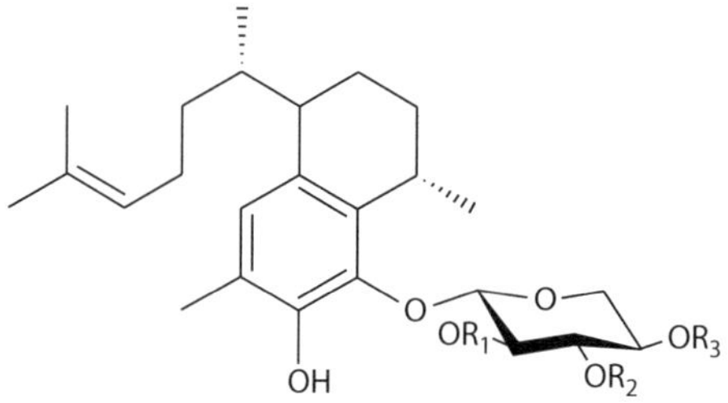

FIGURE 11.42
Seco-pseudopterosins. Seco-pseudopterosin A ($R_1 = R_2 = R_3 = R_4 = H$); B ($R_1 = Ac$, $R_2 = R_3 = R_4 = H$); C ($R_2 = Ac$, $R_1 = R_3 = R_4 = H$) and D ($R_3 = Ac$, $R_1 = R_2 = R_4 = H$).

cyclooxygenase (COX), degranulation of leukocytes, and the consequent liberation of lysosomal enzymes.

Pseudopterosins belong to a class of compounds known as tricyclic diterpene glycosides. Up until now, 26 pseudopterosins (A–Z) have been identified. All known pseudopterosins contain an amphilectane skeleton that features a tricarbocyclic rings possessing four chiral carbons and a sugar moiety (glycoside) attached at either C-9 or C-10 of a catechol subunit on one of the rings. Structural variations are limited to the identity of the glycoside, the degree of its acetylation, and the stereochemistry for the isobutenyl group on C-1. Structurally, they are tricyclic diterpene glycosides, differing in their sugar moiety attached to the catechol, the point of attachment of that sugar to the catechol and by stereochemical differences in the aglycone.

The pseudopterosins represent an important structural class of anti-inflammatory and analgesic agents, with novel anti-inflammatory mechanism and superior analgesic activity compared to pharmaceutical standards such as indomethacin. They do not inhibit PLA2, or COX and cytokine release. Evidence suggests the pseudopterosins block eicosanoid release.

Pseudopterosins are also used as cosmetic additives. At present, partially purified extracts of this sea whip, containing a mixture of pseudopterosins, are currently incorporated into several skin care cosmetic preparations such as Resilience, marketed by Estée Lauder. Due to their excellent anti-inflammatory and analgesic properties (Kijoa and Sawanwong 2004), pseudopterosin extract is used as an additive to prevent irritation caused by exposure to the sun or the chemicals.

Pseudopterosins A–D have been licensed to OsteoArthritis Sciences Inc., for medical use as anti-inflammatory drugs. This pharmaceutical company has completed preclinical tests and developed a potent derivative of pseudopterosin A called methopterosin, which is in clinical phase I/II trial as a wound-healing and anti-inflammatory agent (Haefner 2003, Gross and Konig 2006).

Methopterosin has a variety of important pharmacological properties that make it suitable for application to a number of conditions, including arthritis, psoriasis, and inflammatory bowel disease, among others. Another unique feature of methopterosin is its ability to accelerate wound healing by over 400%, a property of considerable interest in the treatment of burn victims, in postsurgical treatment, and in drug therapies for the many disorders involved in the healing process. The combined anti-inflammatory and wound-healing properties of methopterosin assure that this class of marine-derived drugs will be developed for diverse applications.

11.16.5 Steroids

Very few anti-inflammatory steroids have been reported from marine sponges. The first was contignasterol (50), isolated from the marine sponge *Petrosia contignata*, collected from Papua New Guinea (Burgoyne et al. 1992). The compound has a highly oxygenated sterol configuration with an unusual side chain. Although isolation of the natural product contignasterol (IZP-94005) from the sponge *P. contignata* was first reported in the early 1990s, it took another 10 years for the structural configuration of the compound to be elucidated. It was the first example of an emerging family of sponge steroids that have a number of unusual structural features. Contignasterol (Figure 11.43) was the first steroid from a marine source with a *cis* C/D ring junction, and the cyclic hemiacetal in its side chain, which exists in slow equilibrium with the open chain 22-hydroxy-29-aldehyde form. It also has a keto group in the position C-15 and 3α, 6α, and 7β hydroxyl substituents (Yang and Anderson 2002). Since then, several more 14β sterols have been isolated, all of which possess a ketone functionality at C-15 (Shoji et al. 1992, Kobayashi et al. 1995b, Keyzers et al. 2002).

In contrast to drugs with analogous action, this compound is not an inhibitor of phospholipase A_2, but it inhibits the excretion of histamine by leukocytes in a dose-dependent manner (Takei et al. 1994, Coulsen and O'Donnell 2000). Due to its promising

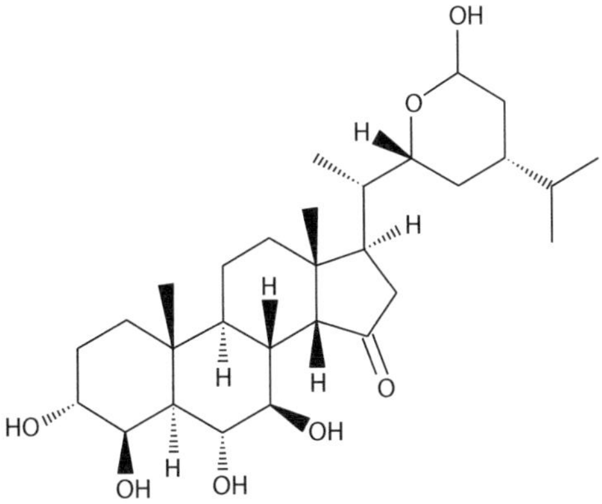

FIGURE 11.43
Contignasterol.

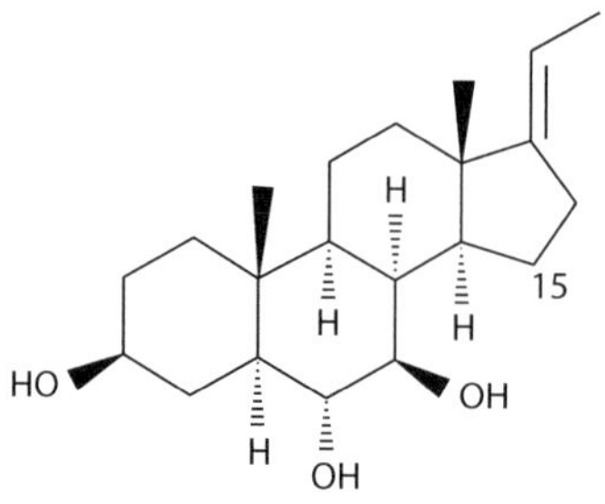

FIGURE 11.44
IPL576,092.

anti-inflammatory activity on in vivo animal models (Bramley et al. 1995), the contignas-terol molecule was used as a lead structure for an analogue synthesis program. IPL576,092 (Figure 11.44) and IPL512,602, synthetic analogues of contignasterol, are in phase II human clinical trials as an anti-inflammatory/anti-asthma agent (Burgoyne et al. 1992, Shen and Burgoyne 2002).

Recently, a novel and promising approach in drug discovery, toward the development of new lead substances, has emerged. It consists in the combination of parts of structur-ally different naturally occurring bioactive products to yield hybrid structures that can, in principle, exceed the activities of their parent compounds (Tietze et al. 2003).

From this perspective and as part of a broad program in the steroid area, Inflazyme in conjunction with Aventis Pharma designed and synthesized the hybrid entities (Figure 11.45), linking the IPL576,092 trihydroxylated tetracyclic nucleus to the conti-gnasterol's (17R,20S,22S,24S)-lactol 5 and manoalide γ-hydroxybutenolide side chains, respectively (Izzo et al. 2004).

This approach was inspired by the perspective of "natural product hybrids" that com-bination of parts of structurally different naturally occurring bioactive products to yield hybrid structures can, in principle, exceed the activities of their parent compounds.

Several structurally related polyhydroxy-steroids, xestobergsterols (Figure 11.46), with unusual *cis*-fused C/D ring junctions and an additional carbocyclic E-ring have also been isolated from marine sources (Shoji et al. 1992). Xestobergsterols A and B, 15-ketosterols, were isolated in 1992 from the sponge *Xestospongia bergquistia* (Shoji et al. 1992). Three years later, xestobergsterol C was isolated from the marine sponge *Ircinia* sp. And the

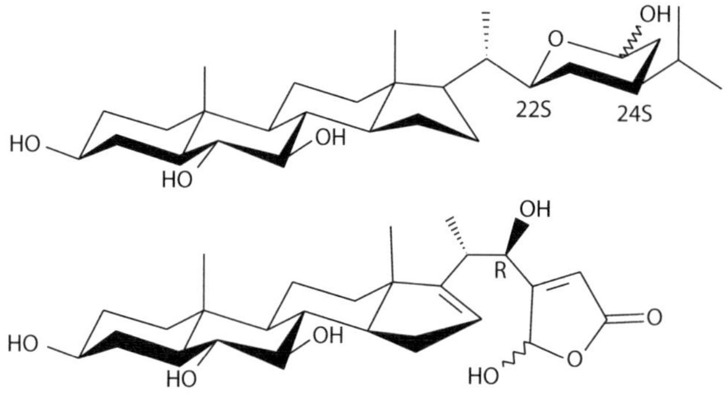

FIGURE 11.45
Hybrid structures of IPL576,092 and manoalide.

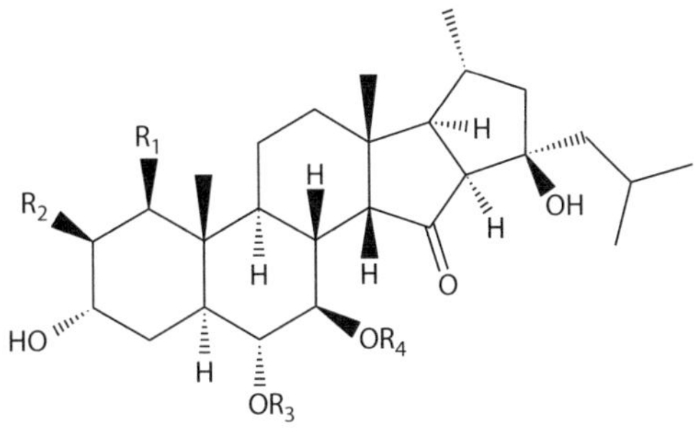

FIGURE 11.46
Xestobergsterols. Xestobergsterol A ($R_1 = R_2 = R_3 = R_4 = H$), B ($R_1 = R_2 = OH$, $R_3 = R_4 = H$) and C ($R_1 = R_3 = R_4 = H$, $R_4 = OH$).

full structures of these xestobergsterols were established (Kobayashi et al. 1995b). Xestobergsterols are strong inhibitors of immunoglobulin E-mediated histamine release, 5000 times more potent than the antiallergic drug disodium cromoglycate (Shoji et al. 1992). It has been reported that the mechanism of action of xestobergsterol A is through strong inhibition of phosphatidylinositol phospholipase C (Takei et al. 1993).

11.16.6 Nitrogenous Anti-Inflammatory Compounds (Alkaloids)

Bisindole alkaloids (Figure 11.47), consisting of two indole moieties connected to each other via heterocyclic units, have been particularly abundant within sponges. Sponge-derived bisindole alkaloids, in particular, a group of rare but structurally related bis(indolyl)imidazole metabolites known as the topsentins (Casapullo et al. 2000, Bao et al. 2007), have established themselves as a class of biologically important natural products in the last few decades. Since topsentin, a bis(indolyl)imidazole, and its analogues were isolated from the sponge *Topsentia genitrix* (*Spongosorites genitrix*) (Bartik et al. 1987, Tsuji et al. 1988), metabolites containing bis(indole) moiety have been found with various carbon skeletons and functionalities. Their biological activities have attracted considerable interest due to remarkably potent and diverse bioactivities including antitumor, antiviral (Puliti et al. 1995, Popov et al. 1999), antifungal, antibacterial, and anti-inflammatory activities (Cimino et al. 1974, Phife et al. 1996, Shin et al. 1999, Bao et al. 2005).

Multiple activities might suggest interaction with multiple receptors or targets. It may be possible that these nonspecific compounds might have multiple ecological targets as well. The biological activity of marine indole alkaloids is clearly a product of the unique

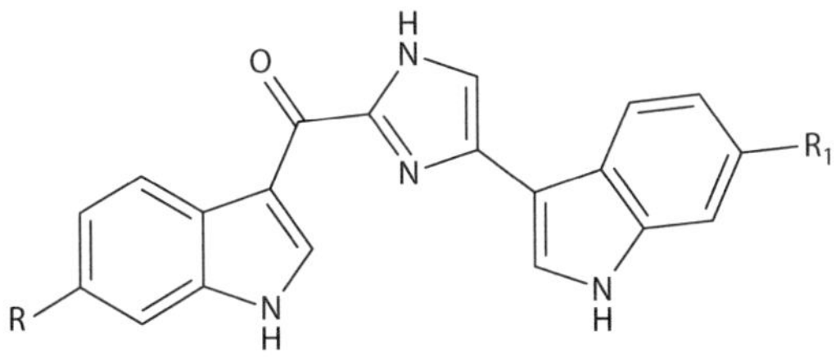

FIGURE 11.47
Bisindole alkaloids. R = R_1 = H Deoxytopsentin; R = OH, R_1 = H Topsentin; R = Br, R_1 = Br Dibromotopsentin; R = H, R_1 = Br Deoxybromotopsentin; R = OH, R_1 = Br Bromotopsentin.

functionality and elements involved in the biosynthesis of marine natural products. Both topsentin and bromotopsentin have been shown to have potent anti-inflammatory activities, comparable or better than the effects of standards such as manoalide, hydrocortisone, or indomethacin (Wylie et al. 1997). It seems that bromination has the potential to increase the biological activity significantly.

11.17 Antiviral

Antiviral compounds are currently of particular interest since viral diseases (e.g., HIV, H1N1, and HSV) have become major human health problems in recent decades. The ability of a virus to rapidly evolve and develop resistance to existing drugs drives the search for new and more effective antiviral drugs. A crucial component in drug discovery continues to be the proven strategy of screening natural products. In the past, structurally diverse compounds produced by terrestrial microorganisms and plants have shown inhibitory activities against various viral diseases (Harnden 1985). However, the repeated isolation and cultivation of the same microbial species from terrestrial environments has led to a number of projects, resulting in isolation of previously identified compounds in recent years. Unlike their terrestrial counterparts, however, the antiviral potential of secondary metabolites produced by marine organisms has not been extensively explored.

11.17.1 Antimetabolites

The discovery of antiviral compounds from marine sources began in 1951 when Bergman reported the isolation of unusual nucleosides, spongothymidine and spongouridine (Figure 11.48) (Bergmann and Feeney 1951, Bergmann and Stempien 1957), from the Caribbean sponge *Tethya crypta* (family Tethyidae). These compounds were nucleosides similar to those forming the building blocks of nucleic acids (DNA and RNA). However, they contained a rare sugar arabinose instead of the typical ribose and desoxyribose residues observed in RNA and DNA. These natural nucleoside analogues were discovered to have unexpected antiviral properties. Examination of their mode of action as reverse transcriptase inhibitors led to the eventual synthesis of a number of important commercially

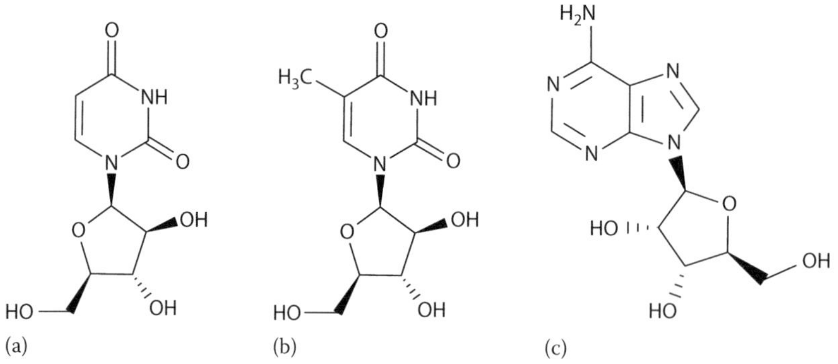

FIGURE 11.48
(a) Spongouridine; (b) spongothymidine; (c) vidarabine.

available antiviral and anticancer drugs. Spongouridine and spongothymidine (Bergmann and Burke 1955) can be considered as the precursors of all nucleoside drugs which act as antimetabolites. In general, antiviral molecules from sponges do not give protection against viruses, but they may result in drugs to treat already infected persons.

This work eventually led to the synthesis of the anti-HIV drug zidovudine (AZT); Ara-C (cytarabine), an anticancer agent; and Ara-A (vidarabine) (Figure 11.48), the first antiviral drug. Vidarabine or Ara-A is a synthetic analogue of spongouridine with improved antiviral activity. Ara-A inhibits viral DNA synthesis by conversion into adenine arabinoside triphosphate which inhibits viral DNA polymerase and DNA synthesis of herpes, vaccinia, and varicella zoster viruses. It was the first nucleoside antiviral to be licensed for the treatment of systematic herpes virus infection and one of the three marine-derived drugs that are currently approved by the FDA in the United States (Mayer et al. 2010).

Since that time, other investigations have uncovered antiviral properties associated with secondary metabolites from other diverse marine organisms, including ascidians (Rinehart et al. 1981, 1987), macroalgae (Cariucci et al. 1999), microalgae (Ohta et al. 1998), cyanobacteria (Patterson et al. 1993), and bacteria (Gustafson et al. 1989, Davidson and Schumacher 1993). However, with marine species estimated to account for at least half of the global biodiversity (De Vries and Hall 1994), the oceans remain relatively unexplored with respect to antiviral drug discovery.

11.17.2 Mycalamides

Perry and coworkers reported the isolation of two potent antiviral and antitumor compounds, mycalamides A (Figure 11.49) and B from the New Zealand marine sponge *Mycale* sp. (Perry et al. 1988, 1990). The structure of the related compound onnamide A from the Japanese sponge *Theonella* sp. has also been described (Sakemi et al. 1988). These three compounds are related to pederin, a toxin originally isolated from the terrestrial blister beetle, *Paederus fuscipes* (Cardani et al. 1965).

Examining the mechanisms involved in the actions of these compounds, Burres and Clement (1989) discovered the inhibition of protein synthesis and translation of RNA into protein in a cell-free lysate of rabbit reticulocytes. A more recent study has described the binding of mycalamide A to the E site of the large ribosomal subunit of *Haloarcula marismortui* and the resulting inhibition of protein synthesis (Gurel et al. 2009).

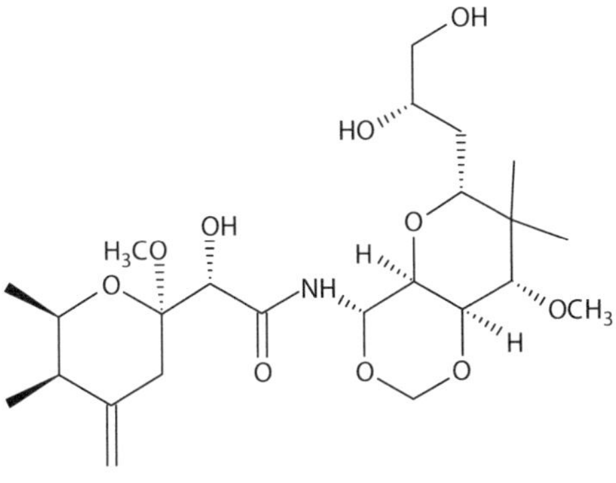

FIGURE 11.49
Mycalamide A.

Acyl, alkyl, and silyl derivatives of the hydroxy and N-amido functionalities of the mycalamides A and B have been prepared, their relative reactivities established, and in vitro P388 leukemia bioassays performed (Thompson et al. 1992). With the availability of the wide range of derivatives described earlier, it was possible to determine some of the features of the mycalamide structure which are essential for determining its biological activity compared to onnamide and pederin. The most notable feature is that methylation of the amide nitrogen together with the 7-OH group causes at least a threefold reduction in activity. The trimethylsilyl (TMS) ethers are all as active as the parent compounds, but this is probably because the TMS ethers are unstable and hydrolyze back to the parent compounds in the assay medium. The more stable tertbutyldimethylsilyl ethers all show marked reduction in activity relative to the comparably substituted O-methyl ethers, an effect which may be attributed to the presence of large, nonpolar substituents. Derivatization of the 7-OH group causes a 10- to 100-fold reduction in activity, whereas methylation of both the 17- and 18-OH groups (as found in pederin) makes the mycalamides as active as pederin. From these observations, it was concluded that the centrally located α-hydroxyamidoacetal functionality is vitally important for the biological activity of the mycalamides.

Four analogues of mycalamide A have recently been reported to bind the nucleoprotein of influenza virus and inhibit its multiplication (Hagiwara et al. 2010).

11.17.3 1,4-Benzoquinones and Avarol

The 1,4-benzoquinone moiety is a common structural feature in a large number of compounds that have received considerable attention, owing to their broad spectrum of biological activities. These include strong activity against mouse lymphoma cells (Müller et al. 1985a, Sarin et al. 1987, Schröder et al. 1989), antiviral activity (Müller et al. 1985b, 1987, De Giulio et al. 1991), anti-inflammatory activity (De Giulio et al. 1991), antipsoriatic properties (Suhadolnik et al. 1989), as well as moderate antifungal and antibacterial activity against Gram-positive strains (Seibert et al. 1985).

Avarol (Figure 11.50), a sesquiterpenoid hydroquinone with a rearranged drimane skeleton, was first isolated from the Red Sea sponge *D. avara* by Minale and coworkers in 1974 (Minale 1974, Müller 1985b). Both avarol and its quinine derivative avarone display moderate antibacterial and antifungal activity and strong antileukemic, cytostatic, and antiviral

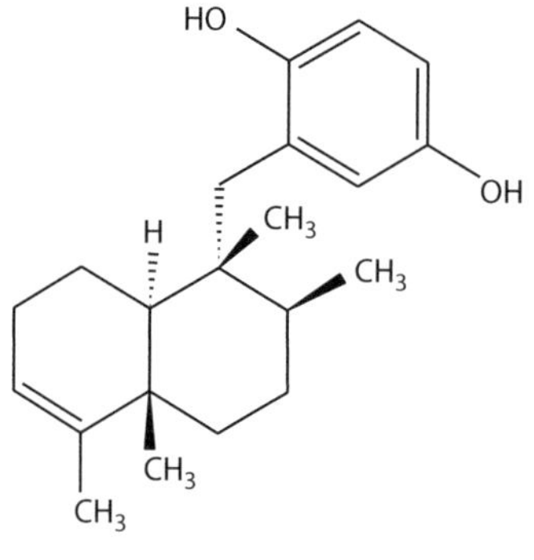

FIGURE 11.50
Avarol.

activity both in vivo and in vitro. Several new derivatives of avarol showing antiviral activities have also been extracted from the Red Sea sponge *Dysidea cinere* (Batke et al. 1988).

Avarol is converted into its corresponding quinone derivative avarone via the semiquinone free radical. The antitumor and the antiviral effects of avarol/avarone may be induced by the drugs, leading to an increase in the intracellular concentrations of superoxide radicals, such as superoxide dismutases and of glutathione peroxidase (Batke et al. 1988).

11.17.4 Cyclic Depsipeptides

The anti-HIV and cytotoxic cyclic depsipeptides, papuamides A–D, were isolated from the sponges *Theonella mirabilis* and *T. swinhoei* that were collected along the north coast of Papua New Guinea (Ford et al. 1999). Depsipeptides are peptides in which one or more of the amide bonds are replaced by ester bonds.

Papuamides are known to strongly inhibit the infection of human T-lymphoblastoid cells by HIV-1RF and also exhibit potent cytotoxicity against a number of human cancer cell lines. These cyclic heptadepsipeptides have a unique structure with a number of unusual amino acids including (2S,3S,4R)-3,4-dimethylglutamine, (2R,3R)-3-hydroxyleucine, β-methoxytyrosine, and 3-methoxyalanine, in addition to glycine, alanine, and threonine. They also contain 2,3-diaminobutanoic acid or 2-amino-2-butenoic acid residues. Papuamides A–D are also the first marine-derived peptides reported to contain 3-hydroxyleucine and homoproline residues and a previously undescribed (4Z,6E)-2,3-dihydroxy-2,6,8-trimethyldeca-(4Z,6E)-dienoic acid moiety N-linked to a terminal glycine residue (Ford et al. 1999).

Two unusual amino acids, β-methoxytyrosine and 3,4-dimethylglutamine, are known as common components of the cyclodepsipeptides callipeltin A (Zampella et al. 1996) and neamphamide A (Oku et al. 2004), which show anti-HIV and antifungal activities.

Papuamides A and B (Figure 11.51) have been evaluated for their anti-HIV activity in cell-based assays (Xie et al. 2008). Activities for both compounds were found to be virtually identical. However, papuamides C and D were found to be less potent. Results suggest that papuamide A shows a direct virucidal mechanism of HIV-1 inhibition. Andjelic and coworkers have shown that papuamide A acts as an entry inhibitor, preventing human immunodeficiency virus infection of host cells, and it has been shown that this inhibition is not specific to R5 or X4 tropic virus (Andjelic et al. 2008). Other papuamides (B–D) were also shown to inhibit viral entry, indicating that the presence of free amino moiety of 2,3-diaminobutanoic acid residue is not required for antiviral activity.

11.17.5 Microspinosamide

Another novel peptide and anti-HIV candidate is the microspinosamide (Figure 11.52) isolated from the sponge *Sidonops microspinosa* (Rashid et al. 2001) in 2001. Microspinosamide is a new cyclic depsipeptide containing 13 amino acids including alanine, tryptophan, arginine, threonine, aspartate, valine, two prolines, tert-leucine, β-methylisoleucine, *N*-methylglutamine, cysteic acid, and a new residue, β-hydroxy-*p*-bromophenylalanine. It is the first naturally occurring peptide containing a beta–hydroxy-p-bromophenylalanine residue. Microspinosamide inhibited the cytopathic effect of HIV-1 infection in an XTT-based in vitro assay (Rashid et al. 2001).

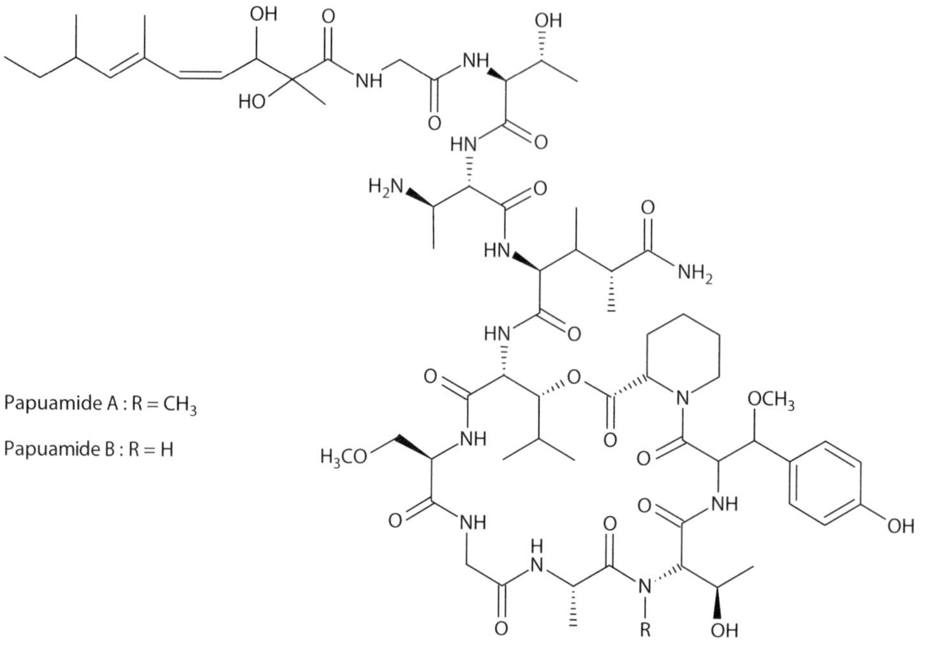

FIGURE 11.51
Papuamides A and B.

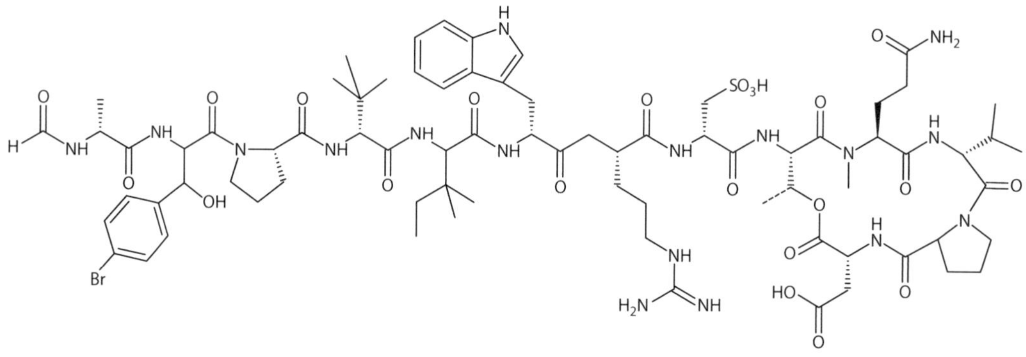

Papuamide A : R = CH₃

Papuamide B : R = H

FIGURE 11.52
Microspinosamide.

11.18 Alkaloids

11.18.1 4-Methylaaptamine

The aaptamines are a small group of biologically active marine alkaloids having a rare 1H-benzo[de]-1,6-naphthyridine skeleton. The parent naphthyridine known as aaptamine was first isolated by Nakamura et al. (1982). Another member of the series, isoaaptamine (N-methylaaptamine), was first reported by Fedoreev et al. (1988), who isolated it from a sponge in the genus *Suberites*. Isoaaptamine was later isolated from *Aaptos aaptos* by two different groups (Kashman et al. 1990, Shen et al. 1997). Seven aaptamines, namely, aaptamine (Fedoreev et al. 1988), isoaaptamine (Shen et al. 1997), 9-demethylaaptamine and 9-demethyloxyaaptamine (Nakamura et al. 1987b), bisdemethylaaptamine (Herlt et al. 2004), bisdemethylaaptamine-9-O-sulfate, and 4-N-methylaaptamine (Coutinho et al. 2002), have been isolated from marine sponges mainly of the genus *Aaptos*. Moreover, aaptamines were isolated from marine sponges of the genus *Suberites* (Kashman et al. 1990), *Hymeniacidon* (Pettit et al. 2004), and *Xestospongia* (Calcul et al. 2003). All these compounds have either an N-methylated or a non-N-methylated 1,6-naphthyridine core fused with a functionalized benzenoid unit. Recently, two C-3-substituted demethyloxy-aaptamines, 3-phenethylamino- and 3-isopentylamino-demethyloxyaaptamines, have been isolated (Khozirah et al. 2009). Some of aaptamines have been reported to have α-adrenoceptor blocking activity (Ohizumi et al. 1984), anti-HIV-1 activity, antimicrobial activity (Gul et al. 2006), antiherpes activity (Souza et al. 2007), sortase A inhibitory activity (Jang et al. 2007), and anticancer activity (Longley et al. 1993, Shen et al. 1999, Bowling et al. 2008).

Aaptamines are marine alkaloids with a unique 1H-benzo[d,e][1,6]naphthyridine structure and interesting biological properties. Alkaloid 4-methylaaptamine was isolated from the marine sponge *Aaptos* sp. The first aaptamines were isolated by Nakamura et al. (1987b) from the marine sponge *A. aaptos*. Later on, it was shown that the presence of these alkaloids is not limited to the genus *Aaptos*. Besides the O-methyl compounds, the new N-methylaaptamine (isoaaptamine) was firstly isolated from sponges of the genus *Suberites* and from the sponge *A. aaptos* (Gul et al. 2006).

The new 1H-benzo[de][1,6]naphthyridine derivative, 4-methylaaptamine, displays potent antiviral activity against HSV-1 replication. It is more potent than acyclovir. The first SAR study of the aaptamines was summarized by Shen et al. (1999). They observed that the phenolic group at the C-9 position was important for cytotoxicity. Acylation of that position led to a decrease in activity.

Although aaptamine and isoaaptamine (Figure 11.53) differ only in the position of one methyl group, its shift from the C-9 position in aaptamine to the N-1 position in isoaaptamine leads to an increase in cytotoxicity. The skeleton of aaptamine bears four positions that could be methylated, two nitrogen atoms and two phenol groups. Therefore, 16 different methyl or demethyl derivatives of the aaptamine scaffold are possible.

11.18.2 Dragmacidin F

Of the many bis(indole) alkaloids found in nature, the dragmacidins have received considerable attention over the past decade due to their wide range of biological and

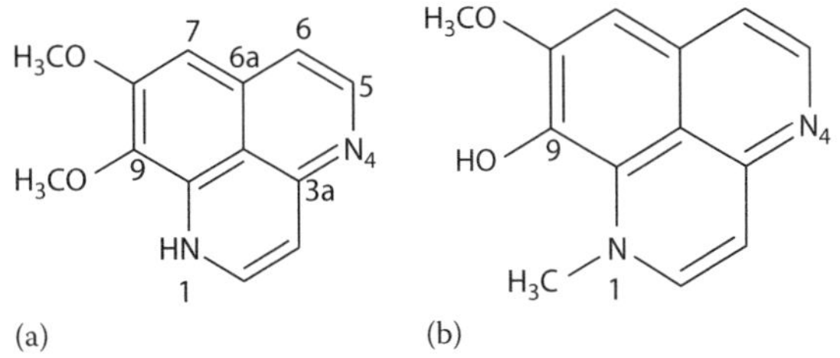

FIGURE 11.53
(a) Aaptamine; (b) isoaaptamine. 9-O-4-Ethylbenzoylisoaaptamine, a novel derivative of isoaaptamine also displays potent activity against HIV-1 with an EC$_{50}$ of 0.47 µg/mL. (From Gul, W. et al., *Bioorg. Med. Chem.*, 14, 8495, 2006.)

pharmacological activities and complex structures (Kohmoto et al. 1988, Morris and Andersen 1990, Wright et al. 1992, Capon et al. 1998, Wright et al. 1999, Cutignano et al. 2000, Jiang and Gu 2000, Feldman and Ngernmeesri 2005).

This structurally elaborate class of bromoindole marine alkaloids was isolated from a variety of deepwater sponges including *Dragmacidon, Halicortex, Spongosorites*, and *Hexadella* and the tunicate *Didemnum candidum* (Kohmoto et al. 1988, Morris and Andersen 1990, Fahy et al. 1991, Capon et al. 1998, Cutignano et al. 2000). The initial dragmacidins A–C identified contained a piperazine linker and displayed modest antifungal, antiviral, and cytotoxic activities. Recently, the structurally more complex aminoimidazole and guanidine-containing pyrazinone dragmacidins D, E, and F were isolated and shown to possess a wide range of interesting biological properties as well. These central pyrazine units are in various oxidization states: piperazine in dragmacidin A–C and pyrazine-2-one in dragmacidin D–F. Dragmacidins A and B have piperazine rings with *trans* configuration. Antiviral bromoindole dragmacidin F was isolated by Cutignano et al. from a marine sponge of the genus *Halicortex* sp. collected off the southern coast of Ustica Island (Italy). Preliminary in vitro pharmacological screening on the ethanol extract of *Halicortex* sp. showed antiherpes activity (Cutignano et al. 2000). The compound demonstrated in vitro antiviral activity against HSV-1 and HIV-1 with an EC_{50} of 96 μM and EC_{50} of 0.9 μM, respectively, and hence is most likely responsible for the antiviral property exhibited by *Halicortex* extracts. The compound has an unprecedented carbon skeleton that is presumed to be derived biosynthetically from dragmacidin D by the cyclization of its partially oxidized form. Total synthesis of (+)-dragmacidin F (Figure 11.54) has been described by Garg et al. (2004).

In addition, dragmacidin F possesses a variety of interesting structural features, including a substituted pyrazinone, the bridged [3.3.1] bicyclic ring system, and the 6-bromoindole fragment which is fused to both the trisubstituted pyrrole and aminoimidazole heterocycles, and the 6-bromoindole fragment.

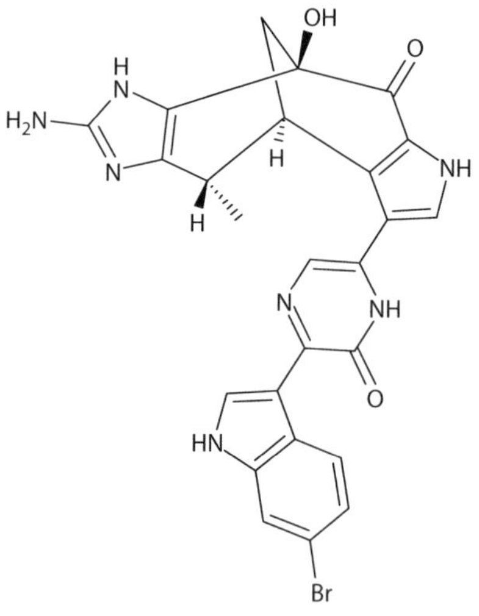

FIGURE 11.54
Dragmacidin F.

11.18.3 Manzamines

Marine invertebrates are rich in β-carboline alkaloids (Blackman et al. 1987, Kearns et al. 1995, Kobayashi et al. 1995a). These natural β-carboline metabolites have been found to possess interesting antitumor and antiviral activities (McNulty and Still 1995). Eudistomins (Rinehart et al. 1984, 1987, Badre et al. 1994) and manzamines (Sakai et al. 1987, Crews et al. 1994), which were isolated from tunicates and sponges, respectively, are of particular interest. The antiviral eudistomins C and E were found to be active against HSV-2, vaccinia virus, and RNA viruses (Munro et al. 1987).

The β-carboline and 3,4-dihydro-β-carboline moieties in manzamines appear to be essential for the biological activity. The SAR revealed that there was a lack of complete correlation between carbon numbers of the side chain and biological activities. However, the negative correlation was present between the alkyl side chain lengths in cytotoxicity tests. The optimal chain length is between 2 and 5 carbons. The optimal chain length for anti-topoisomerase II may be 3 and 5 carbons. The DNA-binding capacity, which favored minor groove binding, was thus influenced by the alkyl substitution on carbazole chromophore and proton donor on β-carboline chromophore (Shen et al. 2011).

Ichiba et al. (1994) reported that manzamine A (Figure 11.55), 8-hydroxymanzamine A, and 8-methoxymanzamine A (Figure 11.56) displayed significant antiviral activities against HSV-II with a minimal inhibitory concentration (MIC) of 0.05, 0.1, and 0.1 g/mL, respectively. Recently, manzamine A, 8-hydroxymanzamine A, and 6-deoxymanzamine X were also found to possess anti-HIV activities against human peripheral blood mononuclear (PBM) cells with EC_{50} of 0.59, 4.2, and 1.6 μM, respectively (Rao et al. 2003).

A more recent study reports the isolation of manzamine A from an undescribed sponge of the genus *Acanthostrongylophora* collected from Manado Bay, Indonesia, together with important oral and intravenous pharmacokinetic properties of manzamine A in rats (Yousaf et al. 2004). This study indicates that it has a low metabolic clearance, a reasonably long pharmacokinetic half-life, and good absolute oral bioavailability, making it a promising lead compound for further development. They also reported the anti-HIV-1 activity of manzamine A, 8-hydroxymanzamine A, 6-deoxymanzamine X, and neokauluamine with an EC_{50} of 4.2, 0.6, 1.6, and 2.3 μM, respectively.

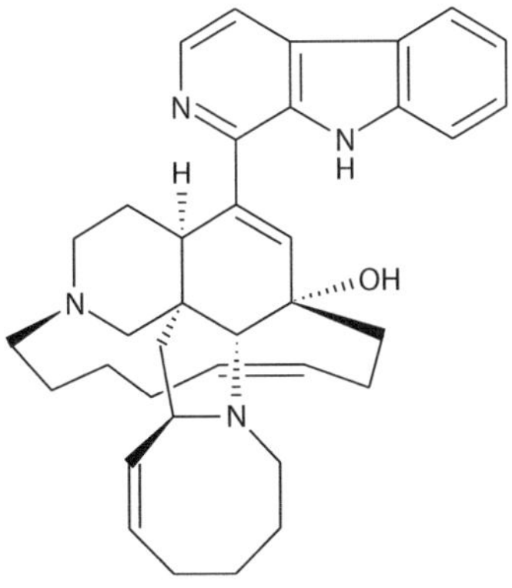

FIGURE 11.55
Manzamine A.

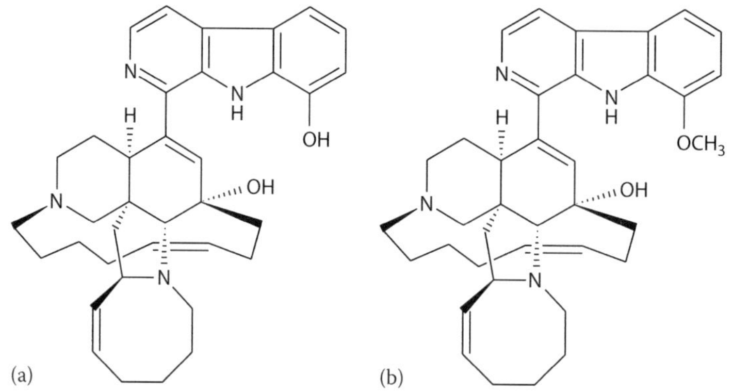

FIGURE 11.56
(a) 8-Hydroxymanzamine A; (b) 8-methoxymanzamine.

11.19 Phenolic Macrolides

11.19.1 Hamigeran B

Hamigerans are a family of metabolites isolated from the poecilosclerid sponge *Hamigera tarangaensis* Bergquist and Fromont (family Anchinoidae, syn. Phorbasidae) (Cambie et al. 2000). Among these natural products, four compounds, hamigeran A, debromohamigeran A, hamigeran B, and 4-bromohamigeran B, are endowed with a unique tricarbocyclic skeleton in which a substituted aromatic nucleus is fused to a hydrindane framework bearing three or more stereogenic centers. Hamigerans are biogenetically quite interesting, and it remains to be established whether they are norditerpenoids or meroterpenoids that arise through mixed biogenesis involving a monoterpenoid moiety. The biological activity profile of hamigerans is impressive, and most of them exhibit moderate in vitro cytotoxicity against P388 leukemia cells. In particular, hamigeran B has interesting biological activity as it exhibits 100% virus inhibition against both herpes and polio viruses with only slight cytotoxicity throughout the host cells (Figure 11.57).

11.19.2 Macrolactins

The macrolactins are polyene macrolides containing a 24-membered lactone ring, isolated from a taxonomically unidentified deep-sea bacterium, *Bacillus amyloliquefaciens* (gorgonian, Junceella juncea, Sanya, China) (Gustafson et al. 1989). Known metabolites were also isolated, including 4-butoxyphenol and, for the first time from a natural source, propoxyphenol and 4-ethoxyphenol. All the known compounds displayed antilarval activity toward *Balanus amphitrite* (Gao et al. 2010). There were a total of 18 isolated macrolactins that have been reported since the first of them, macrolactin A, had been isolated in 1989 (Lu et al. 2008). Macrolactin A (Figure 11.58) showed selective antibacterial activity, inhibited B16-F10 murine melanoma cancer cells in vitro assays, showed significant inhibition of mammalian Herpes simplex viruses (types I and II), and protected T-lymphoblast cells against human HIV viral replication. Macrolactin A was also isolated from a culture broth of *Actinomadura* sp. as a neuronal-cell-protecting substance by Kim et al. (1997), and from a *Bacillus* sp. from a potato-cultivating area (Han et al. 2005). Macrolactin A and macrolactin F

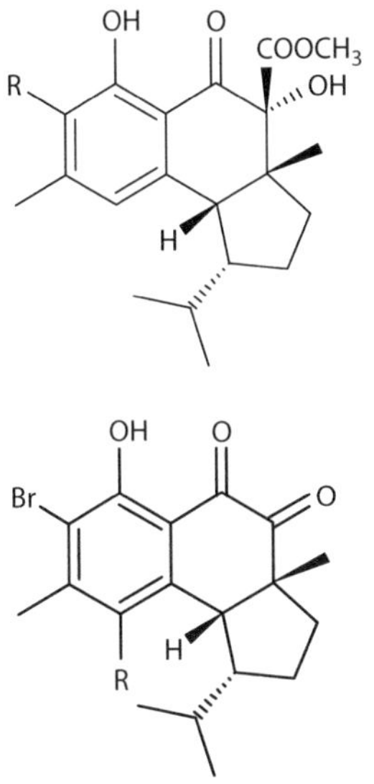

R = Br Hamigeran A

R = H Debromohamigeran A

R = H Hamigeran B

R = Br = 4-bromohamigeran B

FIGURE 11.57
Hamigerans A and B.

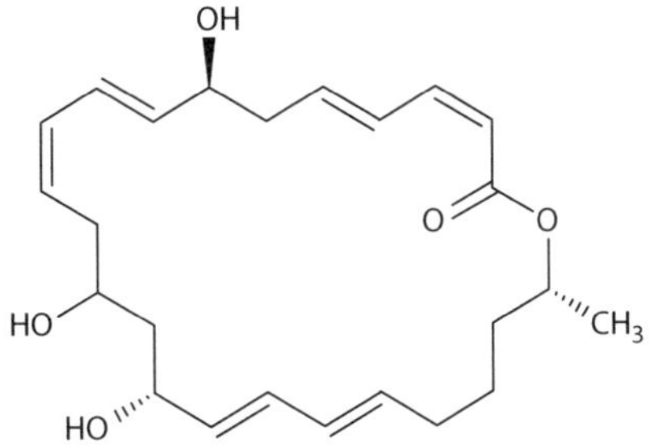

FIGURE 11.58
Macrolactin A.

were both produced by a soil *Streptomyces* sp. and were both found to be squalene synthase inhibitors (Choi et al. 2003).

At least 17 macrolactines are known from a deep-sea *Bacillus*. Some members of this series were already isolated in 1989 by Gustafson et al. (1989), while further compounds were added in 2000 (Jaruchoktaweechai et al. 2000) and 2001 (Nagao et al. 2001). It was found that 24-membered macrolactins were generally produced by the *Bacillus* sp. and exhibited antibacterial, anticancer, and antiviral activities. All macrolactins contain three separate diene structure elements, which were named as macrolactins A–N, 7-O-succinylmacrolactin A, 7-O-succinylmacrolactin F, and 7-O-malonylmacrolactin A, respectively.

Examples of antiviral agents from marine microorganisms are the macrolactins A–F, macrolides from a Gram-positive deep-sea bacterium obtained from a sediment sample obtained from the California coast, and the caprolactins A and B containing a cyclized lysine moiety. They all inhibit the Herpes simplex viruses, and in addition, macrolactin A is effective against HIV.

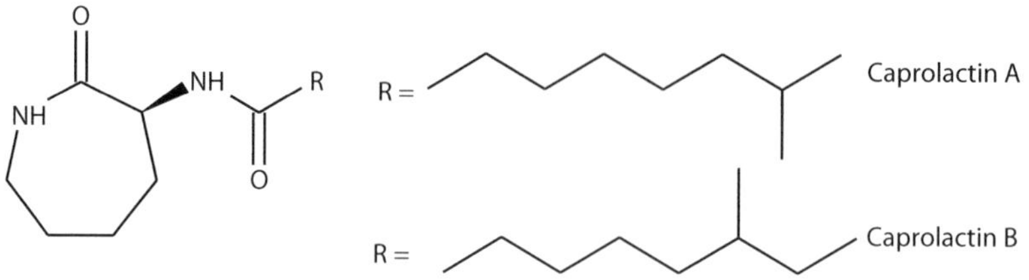

FIGURE 11.59
Caprolactins A and B.

11.19.3 Caprolactins A and B

Caprolactins A and B (Figure 11.59) are new caprolactams from an unidentified Gram-positive bacterium, showing both antiviral and cytotoxic properties. Davidson and coworkers isolated the caprolactins A and B from the fermentation of an unidentified deep-sea sediment bacterium (Davidson and Schumacher 1993). These compounds showed very modest inhibition of HSV-2 at a concentration of 100 μg/mL. Additionally, the caprolactins displayed mild cytotoxicity against human colorectal adenocarcinoma and human epidermoid carcinoma cells at low micromolar concentrations. Both the caprolactins and the macrolactins were obtained by extracting whole-cell culture suspensions with ethyl acetate, so it is unclear to what degree these compounds are extracellular.

Recently, screening assays of the antiviral activity of many extracts have led to the identification of a number of polysaccharides (Chattopadhyay et al. 2007, Mandal et al. 2008, Harden et al. 2009, Yasuhara-Bell and Lu 2010) and diterpenes (El Gamal 2010) having potent inhibitory effects against Herpes simplex virus (HSV) type 1.

References

Adhikari, U., C. G. Mateu, K. Chattopadhyay, C. A. Pujol, E. B. Damonte, and B. Ray. 2006. Structure and antiviral activity of sulfated fucans from *Stoechospermum marginatum*. *Phytochemistry* 67: 2474–2482.
Ahn, K. S., G. Sethi, T.-H. Chao et al. 2007. Salinosporamide A (NPI-0052) potentiates apoptosis, suppresses osteoclastogenesis and inhibits invasion through down-modulation of NF-κB-regulated gene products. *Blood* 10: 2286–2295.
Aicher, T. D., K. R. Buszek, F. G. Fang et al. 1992. Total synthesis of halichondrin B and norhalichondrin B. *J. Am. Chem. Soc.* 114: 3162–3164.
Ajani, J. A., Y. Jiang, J. Faust et al. 2006. A multi-center phase II study of sequential paclitaxel and bryostatin-1 (NSC 339555) in patients with untreated, advanced gastric or gastroesophageal junction adenocarcinoma. *Invest. New Drugs* 24: 353–357.
Albizati, K. F., T. Holman, D. J. Faulkner, K. B. Glaser, and R. S. Jacobs. 1987. Luffariellolide: An anti-inflammatory sesterterpene from the marine sponge *Luffariella sp. Experientia* 43(8): 949–950.
Al-Fadhli, A., S. Wahidulla, and L. D'Souza. 2006. Glycolipids from the red alga *Chondria armata* (Kutz.) Okamura. *Glycobiology* 16: 902–915.
Alhanout, K., S. Malesinki, N. Vidal, V. Peyrot, J. M. Rolain, and J. M. Brunel. 2010. New insights into the antibacterial mechanism of action of squalamine. *J. Antimicrob. Chemother.* 65: 1688–1693.

Alvi, K. A., M. C. Diaz, and P. Crews. 1992. Evaluation of new sesquiterpene quinones from two *Dysidea* sponge species as inhibitors of protein tyrosine kinase. *J. Org. Chem.* 57(24): 6604–6607.

Amador, M. L., J. Jimeno, L. Paz-Ares, H. Cortes-Funes, and M. Hidago. 2003. Progress in the development and acquisition of anticancer agents from marine sources. *Ann. Oncol.* 14: 1607–1615.

Andjelic, C. D., V. Planelles, and L. R. Barrows. 2008. Characterizing the anti-HIV activity of papuamide A. *Mar. Drugs* 6: 528–549.

Ang, K. K., M. J. Holmes, T. Higa, M. T. Hamann, and U. A. Kara. 2000. In vivo antimalarial activity of the beta-carboline alkaloid manzamine A. *Antimicrob. Agent. Chemother.* 44: 1645–1649.

Aoki, S., D. Kong, K. Matsui, R. Rachmat, and M. Kobayashi. 2004. Sesquiterpene aminoquinones, from a marine sponge, induce erythroid differentiation in human chronic myelogenous leukaemia, K562 cells. *Chem. Pharmaceut. Bull.* 52(8): 935–937.

Arena, A., T. L. Maugeri, B. Pavone, D. Iannello, C. Gugliandolo, and G. Bisignano. 2006. Antiviral and immunoregulatory effect of a novel exopolysaccharide from a marine thermotolerant *Bacillus licheniformis*. *Int. Immunopharmacol.* 6: 8–13.

de Arruda, M., C. A. Cocchiaro, C. M. Nelson et al. 1995. LU103793 (NSC D-669356): A synthetic peptide that interacts with microtubules and inhibits mitosis. *Cancer Res.* 55: 3085–3092.

Ashour, M., R. Edrada, R. Ebel et al. 2006. Kahalalide derivatives from the Indian sacoglossan mollusk *Elysia grandifolia*. *J. Nat. Prod.* 69: 1547–1553.

Ata, A., R. G. Kerr, C. E. Moya, and R. S. Jacobs. 2003. Identification of anti-inflammatory diterpenes from the marine gorgonian *Pseudopterogorgia elisabethae*. *Tetrahedron* 59(21): 4215–4222.

Athukorala, Y., W.-K. Jung, T. Vasanthan, and Y. J. Jeon. 2006. An anticoagulative polysaccharide from an enzymatic hydrolysate of Ecklonia cava. *Carbohydr. Polym.* 66: 184–191.

Badre, A., A. Boulanger, E. Abou-Mansom, B. Banaigs, G. Combaut, and C. Francisco. 1994. Eudistomin U and Isoeudistomin U, new alkaloids from the Caribbean Ascidian *Lissoclinum fragile*. *J. Nat. Prod.* 57(4): 528–533.

Bagley, M. C., J. W. Dale, E. A. Merritt, and X. Xiong. 2005. Thiopeptide antibiotics. *Chem. Rev.* 105: 685–714.

Bai, R., M. C. Edler, P. L. Bonate et al. 2009. Intracellular activation and deactivation of tasidotin, an analog of dolastatin 15: Correlation with cytotoxicity. *Mol. Pharmacol.* 75: 218–226.

Bai, R., S. Friedman, G. Pettit et al. 1992. Dolastatin 15, a potent antimitotic depsipeptide derived from *Dolabella auricularia*. Interaction with tubulin and effects of cellular microtubules. *Biochem. Pharmacol.* 43: 2637–2645.

Bai, R., G. Pettit, and E. Hamel. 1990. Dolastatin 10, a powerful cytostatic peptide derived from a marine animal. Inhibition of tubulin polymerization mediated through the Vinca alkaloid binding domain. *Biochem. Pharmacol.* 39: 1941–1949.

Banker, R. and S. Carmeli. 1988. Tenuecyclamides A–D, cyclic hexapeptides from the cyanobacterium *Nostoc spongiaeforme* var. *tenue*. *J. Nat. Prod.* 61: 1248–1251.

Bao, B., Q. Sun, X. Yao, J. Hong, C. O. Lee, H. Y. Cho, K. S. Im, and J. H. Jung. 2007. Bisindole alkaloids of the topsentin and hamacanthin classes from a marine sponge *Spongosorites sp. J. Nat. Prod.* 70(1): 2–8.

Bao, B., Q. Sun, X. Yao, J. Hong, C. O. Lee, C. J. Sim, K. S. Im, and J. H. Jung. 2005. Cytotoxic bisindole alkaloids from a marine sponge *Spongosorites* sp. *J. Nat. Prod.* 68(5): 711–715.

Barr, P. M., H. M. Lazarus, B. W. Cooper et al. 2009. Phase II study of bryostatin 1 and vincristine for aggressive non-Hodgkin lymphoma relapsing after an autologous stem cell transplant. *Am. J. Hematol.* 84: 484–487.

Bartik, K., J.-C. Braekman, D. Daloze, C. Stoller, J. Huysecom, G. Vandevyver, and R. Ottinger. 1987. Topsentins, new toxic bis-indole alkaloids from the marine sponge *Topsentia genitrix*. *Can. J. Chem.* 65(9): 2118–2121.

Batke, E., R. Ogura, P. Vaupel et al. 1988. Action of the antileukemic and anti-HTLV-III (anti-HIV) agent avarol on the levels of superoxide dismutases and glutathione peroxidase activities in L5178y mouse lymphoma cells. *Cell Biochem. Funct.* 6: 123–129.

Beckwith, M., W. Urba, and D. Longo. 1993. Growth inhibition of human lymphoma cell lines by the marine products, dolastatins 10 and 15. *J. Natl Cancer Inst.* 85: 483–488.

Bentley, S. D., K. F. Chater, A. M. Cerdeno-Tarraga et al. 2002. Complete genome sequence of the model actinomycete *Streptomyces coelicolor* A3(2). *Nature* 417: 141–147.

Bérdy, J. 2005. Bioactive microbial metabolites: A personal view. *J. Antibiot. (Tokyo)* 58: 1–26.

Bergmann, W. and D. C. Burke. 1955. Contributions to the study of marine products. XXXIX. The nucleosides of sponges. III. Spongothymidine and spongouridine. *J. Org. Chem.* 20: 1501–1507.

Bergmann, W. and R. J. Feeney. 1951. Contributions to the study of marine products. XXXII. The nucelosides of sponges. I. *J. Org. Chem.* 16: 981–987.

Bergmann, W. and M. F. Stempien Jr. 1957. Contributions to the study of marine products. XLIII. The nucleosides of sponges. V. The synthesis of spongosine. *J. Org. Chem.* 22: 1575–1577.

Bernan, V. S., M. Greenstein, and G. T. Carter. 2004. Mining marine microorganisms as a source of new antimicrobials and antifungals. *J. Med. Chem.* 3: 181–195.

Bewley, C. A., N. D. Holland, and D. J. Faulkner. 1996. Two classes of metabolites from *Theonella swinhoei* are localized in distinct populations of bacterial symbionts. *Experientia* 52: 716–722.

Bhargava, P., J. L. Marshall, W. Dahut et al. 2001. A phase I and pharmacokinetic study of squalamine, a novel antiangiogenic agent, in patients with advanced cancers. *Clin. Cancer Res.* 7: 3912–3919.

Bister, B., D. Bischoff, M. Strobele et al. 2004. Abyssomicin C–a polycyclic antibiotic from a marine Verrucosispora strain as an inhibitor of the p-aminobenzoic acid/tetrahydrofolate biosynthesis pathway. *Angew. Chem. Int. Ed. Engl.* 43: 2574–2576.

Blackman, A.J., D. J. Matthews, and C. K. Narkowicz. 1987. β-Carboline alkaloids from the marine bryozoan *Costaticella hastata*. *J. Nat. Prod.* 50(3): 494–496.

Bourguet-Kondracki, M. L., M. T. Martin, and M. Guyot. 1996. A new β-carboline alkaloid isolated from the marine sponge *Hyrtios erecta*. *Tetrahedron Lett.* 37: 3457–3460.

Bowling, J. J., H. K. Pennaka, K. Ivey et al. 2008. Antiviral and anticancer optimization studies of the DNA-binding marine natural product aaptamine. *Chem. Biol. Drug Des.* 71: 205–215.

Brady, S. F., C. J. Chao, J. Handelsman, and J. Clardy. 2001. Cloning and heterologous expression of a natural product biosynthetic gene cluster from eDNA. *Org. Lett.* 3: 1981–1984.

Bramley, A. M., J. M. Langlands, A. K. Jones, D. L. Burgoyne, Y. Li, R. J. Andersen, and H. Salari. 1995. Effects of IZP-94005 (contignasterol) on antigen-induced bronchial responsiveness in ovalbumin-sensitized guinea-pigs. *Br. J. Pharmacol.* 115(8): 1433–1438.

Broka, C. A. and J. Ehrler. 1991. Enantioselective total syntheses of bengamides B and E. *Tetrahedron Lett.* 32: 5907–5910.

Brunel, J. M., C. Salmi, C. Loncle et al. 2005. Squalamine: A polyvalent drug of the future? *Curr. Cancer Drug Targets* 5: 267–272.

Bull, A. T., J. E. Stach, A. C. Ward, and M. Goodfellow. 2005. Marine actinobacteria: Perspectives, challenges, future directions. *Antonie Leeuwenhoek* 87: 65–79.

Bunker, J. M., L. Wilson, M. A. Jordan, and S. C. Feinstein. 2004. Modulation of microtubule dynamics by tau in living cells: Implications for development and neurodegeneration. *Mol. Biol. Cell.* 15: 2720–2728.

Burgoyne, D. L., R. J. Andersen, and T. M. Allen. 1992. Contignasterol, a highly oxygenated steroid with the "Unnatural" 14β configuration from the marine sponge *Petrusia Cuntignata Thiele*, 1899. *J. Org. Chem.* 57(2): 525–528.

Burres, N. S. and J. J. Clement. 1989. Antitumor activity and mechanism of action of the novel marine natural products mycalamide-A and-B and onnamide. *Cancer Res.* 49: 2935–2940.

Cain, J. M., P. Y. Liu, D. E. Alberta et al. 1992. Phase II clinical and pharmacological study of didemnin B in patients with metastatic breast cancer. *Invest. New Drugs* 10: 113–117.

Calcul, L., A. Longeon, A. Al-Mourabit, M. Guyot, and M. L. Bourguet-Kondracki. 2003. Novel alkaloids of the aaptamine class from an Indonesian marine sponge of the genus *Xestospongia*. *Tetrahedron* 59: 6539–6544.

Cambie, R. C., K. D. Wellington, P. S. Rutledge, and P. R. Bergquist. 2000. Chemistry of sponges. 19. Novel bioactive metabolites from *Hamigera tarangaensis. J. Nat. Prod.* 63(1): 79–85.

Capon, R. J. 1995. *Studies in Natural Products Chemistry, Structure and Chemistry (Part C)*, ed. Atta-ur-Rahman, vol. 15, pp. 289–326. Elsevier Science, New York.

Capon, R. J., F. Rooney, L. M. Murray et al. 1998. Dragmacidins: New protein phosphatase inhibitors from a southern Australian deep-water marine sponge, spongosorites sp. *J. Nat. Prod.* 61: 660–662.

Cardani, C., D. Ghiringhelli, R. Mondelli, and A. Quilico. 1965. The structure of pederin. *Tetrahedron Lett.* 6: 2537–2545.

Cariucci, M. J., M. Ciancia, M. X. Matulewicz, A. S. Cerezo, and E. B. Damonte. 1999. Antiherpetic activity and mode of action of natural carrageenans of diverse structural types. *Antiviral Res.* 43: 93–102.

Carpenter, R. C. 1986. Partitioning herbivory and its effects on coral reef algal communities. *Ecol. Monogr.* 56: 345–363.

Casapullo, A., G. Bifulco, I. Bruno, and R. Riccio. 2000. New bisindole alkaloids of the topsentin and hamacanthin classes from the Mediterranean marine sponge *Rhaphisia lacazei. J. Nat. Prod.* 63(4): 447–451.

Chaplan, S. R., W. A. Eckert III, and N. I. Carruthers. 2010. Drug discovery and development for pain. In *Translational Pain Research: From Mouse to Man*, eds. L. Kruger and A. R. Light, Chapter 18. CRC Press, Boca Raton, FL.

Charan, R. D., G. Schlingmann, J. Janso, V. Bernan, X. Feng, and G. T. Carter. 2004. Diazepinomicin, a new antimicrobial alkaloid from a marine *Micromonospora* sp. *J. Nat. Prod.* 67: 1431–1433.

Chattopadhyay, K., C. G. Mateu, P. Mandal, C. A. Pujol, E. B. Damonte, and B. Ray. 2007. Galactan sulphate of *Grateloupia indica*: Isolation, structural features an antiviral activity. *Phytochemistry* 68(10): 1428–1435.

Cho, J. Y., H. C. Kwon, P. G. Williams, P. R. Jensen, and W. Fenical. 2006. Azamerone, a terpenoid phthalazinone from a marine-derived bacterium related to the genus *Streptomyces* (Actinomycetales). *Org. Lett.* 8: 2471–2474.

Choi, S. W., D. H. Bai, J. H. Yu, and C. S. Shin. 2003. Characteristics of the squalene synthase inhibitors produced by a *Streptomyces* species isolated from soils. *J. Microbiol.* 49(11): 663–668.

Cimino, G., S. De Stefano, and L. Minale. 1974. Scalaradial, a third sesterterpene with the tetracarbocyclic skeleton of scalarin, from the sponge *Cacospongia scalaris. Experientia* 30: 846–847.

Cole, S. P., G. Bhardwaj, J. H. Gerlach et al. 1992. Overexpression of a transporter gene in a multidrug-resistant human lung cancer cell line. *Science* 258: 1650–1654.

Coleman, J. E., B. O. Patrick, R. J. Andersen, and S. J. Rettig. 1996. Hemiasterlin methyl ester. *Acta Cryst. Sec. C* C52: 1525–1527.

Coleman, J. E., E. D. de Silva, F. Kong, R. J. Andersen, and T. M. Allen. 1995. Cytotoxic peptides from the marine sponge *Cymbastela sp. Tetrahedron* 51: 10653–10662.

Coll, J. C. 1992. The chemistry and chemical ecology of octocorals (Coelenterata, Anthozoa, Octocorallia). *Chem. Rev.* 92: 613–631.

Cordell, G. A. 2000. Biodiversity and drug discovery: A symbiotic relationship. *Phytochemistry* 55: 463–480.

Corey, E. J., D. Y. Gin, and R. S. Kania. 1996. Enantioselective total synthesis of ecteinascidin 743. *J. Am. Chem. Soc.* 118: 9202–9203.

Coulson, F. R. and S. R. O'Donnell. 2000. *Inflammation Res.* 49(3): 123–127; Homepage from the company Inflazyme: http://www.inflazyme.com

Coutinho, A. F., B. Chanas, T. M. L. Souza, I. C. P. P. Frugrulhetti, and R. A. Epifanio. 2002. Anti HSV-1 alkaloids from a feeding deterrent marine sponge of the genus *Aaptos. Heterocycles* 57: 1265–1272.

Cragg, G. M., D. J. Newman, and S. S. Yang. 2006. Natural product extracts of plant and marine origin having antileukemia potential. The NCI experience. *J. Nat. Prod.* 69: 488–498.

Crews, P., X.-C. Cheng, M. Adamczeski et al. 1994. 1,2,3,4-Tetrahydro-8-hydroxymanzamines, alkaloids from two different haploslerid sponges. *Tetrahedron* 50: 13567–13574.

Cruz-Monserrate, Z., J. Mullaney, P. Harran, G. R. Pettit, and E. Hamel. 2003. Dolastatin 15 binds in the Vinca domain of tubulin as demonstrated by Hummel-Dreyer chromatography. *Eur. J. Biochem.* 270: 3822–3828.

Cuevas, C., M. Pérez, M. J. Martín et al. 2000. Synthesis of ecteinascidin ET-743 and phthalascidin Pt-650 from cyanosafracin B. *Org. Lett.* 2: 2545–2548.

Cutignano, A., G. Bifulco, I. Bruno, A. Casapullo, L. Gomez-Paloma, and R. Riccio. 2000. Dragmacidin F: A new antiviral bromoindole alkaloid from the Mediterranean sponge *Halicortex* sp. *Tetrahedron* 56(23): 3743–3748.

da Rocha, A. B., R. M. Lopes, and G. Schwartsmann. 2001. Natural products in anticancer therapy. *Curr. Opin. Pharmacol.* 1: 364–369.

da Silva, A. C., J. M. Kratz, F. M. Farias et al. 2006. In vitro antiviral activity of marine sponges collected off Brazilian coast. *Biol. Pharm. Bull.* 29: 135–140.

Dal Piaz, F., A. Casapullo, A. Randazzo, R. Riccio, P. Pucci, G. Marino, and L. Gomez-Paloma. 2002. Molecular basis of phospholipase A2 inhibition by petrosaspongiolide M. *ChemBioChem* 3(7): 664–671.

Das, S., L. R. Ward, and C. Burke. 2008. Prospects of using marine actinobacteria as probiotics in aquaculture. *Appl. Microbiol. Biotechnol.* 81: 419–429.

Davidson, S. K., S. W. Allen, G. E. Lim, G. M. Anderson, and M. G. Haygood. 2001. Evidence for the biosynthesis of bryostatins by the bacterial symbiont "*Candidatus* Endobugula sertula" of the Bryozoan *Bugula neritina. Appl. Environ. Microbiol.* 67: 4531–4537.

Davidson, B. S. and R. W. Schumacher. 1993. Isolation and synthesis of caprolactins A and B, new caprolactams from a marine bacterium. *Tetrahedron* 49(30): 6569–6574.

De Giulio, A., S. De Rosa, G. Strazzulo et al. 1991. Synthesis and evaluation of cytostatic and antiviral activities of 3' and 4'-avarone derivatives. *Antiviral Chem. Chemother.* 2: 223–227.

De Rosa, S., R. Puliti, A. Crispino, A. De Giulio, C. A. Mattia, and L. Mazzarella. 1994. A new scalarane sesterterpenoid from the marine sponge *Cacospongia mollior. J. Nat. Prod.* 57(2): 256–262.

De Silva, E. D. and P. J. Scheuer. 1980. Manoalide, an antibiotic sesterterpenoid from the marine sponge *Luffariella variabilis* (Polejaeff). *Tetrahedron Lett.* 21(17): 1611–1614.

De Silva, E. D. and P. J. Scheuer. 1981. Three new sesterterpenoid antibiotics from the marine sponge *Luffariella variabilis* (Polejaeff). *Tetrahedron Lett.* 22(33): 3147–3150.

De Vries, D. J. and M. R. Hall. 1994. Marine biodiversity as a source of chemical diversity. *Drug Dev. Res.* 33: 161–173.

Degnan, B. M., C. J. Hawkins, M. F. Lavin et al. 1989. New cyclic peptides with cytotoxic activity from the ascidian *Lissoclinum patella. J. Med. Chem.* 32: 1349–1354.

Donia, M. and M. T. Hamann. 2003. Marine natural products and their potential applications as anti-infective agents. *Lancet Infect. Dis.* 3: 338–348.

Donia, M. S., B. J. Hathaway, S. Sudek et al. 2006. Natural combinatorial peptide libraries in cyanobacterial symbionts of marine ascidians. *Nat. Chem. Biol.* 2: 729–735.

Dowlati, A., H. M. Lazarus, P. Hartman et al. 2003. Phase I and correlative study of combination bryostatin 1 and vincristine in relapsed B-cell malignancies. *Clin. Cancer Res.* 9: 5929–5935.

Ducklow, H. W. 1990. The biomass, production and fate of bacteria in coral reefs. In *Ecosystems of the World: Coral Reefs*, ed. Z. Dubinsky, pp. 265–289. Elsevier, New York.

Edrada, R. A., V. Proksch, V. Wray, L. Witte, W. E. G. Müller, and R.W.M. Van Soest. 1996. Four new bioactive manzamine-type alkaloids from the Philippine marine sponge *Xestospongia ashmorica. J. Nat. Prod.* 59: 1056–1060.

El Gamal, A. A. 2010. Biological importance of marine algae. *Saudi Pharm. J.* 18(1): 1–25.

El Sayed, K. A., C. D. Dunbar, T. L. Perry et al. 1997. Marine natural products as prototype insecticidal agents. *J. Agric. Food Chem.* 45: 2735–2739.

El Sayed, K. A., M. Kelly, U. A. Kara et al. 2001. New manzamine alkaloids with potent activity against infectious diseases. *J. Am. Chem. Soc.* 123: 1804–1808.

Elgie, A. W., J. M. Sargenta, P. Altona et al. 1998. Modulation of resistance to ara-C by bryostatin in fresh blast cells from patients with AML. *Leuk. Res.* 22: 373–378.

Engelhardt, K., K. F. Degnes, M. Kemmler et al. 2010. Production of a new thiopeptide antibiotic, TP-1161, by 1 a marine-derived 2 *Nocardiopsis* species. *Appl. Environ. Microbiol.* 76: 4969–4976.

Etcheberrigaray, R., M. Tan, I. Dewachter et al. 2004. Therapeutic effects of PKC activators in Alzheimer's disease transgenic mice. *Proc. Natl Acad. Sci. USA* 101: 11141–11146.

Fahy, E. B., C. M. Potts, D. J. Faulkner, and K. Smith. 1991. 6-Bromotryptamine derivatives from the Gulf of California tunicate *Didemnum candidum. J. Nat. Prod.* 54(2): 564–569.

Fakhr, I., N. Hamdy, M. Radwan, S. El-Batran, and O. El Shabrawy. 2006. Studies on the anti-inflammatory and analgesic effects of extracts from marine sponges. *Nat. Prod. Sci.* 12: 74–78.

Faulkner, D. J. 1991. Marine natural products. *Nat. Prod. Rep.* 8: 97–146.

Faulkner, D. J. 2000. Highlights of marine natural products chemistry (1972–1999). *Nat. Prod. Rep.* 17: 1–6.

Fedoreev, S. A., N. G. Prokofeva, V. A. Denisenko, and N. M. Rebachuk. 1988. Cytotoxic activity of aaptamines derived from Suberitidae sponges. *Khim. Farm. Zh.* 22: 943–946.

Feldman, K. S. and P. Ngernmeesri. 2005. Dragmacidin E synthesis studies. Preparation of a model cycloheptannelated indole fragment. *Org. Lett.* 7(24): 5449–5452.

Feling, R. H., G. O. Buchanan, T. J. Mincer, C. A. Kauffman, P. R. Jensen, and W. Fenical. 2003. Salinosporamide A: A highly cytotoxic proteasome inhibitor from a novel microbial source, a marine bacterium of the new genus Salinospora. *Angew. Chem. Int. Ed.* 42: 355–357.

Fenical, W. 1987. Marine soft corals of the genus *Pseudopterogorgia* : A resource for novel anti-inflammatory diterpenoids. *J. Nat. Prod.* 50(6): 1001–1008.

Fenical, W. 2006. Marine pharmaceuticals: Past, present, and future. *Oceanography* 19: 110–119.

Fenical, W. and P. R. Jensen. 2006. Developing a new resource for drug discovery: Marine actinomycete bacteria. *Nat. Chem. Biol.* 2: 666–673.

Ferrándiz, M. L., M. J. Sanz, G. Bustos, M. Payá, M. J. Alcaraz, and S. De Rosa. 1994. Avarol and avarone, two new anti-inflammatory agents of marine origin. *Eur. J. Pharmacol.* 253(1): 75–82.

Fonseca, G. and G. A. Seoane. 2005. Chemoenzymatic synthesis of enantiopure α-substituted cyclohexanones from aromatic compounds. *Tetrahedron: Asymmetry* 16: 1393–1402.

Ford, P. W., K. R. Gustafson, T. C. McKee et al. 1999. Papuamides A-D, HIV-inhibitory and cytotoxic depsipeptides from the sponges *Theonella mirabilis* and *Theonella swinhoei* collected in Papua New Guinea. *J. Am. Chem. Soc.* 121: 5899–5909.

Furumai, T., K. Takagi, Y. Igarashi, N. Saito, and T. Oki. 2000. Arisostatins A and B, new members of tetrocarcin class of antibiotics from *Micromonospora* sp. TP-A0316. I. Taxonomy, fermentation, isolation and biological properties. *J. Antibiot. (Tokyo)* 53: 227–232.

Furusaki, A., N. Hoshiba, T. Matsumoto, A. Hirano, Y. Iwai, and S. Omura. 1978. X-ray structure of staurosporine: A new alkaloid from a *Streptomyces* strain. *J. Chem. Soc. Chem. Commun.* 18: 800–801.

Fusetani, N. 2000. Introduction. In *Drugs from the Sea*, ed. N. Fusetani, pp. 1–5. Karger, Basel, Switzerland.

Gajate, C., F. An, and F. Mollinedo. 2003. Rapid and selective apoptosis in human leukemic cells induced by aplidine through a Fas/CD95- and mitochondrial-mediated mechanism. *Clin. Cancer Res.* 9: 1535–1545.

Gamble, W. R., N. A. Durso, R. W. Fuller et al. 1999. Cytotoxic and tubulin-interactive hemiasterlins from *Auletta* sp. and *Siphonochalina* spp. sponges. *Bioorg. Med. Chem.* 7: 1611–1615.

Ganguly, A. K., J. L. McCormick, A. K. Saksena, P. R. Das, and T.-M. Chan. 1999. Chemical modifications and structure activity studies of ziracin and related everninomicin antibiotics. *Bioorg. Med. Chem. Lett.* 9: 1209–1214.

Gao, C.-H., X.-P. Tian, S.-H. Qi et al. 2010. Antibacterial and antilarval compounds from marine gorgonian-associated bacterium *Bacillus amyloliquefaciens* SCSIO 00856. *J. Antibiot.* 63: 191–193.

Garcia-Rocha, M., P. Bonay, and J. Avila. 1996. The antitumoral compound kahalalide F acts on cell lysosomes. *Cancer Lett.* 99: 43–50.

Garg, N. K., D. D. Caspi, and B. M. Stoltz. 2004. The total synthesis of (+)-dragmacidin F. *J. Am. Chem. Soc.* 126(31): 9552–9553.

Gennigens, C. and G. Jerusalem. 2011. Trabectedin (ET-743/Yondelis) for treating soft tissue sarcomas and ovarian cancer. *Rev. Med. Liege.* 66: 452–455.

Gerwick, W. H., L. T. Tan, and N. Sitachitta. 2001. Nitrogen-containing metabolites from marine cyanobacteria. In *The Alkaloids*, ed. G. Cordell, pp. 75–184. Academic Press, San Diego, CA.

Giannini, C., C. Debitus, R. Lucas, A. Ubeda, M. Payá, J. N. A. Hooper, and M. V. D'Auria. 2001. New sesquiterpene derivatives from the sponge *Dysidea* species with a selective inhibitor profile against human phospholipase A2 and other leukocyte functions. *J. Nat. Prod.* 64(5): 612–615.

Giannini, C., C. Debitus, I. Posadas, M. Paya, and M. V. D'Auria. 2000. Dysidotronic acid, a new and selective human phospholipase A_2 inhibitor from the sponge *Dysidea* sp. *Tetrahedron Lett.* 41(17): 3257–3260.

Glaser, K. B., M. S. de Carvalho, R. S. Jacobs, M. R. Kernan, and D. J. Faulkner. 1989. Manoalide: Structure-activity studies and definition of the pharmacophore for phospholipase A2 inactivation. *Mol. Pharmacol.* 36(6): 782–788.

Glaser, K. B. and R. S. Jacobs. 1986. Molecular pharmacology of manoalide. Inactivation of bee venom phospholipase A2. *Biochem. Pharmacol.* 35(3): 449–453.

Glaser, K. B. and R. S. Jacobs. 1987. Inactivation of bee venom phospholipase A2 by manoalide. A model based on the reactivity of manoalide with amino acids and peptide sequences. *Biochem. Pharmacol.* 36(13): 2079–2086.

Golakoti, T., J. Ogino, and C. E. Heltzel. 1995. Structure determination, conformational analysis, chemical stability studies, and antitumor evaluation of the Cryptophycins. Isolation of 18 new analogs from *Nostoc* sp, strain GSV 224. *J. Am. Chem. Soc.* 117: 12030–12049.

Gribble, G. and S. Berthel. 1993. *Studies in Natural Products Chemistry*, vol. 12, pp. 365–409. Elsevier Science Publishers, New York.

Gross, H. and G. M. König. 2006. Terpenoids from marine organisms: Unique structures and their pharmacological potential. *Phytochem. Rev.* 5: 115–141.

Groweiss, A., J. J. Newcomer, B. R. O'Keefe, A. Blackman, and M. R. Boyd. 1999. Cytotoxic metabolites from an Australian collection of the sponge *Jaspis* species. *J. Nat. Prod.* 62: 1691–1693.

Gschwend, J. E., W. R. Fair, and C. T. Powell. 2000. Bryostatin 1 induces prolonged activation of extracellular regulated protein kinases and apoptosis of LNCaP cancer cells overexpressing protein kinase c alpha. *Mol. Pharmacol.* 57: 1224–1234.

Gul, W., N. L. Hammond, M. Yousaf et al. 2006. Modification at the C9 position of the marine natural product isoaaptamine and the impact on HIV-1, mycobacterial, and tumor cell activity. *Bioorg. Med. Chem.* 14: 8495–8505.

Gunasekera, S. P., M. Gunasekera, R. E. Longley, and G. K. Schulte. 1990. Discodermolide: A new bioactive polyhydroxylated lactone from the marine sponge *Discodermia dissoluta*. *J. Org. Chem.* 55: 4912–4915.

Gunasekera, S. P., M. Gunasekera, R. E. Longley, and G. K. Schulte. 1991. Discodermolide: A new bioactive polyhydroxylated lactone from the marine sponge *Discodermia dissoluta* [Erratum to document cited in CA113(9):75187b]. *J. Org. Chem.* 56: 1346.

Guo, Y., E. Trivellone, G. Scognamiglio, and G. Cimino. 1998. Misenine, a novel macrocyclic alkaloid with an unusual skeleton from the Mediterranean sponge *Reniera* sp. *Tetrahedron* 54: 541–550.

Gurel, G., G. Blaha, T. Steitz, and P. Moore. 2009. The structures of triacetyloleandomycin and mycalamide A bound to the large ribosomal subunit of *Haloarcula marismortui*. *Antimicrob. Agents Chemother.* 53: 5010–5014.

Gustafson, K., M. Roman, and W. Fenical. 1989. The macrolactins, a novel class of antiviral and cytotoxic macrolides from a deep-sea marine bacterium. *J. Am. Chem. Soc.* 111: 7519–7524.

de Guzman, F. S., B. R. Copp, C. L. Mayne, G. P. Concepcion, G. C. Mangalindan, L. R. Barrows, and C. M. Ireland. 1998. Bolinaquinone: A novel cytotoxic sesquiterpene hydroxyquinone from a Philippine *Dysidea* sponge. *J. Org. Chem.* 63(22): 8042–8044.

Hadaschik, B. A., S. Ettinger, R. D. Sowery et al. 2008. Targeting prostate cancer with HTI-286, a synthetic analog of the marine sponge product hemiasterlin. *Int. J. Cancer* 122: 2368–2376.

Haefner, B. 2003. Drugs from the deep: Marine natural products as drug candidates. *Drug Discov. Today* 8: 536–544.

Hagiwara, K., Y. Kondoh, A. Ueda et al. 2010. Discovery of novel antiviral agents directed against the influenza A virus nucleoprotein using photo-cross-linked chemical arrays. *Biochem. Biophys. Res. Commun.* 394: 721–727.

Hamann, M. T., C. S. Otto, P. J. Scheuer, and D. C. Dunbar. 1996. Kahalalides: Bioactive peptides from a marine mollusk *Elysia rufescens* and its algal diet *Bryopsis* sp. *J. Org. Chem.* 61: 6594–6600.

Hamann, M. T. and P. J. Scheuer. 1993. Kahalalide F: A bioactive depsipeptide from the sacoglossan mollusk *Elysia rufescens* and the green alga *Bryopsis* sp. *J. Am. Chem. Soc.* 115: 5825–5826.

Han, J. S., J. H. Cheng, T. M. Yoon, J. Song, A. Rajkarnikar, W. G. Kim, I. D. Yoo, Y. Y. Yang, and J. W. Suh. 2005. Biological control agent of common scab disease by antagonistic strain *Bacillus* sp. sunhua. *J. Appl. Microbiol.* 99(1): 213–221.

Hao, D., L. A. Hammond, S. G. Eckhardt et al. 2003. A Phase I and pharmacokinetic study of squalamine, an aminosterol angiogenesis inhibitor. *Clin. Cancer Res.* 9: 2465–2471.

Harden, E. A., R. Falshaw, S. M. Carnachan, E. R. Kern, and M. N. Prichard. 2009. Virucidal activity of polysaccharide extracts from four algal species against herpes simplex virus. *Antiviral Res.* 83(3): 282–289.

Harnden, M. R. 1985. *Approaches to Antiviral Agents*. VCH Publishers, Deerfield Beach, FL.

Harried, S. S., C. P. Lee, G. Yang, T. I. Lee, and D. C. Myles. 2003. Total synthesis of the potent microtubule-stabilizing agent (+)-discodermolide. *J. Org. Chem.* 68: 6646–6660.

Harrigan, G. G., G. H. Goetz, H. Luesch, S. Yang, and J. Likos. 2001. Dysideaprolines A–F and Barbaleucamides A–B, novel polychlorinated compounds from a *Dysidea* species. *J. Nat. Prod.* 64: 1133–1138.

Harrigan, G. G., H. Luesch, W. Y. Yoshida et al. 1998. Symplostatin 1: A dolastatin 10 analogue from the marine cyanobacterium *Symploca hydnoides*. *J. Nat. Prod.* 61: 1075–1077.

Harvell, C. D., K. Kim, J. M. Burkholder et al. 1999. Emerging marine diseases—Climate links and anthropogenic factors. *Science* 285: 1505–1510.

Hassan, H. M., M. A. Khanfar, A. Y. Elnagar et al. 2010. Pachycladins A–E, prostate cancer invasion and migration inhibitory Eunicellin-based diterpenoids from the red sea soft coral *Cladiella pachyclados*. *J. Nat. Prod.* 73: 848–853.

Hay, M. E. 1996. Marine chemical ecology: What's known and what's next? *J. Exp. Mar. Biol. Ecol.* 200: 103–134.

Herlt, A., L. Mander, W. Rombang et al. 2004. Alkaloids from marine organisms. Part 8: Isolation of bisdemethylaaptamine and bisdemethylaaptamine-9-O-sulfate from an Indonesian Aaptos sp. marine sponge. *Tetrahedron* 60: 6101–6104.

Hickford, S. J., J. W. Blunt, and M. H. Munro. 2009. Antitumour polyether macrolides: Four new halichondrins from the New Zealand deep-water marine sponge *Lissodendoryx* sp. *Bioorg. Med. Chem.* 17: 2199–2203.

Hirata, Y. and D. Uemura. 1986. Halichondrins-antitumor polyether macrolides from a marine sponge. *Pure Appl. Chem.* 58: 701–710.

Hoffman, M. A., J. A. Blessing, and S. S. Lentz. 2003. A phase II trial of dolostatin-10 in recurrent platinum-sensitive ovarian carcinoma: A Gynecologic Oncology Group Study. *Gynecol. Oncol.* 89: 95–98.

Hogan, P. C. and E. J. Corey. 2005. Proteasome inhibition by a totally synthetic β-lactam related to Salinosporamide A and Omuralide. *J. Am. Chem. Soc.* 127: 15386–15387.

Hongpaisan, J. and D. L. Alkon. 2007. A structural basis for enhancement of long-term associative memory in single dendritic spines regulated by PKC. *Proc. Natl. Acad. Sci. USA* 104: 19571–19576.

Hopper, L. D., S. van Dijk, P. Shannon et al. 2003. Safety and toxicokinetics in a five-day oral toxicity study of a dolastatin-15 analog, ILX651, in beagle dogs [abstract 1749]. *Proc. Am. Assoc. Cancer Res.* 44: 397. http://www.clinicaltrials.gov/

Houge-Frydrych, C. S. V., S. A. Readshaw, and D. J. Bell. 2000. SB-219383, a novel tyrosyl tRNA synthetase inhibitor from *Micromonospora sp.* II. Structure determination. *J. Antibiot.* 53: 351–356.

Hu, J. F., M. T. Hamann, R. Hill, and M. Kelly. 2003. The manzamine alkaloids. *Alkaloids Chem. Biol.* 60: 207–285.

Hughes, C. C., C. A. Kauffman, P. R. Jensen, and W. Fenical. 2010. Structures, reactivities, and antibiotic properties of the marinopyrroles A-F. *J. Org. Chem.* 75: 3240–3250.

Hughes, C. C., J. B. MacMillan, S. P. Gaudencio, P. R. Jensen, and W. Fenical. 2009. The ammosamides, structures of potent cytotoxins from a marine-derived *Streptomyces sp. Angew. Chem. Int. Ed.* 48: 725–727.

Hughes, C. C., A. Prieto-Davo, P. R. Jensen, and W. Fenical. 2008. The marinopyrroles, antibiotics of an unprecedented structure class from a marine *Streptomyces* sp. *Org. Lett.* 10: 629–631.

Hung, D. T., J. B. Nerenberg, and S. L. Schreiber. 1994. Distinct binding and cellular properties of synthetic (+)- and (–)-discodermolides. *Chem. Biol.* 1: 67–71.

Huyck, T. K., W. Gradishar, F. Manuguid, and P. Kirkpatrick. 2011. Fresh from the pipeline: Eribulin mesylate. *Nat. Rev. Drug Discov.* 10: 173–174.

Ichiba, T., J. M. Corgiat, P. J. Scheuer, and K.-M. Borges. 1994. 8-Hydroxymanzamine A, a beta-carboline alkaloid from a sponge, *Pachypellina* sp. *J. Nat. Prod.* 57(1): 168–170.

Ichiba, T., R. Sakai, S. Kohmoto, G. Saucy, and T. Higa. 1988. New manzamine alkaloids from a sponge of the genus *Xestospongia. Tetrahedron Lett.* 29: 3083–3086.

Igarashi, Y., K. Takagi, Y. Kan, K. Fujii, K. Harada, T. Furumai, and T. Oki. 2000. Arisostatins A and B, new members of tetrocarcin class of antibiotics from *Micromonospora* sp. TP-A0316. II. Structure determination. *J. Antibiot. (Tokyo)* 53: 233–240.

Igarashi, Y., M. E. Trujillo, E. Martínez-Molina et al. 2007. Antitumor anthraquinones from an endophytic actinomycete *Micromonospora lupini* sp. *nov. Bioorg. Med. Chem. Lett.* 17: 3702–3705.

Ismet, A., S. Vikinesawary, S. Paramaswari et al. 2004. Production and chemical characterization of antifungal metabolites from *Micromonospora* sp. M39 isolated from mangrove rhizosphere soil. *World J. Microbiol. Biotechnol.* 20: 523–528.

Izzo, I., E. Avallone, M. C. Delia, A. Casapullo, M. Amigo, and F. De Riccardis. 2004. Synthesis of potentially anti-inflammatory IPL576,092-contignasterol and IPL576,092-manoalide hybrids. *Tetrahedron* 60(27): 5587–5593.

Jacobson, P. B., L. A. Marshall, A. Sung, and R. S. Jacobs. 1990. Inactivation of human synovial fluid phospholipase A2 by the marine natural product, manoalide. *Biochem. Pharmacol.* 39(10): 1557–1564.

Jang, K. H., S.-C. Chung, J. Shin et al. 2007. Aaptamines as sortase A inhibitors from the tropical sponge *Aaptos aaptos. Bioorg. Med. Chem. Lett.* 17: 5366–5369.

Janmaat, M. L., J. A. Rodriguez, J. Jimeno, F. A. E. Kruyt, and G. Giaccone. 2005. Kahalalide F induces necrosis-like cell death that involves depletion of ErbB3 and inhibition of Akt signaling. *Mol. Pharmacol.* 68: 502–510.

Jaruchoktaweechai, C., K. Suwanborirux, S. Tanasupawatt, P. Kittakoop, and P. Menasveta. 2000. New macrolactins from a marine *Bacillus* sp. Sc026. *J. Nat. Prod.* 63(7): 984–986.

Jensen, P. R. and W. Fenical. 2005. New natural-product diversity from marine Actinomycetes. In *Natural Products: Drug Discovery and Therapeutic Medicine*, eds. L. Zhang and A. L. Demain, pp. 315–328. Humana Press, Totowa, NJ.

Jiang, B. and X.-H. Gu. 2000. Syntheses and cytotoxicity evaluation of bis(indolyl)thiazole, bis(indolyl) pyrazinone and bis(indolyl)pyrazine: Analogues of cytotoxic marine bis(indole) alkaloid. *Bioorg. Med. Chem.* 8: 363–371.

Jiménez, J. C., A. López-Macià, C. Gracia et al. 2008. Structure-activity relationship of kahalalide F synthetic analogues. *J. Med. Chem.* 51: 4920–4931.

Jimenez, J. I. and P. J. Scheuer. 2001. New lipopeptides from the Caribbean cyanobacterium *Lyngbya majuscula. J. Nat. Prod.* 64: 200–203.

Jones, R. N. and M. S. Barrett. 1995. Antimicrobial activity of SCH 27899, oligosaccharide member of the Everninomycin class with a wide gram-positive spectrum. *Clin. Microbiol. Infect.* 1: 35–43.

Jordan, M. A. 2002. Mechanism of action of antitumor drugs that interact with microtubules and tubulin. *Curr. Med. Chem. Anti-Cancer Agents* 2: 1–17.

Jordan, A., J. A. Hadfield, N. J. Lawrence, and A. T. McGown. 1998. Tubulin as a target for anticancer drugs: Agents which interact with the mitotic spindle. *Med. Res. Rev.* 18: 259–296.

Jordan, M. A., K. Kamath, T. Manna et al. 2005. The primary antimitotic mechanism of action of the synthetic halichondrin E7389 is suppression of microtubule growth. *Mol. Cancer Ther.* 4: 1086–1095.

Jordan, M. A. and L. Wilson. 2004. Microtubules as a target for anticancer drugs. *Nat. Rev. Cancer* 4: 253–265.

Kasanah, N. and M. T. Hamann. 2004. Development of antibiotics and the future of marine microorganism to stem the tide of antibiotic resistance. *Curr. Opin. Invest. Drugs* 5: 827–837.

Kashman, Y., A. Rudi, S. Hirsh et al. 1990. Recent developments in research on metabolites from Red Sea invertebrates. *New J. Chem.* 14: 729–740.

Kavallaris, M., N. M. Verrills, and B. T. Hill. 2001. Anticancer therapy with novel tubulin-interacting drugs. *Drug Resist. Update* 4: 392–401.

Kazlauskas, R., R. O. Lidgard, R. J. Wells, and W. A. Vetter. 1977. A novel hexachloro-metabolite from the sponge *Dysidea herbacea. Tetrahedron Lett.* 36: 3183–3186.

Kazlauskas, R., P. T. Murphy, R. G. Warren, R. J. Wells, and J. F. Blount. 1978. New quinones from a dictyoceratid sponge. *Aust. J. Chem.* 31(12): 2685–2697.

Kearns, P. S., J. C. Coll, and J. A. Rideout. 1995. A new β-carboline dimer from an ascidian, *Didemnum* sp. *J. Nat. Prod.* 58: 1075–1076.

Kehraus, S., G. M. König, A. D. Wright, and G. Woerheide. 2002. Leucamide A: A new cytotoxic heptapeptide from the Australian sponge *Leucetta microraphis. J. Org. Chem.* 67: 4989–4992.

Kelecom, A. 1999. Chemistry of marine natural products: Yesterday, today and tomorrow. *An. Acad. Bras. Ciênc.* 71: 249–263.

Keller, S., G. Nicholson, C. Drahl, E. Sorensen, H.-P. Fiedler, and R. D. Süssmuth. 2007. Abyssomicins G and H and atrop-abyssomicin C from the marine *Verrucosispora* strain AB-18–032. *J. Antibiot.* 60: 391–394.

Kelman, D., Y. Kashman, E. Rosenberg, A. Kushmaro, and Y. Loya. 2006. Antimicrobial activity of red sea corals. *Mar. Biol.* 149: 357–363.

Kerbrat, P., V. Dieras, N. Pavlidis, A. Ravaud, J. Wanders, and P. Fumoleau. 2003. Phase II study of LU 103793 (dolastatin analogue) in patients with metastatic breast cancer. *Eur. J. Cancer* 39: 317–320.

Kernan, M. R., D. J. Faulkner, and R. S. Jacobs. 1987. The luffariellins novel antiinflammatory sesterterpenes of chemotaxonomic importance from the marine sponge *Luffariella variabilis. J. Org. Chem.* 52(14): 3081–3083.

Kernan, M. R., D. J. Faulkner, L. Parkanyi, J. Clardy, M. S. De Carvalho, and R. S. Jacobs. l989. Luffolide, a novel anti-inflammatory terpene from the sponge *Luffariella* sp. *Experientia* 45(4): 388–390.

Keyzers, R. A., P. T. Northcote, and V. Webb. 2002. Clathriol, a novel polyoxygenated 14β steroid isolated from the New Zealand marine sponge *Clathria lissosclera. J. Nat. Prod.* 65(4): 598–600.

Khozirah, S., C. L. Kee, M. R. Zalilawati et al. 2009. Cytotoxic aaptamines from Malaysian *Aaptos aaptos. Mar. Drugs* 7: 1–8.

Kijoa, A. and P. Sawanwong. 2004. Drugs and cosmetics from the sea. *Mar. Drugs* 2(2): 72–82.

Kim, H. H., W. G. Kim, I. J. Ryoo, C. J. Kim, J. E. Suk, and K. H. Han. 1997. Neuronal cell protection activity of macrolactin A produced by *Actinomadura* sp. *J. Microbiol. Biotechnol.* 7(6): 429.

Kim, S., K. LaMontagne, M. Sabio et al. 2004. Depletion of methionine aminopeptidase 2 does not alter cell response to fumagillin or bengamides. *Cancer Res.* 64: 2984–2987.

Kim, S., S. W. Lee, E.-C. Choi, and S. Y. Choi. 2003. Aminoacyl-tRNA synthetases and their inhibitors as a novel family of antibiotics. *Appl. Microbiol. Biotechnol.* 61: 1243–1245.

Kinder, F. R., R. W. Versace, K. W. Bair et al. 2001a. Synthesis and antitumor activity of ester-modified analogues of bengamide B. *J. Med. Chem.* 44: 3692–3699.

Kinder, F. R., S. Wattanasin, R. W. Versace et al. 2001b. Total syntheses of bengamides B and E. *J. Org. Chem.* 66: 2118–2122.

Kobayashi, M., S. Aoki, N. Ohyabu, M. Kuroso, W. Wang, and I. Kitagawa. 1994a. Arenastatin A, a potent cytotoxic depsipeptide from the Okinawan marine sponge *Dysidea arenaria*. *Tetrahedron Lett.* 35: 7969–7972.

Kobayashi, M., Y. C. Chen, S. Aoki, I. Yasuoko, T. Ishida, and I. Kitagawa. 1995a. Four new β carboline alkaloids isolated from two Okinawan marine sponge of *Xestospongia* and *Haliclona* sp. *Tetrahedron* 51: 3727–3736.

Kobayashi, M., M. Kuroso, N. Ohyabu, W. Wang, S. Fujii, and I. Kitagawa. 1994b. The absolute stereostructure of Arenastatin A, a potent cytotoxic depsipeptide from the Okinawan marine sponge *Dysidea arenaria*. *Chem. Pharm. Bull.* 42: 2196–2198.

Kobayashi, J., T. Murayama, Y. Ohizumi, T. Ohta, S. Nozoe, and T. Sasaki. 1989. Metachromin C, a new cytotoxic sesquiterpenoid from the Okinawan marine sponge *Hipposrongia metachromia*. *J. Nat. Prod.* 52(5): 1173–1176.

Kobayashi, J., K. Naitok, T. Sasaki, and H. Shigemori. 1992. Metachromins D-H, new cytotoxic sesquiterpenoids from the Okinawan marine sponge *Hipposrongia metachromia*. *J. Org. Chem.* 57(21): 5773–5776.

Kobayashi, J., H. Shinonaga, H. Shigemori, A. Umeyama, N. Shoji, and S. Arihara. 1995b. Xestobergsterol C, a new pentacyclic steroid from the Okinawan marine sponge *Ircinia sp.* and absolute stereochemistry of xestobergsterol A. *J. Nat. Prod.* 58(2): 312–318.

Kobayashi, J., M. Tsuda, N. Kawasaki, T. Sasaki, and Y. Mikami. 1994c. 6-Hydroxymanzamine A and 3,4-dihydromanzamine A, new alkaloids from the Okinawan marine sponge *Amphimedon* sp. *J. Nat. Prod.* 57: 1737–1740.

Kohmoto, S., Y. Kashman, O. J. McConnell et al. 1988. Dragmacidin, a new cytotoxic bis(indole)alkaloid from a deepwater marine sponge, *Dragmacidon* sp. *J. Org. Chem.* 53: 3116–3118.

Kondo, K., N. Ohnishi, K. Takemoto, H. Yoshida, and K. Yoshida. 1992. Synthesis of optically quadratic nonlinear phenylpyridylacetylenes. *J. Org. Chem.* 57: 1622–1625.

Kondracki, M.-L. and M. Guyot. 1989. Biologically active quinone and hydroquinone sesquiterpenoids from the sponge *Smenospongia* sp. *Tetrahedron* 45(7): 1995–2004.

König, G. M., S. Kehraus, S. F. Seibert, A. Andel-Lateff, and D. Müller. 2006. Natural products from marine organisms and their associated microbes. *ChemBioChem* 7: 229–238.

Koren-Goldshlager, G., Y. Kashman, and M. Schleyer. 1998. Haliclorensin, a novel diamino alkaloid from the marine sponge *Haliclona tulearensis*. *J. Nat. Prod.* 61: 282–284.

Kuzirian, A. M., H. T. Epstein, C. J. Gagliardi et al. 2006. Bryostatin enhancement of memory in *Hermissenda*. *Biol. Bull.* 210: 201–214.

Kuznetsov, G., M. J. Towle, H. Cheng et al. 2004. Induction of morphological and biochemical apoptosis following prolonged mitotic blockage by halichondrin B macrocyclic ketone analog E7389. *Cancer Res.* 64: 5760–5766.

Kwok, J. M., S. S. Myatt, C. M. Marson, R. C. Coombes, D. Constantinidou, and E. W. Lam. 2008. Thiostrepton selectively targets breast cancer cells through inhibition of forkhead box M1 expression. *Mol. Cancer Ther.* 7: 2022–2032.

Lam, K. S. 2006. Discovery of novel metabolites from marine actinomycetes. *Curr. Opin. Microbiol.* 9: 245–251.

Leusch, H., G. G. Harrigan, G. Goetz, and F. D. Horgen. 2002. The cyanobacterial origin of potent anticancer agents originally isolated from sea hares. *Curr. Med. Chem.* 9: 1791–1806.

Ling, T., E. Poupon, E. J. Rueden, S. H. Kim, and E. A. Theodorakis. 2002. Unified synthesis of quinine sesquiterpenes based on a radical decarboxylation and quinone addition reaction. *J. Am. Chem. Soc.* 124(41): 12261–12267.

Linington, R. G., J. Gonzáles, L. D. Ureña, L. I. Romero, E. Ortega-Barría, and W. H. Gerwick. 2007. Venturamides A and B: Antimalarial constituents of the Panamanian marine cyanobacterium *Oscillatoria* sp. *J. Nat. Prod.* 70: 397–401.

Lo, M. C., A. Aulabaugh, G. Krishnamurthy et al. 2004. Probing the interaction of HTI-286 with tubulin using a stilbene analogue. *J. Am. Chem. Soc.* 126: 9898–9899.

Lombardo, D. and E. A. Dennis. 1985. Cobra venom phospholipase A2 inhibition by manoalide. A novel type of phospholipase inhibitor. *J. Biol. Chem.* 260(12): 7234–7240.

Longley, R. E., O. J. McConnell, E. Essich, and D. Harmody. 1993. Evaluation of marine sponge metabolites for cytotoxicity and signal transduction activity. *J. Nat. Prod.* 56: 915–920.

Look, S. and W. Fenical. 1987. The seco-pseudopterosins, new anti-inflammatory diterpene-glycosides from a Caribbean gorgonian octocoral of the genus *Pseudopterogorgia*. *Tetrahedron* 43(15): 3363–3370.

Look, S. A., W. Fenical, R. S. Jacobs, and J. Clardy. 1986a. The pseudopterosins: Anti-inflammatory and analgesic natural products from the sea whip *Pseudopterogorgia elisabethae*. *Proc. Natl Acad. Sci. USA* 83(17): 6238–6240.

Look, S., W. Fenical, G. Matsumoto, and J. Clardy. 1986b. The pseudopterosins: A new class of anti-inflammatory and analgesic diterpene pentosides from the marine sea whip *Pseudopterogorgia elisabethae* (Octocorallia). *J. Org. Chem.* 51(26): 5140–5145.

Lopanik, N., N. Lindquist, and N. Targett. 2004. Potent cytotoxins produced by a microbial symbiont protect host larvae from predation. *Oecologia* 139: 131–139.

Lopez-Macia, A., J. C. Jimenez, M. Royo, E. Giraet, and F. Albericio. 2001. Synthesis and structure determination of kahalalide F. *J. Am. Chem. Soc.* 123: 11398–11401.

Lu, X. L., Q. Z. Xu, X. Y. Liu, X. Cao, K. Y. Ni, and B. H. Jiao. 2008. Marine drugs-macrolactins. *Chem. Biodivers.* 5(9): 1669–1674.

Lucas, R., C. Giannini, M. V. D'auria, and M. Pay'a. 2003. Modulatory effect of bolinaquinone, a marine sesquiterpenoid, on acute and chronic inflammatory processes. *J. Pharmacol. Exp. Ther.* 304: 1172–1180.

Lucas-Elio, P., P. Hernandez, A. Sanchez-Amat, and F. Solano. 2005. Purification and partial characterization of marinocine, a new broad-spectrum antibacterial protein produced by *Marinomonas mediterranea*. *Biochim. Biophys. Acta* 1721: 193–203.

Luesch, H., R. E. Moore, V. J. Paul, S. L. Mooberry, and T. H. Corbett. 2001. Isolation of dolastatin 10 from the marine cyanobacterium Symploca species VP642 and total stereochemistry and biological evaluation of its analogue symplostatin 1. *J. Nat. Prod.* 64: 907–910.

Macherla, V. R., J. N. Liu, M. Sunga et al. 2007. Lipoxazolidinones A, B, and C: Antibacterial 4-oxazolidinones from a marine actinomycete isolates from a Guam marine sediment. *J. Nat. Prod.* 70: 1454–1457.

Maldonado, L. A., W. Fenical, P. R. Jensen et al. 2005. *Salinispora arenicola* gen. nov., sp. nov. and *Salinispora tropica* sp. nov., obligate marine actinomycetes belonging to the family *Micromonosporaceae*. *Int. J. Syst. Evol. Microbiol.* 55: 1759–1766.

Mallams, A. K., M. S. Puar, and R. R. Rossman. 1981. Kijanimicin. 1. Structures of the individual sugar components. *J. Am. Chem. Soc.* 103: 3938–3940.

Mandal, P., C. A. Pujol, M. J. Carlucci, K. Chattopadhyay, E. B. Damonte, and B. Ray. 2008. Antiherpetic activity of a sulfated xylomannan from *Scinaia hatei*. *Phytochemistry* 69(11): 2193–2199.

Marks, R. S., D. L. Graham, J. A. Sloan et al. 2003. A phase II study of the dolastatin 15 analogue LU 103793 in the treatment of advanced non-small cell lung cancer. *Am. J. Clin. Oncol.* 26: 336–337.

Matsubara, K., C. Xue, X. Zhao, M. Mori, T. Sugawara, and T. Hirata. 2005. Effects of middle molecular weight fucoidans on in vitro and ex vivo angiogenesis of endothelial cells. *Int. J. Mol. Med.* 15: 695–699.

Mayer, A. M., K. B. Glaser, C. Cuevas et al. 2010. The odyssey of marine pharmaceuticals: A current pipeline perspective. *Trends Pharmacol. Sci.* 31: 255–265.

Mayer, A. M. S., M. L. Hall, S. M. Lynch, S. P. Gunasekera, S. H. Sennett, and S. A. Pomponi. 2005. Differential modulation of microglia superoxide anion and thromboxane B2 generation by the marine manzamines. *BMC Pharmacol.* 5: 6–18.

Mayer, A. M. S., P. B. Jacobson, W. Fenical, R. S. Jacobs, and K. B. Glaser. 1998. Pharmacological characterization of the pseudopterosins: novel anti-inflammatory natural products isolated from the Caribbean soft coral, *Pseudopterogorgia elisabethae*. *Life Sci.* 62(5): 401–407.

Mayer, A. M. S. and V. K. B. Lehmann. 2000. Marine pharmacology. *The Pharmacologist* 42: 62–69.

McAlpine, J. B., A. H. Banskota, R. D. Charan et al. 2008. Biosynthesis of diazepinomicin/ECO-4601, a Micromonospora secondary metabolite with a novel ring system. *J. Nat. Prod.* 71: 1585–1590.

McClintock, J. B. and B. J. Baker (eds). 2001. *Marine Chemical Ecology*. CRC Press, Boca Raton, FL.

McConkey, G. A., M. J. Rogers, and T. F. McCutchan. 1997. Inhibition of *Plasmodium falciparum* protein synthesis. Targeting the plastid-like organelle with thiostrepton. *J. Biol. Chem.* 272: 2046–2049.

McNulty, J. and I. W. J. Still. 1995. Selective methylation and stereoselective reduction of a β-carboline to a N(2)-methyl-1,2,3,4-tetrahydro-β-carboline. *Tetrahedron Lett.* 36(44): 7965–7966.

Mehla, R., S. Bivalkar-Mehla, R. Zhang et al. 2010. Bryostatin modulates latent HIV-1 infection via PKC and AMPK signaling but inhibits acute infection in a receptor independent manner. *PLoS ONE* 5: e11160.

Mendola, D. 2000. Aquacultural production of bryostatin 1 and ecteinascidin 743. In *Drugs from the Sea*, ed. N. Fusetani, pp. 120–133. Karger, Basel, Switzerland.

Michelle, S., S. Teisan, G. Tsueng, M. Venkat, and L. Kin. 2008. Seawater requirement for the production of lipoxazolidinones by marine actinomycete strain NPS8920. *J. Ind. Microbiol. Biotechnol.* 35: 761–765.

Mickel, S. J., G. H. Sedelmeier, D. Niederer et al. 2004a. Large-scale synthesis of the anticancer marine natural product (+)-discodermolide. Part 1: Synthetic strategy and preparation of a common precursor. *Org. Proc. Res. Dev.* 8: 92–100.

Mickel, S. J., G. H. Sedelmeier, D. Niederer et al. 2004b. Large-scale synthesis of the anticancer marine natural product (+)-discodermolide. Part 2: Synthesis of fragments C1-6 and C9–14. *Org. Proc. Res. Dev.* 8: 101–106.

Mickel, S. J., G. H. Sedelmeier, D. Niederer et al. 2004c. Large-scale synthesis of the anticancer marine natural product (+)-discodermolide. Part 3: Synthesis of fragment C15-21. *Org. Proc. Res. Dev.* 8: 107–112.

Mickel, S. J., G. H. Sedelmeier, D. Niederer et al. 2004d. Large-scale synthesis of the anticancer marine natural product (+)-discodermolide. Part 4: Preparation of fragment C7-24. *Org. Proc. Res. Dev.* 8: 113–121.

Mickel, S. J., G. H. Sedelmeier, D. Niederer et al. 2004e. Large-scale synthesis of the anticancer marine natural product (+)-discodermolide. Part 5: Linkage of fragments C1-6 and C7-24 and finale. *Org. Proc. Res. Dev.* 8: 122–130.

Minale, L., R. Riccio, and G. Sodano. 1974. Avarol a novel sesquiterpenoid hydroquinone with a rearranged drimane skeleton from the sponge *Dysidea avara*. *Tetrahedron Lett.* 15(38): 3401–3404.

Mincer, T. J., P. R. Jensen, C. A. Kauffman, and W. Fenical. 2002. Widespread and persistent populations of a major new marine actinomycete taxon in ocean sediments. *Appl. Environ. Microbiol.* 68: 5005–5011.

Mita, A., A. C. Lockhart, T.-L. Chen et al. 2004. A phase I pharmacokinetic (PK) trial of XAA296A (Discodermolide) administered every 3 wks to adult patients with advanced solid malignancies. *J. Clin. Oncol.* 22(14S, July 15 Supplement): 2025.

Miyazaki, K., M. Kobayashi, T. Natsume et al. 1995. Synthesis and antitumor activity of novel dolastatin 10 analogs. *Chem. Pharm. Bull. (Tokyo)* 43: 1706–1718.

Molinski, T. F. 2004. Antifungal compounds from marine organisms. *Curr. Med. Chem. Anti-Infective Agents* 3: 197–220.

Molinski, T. F., D. S. Dalisay, S. L. Lievens, and J. P. Saludes. 2009. Drug development from marine natural products. *Nat. Rev. Drug Discov.* 8: 69–85.

Montgomery, D. and C. F. Zukoshi. 1985. Didemnin B: A new immunosuppressive cyclic peptide with potent activity in vitro and in vivo. *Transplantation* 40: 49–56.

Moore, K. S., S. Wehrli, H. Roder et al. 1993. Squalamine: An aminosterol antibiotic from the shark. *Proc. Natl Acad. Sci. USA* 90: 1354–1358.

Morimoto, M., M. Fukui, S. Ohkubo, T. Tamaoki, and F. Tomita. 1982. Tetrocarcins, new antitumor antibiotics. 3. Antitumor activity of tetrocarcin A. *J. Antibiot. (Tokyo)* 35: 1033–1037.

Morris, S. A. and R. J. Andersen. 1990. Brominated bis(indole)alkaloids from the marine sponge *Hexadella* sp. *Tetrahedron* 46: 715–720.

Motti, C. A., M.-L. Bourguet-Kondracki, A. Longeon, J. R. Doyle, L. E. Llewellyn, D. M. Tapiolas, and P. Yin. 2007. Comparison of the biological properties of several marine sponge-derived sesquiterpenoid quinones. *Molecules* 12(7): 1376–1388.

Mross, K., K. Herbst, W. E. Berdel et al. 1996. Phase I clinical and pharmacokinetic study of LU103793 (cemadotin hydrochloride) as an intravenous bolus injection in patients with metastatic solid tumors. *Onkologie* 19: 490–495.

Müller, W. E. G., A. Maidhof, R. K. Zahn et al. 1985a. Potent antileukemic activity of the novel cytostatic agent avarone and its analogues in vitro and in vivo. *Cancer Res.* 45: 4822–4826.

Müller, W. E. G., D. Sladić, R. K. Zahn et al. 1987. Avarol-induced DNA strand breakage in vitro and in Friend erythroleukemia cells. *Cancer Res.* 47: 6565–6571.

Müller, W. E. G., R. K. Zahn, M. J. Gašić et al. 1985b. Avarol, a cytostatically active compound from the marine sponge *Dysidea avara. Comp. Biochem. Physiol. C* 80: 47–52.

Munro, M. H. G., J. W. Blunt, E. J. Dumdei et al. 1990. The discovery and development of marine compounds with pharmaceutical potential. *J. Biotechnol.* 70: 15–25.

Munro, M. H. G., R. T. Luibrand, and J. W. Blunt, 1987. The search for antiviral and anticancer compounds from marine organisms. In *Bioorganic Marine Chemistry*, ed. P. J. Scheuer, vol. 1, pp. 103–105. Springer-Verlag, New York.

Mutter, R. and M. Wills. 2000. Chemistry and clinical biology of the bryostatins. *Bioorg. Med. Chem.* 8: 1841–1860.

Nagai, K., K. Kamigiri, N. Arao et al. 2003. YM-266183 and YM-266184, novel thiopeptide antibiotics produced by *Bacillus cereus* isolated from a marine sponge. I. Taxonomy, fermentation, isolation, physico-chemical properties and biological properties. *J. Antibiot. (Tokyo)* 56: 123–128.

Nagao, T., K. Adachi, M. Sakai, M. Nishijima, and H. Sano. 2001. Novel macrolactins as antibiotic lactones from a marine bacterium. *J. Antibiot. (Tokyo)* 54(4): 333–339.

Nakamura, H., S. Deng, J. Kobayashi et al. 1987a. Physiologically active marine natural products from Porifera. XV. Keramamine-A and -B, novel antimicrobial alkaloids from the Okinawan marine sponge *Pellina* sp. *Tetrahedron Lett.* 28: 621–624.

Nakamura, H., J. Kobayashi, Y. Ohizumi, and Y. Hirata. 1982. Isolation and structure of aaptamine a novel heteroaromatic substance possessing α-blocking activity from the sea sponge *Aaptos aaptos. Tetrahedron Lett.* 23: 5555–5558.

Nakamura, H., J. Kobayashi, Y. J. Ohizumi, and Y. J. Hirata. 1987b. Aaptamines. Novelbenzo[de][1,6]naphthyridines from the Okinawan marine sponge *Aaptos aaptos. Chem. Soc. Perkin Trans.* 1: 173–176.

Nakashima, T., M. Miura, and M. Hara. 2000. Tetrocarcin A inhibits mitochondrial functions of Bcl-2 and suppresses its anti-apoptotic activity. *Cancer Res.* 60: 1229–1235.

Nerenberg, J. B., D. T. Hung, P. K. Somers, and S. L. Schreiber. 1993. Total synthesis of the immunosuppressive agent (–)-discodermolide. *J. Am. Chem. Soc.* 115: 12621–12622.

Nevalainen, T. J., R. J. Quinn, and J. N. Hooper. 2004. Phospholipase A2 in porifera. *Comp. Physiol. Ecol.* 137(3): 413–420.

Newman, D. J. and G. M. Cragg. 2004a. Marine natural products and related compounds in clinical and advanced preclinical trials. *J. Nat. Prod.* 67(8): 1216–1238.

Newman, D. J. and G. M. Cragg. 2004b. Advanced preclinical and clinical trials of natural products and related compounds from marine sources. *Curr. Med. Chem.* 11: 1693–1713.

Newman, D. J. and G. M. Cragg. 2007. Natural products as sources of new drugs over the last 25 years. *J. Nat. Prod.* 70: 461–477.

Newman, D. J., G. M. Cragg, and K. M. Snader. 2003. Natural products as sources of new drugs over the period 1981–2002. *J. Nat. Prod.* 66: 1022–1037.

Nieman, J. A., J. E. Coleman, D. J. Wallace et al. 2003. Synthesis and antimitotic/cytotoxic activity of hemiasterlin analogues. *J. Nat. Prod.* 66: 183–199.

Niu, C., D. Smith, A. Zask et al. 2004. Tubulin inhibitors. Synthesis and biological activity of HTI-286 analogs with B-segment heterosubstituents. *Bioorg. Med. Chem. Lett.* 14: 4329–4332.

Nolan, F. C. and T. Cross. 1988. Isolation and screening of actinomycetes. In *Actinomycetes in Biotechnology*, eds. M. Goodfellow, S. T. Williams, and M. Modarski, pp. 1–32. Academic Press, London, U.K.

Nunes, M., J. Kaplan, J. Wooters et al. 2005. Two photoaffinity analogues of the tripeptide, hemiasterlin, exclusively label α-tubulin. *Biochemistry* 44: 6844–6857.

Ogino, J., R. E. Moore, G. M. L. Patterson, and C. D. Smith. 1996. Dendroamides, new cyclic hexa-peptides from a blue-green alga. Multidrug-resistance reversing activity of dendroamide A. *J. Nat. Prod.* 59: 581–586.

Ohizumi, Y., A. Kajiwara, H. Nakamura, and J. Kobayashi. 1984. α-Adrenoceptor blocking action of aaptamine, a novel marine natural product, in vascular smooth muscle. *J. Pharm. Pharmacol.* 36: 785–786.

Ohta, S., F. Ono, Y. Shiomi et al. 1998. Anti-herpes simplex virus substances produced by the marine green alga, *Dunaliella primolecta*. *J. Appl. Phycol.* 10: 349–355.

Okouneva, T., O. Azarenko, L. Wilson, B. A. Littlefield, and M. A. Jordan. 2008. Inhibition of centromere dynamics by eribulin (E7389) during mitotic metaphase. *Mol. Cancer Ther.* 7: 2003–2011.

Okouneva, T., B. T. Hill, L. Wilson, and M. A. Jordan. 2003. The effects of vinflunine, vinorelbine, and vinblastine on centromere dynamics. *Mol. Cancer Ther.* 2: 427–436.

Oku, N., K. R. Gustafson, L. K. Cartner et al. 2004. Neamphamide A, a new HIV-inhibitory depsipeptide from the Papua New Guinea marine sponge *Neamphius huxleyi*. *J. Nat. Prod.* 67: 1407–1411.

Olano, C., C. Méndez, and J. A. Salas. 2009. Antitumor compounds from marine actinomycetes. *Mar. Drugs* 7: 210–248.

Omura, S., H. Ikeda, J. Ishikawa et al. 2001. Genome sequence of an industrial microorganism *Streptomyces avermitilis*: Deducing the ability of producing secondary metabolites. *Proc. Natl Acad. Sci. USA* 98: 12215–12220.

Omura, S., Y. Iwai, A. Hirano et al. 1977. A new alkaloid AM-2282 of *Streptomyces* origin. Taxonomy, fermentation, isolation and preliminary characterization. *J. Antibiot.* 30: 275–282.

Omura, S., Y. Sasaki, Y. Iwai, and H. Takeshimi. 1995. Staurosporine, a potentially important gift from a micro-organism. *J. Antibiot.* 48: 535–548.

Orjala, J. and W. H. Gerwick. 1996. Barbamide, a chlorinated metabolite with molluscicidal activity from the Caribbean cyanobacterium *Lyngbya majuscule*. *J. Nat. Prod.* 59: 427–430.

Oz, H. S., W. T. Hughes, J. E. Rehg, and E. K. Thomas. 2000. Effect of CD40 ligand and other immuno-modulators on *Pneumocystis carinii* infection in rat model. *Microb. Pathog.* 29: 187–190.

Paterson, I., O. Delgado, G. J. Florence et al. 2005. A second-generation total synthesis of (+)-discodermolide: The development of a practical route using solely substrate-based stereocontrol. *J. Org. Chem.* 70: 150–160.

Paterson, I. and I. Lyothier. 2004. Total synthesis of (+)-discodermolide: An improved endgame exploiting a Still-Gennari-type olefination with a C1-C8 β-ketophosphonate fragment. *Org. Lett.* 6: 4933–4936.

Patterson, G. M. L., K. K. Baker, C. L. Baldwin et al. 1993. Antiviral activity of cultured blue-green algae (*Cyanophyta*). *J. Phycol.* 29: 125–130.

Paul, V. J. 1992. *Ecological Roles of Marine Natural Products*. Cornell University Press, Ithaca, NY.

Pawlik, J. R. 1993. Marine invertebrate chemical defenses. *Chem. Rev.* 93: 1911–1922.

Peláez, F. 2006. The historical delivery of antibiotics from microbial natural products-can history repeat? *Biochem. Pharmacol.* 71: 981–990.

Peng, J., S. Kudrimoti, S. Prasanna et al. 2010. Structure-activity relationship and mechanism of action studies of manzamine analogues for the control of neuroinflammation and cerebral infections. *J. Med. Chem.* 53: 61–76.

Peng, J., K. V. Rao, Y.-M. Choo, and M. T. Hamann. 2008. Manzamine alkaloids. In *Modern Alkaloids: Structure, Isolation, Synthesis and Biology*, eds. E. Fattorusso and O. Taglialatela-Scafati, pp. 189–232. Wiley-VCH Verlag GmbH & Co. KGaA, Weinheim, Germany.

Peng, J., X. Shen, K. A. El Sayed et al. 2003. Marine natural products as prototype agrochemical agents. *J. Agric. Food Chem.* 51: 2246–2252.

Perry, N. B., J. W. Blunt, M. H. G. Munro, and L. K. Pannell. 1988. Mycalamide A, an antiviral com-pound from a New Zealand sponge of the genus Mycale. *J. Am. Chem. Soc.* 110: 4850–4851.

Perry, N. B., J. W. Blunt, M. H. G. Munro, and A. M. Thompson. 1990. Antiviral and antitumor agents from a New Zealand sponge, *Mycale* sp. 2. Structures and solution conformations of mycal-amides A and B. *J. Org. Chem.* 55: 223–227.

Pettit, G. R., J. F. Day, J. L. Hartwell, and H. B. Wood. 1970. Antineoplastic components of marine animals. *Nature* 227: 962–963.

Pettit, G. R., C. L. Herald, D. L. Doubek, D. L. Herald, E. Arnold, and J. Clardy. 1982. Isolation and structure of bryostatin 1. *J. Am. Chem. Soc.* 104: 6846–6848.

Pettit, G. R., H. Hoffmann, J. McNulty et al. 2004. Antineoplastic agents. 380. Isolation and X-ray crystal structure determination of isoaaptamine from the Republic of Singapore Hymeniacidon sp. and conversion to the phosphate prodrug hystatin. *J. Nat. Prod.* 67: 506–509.

Pettit, G. R., Y. Kamano, C. Dufresne et al. 1989a. Isolation and structure of the cytostatic linear depsipeptide dolastatin 15. *J. Org. Chem.* 54: 6005–6006.

Pettit, G. R., Y. Kamano, C. L. Herald et al. 1987. The isolation and structure of a remarkable marine animal antineoplastic constituent: Dolastatin 10. *Am. Chem. Soc.* 109: 6883–6885.

Pettit, G. R., S. B. Singh, F. Hogan et al. 1989b. The absolute configuration and synthesis of natural (-)-dolastatin 10. *J. Am. Chem. Soc.* 111: 5463–5465.

Phife, D. W., R. A. Ramos, M. Feng, I. King, S. P. Gunasekera, A. Wright, M. Patel, J. A. Pachter, and S. J. Coval. 1996. Marine sponge bis(indole) alkaloids that displace ligand binding to α1 adrenergic receptors. *Bioorg. Med. Chem. Lett.* 6(17): 2103–2106.

Pitot, H. C., E. A. McElroy Jr., J. M. Reid et al. 1999. Phase I trial of dolastatin-10 (NSC 376128) in patients with advanced solid tumors. *Clin. Cancer Res.* 5: 525–531.

Pommier, Y., G. Kohlhagen, C. Bailly, M. Waring, A. Mazumder, and K. W. Kohn. 1996. DNA sequence- and structure-selective alkylation of guanine N2 in the DNA minor groove by ecteinascidin 743, a potent antitumor compound from the Caribbean tunicate *Ecteinascidia turbinata*. *Biochemistry* 35: 13303–13309.

Pommier, A., V. Stepanenko, K. Jarowicki, and P. J. Kocienski. 2003. Synthesis of (+)-manoalide via a copper(I)-mediated 1.2-metalate rearrangement. *J. Org. Chem.* 68(10): 4008–4013.

Popov, A. M., S. I. Stekhova, N. K. Utkina, and N. M. Rebachuk. 1999. Antimicrobial and cytotoxic activity of sesquiterpenequinones and brominated diphenyl esters isolated from marine sponges. *J. Pharm. Chem.* 33(2): 71–73.

Potts, B. C. and D. J. Faulkner. 1992. Phospholipase A$_2$ inhibitors from marine organisms. *J. Nat. Prod.* 55(12): 1707–1717.

Potts, B. C. M., D. J. Faulkner, M. S. De Carvalho, and R. S. Jacobs. 1992. Chemical mechanism of inactivation of bee venom phospholipase A2 by the marine natural products manoalide, luffariellolide, and scalaradial. *J. Am. Chem. Soc.* 114(13): 5093–5100.

Proksch, P., R. Edrada, and R. Ebel. 2002. Drugs from the seas—Current status and microbiological implications. *Appl. Microbiol. Biotechnol.* 59: 125–134.

Puliti, R., S. De Rosa, C. A. Mattia, and L. Mazzarella. 1990. Structure and stereochemistry of an acetate derivative of cacospongionolide a new antitumoral sesterterpenoid from marine sponge *Cacospongia mollior*. *Acta Crystallogr. C Cryst. Struct. Commun.* 46(8): 1533–1536.

Puliti, R., C. A. Mattia, and L. Mazzarella. 1995. Scalaradial, a sesterterpenoid metabolite from the marine sponge *Cacospongia mollior*. *Acta Crystallogr. Sect. C* 51: 1703–1707.

Quinoa, E., M. Adamczeski, P. Crews, and G. J. Bakus. 1986. Bengamides, heterocyclic anthelmintics from a Jaspidae marine sponge. *J. Org. Chem.* 51: 4494–4497.

Rademaker-Lakhai, J. M., S. Horenblas, W. Meinhardt et al. 2005. Phase I clinical and pharmacokinetic study of Kahalalide F in patients with advanced androgen refractory prostate cancer. *Clin. Cancer Res.* 11: 1854–1862.

Randazzo, A., C. Debitus, L. Minale et al. 1998. Petrosaspongiolides M-R: New potent and selective phospholipase A2 inhibitors from the new Caledonian marine sponge *Petrosaspongia nigra*. *J. Nat. Prod.* 61(5): 571–575.

Rao, K. V., N. Kasanah, S. Wahyuono, B. L. Tekwani, R. F. Schinazi, and M. T. Hamann. 2004. Three new manzamine alkaloids from a common Indonesian sponge and their activity against infectious and tropical parasitic diseases. *J. Nat. Prod.* 67: 1314–1318.

Rao, K. V., B. D. Santarsiero, A. D. Mesecar, R. F. Schinazi, B. L. Tekwani, and M. T. Hamann. 2003. New manzamine alkaloids with activity against infectious and tropical parasitic diseases from an Indonesian sponge. *J. Nat. Prod.* 66: 823–828.

Rashid, M.A., K. R. Gustafson, L. K. Cartner, N. Shigematsu, L. K. Pannell, and M. R. Boyd. 2001. Microspinosamide, a new HIV-inhibitory cyclic depsipeptide from the marine sponge *Sidonops microspinosa. J. Nat. Prod.* 64(1): 117–121.

Rath, J.-P., S. Kinast, and M. E. Maier, 2005. Synthesis of the full functionalized core structure of the antibiotic abyssomicin C. *Org. Lett.* 7: 3089–3092.

Ray, A., T. Okouneva, T. Manna et al. 2007. Mechanism of action of the microtubule-targeted antimitotic depsipeptide tasidotin (formerly ILX651) and its major metabolite tasidotin C-carboxylate. *Cancer Res.* 67: 3767–3776.

Rechter, S., T. Konig, S. Auerochs et al. 2006. Antiviral activity of arthrospira-derived spirulan-like substances. *Antiviral Res.* 72: 197–206.

Reynolds, L. J., B. P. Morgan, G. A. Hite, E. D. Mihelich, and E. A. Dennis. 1988. Phospholipase A-2 inhibition and modification by manoalogue. *J. Am. Chem. Soc.* 110(15): 5172–5177.

Rheinheimer, I. G. 1992. *Aquatic Microbiology.* John Wiley, New York.

Riedlinger, J., A. Reicke, H. Zähner et al. 2004. Abyssomicins, inhibitors of the para-aminobenzoic acid pathway produced by the marine *Verrucosispora* strain AB-18-032. *J. Antibiot.* 57: 271–279.

Rinehart Jr., K. L., J. B. Gloer, J. C. Cook, S. A. Mizsac, and T. Scahill. 1981. Structures of the didemnins, antiviral and cytotoxic depsipeptides from a Caribbean tunicate. *J. Am. Chem. Soc.* 103: 1857–1859.

Rinehart, K. L., T. G. Holt, N. L. Fregeau et al. 1990. Ecteinascidins 729, 743, 745, 759A, 759B, and 770: Potent antitumor agents from the Caribbean tunicate *Ecteinascidia turbinate. J. Org. Chem.* 55: 4512–4515.

Rinehart Jr., K. L., J. Kobayashi, G. C. Harbour et al. 1987. Eudistomins A-Q, β-carbolines from the antiviral Caribbean tunicate *Eudistoma olivaceum. J. Am. Chem. Soc.* 109(11): 3378–3387.

Rinehart Jr., K. L., J. Kobayashi, G. C. Harbour, R. G. Hughes Jr., S. A. Mizsak, and T. A. Scahill. 1984. Eudistomins C, E, K, and L, potent antiviral compounds containing a novel oxathiazepine ring from the Caribbean tunicate *Eudistoma olivaceum. J. Am. Chem. Soc.* 106(5): 1524–1526.

Rodriguez, A. D. and N. Martinez. 1993. Marine antitumor agents: 14-deoxycrassin and pseudoplexaurol, new cembranoid diterpenes from the Caribbean gorgonian *Pseudoplexaura porosa. Experientia* 49: 179–181.

Rogers, M. J., E. Cundliffe, and T. F. McCutchan. 1998. The antibiotic micrococcin is a potent inhibitor of growth and protein synthesis in the malaria parasite. *Antimicrob. Agents Chemother.* 42: 715–716.

Rohwer, F., V. Seguritan, F. Azam, and N. Knowlton. 2002. Diversity and distribution of coral-associated bacteria. *Mar. Ecol. Prog. Ser.* 243: 1–10.

Ruzicka, Z. L. 1953. The isoprene rule and the biogenesis of terpenic compounds. *Experientia* 9: 357–367.

Sakai, R., T. Higa, C. W. Jefford, and G. Bernardinelli. 1986. Manzamine A; an antitumor alkaloid from a sponge. *J. Am. Chem. Soc.* 108: 6404–6405.

Sakai, R., S. Kohmoto, T. Higa, C. W. Jefford, and G. T. Bernardinelli. 1987. Manzamine B and C, two novel alkaloids from the sponge *Haliclona* sp. *Tetrahedron Lett.* 28(45): 5493–5496.

Sakemi, S., T. Ichiba, S. Kohmoto, G. Saucy, and T. Higa. 1988. Isolation and structure elucidation of onnamide A, a new bioactive metabolite of a marine sponge, *Theonella* sp. *J. Am. Chem. Soc.* 110: 4851–4853.

Salmi, C. and J. M. Brunel. 2007. Therapeutic potential of cationic steroid antibacterials. *Expert Opin. Investig. Drugs* 16: 1143–1157.

Salmoun, M., C. Devijver, D. Daloze et al. 2000. New sesquiterpene/quinones from two sponges of the genus *Hyrtios. J. Nat. Prod.* 63(4): 452–456.

Sammarco, P. W. and J. C. Coll. 1992. Chemical adaptations in the Octocorallia: Evolutionary perspectives. *Mar. Ecol. Prog. Ser.* 88: 93–104.

Sapi, J. and Massiot, G. 1995. *The Alkaloids*, vol. 47, pp. 173–226. Academic Press, New York.

Sarabia, F. and A. Sanchez-Ruiz. 2005. A diversity-oriented synthetic approach to bengamides. *Tetrahedron Lett.* 46: 1131–1135.

Sarin, P. S., D. Sun, A. Thornton, and W. Muller. 1987. Inhibition of replication of the etiologic agent of acquired immune deficiency syndrome (human T-lymphotropic retrovirus/lymphadenopathy-associated virus) by avarol and avarone. *J. Natl Cancer Inst.* 78: 663–666.

Schmidt, E. W., J. T. Nelson, D. A. Rasko et al. 2005. Patellamide A and C biosynthesis by a microcin-like pathway in *Prochloron didemni*, the cyanobacterial symbiont of *Lissoclinum patella*. *Proc. Natl Acad. Sci. USA* 120: 7315–7320.

Schröder, H. C., R. Wenger, H. Gerner et al. 1989. Suppression of the modulatory effects of the anti-leukemic and anti-human immunodeficiency virus compound avarol on gene expression by tryptophan. *Cancer Res.* 49: 2069–2076.

Schwartz, R. E., C. F. Hirsch, D. F. Sesin, J. E. Flor, M. Chartrain, and R. E. Fromtling. 1990. Pharmaceuticals from cultured algae. *J. Ind. Microbiol.* 5: 113–124.

Seibert, G., W. Raether, N. Dogovic, M. J. Gasic, R. K. Zahn, and W. E. G. Müller. 1985. Antibacterial and antifungal activity of avarone and avarol. *Zbl. Bakt. Hyg.* A260: 379–386.

Selinsky, B. S., Z. Zhou, K. G. Fojtik, S. R. Jones, N. R. Dollahon, and A. E. Shinnar. 1998. The aminos-terol antibiotic squalamine permeabilizes large unilamellar phospholipid vesicles. *Biochim. Biophys. Acta* 1370: 218–234.

Shaha, S. P., J. Tomic, Y. Shi et al. 2009. Prolonging microtubule dysruption enhances the immunoge-nicity of chronic lymphocytic leukaemia cells. *Clin. Exp. Immunol.* 158: 186–198.

Shen, Y. and D. L. Burgoyne. 2002. Efficient synthesis of IPL576,092: A novel anti-asthma agent. *J. Org. Chem.* 67(11): 3908–3910.

Shen, Y.-C., Y.-T. Chang, C.-L. Lin et al. 2011. Synthesis of 1-substituted carbazolyl-1,2,3,4-tetrahydro- and carbazolyl-3,4-dihydro-β-carboline analogs as potential antitumor agents. *Mar. Drugs* 9: 256–277.

Shen, Y.-C., C.-C. Chein, P.-W. Hsiehand, and C.-Y. Duh. 1997. Bioactive constituents from marine sponge *Aaptos aaptos*. *Taiwan Shuichan Xuehuikan* 24: 117–125.

Shen, Y.-C., T. T. Lin, J. H. Sheu, and C.-Y. Duh. 1999. Structures and cytotoxicity relationship of isoaaptamine and aaptamine derivatives. *J. Nat. Prod.* 62(9): 1264–1267.

Sheridan, C. 2006. Antibiotics au naturel. *Nat. Biotechnol.* 24: 1494–1496.

Shigeo, K., F. Shinya, and I. Sachihiko. 1985. Total synthesis of manoalide and seco-manoalide. *Tetrahedron Lett.* 26(47): 5827–5830.

Shin, H. C., H. J. Hwang, K. J. Kang, and B. H. Lee. 2006. An antioxidative and anti-inflammatory agent for potential treatment of osteoarthritis from *Ecklonia cava*. *Arch. Pharmacol. Res.* 29: 165–171.

Shin, J., Y. Seon, K. W. Cho, J.-R. Rho, and C. J. Sim. 1999. New bis(indole) alkaloids of the topsentin class from the sponge *Spongosorites genitrix*. *J. Nat. Prod.* 62(4): 647–649.

Shoji, N., A. Umeyama, K. Shin et al. 1992. Two unique pentacyclic steroids with *cis* C/D ring junc-tion from *Xestospongia bergquistia* Fromont, powerful inhibitors of histamine release. *J. Org. Chem.* 57(11): 2996–2997.

Sills, Jr. A. K., J. I. Williams, B. M. Tyler et al. 1998. Squalamine inhibits angiogenesis and solid tumor growth in vivo and perturbs embryonic vasculature. *Cancer Res.* 58: 2784–2792.

Simpson, T. J. 1987. Applications of multinuclear NMR to structural and biosynthetic studies of polyketide microbial metabolites. *Chem. Soc. Rev.* 16: 123–160.

Smith, C. D., X. Zhang, S. L. Mooberry, G. M. L. Patterson, and R. E. Moore. 1994. Cryptophycin: A new antimicrotubule agent active against drug-resistant cells. *Cancer Res.* 54: 3779–3784.

Smyth, J., M. E. Boneterre, J. Schellens et al. 2001. Activity of the dolastatin analogue, LU103793, in malignant melanoma. *Ann. Oncol.* 12: 509–511.

Sneader, W. 2005. *Drug Discovery: A History*, p. 258. Wiley, New York.

Soria-Mercado, I. E., A. Prieto-Davo, P. R. Jensen, and W. Fenical. 2005. Antibiotic terpenoid chloro-dihydroquinones from a new marine actinomycete. *J. Nat. Prod.* 68: 904–910.

Soriente, A., M. M. DeRosa, A. Scettri, G. Sodano, M. C. Terencio, M. Payá, and M. J. Alcaraz. 1999. Manoalide. *Curr. Med. Chem.* 6(5): 415–431.

Souza, T. M. L., J. L. Abrantes, R. A. Epifanio et al. 2007. The alkaloid 4-methylaaptamine isolated from the sponge *Aaptos aaptos* impairs Herpes simplex virus type 1 penetration and immediate-early protein synthesis. *Planta Med.* 73: 200–205.

Spitaler, M., I. Utz, W. Hilbe, J. Hofmann, and H. H. Grunicke. 1998. PKC-independent modulation of multidrug resistance in cells with mutant (V185) but not wild-type (G185) p-glycoprotein by bryostatin 1. *Biochem. Pharmacol.* 56: 861–869.

Stefanska, A. L., N. J. Coates, L. M. Mensah, A. J. Pope, S. J. Ready, and S. R. Warr. 2000. SB-219383, a novel tyrosyl tRNA synthetase inhibitor from *Micromonospora* sp. I. Fermentation, isolation and properties. *J. Antibiot.* 53: 345–350.

Stephenson, K., V. Prasad, S. Weitman et al. 2004. ILX651 disrupts microtubule assembly by two mechanisms [abstract 5616]. *Proc. Am. Assoc. Cancer Res.* 45: 1297.

Subbaraju, G. V., T. Golakoti, G. M. L. Patterson, and R. E. Moore. 1997. Three new cryptophycins from *Nostoc* sp. GSV 224. *J. Nat. Prod.* 60: 302–305.

Suhadolnik, R., S. Pornbanlualap, D. C. Baker, K. N. Tiwari, and A. K. Hebbler. 1989. Stereospecific 2'-amination and 2'-chlorination of adenosine by Actinomadura in the biosynthesis of 2'-amino-2'-deoxyadenosine and 2'-chloro-2'-deoxycoformycin. *Arch. Biochem. Biophys.* 270: 374–382.

Sumioka, A., D. Yan, and S. Tomita. 2010. TARP phosphorylation regulates synaptic AMPA receptors through lipid bilayers. *Neuron* 66: 755–767.

Sun, M. K. and D. L. Alkon. 2005. Dual effects of bryostatin-1 on spatial memory and depression. *Eur. J. Pharm.* 512: 43–51.

Sun, M. K. and D. L. Alkon. 2006. Bryostatin-1: Pharmacology and therapeutic potential as a CNS drug. *CNS Drug Rev.* 12: 1–8.

Sun, M. K., J. Hongpaisan, and D. L. Alkon. 2009. Postischemic PKC activation rescues retrograde and anterograde long-term memory. *Proc. Natl Acad. Sci. USA* 106: 14676–14680.

Takei, M., D. L. Burgoyne, and R. J. Andersen. 1994. Effect of contignasterol on histamine release induced by anti-immunoglobulin from rat peritoneal mast cells. *J. Pharmaceut. Sci.* 83(9): 1234–1234.

Takei, M., A. Umeyama, N. Shoji, S. Arihara, and K. Endo. 1993. Mechanism of inhibition of IgE-dependent histamine release from rat mast cells by xestobergsterol A from the Okinawan marine sponge *Xestospongia bergquistia*. *Experientia* 49(2): 145–149.

Talpir, R., Y. Benayahu, Y. Kashman, L. Panell, and M. Schleyer. 1994. Hemiasterlin and geodiamolide TA; two new cytotoxic peptides from the marine sponge *Hemiasterella minor* (Kirkpatrick). *Tetrahedron Lett.* 35: 4453–4456.

Tamaoki, T., H. Nomoto, I. Takahashi, Y. Kato, M. Morimoto, and F. Tomita. 1986. Staurosporine, a potent inhibitor of phospholipid/Ca++ dependent protein kinase. *Biochem. Biophys. Res. Commun.* 135: 397–402.

Tanaka, Y. T. and S. Omura. 1993. Agroactive compounds of microbial origin. *Annu. Rev. Microbiol.* 47: 57–87.

Taylor, S. A., P. Goodman, W. J. Stuckey, R. L. Stephens, and E. R. Gaynor. 1992. Phase II evaluation of didemnin B in advanced adenocarcinoma of the kidney A Southwest Oncology Group study. *Invest. New Drugs* 10: 55–56.

Terakubo, S., H. Takemura, H. Yamamoto et al. 2001. Antimicrobial activity of everninomicin against clinical isolates of *Enterococcus* spp., *Staphylococcus* spp., and *Streptococcus* spp. tested by Etest. *J. Infect. Chemother.* 7: 263–266.

Thakur, A. N., N. L. Thakur, M. M. Indap, R. A. Pandit, V. V. Datar, and W. E. Muller. 2005. Antiangiogenic, antimicrobial, and cytotoxic potential of sponge-associated bacteria. *Mar. Biotechnol. (NY)* 7: 245–252.

Thale, Z., F. R. Kinder, K. W. Bair et al. 2001. Bengamides revisited: New structures and antitumor studies. *J. Org. Chem.* 66: 1733–1741.

The World Health Report. 2000. *Health System: Improving Performance*. World Health Organization, Geneva, Switzerland.

Thomas, T. R. A., D. P. Kavlekar, and P. A. LokaBharathi. 2010. Marine drugs from sponge-microbe association–A review. *Mar. Drugs* 8: 1417–1468.

Thompson, A. M., J. W. Blunt, H. G. Murray, Munro, N. B. Perry, and L. K. Pannell. 1992. Chemistry of the mycalamides, antiviral and antitumour compounds from a marine sponge. Part 3. Acyl, alkyl and silyl derivatives. *J. Chem. Soc. Perkin Trans.* 1: 1335–1342.

Tietze, L. F., H. P. Bell, and S. Chandrasekhar. 2003. Natural product hybrids as new leads for drug discovery. *Angew. Chem. Int. Ed*. 42: 3996–4028.

Tilvi, S. and C. G. Naik. 2007. Tandem mass spectrometry of kahalalides: Identification of two new cyclic depsipeptides, kahalalide R and S from *Elysia grandifolia*. *J. Mass. Spectrom*. 42: 70–80.

Todorova, A. K., F. Jüttner, A. Linden, T. Pluess, and W. von Philipsborn. 1995. Nostocyclamide: A new macrocyclic, thiazole-containing allelochemical from *Nostoc* sp. 31 (cyanobacteria). *J. Org. Chem*. 60: 7891–7895.

Tomita, F., T. Tamaoki, K. Shirahat et al. 1980. Novel antitumor antibiotics, tetrocarcins. *J. Antibiot. (Tokyo)* 33: 668–670.

Towle, M. J., K. A. Salvato, J. Budrow et al. 2001. In vitro and in vivo anticancer activities of synthetic macrocyclic ketone analogues of halichondrin B. *Cancer Res*. 61: 1013–1021.

Trimurtulu, G., I. Ohtani, and G. M. L. Patterson. 1994. Total Structures of cryptophycins, potent antitumor depsipeptides from the blue-green alga *Nostoc* sp. strain GSV 224. *J. Am. Chem. Soc*. 116: 4729–4737.

Tsuda, M. and J. Kobayashi. 1997. Structures and biogenesis of manzamine and related alkaloids. *Heterocycles* 46: 765–794.

Tsuji, S., K. L. Rinehart, S. P. Gunasekera et al. 1988. Topsentin, bromotopsentin, and dihydrode-oxybromotopsentin: Antiviral and antitumor bis(indolyl)imidazoles from Caribbean deep-sea sponges of the family Halichondriidae. Structural and synthetic studies. *J. Org. Chem*. 53(23): 5446–5453.

Uemura, D., K. Takahashi, T. Yamamoto et al. 1985. Norhalichondrin A: An antitumor polyether macrolide from a marine sponge. *J. Am. Chem. Soc*. 107: 4796–4798.

Vaishampayan, U., M. Glode, W. Du et al. 2000. Phase II study of dolastatin 10 in patients with hormone-refractory metastatic prostate adenocarcinoma. *Clin. Cancer Res*. 6: 4205–4208.

van Kestren, C., M. M. de Vooght, L. López-Lázaro et al. 2003. Yondelis (trabectedin, ET-743): The development of an anticancer agent of marine origin. *Anti-Cancer Drugs* 14: 487–502.

Villalona-Calero, M. A., S. D. Baker, L. Hammond et al. 1998. Phase I and pharmacokinetic study of the water-soluble dolastatin 15 analog LU103793 in patients with advanced solid malignancies. *J. Clin. Oncol*. 16: 2770–2779.

Wagman, G. H., R. D. Gannon, and M. J. Weinstein. 1969. Production of vitamin B12 by micromonos-pora. *Appl. Microbiol*. 17(4): 648–649.

Walker, G., P. Brown, A. K. Forrest, P. O'Hanlon, and J. E. Pons. 1993. Chemistry of antibacterials/antibiotics. In *Recent Advances in the Chemistry of Anti-Infective Agents*, eds. P. H. Bentley and R. Ponsford, p. 106. Royal Society of Chemistry, London, U.K.

Wall, N. R., R. M. Mohammad, and A. M. Al-Katib. 1999. Bax:Bcl-2 ratio modulation by bryostatin 1 and novel antitubulin agents is important for susceptibility to drug induced apoptosis in the human early pre-B acute lymphoblastic leukemia cell line. *Reh. Leuk. Res*. 23: 881–888.

Wang, J. H., J. Kong, W. Li et al. 2006. A beta-galactose-specific lectin isolated from the marine worm *Chaetopterus variopedatus* possesses anti-HIV-1 activity. *Comp. Biochem. Physiol. C Pharmacol*. 142: 111–117.

Watanabe, J., T. Natsume, and M. Kobayashi. 2007. Comparison of the antivascular and cytotoxic activities of TZT-1027 (Soblidotin) with those of other anticancer agents. *Anticancer Drugs* 18: 905–911.

Wehrli, S. L., K. S. Moore, H. Roder, S. Durell, and M. Zasloff. 1993. Structure of the novel steroidal antibiotic squalamine determined by two-dimensional NMR spectroscopy. *Steroids* 58: 370–378.

Wender, P. A., J.-M. Kee, and J. M. Warrington. 2008. Practical synthesis of prostratin DPP and their analogs, adjuvant leads against latent HIV. *Science* 320: 649–652.

Wilson, L., D. Panda, and M. A. Jordan. 1999. Modulation of microtubule dynamics by drugs: A paradigm for the actions of cellular regulators. *Cell Struct. Funct*. 24: 329–335.

Winter, J. M., A. L. Jansma, T. M. Handel, and B. S. Moore. 2009. Formation of the pyridazine natural product azamerone by biosynthetic rearrangement of an aryl diazoketone. *Angew. Chem. Int. Ed*. 48: 767–770.

Wolff, I., U. Bruntsch, F. Cavalli, J. de Jonk, I. M. von Broen, and C. Sessa. 1996. Phase I clinical and pharmacokinetic study of the dolastatin analogue LU103793 on a weekly × 4 schedule. *Ann. Oncol.* 7(suppl 5): 124.

Wright, A. E., D. A. Forleo, G. P. Gunawardana, S. P. Gunasekera, F. E. Koehn, and O. J. McConnell. 1990. Antitumor tetrahydroisoquinoline alkaloids from the colonial ascidian *Ecteinascidia turbinate*. *J. Org. Chem.* 55: 4508–4512.

Wright, A. E., S. A. Pomponi, S. S. Cross, and P. McCarthy. 1992. A new bis-(indole)alkaloid from a deep-water marine sponge of the genus *Spongosorites*. *J. Org. Chem.* 57: 4772–4775.

Wright, A. E., S. A. Pomponi, and R. S. Jacobs. 1999. Compounds and methods of use for treatment of neurogenic inflammation. *PCT Int. Appl.* 29: WO 9942092.

Wylie, B. L., N. B. Ernst, K. J. S. Grace, and R. S. Jacobs. 1997. Marine natural products as phospholipase A$_2$ inhibitors. In: *Phospholipase A$_2$: Basic and Clinical Aspects in Inflammatory Diseases,* Eds. W. Uhl, T. J. Nevaleinen, and M. W. Büchler, Karger, Basel, Vol. 24, pp. 146–152.

Xie, W., D. Ding, W. Zi, G. Li, and D. Ma. 2008. Total synthesis and structure assignment of papuamide B, a potent marine cyclodepsipeptide with anti-HIV properties. *Angew. Chem. Int. Ed.* 47: 2844–2848.

Xu, D. D., L. Waykole, J. V. Calienni et al. 2003. An expedient synthesis of LAF389, a bengamide B analogue. *Org. Process Res. Dev.* 796: 856–865.

Yamashita, A., E. B. Norton, J. A. Kaplan et al. 2004. Synthesis and activity of novel analogs of hemiasterlin as inhibitors of tubulin polymerization: Modification of the A segment. *Bioorg. Med. Chem. Lett.* 14: 5317–5322.

Yang, L. and R. J. Andersen. 2002. Absolute configuration of the antiinflammatory sponge natural product contignasterol. *J. Nat. Prod.* 65(12): 1924–1926.

Yasuhara-Bell, J. and Y. Lu. 2010. Marine compounds and their antiviral activities. *Antiviral Res.* 86(3): 231–240.

Yeung, T., G. E. Gilbert, J. Shi, J. Silvius, A. Kapus, and S. Grinstein. 2008. Membrane phosphatidyl-serine regulates surface charge and protein localization. *Science* 319: 210–213.

Yim, J. H., E. Son, S. Pyo, and H. K. Lee. 2005. Novel sulfated polysaccharide derived from redtide microalga *Gyrodinium impudicum* strain KG03 with immunostimulating activity in vivo. *Mar. Biotechnol. (NY)* 7: 331–338.

Young, R. N. 1999. Importance of biodiversity to the modern pharmaceutical industry. *Pure Appl. Chem.* 71: 1655–1661.

Yousaf, M., K. A. El Sayed, K. V. Rao et al. 2002. 12,34-Oxamanzamines, novel biocatalytic and natural products from manzamine producing Indo-Pacific sponges. *Tetrahedron* 58: 7397–7402.

Yousaf, M., N. L. Hammond, J. Peng et al. 2004. New manzamine alkaloids from an Indo-Pacific sponge. Pharmacokinetics, oral availability, and the significant activity of several manzamines against HIV-I, AIDS opportunistic infections, and inflammatory diseases. *J. Med. Chem.* 47: 3512–3517.

Yu, M., B. Littlefield, and Y. Kishi. 2005. Discovery of E7389, a fully synthetic macrocyclic ketone analog of halichondrin B. In *Anticancer Agents from Natural Products,* eds. G. M. Cragg, D. G. I. Kingston, and D. J. Newman, pp. 241–265. Taylor & Francis Group, Boca Raton, FL.

Yun, S. S. and W. Li. 2007. Identification of squalamine in the plasma membrane of white blood cells in the sea lamprey, *Petromyzon marinus. J. Lipid Res.* 48: 2579–2586.

Zampella, A., M. V. D'Auria, L. Gomez-Paloma et al. 1996. Callipeltin A, an anti-HIV cyclic depsipeptide from the New Caledonian Lithistida sponge *Callipelta* sp. *J. Am. Chem. Soc.* 118: 6202–6209.

Zarai, Z., A. B. Bacha, H. Horchani, S. Bezzine, N. Zouari, and Y. Gargouri. 2010. A novel hepato-pancreatic phospholipase A2 from *Hexaplex trunculus* with digestive and toxic activities. *Arch. Biochem. Biophys.* 494(2): 121–129.

Zask, A., G. Birnberg, K. Cheung et al. 2004a. Synthesis and biological activity of analogues of the antimicrotubule agent N,β,β- trimethyl-l-phenylalanyl-N1-[(1S,2E)-3-carboxy- 1-isopropylbut-2-enyl]-N1,3-dimethyl-l-valinamide (HTI-286). *J. Med. Chem.* 47: 4774–4786.

Zask, A., G. Birnberg, K. Cheung et al. 2004b. D-piece modifications of the hemiasterlin analog HTI-286 produce potent tubulin inhibitors. *Bioorg. Med. Chem. Lett.* 14: 4353–4358.

Zasloff, M., A. P. Adams, B. Beckerman et al. 2011. Squalamine as a broad-spectrum systemic antiviral agent with therapeutic potential. *Proc. Natl Acad. Sci. USA* 108: 15978–15983.

Zewail-Foote, M. and L. H. Hurley. 1999. Ecteinascidin 743: A minor groove alkylator that bends DNA toward the major groove? *J. Med. Chem.* 42: 2493–2497.

12

Environmental and Human Impact on Marine Microorganism—Synthesized Nanoparticles

L. Karthik, Gaurav Kumar, and K.V. Bhaskara Rao

CONTENTS

12.1 Marine Microorganisms

The biological and chemical diversity of the marine environment has been the source of unique chemical compounds with the potential for industrial development as pharmaceuticals, cosmetics, nutritional supplements, molecular probes, enzymes, fine chemicals, and agrichemicals (Ireland et al. 1993). The oceans represent a virtually untapped resource for the discovery of even more novel compounds with useful activity. Even though the commercial success stories in biotechnology are familiar, such stories in marine biotechnology are far less familiar and far fewer (Zilinskas et al. 1995). In the last decade, there has been a continuous effort to learn more about the still largely unexplored realm of marine-related products.

Besides microorganisms like bacteria, fungi, and actinobacteria, many other marine organisms such as fishes, prawns, crabs, snakes, plants, and algae have also been studied to tap the arsenal of the marine world. Properties like high salt tolerance, hyperthermostability, barophilicity, cold adaptivity, and ease in large-scale cultivation are the key interests of scientists. These properties may not be expected in terrestrial sources as marine organisms thrive in habitats such as hydrothermal vents, oceanic caves, and some areas where high pressure and absence of light are obvious (Ghosh 2004).

Marine bioactive compounds are organic compounds produced by prokaryotes and eukaryotes. The organic compound was helping the host organism to protect them against predators. So far, less than 1.0% of the total marine organisms producing bioactive metabolites are known. The seawater has bactericidal properties and it endorses the production of antibiotics by planktonic algae and bacteria, respectively.

12.2 What Are Nanoparticles?

Nanotechnology is a rapidly developing field. Nanotechnology refers to the synthesis and applications of nanoparticles (NPs). "Nano" is derived from the Greek word "nanos," which means dwarf or extremely small. NPs have a size of one billionth of a meter (i.e., 10^{-9} m). Particles of size between 1 and 100 nm are termed NPs. The double helical DNA is measured to be 2.5 nm. The NPs are drawing the attention of scientists because of their unique properties. The properties of the materials change with respect to their size (Buzea et al. 2007).

The term "nanotechnology" was first used by the Japanese scientist Norio Taniguchi in 1974. He was a professor in Tokyo Science University. He has mentioned in a paper that "Nano-technology mainly consists of the processing of separation, consolidation and deformation of materials by one atom one molecule." Dr. K. Eric Drexler gave the appropriate definition and technological significance of nanotechnology in the 1980s in his speeches and books.

12.2.1 Synthesis of Nanoparticles

There are several methods for synthesizing NPs physically, chemically, and biologically.

12.2.1.1 Physical Synthesis

In physical synthesis, two methods are employed. They are planetary ball milling and pyrolysis.

12.2.1.1.1 Planetary Ball Milling

Planetary ball milling is generally known as mechanical alloying and widely used for NP preparation. It is capable of producing solid–solid, solid–liquid, and solid–gas chemical reactions. It can be used for large-scale production. The important parameters for the mechanical milling process are milling time, milling speed, charge ratio, temperature, nature of milling, atmosphere, chemical composition of the powder mixture, milling machine, etc. In this method the particles are ground by a size-reducing mechanism and air classified to get the oxidized NPs (Goya 2004).

12.2.1.1.2 Pyrolysis

In pyrolysis, an organic precursor is forced through an orifice using high pressure and burned. Then the ash is air classified to get the oxidized NPs. In both of the aforementioned methods, the major disadvantage is high consumption of energy to maintain pressure and temperature. It is highly cost-effective (Grimm et al. 1997).

12.2.1.2 Chemical Synthesis

In wet-chemical methods, the NPs were produced in a liquid medium that contains reducing agents like sodium borohydride or potassium bitartrate or hydrazine. The agglomeration of NPs is protected by adding stabilizing agents like sodium dodecyl benzyl sulfate or polyvinyl pyrrolidone. The chemical synthesis methods are cost-effective, but the major disadvantage is usage of toxic solvents, resulting in the formation of hazardous by-products (Kaushik et al. 2010).

12.2.1.3 Biological Synthesis

There are many drawbacks in both the physical and chemical synthesis. The synthesis of metal NPs by physical and chemical methods has many disadvantages like costliness and high energy input, and toxicity of the chemicals used, side effects, and harmful by-products, respectively. Hence, an alternative method by which the abovesaid disadvantages could be overcome has to be developed in order to yield safer products in a cost-effective method. Plants, bacteria, yeast, fungi, viruses, algae, etc., were reported to synthesize NPs in an eco-friendly method (Kaushik et al. 2010). Hence, there is an ever-increasing need to develop the high-yield, low-cost, environment-friendly method for the production of NPs, and the biological method is much suitable for the NP synthesis. Both the unicellular and multicellular organisms are known for their capacity of intracellular or extracellular production of metallic NPs. The major advantages of biological synthesis are cost-effectiveness and nontoxicity.

12.2.2 Reports on Biological Synthesis of NPs in Indian Scenario

12.2.2.1 Silver NP Synthesis

Silver NPs (AgNPs) were synthesized by *Candida glabrata* and *Fusarium oxysporum*. The NPs were spherical in shape and the size was in the range of 45–60 and 75–100 nm, respectively. The NPs exhibited antimicrobial activity against *Staphylococcus aureus*, *Escherichia coli*, *Klebsiella pneumoniae*, *Bacillus subtilis*, *Enterococcus faecalis*, and *Pseudomonas aeruginosa*. The antibacterial activity increased with the increase in concentration (Namasivayam et al. 2011). *Cladosporium cladosporioides* were reported to synthesize AgNPs extracellularly.

The extracellular synthesis made the harvest of the AgNPs easier and the quantity was also large. The NPs were crystalline in nature when analyzed by x-ray diffraction (XRD). Transmission electron microscopy (TEM) images were used to confirm the size and it measured about 10–100 nm. Fungal proteins, polysaccharides, and organic acids enhanced the synthesis (Balaji et al. 2009).

Multidrug-resistant pathogens pose a serious threat in the field of medicine. Silver has antimicrobial activity. AgNPs synthesized by *S. aureus* showed inhibitory effect on the multidrug-resistant pathogenic strains. The AgNPs were active against many pathogens subsuming methicillin-resistant *Staphylococcus aureus* (MRSA) and methicillin-resistant *Staphylococcus epidermidis* (MRSE). The advances in generating AgNPs have made possible a revival of the use of silver as a powerful bactericide. The present research work mostly emphasized MRSA and MRSE, because they are found to be resistant to a wide range of broad-spectrum antibiotics. The extracellular synthesis would make the process easier for downstream processing (Nanda and Saravanan 2009). Biologically, AgNPs were synthesized when silver nitrate was exposed to the fungi *F. oxysporum*. The synthesis was extracellular as the fungi excreted the enzyme that reduced the silver nitrate into silver ions. The silver ions were reduced by an NADH-dependent reductase. Upon characterization, the AgNPs were of 5–50 nm in size. The NPs were spherical and triangular in shape (Ahmad et al. 2003a).

Fusarium solani, a phytopathogen, was reported to synthesize AgNPs extracellularly. The size of AgNPs was 5–35 nm. Upon characterization using Fourier transform infrared spectroscopy (FTIR), it was found that the presence of proteins as capping agents increased the stability (Ingle et al. 2008). *Aspergillus fumigatus* was reported to synthesize AgNPs. The synthesis occurred in a few minutes upon the addition of substrate. The filamentous fungus, *A. fumigatus*, has shown potential for extracellular synthesis of fairly monodispersed AgNPs in the range of 5–25 nm (Bhainsa and Souza 2006). Silver-tolerant yeast strain MYK3 synthesized AgNPs extracellularly. The size was about 2–5 nm (Kowshik et al. 2003). AgNPs and gold NPs (AuNPs) were reported to be synthesized by the fungi *Verticillium* sp. The synthesis was intracellular as the NPs accumulated within the fungal biomass. The AgNPs were 25–12 nm in size and adhered to the cytoplasmic membrane.

12.2.2.2 Zinc Oxide, Titanium Dioxide, and BaTiO₃

Zinc oxide (ZnO) NPs with the size of 2–18 nm were synthesized using a natural surfactant. The ZnO particles showed antibacterial and antifungal activity (Sharma et al. 2010). $BaTiO_3$ NPs were synthesized using *Lactobacillus* sp. in an economical method. The synthesis was also environment-friendly. The synthesized NPs were characterized using XRD and TEM. The size was found to be 20–80 nm (Jha and Prasad 2009). Titanium dioxide (TiO_2) NPs synthesized by *Lactobacillus* and baker's yeast (*Saccharomyces cerevisiae*). The NPs were characterized by XRD and TEM. The size was measured to be 8–35 nm. The reaction might involve the action of membrane-bound oxidoreductase (Jha et al. 2009).

12.2.2.3 Gold Nanoparticles

An alkalotolerant actinomycete, *Rhodococcus* sp., produced intracellular AuNPs with good monodispersity. The NPs were concentrated on the cytoplasmic membrane and cell wall. The size of AuNPs was of 5–15 nm (Ahmad et al. 2003b). The extremophilic actinomycete

Thermomonospora sp. reduced the $AuCl_4$- ions into Au0 NPs extracellularly. The NPs were spherical in shape with an average size of 8 nm (Sastry et al. 2003).

12.2.3 Reports on Biological Synthesis in International Scenario

12.2.3.1 Silver and Gold

Candida guilliermondii was reported to synthesize AuNPs and AgNPs. The NPs exhibited antimicrobial property against pathogens. The sizes of the synthesized AuNPs and AgNPs were 50–70 and 10–20 nm, respectively (Mishra et al. 2011). AgNPs were synthesized in a green method by using *Streptomyces hygroscopicus*. The biologically synthesized AgNPs showed a greater antimicrobial activity against gram-positive and gram-negative bacteria and also the yeast pathogens. Upon characterization, they were of 20–30 nm in size. The advantages of the biological synthesis were high biosafety, eco-friendliness, and nontoxicity. Further the AgNPs showed antimicrobial activity against many clinically important pathogens (Sadhasivam et al. 2010).

A filamentous fungus, *Neurospora crassa*, was reported to synthesize AgNPs and AuNPs when exposed to the respective precursors. It was observed that *N. crassa* was a potential nanofactory for the synthesis of metal NPs. The advantage is that this is a nonpathogenic organism. Apart from that, the organism has a fast growth rate, rapid reduction of metals, etc. The fast and easy method was for the production of mono- and bimetallic Ag/AuNPs using *N. crassa* (Castro et al. 2011). Using the culture supernatants of *K. pneumoniae*, *E. coli*, and *Enterobacter cloacae* (Enterobacteriaceae), a rapid synthesis of AgNPs had been reported. The synthesis was rapid that the result was observed within 5 min of the addition of the precursor. This method remained an economical means of synthesis (Shahverdi et al. 2007).

Various organisms including bacteria, fungi, and yeasts were reported to synthesize AuNPs of different sizes and shapes. The most promising results were obtained with the yeast *Pichia jadinii* and the fungal cultures *Verticillium luteoalbum* and Isolate 6–3. The NPs were analyzed using TEM and SEM. NPs with a size of approximately 100 nm were accumulated intracellularly (Gericke and Pinches 2006). *F. oxysporum* was used to synthesize the AgNPs. The synthesized NPs were proven to be an antibacterial agent. The AgNPs were incorporated onto the silk and cotton cloths and checked for the antibacterial activity. It was reported that the cotton cloth incorporated with silver exhibited the antibacterial activity against *S. aureus*, thus making the cotton cloth sterile (Marcato et al. 2005).

12.2.3.2 Zinc Oxide and Zinc Phosphate

ZnO NPs have been synthesized using an eco-friendly method, by decomposing bacterial cellulose (BC) infiltrated with zinc acetate aqueous solution at high temperature. A BC membrane was obtained from *Acetobacter xylinum* cultures. Upon characterization, the NPs were well dispersed with the size of 20–50 nm (Hu et al. 2010). Zinc phosphate NPs were synthesized through biomineralization by chemical precipitation using yeast cells. The NPs were characterized and the size was found to be 80–200 nm in length and 10–80 nm in width (Yan et al. 2009).

12.2.4 Characterization of Nanoparticles

The physicochemical characterization of the NPs is important to study their applications. Hence, sample preparation, selection of instrument, and application are listed in Table 12.1.

TABLE 12.1

Characterization of Metal Nanoparticles

Instruments	Sample Preparation	Application	Mechanism
Electronic, optical analysis			
UV–visible spectroscopy	Microbial supernatant	Finds out the absorbance of metal NPs	Magnitude, wavelength, and bandwidth of the plasmon resonance associated with the particle size, shape, and material composition
UV photoelectron spectroscopy	Microbial supernatant	Band structure of the NPs has been evaluated	Measurement of kinetic energy spectra of photoelectrons emitted by molecules
Structural analysis			
SEM/FESEM	Liquid or solid	It is used to view the dispersion of NPs	3D images (up to ×300,000). Surface structure of nanocomposite, fracture surface, and nanocoating can be observed with good clarity
TEM/HRTEM	Supernatant	Dispersion, distribution, exfoliation, intercalation, and orientation of NPs can be visualized	Crystallographic structure of a sample at an atomic scale, highest resolution achieved at 0.8 Å
SPM	Supernatant thin film	Topology view of NPs (structure, properties, and surfaces of NPs)	Quantitatively measuring the nanometer scale surface roughness
XRD	Powder	It provides the information about crystal, crystal size, orientation of crystal, and phase composition in semicrystalline polymer	It is produced when electrically charged particles of sufficient energy are decelerated
Chemical analysis			
XPS	Powder	Quantitate the elements that are present within 10 nm of the sample surface, chemical state, and electronic state of elements	Kinetic energy and the number of electron escaping from the surface of the material
EDX	Supernatant	The amount of NPs near and at the surface can be estimated	It is connected with SEM. When element crosses the electron beam, it shows the image of each elements
Temperature-programmed desorption	Supernatant	Characterizing the acid sites on oxide surfaces	The surface is heated and the energy transferred to the adsorbed species

TABLE 12.1 (continued)

Characterization of Metal Nanoparticles

Instruments	Sample Preparation	Application	Mechanism
Vibrational analysis			
FTIR	Powder	To find out the functional group of the molecule responsible for synthesis of NPs	It acquires spectrum of light emitted by the molecule and this emission could be induced by various processes
Raman spectroscopy	Supernatant	It provides the fingerprint of the molecule and orientation of the crystal	When light passes to the molecules, it interacts with the electron cloud of the bond of that molecule
Particle size analyzer			
Dynamic light scattering	Supernatant	Size distribution of the NPs can be estimated	Due to the bombardment of the particle, it induces the motion and its exposure with laser. The intensity of the scattered light fluctuation depends on the particle size

12.3 Impact of Metal Nanoparticles on Human Health

Metal NPs find applications in many fields like biosensors, biolabeling (Cho et al. 2005), antimicrobial therapy, and drug delivery (Mishra et al. 2011). NPs made of semiconducting material that may also be termed quantum dots (usually 10 nm or even less in size) are used in biomedical applications as drug carriers or imaging agents. Semisolid and soft NPs have been manufactured. A prototype NP of semisolid nature is the liposome. Various types of liposome NPs are currently used clinically as delivery systems for anticancer drugs and vaccines. Nanotechnology has a promising future in many fields including medicine. NPs help in the detection and treatment of cancers (Fortina et al. 2007).

12.3.1 Silver Nanoparticles

The oldest detail of silver as an antimicrobial came from Herodotus in 450 BC. He told that the King of Persia kept boiled water in flagons of silver to keep the water fresh. Ancient Romans kept silver pieces at the bottom of milk containers. In the seventeenth and eighteenth centuries, silver nitrate was used to treat open wounds mainly caused by burns. In 1869, it was reported that *Aspergillus niger* could not grow in silver-lined vessels (Klasen 2000)

In the year 1880, silver nitrate solution was used to protect the newborns from the common eye infection called ophthalmia neonatorum, and a similar treatment is still used (Forbes 1971). In the late 1940s, silver sulfadiazine was used as the standard treatment for the wounds caused by burns. Before the twentieth century, the silver was processed by grinding and reducing it to fine powder. This presented a drawback that the fine silver powder does not stay suspended in the solution for long. In nanoparticulate form, they are mixed with a liquid base; this permits for solution dispensation of tiny, crystalline metallic particles. This also increases the surface area greatly and this allows the mainstream of silver atoms to react more. Even U.S. silver dollar were once placed in milk jugs for prevention of microbe growth and this is a great example of the antimicrobial activity of silver. This coin contains 26.96 g of coin silver; it is 40 mm in diameter and approximately 27.70 cm² in surface area. If the same silver coin were divided into particles 1 nm in diameter, the total surface area of those particles would increase 11,400 m², i.e., 4.115 million times greater than the normal surface area of the silver dollar, and it will be a more effective antimicrobial agent as compared to the coin as a whole.

The silver ion and silver-based compounds are highly toxic to microorganisms, and show strong biocidal effects against 16 species of bacteria and fungi. The silver toxicity machinery mainly relies on the interaction between the metal and cellular membranes. The silver binds either to membrane-bound proteins or to the lipid bilayer of the plasma membrane, and thereby destabilizes the membrane, causing ion leakage and cell rupture. And inside the cell, silver binds to mitochondrial membranes and disrupts the function; it also interferes with the energy (ATP)-yielding reactions of the respiratory chain. Silver binds specifically to cellular enzymes and DNA interferes with their functions. An AgNP can directly insert into the yeast membrane; it is very small, it may destabilize the membrane and release silver ions locally from the silver particle directly into the microbe. This mechanism can overcome the limitation of biotoxicity to the host as much smaller amounts are needed. The mode of action of nanoparticulate silver is thought to be similar to that of silver ions (Lansdown 2010).

Silver has been used as antimicrobial agent since ancient days. As antibacterial agents, AgNPs have a wide range of applications from disinfecting medical devices and home appliances to water treatment (Li et al. 2007). Silver is widely used in topical gels and impregnated into bandages because of its wide-spectrum antimicrobial activity (Slawson et al. 1992). Alginate, a naturally occurring biopolymer, is used in wound management procedures (Hermans 2006). Silver sulfadiazine is used to treat burns. Silver inhibits the growth of bacteria and fungi on clothing (Lansdown 2010). AgNPs have many important applications that include spectrally selective coating for solar energy absorption and intercalation material for electrical batteries, as optical receptors (McFarland and Duyne 2003), polarizing filters, catalysts in chemical reaction (Jiang et al. 2005), and biolabeling (Hayat 1989). The antibacterial action of silver electrodes increases when coated with silver nanorods (Akhavan and Ghaderi 2009). Currently AgNPs have found applications in catalysis, optics, and electronics and as antibacterial/antifungal agents in biotechnology and bioengineering, textile engineering, water treatment, and silver-based consumer products.

12.3.2 Zinc Oxide Nanoparticles

ZnO particles have been found to have superior ultraviolet (UV) blocking properties and hence used in the preparation of sunscreen lotions and are completely photostable (Mitchnick et al. 1999). ZnO NPs dispersed in industrial coatings to protect wood, plastic, and textiles from exposure to UV rays. ZnO has high refractive index, high thermal conductivity, binding, antibacterial, and UV-protection properties. Consequently, it is added into various materials and products, including plastics, ceramics, glass, cement, rubber, lubricants (Hernandez Battez et al. 2008), paints, ointments, adhesive, sealants, pigments, foods, batteries, ferrites, and fire retardants. ZnO has antibacterial and deodorizing property (Padmavathy et al. 2008) and is used in topical agents like baby powders, band aid, and shampoos (Hughes and McLean 1988; Harding 2007). It is also used in cigarette filters, in food additives, used as pigments in paints, in electric field emitters and other electronics (Look 2001; Kucheyev 2003; Li et al. 2004), and as biosensors. It is also used in rubber manufacturing (Brown 1957, 1976) and concrete industry (Brown 1957) and also added to various materials like cotton fabric, rubber, and food packaging (Saito 1993).

12.3.3 Titanium Dioxide Nanoparticles

TiO_2 is used as white pigment in cosmetics, food coloring, tattooing, etc., as opacifier in paints, coatings, plastics, papers, inks, foods, medicines (i.e., pills and tablets), as well as in most of the toothpastes. It is used as sunscreen and thickener in cosmetics and topical products. TiO_2, particularly in the anatase form, serves as a photocatalyst under UV light. TiO_2 has sterilizing, deodorizing, and antifouling properties. It is used as a photocatalyst, protein (Jones et al. 2007), circuit element, solar cells (Lewis 2009), semiconductor (Earle 1942), cleaver in dielectric mirrors (Paschotta 2009), etc. Apart from these, titanium oxide reduces the airborne pollutants (Hogan 2004) and is also used as an antifogging agent.

12.3.4 Gold Nanoparticles

AuNPs have been widely known for many centuries. Until the 1990s, AuNPs were able to be synthesized in aqueous solutions with little functionalization of the NP due to the synthetic procedures that existed. In 1994, Brust–Schiffrin developed a synthetic technique for the production of AuNPs (Brust et al. 1994). Murray further developed this synthesis to get many different functional groups and with various sizes of AuNPs. Gold colloid research is not new but has been gradually researched over the previous century and a half (Daniel and Astruc 2004). In 1685, gold colloid's preparation was published by Andreas Cassius in *De Auro*, which went on to bring fame to his name, whereas preparation of soluble gold became known as "purple of Cassius" (Hunt 1976). Gold colloids have been used widely in biological applications such as treatment of arthritis (Visuthikosol and Kumpolpunth 1981) and carcinoma (Fountain and Malkasian 1981) and in imaging of proteins and DNA. In ancient China, gold powder was used extensively in medicine, painting, and clothing; to promote long life; and as an antibiotic (Huaizhi and Ning 2003). Research in recent years has allowed for the designing of AuNPs for DNA recognition.

Based on human welfare, we covered four important types of metal NPs and their roles and applications in human health, for example, ranging from identification of a cancer to chemotherapy. Hence, some of the biological syntheses of NPs and their applications are reported here.

12.4 Biological Synthesis of NPs Using Marine Microorganisms and Their Impact on Human Health Care

In this topic, we have covered the metallic NPs synthesized by using marine microorganisms as it is less studied. It is more important to human health-care system. When compared to terrestrial microorganisms, their marine counterparts show less toxic effects.

Generally the molecules produced by microorganisms help to synthesize and stabilize the NPs, and in some condition they can act as antigens; hence, using marine microorganism is safer to synthesize NPs because it is not pathogenic to humans. Most of the studies reported on antimicrobial activity of NPs; hence, in future it can be a promising source for combination therapy and drug resistance occurrences should be less.

12.4.1 Marine Bacteria

Marine bacteria attractive to attention from researchers because they are enriched with bioactive compounds with unique biological properties (Fenical 1993). Until now, marine *Pseudomonas, Pseudoalteromonas, Bacillus,* and *Vibrio* isolated from seawater, sediments, algae, and marine invertebrates are known to produce bioactive agents. They are able to produce indole derivatives (quinines and violacein), alkaloids (prodiginines and tambjamines), polyenes, macrolides, peptides, and terpenoids. In 1947, Rosenfeld and Zobell observed marine bacteria producing bioactive substances. In 1966, Burkholder et al. reported the first documented bioactive marine bacterial metabolite, brominated pyrrole antibiotic.

Laatsch (2005) compared the 250 marine bacterial metabolites and 150 isolated from terrestrial bacteria between 2000 and 2005. Bioactive compounds from marine microorganisms show promising biological activities; it is difficult to point out any particular bioactive agent that has readily been commercialized as a medicine. Currently, 13 bioactive compounds from marine microorganisms are in different phases of clinical trials and a large number of others are under preclinical investigations (Mayer et al. 2010), highlighting the importance of bioactive natural compounds. Marine *Pseudomonas* sp. ram bt-1 were synthesizing monodisperse AgNPs intracellularly, and they are quite stable in solution for months. The AgNPs have different morphological shapes such as spherical to triangular ranging from 20 to 100 nm in size (Rammohan and Balakrishnan 2011). In 2010, Kathiresan et al. reported 45 kDa proteins from *E. coli* synthesizing spherical-shaped AgNPs, ranging in size from 5 to 20 nm. It shows antibacterial activity against certain clinical pathogens and they also reported the polyvinyl alcohol enhancing antimicrobial activity. Magnetotactic bacteria synthesize magnetic iron nanominerals with size ranging from 50 to 100 nm. These bacteria occur in the oxic–anoxic transition zone of a water column (Chen et al. 2010). Hence, the studies on marine bacteria–mediated NP synthesis are therefore essential.

12.4.2 Marine Fungi

The biomedical application of marine fungi is less studied compared to terrestrial fungi as a major biomedicinal resource (penicillin from *Penicillium*). In 1980, Schiehser confirmed that marine fungi are important resource for unique metabolites (lactone, leptosphaerin from *Leptosphaeria oraemaris*). Later, Shin and Fenical (1987) isolated gliovictin from marine fungus *Asteromyces cruciatus*. So far, more than 20 useful bioactive compounds have been derived from marine fungi. Kathiresan et al. (2009) reported extracellular synthesis of silver NPs using marine fungus, *Penicillium fellutanum*. They achieved maximum level of synthesized NPs, when the culture filtrate was treated with 1.0 mM AgNO$_3$, maintained at 0.3% NaCl and pH 6.0, incubated at 5°C for 24 h. The size and shape of the NPs was spherical shape and 5 to 25 nm respectively. They also reported extracellular biosynthesis of antimicrobial AgNPs by *A. niger* AUCAS 237 derived from a coastal mangrove sediment of southeast India. The size ranges from 5 to 35 nm. The antimicrobial activity of AgNPs from *A. niger* was reported. Bhimba et al. (2011) observed marine fungi *Hypocrea lixii* MV1 isolated from mangrove sediment soil synthesizing antibacterial AgNPs. This research team highlighted the possibility of using marine fungi for the synthesis of antimicrobial AgNPs.

12.4.3 Marine Yeast

The terrestrial distributed yeast is important in food industry, production of biofuel, biocontrol of fungi in agriculture, and other applications in biotechnology. The aquatic distributed yeast has different metabolic attributes when compared to terrestrial yeast (Kutty and Philip 2008). Zhenming et al. (2006) found that marine yeasts could produce bioactive substances with potential application in mariculture, food, pharmaceutical, cosmetic, and chemical industries and environmental protection. Marine yeast *Yarrowia lipolytica* has been demonstrated for intracellular synthesis of AuNPs. In acidic pH, NPs with a size of 15 nm were synthesized. The reductases or proteases may be responsible for the reduction of the gold salt into NPs (Agnihotri et al. 2009). Out of 12 species of marine yeasts, *Pichia capsulata* exhibited synthesis of AgNPs within minutes. This work reveals that using marine yeasts achieves a faster rate of AgNP synthesis (Subramanian et al. 2010).

Seshadri et al. (2011) reported the intracellular synthesis of stable lead sulfide (PbS) NPs by a marine yeast, *Rhodosporidium diobovatum*. PbS NPs were cubic in structure with their size ranging from 2–5 nm. The overall recovery of PbS NPs was 90%.

Dinesh et al. (2011) observed that the extracellular biosynthesis of AgNPs was performed by using marine yeast *Candida* sp. VITDKGB. The AgNPs of around 87 nm were formed. Biologically synthesized AgNPs were further examined for antimicrobial activity against multidrug-resistant *S. aureus* and *K. pneumoniae*. *S. aureus* formed a 14.66 ± 1.52 mm zone of inhibition with an MIC value of 20 µg/mL, whereas *K. pneumoniae* formed a 12.33 ± 0.57 mm zone of inhibition with an MIC value of 40 µg/mL.

12.4.4 Marine Algae

So far, 25% of isolated marine algae were only evaluated for their biological activity. They are classified into two types, namely microalgae and macroalgae. Microalgae are a potential source of bioactive compounds, particularly chemotherapy agents for treatment of cancer (Moore et al. 1988). In 1961, Sieburth reported *Phaeocystis pouchetii* producing antibiotics such as acrylic acid, and it was transferred to the food chain of marine animals like Antarctic penguins. Macroalgae produce many beneficial products for example, 1,4-diacetoxy-butadiene from green algae, halogenated lipids from the red algae *Laurencia* sp, prostaglandin from *Gracilaria lichenoides*, brown algae, green algae, etc. (Satoh et al. 1987). In Japan, Nakagawa et al. (1987) observed that Ulva meal–supplemented black sea bream showed high growth rate and resistance against diseases. *Porphyra yezoensis* producing polysaccharide fractions induce the phagocytic function (Yoshizawa et al. 1995).

AuNPs were synthesized using extracellular extract of *Sargassum wightii* and monodispersity was achieved in a short duration. The size was in the range of 8–12 nm. *Sargassum* synthesizes highly stable AuNPs (Singaravelu et al. 2009). It is also used in Chinese medicine in the treatment of cancer, goiters, testicular pain and swelling, edema, urinary infections, and sore throat. In the future, this combination treatment may be a powerful tool in the field of medicine.

The potential of the brown alga *Turbinaria conoides* in biosorption and bioreduction of Au (III) was explored. The proposed mechanism was electrostatic interactions between gold anions and algal functional groups (polysaccharides) for biosorption (Vijayaraghavan et al. 2011). Shakibaie et al. (2010) carried out similar kind of work;

AuNPs were synthesized using *Tetraselmis suecica*. A polysaccharide isolated from *Porphyra vietnamensis* was used to synthesize AgNPs. The average particle size was found to be 13 ± 3 nm. The synthesized AgNPs revealed strong antibacterial activity against gram-negative bacteria (5 µg/mL) as compared to gram-positive bacteria (15 µg/mL) (Venkatpurwar and Pokharkar 2011). Rajasulochana et al. (2010) reported AuNP synthesis using *Kappaphycus alvarezii*. It is a rapid extracellular synthesis of spherical morphology AuNPs. This is not toxic to algal cells. Vivek et al. (2011) reported antifungal activity of the synthesized AgNPs using the aqueous extract of red seaweed *Gelidiella acerosa*. The antifungal effects of these NPs showed promising results when compared with standard antifungal drug. Hence, further investigation for clinical applications is necessary.

12.4.5 Marine Cyanobacteria

Bioactive compounds from marine cyanobacteria have a wide range of applications. In marine natural compounds, approximately 40% are of cyanobacterial origin (Blunt et al. 2008). In the literature, more than 300 nitrogen-containing natural products have been reported. The majority of these compounds belong to either the polypeptide or the mixed polyketide–polypeptide structural class. The compounds isolated from marine cyanobacteria acquire important biological activities, ranging from antimitotic to antimicrobial (hectochlorin, lyngbyabellins, apratoxins, and aurilides) (Tan and Goh 2009).

Marine cyanobacterium *Oscillatoria willei* NTDM01 has reduced silver ions, and its size ranges from 100 to 200 nm. The advantages of cyanobacteria-mediated NPs are easy availability, low-cost cyanobacterial biomass production, and ease of separation (Ali et al. 2011).

Phormidium tenue produces C-phycoerythrin used for the biosynthesis of cadmium sulfide (CdS) NPs. The size of the NPs was 5 nm. In the future, the C-phycoerythrin-labeled CdS NPs can be used for biolabeling. Based on the review of literature, only two reports are available and freshwater cyanobacteria–mediated NP synthesis reports are also few (Mubarak et al. 2012).

12.4.6 Marine Actinobacteria

An extensive survey was conducted on distribution of marine actinobacteria in the sediments of North Sea and Atlantic Ocean. This study reported that the marine actinobacteria are the best sources for isolation of unique bioactive compounds compared to terrestrial ones (Weyland 1969). The marine actinobacteria have different characteristics than those of their terrestrial counterparts. Almost 80% of the world's antibiotics are known to come from actinomycetes, mostly from the genera *Streptomyces* and *Micromonospora*. Due to this property, marine actinobacteria have received attention. It has been proposed that these antimicrobials are used in competition between microorganisms, offering an advantage to the producer strains (Jensen et al. 2005; Karthik et al. 2010).

The extracellular synthesis of AgNPs has been investigated using the marine actinobacteria *Streptomyces* sp. LK-3. Upon various characterizations, spherical AgNPs were found within a size range of 1–81 nm (Figure 12.1). The NPs showed antibacterial activity against multidrug-resistant pathogenic strains. The AgNPs showed a zone of inhibition around 18 mm. It also showed larvicidal activity. The development of an eco-friendly method to synthesize metal NPs would further promote the interest in the synthesis and application of metal NPs (Karthik et al. 2012a). The extracellular synthesis of TiO_2 NPs has been investigated using the marine actinobacteria *Streptomyces* sp. LK-3. TiO_2 NPs were found within the size range of 3.5–92 nm. The morphology was found to be spherical and oval.

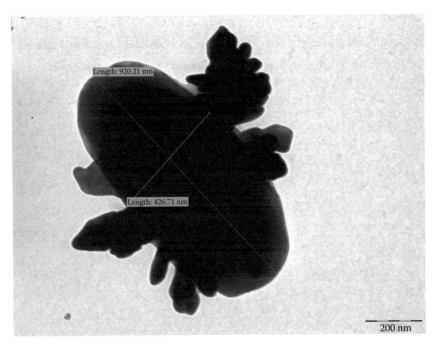

FIGURE 12.1
TEM image of AgNPs with *Streptomyces* sp LK-3.

2,3,4-Trisubstituted quinolines have been synthesized by using TiO_2 NPs in good yields. This procedure is cost-effective and environmentally benign. TiO_2 is an efficient catalyst and reusable (Karthik et al. 2012b). *Streptomyces* sp. LK-3 (JF710608)–synthesized AuNPs were found within the size range of 5–17.3 nm. Au NP treatment in *Plasmodium berghei* ANKA (PbA)–infected mice delayed the rise of parasitemia compared to PbA infection 8 days postinfection. The incidence of chromosomal aberration in human PBL was not affected by treatment with the AuNP. The results obtained suggest that the AuNP possesses antimalarial activity and could be considered as a potential source for antimalarial drug development (Karthik et al. 2012c). The extracellular synthesis of ZnO NPs has been investigated using the marine actinobacteria *Streptomyces roseiscleroticus*. Upon various characterizations, ZnO NPs were found within a size range of 3.6–95 nm. The zone of inhibition exhibited by ZnO NPs against MRSA was 15 mm (Bhargavi et al. 2011). AgNPs have been synthesized intra- and extracellularly from two isolates of marine actinomycetes, *Streptomyces parvulus* SSNP11 and *Streptomyces albidoflavus* CNP10. The size of the NPs was 2–100 nm in addition to variation in antimicrobial activity (Prakasham et al. 2011). In another report, a glycolipid from *Brevibacterium casei* MSA19 was found to synthesize AgNPs. It was uniform and stable for up to 2 months. Therefore, glycolipid acts as a "green" stabilizer of NPs (Kiran et al. 2010).

The biosynthesis of AgNPs was carried out by using actinobacteria isolated from salt pan soils (*Streptomyces* SRBVIT). The synthesized NPs were characterized and the average size of NP was 13.8 nm. The anti-dermatophytic activity of AgNPs was analyzed and it showed activity toward *Trichophyton rubrum* and *Trichophyton mentagrophytes*. The MIC test showed highest inhibition for *T. rubrum* (100 µg/mL) and *T. mentagrophytes* (200 µg/mL). Cytotoxicity effects of biosynthesized AgNPs are investigated with the help of a brine shrimp assay (Sathish et al. 2012).

12.5 Environmental Impact on Biologically Synthesized Nanoparticles

The engineered NPs are more toxic. This has already been reported in several research papers. However, in biologically synthesized NPs, the toxic effect will be less because the attached biomolecules from microorganisms can nullify the toxicity. In our lab, we carried out some preliminary studies; in these studies we observed less toxicity of marine actinobacteria–synthesized AgNPs in plants, earthworms, and fish (data not shown). Hence, the NPs synthesized by microbes, especially marine microorganism–synthesized NPs, should be focused more.

12.6 Conclusion

Diverse natural products have been isolated from marine microorganisms. A number of these molecules are responsible for NP synthesis and are a potential source of novel pharmaceuticals. However, research on the NP synthesis and their role in antimicrobial activity are still in their infancy. This chapter showed that only a handful of marine microorganisms have been investigated with regard to their NP synthesis and their application. This chapter also highlighted the number of marine actinobacteria–mediated NP synthesis research conducted at our laboratory. Research on NP synthesis using marine microorganism compounds is important to find a new drug formulation to avoid drug resistance. In the future, it can be used as a natural drug delivery system. Furthermore, such research can lead to potential applications in medical biotechnology.

References

Agnihotri, M., S. Joshi, A. Ravi Kumar, S. Zinjarde, and S. Kulkarni. 2009. Biosynthesis of gold nanoparticles by the tropical marine yeast *Yarrowia lipolytica* NCIM 3589. *Materials Letters* 63 (15):1231–1234.

Ahmad, A., M. Priyabrata, and S. Satyajyoti. 2003a. Extracellular biosynthesis of silver nanoparticles using the fungus *Fusarium oxysporum*. *Colloids and Surfaces B: Biointerfaces* 28:313–318.

Ahmad, A., S. Senapati, M. I. Khan, R. Kumar, R. Ramani, V. Srinivas, and M. Sastry. 2003b. Intracellular synthesis of gold nanoparticles by a novel alkalotolerant actinomycete, *Rhodococcus* species. *Nanotechnology* 14 (7):824–828.

Akhavan, O. and Ghaderi, E. 2009. Enhancement of antibacterial properties of Ag nanorods by electric field. *Science and Technology of Advanced Materials* 10 (1):015003.

Ali, D. M., M. Sasikala, M. Gunasekaran, and N. Thajuddin. 2011. Biosynthesis and characterization of silver nanoparticles using marine cyanobacterium, *Oscillatoria willei* NTDM01 Digest. *Journal of Nanomaterials and Biostructures* 6 (2):385–390.

Balaji, D. S., S. Basavaraja, and R. Deshpandeb. 2009. Extracellular biosynthesis of functionalized silver nanoparticles by of *Cladosporium cladosporioides* fungus. *Colloids and Surfaces B: Biointerfaces* 68 (1):88–92.

Bhainsa, K. C. and S. F. D'Souza. 2006. Extracellular biosynthesis of silver nanoparticles using the fungus *Aspergillus fumigatus*. *Colloids and Surfaces B: Biointerfaces* 47 (2):160–164.

Bhargavi, G., L. Karthik, G. Kumar, and K. V. Bhaskara Rao. 2011. Marine actinobacterial mediated ZnO nanoparticles synthesis. Presented at *National Conference on Aquatic Biotoxins—2011*, Cuddalore, India, pp. 79–101.

Bhimba, V. B., N. Nath, and P. Sinha. 2011. Characterization and antibacterial analysis of silver nanoparticles synthesized by the marine fungi *Hypocrea lixii* MV1 isolated from mangrove sediment soil. *Journal of Pharmacy Research* 4 (2):477–479.

Blunt, J. W., B. R. Copp, W. P. Hu, M. H. Munro, P. T. Northcote, and M. R. Prinsep. 2008. Marine natural products. *Natural Product Reports* 25:35–94.

Brown, H. E. 1957. *Zinc Oxide Rediscovered*. The New Jersey Zinc Company, New York.

Brown, H. E. 1976. *Zinc Oxide Properties and Applications*. International Lead Zinc Research Organization, New York.

Brust, M., M. Walker, D. Bethell, D. J. Schiffrin, and R. Whyman. 1994. Synthesis of thiol-derivatized gold nanoparticles in a 2-phase liquid-liquid system. *Journal of the Chemical Society—Chemical Communications* 7 (7):801–802.

Burkholder, P. R., R. M. Pfister, and F. P. Leitz. 1966. Production of a pyrrole antibiotic by a marine bacterium. *Applied Microbiology* 14:649.

Buzea, C., Pacheco, I., and K. Robbie. 2007. Nanomaterials and nanoparticles: Sources and toxicity. *Biointerphases* 2 (4):17–71.

Castro, E. L., A. R. N. Vilchis, and M. B. Avalos. 2011. Biosynthesis of silver, gold and bimetallic nanoparticles using the filamentous fungus *Neurospora crassa*. *Colloids and Surfaces B: Biointerfaces* 83 (1):42–48.

Chen, L., D. A. Bazylinski, and B. H. Lower. 2010. Bacteria that synthesize nano-sized compasses to navigate using Earth's geomagnetic field. *Nature Education Knowledge* 1 (10):14.

Cho, K. H., J. E. Park, T. Osaka, and S. G. Park. 2005. The study of antimicrobial activity and preservative effects of nanosilver ingredient. *Electrochimica Acta* 51:956–960.

Daniel, M. C. and D. Astruc. 2004. Gold nanoparticles: Assembly, supramolecular chemistry, quantum-size-related properties, and applications toward biology, catalysis, and nanotechnology. *Chemical Reviews* 104 (1):293–346.

Dinesh Kumar, S., L. Karthik, K. Gaurav, and K. V. Bhaskara Rao. 2011. Biosynthesis of silver nanoparticles from marine yeast and their antimicrobial activity against multidrug resistant pathogens. *Pharmacologyonline* 3:1100–1111.

Earle, M. D. 1942. The electrical conductivity of titanium dioxide. *Physical Reviews* 61 (1–2):56–62.

Fenical, W. 1993. Chemical studies of marine bacteria: Developing a new resource. *Chemical Reviews* 93 (5):1673–1683.

Forbes, G. B. and G. M. Forbes. 1971. Silver nitrate and the eye of the newborn - Credé's contribution to preventive medicine. *American Journal of Diseases of Children* 121:1–4.

Fortina, P., L. K. Kricka, D. J. Graves et al. 2007. Applications of nanoparticles to diagnostics and therapeutics in colorectal cancer. *Trends in Biotechnology* 25 (4):145–152.

Fountain, K. S. and G. D. Malkasian. 1981. Radioactive colloidal gold in the treatment of endometrial cancer—Mayo clinic experience, 1952–1976. *Cancer* 47 (10):2430–2432.

Gericke, M. and A. Pinches. 2006. Biological synthesis of metal nanoparticles. *Hydrometallurgy* 83:132–140.

Ghosh, D. 2004. Bioprospecting in the deltaic sundarbans for marine microorganisms producing commercially important bioactive compounds. PhD dissertation. Jadavpur University, Kolkata, India.

Goya, G. F. 2004. Magnetic interactions in ball-milled spinel ferrites. *Journal of Materials Science* 39:5045–5049.

Grimm, S., M. Schultz, S. Barth, and R. Muller. 1997. Flame pyrolysis—A preparation route for ultrafine pure c-Fe_2O_3 powders and the control of their particle size and properties. *Journal of Materials Science* 32:1083–1092.

Harding, F. J. 2007. *Breast Cancer: Cause—Prevention—Cure*. Tekline Publishing, Devon, England.

Hayat, M. A. 1989. *Colloidal Gold: Principles, Methods and Applications*. Academic Press, San Diego, CA.

Hermans, M. H. 2006. Silver-containing dressings and the need for evidence. *The American Journal of Nursing* 106 (12):60–68.

Hernandez Battez, A., R. Gonzalez, J. Viesca et al. 2008. CuO, ZrO$_2$ and ZnO nanoparticles as anti-wear additive in oil lubricants. *Wear* 265 (3–4):422–428.

Hogan, J. 2004. Smog-busting paint soaks up noxious gases in the World Wide Web http://www.newscientist.com (accessed March 12, 2012).

Hu, W., S. Chen, B. Zhou, and H. Wang. 2010. Facile synthesis of ZnO nanoparticles based on bacterial cellulose. *Materials Science and Engineering B* 170:88–92.

Huaizhi, Z. and Y. Ning. 2003. Techniques used for the preparation and application of gold powder in ancient China. *Gold Bulletin* 33 (3):103–105.

Hughes, G. and N. R. McLean. 1988. Zinc oxide tape: A useful dressing for the recalcitrant finger-tip and soft-tissue injury. *Archives of Emergency Medicine* 5 (4):223–227.

Hunt, L. B. 1976. The true story of purple of Cassius. *Gold Bulletin* 9 (4):134–139.

Ingle, A., M. Rai, A. Gade, and A. Bawaskar. 2008. *Fusarium solani*: A novel biological agent for the extracellular synthesis of silver nanoparticles. *Journal of Nanoparticle Research* 11 (8):2079–2085.

Ireland, C. M., B. R. Copp, M. D. Foster, L. A. McDonald, D. C. Radisky, and J. C. Swersey. 1993. Biomedical potential of marine natural products. In: *Marine Biotechnology. Pharmaceutical and Bioactive Natural Products*, eds. D. H. Attaway and O. R. Zaborsky, pp. 1–43. Plenum press, New York.

Jensen, P. R., T. J. Mincer, P. G. Williams, and W. Fenical. 2005. Marine actinomycete diversity and natural product discovery. *Antonie Leeuwenhoek* 87:43–48.

Jha, A. K. and K. Prasad. 2009. Ferroelectric BaTiO$_3$ nanoparticles: Biosynthesis and characterization, *Colloids and Surfaces B: Biointerfaces* 75 (1):330–334.

Jha, A. K., K. Prasad, and A. R. Kulkarni. 2009. Synthesis of TiO$_2$ nanoparticles using microorganisms. *Colloids and Surfaces B: Biointerfaces* 71 (2):226–229.

Jiang, Z. J., C. Y. Liu, and L. W. Sun. 2005. Catalytic properties of silver nanoparticles supported on silica spheres. *The Journal of Physical Chemistry B* 109 (5):1730–1735.

Jones, B. J., M. J. Vergne, D. M. Bun, L. E. Locascio, and M. A. Hayes. 2007. Cleavage of peptides and proteins using light-generated radicals from titanium dioxide. *Analytical Chemistry* 79 (4):1327–1332.

Karthik, L., K. Gaurav, and K. V. Bhasakara Rao. 2010. Diversity of marine actinomycetes from Nicobar marine sediments and its anti fungal activity. *International Journal of Pharmacy and Pharmaceutical Sciences* 2:199–203.

Karthik, L., K. Gaurav, K. V. Bhaskara Rao et al. 2012a. Larvicidal efficacy of marine actinobacteria mediated biosynthesis of silver nanoparticles using *Streptomyces* sp LK-3 against *Rhipicephalus (Boophilus) microplus* and *Haemaphysalis bispinosa* (Manuscript in preparation).

Karthik, L., K. Gaurav, and K. V. Bhaskara Rao. 2012b. Marine actinobacterial mediated titanium dioxide nanoparticles synthesis. Presented at *International Conference on Nano Science and Technology*, Hyderabad, India, p. 285.

Karthik, L., K. Gaurav, and K. V. Bhaskara Rao. 2012c. Marine actinobacterial mediated gold nanoparticles synthesis and their antimalarial activity. Presented at *International Conference on Nano Bio 2012*, Kochi, India, p. 295.

Kathiresan, K., N. M. Alikunhi, S. M. Pathmanaban, A. Nabikhan, and S. Kandasamy. 2010. Analysis of antimicrobial silver nanoparticles synthesized by coastal strains of *Escherichia coli* and *Aspergillus niger*. *Canadian Journal of Microbiology* 56:1050–1059.

Kathiresan, K., S. Manivannan, M. A. Nabeel, and B. Dhivya. 2009. Studies on silver nanoparticles synthesized by marine fungus, *Penicillium fellutanum* isolated from coastal mangrove sediments. *Colloids and Surfaces B: Biointerfaces* 71:133–137.

Kaushik, N. T., S. M. Snehit, and Y. P. Rasesh. 2010. Biological synthesis of metallic nanoparticles. *Nanomedicine: Nanotechnology, Biology and Medicine* 6 (2):257–262.

Kiran, G. S., A. Sabu, and J. Selvin. 2010. Synthesis of silver nanoparticles by glycolipid biosurfactant produced from marine *Brevibacterium casei* MSA19. *Journal of Biotechnology* 148:221–225.

Klasen, H. J. 2000. A historical review of the use of silver in the treatment of burns. II. Renewed interest for silver. *Burns* 26 (2):131–138.

Kowshik, M., S. Ashtaputre, S. Kharrazi et al. 2003. Extracellular synthesis of silver nanoparticles by a silver-tolerant yeast strain MKY3. *Nanotechnology* 14 (1):95–100.

Kucheyev, S. O. 2003. Ion-beam-produced structural defects in ZnO. *Physical Reviews B* 67 (9):094115.

Kutty, S. N. and R. Philip. 2008. Marine yeasts—A review. *Yeast* 25:465–483.

Laatsch, H. 2005. Marine bacterial metabolites in the World Wide Web 2005. http://wwwuser.gwdg.de/~ucoc/laatsch/Reviews Books Patents/R30 Marine BacterialMetabolites.pdf (accessed March 12, 2012).

Lansdown, A. B. G. 2010. *Silver in Healthcare: Its Antimicrobial Efficacy and Safety in Use.* Royal Society of Chemistry, London, U.K., p. 159.

Lewis, N. 2009. Nanocrystalline TiO$_2$ in the World Wide Web. Research. California Institute of Technology. http://nsl.caltech.edu/research.nt.html (accessed March 12, 2012).

Li, M., H. Bala, X. Lv, X. Ma, F. Sun, L. Tang, and Z. Wang. 2007. Direct synthesis of monodispersed ZnO nanoparticles in an aqueous solution. *Materials Letters* 61:690–693.

Li, Y. B., Y. Bando, and D. Golberg. 2004. ZnO nanoneedles with tip surface perturbations: Excellent field emitters. *Applied Physics Letters* 84 (18):3603.

Look, D. 2001. Recent advances in ZnO materials and devices. *Materials Science and Engineering B* 80 (1–3):383–387.

Marcato, P. D., E. De Souza, E. Alves, and N. Duran. 2005. Antibacterial activity of silver nanoparticles synthesized by *Fusarium oxysporum* strain. Paper presented at *Fourth Mercosur Congress on Process Systems Engineering*, Rio de Janeiro, Brasil, pp. 1–5.

Mayer, A. M. S., K. B. Glaser, and C. Cuevasetal. 2010. Theodyssey of marine pharmaceuticals: A current pipeline perspective. *Trends in Pharmacological Sciences* 31 (6):255–265.

McFarland, A. D. and R. P. V. Duyne. 2003. Single silver nanoparticles as real-time optical sensors with zep-tomole sensitivity. *Nano Letters* (8):1057–1062.

Mishra, A., S. K. Tripathy, and S. I. Yun. 2011. Bio-synthesis of gold and silver nanoparticles from *Candida guilliermondii* and their antimicrobial effect against pathogenic bacteria. *Journal of Nanoscience Nanotechnology* 11 (1):243–248.

Mishra, G. P., M. Bagui, V. Tamboli, and A. K. Mitra, 2011. Recent applications of liposomes in ophthalmic drug delivery. *Journal of Drug Delivery*, Vol. 2011, Article ID 863734, 14 pages. doi: 10.1155/2011/863734.

Mitchnick, M. A., D. Fairhurst, and S. R. Pinnell. 1999. Microfine zinc oxide (Z-cote) as a photostable UVA/UVB sunblock agent. *Journal of the American Academy of Dermatology* 40 (1):85–90.

Moore, R. E., G. M. L. Patterson, and W. W. Garmichael. 1988. New pharmaceuticals from cultured blue-green algae. In: *Biomedical Importance of Marine Organisms*, ed. D. G. Fautin, pp. 143–150. Academy of Science, San Francisco, CA.

Mubarak, D., V. Ali, N. Gopinath, N. Rameshbabu, and N. Thajuddin. 2012. Synthesis and characterization of CdS nanoparticles using C-phycoerythrin from the marine cyanobacteria. *Materials Letters* 74 (1):8–11.

Nakagawa, H., S. Kasahara, and T. Sugiyama. 1987. Effect of Ulva meal supplementation on the lipid metabolism of black sea bream. *Aquaculture* 62:109–121.

Namasivayam, S. K. R., S. Ganesh, and Avimanyu. 2011. Evaluation of anti-bacterial activity of silver nanoparticles synthesized from *Candida glabrata* and *Fusarium oxysporum*. *International Journal of Medical Research* 1 (3):131–136.

Nanda, A. and M. Saravanan. 2009. Biosynthesis of silver nanoparticles from *Staphylococcus aureus* and its antimicrobial activity against MRSA and MRSE. *Nanomedicine* 5 (4):452–456.

Padmavathy, N., R. Vijayaraghavan, and R. Rajagopalan. 2008. Enhanced bioactivity of ZnO nanoparticles—An antimicrobial study. *Science and Technology of Advanced Materials* 9 (3):035004.

Paschotta, R. 2009. Bragg mirrors in the World Wide Web. *Encyclopedia of Laser Physics and Technology*. RP Photonics. http://www.rp-photonics.com/bragg_mirrors.html (accessed March 12, 2012).

Prakasham, R. S., B. S. Kumar, Y. S. Kumar, and G. S. Shanker. 2011. Synthesis and characterization of silver nanoparticles from marine *Streptomyces* species. Paper presented at the *World Congress on Biotechnology*, Hyderabad, India, p. 1.

Rajasulochana, P., R. Dhamotharan, P. Murugakoothan, S. Murugesan, and P. Krishnamoorthy. 2010. Biosynthesis and characterization of gold nanoparticles using the alga *Kappaphycus alvarezii*. *International Journal of Nanoscience* 9 (5):511–516.

Rammohan, M. and K. Balakrishnan. 2011. Rapid synthesis and characterization of silver nano particles by novel *Pseudomonas sp.* ."ram bt – 1". *Journal of Ecobiotechnology* 3 (1):24–28.

Rosenfeld, W. D. and C. Zobell. 1947. Antibiotic production by marine microorganisms. *Journal of Bacteriology* 54:393–398.

Sadhasivam, S., S. Parthasarathi, and Y. Kyusik. 2010. Biosynthesis of nanoparticles by *Streptomyces hygroscopicus* and antimicrobial activity against medically important pathogenic microorganisms. *Colloids and Surfaces B: Biointerfaces* 81:358–362.

Saito, M. 1993. Antibacterial, deodorizing, and UV absorbing materials obtained with zinc oxide (ZnO) coated fabrics. *Journal of Industrial Textiles* 23 (2):150–164.

Sastry, M., A. Ahmad, M. I. Khan, and R. Kumar. 2003. Biosynthesis of metal nanoparticles using fungi and actinomycete. *Current Science* 85 (2):162–170.

Sathish Kumar, S. R. and K. V. Bhaskara Rao. 2012. Biosynthesis of silver nanoparticles using marine actinobacteria and their anti-dermatophytic activity. Presented at *International conference on Nano Bio 2012*, Kochi, India, p. 296.

Satoh, K., H. Nakagawa, and S. Kasahara. 1987. Effect of Ulva meal supplementation of disease resistance red sea bream. *Nippon Suisan Gakkaishi* 53:1115–1120.

Schiehser, G. A. 1980. The isolation and structure of leptosphaerin: A metabolite of the marine Ascomycete, Leptosphaeria oraemaris. PhD dissertation. Oregon State University, Corvallis, OR.

Seshadri, S., K. Saranya, and M. Kowshik. 2011. Green synthesis of lead sulfide nanoparticles by the lead resistant marine yeast *Rhodosporidium diobovatum*. *Biotechnology Progress* 27:1464–1469.

Shahverdi, A. R., S. Minaeian, H. R. Shahverdi, H. Jamalifar, and A. A. Nohi. 2007. Rapid synthesis of silver nanoparticles using culture supernatants of *Enterobacteriaceae*: A novel biological approach. *Process Biochemistry* 42:919–923.

Shakibaie, M., H. Forootanfar, K. Mollazadeh-Moghaddam et al. 2010. Green synthesis of gold nanoparticles by the marine microalga *Tetraselmis suecica*. *Biotechnology and Applied Biochemistry* 57:71–75.

Sharma, D., J. Rajput, B. S. Kaith, M. Kaur, and S. Sharma. 2010. Synthesis of ZnO nanoparticles and study of their antibacterial and antifungal properties. *Thin Solid Films* 519 (3):1224–1229.

Shin, J. and W. Fenical. 1987. Isolation of gliovictin from the marine deuteromycete *Asteromyces cruciatus*. *Phytochemistry* 26:33–47.

Sieburth, J. M. 1961. Antibiotic properties of acrylic acid, a factor in the gastrointestinal antibiosis of polar marine animals. *Journal of Bacteriology* 82:72–79.

Singaravelu, G., J. S. Arockiamary, V. Ganesh Kumar, and K. Govindaraju. 2009. A novel extracellular synthesis of monodisperse gold nanoparticles using marine alga, *Sargassum wightii* Greville. *Colloids and Surfaces B: Biointerfaces* 57 (1):97–101.

Slawson, R. M., M. I. Van Dyke, H. Lee, and J. T. Trevors. 1992. Germanium and silver resistance, accumulation, and toxicity in microorganisms. *Plasmid* 27 (1):72–79.

Subramanian, M., N. M. Alikunhi, and K. Kandasamy. 2010. In vitro synthesis of silver nanoparticles by marine yeasts from coastal mangrove sediment. *Advanced Science Letters* 3:428–433.

Tan, L. T. and B. P. L. Goh. 2009. Chemical ecology of marine cyanobacterial secondary metabolites: A mini-review. *Journal of Coastal Development* 13 (1):1–9.

Venkatpurwar, V. and V. Pokharkar. 2011. Green synthesis of silver nanoparticles using marine polysaccharide: Study of *in-vitro* antibacterial activity. *Materials Letters* 65 (6):999–1002.

Vijayaraghavan, K., A. Mahadevana, M. Sathish Kumar, S. Pavagadhi, and R. Balasubramanian. 2011. Biosynthesis of Au(0) from Au(III) via biosorption and bioreduction using brown marine alga *Turbinaria conoides*. *Chemical Engineering Journal* 167:223–227.

Visuthikosol, V. and S. Kumpolpunth. 1981. Intra-articular radioactive colloidal gold (Au-198) in the treatment of rheumatoid-arthritis. *Journal of the Medical Association of Thailand* 64 (9):419–427.

Vivek, M., S. K. Palanisamy, S. Sesurajan, and S. Sudha. 2011. Biogenic silver nanoparticles by *Gelidiella acerosa* extract and their antifungal effects. *Avicenna Journal of Medical Biotechnology* 3 (3):143–148.

Weyland, H. 1969. Actinomycetes in North Sea and Atlantic Ocean sediments. *Nature* 23:858.

Yan, S., W. He, C. Sun et al. 2009. The biomimetic synthesis of zinc phosphate nanoparticles. *Dyes and Pigments* 80:254–258.

Yoshizawa, Y., A. Ametani, J. Tsunehiro et al. 1995. Macrophage stimulating activity of the polysaccharide fraction from marine alga *Porphyra yezoensis*: Structure—Function relationship and improved solubility. *Bioscience, Biotechnology, and Biochemistry* 59 (10):1933–1937.

Zhenming, C. H. I., L. Zhiqiang, G. Lingmei, G. Fang, M. Chunling, W. Xianghong, and L. Haifeng. 2006. Marine Yeasts and their applications in mariculture. *Journal of Ocean University of China* 5 (3):251–256.

Zilinskas, R. A., R. R. Colwell, D. W. Lipton, and R. T. Hill. 1995. The global challenge of marine biotechnology: A status report on the United States, Japan, Australia and Norway. Maryland Sea Grant Publication, College Park, MD, 1995.

13

Biosynthesis and Characterization of Different Nanoparticles and Its Larvicidal Activity against Human Disease Vectors

Arivarasan Vishnu Kirthi, Chidambaram Jayaseelan, and Abdul Abdul Rahuman

CONTENTS

13.1 Introduction

Vector control is a serious concern in developing countries like India. Mosquitoes are the most important single group of insects in terms of public health importance, which transmit a number of diseases, such as malaria, filariasis, dengue, and Japanese encephalitis (JE), causing millions of deaths every year. There is an urgent need to check the proliferation of the population of vector mosquitoes in order to reduce vector-borne diseases by appropriate control methods (Kuppusamy and Murugan 2009). Mosquito-borne diseases have an economic impact, including loss in commercial and labor outputs, particularly in countries with tropical and subtropical climates; however, no part of the world is free from vector-borne diseases (Fradin and Day 2002). Nowadays, the control of vector-borne diseases is more difficult due to the increased resistance of mosquito populations to synthetic insecticides and even to microbial control agents and because of the resistance of malarial parasites to chemotherapeutic drugs and some economic issues (Shelton et al. 2007). Control of mosquito populations is most effective when the aquatic stage is targeted because that is the stage where they are most concentrated and immobile (Cetin et al. 2010). Although effective, repeated use of these controlling agents has fostered several environmental and health concerns, including disruption of natural biological control systems, outbreaks of other insect species, widespread development of resistance, and undesirable effects on nontarget organisms (Isman 2006).

13.1.1 Vector-Borne Diseases

13.1.1.1 Malaria

Malaria is the world's most dreadful tropical disease. Malaria is one of the most common vector-borne diseases widespread in tropical and subtropical regions, including parts of the America, Asia, and Africa (WHO 2007). Worldwide, there were about 247 million malaria cases with 0.881 million deaths reported in 2006 (WHO 2008a). Mosquito-borne diseases are endemic in more than over 100 countries, causing mortality of nearly two million people every year, and at least 1 million children die of such diseases each year, leaving as many as 2100 million people at risk around the world (Kager 2002). As reported recently, 406 million Indians were at risk of stable *Plasmodium falciparum* transmission in 2007 with an uncertainty point estimate of 101.5 million clinical cases (95% CI 31.0–187.0 million cases; Hay et al. 2010).

13.1.1.2 Anopheles stephensi

Anopheles stephensi is the major malaria vector in India with an annual incidence of 300–500 million clinically manifest cases and a death toll of 1.1–2.7 million; malaria is still one of the most important communicable diseases. Currently, about 40% of the world's population lives in areas where malaria is endemic (Wernsdorfer and Wernsdorfer 2003).

13.1.1.3 Anopheles subpictus

Anopheles subpictus is a complex isomorphic sibling species and is recognized as a vector of malaria, some helminth and arboviruses (Chandra et al. 2010). *A. subpictus* is recognized as a primary or secondary vector of malaria, a disease of great socioeconomic importance in different parts of the world (Panicker et al. 1981; Kulkarni 1983; Chatterjee and Chandra

2000). It breeds profusely in water collections and fallow rice fields of southern India, where the larval incidence is high throughout the year (Dhanda and Kaul 1980).

13.1.2 Lymphatic Filariasis and Japanese Encephalitis

Lymphatic filariasis (LF) caused by the mosquito-borne, lymphatic-dwelling nematodes *Wuchereria bancrofti* and *Brugia malayi* are still a common tropical parasitic disease. Of the estimated 120 million people affected by this disease in the world, one-third lives in India. LF is next to malaria as the most important vector-borne disease in India. Approximately 420 million people reside in endemic areas and 48.11 million are infected (Ramaiah et al. 2000). Six union territories in India were identified to be endemic with about 553 million people exposed to the risk of infection; and of them, about 146 million live in urban and the remaining in rural areas. About 31 million people are estimated to be the carriers of microfilaria, and over 23 million suffer from filarial disease manifestations in India (WHO 2005). *W. bancrofti* accounts for ~90% of the disease burden, while *B. malayi* contributes the remaining ~10% (Anitha and Shenoy 2001). India contributes about 40% of the total global burden and accounts for about 50% of the people at the risk of infection. Of the people exposed to the risk of infection, individuals with microfilaremia, suffering from lymphedema, and hydrocele cases in the globe, India alone accounts for 39.0%, 37.9%, 46.4%, and 48.1%, respectively (Michael et al. 1996).

Japanese encephalitis (JE) outbreaks occur frequently in 14 Asian countries with about 3060 million people at risk of infection (Sabesan 2003). JE is a major public health concern due to its high epidemic potential, high case fatality, and neuropsychiatric sequelae among survivors. The estimated global burden of JE was 709,000 disability-adjusted life year lost in 2003 (WHO 2004). Approximately 2 billion people live in countries where JE presents a significant risk to humans and animals, particularly in China and India, with at least 700 million potentially susceptible children (Gould et al. 2008).

13.1.3 *Culex tritaeniorhynchus*

Culex tritaeniorhynchus Giles is an important vector of JE in India and Southeast Asian countries (Suman et al. 2008). JE is endemic in few states of India and highly endemic in few districts of Tamil Nadu, Southern India (Reuben and Gajanana 1997). Keiser et al. (2005) have reported that approximately 1.9 billion people currently live in rural JE-prone areas of the world, the majority of them live in China (766 million) followed by India (646 million).

13.1.4 *Culex quinquefasciatus*

Culex quinquefasciatus is a vector of LF that is one of the widely distributed tropical diseases (Michael et al. 1996). Larvae of *C. quinquefasciatus* vector species are commonly found in partially blocked drains and ditches soakaway pits, septic tanks, and in village pots, especially the abandoned ones in which the water is polluted and unfit for drinking. Mosquito is associated with urbanization and towns with poor and inadequate drainage and sanitation. Thenmozhi et al. (2006) reported this species as a vector of JE virus in Cuddalore, an area of Tamil Nadu, where the disease is endemic. *W. bancrofti* is the most predominant filarial nematode, which is usually characterized by progressive debilitating swelling at the extremities, scrotum, or breast of an infected individual (Myung et al. 1998).

13.1.5 Yellow Fever

Liver failure causes jaundice which is also known as yellow fever. It causes yellowing of the skin and the whites of the eyes. About half of the patients in the toxic phase die within 10–14 days. Persons recovering from yellow fever have lifelong immunity against reinfection. Yellow fever is difficult to recognize, especially during the early stages, and can be easily confused with diseases including malaria, typhoid, rickettsial diseases, hemorrhagic viral fevers, dengue fever, and viral hepatitis.

13.1.6 *Aedes* Species

Aedes aegypti and *Aedes albopictus* act as a vector for the arboviruses that are responsible for causing yellow fever and dengue fever. The number of these cases has increased sharply in recent years (Maheswaran and Ignacimuthu 2011). Fifty million dengue infections are reported in tropical and subtropical countries annually (WHO 2008a,b). *A. aegypti* is more widely dispersed now than any time in the past, placing billions of humans at risk of infection.

The control of mosquito larvae worldwide depends primarily on continued applications of organophosphates such as temephos and fenthion, and insect growth regulators such as diflubenzuron and methoprene (Yang et al. 2002). Mosquitoes in the larval stage are attractive targets for pesticides because mosquitoes breed in water, and thus, it is easy to deal with them in this habitat. Recently, concerns increased with respect to public health and environmental security requiring detection of natural products that may be used against insect pests (Karunamoorthi et al. 2008). As mosquitoes are known to be a carrier of a series of infectious diseases, the problem of their control is considered to be presently challenging. Use of chemical larvicides is not sufficiently effective and, sometimes, leads to tolerance of mosquito larvae.

13.2 Nanotechnology

Nanotechnology involves the production, manipulation, and use of materials ranging in size from less than a micron to that of individual atoms. Although nanomaterials may be synthesized using chemical approaches, it is now possible to include the use of biological materials. Development of biologically inspired experimental processes for the synthesis of NPs is evolving into an important branch of nanotechnology. Production of NPs can be achieved through different methods. Chemical approaches are the most popular methods for the production of NPs. However, some chemical methods cannot avoid the use of toxic chemicals in the synthesis protocol. Biological methods of NPs synthesis using microorganisms (Nair and Pradeep 2002), enzyme (Wilner et al. 2006), and plant or plant extract have been suggested as possible ecofriendly alternatives to chemical and physical methods. Biosynthetic methods have been investigated as an alternative to chemical and physical ones. These methods can be divided into two categories depending on the place where the NPs or nanostructures are created as many microorganisms can provide inorganic materials either intra- or extracellularly (Mann 1996). For example, bacteria *Pseudomonas stutzeri* isolated from silver mine materials is able to reduce Ag^+ ions and accumulates Ag NPs, the size of such NPs being in the range 16–40 nm, with the average diameter of 27 nm (Joerger et al. 2001). The biosynthesis of NPs as an emerging highlight of the intersection of nanotechnology and biotechnology has received increasing attention due to a growing need to develop environmentally benign technologies in material synthesis (Kalishwaralal et al. 2008). The biological synthesis of NPs germinated from the experiments on biosorption of metals with Gram-negative and Gram-positive bacteria. The synthesized molecules were not identified as NPs but as aggregates (Mullen et al. 1989). Currently, there is a growing need to develop environmentally benign NP synthesis processes that do not use toxic chemicals in the synthesis protocol. As a result, researchers in the field of NP synthesis and assembly have turned to biological systems for inspiration. Though nanobiotechnology is at its infancy, various examples through which this technology and their use have been explained in this chapter would attract the attention of people toward its applications. Among these studies, a few have shown that different kinds of reductases of these organisms might be involving in the mechanism of NP production and attribute them various shape and size. However, the elucidation of exact mechanism of NP production using living organisms needs much more experimentations.

13.2.1 Properties of Nanoparticles

Nanomaterials are the raw engineered, sub-100 nm particles or structures and include NPs, fullerenes, and other carbon-based molecules, such as carbon nanotubes, quantum dots, dendrimers, nanoporous materials, and biological NPs. The size of a particle decreases to the nanoscale, the physical properties of the particle are altered, and rules of quantum mechanics, which determine the behavior of matter and light at the atomic and subatomic level, begin to dominate as particles shrink to the nanoscale. This means nano-sized particles, particularly at the lower end of the nanoscale, have optical, electrical, and magnetic properties that differ substantially from larger particles of the same compounds (Dowling et al. 2004), and it is these factors that lend themselves to new potential applications in electronics, data storage, and solar cells. NPs include ultrafine particles of metals, metal oxides, nonmetals, and ceramics. Metal NPs and nano-alloys are usually produced via reduction or co-reduction of metal salts (Masala and Seshadri 2004).

13.2.2 Types of Nanoparticles

NPs can be broadly grouped into two, namely, organic and inorganic NPs. Organic NPs may include carbon NPs (fullerenes) while some of the inorganic NPs may include magnetic NPs, noble metal NPs (like gold and silver), and semiconductor NPs (like TiO_2 and ZnO). Inorganic nanomaterials have been widely used for cellular delivery due to their versatile features like wide availability, rich functionality, good biocompatibility, capability of targeted drug delivery, and controlled release of drugs (Xu et al. 2006). For example, mesoporous silica when combined with molecular machines proved to be excellent imaging and drug-releasing systems. Au NPs have been used extensively in imaging, as drug carriers and in thermotherapy of biological targets (Cheon and Horace 2009).

13.2.2.1 Silver Nanoparticles

The bactericidal effect of Ag NPs is due to their small size and high-surface-area-to-volume ratio, which allows them to interact closely with microbial membranes (Morones et al. 2005). Smaller particles with a larger surface area have effective antibacterial activity (Baker et al. 2005). Silver acts as a nonspecific biocidal agent and is able to act strongly against a broad spectrum of bacterial and fungal species including antibiotic-resistant strains (Agarwal et al. 2010). Metal NPs are well known to display characteristic size-dependent properties different from those of their bulk counterparts, and the most significant effects occur in the 1–10 nm range. These NPs elicit considerable interest due to their high dispersion and the manifestation of quantum effects (Alivisatos 1996). Silver has been used for centuries as an antimicrobial agent, and on the basis of its well-documented efficacy, it is still in use today to treat burns and to prevent infection (Edwards-Jones 2009). Based on its antimicrobial activity, silver has become one of the most prominent nanomaterials, in many consumer products, such as disinfectants, deodorants, room spray, bedding, washing machines, humidifiers, shampoo, kitchen tools, toys, and fabrics (Zanette et al. 2011).

13.2.2.2 Titanium Dioxide Nanoparticles

TiO_2 is a well-known semiconductor with photocatalytic properties and is widely used for water and air remediation. It has proven to be highly effective in the nonselective degradation of organic contaminants due to high decomposition and mineralization rates (Pelaez et al. 2009). Moreover, TiO_2 NPs possess interesting optical, dielectric, antimicrobial, antibacterial, chemical stability, and catalytic properties, which leads to industrial applications such as pigment, fillers, catalyst supports, and photocatalyst. Recently, NP synthesis was achieved with bacteria, fungi, actinomycetes, and use of plant extract such as *Camellia sinensis*, *Coriandrum sativum*, *Nelumbo nucifera*, *Ocimum sanctum*, and several others, which is compatible with the green chemistry principles. Among the various biosynthetic approaches, the use of plant extracts has advantages such as easy availability and handling and a broad viability of metabolites (Sundrarajan and Gowri 2011).

13.2.2.3 Gold Nanoparticles

Soni and Prakash (2012) synthesized the Ag and Au NPs using *Candida tropicum*; the Au NPs used as an efficacy enhancer have shown mortality at three times higher concentration than the Ag NPs. Guirgis et al. (2012) have reported a simple and sensitive immunoassay that successfully detects malaria antigens in infected blood cultures. This homogeneous assay is based on the fluorescence quenching of cyanine 3B (Cy3B)-labeled recombinant *P. falciparum* heat shock protein 70(Pf Hsp70) upon binding to Au NPs functionalized with an anti-Hsp70 monoclonal antibody.

13.2.3 Synthesis of Nanoparticles

13.2.3.1 Green Synthesis

The need for biosynthesis of NPs rose as the physical and chemical processes were costly. So in the search for cheaper pathways for NP synthesis, scientists used microorganisms and then plant extracts for synthesis. Nature has devised various processes for the synthesis of nano- and micro-length scaled inorganic materials, which have contributed to the development of relatively new and largely unexplored area of research based on the biosynthesis of nanomaterials (Mohanpuria et al. 2008).

The assessments of the antiparasitic activities of synthesized TiO_2 NPs using leaf aqueous extract of *Catharanthus roseus* against the adults of hematophagous fly *Hippobosca maculata* Leach (Diptera: Hippoboscidae) and sheep-biting louse *Bovicola ovis* (Velayutham et al. 2011). Santhoshkumar et al. (2011) studied the larvicidal potential of the hexane, chloroform, ethyl acetate, acetone, methanol, and aqueous leaf extracts of *Nelumbo nucifera* and synthesized Ag NPs using aqueous leaf extract against fourth instar larvae of *A. subpictus* and *C. quinquefasciatus*. Marimuthu et al. (2011) have reported the antiparasitic efficacies of synthesized Ag NPs using aqueous leaf extract of *Mimosa pudica* against the larvae of malaria vector *A. subpictus*, filariasis vector *C. quinquefasciatus*, and *Rhipicephalus (Boophilus) microplus*. The acaricidal and larvicidal activities were reported against the larvae of *Haemaphysalis bispinosa* and larvae of hematophagous fly *H. maculata* and against the fourth instar larvae of malaria vector *A. stephensi* and JE vector *C. tritaeniorhynchus* of synthesized Ag NPs utilizing aqueous leaf extract from *Musa paradisiaca* (Jayaseelan et al. 2012a). The aqueous plant extracts and synthesized Ag NPs were tested against head lice and vectors and the direct contact method was conducted to determine the potential of pediculocidal activity (Jayaseelan et al. 2011). Jayaseelan et al. (2012b) have determined the efficacy of synthesized Ag NPs utilizing aqueous leaf extract of *Ocimum canum* against the larvae of *Hyalomma anatolicum* and *Hyalomma marginatum*. Recently much work has been done with regard to plant-assisted reduction of metal NPs and the respective role of phytochemicals. The main phytochemicals responsible have been identified as terpenoids, flavones, ketones, aldehydes, amides, and carboxylic acids in the light of IR spectroscopic studies. The main water-soluble phytochemicals like flavones, organic acids, and quinones are responsible for immediate reduction of metal NPs. The phytochemicals present in *Bryophyllum* sp. (xerophytes), *Cyprus* sp. (mesophytes), and *Hydrilla* sp. (hydrophytes) were studied for their role in the synthesis of Ag NPs. The Xerophytes were found to contain emodin, an anthraquinone that could undergo redial tautomerization leading to the formation of Ag NPs. The mesophyte studied contained three types of benzoquinones, namely, cyperoquinone, dietchequinone, and remirin. It was suggested that gentle warming followed by subsequent incubation resulted in the activation of quinones leading to particle size reduction. Catechol and protocatechaldehyde were reported in the hydrophyte studied along with other phytochemicals. It was reported that catechol under alkaline conditions gets transformed into protocatechaldehyde and finally into protocatechuic acid. Both these processes liberated hydrogen, which was suggested that it played a role in the synthesis of the NPs. The size of the NPs synthesized using xerophytes, mesophytes, and hydrophytes was in the range of 2–5 nm (Jha et al. 2009).

13.2.3.2 Bacterial Synthesis

Kirthi et al. (2011) have reported a low-cost, new material, ecofriendly, and reproducible microbes *Bacillus subtilis*–mediated biosynthesis of TiO_2 NPs. TiO_2 NPs were synthesized from titanium as a precursor, using the bacterium *B. subtilis*. Jayaseelan et al. (2012c) described a new, cost-effective, and simple procedure for biosynthesis of zinc oxide nanoparticles (ZnO NPs) using reproducible bacteria *Aeromonas hydrophila* as ecofriendly reducing and capping agent. The use of a specific enzyme α-NADPH-dependent nitrate reductase in the *in vitro* synthesis of NPs is important because this would do away with the downstream processing required for the use of these NPs in homogeneous catalysis and other applications such as nonlinear optics. During the catalysis, nitrate is converted to nitrite, and an electron will be shuttled to the incoming silver ions. This has been excellently described in the organism *Bacillus licheniformis*, which is known to secrete the cofactor NADH- and NADH-dependent enzymes, especially nitrate reductase, that might be responsible for the bioreduction of Ag^+ to Ag^0 and the subsequent formation of Ag NPs.

13.2.3.3 Fungal Synthesis

Anil Kumar et al. (2007) have directly used the purified nitrate reductase from the organism *Fusarium oxysporum* for the synthesis of Ag NP in test tube. Their reaction mixture contained only the enzyme nitrate reductase, silver nitrate, and NADPH. Slowly, the reaction mixture turned brown with all the characteristics of Ag NPs. Several strains of *Fusarium*, namely, *F. oxysporum* (Duran et al. 2005), *Aspergillus fumigatus,* and *Aspergillus flavus*, were used for successful production of metal NPs (Vighneshwaran et al. 2007). Recently, white rot fungus *Coriolus versicolor* has also been used for the synthesis of stable Ag NPs (Sanghi and Verma 2009). Kowshik et al. (2003) have identified yeast, *Torulopsis* spp. being capable of intracellular synthesis of PbS crystallite when exposed to aqueous Pb^{2+} ions and CdS NPs synthesized intracellularly by using *Schizosaccharomyces pombe*. The filamentous fungus *A. fumigatus* has been known for rapid extracellular synthesis of fairly monodispersed Ag NPs ranging from 5 to 25 nm. Hence, this system could be suitable for developing a biological process for mass scale production. Furthermore, the extracellular synthesis would make the process simpler and easier for downstream processing. In future, it might be important to understand the biochemical and molecular mechanism of the synthesis of the NPs by the cell filtrate in order to achieve better control over size and polydispersity of the NPs (Bhainsa and D'Souza 2006).

13.2.3.4 Actinobacteria Synthesis

Besides the eubacteria, actinomycetes also play a key role in fabrication of anisotropic metal NPs. The extremophilic actinomycete *Thermospora* reduced Au ions in an extracellular mechanism and yielded polydispersed Au NPs (Sastry et al. 2003). The reduction of metal ions as well as stability of the NPs is achieved by an enzymatic process and results in the efficient synthesis of 50 nm in diameter (Matsunaga and Takeyama 1998). The extracellular synthesis of TiO_2 and Au NPs has been investigated using novel marine actinobacteria *Streptomyces sp* LK-3 (JF710608) (Karthik et al. 2012a,b). Intracellular synthesis of Au has been observed more accurately and found concentrated on the cytoplasmic membrane rather than on the cell wall of alkalotolerant actinomycete *Rhodococcus*. Ahmad et al. (2003a) have observed that the extremophilic actinomycete *Thermomonospora* sp. when exposed to gold ions reduced the metal ions extracellularly, yielding Au NPs with a much improved polydispersity. Based on the hypothesis, alkalotolerant *Rhodococcus* sp. has been used for intracellular synthesis of good quality monodisperse Au NPs. They observed that the concentration of NPs was more on the cytoplasmic membrane than on the cell wall. This could be due to reduction of the metal ions by enzymes present in the cell wall and on the cytoplasmic membrane but not in the cytosol. These metal ions were not toxic to the cells, which are producing them, as they continued to multiply even after the biosynthesis of Au NPs (Ahmad et al. 2003b).

13.2.4 Characterization of Nanoparticles

Nanomaterials, characterized by at least one dimension in the nanometer range, can be considered to institute a bridge among single molecules and infinite bulk systems. Besides individual nanostructures involving clusters, NPs, quantum dots, nanowires, and nanotubes, collections of these nanostructures as arrays and superlattices were the vital interest of nanomaterial researchers. The structure and properties of nanomaterials differ significantly from those of atoms and molecules as well as those of bulk materials. Many topics were found in the emerging area of nanoscience, which include structure, energetics, response, dynamics, and a variety of other properties and there is a large chemical component in each of these aspects.

Metal NPs are of much importance due to their high specific surface area and a high fraction of surface atoms. They have been studied in great extent because of their unique and biomedicinal properties (Biswas et al. 2004; Wang et al. 2004; Govindaraju et al. 2009). Today, from simple prokaryotes to complex eukaryotic organisms are harvested for the fabrication of NPs. Biological systems possess a unique property to be self-organized and synthesize molecules that have highly selective properties. These properties make them prospective candidates that can be harvested to synthesize nanoscale particles used in sensors and other devices (Cui and Gao 2003).

In terms of physicochemical properties, traditional small-molecule drugs are characterized by their molecular weight, chemical composition, purity, solubility, and stability. These properties influence biological activity, as it may depend on parameters such as particle size, size distribution, surface area, surface charge, surface functionality, shape, and aggregation state. Methods are presented for determining NP size in solution by DLS, molecular weight via mass spectrometry, surface charge through zeta-potential measurement, and topology by atomic force microscopy (AFM). Methods are also presented for transmission electron microscopy (TEM) and scanning electron microscopy (SEM) examination of NP samples, and elemental identification using energy dispersive X-ray (EDX) spectroscopy.

13.2.4.1 X-Ray Diffraction Analysis

X-ray diffraction analysis (XRD) offers unparalleled accuracy in the measurement of atomic spacings and is the technique of choice for determining strain states in thin films. XRD is noncontact and nondestructive, which makes it ideal for in situ studies. The intensities measured with XRD can provide quantitative, accurate information on the atomic arrangements at interfaces. Materials composed of any element can be successfully studied with XRD, but XRD is not most sensitive to high-Z elements, due to the diffracted intensity. One of the most important uses of XRD is phase identification. Although other techniques yield film stoichiometries, XRD provides positive phase identification, which is done by comparing the measured d-spacings in the diffraction pattern and integrated intensities with known standards in the JCPDS Powder Diffraction File (Joint Committee on Powder Diffraction Standards, Swarthmore, Pennsylvania 1980). Other excellent methods of phase identification include TEM and electron diffraction.

13.2.4.2 Fourier Transform Infrared Spectroscopy

Fourier transform infrared (FT-IR) spectroscopy is used to probe the chemical composition of the surface of the Ag NPs and the local molecular environment of the capping agents on the NPs. The qualitative aspects of infrared spectroscopy are one of the most powerful attributes of this diverse and versatile analytical technique.

Analytical methods have inherent trade-offs between spatial resolution versus the number and type of components that may be analyzed. High spatial resolution histochemistry can reveal the location of target components in subcellular compartments, whereas high biochemical resolution analyses require bulk samples. FT-IR spectroscopy bridges this gap by providing noninvasive biochemical characterization with spatial resolution at the subcellular level (Szeghalmi et al. 2007).

13.2.4.3 Field Emission Scanning Electron Microscope Analysis

The resolution of the SEM can approach a few nm, and it can operate at magnifications of about 10X–300,000X. Not only topographical information is produced in the SEM, but information concerning the composition near surface regions of the material is provided as well. Nanotechnology has strongly driven the development of recent electron microscopy, with demands not only for increasing resolution but also for more information from the sample. In standard electron microscopes, electrons are mostly generated by heating a tungsten filament (electron gun). In a field emission (FE) electron microscope, the emission of electrons is caused by a strong electric field. An extremely thin and sharp tungsten needle (tip diameter 10–100 nm) works as a cathode. The FE source reasonably combines with SEMs whose development has been supported by advances in secondary electron detector technology. The acceleration voltage between cathode and anode is commonly in the order of magnitude of 0.5–30 kV, and the apparatus requires an extreme vacuum (~10–6 Pa) in the column of the microscope (Yao and Kimura 2007).

13.2.4.4 Energy Dispersive X-Ray Spectroscopy

EDX microanalysis is a technique used for identification of the elemental composition of a specimen. The detection of NPs in tissue is a common problem in biodistribution and toxicity studies. High-resolution TEM can be employed to detect NPs based on morphology; however, TEM alone cannot conclusively identify NPs. Indeed, micrographs are often ambiguous due to particle aggregation, contamination, or morphology change after cellular uptake. EDX can be used to confirm the composition and distribution of the NPs through spectrum and elemental mapping.

13.2.4.5 Transmission Electron Microscopy

TEM is used to characterize the microstructure of materials with very high spatial resolution. Information about the morphology, crystal structure and defects, crystal phases and composition, and magnetic microstructure can be obtained by a combination of electro-optical imaging (sub-Ångstrom in the Titan, 2.5 Å point resolution in the Tecnai), electron diffraction, and small probe capabilities. Further, the Titan provides significant in situ capabilities, allowing for the investigation of how material structure can evolve due to different environmental factors. The trade-off for this diverse range of structural information and high resolution includes the challenge of producing very thin samples for electron transmission.

13.2.4.6 Atomic Force Microscopy

Atomic force microscopy (AFM) was developed to overcome a basic drawback with scanning tunneling microscopy (STM)—that it can only image conducting or semiconducting surfaces. The AFM, however, has the advantage of imaging almost any type of surface, including polymers, ceramics, composites, glass, and biological samples. Resolution is limited to about 1 μm, and only images and size measurements from features lying in the surface (x–y) plane are obtainable. AFM provides a number of advantages over conventional microscopy techniques. AFMs probe the sample and make measurements in three dimensions, x, y, and z (normal to the sample surface), thus enabling the presentation of three-dimensional images of a sample surface. This provides a great advantage over any microscope available previously. With good samples (clean, with no excessively large surface features), resolution in the x–y plane ranges from 0.1 to 1.0 nm and 0.01 nm in z direction (atomic resolution). AFMs require neither a vacuum environment nor any special sample preparation and they can be used in either an ambient or liquid environment. With these advantages, AFM has significantly impacted the fields of materials science, chemistry, biology, physics, and the specialized field of semiconductors.

13.2.4.7 Dynamic Light Scattering Analysis

One technique that can provide an accurate measure of NP hydrodynamic size is dynamic light scattering (DLS). In DLS, the NP solution is illuminated by a monochromatic laser, and its scattering intensity is recorded with a photon detector at a fixed or variable scattering angle. The scattered intensity is time dependent when observed on a microsecond times-cale due to the Brownian motion of the NPs. Although particle size is the primary deter-minant of the measured diffusion coefficient, sample handling and preparation can impact these measurements and thus influence the determined size. The size similarity of NPs to biological moieties is believed to impart many of their unique medical properties. NPs with a zeta-potential between –10 and +10 mV are considered approximately neutral, while NPs with zeta-potentials of greater than +30 mV or less than –30 mV are considered strongly cationic and strongly anionic, respectively. The electrostatic potential changes very quickly (and linearly) from its value at the surface through the first layer of counter ions and then changes more or less exponentially through the diffuse layer. The junction between the bound charges and the diffuse layer is again marked by the broken line. The surface, which separates the bound charge from the diffuse charge around the particle, marks where the solution and the particle move in opposite directions when an external field is applied.

13.3 Conclusion

A naturally motivated investigational practice for the biosynthesis of metal NPs is now established as an emerging area of nanoscience research and development. The biosynthe-sis of NPs using biomaterials is advantageous over chemical and physical methods because it is a cost-effective and environment-friendly method, since it does not involve the use of high pressure, energy, temperature, and toxic chemicals. The biosynthetic method devel-oped for producing Ag, TiO_2, and Au NPs has distinct advantages over chemical methods such as high biosafety and being ecofriendly and nontoxic to the environment. We have explained the biological materials for biosynthesis of metal and metal oxide NPs, which could be an excellent bioreductant and easily available source for synthesis of Ag, Au, and TiO_2 NPs. The biomaterials appear to be environmentally friendly, and therefore, this protocol could be used for the rapid production of metal and metal oxide NPs. Instead of using toxic chemicals for the reduction and stabilization of metallic NPs, the use of various biological entities has received considerable attention in the field of nanobiotechnology. As nature makes optimum use of materials and space, many inorganic materials are produced in biological systems. Similar to such natural processes, plants, fungi, and bacteria were found to be of great success for the synthesis of metal NPs. Though various biocontrol measures are in vogue, their effective control of vectors has not been hitherto highlighted, whereas possibilities of biosynthesis of metal and metal oxide NPs using biomaterials have been fragmentally documented.

References

Agarwal, A., T. L. Weis, M. J. Schurr, N. G. Faith, C. J. Czuprynski, J. F. McAnulty, C. J. Murphy, and N. L. Abbott. 2010. Surfaces modified with nanometer-thick silver-impregnated polymeric films that kill bacteria but support growth of mammalian cells. *Biomaterials* 31:680–690.

Ahmad, A., S. Senapati, M. I. Khan, R. Kumar, R. Ramani, V. Srinivas, and M. Sastry. 2003a. Intracellular synthesis of gold nanoparticles by a novel alkalotolerant actinomycete, *Rhodococcus* species. *Nanotechnology* 14:824–828.

Ahmad, A., S. Senapati, M. I. Khan, R. Kumar, and M. Sastry. 2003b. Extracellular biosynthesis of monodisperse gold nanoparticles by a novel extremophilic actinomycete, *Thermomonospora* sp. *Langmuir* 19:3550–3553.

Alivisatos, A. P. 1996. Perspectives on the physical chemistry of semiconductor nanocrystals. *The Journal of Physical Chemistry* 31(100):13226–13239.

Anil Kumar, S., M. K. Abyaneh, S. W. Gosavi Sulabha, A. Ahmad, and M. I. Khan. 2007. Nitrate reductase-mediated synthesis of silver nanoparticles from $AgNO_3$. *Biotechnology Letters* 29:439–445.

Anitha, K. and R. K. Shenoy. 2001. Treatment of lymphatic filariasis: Current trends. *Indian Journal of Dermatology, Venereology and Leprology* 67(2):60–65.

Baker, C., A. Pradhan, L. Pakstis, D. J. Pochan, and S. I. Shah. 2005. Synthesis and antibacterial properties of silver nanoparticles. *Journal of Nanoscience and Nanotechnology* 5(2):244–249.

Bhainsa, C. K. and S. F. D'Souza. 2006. Extracellular biosynthesis of silver nanoparticles using the fungus *Aspergillus fumigatus*. *Colloids and Surfaces B: Biointerfaces* 47(2):160–164.

Biswas, T. K., L. N. Maity, and B. Mukherjee. 2004. Wound healing potential of *Pterocarpus santalinus* Linn: a pharmacological evaluation. *The International Journal of Lower Extremity Wounds* 3(3):143–150.

Cetin, H., A. Yanikoglu, and J. E. Cilek. 2010. Larvicidal activity of selected plant hydrodistillate extracts against the house mosquito, *Culex pipiens*, a West Nile virus vector. *Parasitology Research* 108(4):943–948.

Chandra, G., I. Bhattacharjee, and S. Chatterjee. 2010. A review on *Anopheles subpictus* Grassi– a biological vector. *Acta Tropica* 115(2):142–154.

Chatterjee, S. N. and G. Chandra. 2000. Role of *Anopheles subpictus* as a primary vector of malaria in an area in India. *Japanese Journal of Tropical Medicine and Hygiene* 28(3):177–181.

Cheon, J. and G. Horace. 2009. Inorganic nanoparticles for biological sensing, imaging and therapeutics. *Journal of Materials Chemistry* 19:6249–6250.

Cui, D. and H. Gao. 2003. Advance and prospects of bionanomaterials. *Biotechnology Progress* 19:683–692.

Dhanda, V. and H. N. Kaul. 1980. Mosquito vectors of Japanese encephalitis virus and their bionomics in India. *Indian National Science Academy* 46:759–768.

Dowling, A., R. Clift, N. Grobert, D. Hutton, R. Oliver, O. O'Neill, J. Pethica, N. Pidgeon, J. Porritt, J. Ryan, A. Seaton, S. Tendler, M. Welland, and R. Whatmore. 2004. Nanoscience and nanotechnologies: Opportunities and uncertainties. The Royal Society, The Royal Academy of Engineering, London, U.K., July 29, 2004.

Duran, N., D. P. Marcato, L. O. Alves, H. G. Desouza, and E. Esposito. 2005. Mechanistic aspects of biosynthesis of silver nanoparticles by several *Fusarium oxysporum* strains. *Journal of Nanobiotechnology* 3:8.

Edwards-Jones, V. 2009. The benefits of silver in hygiene, personal care and healthcare. *Letters in Applied Microbiology* 49(2):147–52.

Fradin, M. S. and J. F. Day. 2002. Comparative efficacy of insect repellents against mosquitoes bites. *New England Journal of Medicine* 347:13–18.

Gould, E. A., T. Solomon, and J. S. Mackenzie. 2008. Does antiviral therapy have a role in the control of Japanese encephalitis? *Antiviral Research* 78:140–914.

Govindaraju, K., V. Kiruthiga, V. Ganesh kumar, and G. Sigaravelu. 2009. Extracellular synthesis of silver nanoparticles by a marine alga, *Sargassum wightii Grevilli* and their antibacterial effects. *Journal of Nanoscience and Nanotechnology* 9(9): 5497–5501.

Guirgis, B. S., C. Sá e Cunha, I. Gomes, M. Cavadas, I. Silva, G. Doria, G. L. Blatch, P. V. Baptista, E. Pereira, H. M. Azzazy, M. M. Mota, M. Prudêncio, and R. Franco. 2012. Gold nanoparticle-based fluorescence immunoassay for malaria antigen detection. *Analytical and Bioanalytical Chemistry* 402:1019–1027.

Hay, S. I., P. W. Gething, and R. W. Snow. 2010. India's invisible malaria burden. *Lancet* 376:1716–1717.

Isman, M. B. 2006. Botanical insecticides, deterrents, and repellents in modern agriculture and an increasingly regulated world. *Annual Review of Entomology* 51:45–66.

Jayaseelan, C., A. A. Rahuman, G. Rajakumar, T. Santhoshkumar, A. V. Kirthi, S. Marimuthu, A. Bagavan, C. Kamaraj, A. A. Zahir, G. Elango, K. Velayutham, K. V. Rao, L. Karthik, and S. Raveendran. 2012a. Efficacy of plant-mediated synthesized silver nanoparticles against hematophagous parasites. *Parasitology Research* 111(2):921–933.

Jayaseelan, C. and A. A. Rahuman. 2012b. Acaricidal efficacy of synthesized silver nanoparticles using aqueous leaf extract of *Ocimum canum* against *Hyalommaanatolicum anatolicum* and *Hyalomma marginatum* isaaci (Acari: Ixodidae). *Parasitology Research* 111(3):1369–1378.

Jayaseelan, C., A. A. Rahuman, A. V. Kirthi, S. Marimuthu, T. Santhoshkumar, A. Bagavan, K. Gaurav, L. Karthik, and K. V. Rao. 2012c. Novel microbial route to synthesize ZnO nanoparticles using *Aeromonas hydrophila* and their activity against pathogenic bacteria and fungi. *Spectrochimica Acta Part A: Molecular and Biomolecular Spectroscopy* 90:78–84.

Jayaseelan, C., A. A. Rahuman, G. Rajakumar, A. V. Kirthi, T. Santhoshkumar, S. Marimuthu, A. Bagavan, C. Kamaraj, A. A. Zahir, and G. Elango. 2011. Synthesis of pediculocidal and larvicidal silver nanoparticles by leaf extract from heartleaf moonseed plant, *Tinospora cordifolia* miers. *Parasitology Research* 109(1):185–194.

Jha, A. K., K. Prasad, K. Prasad, and A. R. Kulkarni. 2009. Plant system: Nature's nano factory. *Colloids and Surfaces B: Biointerfaces* 73:219–223.

Joerger, K. T., R. Joerger, E. Olsson, and C. Granqvist. 2001. Bacteria as workers in the living factory: Metal-accumulating bacteria and their potential for materials science. *Trends in Biotechnology* 19(1):15–20.

Joint Committee on Powder Diffraction Standards, Powder Diffraction File 21–1272, Swarthmore, PA, 1980.

Kager, P. A. 2002. Malaria control: Constraints and opportunities. *Tropical Medicine and International Health* 7:1042–1046.

Kalishwaralal, K., V. Deepak, S. Ramkumarpandian, H. Nellaiah, and G. Sangiliyandi. 2008. Extracellular biosynthesis of silver nanoparticles by the culture supernatant of *Bacillus licheniformis. Materials Letters* 62:4411–4413.

Karthik, L., G. Kumar, and K. V. Bhaskara Rao. 2012a. Marine actinobacterial mediated titanium dioxide nanoparticles synthesis. Paper presented at the *International Conference on Nano Science and Technology (ICONSAT-2012)*, Hyderabad, India.

Karthik, L., G. Kumar, and K. V. Bhaskara Rao. 2012b. Marine actinobacterial mediated gold nanoparticles synthesis and their antimalarial activity. Paper presented at the *International Conference on NanoBio 2012*, Kochi, India.

Karunamoorthi, K., S. Ramanujam, and R. Rathinasamy. 2008. Evaluation of leaf extracts of *Vitex negundo* L. (Family: Verbenaceae) against larvae of *Culex tritaeniorhynchus* and repellent activity on adult vector mosquitoes. *Parasitology Research* 103(3):545–550.

Keiser, J., M. F. Maltese, T. E. Erlanger, R. Bos, M. Tanner, B. H. Singer, and J. Utzinger. 2005. Effect of irrigated rice agriculture on Japanese encephalitis, including challenges and opportunities for integrated vector management. *Acta Tropica* 95:40–57.

Kirthi, A. V., A. A. Rahuman, G. Rajakumar, S. Marimuthu, T. Santhoshkumar, C. Jayaseelan, G. Elango, A. A. Zahir, C. Kamaraj, and A. Bagavan. 2011. Biosynthesis of titanium dioxide nanoparticles using bacterium *Bacillus subtilis. Materials Letters* 65(18):2745–2747.

Kowshik, M., S. Ashtaputre, S. Kharrazi, W. Vogel, J. Urban, S. Kulkarni, and K. Paknikar. 2003. Extracellular synthesis of silver nanoparticles by a silver-tolerant yeast strain MKY3. *Nanotechnology* 14:95–100.

Kulkarni, S. M. 1983. Detection of sporozoites in *Anopheles subpictus* in Baster district, Madhya Pradesh. *Indian Journal of Malariology* 20:159–160.

Kuppusamy, C. and K. Murugan. 2010. Effects of *Andrographis paniculata* Nees on growth, development and reproduction of malarial vector *Anopheles stephensi* Liston (Diptera: Culicidae). *Tropical Biomedicine* 27(3):509–516.

Maheswaran, R. and S. Ignacimuthu. 2011. A novel herbal formulation against dengue vector mosquitoes *Aedes aegypti* and *Aedes albopictus*. *Parasitology Research* 110:1801–1813.

Mann, S. 1996. *Biomimetic Materials Chemistry*. VCH, New York.

Marimuthu, S., A. A. Rahuman, G. Rajakumar, T. Santhoshkumar, A. V. Kirthi, C. Jayaseelan, A. Bagavan, A. A. Zahir, G. Elango, and C. Kamaraj. 2011. Evaluation of green synthesized silver nanoparticles against parasites. *Parasitology Research* 108(6):1541–1549.

Masala, O. and R. Seshadri. 2004. Synthesis routes for large volumes of nanoparticles. *Annual Review of Materials Research* 34:41–81.

Matsunaga, T. and H. Takeyama. 1998. Biomagnetic nanoparticle formation and application. *Supramolecular Science* 5:391–394.

Michael, E., D. A. Bundy, and B.T. Grenfell. 1996. Re-assessing the global prevalence and distribution of lymphatic filariasis. *Parasitology* 112(4):409–428.

Mohanpuria, P., K. N. Rana, and S. K. Yadav. 2008. Biosynthesis of nanoparticles: Technological concepts and future applications. *Journal of Nanoparticle Research* 10:507–517.

Morones, J. R., J. L. Elechiguerra, A. Camacho, K. Holt, J. B. Kouri, J. T. Ramirez, and M. J. Yacaman. 2005. The bactericidal effect of silver nanoparticles. *Nanotechnology* 16:2346–2353.

Mullen, M. D., D. C. Wolf, F. G. Ferris, T. J. Beveridge, C. A. Flemming, and G. W. Bailey. 1989. Bacterial sorption of heavy metals. *Applied and Environmental Microbiology* 55:3143–3149.

Myung, K., A. Massougbodji, S. Ekoue, P. Atchade, V. Kiki-Fagla, and A. D. Klion. 1998. Lymphatic filariasis in a hyper endemic region: A ten-year, follow-up panel survey. *The American Journal of Tropical Medicine and Hygiene* 59(2):222–226.

Nair, B. and T. Pradeep. 2002. Coalescence of nanoclusters and formation of submicron crystallites assisted by *Lactobacillus* strains. *Crystal Growth and Design* 2:293–298.

Panicker, K. N., M. GeethaBai, U. S. B. Rao, K. Viswam, and U. Suryanarayanamurthy. 1981. *An. subpictus* vector of malaria in coastal villages of South-East India. *Current Science* 50:694–695.

Pelaez, M., A. de la Cruz, E. Stathatos, P. Falaras, and D. D. Dionysiou 2009. Visible light-activated N-F-codoped TiO_2 nanoparticles for the photocatalytic degradation of microcystin-LR in water. *Catalysis Today* 144(2):19–25.

Ramaiah, K. D., P. K. Das, E. Michael, and H. Guyatt. 2000. The economic burden of lymphatic filariasis in India. *Parasitology Today* 16(6):251–253.

Reuben, R. and A. Gajanana. 1997. Japanese encephalitis in India. *Indian Journal of Pediatrics* 64:243–251.

Sabesan, S. 2003. Forecasting mosquito abundance to prevent Japanese encephalitis. *Current Science* 84(9):1172–1173.

Sanghi, R. and P. Verma. 2009. Biomimetic synthesis and characterization of protein capped silver nanoparticles. *Bioresource Technology* 100(1):501–504.

Santhoshkumar, T., A. A. Rahuman, G. Rajakumar, S. Marimuthu, A. Bagavan, C. Jayaseelan, A. A. Zahir, G. Elango, and C. Kamaraj. 2011. Synthesis of silver nanoparticles using *Nelumbo nucifera* leaf extract and its larvicidal activity against malaria and filariasis vectors. *Parasitology Research* 108(3):693–702.

Sastry, M., A. Ahmad, M. I. Khan, and R. Kumar. 2003. Biosynthesis of metal nanoparticles using fungi and actinomycetes. *Current Science* 85:162–170.

Shelton, A. M., P. Wang, J. Z. Zhao, and R. T. Roush. 2007. Resistance to insect pathogens and strategies to manage resistance: An update. In: L. A. Lacey and H. K. Kaya (eds), *Field Manual of Techniques in Invertebrate Pathology*. Springer-Verlag, New York.

Soni, N. and S. Prakash. 2012. Efficacy of fungus mediated silver and gold nanoparticles against *Aedes aegypti* larvae. *Parasitology Research* 110:175–184.

Suman, D. S., A. R. Shrivastava, B. D. Parashar, S. C. Pant, O. P. Agrawal, and S. Prakash. 2008. Scanning electron microscopic studies on egg surface morphology and morphometric of *Culex tritaeniorhynchu*s and *Culex quinquefasciatus* (Diptera: Culicidae). *Parasitology Research* 104:173–176.

Sundrarajan, M. and S. Gowri. 2011. Green synthesis of titanium dioxide nanoparticles by *Nyctanthes arbor-tristis* leaves extract. *Chalcogenide Letters* 8(8):447–451.

Szeghalmi, A., S. Kaminskyj, and K. M. Gough. 2007. A synchrotron FTIR micro spectroscopy investigation of fungal hyphae grown under optimal and stressed conditions. *Analytical and Bioanalytical Chemistry* 387(5):1779–1789.

Thenmozhi, V., R. Rajendran, K. Ayanar R. Manavalan, and B. K. Tyagi. 2006. Long-term study of Japanese encephalitis virus infection in *Anopheles subpictus* in Cuddalore district, Tamilnadu, South India. *Tropical Medicine and International Health* 11(3):288–293.

Velayutham, K., A. A. Rahuman, G. Rajakumar, T. Santhoshkumar, S. Marimuthu, C. Jayaseelan, A. Bagavan, A. V. Kirthi, C. Kamaraj, A. A. Zahir, and G. Elango. 2011. Evaluation of *Catharanthus roseus* leaf extract-mediated biosynthesis of titanium dioxide nanoparticles against *Hippobosca maculata* and *Bovicola ovis*. *Parasitology Research*. doi: 10.1007/s00436–011–2676-x.

Vigneshwaran, N., A. A. Kathe, P. V. Varadarajan, R. P. Nachane, and R. H. Balasubramanya. 2007. Silver-protein (core-shell) nanoparticle production using spent mushroom substrate. *Langmuir* 23(13):7113–7117.

Wang, C., N. T. Fynn, and R. Langer. 2004. Controlled structure and properties of thermo responsive nanoparticle–hydrogel composites. *Advanced Materials* 13:1074–1079.

Wernsdorfer, G. and W. H. Wernsdorfer. 2003. Malaria at the turn from the 2nd to the 3rd millennium. *Wien Klin Wochenschr* 115(3):2–9.

WHO. 2004. *First Meeting of the Regional Technical Advisory Group on Malaria*, Manesar, Haryana, India, SEA-MAL 239, pp. 1–38.

WHO. 2005. *Sixth Meeting of the Technical Advisory Group on the Global Elimination of Lymphatic Filariasis*, Geneva, Switzerland. *Weekly Epidemiological Record* 80:401–408.

WHO. 2007. Global malaria programme. In: WHO Global Malaria Programme. Available at http://www.who.int/malaria/

WHO. 2008a. World malaria report. In: WHO/HTM/GMP/2008.1, Geneva, Switzerland, p. 215. Available at http://www.who.int/malaria/wmr2008/malaria2008.pdf

WHO. 2008b. Global programme to eliminate lymphatic filariasis. *Weekly Epidemiological Record* 83:333–341.

Willner, I., R. Baron, and B. Willner. 2006. Growing metal nanoparticles by enzymes. *Advanced Materials* 18:1109–1120.

Xu, Z. P., Q. H. Zeng, G. Q. Lu, and A. B. Yu. 2006. Inorganic nanoparticles as carriers for efficient cellular delivery. *Chemical Engineering Science* 61:1027–1040.

Yang, Y. C., S. G. Lee, H. K. Lee, M. K. Kim, S. H. Lee, and H. S. Lee. 2002. A piper dine amide extracted from *Piper longum* L. fruit shows activity against *Aedes aegypti* mosquito larvae. *Journal of Agricultural and Food Chemistry* 50:3765–3767.

Yao, H. and K. Kimura. 2007. Field emission scanning electron microscopy for structural characterization of 3D gold nanoparticle super lattices. In: *Modern Research and Educational Topics in Microscopy,* A. Méndez-Vilas and J. Díaz (eds), FORMATEX, Spain, pp. 568–575.

Zanette, C., M. Pelin, M. Crosera, G. Adami, M. Bovenzi, F. F. Larese, and C. Florio. 2011. Silver nanoparticles exert a long-lasting ant proliferative effect on human keratinocyte HaCaT cell line. *Toxicology in Vitro* 25(5):1053–1060.

14

Mussel-Derived Adhesive Biomaterials

Dong Soo Hwang,* Yoo Seong Choi,* and Hyung Joon Cha

CONTENTS

14.1 Introduction

Marine-fouling invertebrates (e.g., mussel, barnacle, sandcastle worm, hydroid, and sea star) form a strong attachment to the marine substratum against mechanical stresses arising from the tide, buoyancy, and drag using their special physical and chemical underwater adhesives (Waite and Tanzer, 1981; Kamino et al., 2000; Stewart et al., 2004; Santos et al., 2005). There are many unveiled lessons to learn from these organisms, and indeed, underwater adhesives from these marine organisms have been investigated as a source of potential underwater

---

* The authors have contributed equally to this chapter.

adhesives because of their fascinating properties. These properties include strong adhesion to various material substrates, water displacement, biocompatibility, and controlled biodegradability (Holten-Andersen and Waite, 2008). In addition, the marine environment has much in common with the human body; both systems are naturally saline and experience varied fluid flow, macromolecule-mediated fouling, and degradation of organic constituents via cell-level activities (Holten-Andersen and Waite, 2008). These are just a few examples of matching biological and mechanical events present in both the human body and marine environment. Therefore, an understanding of how adhesives are produced by marine organisms will inspire new paradigms for the design and engineering of adhesives for medical use.

The mussel is one of the best model systems to understand how marine organisms anchor to the marine substratum effectively, due to lots of advanced researches on their biochemistry, physics, and mechanics (Waite, 2005; Lee et al., 2011). Using fundamental research on mussel adhesion, there have been many attempts to translate insights from mussel adhesion to biomedical materials. Therefore, the review here is to describe the mechanism of mussel adhesion and its production and application as a biomedical adhesive material.

14.2 Mussel Adhesion Mechanism

14.2.1 Mussel Byssus

Investigation of mussel adhesion most likely began with the studies by Brown in 1950–1952 (Brown, 1952) and Smyth (1954), and detailed investigations by Pujol (1967), Tamarin (1975), and Tamarin et al. (1976) followed. Modern interdisciplinary investigations that integrate biochemistry, molecular biology, and biomechanics of mussel adhesion in detail have been performed chiefly by Waite and his colleagues (1976 to date), and these authors provide a comprehensive picture of the mussel adhesion system. Because the Waite research group has focused primarily on the *Mytilus* species, we describe and review mussel adhesion devoted to the findings from the *Mytilus* species.

The mussel fabricates and utilizes what is called a byssus, which is a bundle of threads used to adhere the organism to the substratum. The individual thread is called a byssal thread (Figure 14.1, inset) (Hwang et al., 2010a). At the end of individual byssal thread, there is an adhesive plaque where underwater adhesion between the byssal thread and substratum occurs. Byssal thread is composed primarily of proteins (slightly greater than 90%) and some trace levels of carbohydrates, lipids, and metal ions. Therefore, most research on mussel adhesion has focused on the adhesive proteins. One intriguing finding from byssus is that the adhesive plaque has three times as much calcium and 10^4 times as much iron as standard seawater, which implies the existence of an interaction between mussel adhesive proteins and these metal ions (Sun and Waite, 2005). Byssal threads are synthesized by the mussel foot, an extendable tonguelike organ, in which the protein precursors that compose the byssal thread are stored prior to thread formation. This is the reason why mussel fp is often considered when researchers describe mussel adhesive proteins. When a mussel makes a new thread, its foot emerges from its shell, finds a favorite spot for anchoring, and secretes the precursors for byssus into a groove running along the length of the ventral side of the foot. Muscular contractions of the foot around the groove follow, and the precursors assemble as a thread within 10 min (Waite, 1992). A byssus is composed of approximately 25–30 different types of precursor proteins, and 10 of them have been characterized in biochemical and molecular biological studies (Table 14.1). The precursor proteins are classified

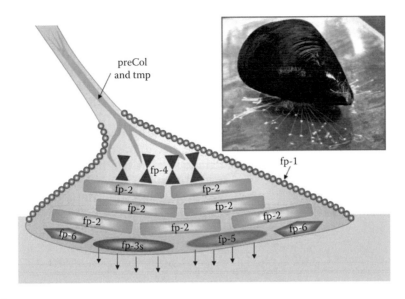

FIGURE 14.1
Byssal plaque proteins of *Mytilus*. A mussel (*Mytilus galloprovincialis*, inset) is shown attached to a sheet of mica. One of its plaques (red circle) is enlarged as a schematic drawing to illustrate the approximate distribution of proteins. (Adapted from Hwang, D.S., Zeng, H.B., Masic, A., Harrington, M.J., Israelachvili, J.N., and Waite, J.H., Protein- and metal-dependent interactions of a prominent protein in mussel adhesive plaques, *J. Biol. Chem.*, 285, 25850–25858. Copyright 2010, American Society for Biochemistry and Molecular Biology.)

TABLE 14.1

fps Diversity in the Adhesive Plaque

Protein	Species	Mass (kDa)	pI	Dopa (mol%)	Features	Reference
fp-1	*M. edulis*	~110	10.5	13	Coating protein, iron binding, decapeptide (AKPSY**O*O**TY*K)	Waite (1983), Taylor et al. (1994b)
fp-2	*M. edulis*	~45	9.5	3	Bulk adhesive, EGF motif, metal binding (calcium, iron)	Vovelle (1965), Rzepecki and Waite (1992), Inoue et al. (1995)
fp-3	*M. edulis*	5~6	NA	~20	Adhesive primer, hydroxyarginine	Inoue et al. (1996)
fp-4	*M. californianus*	~90	NA	4	Load-bearing junction, decapeptide (HVHTHRVLHK), copper binding, undecapeptide (DDHVNDIAQTA), calcium binding	Zhao and Waite (2006a)
fp-5	*M. edulis*	~9	9	~30	Adhesive primer, phosphoserine	Waite and Qin (2001)
fp-6	*M. californianus*	~11	9.5	~4	Antioxidant	Zhao and Waite (2006a)

as byssal prepolymerized collagens (PreCols) (Coyne et al., 1997), thread matrix proteins (tmps) (Sagert and Waite, 2009), and fps (Filpula et al., 1990; Rzepecki and Waite, 1992; Inoue et al., 1995, 1996; Papov et al., 1995; Waite and Qin, 2001; Zhao and Waite, 2006a,b) based on their roles and biochemistries. PreCols and tmps comprise the byssal thread filler and matrix, respectively, whereas fps is found in the adhesive plaque and acts an adhesive pad for underwater adhesion (Figure 14.1). Here, as we focus on mussel adhesion, we review only fps in detail.

To date, six types of fps have been isolated from the *Mytilus* genus, and 3,4-dihydroxy-phenylalanine (DOPA), a hydroxylated tyrosine, due to posttranslational modification of its benzene ring, is found in all of the identified fps, which implies that it may play an important role in mussel adhesion and byssus assembly (Figure 14.2, Table 14.1) (Deming, 1999). Most fps mentioned in this review were isolated from the mussel *Mytilus edulis*, unless otherwise mentioned.

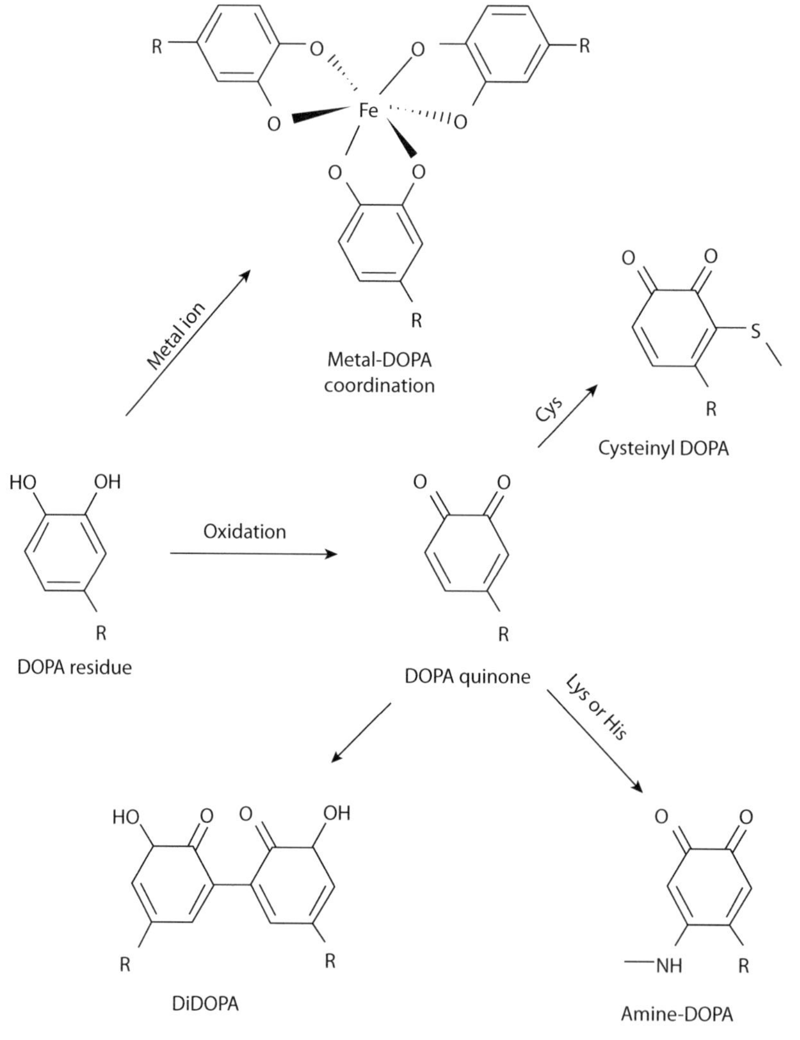

FIGURE 14.2
DOPA cross-linking mechanism.

14.2.2 Foot Proteins

14.2.2.1 fp-1

fp-1 (~108 kDa) is a mussel coating protein that is composed of 50–80 repeats of a tandem decapeptide (e.g., AKPSYO*OTY*K from *M. edulis fp-1*; **O**, *trans*-4-hydroxyproline; **O***, *trans*-2,3-*cis*-3,4-dihydroxy proline; **Y***, DOPA) (Filpula et al., 1990; Taylor et al., 1994b). Circular dichroism (CD) and 2D-NMR solution structure analysis of fp-1 suggest that the fp-1 decapeptide has a trans-polyproline type II helix secondary structure (Kanyalkar et al., 2002). fp-1 is the only known biopolymer that is distributed uniformly in the cuticle of byssal thread and its adhesive plaque and has been suggested to be a coating protein (Lin et al., 2007). A byssal coating made from fp-1 has two critical mechanical properties that rarely coexist in the same coating material: high hardness (and stiffness) and high extensibility (Holten-Andersen et al., 2007). Cohesive energy, the attraction between molecules of the same substance, in coating materials is one of the most important factors that determine the mechanical properties of a coating. Thus, understanding the cohesive force of fp-1 could enable mimicking of the protective coating of *Mytilus* species (Pocius, 2002). Unexpectedly, fp-1 coats two opposed surfaces in the surface force apparatus (SFA, nanomechanical tool to measure a force between two surfaces) but does not contribute to any cohesive bridges between the two surfaces in 0.1 M sodium acetate buffer (pH 5.5–7.0, 0.25 M KNO_3) (Lin et al., 2007; Zeng et al., 2010) This implies that the cohesive strength of *Mytilus* byssal cuticle is mediated by fp-1 and other molecules existing in the cuticle. Recently, a secondary ion mass spectrometry (SIMS) study on *Mytilus* byssal cuticle revealed the *Mytilus* byssal cuticle contains extraordinary levels of Fe, and resonance Raman microscopy on the thin sections of the cuticle has directly confirmed the presence of catechol–Fe^{3+} complexes in the cuticle (Holten-Andersen et al., 2009; Harrington et al., 2010). Therefore, Fe^{3+}-mediated bridging between two DOPA-containing fp-1 layers was investigated. In the presence of low Fe^{3+} (~10 μM), significant and reversible cohesion ($F_{ad}/R \sim -6$ mN/m) occurred immediately when two layers of fp-1 were brought into contact and separated, and the cohesion increased to $F_{ad}/R \sim -20$ mN/m for 100 min contact times (Figure 14.3) (Hwang et al., 2010a). Resonance Raman peaks at 550, 596, and 637 cm^{-1}, which are indicative of catechol–Fe complexes, were detected in mica sandwiches of fp-1 films with 10 μM Fe^{3+}, as was prepared for SFA experiments. However, at 10-fold higher concentrations (100 μM Fe^{3+}), cohesion disappeared, again suggesting that moderate levels of Fe^{3+} are required to form catechol–Fe^{3+} complexes. The fp-1 cohesion mediated by Fe^{3+} was reversible even after more than 10 separations in aqueous buffer, and contact times of 100 min (~ –20 mN/m) reached half the adhesion energy between biotin and avidin layers immobilized in the lipid bilayer (~ –40 mN/m). These results suggest that the interaction between Fe^{3+} and DOPA in fp-1 is one of the main contributors to the extraordinary mechanical properties of the *Mytilus* byssal cuticle.

14.2.2.2 fp-2

fp-2 (~45 kDa), the most abundant protein in adhesive plaque (~25% w/w), has 11 repeats of an epidermal growth factor (EGF) domain containing approximately two DOPA residues and a calcium binding motif that has a known consensus amino acid sequence of Cys_3-x-Asx-x-x-x-Tyr-x-Cys_4 (Rzepecki and Waite, 1992; Inoue et al., 1995). As observed in fp-1 cohesion experiments, fp-2 also shows strong cohesion mediated by Fe^{3+}–DOPA complexes, using SFA and resonance Raman microscopy (Hwang et al., 2010a). The addition

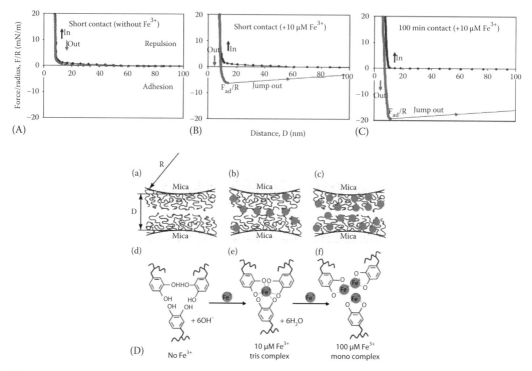

FIGURE 14.3

Cohesion of fp-1 films measured using SFA. (A) Without Fe^{3+}, no interaction occurs after contact. (B) Addition of 10 μMFe^{3+} results in an immediate interaction evident by the jump-out peaking at 7 mN/m. (C) A 100 min contact increases the interaction to 20 mN/m. (D) Schematic showing two opposed symmetric fp-1 films on mica (a) without Fe^{3+}, (b) with 10-μMFe^{3+}, and (c) with 100-μMFe^{3+}. Also shown are the suggested chemical interactions between Dopa and Fe^{3+}: (d) no Fe^{3+}, (e) tris-Dopa–Fe^{3+} complexes, and (f) mono-Dopa–Fe^{3+} complexes. (Adapted from Zeng, H., Hwang, D.S., Israelachvili, J.N., and Waite, J.H., Strong reversible Fe^{3+}-mediated bridging between dopa-containing protein films in water, *Proc. Natl Acad. Sci. USA*, 107, 12850–12853. Copyright 2010 National Academy of Sciences, USA.)

of micromolar levels of calcium also induces moderate cohesion, suggesting that calcium ions in byssus make a bridge between calcium binding sites of fp-2 (Hwang et al., 2010a). In the presence of metal ions, fp-2 adhesion is reversible without diminishing adhesion, suggesting that the metal ions-fp-2 interaction is reversible in water.

14.2.2.3 fp-3

fp-3 (5–7 kDa) is the most polymorphic protein (>20 variants) of the fps, and it participates in adhesion between the adhesive plaque and the substratum (Zhao and Waite, 2006a; Lee et al., 2011). *In situ* MALDI–TOF (matrix-assisted laser desorption ionization) has revealed that fp-3 is the most abundant protein in the interface between the adhesive plaque and substratum (i.e., footprint) (Zhao and Waite, 2006a; Lee et al., 2011). The polymorphism is likely to originate from multiple genes and gene copies of fp-3 or alternative splicing. The fp-3 family is all positively charged and DOPA rich, with typically 10–20 mol% DOPA content. Hydroxyarginine is one of the distinctive features of fp-3, but its function remains unclear. fp-3 adheres to various types of substrates, including mica, polystyrene, poly(methylmethacrylate), SiO_2, and TiO_2. The solution structure of fp-3, by

CD analysis, is an unstructured extended coil structure that is well adapted to adhere to a variety of surfaces.

14.2.2.4 fp-4

The only available cDNA sequence of fp-4 originates from *Mytilus californianus* (Zhao and Waite, 2006b; Lee et al., 2011). Its mass, determined by MALDI–TOF, is approximately 94 kDa, and it contains 22 mol% histidine and 2 mol% DOPA. The deduced protein sequence reveals 35 tandem repeats of a histidine-rich decapeptide (HVHTHRVLHK) and an aspartic acid-rich undecapeptide (DDHVNDIAQTA), which is repeated 16 times in fp-4. The histidine-rich decapeptide binds only copper ions with high capacity when it is incubated with Fe^{3+}, Co^{2+}, Ni^{2+}, Zn^{2+}, and Cu^{2+}. In contrast, the aspartic acid–rich undecapeptide preferentially binds Ca^{2+}. In byssus, fp-4 locates to a junction between the byssal thread and the adhesive plaque. Therefore, it has been suggested that fp-4 interacts with pre-Cols via Cu^{2+}–histidine complexes and with fp-2 via Ca^{2+}–Ca^{2+} binding-motif interactions (Zhao and Waite, 2006b).

14.2.2.5 fp-5

fp-5 (~9 kDa) is also abundant in the adhesion interface, and it functions in the adhesive plaque as an adhesive primer (Waite and Qin, 2001). fp-5 has the highest DOPA content of all fps (25~30 mol%), and glycine, lysine, and phosphoserine are also abundant in fp-5. High mole% glycine (~20) implies that fp-5 has a flexible structure that is transformed easily for surface adhesion. Recombinant fp-5 showed stronger adhesion than Cell-Tak™, a mixture of fp-1 and fp-2, in air using atomic force microscopy (AFM) (Hwang et al., 2004), but its adhesion in aqueous solutions requires further research.

14.2.2.6 fp-6

fp-6 (~11 kDa) has been fully sequenced from *M. californianus* only (Zhao and Waite, 2006a; Lee et al., 2011). As with fp-3 and fp-5, it is also an interfacial protein located between the plaque and substratum. It contains high levels of lysine, tyrosine, and glycine and cysteine, but its DOPA content is extremely low (~2 mol%) compared with fp-3 and fp-5. The intriguing role of fp-6 in the adhesive plaque is as an "antioxidant" (Yu et al., 2011). The DOPA residues in adhesive primers, for example, fp-3 and fp-5, are oxidized to DOPA quinone (Figure 14.2) when they are exposed to oxidants or buffers of neutral or basic pHs (>6), which results in reduced adhesion to the target surface. Thus, fp-3 and fp-5 may lose their adhesiveness due to DOPA oxidation during their secretion from mussel foot to seawater (~pH 8.2) for underwater adhesion. However, in practice, fp-6 can effectively reduce the DOPA quinones in fp-3 and fp-5 back to DOPA by coupling with a half reaction resulting in the oxidation of two thiols (cysteines) in fp-6 to form a disulfide bond, thereby protecting DOPA residues in fp-3 and fp-5 for surface adhesion (Yu et al., 2011).

14.2.3 Two Key Mechanisms for Mussel Adhesion: Complex Coacervation and DOPA Chemistry

Mussel-mediated secretion and application of adhesive to target surfaces appears to utilize complex coacervation and L-3,4-dihydroxyphenyl alanine (DOPA) chemistry (Hwang et al., 2010b).

14.2.3.1 Complex Coacervation

Complex coacervation is a fluid–fluid phase separation, typically involving two oppositely charged polyelectrolytes in aqueous solution, which results in a dense coacervate phase and a dilute equilibrium phase (Figure 14.4) (Bungenberg de Jong, 1932, 1949). Complex coacervation was suggested as the origin of life by a Russian scientist, Alexander Oparin, as a means to separate combinations of biomolecules from the surrounding medium (Oparin, 1924). More simply put, cationic and anionic polymers interact at a certain pH range where their net charge is mutually neutralized to form a liquid droplet, a polymer-rich phase called a complex coacervate (Figure 14.4A). Via coalescence, coacervates can grow from micro- to mesodroplets and, eventually, phase separate from solution (Figure 14.4B). Phase-separated coacervates remain fluid unless triggered. Physical properties of complex coacervate are influenced by pH, ionic strength, shapes of polyelectrolyte, and types of charged group, but systematic studies are lacking (Hwang et al., 2010b). One common feature of complex coacervates is their very low interfacial energy (<3 mJ/m^2) in aqueous solution, and it is this property that enables the coacervate not only to coalesce with each other but also to engulf a variety of particles in solution. Consequently, coacervates have been utilized as encapsulants for flavors, oils, explosives, and cells (de Kruif et al., 2004). It was recently reported that marine sandcastle worms utilize DOPA-containing complex coacervate adhesive for their adhesion, and many researchers speculate that mussel adhesive is also secreted in a complex coacervation form (Zhao et al., 2005; Hwang et al., 2010b; Lim et al., 2010). Complex coacervation has many advantages as an underwater-adhesive material process:

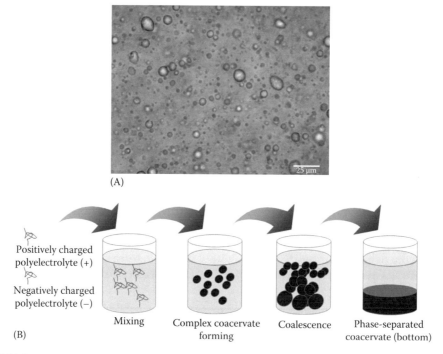

FIGURE 14.4

(A) Light microscopy image of coacervated microdroplet of hyaluronic acid and recombinant mussel fp-151. Scale bar is 25 μm. (B) Complex coacervation process.

1. Complex coacervate is the result of liquid–liquid phase separation, and the coacervate is not easily diluted out by diffusion when it is in water phase. Most mussel and tubeworm adhesive proteins discovered to date are polyelectrolytes (Zhao et al., 2005) that lack secondary structure and contain hydrophilic primary sequences with high charge densities. Secreting highly soluble polyelectrolytes directly into seawater where they will be quickly diluted by diffusion appears counterproductive to underwater adhesion. However, coacervates of oppositely charged polyelectrolytes usually undergo a fluid–fluid phase separation at certain pHs, and an adhesive in coacervate remains as a condensed liquid that does not disperse into the seawater (Zhao et al., 2005).

2. The polyelectrolyte concentration in a dense coacervate phase can reach 0.5–4 g/mL depending on the polyelectrolyte system and mixing ratio. This concentration range is sufficiently viscous for practical adhesive applications (Kausik et al., 2009; Hwang et al., 2010b; Lim et al., 2010).

3. A coacervate phase has extremely low interfacial energy. One of the most significant properties affecting adhesive performance is the ability to "wet" a surface, which depends critically upon interfacial energy. Recent studies by (Hwang et al., 2010b) and (Spruijt et al., 2010) measured interfacial energies of coacervates to water, and they ranged from 0.1 to 3 mJ/m². They found that the interfacial energy range of coacervates to water is extremely low when compared with that of mineral oil to water (10–50 mJ/m²) (Kim and Burgess, 2001). Lim et al. have also reported bulk-scale adhesive properties of coacervated recombinant hybrid mussel adhesive proteins (Lim et al., 2010). Therefore, the coacervate adhesives of mussel and sandcastle can spread readily over the target wet surfaces and fill gaps in a rough surface in seawater.

4. A coacervate phase maintains proper rheological properties of an adhesive, such as low viscosity, shear thinning behavior, and high diffusion coefficient. To better understand adhesive underwater processing, marine adhesives have been approximated by combining a recombinant mussel fp-151 (a polycation) with hyaluronic acid (a polyanion) in vitro at pH 5, and viscosity and bulk-scale adhesive strength were measured by SFA and shear strength test, respectively (Kausik et al., 2009; Hwang et al., 2010b). Viscosity measurements of the coacervate, which was produced at the optimal ratio where the coacervate charge is approximately neutral and at two suboptimal mixing ratios (positively charged coacervates or negatively charged coacervates), revealed that whereas the optimal ratio showed shear thinning, both suboptimal mixing ratios showed robust shear thickening. These results have intriguing biological implications. During secretion of adhesive, the coacervate adhesive should pass from the cells to a conducting tubule (~40–60 μm) and is dispensed via pores of 20–30 μm in diameter. Fluid flow rate through a tube is inversely proportional to the forth power of the tube radius. Therefore, shear thinning in the coacervate (the optimal coacervate charge balance, i.e., neutral) would improve its flow through the pores, whereas immature coacervate mixtures (the positively charged coacervates or negatively charged coacervates) with shear thickening would effectively clog the pores (Figure 14.5). Coacervates also contain very high protein concentrations without a significant compromise in solute diffusion coefficients, and it thus beneficial for uniform cross-linking reactions when the adhesive is required to transform into a solid phase.

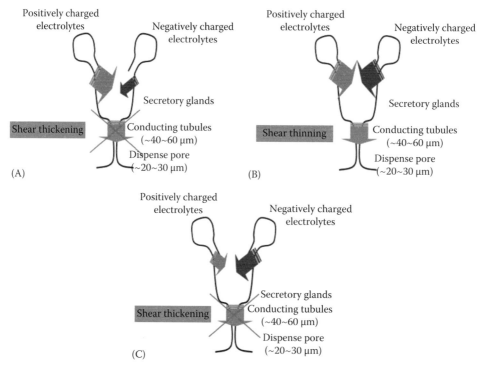

FIGURE 14.5
Viscosity properties of mussel-inspired coacervate. (A) Positively charged coacervate, (B) neutralized coacervate, (C) negatively charged coacervate.

5. Complex coacervate is formed in aqueous solution at moderate pH, thereby avoiding nonbiocompatible solvents and exothermic polymerization chemistries, which is one of the most important properties promoting the use of coacervate adhesive in biomedical fields.

Thus, the secreted marine adhesives and coatings in seawater are highly concentrated liquids that spread readily over the target wet surfaces, fill gaps and rough surface, and do not disperse into the seawater.

14.2.3.2 DOPA Chemistry

Following the coacervation of adhesive materials, the stabilization and cross-linking of coacervate is required. When mussels secrete their adhesive materials, they exploit pH-sensitive DOPA chemistry. DOPA, an essential factor for marine adhesives and coatings, is not easily cross-linked when DOPA-containing coacervate is stored in mussel secretory granules at pH 5.5. However, in aerated solution at pH 7, DOPA has a redox potential of $E_o = +0.65$ V, in which two half reactions are coupled: $1/2O_2^+ 2e^- + 2H^+ \leftrightarrow H_2O$ and DOPA $\leftrightarrow$ DOPA quinone $+ 2e^- + 2H^+$ (Holten-Andersen and Waite, 2008). The oxidizing power of O_2 drives the production of DOPA quinone effectively at pHs greater than 7. Due to the coupling reaction of DOPA quinone, 5- and 2-S-cysteinyl DOPA cross-linking was detected in green mussel coating and 5,-5-diDOPA was detected in blue mussel byssus (Figure 14.2) (Zhao and Waite, 2005, 2006a). DOPA also has strong coordination chemistry with metal ions (Weinbreck et al., 2004; Lee et al., 2006; Hwang et al., 2010a; Zeng et al., 2010). fp-1 and its decapeptide analog were shown to form bis- and triscatecholate complexes with Fe^{3+} at pH 7.5 with log stability constants greater than 40 (Taylor et al., 1994a, 1996). Therefore, DOPA is oxidized and cross-linked via DOPA quinine oxidation or DOPA–metal ion coordination at pH 8.2 (pH of seawater, Figure 14.4). As a result, DOPA plays dual roles in interfacial adhesion of the coacervate phase with substrate and in cohesive cross-linking dense coacervate phases. Furthermore, DOPA showed a strong interaction with metal oxides and metal surfaces, which are common medical implant materials, and it would be a more biocompatible cross-linker because it is a metabolite found in the human body.

14.3 Production of Mussel Adhesive Proteins

Production capability and superior properties are very important for practical applications of mussel adhesive proteins. The natural proteins were initially extracted to study their biochemical properties; however, limited productivity hampered investigation of bulk-scale adhesive properties and biomedical and industrial applications. Thus far, extracts of mussel adhesive proteins containing primarily fp-1 and fp-2 are used commercially as a cell and tissue adhesive (Cell-Tak, BD Biosciences) (Hwang et al., 2004). Recombinant protein approaches using cDNAs or synthetic constructs of mussel adhesive protein have been used to obtain practical amounts of the proteins in various bacterial, yeast, insect, plant, and mammalian cell expression systems.

14.3.1 Extraction of Natural Mussel Adhesive Proteins

Mussel adhesive proteins show basic properties due to the biased amino acid composition of DOPA and basic amino acids. Thus, the proteins could be extracted from mussel feet using acid solutions. Mussel polyphenolic proteins that contain DOPA and hydroxyproline (hyp) were firstly described by Waite (1983). The process provided an acid-soluble extract of the DOPA-containing proteins, and a soluble borate complex of the proteins was formed at pH 7.0–9.0; thus, acid-extracted impurities were removed. The complex was then separated and treated with acetic acid solution to obtain DOPA-containing proteins. In addition, the adhesive proteins were purified based on their solubility in dilute perchloric acid and on differential precipitation with acetone containing approximately 0.3 N HCl (Pardo et al., 1990). These methods isolate the easily extractable fp-1 and fp-2; however, it is difficult to obtain individual adhesive proteins with high purity and yield, and the process is labor intensive and time-consuming. Approximately 10,000 mussels are required to produce 1 g of the most easily extractable fp-1 protein (Strausberg and Link, 1990; Hwang et al., 2007b). Similarly, fp-3, fp-4, fp-5, and fp-6 have also been extracted from mussel feet and used for biochemical analysis, although feasible production of the natural proteins has not been successful until recently (Papov et al., 1995; Waite and Qin, 2001; Zhao and Waite, 2006a,b; Kim et al., 2008).

14.3.2 Recombinant Production of Mussel Adhesive Proteins

Due to highly limited production processes, natural extraction appears unfeasible for bulk-scale practical applications of the protein, although the adhesive properties, such as versatile adhesion in wet environments, biodegradability, and biocompatibility, have come to be recognized as very attractive. Recombinant DNA technology has been considered as a solution for obtaining large amounts of adhesive proteins for bulk-scale adhesion and practical applications. Recombinant protein expression systems have been used in various host cells, and the technology has greatly improved for mass production of target proteins. cDNAs of mussel adhesive proteins were introduced heterologously into various vector systems, and their overexpression has been attempted, with partial success. Synthetic constructs of the mussel adhesive components have also been prepared as an alternative approach for obtaining large amounts of adhesive proteins, and the initial low production and purification yields have now been greatly improved, and the resulting proteins have been applied practically.

14.3.2.1 Recombinant Expression of Mussel Adhesive Protein cDNAs

A technique for cloning and expressing recombinant *M. edilus* fp-1 and fp-2 from cDNA clones in *S. cerevisiae* has been patented; however, experimental results following expression of the recombinant proteins were not described in the patents (Silverman and Roberto, 2006, 2007). Expression of fp-1 from *M. galloprovincialis* was attempted in transgenic tobacco plants due to the similarity with repetitive plant cell wall proteins (Marks, 1999); however, production levels and adhesion ability were not reported. Mussel foot cells from *M. galloprovincialis* were cultured in Petri dishes to produce adhesive proteins; however, the production details were similarly not reported (Takeuchi et al., 1999).

Recombinant fp-3 variant A was expressed in *E. coli* using the IPTG-inducible *trc* promoter system (Hwang et al., 2005). Because the production level was relatively low (approximately 1 mg/L), only microscale adhesion tests were performed using quartz crystal microbalance (QCM) analysis and modified AFM. The adsorption abilities were comparable with those of Cell-Tak. Recombinant fp-5 from *M. galloprovincialis* was also produced in *E. coli* by the same research group (Hwang et al., 2004). The production faced difficulties, such as low production yield and low postpurification solubility; thus, microscale adhesive properties were only reported similar to the recombinant fp-3, and the feasibility of the recombinant fp-5 as a cell adhesion biomaterial was investigated (Hwang et al., 2004, 2007a). Recently, these limitations were overcome by *E. coli*–based codon optimization and application of a different vector system (Choi et al., 2011). Approximately 40% of total resulting proteins were soluble in 4.5 L cultures, and ~50 mg/L of the purified recombinant fp-5 was obtained (Figure 14.6A). Thus, there has been partial success in the expression of recombinant mussel adhesive protein cDNA. However, it can be expected that recent development of recombinant protein technology will increase the possibility of successful expression of mussel adhesion proteins cDNAs for practical applications.

14.3.2.2 Recombinant Expression of Synthetic Constructs of Mussel Adhesive Proteins

Partial tandem repeats of fp-1 (20–100 kDa) were produced in *S. cerevisiae*, and approximately 2%–5% of the total cell protein produced was the recombinant protein (Filpula et al., 1990). Adhesive tests revealed a water-resistant bonding following in vitro modification of tyrosine residues to DOPA and DOPA quinone. Twenty decapeptide repeats were expressed in *E. coli* using a T7 promoter system (Salerno and Goldberg, 1993) and were 60% of total cell proteins produced, and six decapeptide repeats were similarly expressed in *E. coli*, which produced 10 mg/L product, and the structure was investigated using

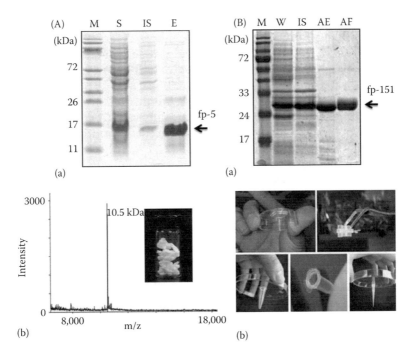

FIGURE 14.6

Bulk-scale production of recombinant mussel adhesive proteins. (A) Recombinant fp-5. (a) Tricine–SDS–PAGE analysis for expression and purification of recombinant fp-5. Lanes: M, protein molecular weight marker; S, soluble fraction of cell lysate; IS, insoluble fraction of cell lysate; E, purified recombinant fp-5. (b) MALDI–TOF MS analysis and lyophilized power of purified fp-5. (B) Recombinant fp-151. (a) SDS–PAGE analysis for expression and purification of fp-151. Lanes: M, protein molecular weight marker; W, whole cell sample; IS, insoluble fraction of cell lysate; AE, fraction extracted with 25% (v/v) acetic acid; AF, eluted fraction using affinity chromatography. (b) Adhesion of laboratory plastic consumables using recombinant fp-151. (From Choi, Y.S., Kang, D.G., Lim, S., Yang, Y.J., Kim, C.S., and Cha, H.J., Recombinant mussel adhesive protein fp-5 (MAP fp-5) as a bulk bioadhesive and surface coating material, *Biofouling*, 27, 729–737, Copyright 2011 Taylor & Francis; From *Biomaterials*, 28, Hwang, D.S., Gim, Y., Yoo, H.J., and Cha, H.J., Practical recombinant hybrid mussel bioadhesive fp-151, 3560–3568. Copyright 2007, with permission from Elsevier.)

CD spectrometry and NMR (Kitamura et al., 1999). However, the functional adhesive properties of the partial gene constructs of fp-1 have not been fully addressed.

Hybrid recombinant mussel adhesive proteins were designed to improve the production level and purification yield of natural mussel adhesive proteins, and this approach has greatly expanded the practical applications of mussel adhesive proteins. First, recombinant fp-151, which comprises six fp-1 decapeptide repeats at both termini of fp-5, was constructed and overexpressed successfully in *E. coli* (Hwang et al., 2007b) (Figure 14.6B). The production yield was approximately 100 mg/L in the laboratory in 5 L cultures and approximately 1 g/L in a pilot-scale fed-batch bioreactor culture, and the protein showed approximately 300 g/L solubility in aqueous solution. fp-151 was also expressed solubly in insect Sf-9 cells (Lim et al., 2011). The insect-derived mussel adhesive protein contained DOPA residues and hyp converted by in vivo posttranslational modification; thus, additional in vitro tyrosinase modification was not required. However, low production yields hampered investigation of bulk-scale adhesive properties. Recombinant fp-353 was also designed as a fusion protein with fp-3A at each terminus of fp-5 (Gim et al., 2008). Similar to fp-151, fp-131 was expressed as an inclusion body; thus, host-cell growth inhibition did not occur, and the greatly enhanced solubility and productivity enabled bulk-scale adhesion measurement and cell adhesion analyses. Recently, another hybrid mussel adhesive protein, fp-131, containing six fp-1 decapeptide repeats at both termini of fp-3 variant A, was designed and successfully overexpressed in *E. coli* (Lim et al., 2010).

In addition, functional peptides and domains were fused with recombinant mussel adhesive proteins to introduce biofunctionality and adhesive properties into adhesive proteins. Firstly, the Arg-Gly-Asp (RGD) peptide sequence was introduced into the C-termini of fp-151 resulting in the fusion protein fp-151-RGD, which was produced with high production yield, simple purification, and improved solubility, similar to fp-151 (Hwang et al., 2007c). The RGD sequence is known as the most effective cell-recognition motif that stimulates cell adhesion by integrin signaling primarily (Ruoslahti, 1996). fp-151-RGD showed superior cell adhesion and spreading abilities in various mammalian cell types when compared with Cell-Tak and poly-L-lysine, and the fused RGD peptide also efficiently triggered integrin-mediated adhesion and signaling for enhanced cell spreading, proliferation, and survival (Ohkawa et al., 2004; Hwang et al., 2007c; Kim et al., 2010). This approach was then applied to other functional peptides originating from essential recognition sites of extracellular matrix (ECM) proteins for cellular signaling. Fusion proteins containing fp-151 with functional peptides of fibronectin, laminin, and collagen were also overexpressed in *E. coli* and applied as surface coating for the preparation of artificial ECM in tissue engineering (Choi et al., 2010; Kim et al., 2012). All fusion proteins enhanced cell attachment, proliferation, spreading, viability, and differentiation; thus, it is likely that the fusion approach is a feasible option for preparation of other multifunctional biomaterials with adhesive properties.

Overall, synthetic constructs of mussel adhesive proteins based on hybrid and fusion strategies have been successful in producing the proteins and provide the ability to apply the adhesive biomaterials to various application fields. In particular, research and applications have been initially concentrated on biomaterials for tissue engineering and biomedical engineering use due to the economic implications and functional performance.

14.3.3 Bulk-Scale Adhesive Strength of Mussel Adhesive Proteins

At least 100 mg of adhesive protein is required to conduct small-scale and conventional bulk tests, including tensile strength analysis for obtaining mechanical properties as adhesive biomaterials (Silverman and Roberto, 2007). Thus, few reports are available that measure the bulk adhesive strength of mussel adhesive proteins due to their very limited abundance. Thus far, the shear strength has only been reported for mussel foot extract (composed primarily of fp-1 and fp-2; on porcine skin, ~0.33 MPa under dry conditions and ~1 MPa under humid conditions) (Ninan et al., 2003), 10 repeats of fp-1 decapeptide (~0.3 MPa compressive shear strength on aluminum) (Yamamoto, 1987), tyrosinase-modified recombinant fp-5 (~1.11 MPa on aluminum adherents) (Choi et al., 2011), tyrosinase-modified recombinant fp-151 (0.42–1.98 MPa on aluminum) (Hwang et al., 2007b; Cha et al., 2009; Lim et al., 2010), and tyrosinase-modified recombinant fp-131 (1,87 MPa on aluminum) (Gim et al., 2008). However, recombinant mussel adhesive proteins are expected to be used chiefly for practical applications due to their productivity and biocompatibility. The sacrifice of large numbers of mussels (1 g adhesive protein per 10,000 mussels) is neither environmentally friendly nor economically viable (Silverman and Roberto, 2007), and synthetic polypeptide mimetics of fp-1 have not shown similar biocompatibility to naturally occurring mussel adhesive proteins (Cha et al., 2008).

Moreover, the solubility and high productivity of recombinant mussel adhesive proteins has accelerated applied research. Recombinant fp-151 showed approximately 330 g/L solubility in both water and 5% acetic acid, whereas 650 g/L was reported for recombinant fp-5 in 50 mM sodium acetate buffer (pH 5.5) (Hwang et al., 2007b). However, the solubility was greatly reduced at pHs above 7 due to their basic properties. This is similar to naturally occurring mussel adhesive proteins, which are soluble below pH 6 but show discolored precipitates at pH 7.5–8.5 (Hwang et al., 2007b; Lin et al., 2007). The solubility appeared to depend upon the initial protein concentration and the solubility behavior of a highly charged polyion because protein solubility is affected by the properties of the protein itself and extrinsic factors (Choi et al., 2011). In addition, complex coacervates using recombinant mussel adhesive proteins and anionic partners, such as hyaluronic acid, were formed based on the cationic properties and the productivity. The complex coacervates are formed by liquid–liquid phase separation in water, are dependent upon concentration, have very low interfacial tension, behave like viscous particles, and are efficient for formulation for practical applications (Hwang et al., 2010b; Lim et al., 2010; Choi et al., 2011). The complex coacervates showed approximately twofold higher adhesive properties compared with the solubilized protein power (~3.17 MPa for coacervates of the modified recombinant fp-151 and hyaluronic acid, ~4.00 MPa for coacervates of the modified fp-131 and hyaluronic acid, and ~1.73 MPa for coacervates for the modified fp-5 and hyaluronic acid).

14.4 Applications of Mussel Adhesive Proteins as the Next Generation of Biomaterials

Ultimately, we expect that mussel adhesive proteins can be used as bioadhesives for binding items together in dry and wet environments, given their bulk-scale adhesive properties and biocompatibility. Moreover, mussel adhesive proteins will be utilized in various biomedical and industrial fields in the near future, given their diverse adhesive properties even in wet conditions, environmentally friendly properties, and high biocompatibility and high productivity and economical cost. Recent results have shown the high potential of adhesive biomaterials as cell and tissue adhesives and ECM and scaffold-coating materials for tissue engineering, immobilizing agents for biochip preparation, gene and drug delivery carriers, and skin and bone adhesives.

Recently, a layer-by-layer technology using mussel adhesive proteins and glycosaminoglycans (GAGs) was developed, where GAGs, such as hyaluronic acid, heparin sulfate, chondroitin sulfate, and dermatan sulfate, were used for many cell signaling events (Choi et al., 2012). GAGs were simply coated onto various surfaces using recombinant mussel adhesive proteins, and enhanced cellular behavior was observed on the functionalized surfaces. The results suggested that negatively charged ECM molecules and ECM peptides could be efficiently immobilized and utilized in various tissue engineering and medical implantation applications (Figure 14.7). Moreover, novel, functional nanofibrous scaffolds based on recombinant mussel adhesive proteins were fabricated, which provided a mechanically durable structural backbone with the functionality of bioactive peptides (Figure 14.8) (Kim et al., 2012). Moreover, facile functionalization of the nanofiber surfaces with various biomolecules was achieved using the adhesive and charged properties of mussel adhesive proteins, without surface modifications. These 2D and 3D strategies

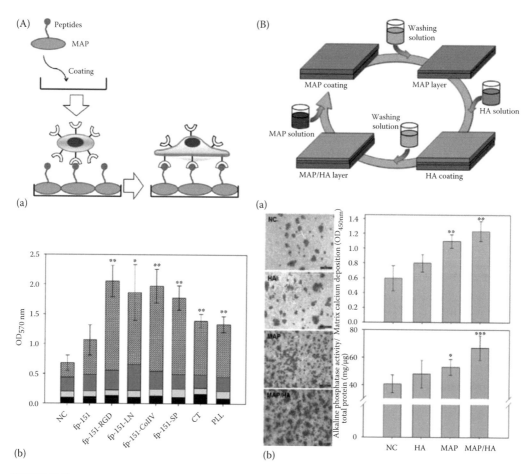

FIGURE 14.7
Facile surface functionalization of ECM molecules using mussel adhesive proteins. (A) Immobilization of biofunctional peptides originating from ECM proteins using mussel adhesive proteins. (a) Schematic diagram of the coating of ECM peptides. (b) Proliferation of 3T3-L1 cells on fp-151-peptide-coated surfaces. (B) Immobilization of GAGs using mussel adhesive proteins. (a) Schematic diagram of the coating of ECM GAGs. (b) The differentiation of MC3T3-E1 preosteoblast cells on bare (NV), solely HA-treated (HA), solely MAP-coated (MAP), and HA-immobilized-MAP-coated (MAP/HA) titanium surfaces. (From *Biomaterials*, 31, Choi, B.H., Choi, Y.S., Kang, D.G., Kim, B.J., Song, Y.H., and Cha, H.J., Cell behavior on extracellular matrix mimic materials based on mussel adhesive protein fused with functional peptides, 8980–8988. Copyright 2010, with permission from Elsevier; Choi, B.H., Choi, Y.S., Hwang, D.S., and Cha, H.J., Facile surface functionalization with glycosaminoglycans by direct coating with mussel adhesive protein. *Tissue Eng. Part C Methods*, 18, 71–79. Copyright 2012 Mary Ann Liebert, Inc. publishers.)

and the aforementioned cell adhesion abilities of mussel adhesive proteins have greatly accelerated the practical use of mussel adhesive proteins for the cell adhesion and tissue engineering fields.

The BC domain of protein A (antibody-binding protein, used as an antibody immobilizing linker) was fused with the N-termini of fp-5, which was overexpressed satisfactorily in *E. coli* (Kim et al., 2011). The fp-5 of the fusion protein enabled direct coating, without any modifications, onto diverse surfaces including glass, polymers, and metals, and the BC domain showed excellent antibody binding to the surfaces. This new strategy for effective and simple immobilization of antibodies onto diverse unmodified surfaces

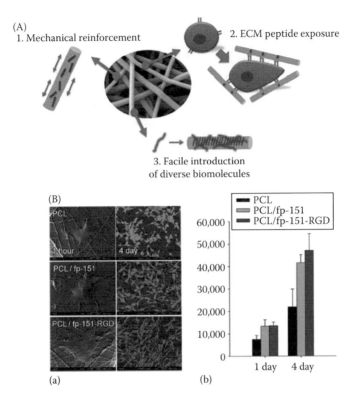

FIGURE 14.8
Reinforced multifunctional nanofibrous scaffolds using mussel adhesive proteins. (A) Schematic representation of various functionalized MAP-based nanofibrous scaffolds. (B) (a) Morphology of MC3T3-E1 cells on the surface of PCL, PCL/fp-151, and PCL/fp-151-RGD nanofibers after 1 h and 4 days in the culture. (b) Attached cell numbers as determined by direct cell counting after 1 and 4 days in the culture. (Kim, B.J., Choi, Y.S., and Cha, H.J.: Reinforced multifunctionalized nanofibrous scaffolds using mussel adhesive proteins. *Angew. Chem. Int. Edn. Eng.* 2012. 51. 675–678. Copyright Wiley-VCH Verlag GmbH & Co. KGaA. Reproduced with permission.)

showed the high potential of mussel adhesive proteins as linking materials and can be successfully applied to prepare biochip surfaces permitting antigen–antibody interactions (Figure 14.9). It is expected that similar strategies may be utilized to efficiently immobilize other biomolecules onto various surfaces.

In addition, the potential use of fp-151 as a gene delivery material was investigated, in view of its similar basic amino acid composition to histone proteins (Hwang et al., 2009). fp-151 exhibited efficient DNA binding ability and transfection efficiency in mammalian cells, which demonstrates the potential of using mussel adhesive proteins as gene delivery carriers. Complex coacervates of mussel adhesive proteins have also been used in micro-encapsulation to initially protect and subsequently release encapsulated biologically active compounds, such as hydrophobic drugs and food ingredients (Lim et al., 2010). As a model of microencapsulation, red pepper seed oil was used due to the ease of monitoring the encapsulation using fluorescence, and interfacial coacervations of approximately 1–30 μm in diameter formed spontaneously. These results suggest that the microencapsulation system could be a useful component of the development of new adhesive biomaterials, including self-adhesive microencapsulated drug carriers.

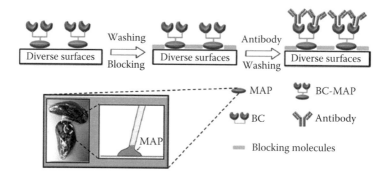

FIGURE 14.9

Schematic representation of simple and efficient antibody immobilization on diverse surfaces coated with BC-MAP. (Kim, C.S., Choi, Y.S., Ko, W., Seo, J.H., Lee, J., and Cha, H.J.: A mussel adhesive protein fused with the BC domain of protein A is a functional linker material that efficiently immobilizes antibodies onto diver surfaces. *Adv. Funct. Mater.* 2011. 21. 4101–4108. Copyright Wiley-VCH Verlag GmbH & Co. KGaA. Reproduced with permission.)

14.5 Concluding Remarks

Marine mussels attach rapidly to various solid surfaces in wave-swept seashores. The superior properties of the adhesives, such as strong adhesion with flexibility, biocompatibility, and biodegradability, have resulted in their consideration as very promising biomaterials. Isolation of the mussel adhesive protein and biochemical studies have greatly increased the potential for their use as the next generation of biomaterials, and bulk-scale productions have accelerated practical applications, especially in the biomedical and tissue engineering fields. In particular, bioadhesive preparation and formulation for multifunctional biomaterials will be enabled by recent technological improvements in production of recombinant synthetic constructs from mussel adhesive proteins. This strategy will be expanded to discover new biomaterial and mimic natural materials successfully.

References

Brown, C.H., 1952. Some structural proteins of *Mytilus edulis*. *Quarterly Journal of Microscopic Science*, 93, 487–502.

Bungenberg De Jong, H.G., 1932. Die Koazervation und ihre. Bedeutung für die Biologie. *Protoplasma*, 15, 110.

Bungenberg De Jong, H.G., 1949. *Colloid Science*. Elsevier, Amsterdam, the Netherlands.

Cha, H.J., Hwang, D.S., and Lim, S., 2008. Development of bioadhesives from marine mussels. *Biotechnology Journal*, 3, 631–638.

Cha, H.J., Hwang, D.S., Lim, S., White, J.D., Matos-Perez, C.R., and Wilker, J.J., 2009. Bulk adhesive strength of recombinant hybrid mussel adhesive protein. *Biofouling*, 25, 99–107.

Choi, B.H., Choi, Y.S., Hwang, D.S., and Cha, H.J., 2012. Facile surface functionalization with glycosaminoglycans by direct coating with mussel adhesive protein. *Tissue Engineering Part C Methods*, 18, 71–79.

Choi, B.H., Choi, Y.S., Kang, D.G., Kim, B.J., Song, Y.H., and Cha, H.J., 2010. Cell behavior on extracellular matrix mimic materials based on mussel adhesive protein fused with functional peptides. *Biomaterials*, 31, 8980–8988.

Choi, Y.S., Kang, D.G., Lim, S., Yang, Y.J., Kim, C.S., and Cha, H.J., 2011. Recombinant mussel adhesive protein fp-5 (MAP fp-5) as a bulk bioadhesive and surface coating material. *Biofouling*, 27, 729–737.

Coyne, K.J., Qin, X.X., and Waite, J.H., 1997. Extensible collagen in mussel byssus: A natural block copolymer. *Science*, 277, 1830–1832.

De Kruif, C.G., Weinbreck, F., and De Vries, J., 2004. Complex coacervation of proteins and anionic polysaccharides. *Current Opinions in Colloid Interface Science*, 9, 340–349.

Deming, T.J., 1999. Mussel byssus and biomolecular materials. *Current Opinions in Chemical Biology*, 3, 100–105.

Filpula, D.R., Lee, S.M., Link, R.P., Strausberg, S.L., and Strausberg, R.L., 1990. Structural and functional repetition in a marine mussel adhesive protein. *Biotechnology Progress*, 6, 171–177.

Gim, Y., Hwang, D.S., Lim, S., Song, Y.H., and Cha, H.J., 2008. Production of fusion mussel adhesive fp-353 in *Escherichia coli*. *Biotechnology Progress*, 24, 1272–1277.

Harrington, M.J., Masic, A., Holten-Andersen, N., Waite, J.H., and Fratzl, P., 2010. Iron-clad fibers: A metal-based biological strategy for hard flexible coatings. *Science*, 328, 216–220.

Holten-Andersen, N., Fantner, G.E., Hohlbauch, S., Waite, J.H., and Zok, F.W., 2007. Protective coatings on extensible biofibres. *Nature Materials*, 6, 669–672.

Holten-Andersen, N., Mates, T.E., Toprak, M.S., Stucky, G.D., Zok, F.W., and Waite, J.H., 2009. Metals and the integrity of a biological coating: The cuticle of mussel byssus. *Langmuir*, 25, 3323–3326.

Holten-Andersen, N. and Waite, J.H., 2008. Mussel-designed protective coatings for compliant substrates. *Journal of Dental Research*, 87, 701–709.

Hwang, D.S., Gim, Y., and Cha, H.J., 2005. Expression of functional recombinant mussel adhesive protein type 3A in *Escherichia coli*. *Biotechnology Progress*, 21, 965–970.

Hwang, D.S., Gim, Y., Kang, D.G., Kim, Y.K., and Cha, H.J., 2007a. Recombinant mussel adhesive protein Mgfp-5 as cell adhesion biomaterial. *Journal of Biotechnology*, 127, 727–735.

Hwang, D.S., Gim, Y., Yoo, H.J., and Cha, H.J., 2007b. Practical recombinant hybrid mussel bioadhesive fp-151. *Biomaterials*, 28, 3560–3568.

Hwang, D.S., Kim, K.R., Lim, S., Choi, Y.S., and Cha, H.J., 2009. Recombinant mussel adhesive protein as a gene delivery material. *Biotechnology and Bioengineering*, 102, 616–623.

Hwang, D.S., Sim, S.B., and Cha, H.J., 2007c. Cell adhesion biomaterial based on mussel adhesive protein fused with RGD peptide. *Biomaterials*, 28, 4039–4046.

Hwang, D.S., Yoo, H.J., Jun, J.H., Moon, W.K., and Cha, H.J., 2004. Expression of functional recombinant mussel adhesive protein Mgfp-5 in *Escherichia coli*. *Applied and Environmental Microbiology*, 70, 3352–3359.

Hwang, D.S., Zeng, H.B., Masic, A., Harrington, M.J., Israelachvili, J.N., and Waite, J.H., 2010a. Protein- and metal-dependent interactions of a prominent protein in mussel adhesive plaques. *Journal of Biological Chemistry*, 285, 25850–25858.

Hwang, D.S., Zeng, H.B., Srivastava, A., Krogstad, D.V., Tirrell, M., Israelachvili, J.N., and Waite, J.H., 2010b. Viscosity and interfacial properties in a mussel-inspired adhesive coacervate. *Soft Matter*, 6, 3232–3236.

Inoue, K., Takeuchi, Y., Miki, D., and Odo, S., 1995. Mussel adhesive plaque protein gene is a novel member of epidermal growth factor-like gene family. *Journal of Biological Chemistry*, 270, 6698–6701.

Inoue, K., Takeuchi, Y., Miki, D., Odo, S., Harayama, S., and Waite, J.H., 1996. Cloning, sequencing and sites of expression of genes for the hydroxyarginine-containing adhesive-plaque protein of the mussel *Mytilus galloprovincialis*. *European Journal of Biochemistry*, 239, 172–176.

Kamino, K., Inoue, K., Maruyama, T., Takamatsu, N., Harayama, S., and Shizuri, Y., 2000. Barnacle cement proteins. Importance of disulfide bonds in their insolubility. *Journal of Biological Chemistry*, 275, 27360–27365.

Kanyalkar, M., Srivastava, S., and Coutinho, E., 2002. Conformation of a model peptide of the tandem repeat decapeptide in mussel adhesive protein by NMR and MD simulations. *Biomaterials*, 23, 389–396.

Kausik, R., Srivastava, A., Korevaar, P.A., Stucky, G., Waite, J.H., and Han, S., 2009. Local water dynamics in coacervated polyelectrolytes monitored through dynamic nuclear polarization-enhanced H NMR. *Macromolecules*, 42, 7404–7412.

Kim, H.C. and Burgess, D.J., 2001. Prediction of interfacial tension between oil mixtures and water. *Journal of Colloidal Interface Science*, 241, 509–513.

Kim, B.J., Choi, Y.S., and Cha, H.J., 2012. Reinforced multifunctionalized nanofibrous scaffolds using mussel adhesive proteins. *Angewandte Chemie International Edition English*, 51, 675–678.

Kim, B.J., Choi, Y.S., Choi, B.H., Lim, S., Song, Y.H., and Cha, H.J., 2010. Mussel adhesive protein fused with cell adhesion recognition motif triggers integrin-mediated adhesion and signaling for enhanced cell spreading, proliferation, and survival. *Journal of Biomedical Material Research A*, 94, 886–892.

Kim, C.S., Choi, Y.S., Ko, W., Seo, J.H., Lee, J., and Cha, H.J., 2011. A mussel adhesive protein fused with the BC domain of protein A is a functional linker material that efficiently immobilizes antibodies onto diver surfaces. *Advanced Functional Materials*, 21, 4101–4108.

Kim, D., Hwang, D.S., Kang, D.G., Kim, J.Y.H., and Cha, H.J., 2008. Enhancement of mussel adhesive protein production in *Escherichia coli* by co-expression of bacterial hemoglobin. *Biotechnology Progress*, 24, 663–666.

Kitamura, M., Kawakami, K., Nakamura, N., Tsumoto, K., Uchiyama, H., Ueda, Y., Kumagai, I., and Nakaya, T., 1999. Expression of a model peptide of a marine mussel adhesive protein in Escherichia coli and characterization of its structural and functional properties. *Journal of Polymer Science Part A: Polymer Chemistry*, 37, 729–736.

Lee, B.P., Messersmith, P.B., Israelachvili, J.N., and Waite, J.H., 2011. Mussel-inspired adhesives and coatings. *Annual Review of Materials Research*, 41, 99–132.

Lee, H., Scherer, N.F., and Messersmith, P.B., 2006. Single-molecule mechanics of mussel adhesion. *Proceedings of the National Academy of Sciences of the United States of America*, 103, 12999–13003.

Lim, S., Choi, Y.S., Kang, D.G., Song, Y.H., and Cha, H.J., 2010. The adhesive properties of coacervated recombinant hybrid mussel adhesive proteins. *Biomaterials*, 31, 3715–3722.

Lim, S., Kim, K.R., Choi, Y.S., Kim, D.K., Hwang, D., and Cha, H.J., 2011. In vivo post-translational modifications of recombinant mussel adhesive protein in insect cells. *Biotechnology Progress*, 27, 1390–1396.

Lin, Q., Gourdon, D., Sun, C., Holten-Andersen, N., Anderson, T.H., Waite, J.H., and Israelachvili, J.N., 2007. Adhesion mechanisms of the mussel foot proteins mfp-1 and mfp-3. *Proceedings of the National Academy of Sciences of the United States of America*, 104, 3782–3786.

Marks, P., 1999. Mussel power. *New Scientist*, 164, 12.

Ninan, L., Monahan, J., Stroshine, R.L., Wilker, J.J., and Shi, R., 2003. Adhesive strength of marine mussel extracts on porcine skin. *Biomaterials*, 24, 4091–4099.

Ohkawa, K., Nishida, A., Yamamoto, H., and Waite, J.H., 2004. A glycosylated byssal precursor protein from the green mussel *Perna viridis* with modified dopa side-chains. *Biofouling*, 20, 101–115.

Oparin, A.I., 1924. *The Origin of the Life*. Moscow Worker publisher, Moscow, Russia.

Papov, V.V., Diamond, T.V., Biemann, K., and Waite, J.H., 1995. Hydroxyarginine-containing polyphenolic proteins in the adhesive plaques of the marine mussel *Mytilus edulis*. *Journal of Biological Chemistry*, 270, 20183–20192.

Pardo, J., Gutierrez, E., Saez, C., Brito, M., and Burzio, L.O., 1990. Purification of adhesive proteins from mussels. *Protein Experimental Purification*, 1, 147–150.

Pocius, A.V., 2002. *Adhesion and Adhesives Technology*. Hanser, Munich, Germany.

Pujol, J.P., 1967. Les complex byssogene des mollusques bivalves. Histochimie comparee des secretions chez *Mytilus edulis* L. et *pinna nobilis*. *Bulletin de la Société linnéenne de Normandie*, 8, 308–332.

Ruoslahti, E., 1996. RGD and other recognition sequences for integrins. *Annual Review of Cell and Developmental Biology*, 12, 697–715.

Rzepecki, L.M. and Waite, J.H., 1992. Characterization of a cystine-rich polyphenolic protein family from the blue mussel *Mytilus edulis L. Biology Bulletin*, 183, 123–137.

Sagert, J. and Waite, J.H., 2009. Hyperunstable matrix proteins in the byssus of *Mytilus galloprovincialis. Journal of Experimental Biology*, 212, 2224–2236.

Salerno, A.J. and Goldberg, I., 1993. Cloning, expression, and characterization of a synthetic analog to the bioadhesive precursor protein of the sea mussel *Mytilus edulis. Applied Microbiology and Biotechnology*, 39, 221–226.

Santos, R., Gorb, S., Jamar, V., and Flammang, P., 2005. Adhesion of echinoderm tube feet to rough surfaces. *Journal of Experimental Biology*, 208, 2555–2567.

Silverman, H.G. and F.F. Roberto, 2006. Cloning and expression of recombinant adhesive protein Mefp-2 of the Blue Mussel, *Mytilus edulis.* US Patent: 6,987,170.

Silverman, H.G. and Roberto, F.F., 2007. Understanding marine mussel adhesion. *Marine Biotechnology (NY)*, 9, 661–681.

Smyth, J.D., 1954. A technique for the histochemical demonstration of polyphenol oxidase and its application to egg shell formation in helminths and byssus formation in *Mytilus. Quarterly Journal of Microscopical Science*, 95, 139–152.

Spruijt, E., Sprakel, J., Stuart, M.A.C., and Van Der Gucht, J., 2010. Interfacial tension between a complex coacervate phase and its coexisting aqueous phase. *Soft Matter*, 6, 172–178.

Stewart, R.J., Weaver, J.C., Morse, D.E., and Waite, J.H., 2004. The tube cement of *Phragmatopoma californica*: A solid foam. *Journal of Experimental Biology*, 207, 4727–4734.

Strausberg, R.L. and Link, R.P., 1990. Protein-based medical adhesives. *Trends Biotechnology*, 8, 53–57.

Sun, C. and Waite, J.H., 2005. Mapping chemical gradients within and along a fibrous structural tissue, mussel byssal threads. *Journal of Biological Chemistry*, 280, 39332–39336.

Takeuchi, Y., Inoue, K., Miki, D., Odo, S., and Harayama, S., 1999. Cultured mussel foot cells expressing byssal protein genes. *Journal of Experimental Zoology*, 283, 131–136.

Tamarin, A., 1975. An ultrastructural study of byssus stem formation in *Mytilus californianus, Journal of Morphology*, 145, 151–177.

Tamarin, A., Lewis, P., and Askey, J., 1976. The structure and formation of the byssus attachment plaque in *Mytilus. Journal of Morphology*, 149, 199–221.

Taylor, S.W., Chase, D.B., Emptage, M.H., Nelson, M.J., and Waite, J.H., 1996. Ferric ion complexes of a DOPA-containing adhesive protein from *Mytilus edulis. Inorganic Chemistry*, 35, 7572–7577.

Taylor, S.W., Luther, G.W., and Waite, J.H., 1994a. Polarographic and spectrophotometric Investigation of iron(III) complexation to 3,4-dihydroxyphenylalanine-containing peptides and proteins from *Mytilus-Edulis. Inorganic Chemistry*, 33, 5819–5824.

Taylor, S.W., Waite, J.H., Ross, M.M., Shabanowitz, J., and Hunt, D.F., 1994b. Trans-2,3-cis-3,4-dihydroxyproline, a new naturally-occurring amino-acid, is the 6th residue in the tandemly repeated consensus decapeptides of an adhesive protein from *Mytilus-Edulis. Journal of the American Chemical Society*, 116, 10803–10804.

Vovelle, J., 1965. The tube of Sabellaria alveolata. *Archives de zoologie expérimentale et générale*, 106, 1–187.

Waite, J.H., 1976. Rosewood polyphenol alter phenoloxidase activity from the mantles of the marine bivalve mollusc *Moliolus demissus. Pesticide Biochemistry and Physiology*, 6, 239–242.

Waite, J.H., 1983. Evidence for a repeating 3,4-dihydroxyphenylalanine- and hydroxyproline-containing decapeptide in the adhesive protein of the mussel, *Mytilus edulis L. Journal of Biological Chemistry*, 258, 2911–2915.

Waite, J.H., 1992. The formation of mussel byssus: Anatomy of a natural manufacturing process. *Results and Problems in Cell Differentiation*, 19, 27–54.

Waite, J.H., Andersen, N.H., Jewhurst, S., and Sun, C.J., 2005. Mussel adhesion: Finding the tricks worth mimicking. *Journal of Adhesion*, 81, 297–317.

Waite, J.H. and Qin, X., 2001. Polyphosphoprotein from the adhesive pads of *Mytilus edulis. Biochemistry*, 40, 2887–2893.

Waite, J.H. and Tanzer, M.L., 1981. Polyphenolic substance of *Mytilus edulis*: Novel adhesive containing L-dopa and hydroxyproline. *Science*, 212, 1039–1040.

Weinbreck, F., Minor, M., and De Kruif, C.G., 2004. Microencapsulation of oils using whey protein/ gum Arabic coacervates. *Journal of Microencapsulation*, 21, 667–679.

Yamamoto, H., 1987. Synthesis and adhesive studies of marine polypeptides. *Journal of the Chemical Society, Perkin Transactions*, 1, 613–618.

Yu, J., Wei, W., Danner, E., Ashley, R.K., Israelachvili, J.N., and Waite, J.H., 2011. Mussel protein adhesion depends on interprotein thiol-mediated redox modulation. *Nature Chemical Biology*, 7, 588–590.

Zeng, H., Hwang, D.S., Israelachvili, J.N., and Waite, J.H., 2010. Strong reversible Fe^{3+}-mediated bridging between dopa-containing protein films in water. *Proceedings of the National Academy of Sciences of the United States of America*, 107, 12850–12853.

Zhao, H., Sun, C., Stewart, R.J., and Waite, J.H., 2005. Cement proteins of the tube-building polychaete Phragmatopoma californica. *Journal of Biological Chemistry*, 280, 42938–42944.

Zhao, H. and Waite, J.H., 2005. Coating proteins: structure and cross-linking in fp-1 from the green shell mussel *Perna canaliculus*. *Biochemistry*, 44, 15915–15923.

Zhao, H. and Waite, J.H., 2006a. Linking adhesive and structural proteins in the attachment plaque of *M. californianus*. *Journal of Biological Chemistry*, 281, 26150–26158.

Zhao, H. and Waite, J.H., 2006b. Proteins in load-bearing junctions: the histidine-rich metal-binding protein of mussel byssus. *Biochemistry*, 45, 14223–14231.

Part II

Biological Activities of Marine Biomaterials

15

Biological Applications of Marine Biomaterials

A. Malshani Samaraweera and Janak K. Vidanarachchi

CONTENTS

15.1 Anticancer Properties

Cancer is one of the major causes for deaths in the world with increasing threats due to life-style and global environmental changes. The World Health Organization (WHO) predicts that there will be more than 11 million cancer-related deaths per annum by 2030. Moreover, certain defects in existing anticancer drugs like cytotoxicity to both cancer and healthy cells need to be addressed. Thus, production and invention of new anticancer drugs is essential to solve these problems. Therefore, the scientists around the globe focus on sea where it is believed as a source of many untapped natural resources wherein over 70% of the earth surface is covered. Large numbers of novel compounds isolated from diverse marine macro- and microorganisms have been reported to exert anticancer activity (Table 15.1). These compounds known to act by activation of P53 anti-proliferative gene, inducing apoptosis, affecting the tubulin–microtubule equilibrium, or inhibiting angiogenesis, where few mode of actions are described in this chapter (Vidanarachchi et al., 2010; Zheng et al., 2011).

15.1.1 Marine Anticancer Apoptosis-Inducing Compounds

Apoptosis is a naturally occurring and evolutionary conserved process by which cells that are no longer useful are directed to death (Danial and Korsmeyer, 2004). Thus, selective induction of apoptosis and modulation of apoptotic pathways and by chemical agents are promising approaches for cancer therapy.

TABLE 15.1

Marine Organisms with Potential Anticancer Activity, Their Source of Origin, and Active Compound

Group	Organism	Active Compound	Biological Activity	Reference
Sponge	*Leiodermatium* species	Synthesis of macrolide (−)-dictyostatin	Spindle formation in mitosis	Paterson et al. (2011)
Sponge	*Pseudoaxinella flava*	Isonitrile diterpenes	Cytotoxic	Lamoral-Theys et al. (2011)
Sponge	*Polymastia janeirensis*	Aqueous and organic extracts	Cytotoxic	Frota et al. (2009)
Sponge	*Ianthella* sp.	C29 sterols with a cyclopropane ring at C-25 and C-26(petrosterol-3,6-dione; 5a,6aepoxy-petrosterol; petrosterol)	Apoptosis induction	Tung et al. (2009)
Sponge	*Candidaspongia* sp.	A polyketide—candidaspongiolide	Cytotoxic	Trisciuoglio et al. (2008)
Sponge	*D. elegans*	A sesquiterpene aminoquinone—smenospongine	Apoptosis	Kong et al. (2008)
Sponge	*Jaspis* sp.	Isomalabaricane-type triterpene—jaspolide B	Apoptosis, cell cycle arrest, microtubule disassembly	Wei et al. (2008)
Sponge	*Oceanapia sagittaria*	The pyridoacridine alkaloids—kuanoniamines A and C	Antitumor	Kijjoa et al. (2007)
Brown alga	*Laminaria japonica*	Polysaccharide WPS-2-1	Antitumor	Peng et al. (2012)
Tunicate	*Eudistoma vannamei*	Dichloromethane extract	Apoptosis	Jimenez et al. (2008)
Tunicate	*Eudistoma* cf. *rigida*	A macrolide—iejimalide B	Apoptosis	Wang et al. (2008)
Marine actinomycete	*Nocardia dassonvillei* (BM-17)	Secondary metabolite, N-(2-hydroxyphenyl)-2-phenazinamine (NHP)	Cytotoxic	Gao et al. (2012)
Sponge-associated actinomycetes	*Streptomyces* sp.	Cell-free extracts of actinomycetes	Anticancer	Ravikumar et al. (2010)
Marine actinomycete	*Nocardiopsis* sp. 03N67	*Cyclo*-(1-Pro-1-Met)	Anti-angiogenesis activity	Shin et al. (2010)
Marine cyanobacterium	*Lyngbya* sp.	Biselyngbyaside (1)	Protein kinase inhibition	Teruya et al. (2009)
Marine diatom	*P. tricornutum*	Two monogalactosyl diacylglycerols-1 ($C_{45}H_{70}O_{10}$) and 2 ($C_{45}H_{68}O_{10}$)	Apoptosis	Andrianasolo et al. (2008)

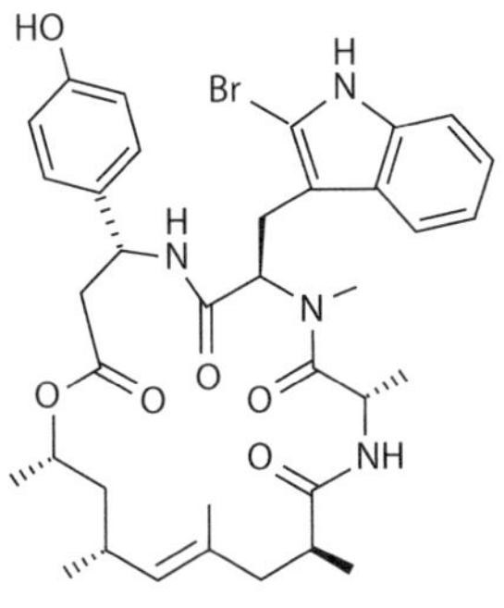

FIGURE 15.1
Chemical structure of the parent jaspamide (jasplakinolide).

Among different marine organisms, compounds isolated from sponges are widely studied for apoptosis-induced anticancer activity within the scientific community (Table 15.1). For example, a cyclic depsipeptide jaspamide (jasplakinolide) (Figure 15.1), isolated from marine sponge *Jaspis splendens* (family Jaspidae) is known to induct apoptosis through a caspase-3-like protease-dependent pathway in human leukemia Jurkat T cells upon examination with fluorescent substrate with N-acetyl-Asp-Glu-Val-Asp-7-amino-4-methylcoumarin (DEVD-MAC) (Odaka et al., 2000). Furthermore, two derivatives of jaspamide (jaspamide 1), jaspamide-Q (jaspamide 2), and jaspamide-R (jaspamide 3), separated from the crude methanolic extract of the same organism, inhibited the growth of mouse lymphoma (L5178Y) cell line in vitro with IC_{50} values of <0.1 µg/mL (Ebada et al., 2009). Moreover, apoptosis-inducing compounds isolated from marine sponges have been extensively reviewed by Essack et al. (2011). Certain compounds such as tedanolide macrolides usually have the potential cytotoxic activity associated with inhibition of protein synthesis. A polyketide from marine sponge (Table 15.1) triggered caspase 12, protein kinase PKR, and inhibitory phosphorylation of eukaryotic initiation factor-2 (eIF2)-α (Trisciuoglio et al., 2008). However, the compound inhibited protein synthesis in both cancer and normal human fibroblasts similar to its chemical group. Interestingly, it induced eIF2α phosphorylation and apoptosis only in cancer cells.

A specific feature of most of the tumor cells is the evolvement of genetic mutations that activate resistance to apoptosis, which endures the tumor growth. For example, majority of human cancers with defects in apoptosis have the pathway disabled upstream of *Bax* and *Bak*. Therefore, a cell-based assay had been carried out to explore the apoptosis induction ability of galactolipids from marine diatom *Phaeodactylum tricornutum* (Table 15.1) for the first time by Andrianasolo et al. (2008), with disabled apoptosis function through specific genetic deletion of both *Bax* and *Bak*. Interestingly, the compounds isolated from methanol extract of *P. tricornutum* specifically induced apoptosis upstream of *Bax* and *Bak* and may have a potential to use as anticancer agents that exploit the apoptosis pathway in tumor cells.

Cytotoxicity to cancer as well as non-cancer cells is a major drawback of potential anticancer compounds. Therefore, nonspecifically toxic compounds can be eliminated by identifying compounds that indiscriminately kill both apoptosis-competent and apoptosis-defective cells.

15.1.2 Marine Anticancer Compounds Affecting Tubulin–Microtubulin Equilibrium

Microtubules are essential in development and maintenance of the cell shape, in transport of vesicles and mitochondria through cells in cell signaling, and in mitosis. They are long,

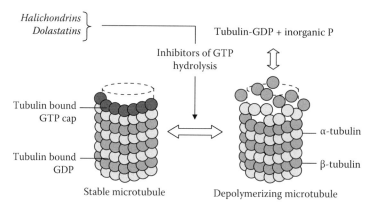

FIGURE 15.2
Polymerization dynamics of microtubule structure through assembly and disassembly of α- and β-tubulin subunits.

filamentous polymers composed of altering α- and β-tubulin subunits along the longitudinal axis (Figure 15.2). Shrinking or elongation of the filamentous polymer through assembly or disassembly of α- and β-tubulin subunits (dynamic instability) is essential in chromosomal segregation in mitosis. Hence, mitotic spindle microtubules can be used as a successful target in chemotherapy to arrest cells at mitosis and thereby to retard cell proliferation. In other words, this is attained via increasing or decreasing the cellular microtubule mass or by suppression of microtubule dynamics during mitotic spindle formation, which essentially blocks the cell division and induction of apoptotic cell death. Introduction of drugs such as vinca alkaloids, paclitaxel, and vinblastine, which are used in clinical oncology, has confirmed the importance of microtubule-targeted drugs as anticancer compounds.

Halichondrins have been studied extensively for anticancer activity based on their ability to restrain the microtubule dynamics. For example, halichondrin-B isolated from marine sponge *Halichondria okadai* inhibits guanosine triphosphate (GTP) hydrolysis (Figure 15.2), which provides energy for polymerization dynamics upon hydrolysis. Once the tubulin-bound GTP is hydrolyzed to tubulin–guanosinediphosphate (GDP) and inorganic phosphate, the microtubule structure is destabilized and initiates the depolymerization that shortens the microtubule structure, which is essential for chromosomal segregation. Furthermore, to exert the antimitotic effect, the drugs must bind directly to the microtubule structure. It was found that both halichondrin-B and homohalichondrin-B (from the sponges of the genera Axinella) inhibit vinca alkaloid binding to tubulin (Bai et al., 1991). Further, a synthetic analog of halichondrin-B, eribulin, binds both with soluble tubulin and microtubules with higher affinity for microtubule plus ends (Smith et al., 2010).

The short supply of halichondrins has remained as a major obstacle for extensive studies on anticancer activity, until the synthesis of eribulin mesylate (E7389), a synthetic analog of halichondrin-B. Eribulin is under phase III clinical trials for the treatment of the cancer showing its impending use in oncology (Smith et al., 2010).

Dolastatins are naturally occurring microtubule depolymerizing peptides that exert their effects by binding at or near the vinca-binding site on tubulin (Risinger et al., 2009). A microtubule assembly inhibition similar to dolastatin-10 was reported from diazonamide-A, a peptide isolated from marine ascidian *Diazona angulata* that exhibited potential anticancer activity via inhibiting tubulin-dependent GTP hydrolysis

(Cruz-Monserrate et al., 2003). Moreover, the same authors revealed that though diazon-amide-A exhibits microtubule assembly inhibition similar to dolastatin-10, the remaining biochemical properties resembles dolastatin-15. Therefore, it is believed that dolastatin-10 binds avidly to tubulin, where dolastatin-15 has a much weaker binding with tubulin.

15.1.3 Marine Anticancer Compounds That Inhibit Angiogenesis

Angiogenesis is the formation of new blood vessels from the preexisting vessels, with a cascade of events, involving basement membrane dissolution, endothelial cell proliferation, migration, and new basement membrane formation. This process is activated largely and momentarily during reproduction, development, and wound healing, which otherwise is under a suppressed condition. Generally, both vasculogenesis (during embryogenesis) and angiogenesis (in the adult) are regulated by vascular endothelial growth factor (VEGF). Moreover, protein kinase Cα (PKCα) is essential for the VEGF-induced proliferation of endothelial cells. However, this cascade of events also activates during tumor growth where a correlation between VEGF expression and tumor vascularity has been noted (Keshet and Ben-Sasson, 1999). Moreover, necessity of tumor vascularity for tumor growth is proven by the fact that tumor growth inhibition beyond 1 mm^3 due to lack of proper oxygen and nutrition supply (Folkman, 1971). Therefore, anti-angiogenetic compounds can be used as prime chemotherapeutic agents via suppression of both VEGF signal pathway and inhibition of VEGF-specific endothelial cell tyrosine kinase receptors (Wahl et al., 2011).

Inhibition of the phosphorylation activity of PKCα and its translocation from the cytosol to the membrane was inhibited by a marine sponge-derived macrocyclic lactone polyether, spongistatin-1. In vitro studies of endothelial cells and in vivo studies of mouse cornea pocket assay using spongistatin-1 inhibited angiogenesis at nano-molar concentrations (in vivo neovascularization 10 μg/kg). Another compound with marine sponge origin, smenospongine (Figure 15.3), a sesquiterpene aminoquinone from *Dactylospongia elegans*, exhibited antitumor activity against 39 human solid cancer cell lines in vitro (Kong et al., 2011). Moreover, the authors have revealed that the antitumor effect of the compound is due to both inhibitions of angiogenesis on endothelial cells and direct inhibition of tumor cell growth. At present, compounds from diverse groups of marine organisms with anti-angiogenesis properties are being identified extensively. Moreover, PKC and other kinase inhibitors isolated from marine sponge are reviewed recently by Skropeta et al. (2011).

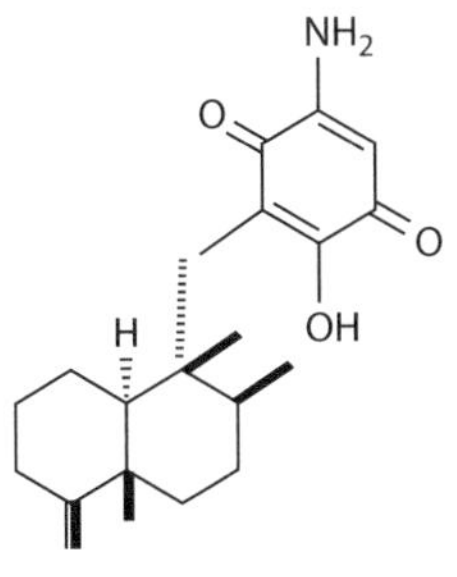

FIGURE 15.3
Chemical structure of smenospongine.

15.2 Anticoagulant/Antithrombotic Properties

Hemostasis mechanism in the body ensures the control of blood coagulation by balanced generation of thrombin, the protein that is responsible for the formation of fibrin net against bleeding. Dysfunction of coagulation and platelet aggregation may lead to inflammation, cardiovascular disturbances, venous thrombosis, thromboembolism, and other pathologies. At present, vascular disturbances are among the major causes of mortality and morbidity in the world.

Heparin is the anticoagulant of choice among several other anticoagulant drugs since its identification from about 50 years. Heparin is normally extracted from mucosal tissues of meat animals such as porcine intestine and bovine lung, and therefore, availability of heparin is limited. On the other hand, undesirable effects of heparin have been reported like bleeding, heparin-induced thrombocytopenia (HIT), heparin-associated osteoporosis (HAO), eosinophilia, skin reactions, allergic reactions, and alopecia (Walenga and Bick, 1998). Other than low availability and side effects, risk of zoonoses and religious issues due to animal origin associated with heparin need to be addressed. Hence, natural novel compounds with anticoagulant properties need to be identified to replace heparin.

Anticoagulant activity of heparin is mediated by specific plasma cofactors, antithrombin, and heparin cofactor II, and the major inhibitors of coagulation enzymes are thrombin and factor Xa (Melo et al., 2004). The blood coagulation cascade system consists of intrinsic, extrinsic, and a final common pathway that is associated with more than 13 plasma serine proteases or blood coagulating factors (Figure 15.4) (Samarakoon and Jeon, 2012). A diverse group of sulfated polysaccharides (SPs) isolated from seaweeds, including galactans

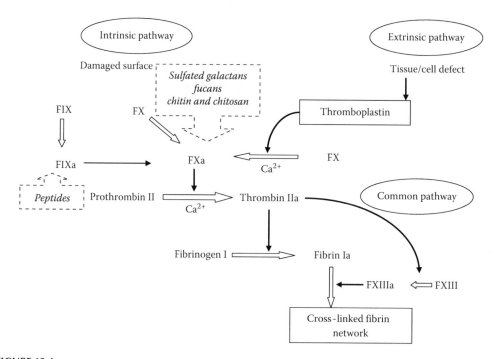

FIGURE 15.4
Schematic representation of blood clotting and involvement of marine materials for anticoagulation (all serine proteases and blood coagulation factors are not given).

TABLE 15.2

Marine Organisms with Potential Anticoagulation Activity, Their Source of Origin, and Active Compound

Group	Organism	Active Compound	Reference
Marine algae	*Canistrocarpus cervicornis*	Dolastane diterpene	Moura et al. (2011)
Brown seaweed	*E. cava*	SP	Wijesinghe et al. (2011)
Brown algae	*Ca. cervicornis*	Heterofucans (fucose, glucuronic acid, galactose, and sulfate)	Camara et al. (2011)
Red algae	*Lomentaria catenata*	A highly sulfated proteoglycan	Pushpamali et al. (2007)
Green algae	*M. latissimum*	SP	Zhang et al. (2008)
Green algae	*Ulva conglobata*	SPs	Mao et al. (2005)
Sea cucumbers	*Pearsonothuria graeffei* *Stichopus tremulus* *Holothuria vagabunda* *I. badionotus*	Fucosylated chondroitin sulfates	Chen et al. (2011)
Sea cucumber	*I. badionotus*	Sulfated fucan	Chen et al. (2012)

(e.g., agarans, carrageenans), ulvans, and fucans, and from invertebrates tissues, mainly sulfated glycosaminoglycans, have been extensively studied in the past for anticoagulant activity (Table 15.2). A probable reason for this may be due to the structural similarities between SP from marine algae and heparin (Lee et al., 2008). An anticoagulant activity similar to heparin, that is, by inhibition of thrombin and factor Xa, was exhibited by a sulfated galactan isolated from red algae *Botryocladia occidentalis* (Melo et al., 2008).

Anticoagulant activity of SPs depends on the sugar composition, molecular weight, proportion of sulfation, and position of the sulfate group along the macromolecule backbone/distribution of sulfate groups in the repeating units (Jiao et al., 2011). Shanmugam and Mody (2000) reported that carrageenans with higher molecular weight and higher sulfur content showed better anticoagulant activity than those with low molecular weight and low sulfur content. An SP (725.4 kDa) from the green alga *Monostroma latissimum* and its fragments (216.4–61.9 kDa) prepared by H_2O_2 degradation showed similar anticoagulant activities in prolonged activated partial thromboplastin time (APTT) and prothrombin time (PT) (Zhang et al., 2008). However, fragments with lower molecular size showed reduced anticoagulant activities (Zhang et al., 2008).

Fucoidans and galactans from brown algae and red seaweeds, respectively, are potent compounds as anticoagulants. The structure of a sulfated galactan isolated from marine red alga *Gelidium crinale* is composed of repeating structure -4-α-Gal$p$-(1 → 3)-β-Gal$p$1 → but with a variable sulfation pattern, where 15% of the total α-units are 2,3-disulfated and another 55% are 2-sulfated (Pereira et al., 2005). Comparison of anticoagulant activity of the sulfated galactan of *G. crinale* with a similar polysaccharide but with higher 2,3-disulfated α-units from red algae *B. occidentalis* exhibited venous thrombosis at low doses (0.5 mg/kg of body weight) compared to *G. crinale* (>1.0 mg/kg of body weight), proving the highly SP has better anticoagulant activity (Fonseka et al., 2008). Furthermore, brown seaweed *Ecklonia cava* exhibited good anticoagulant properties comparable with commercially available fucoidan both in vivo and in vitro.

The molecular weight is also known to influence on the anticoagulant activity. Sulfated galactan from *B. occidentalis* inhibits thrombin and factor Xa at low doses, whereas it activates factor XII at high doses in venous thrombosis (Melo et al., 2008). Moreover, the low molecular weight (~5 kDa) fraction of the sulfated galactan had no effect on factor XII activation and inhibition of antithrombin and heparin cofactor II (Melo et al., 2008). Anticoagulant activity of sulfated galactan from *B. occidentalis* is due to its ability to enhance thrombin and factor Xa inhibition by antithrombin and/or heparin cofactor II.

Similar to SPs, 6-O-sulfated chitosan strongly inhibited blood coagulation compared to compounds, 2,3-disulfate and 3-sulfate which consist of selectively introduced sulfate groups at O-2 and/or O-3 (Nishimura et al., 1998). Further, a chitosan polysulfate produced by modification of chitosan from crab shells using semiheterogeneous conditions prolonged thrombin time (TT) similar to heparin (inhibit factor Xa by promoting antithrombin III activity) (Vongchan et al., 2003).

Other than the SPs from marine algae, anticoagulant activities of SPs from other marine organisms have been reported. Chondroitin sulfates and fucan are two types of acidic polysaccharides found in major edible portion of sea cucumbers (Chen et al., 2011). Among these two compounds, fucan is better in terms of anticoagulant activity compared to heparin and fucosylated chondroitin sulfate isolated from sea cucumber *Isostichopus badionotus*. Moreover, these two compounds exert different mechanism of actions, where fucan potentiation of antithrombin acts on thrombin and factor Xa, whereas the fucosylated chondroitin sulfate acts mainly through heparin cofactor II (Chen et al., 2012). Similar to SPs, the site of sulfation and position of the glycosidic linkage of fucosylated chondroitin sulfate are important structural requirements to interact with the coagulation cascade. Chen et al. (2011) assessed the effect of different sulfation patterns of fucose on anticoagulant activities isolated from four sea cucumbers (Table 15.2) by APTT and TT. Three different sulfation patterns, 4-O-mono-, 2,3-O-di-, and 2,4-O-disulfation, were identified from fucosylated chondroitin sulfates, with varying anticoagulant activities where 2,4-O-disulfation has been identified with highest anticoagulant activity.

In addition to marine polysaccharides, few marine peptides also are known to exert the anticoagulant activity. For example, a marine peptide isolated from the marine echiuroid worm, *Urechis unicinctus* (order Urechidae), acts against the blood coagulation factor IXa (FIXa) (Jo et al., 2008).

15.3 Anti-Inflammatory Activity

Cornelius Celsus, a Roman encyclopedist of ancient times, is the first person to record the signs of inflammation as redness and swelling with heat and pain (Ferrero-Miliani et al., 2006). Nowadays, it is believed that inflammation is part of the nonspecific immune response with a cascade of biochemical events that occurs in reaction to any type of injurious stimuli (pathogens, damaged cells, irritants) in order to protect the organism and to initiate the healing process. The principal signs of inflammation are increased blood flow, elevated cellular metabolism, vasodilatation, release of soluble mediators, extravasation of fluids, and cellular influx (Ferrero-Miliani et al., 2006). Inflammation can be categorized as acute inflammation and chronic inflammation where prolonged inflammation can lead to variety of disorders as cancer, cardiovascular and pulmonary disorders, arthritis, diabetes, and Alzheimer's disease. For example, in Alzheimer's disease, accumulation of microglia around plaques and activation of complement cascade may damage neurons and aggravate the pathological process underlying the disease (Veld et al., 2001). Similarly, in rheumatoid arthritis, chronic synovial inflammation due to infiltration of leukocyte into the joint space leads to progressive cartilage and bone destruction (Tarrant and Patel, 2006). Thus, drugs have been targeted to reduce the accumulation of macrophages in the tissues.

Among different algae, anti-inflammatory effect of green algae of genus Caulerpa has been studied extensively, due to its ability to avoid excessive inflammation minimizing the cell migration to the inflammatory region. For example, aqueous, methanolic, acetate, hexanic, and chloroform extracts of *Caulerpa mexicana* minimized the leukocyte migration to the peritoneal cavity in chemically induced inflammation in vitro (Bitencourt et al., 2011; Matta et al., 2011). Furthermore, some extracts of *C. mexicana* showed better anti-inflammatory properties than the commercial product. For example, the aqueous extract of *C. mexicana*, a dose of 0.4 mg/kg, reduced xylene-induced ear edema by 84.83% after 15 min of the treatment compared to dexamethasone (dose of 05 mg/kg, by 70.60%, after 15 min), showing better anti-inflammatory properties than the control (Bitencourt et al., 2011).

However, identification and isolation of respective anti-inflammatory active compounds are essential in drug development. A such compound isolated from the lipid extract of *Caulerpa racemosa*, caulerpin (a bisindole alkaloid), showed high anti-inflammatory activity, which confirmed on a capsaicin-induced ear edema and carrageenan-induced peritonitis models, which reduces the number of leukocytes in peritoneal exudates (Souza et al., 2009).

Other than the discovery of marine organisms and different compounds with anti-inflammatory property (Table 15.3), scientists investigated the mechanism of action of these active compounds, which is crucially important for drug development. NF-κB signaling plays a key role in regulating inflammatory reaction cascade that coordinates the expression of

TABLE 15.3

Marine Organisms with Potential Anti-Inflammatory Property, Their Source of Origin, and Active Compound

Group	Organism	Active Compound	Reference
Green algae	*C. mexicana*	Aqueous, methanolic extracts	Bitencourt et al. (2011) Matta et al. (2011)
Green algae	*C. mexicana* *Caulerpa sertularioides*	Methanolic, acetate, hexanic and chloroform extracts	Matta et al. (2011)
Brown algae	*E. cava*	Dichloromethane, ethanol, and boiling water extracts	Kang et al. (2012a)
Brown algae	*Padina gymnospora*	Sulfated fucans	Marques et al. (2012)
Green algae	*Codium fragile*	Methanol extract	Kang et al. (2012b)
Brown algae	*E. cava*	Phlorotannins- 6,6-bieckol	Yang et al. (2012)
Brown algae	*L. japonica*	n-hexane fraction	Lee et al. (2012)
Brown algae	*Fucus vesiculosus* *Macrocystis pyrifera* *L. japonica*	Fucoidans	Myers et al. (2010)
Sponge	*Theonella swinhoei*	Cyclopeptides—perthamides A to K	Festa et al. (2009), Festa et al. (2012)
Sponge	*T. swinhoei*	Peptides—solomonamides A and B	Festa et al. (2011)
Sponge	*Dysidea* cf. *cristagalli*	Sesquiterpene—quinone	McNamara et al. (2005)

pro-inflammatory enzymes and cytokines including iNOS, cyclooxygenase-2 (COX-2), and tumor necrosis factor-α (TNFα). COX-2 is the key enzyme regulating the production of prostaglandins, the central mediators of inflammation. For example, neorogioltriol, a tricyclic brominated diterpenoid isolated from the organic extract of red algae *Laurencia glandulifera*, inhibited TNFα production, COX-2 release, and production of NO in an LPS-treated Raw264.7 cells (Chatter et al., 2011). Moreover, pretreatment with neorogioltriol, prior to LPS stimulation, significantly decreases NF-κB transactivation. However, it is observed that high concentrations of neorogioltriol failed to inhibit expression of certain NF-κB-dependent genes, such as COX-2, where release of COX-2 was inhibited at concentrations below 62.5 μM (Chatter et al., 2011).

15.4 Antiviral Activity

Viral-induced emerging and reemerging diseases are threats to the human survival. For example, acquired immunodeficiency syndrome (AIDS), which is caused by human immunodeficiency virus (HIV), is a major health problem in many parts of the world and is considered a pandemic disease. In 2009, WHO estimated that there are 33.4 million people worldwide living with HIV/AIDS, 2.7 million new HIV infections per year and 2.0 million annual deaths due to AIDS (World Health Organization, 2009). Considering the influenza viruses, type A, B, and C of the family Orthomyxoviridae, type A accounted for the human pandemic diseases worldwide during the last century. Other than that, viral infections to livestock or marine fish may markedly reduce the human food supply. For example, a viral strain with swine origin was declared by WHO as H1N1, in 2009. On the other hand, these new viral strains among livestock have the possibility to become zoonoses, which ultimately cause human deaths.

It is a known fact that the currently available drugs could keep the infection dormant in HIV-positive patients but unable to eliminate the virus (Pinti et al., 2006). Though there are a number of antivirals used clinically, resistance development due to viral intracellular replicative nature and readily mutating genome and side effects caused by classical antiviral drugs emphasize the need for alternative drugs including novel mode of action (Yasuhara-Bell et al., 2010). It is estimated that around 10^{23} of viral infections occur in marine environments every second (Dang et al., 2011). Thus, it is believed that large number of antiviral agents has evolved in marine organisms to protect them from viruses, which are abundant in oceans. These novel marine compounds with potent antiviral activity are being discovered from number of marine organisms against viral infections such as HIV, influenza virus, herpes simplex virus (HSV), vesicular stomatitis virus (VSV), human cytomegalovirus (HCMV), and human influenza virus (Table 15.4). Preliminary studies based on crude extracts helpful to identify the organisms with antiviral potential, isolation of chemical compounds, and identification of their mode of action are important for development of drugs.

Considering the mode of action of antiviral compounds, they can be broadly categorized in to two groups as compounds that block the cellular receptors utilized by the virus to enter into the cells and compounds that inhibit the viral replication after the cell is infected (Figure 15.5).

TABLE 15.4

Marine Organisms with Potential Antiviral Activity, Their Source of Origin, and Active Compound

Group	Organism	Compound	Virus	Reference
Sponge	*Celtodoryx girardae*	Exopolysaccharides	—	Rashid et al. (2009)
Sponge	*Erylus discophorus*	Sulfated polysaccharide (>2000 kDa)	Anti-HIV-1	Esteves et al. (2011)
Sea snail/ Gastropod mollusk (Family Haliotidae)	Greenlip abalone	Peptide, lipophilic and non-lipophilic extracts	HSV-1	Dang et al. (2011)
Brown algae	*E. cava*	Phlorotannin	Anti-human influenza virus	Ryu et al. (2011)
Marine algae	*U. pinnatifida* *S. rugosum* *Gi. atropurpurea* *Pl. cartilagineum*	Polysaccharide extracts	HSV types 1 and 2	Harden et al. (2009)
Antarctic red algae	*Gigartina skottsbergii*	Extracts	Influenza virus	Maschek et al. (2011)
Red microalgae	*Gyrodinium impudium*	SP p-KG03	Influenza A virus	Kim et al. (2012)

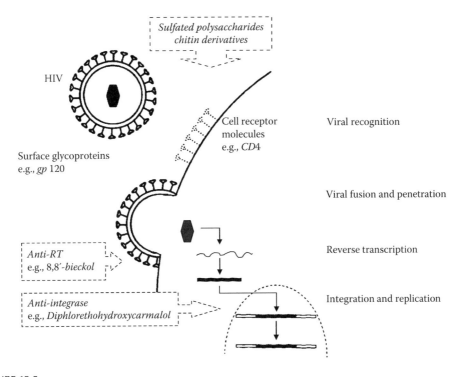

FIGURE 15.5
Schematic representation of HIV entry and replication and involvement of marine materials for anti-HIV activity in different steps.

15.4.1 Inhibition of Viral Attachment to Host by Marine Antiviral Materials

SPs are considered as an emerging class of anti-HIV compounds that serve as a mimetic for cellular receptors of viruses, preventing the adherence and subsequent entry and infection of virus particles (Bandyopadhyay et al., 2011). Accordingly, the SPs have the ability to interact with envelope glycoproteins of viral particles at the initial stage of infection, by formation of a stable virion-SP complex where viral attachment sites to host at the viral envelope are occupied by the SP (Damonte et al., 2004). This was confirmed by a real-time PCR carried out to detect the presence of viral DNA in a cell monolayer incubated with SP prior to infection; hence, it is believed that the binding sites were occupied by the SP (Harden et al., 2009).

A highly charged molecule may interfere with electrostatic interactions between the positively charged region of the viral glycoprotein and the negatively charged chains of the cell surface glycoprotein receptor (Ghosh et al., 2009). However, the antiviral activity of SPs is not only due to charge density and chain length but also due to their complex structural features, such as degree of sulfation, molecular weight, distribution of sulfate groups in the polysaccharide, constituent sugars, molecular conformation, and stereochemistry (Damonte et al., 2004; Harden et al., 2009). Nevertheless, degree of sulfation is the main important parameter for the antiviral activity of the polymer (i.e., the number of sulfate groups per monosaccharide residue) (Ghosh et al., 2009). The predominant reason behind the strong antiviral activity and degree of sulfation can be due to the similarity between the receptor molecules for viruses in cells and SPs. For example, heparin sulfate serves as an initial receptor for many different viruses, where SPs can mimic the activity of heparin sulfate (Bandyopadhyay et al., 2011). In general, SPs with a sulfate content higher than 20% (mol%) have shown potent antiviral activity (Ghosh et al., 2009).

With increasing molecular weight and degree of sulfation, increased antiviral activity of SPs has been reported (Bouhlal et al., 2011). For example, high molecular weight sulfated fucan (670 kDa) was more potent against HSV-1 and HSV-2 compared with the hydrolyzed sample (44 kDa). Moreover, the activity of unhydrolyzed sample is higher in the plaque reduction assay when added prior to infection (Harden et al., 2009). Conversely, polysaccharides containing high amount of uronic acid residues, such as alginic acid and carboxyl groups, retard the antiviral activity (Ghosh et al., 2009). For example, even the sulfated xylogalactofucan from a marine alga *Sphacelaria indica* showed lower antiviral activity than both sulfated alginate and acyclovir (the control) (Bandyopadhyay et al., 2011).

Valuable insight to the sulfation position on anti-HIV activity was revealed by studies conducted by Nishimura et al. (1998) on regioselective synthesis of sulfated analogs of chitin and chitosan. Study on structure and biological activity of chitin and chitosan revealed that selective sulfation at 0–2 and/or 0–3 showed much higher inhibitory effect on infection of AIDS virus in vitro. Moreover, 23-S product (2,3-disulfate) completely inhibited the infection of HIV to T lymphocytes at concentrations as low as EC_{50} 0.28 μg/mL without significant cytotoxicity. Similar to SPs from marine alga, sulfation position strongly affects the activity of these chitin derivatives. For example, 6-O sulfated derivative (6-sulfate) had lower anti-HIV activity compared to O-2 and O-3 derivatives (3-sulfate and 2,3-disulfate).

Studies on mode of action reveal that SP needs to be present prior to adsorption of the virus in order to exert their antiviral effect. For example, the SPs from red algae *Sphaerococcus coronopifolius* and *Boergeseniella thuyoides* exert anti-HSV-1 activity only if present during the first 2 h after viral infection. Furthermore, they interfered mainly in the very early stages of HSV type 1 replication on Vero cells in vitro at EC_{50} of 4.1 and 17.2 μg/mL (Bouhlal et al., 2011). Harden et al. (2009) also confirmed extracts from *Undaria pinnatifida, Splachnidium rugosum, Gigartina atropurpurea, Plocamium cartilagineum* have potent anti-HSV-1 and HSV-2 activity when added during the first hour of viral infection but was ineffective if added later.

Moreover, drugs targeting a specific biological activity needed to be lacking other inhibitory or side effects on the biological system. Though chitin and its derivatives, 3-sulfate and 2,3-disulfate, exert strong anti-HIV activity, they had little effect on generating the anticoagulant activity indicating the possibility of developing drugs with less side effects (Nishimura et al., 1998).

15.4.2 Inhibition of Viral Replication by Marine Antiviral Materials

The HIV-1 genome encodes three essential enzymes for replication cycle, reverse transcriptase (RT), integrase, and protease (Princen and Schols, 2005). Considering the anti-HIV drugs, there are three major classes as nucleoside reverse transcriptase inhibitors (NRTI), non-nucleoside reverse transcriptase inhibitors (NNRTI), and protease inhibitors (Tandon and Chhor, 2005).

Dollabelane diterpene, isolated from the marine alga *Dictyota pfaffii* (dolabelladienetriol), is known to exert its anti-HIV effect by inhibiting the enzyme RT, which is an enzyme encoded by HIV-1 genome for replication (Cirne-Santos et al., 2008). Moreover, studies done by the same authors with classical antiretroviral agents indicate that dolabelladienetriol is an NNRTI. Usually, NRTI can alter mitochondrial function by inhibiting the mitochondrial DNA polymerase gamma, the enzyme responsible for replication of mitochondrial DNA that could lead to a variety of side effects (Pinti et al., 2006). Since dollabelane diterpene is not an NRT inhibitor, there is a potential to use it as an antiviral agent in the future.

Though the major antiviral activity of SP is exerted via interacting with surface glycoproteins of HIV, some SPs are known to exert virucidal activity via inhibiting replication of viral in vitro (Nishimura et al., 1998). For example, *N*-carboxymethyl chitosan *N,O*-sulfate, a polysaccharide derived from *N*-carboxymethyl chitosan by a random sulfation reaction, exerts anti-HIV activity by competitive inhibition of HIV-I RT through inhibiting viral adsorption to the CD4 receptor (Sosa et al., 1991).

Another group with potent antiviral activity from marine origin is the phlorotannins, which can be found exclusively in brown marine algae. They are a group of phenolic compounds, formed by polymerization of phloroglucinol (1,3,5-trihydroxybenzene) monomer units in range of ways that derive compounds as phloroglucinol, eckol, dieckol, etc. Among marine brown algae, *E. cava* has been extensively studied for various biological activities, especially antiviral activity due to its richness of phlorotannin and its derivatives (Li et al., 2011). Ahn et al. (2004) had explored the inhibitory effect of 8,8-bieckol and dieckol on HIV-1 RT and protease in vitro. Nevertheless, the compounds are dimers of eckol; 8-8′-bieckol (IC_{50} 0.51 μM) showed 10-fold greater inhibitory activity against HIV-1 RT than 8,4′-dieckol (IC_{50} 5.3 μM). Moreover, the two compounds, bieckol and dieckol, consist of biaryl and diphenyl ether linkages, respectively. Ahn et al. (2004) had pointed out that difference in inhibition activity is due to the steric hindrance of the hydroxyl and aryl groups near the biaryl linkage of bieckol. Further, 8,8′-bieckol showed selective inhibition of RT over protease, whereas the inhibitory effect of bieckol was comparable to that of NNRTI, nevirapine (IC_{50} 0.28 μM). Furthermore, the molecular mechanics of this compound against HIV-I RT revealed that 8,8-bieckol binds to HIV-I RT only after the template/primer initially binds to the enzyme, displaying noncompetitive type of HIV inhibition. Hence, 8-8′-bieckol can be considered as an NNRTI against HIV-I.

TABLE 15.5

Marine Organisms with Potential NA Inhibitory Activity, Their Source of Origin, and Active Compound

Group	Organism	Active Compound	Chemical Group	Reference
Sponge	*Erylus nobilis*	Nobiloside	Penasterol trisaccharide	Takada et al. (2002)
Sponge	*Discodermia calyx*	Calceramides A–C	Sulfated ceramides	Nakao et al. (2001)
Fungus	*Phoma herbarum*	Arthropsadiol C and massarilactone H	Polyketides	Zhang et al. (2012)
Mangrove-derived fungus	—	Synthetic aromatic ether analog, **1–32**	—	Li et al. (2011)

The ethyl acetate fraction of *Ishige okamurae* inhibited the HIV-I RT and integrase activity showing the potential anti-HIV activity (93% inhibition at a concentration of 100 μg/mL) (Ahn et al., 2006). The bioassay-directed isolation afforded a diphlorethohydroxycarmalol, which exhibited inhibitory effects on HIV-I RT and integrase with IC_{50} values of 9.1 and 25.2 μM, respectively. Diphlorethohydroxycarmalol is a carmalol derivative, which consists of two phloroglucinol and one hydroxydibenzodioxin moiety. The authors suggested that the free hydroxyl groups play a key role in the anti-HIV-I RT and anti-integrase activities of diphlorethohydroxycarmalol. HIV-1 RT and HIV-1 integrase is responsible for the conversion of single-stranded viral genome into double-stranded proviral DNA and incorporation of resulting double-stranded DNA product to host genome, respectively.

15.4.3 Inhibition of Viral Spread by Marine Antiviral Compounds

Usually, all influenza viruses bear two surface glycoproteins, a hemagglutinin and a neuraminidase (NA) that is specific to a particular strain of influenza. The hemagglutinins being sialic acid receptor-binding molecules mediate the entry of the virus to target cells, where NA cleaves the sialic acid residues and facilitate the virus release and thereby invasion of new cells (Moscona, 2005). Hence, without NA, the infection will be limited to one round of replication, which is hardly enough to cause the disease (Moscona, 2005). Thus, marine compounds with potential NA inhibitory activity can be utilized as therapeutic agents against influenza virus (Table 15.5). Phlorotannins isolated from the ethanol extract of *E. cava* exhibited influenza virus NA inhibitory activity (72.1% inhibition at 30 μg/mL), where phlorotannin derivatives, phloroglucinol, eckol, 7-phloroeckol, phlorofucofuroeckol, and dieckol, were identified as selective NA inhibitors and phlorofucofuroeckol and dieckol exhibited the most potent inhibitory activity against the virus in vitro.

15.5 Conclusion

Owing to the unique physicochemical properties of these marine-derived compounds, there are enormous potential biological applications as anticancer, anticoagulant, anti-inflammation, and antiviral agents. Further, diverse groups of marine compounds such as polysaccharides, fatty acids, polyphenols, proteins or peptides, vitamins, and certain enzymes are still being discovered, showing that threats to the human well-being can be solved from the same place that life originated.

References

Ahn, M.J., Yoon, K.D., Kim, C.Y. et al. (2006). Inhibitory activity on HIV-1 reverse transcriptase and integrase of a carmalol derivative from a brown Alga, *Ishigeokamurae*. *Phytother Res.* 20(8):711–713.

Ahn, M.J., Yoon, K.D., Min, S.Y. et al. (2004). Inhibition of HIV-1reverse transcriptase and protease by phlorotannins from the brown alga, *Ecklonia cava*. *Biol. Pharm. Bull.* 27:544–547.

Andrianasolo, E.H., Haramaty, L., Vardi, A. et al. (2008). Apoptosis-inducing galactolipids from a Cultured Marine Diatom, *Phaeodactylum tricornutum*. *J. Nat. Prod.* 71(7):1197–1201.

Bai, R., Paull, K.D., Herald, C.L. et al. (1991). Halichondrin B and homohalichondrin B, marine natural products binding in the vinca domain of tubulin. *J. Biol. Chem.* 266(24):15882–15889.

Bandyopadhyay, S.S., Navid, M.H., Ghosh, T. et al. (2011). Structural features and in vitro antiviral activities of sulfated polysaccharides from *Sphacelaria indica*. *Phytochemistry* 72:276–283.

Bitencourt, M.A.O., Dantas, G.R., Lira, D.P. et al. (2011). Aqueous and methanolic extracts of *Caulerpa mexicana* suppress cell migration and ear edema induced by inflammatory agents. *Mar. Drugs* 9:1332–1345.

Bouhlal, R., Haslin, C., Chermann, J.C. et al. (2011). Antiviral activities of sulfated polysaccharides isolated from *Sphaerococcus coronopifolius* (*Rhodophytha, Gigartinales*) and *Boergeseniella thuyoides* (*Rhodophyta, Ceramiales*). *Mar. Drugs* 9:1187–1209.

Camara, R.B.G., Costa, L.S., Fidelis, G.P. et al. (2011). Heterofucans from the brown seaweed *Canistrocarpus cervicornis* with anticoagulant and antioxidant activities. *Mar. Drugs* 9:124–138.

Chatter, R., Othman, R.B., Rabhi, S. et al. (2011). In vivo and in vitro anti-inflammatory activity of neorogioltriol, a new diterpene extracted from the red algae *Laurencia glandulifera*. *Mar. Drugs* 9:1293–1306.

Chen, S., Hu, Y., Ye, X. et al. (2012). Sequence determination and anticoagulant and antithrombotic activities of a novel sulfated fucan isolated from the sea cucumber *Isostichopus badionotus*. *Biochim. Biophys. Acta* 1820(7):989–1000.

Chen, S., Xue, C., Yin, L. et al. (2011). Comparison of structures and anticoagulant activities of fucosylated chondroitin sulfates from different sea cucumbers. *Carbohydr. Polym.* 83:688–696.

Cirne-Santos, C.C., Souza, T.M.L., Teixeira, V.L. et al. (2008). The dolabellane diterpene dolabelladienetriol is a typical noncompetitive inhibitor of HIV-1 reverse transcriptase enzyme. *Antiviral Res.* 77:64–71.

Cruz-Monserrate, Z., Vervoort, H.C., Bai, R. et al. (2003). Diazonamide A and a synthetic structural analog: Disruptive effects on mitosis and cellular microtubules and analysis of their interactions with tubulin. *Mol. Pharmacol.* 63(6):1273–1280.

Damonte, E.B., Matulewicz, M.C., and Cerezo, A.S. (2004). Sulfated seaweed polysaccharides as antiviral agents. *Curr. Med. Chem.* 18:2399–2419.

Dang, V.T., Benkendorff, K., and Speck, P. (2011). In vitro antiviral activity against herpes simplex virus in the abalone *Haliotis laevigata*. *J. Gen. Virol.* 92:627–637.

Danial, N.N. and Korsmeyer, S.J. (2004). Cell death: Critical control points. *Cell* 116:205–219.

Ebada, S.S., Wray, V., Voogd, N.J. et al. (2009). Two new jaspamide derivatives from the marine sponge *Jaspis splendens*. *Mar. Drugs* 7:435–444.

Essack, M., Bajic, V.B., and Archer, J.A.C. (2011). Recently confirmed apoptosis-inducing lead compounds isolated from marine sponge of potential relevance in cancer treatment. *Mar. Drugs* 9:1580–1606.

Esteves, A.I.S., Nicolai, M., Humanes, M. et al. (2011). Sulfated polysaccharides in marine sponges: Extraction methods and anti-HIV activity. *Mar. Drugs* 9:139–153.

Ferrero-Miliani, L., Nielsen, O.H., Andersen, P.S. et al. (2006). Chronic inflammation: Importance of NOD2 and NALP3 in interleukin-1β generation. *Clin. Exp. Immunol.* 147:227–235.

Festa, C., Marino, S.D., D'Auria, M.V. et al. (2012). Anti-inflammatory cyclopeptides from the marine sponge *Theonella swinhoei*. *Tetrahedron* 68:2851–2857.

Festa, C., Marino, S.D., Sepe, V. et al. (2009). Perthamides C and D, two new potent anti-inflammatory cyclopeptides from a Solomon Lithistid sponge *Theonella swinhoei*. *Tetrahedron* 65:10424–10429.

Festa, C., Marino, S.D., Sepe, V. et al. (2011). Solomonamides A and B, new anti-inflammatory peptides from *Theonella swinhoei*. *Org. Lett.* 13(6):1532–1535.

Folkman, J. 1971. Tumor angiogenesis: Therapeutic implications. *N. Engl. J. Med.* 285:1182–1186.

Fonseka, R.J., Oliveira, S.N., Melo, F.R. et al. (2008). Slight differences in sulfation of algal galactans account for differences in their anticoagulant and venous antithrombotic activities. *Thromb. Haemost.* 99(3):539–545.

Frota, M.L.C., Braganhol, E., Canedo, A.D. et al. (2009). Brazilian marine sponge *Polymastia janeirensis* induces apoptotic cell death in human U138MG glioma cell line, but not in a normal cell culture. *Invest. New Drugs* 27:13–20.

Gao, X., Lu, Y., Xing, Y. et al. (2012). A novel anticancer and antifungus phenazine derivative from a marine actinomycete BM-17. *Microbiol. Res.* doi:10.1016/j.micres.2012.02.008.

Ghosh, T., Chattopadhyay, K., Marschall, M. et al. (2009). Focus on antivirally active sulfated polysaccharides: From structure–activity analysis to clinical evaluation. *Glycobiology* 19(1):2–15.

Harden, E.A., Falshaw, R., Carnachan, S.M. et al. (2009). Virucidal activity of polysaccharide extracts from four algal species against herpes simplex virus. *Antiviral Res.* 83(3):282–289.

Jiao, G., Guangli, Y., Zhang, J. et al. (2011). Chemical structures and bioactivities of sulfated polysaccharides from marine algae. *Mar. Drugs* 9:196–223.

Jimenez, P.C., Wilke, D.V., Takeara, R. et al. (2008). Cytotoxic activity of a dichloromethane extract and fractions obtained from *Eudistoma vannamei* (Tunicata: Ascidiacea). *Comp. Biochem. Physiol. A: Mol. Integr. Physiol.* 151(A):391–398.

Jo, H.Y., Jung, W.K., and Kim, S.K. (2008). Purification and characterization of a novel anticoagulant peptide from marine echiuroid worm, *Urechis unicinctus*. *Process Biochem.* 43(2):179–184.

Kang, J.Y., Choi, J.S., Park, N.G. et al. (2012a). In vivo antipyretic, analgesic, and anti-inflammatory activities of the brown alga *Ecklonia cava* extracts in Mice. *Fish Aquat. Sci.* 15(1):73–76.

Kang, C.H., Choi, Y.H., Park, S.Y. et al. (2012b). Anti-inflammatory effects of methanol extract of *Codium fragile* in lipopolysaccharide-stimulated RAW 264.7 cells. *J. Med. Food* 15(1):44–50.

Keshet, E. and Ben-Sasson, S. (1999). Anticancer drug targets: Approaching angiogenesis. *J. Clin. Invest.* 104(11):1497–1501.

Kijjoa, A., Wattanadilok, R., Campos, N. et al. (2007). Anticancer activity evaluation of kuanoniamines A and C isolated from the marine sponge *Oceanapia sagittaria*, collected from the Gulf of Thailand. *Mar. Drugs* 5:6–22.

Kim, M., Yim, J.H., Kim, S.Y. et al. (2012). In vitro inhibition of influenza A virus infection by marine microalga-derived sulfated polysaccharide p-KG03. *Antiviral Res.* 93(2):253–259.

Kong, D., Aoki, S., Sowa, Y. et al. (2008). Smenospongine, a sesquiterpene aminoquinone from a marine sponge, induces G1 arrest or apoptosis in different leukemia cells. *Mar. Drugs* 6:480–488.

Kong, D., Yamori, T., Kobayashi, M. et al. (2011). Antiproliferative and antiangiogenic activities of smenospongine, a marine sponge sesquiterpene aminoquinone. *Mar. Drugs* 9:154–161.

Lamoral-Theys, D., Fattorusso, E., Mangoni, A. et al. (2011). Evaluation of the antiproliferative activity of diterpene isonitriles from the sponge *Pseudoaxinella flava* in apoptosis-sensitive and apoptosis-resistant cancer cell lines. *J. Nat. Prod.* 74(10):2299–2303.

Lee, S.H., Athukorala, Y., Lee, J.S. et al. (2008). Simple separation of anticoagulant sulfated galactan from marine red algae. *J. Appl. Phycol.* 20:1053–1059.

Lee, J.Y., Lee, M.S., Choi, H.J. et al. (2012). Hexane fraction from *Laminaria japonica* exerts anti-inflammatory effects on lipopolysaccharide-stimulated RAW 264.7 macrophages via inhibiting NF-kappaB pathway. *Eur. J. Nutr.* Doi 10.1007/s00394-012-0345-1.

Li, J., Zhang, D., Zhu, X. et al. (2011). Studies on synthesis and structure-activity relationship (SAR) of derivatives of a new natural product from marine fungi as inhibitors of influenza virus neuraminidase. *Mar. Drugs* 9:1887–1901.

Mao, W., Zang, X., Li, Y. et al. (2005). Sulfated polysaccharides from marine green algae *Ulva conglobata* and their anticoagulant activity. *J. Appl. Phycol.* 18(1):9–14.

Marques, C.T., Azevedo, T.C.G., Nascimento, M.S. et al. (2012). Sulfated fucans extracted from algae *Padina gymnospora* have anti-inflammatory effect. *Braz. J. Pharmacol.* 22(1):115–122.

Maschek, J.A., Bucher, C.J., Olphen, A.V. et al. (2011). The pursuit of potent anti-influenza activity from the Antarctic red marine alga *Gigartina skottsbergii. Recent Adv. Phytochem.* 41:1–12.

Matta, C.B.B., Souza, E.T., Queiroz, A.C. et al. (2011). Antinociceptive and anti-inflammatory activity from algae of the genus *Caulerpa. Mar. Drugs* 9:307–318.

McNamara, C.E., Larsen, L., Perry, N.B. et al. (2005). Anti-inflammatory sesquiterpene-quinones from the New Zealand sponge *Dysidea* cf. *cristagalli. J. Nat. Prod.* 68:1431–1433.

Melo, F.R. and Mourão, P.A.S. (2008). An algal sulfated galactan has an unusual dual effect on venous thrombosis due to activation of factor XII and inhibition of the coagulation proteases. *Vet. Comp. Orthopaed.* 99(3):531–538.

Melo, F.R., Pereira, M.S., Foguels, D. et al. (2004). Antithrombin-mediated anticoagulant activity of sulfated polysaccharides. *J. Biol. Chem.* 279(20):20824–20835.

Moscona, A. (2005). Neuraminidase inhibitors for influenza. *N. Engl. J. Med.* 353:1363–1373.

Moura, L.A., Bianco, E.M., Pereira, R.C. et al. (2011). Anticoagulation and antiplatelet effects of a dolastane diterpene isolated from the marine brown alga *Canistrocarpus cervicornis. J. Thromb. Thrombolysis* 31:235–240.

Myers, S.P., O'Connor, J., Fitton, J.H. et al. (2010). A combined phase I and II open label study on the effects of a seaweed extract nutrient complex on osteoarthritis. *Biologics* 4:33–44.

Nakao, Y., Takada, K., Matsunaga, S. et al. (2001). Calceramides A-C: Neuraminidase inhibitory sulfated ceramides from the marine sponge *Discodermia calyx. Tetrahedron* 57:3013–3017.

Nishimura, S.I., Kai, H., Shinada, K. et al. (1998). Regioselective syntheses of sulfated polysaccharides: Specific anti-HIV-1 activity of novel chitin sulfates. *Carbohydr. Res.* 306:427–433.

Odaka, C., Sanders, M.L., and Crews, P. (2000). Jasplakinolide induces apoptosis in various transformed cell lines by a caspase-3-like protease-dependent pathway. *Clin. Diagn. Lab. Immunol.* 7(6):947–952.

Paterson, I., Britton, R., Delgado, O. et al. (2011). Total synthesis of (−)-dictyostatin, a microtubule-stabilising anticancer macrolide of marine sponge origin. *Tetrahedron* 66:6534–6545.

Peng, Z., Liu, M., Fang, Z. et al. (2012). Composition and cytotoxicity of a novel polysaccharide from brown alga (*Laminaria japonica*). *Carbohydr. Polym.* 89(4):1022–1026.

Pereira, M.G., Benevides, N.M.B., Melo, M.R.S. et al. (2005). Structure and anticoagulant activity of a sulfated galactan from the red alga, *Gelidium crinale*. Is there a specific structural requirement for the anticoagulant action? *Carbohydr. Res.* 340(12):2015–2023.

Pinti, M., Salomoni, P., and Cossarizza, A. (2006). Anti-HIV drugs and the mitochondria. *Biochimica et Biophysica Acta* 1757:700–707.

Princen, K. and Schols, D. (2005). HIV chemokine receptor inhibitors as novel anti-HIV drugs. *Cytokine Growth Factor Rev.* 16:659–677.

Pushpamali, W.A., Nikapitiya, C., Zoyza, M.D. et al. (2007). Isolation and purification of an anticoagulant from fermented red seaweed *Lomentaria catenata. Carbohydr. Polym.* 73:274–279.

Rashid, Z.M., Lahaye, E., Defer, D. et al. (2009). Isolation of a sulphated polysaccharide from a recently discovered sponge species (*Celtodoryx girardae*) and determination of its anti-herpetic activity. *Int. J. Biol. Macromol.* 44:286–293.

Ravikumar, S., Gnanadesigan, M., Thajuddin, N. et al. (2010). Anticancer property of sponge associated *Actinomycetes* along Palk Strait. *J. Pharm. Res.* 3(10):2415–2417.

Risinger, A.L., Glies, F.J., and Mooberry, S.L. (2009). Microtubule dynamics as a target in oncology. *Cancer Treat. Rev.* 35(3):255–261.

Ryu, Y.B., Jeong, H.J., Yoon, S.Y. et al. (2011). Influenza virus neuraminidase inhibitory activity of phlorotannins from the edible brown alga *Ecklonia cava. J. Agric. Food Chem.* 59(12):6467–6473.

Samarakoon, K. and Jeon, Y.J. (2012). Bio-functionalities of proteins derived from marine algae—A review. *Food Res. Int.* 48(2):948–960.

Shanmugam, M. and Mody, K.H. (2000). Heparinoid-active sulfated polysaccharides from marine algae as potential blood anticoagulant agents. *Curr. Sci.* 79:1672–1683.

Shin, H.J., Mondol, M.A.M., Yu, T.K. et al. (2010). An angiogenesis inhibitor isolated from a marine-derived actinomycete, *Nocardiopsis* sp. 03N67. *Phytochem. Lett.* 3(4):194–197.

Skropeta, D., Pastro, N., and Zivanovic, A. (2011). Kinase inhibitors from marine sponges. *Mar. Drugs* 9(10):2131–2154.

Smith, J.A., Wilson, L., Azarenko, O. et al. (2010). Eribulin binds at microtubule ends to a single site on Tubulin to suppress dynamic instability. *Biochemistry* 49(6):1331–1337.

Sosa, M.A., Fazely, F., Koch, J.A. et al. (1991). N-carboxymethylchitosan-N,O-sulfate as an anti-HIV-1 agent. *Biochem. Biophys. Res. Commun.* 174(2):489–496.

Souza, E.T., Lira, D.P., Queiroz, A.C. et al. (2009). The antinociceptive and anti-inflammatory activities of Caulerpin, a bisindole alkaloid isolated from seaweeds of the genus *Caulerpa*. *Mar. Drugs* 7:689–704.

Takada, K., Nakao, Y., Matsunaga, S. et al. (2002). Nobiloside, a new neuraminidase inhibitory triterpenoidal saponin from the marine sponge *Erylus nobilis*. *J. Nat. Prod.* 65(3):411–413.

Tandon, V.K. and Chhor, R.B. (2005). Current status of anti-HIV agents. *Curr. Med. Chem.* 4:3–28.

Tarrant, T.K. and Patel, D.D. (2006). Chemokines and leukocyte trafficking in rheumatoid arthritis. *Pathophysiology* 13(1):1–14.

Teruya, T., Sasaki, H., Fukazawa, H. et al. (2009). Bisebromoamide, a potent cytotoxic peptide from the marine cyanobacterium *Lyngbya* sp.: Isolation, stereostructure, and biological activity. *Org. Lett.* 11(21):5062–5065.

Trisciuoglio, D., Uranchimeg, B., Cardellina, J.H. et al. (2008). Induction of apoptosis in human cancer cells by candidaspongiolide, a novel sponge polyketide. *J. Natl Cancer Inst.* 100(17):1233–1246.

Tung, N.H., Minh, C.V., Ha, T.T. et al. (2009). C_{29} sterols with a cyclopropane ring at C-25 and 26 from the Vietnamese marine sponge *Ianthella* sp. and their anticancer properties. *Bioorg. Med. Chem. Lett.* 19:4584–4588.

Veld, B.A., Ruitenberg, A., Hofman, A. et al. (2001). Nonsteroidal antiinflammatory drugs and the risk of Alzheimer's disease. *N. Engl. J. Med.* 345(21):1515–1521.

Vidanarachchi, J.K., Kurukulasooriya, M.S., and Kim, S.K. (2010). Chitin, chitosan, and their oligosaccharides in food industry. In *Chitin, Chitosan, Oligosaccharides and Their Derivatives*, S. K. Kim, Ed., pp. 543–560. Taylor & Francis Group, New York.

Vongchan, P., Sajomsang, W., Kasinrerk, W. et al. (2003). Anticoagulant activities of the chitosan polysulfate synthesized from marine crab shell by semi-heterogeneous conditions. *Science Asia.* 29:115-120.

Wahl, O., Oswald, M., Tretzel, L. et al. (2011). Inhibition of tumor angiogenesis by antibodies, synthetic small molecules and natural products. *Curr. Med. Chem.* 18(21):3136–3155.

Walenga, J.M. and Bick, R.L. (1998). Heparin-induced thrombocytopenia, paradoxical thromboembolism, and other side effects of heparin therapy. *Med. Clin. North Am.* 82(3):635–658.

Wang, W.L.W., McHenry, P., Jeffrey, R. et al. (2008). Effects of iejimalide B, a marine macrolide, on growth and apoptosis in prostate cancer cell lines. *J. Cell. Biochem.* 105:998–1007.

Wei, S.Y., Li, M., Tang, S.A. et al. (2008). Induction of apoptosis accompanying with G1 phase arrest and microtubule disassembly in human hepatoma cells by jaspolide B, a new isomalabaricane-type triterpene. *Cancer Lett.* 262:114–122.

Wijesinghe, W.A.J.P., Athukorala, Y., and Jeon, Y.J. (2011). Effect of anticoagulative sulfated polysaccharide purified from enzyme-assistant extract of a brown seaweed *Ecklonia cava* on Wistar rats. *Carbohydr. Polym.* 86:917–921.

World Health Organization. (2009). *AIDS Epidemic Update*. UNAIDS, Geneva, Switzerland.

Yang, Y.I., Shin, H.C., Kim, S.H. et al. (2012). 6,6'-Bieckol, isolated from marine alga Ecklonia cava, suppressed LPS-induced nitric oxide and PGE2 production and inflammatory cytokine expression in macrophages: The inhibition of NFκB. *Int. Immunopharmacol.* 12:510–517.

Yasuhara-Bell, J., Yang, Y., Barlow, R. et al. (2010). In vitro evaluation of marine-microorganism extracts for anti-viral activity. *Virol. J.* 7:182. http://www.biomedcentral.com/content/pdf/1743-422X-7-182.pdf

Zhang, G.F., Han, W.B., Cui, J.T. et al. (2012). Neuraminidase inhibitory polyketides from the marine-derived fungus *Phoma herbarum. Planta Med.* 78(1):76–78.

Zhang, H.J., Mao, W.J., Fang, F. et al. (2008). Chemical characteristics and anticoagulant activities of a sulfated polysaccharide and its fragments from *Monostroma latissimum. Carbohydr. Polym.* 71(3):428–434.

Zheng, L.H., Wang, Y.J., Sheng, J. et al. (2011). Antitumor peptides from marine organisms. *Mar. Drugs* 9:1840–1859.

16

Health Benefits of Sulfated Polysaccharides from Marine Algae

Se-Kwon Kim, Dai-Hung Ngo, Thanh-Sang Vo, and Dai-Nghiep Ngo

CONTENTS

16.1 Introduction

Marine algae are the most abundant source of nonanimal sulfated polysaccharides (SPs) in nature. In recent years, various SPs isolated from marine algae have attracted much attention in nutraceutical/functional food, cosmetic/cosmeceutical, and pharmaceutical applications. SPs include a complex group of macromolecules with a wide range of important biological activities such as antioxidant, anticoagulant, anticancer, antiviral, and anti-inflammation (Costa et al. 2010). SPs are commonly found in three major groups of marine algae, red algae (Rhodophyceae), brown algae (Phaeophyceae), and green algae (Chlorophyceae). The major SPs of red algae are galactans commercially known as agar and carrageenan, and those of brown algae are fucans, including fucoidan, sargassan, ascophyllan, and glucuronoxylofucan. On the other hand, the major SPs of green algae are usually sulfated heteropolysaccharides that contain galactose, xylose, arabinose, mannose, glucuronic acid, or glucose (Jiao et al. 2011). This chapter focuses on SPs derived from marine algae and presents an overview of their biological activities with potential health benefits.

16.2 Potential Health Benefits of SPs Derived from Marine Algae

16.2.1 Antioxidant Activity

Humans are impacted by many free radicals both from inside our body and surrounding environment, particularly reactive oxygen species (ROS) generated in living organisms during metabolism. It is produced in the forms of H_2O_2, superoxide radical, hydroxyl radical, and nitric oxide (NO). In addition, oxidative stress may cause inadvertent enzyme activation and oxidative damage to cellular systems. Antioxidants can decrease oxidative stress-induced carcinogenesis by a direct scavenging of ROS. Recently, SPs including fucoidan and laminaran from a number of seaweeds have appreciable antioxidant capability (Wang et al. 2008). Antioxidant activity of SPs has been determined by various methods such as 1,1-diphenyl-2-picrylhydrazyl (DPPH) radical scavenging, ferric-reducing antioxidant power (FRAP), lipid peroxide inhibition, NO scavenging, ABTS radical scavenging, and superoxide and hydroxyl radical scavenging assays.

Xue et al. (1998) reported that several marine-derived SPs have antioxidative activities in phosphatidylcholine-liposomal suspension and organic solvents. According to Kim et al. (2007) the SP of brown alga *Sargassum fulvellum* is a more potent NO scavenger than commercial antioxidants such as butylated hydroxyanisole (BHA) and α-tocopherol. Antioxidant activity of SP depends on their structural features such as sulfation level, distribution of sulfate groups along the polysaccharide backbone, molecular weight, sugar composition, and stereochemistry (Ghosh et al. 2004). Antioxidant properties of carrageenans (Rocha et al. 2007) and ulvans (Qi et al. 2005) also appeared related to sulfate content. In the latter study, low molecular weight and high sulfate content derivatives of ulvans showed improved antioxidant activities (Sun et al. 2009). Interestingly, metal chelating, free radical, and hydroxyl radical scavenging activities of fucan fractions appear to relate to their ratio of sulfate content/fucose (Wang et al. 2010).

Fucans from *Fucus vesiculosus* exhibited considerable FRAP (Ruperez et al. 2002) and superoxide radical scavenging property (Rocha et al. 2007). In addition, a positive correlation has reported for sulfate content, superoxide radical, and hydroxyl radical scavenging assays in fucoidan fractions obtained from brown alga *Laminaria japonica* (Zhao et al. 2005; Wang et al. 2009). Furthermore, fucoidan has shown the highest antioxidant activity followed by alginate and laminaran from brown alga *Turbinaria conoides* according to FRAP and DPPH assays (Chattopadhyay et al. 2010). Besides, in vivo antioxidant activity of SP derived from marine red alga *Porphyra haitanensis* in aging mice has been reported (Zhang et al. 2003). These evidences suggest that among various naturally occurring substances, SP proves to be one of the useful candidates in search for effective, nontoxic substances with potential antioxidant activity. SPs are byproducts in the preparation of alginates from edible brown seaweeds and could be used as a rich source of natural antioxidants with potential application in the food industry as well as cosmetic and pharmaceutical industries.

16.2.2 Anti-Human Immunodeficiency Virus

Human immunodeficiency virus type-1 (HIV-1) is the cause of acquired immunodeficiency syndrome (AIDS), a major human viral disease with about 33.2 million people infected worldwide up to 2008. Antiviral agents that interfere with HIV at different stages of viral replication have been developed (Vo and Kim 2010). Marine algae-derived SPs have great

TABLE 16.1

Anti-HIV SPs from Marine Algae

SPs	Major Sugars	Source	References
Sulfated glucuronogalactan	Galactose	Red algae *Schizymenia dubyi*	Bourgougnon et al. (1996)
Sulfated polymannoroguluronate	Mannuronate	Brown algae	Meiyu et al. (2003)
Sulfated polymannuronate	Mannuronate	Brown algae	Liu et al. (2005)
Sulfated galactans	Galactose, xylose	Red algae *Grateloupia filicina*, *Grateloupia longifolia*	Wang et al. (2007)
Sulfated fucans	Fucose	Brown algae *D. mertensii*, *L. variegate*, *F. vesiculosus*, *S. schroederi*	Queiroz et al. (2008)
Galactofucan	Fucose, galactose	Brown algae *A. utricularis*	Trinchero et al. (2009)

potential for the development of new generation of anti-HIV therapeutics, as reported by several studies (Table 16.1).

Marine algae contain significant quantities of complex structural SPs that have been shown to inhibit the replication of enveloped viruses including members of the togavirus, arenavirus, flavivirus, orthopoxvirus, rhabdovirus, and herpesvirus families (Witvrouw and De Clercq 1997). The chemical structure including the degree of sulfation, constituent sugars, molecular weight, conformation, and dynamic stereochemistry is affecting the antiviral activity of algal SPs (Adhikari et al. 2006). Moreover, SPs may inhibit the attachment of viruses with target molecules on the cell surface. The viral attachment peptides are highly conserved regions within rather variable scaffolds of viral surface glycoproteins. These peptides are poorly subject to alterations by the natural antigenic drift of viruses. Likewise, they are not expected to represent frequent sites of drug-induced resistant mutation. Therefore, SPs that are directed toward these target peptides are preferred candidates for antiviral drug development (Ghosh et al. 2009).

A number of SPs from red algae have exhibited an appreciable HIV-1 inhibitory activity. Bourgougnon et al. (1996) determined anti-HIV activity of the sulfated glucuronogalactan from *Schizymenia dubyi*. As shown in their study, the syncytial formation and HIV-associated RT in vitro were completely suppressed with 5 μg/mL of this polysaccharide. They suggested that the mechanism of action in vitro of this polysaccharide has been mainly attributed to the inhibition of virus–host cell attachment or an early step of HIV infection. Moreover, antiretroviral activity of sulfated galactans from *Grateloupia filicina* (GFP) and *Grateloupia longifolia* (GLP) was investigated with a primary isolate of HIV-1 and human peripheral blood mononuclear cells (Wang et al. 2007). These results show that both GFP and GLPE (the 1,4-α-D-glucan-glucanohydrolase digest of GLP) had potent anti-HIV-1 activity when added at the time of infection and 2 h post-infection (EC$_{50s}$ 0.010–0.003 μM and EC$_{90s}$ 0.87–0.33 μM, respectively) with low cytotoxicity. EC$_{50}$ and EC$_{90}$ is a measure of anti-HIV activity being the concentration required to inhibit 50% and 90% HIV p24 core protein production 7 days post infection, respectively.

In addition, brown algae are also known to produce a variety of interesting SPs, which have been found to exhibit anti-HIV activity with different mechanisms of action. Sulfated polymannuroguluronate (SPMG) from brown algae is rich in 1,4-linked β-D-mannuronate, with 1.5 sulfate and 1.0 carboxyl groups averaging each sugar residue (Miao et al. 2005). Marine SPMG involved in inhibition of HIV-1 entry was investigated by Meiyu et al. (2003). Results indicated that binding of SPMG either to soluble oligomeric rgp120 or to complexed rgp120–sCD4 mainly resided in V3 loop region. The V3 loop of gp120 is considered as a positively charged region, which is targeted by negatively charged polysaccharides. In addition, the preincubation of SPMG with rgp120 triggered partial suppression of rgp120 binding to sCD4. Thus, they have suggested that SPMG either shared common binding sites on gp120 with sCD4 or masked the docking sites of gp120 for sCD4. Finally, SPMG showed less accessibility for sCD4 when sCD4 was precombined with rgp120, though SPMG multivalently bound to sCD4 with relatively low affinity. However, SPMG may suppress the multivalent binding of rgp120 to sCD4 receptor when SPMG is added either prior to or after the interaction of rgp120 with sCD4. These effective suppressions indicate that SPMG is endowed with both preventive and therapeutic potential on HIV-1 entry.

The sulfated fucans from the brown seaweed species *Dictyota mertensii*, *Lobophora variegata*, *Spatoglossum schroederi*, and *F. vesiculosus* were reported to inhibit HIV reverse transcriptase (RT) by Queiroz et al. (2008). They have indicated that the galactofucan fraction from *L. variegata*, which is rich in galactose, fucose, and glucose with a lower sulfate content, had a marked inhibitory effect on RT, with 94% inhibition for synthetic polynucleotides at concentration of 1.0 μg/mL. On the other hand, fucan A from *S. schroederi* and *D. mertensii*, which mainly contain fucose with a lower sulfate level, showed a high inhibitory effect on RT enzyme at 1.0 mg/mL with 99.03% and 99.3% inhibition, respectively. Meanwhile, fucan B from *S. schroederi*, which contained galactose, fucose, and high sulfate level, showed a lower inhibitory activity (53.9%) at the same concentration. Taking another approach, they purified a fucan fraction from *F. vesiculosus*, a homofucan containing only sulfated fucose with high sulfate content, which exhibited high inhibitory activity of HIV on RT. This fraction inhibited 98.1% of the reaction with poly(rA)-oligo(dT) at a concentration of 0.5 mg/mL. In addition, they modified SPs by carboxyreduction and desulfation to determine the structure–activity relationship. These modified conditions reduced the inhibitory activities of these polysaccharides for RT approximately fourfold. From these results, they have suggested that fucan activity is dependent on both the ionic changes and the sugar rings that act to spatially orientate the charges in a configuration and recognizes the enzyme, thus determining the specificity of the binding.

In the recent study, Trinchero et al. (2009) have shown that galactofucan fractions from the brown algae *Adenocystis utricularis* exhibited anti-HIV-1 activity in vitro. Among five fractions, EA1-20 and EC2-20 had a strong effect to inhibit HIV-1 replication in vitro with low IC_{50} values (0.6 and 0.9 μg/mL, respectively). Additionally, EA1-20 and EC2-20 exposed the capacity against wild-type and drug-resistant HIV-1 strains. For active fractions, it was also shown that the inhibitory effect was not due to an inactivating effect on the viral particles but rather to a blockade of early events of viral replication. Based on these results, seaweed-derived SPs are regarded as good candidates for further studies on prevention of HIV-1 infection.

16.2.3 Antiallergic Activity

Allergy, also referred to atopy, is caused by an exaggerated reaction of the immune system to harmless environmental substances, such as animal dander, house dust mites, foods, pollen, insects, and chemical agents. In the recent study, fucoidan from *Undaria pinnatifida* reduced the concentrations of both interleukin-4 (IL-4) and IL-13 in bronchoalveolar lavage fluid and inhibited the increase of antigen-specific immunoglobulin E (IgE) in ovalbumin (OVA)-induced mouse airway hypersensitivity (Maruyama et al. 2005). Yanase et al. (2009) have reported that the peritoneal injection of fucoidan inhibited the increase of plasma IgE via suppressing a number of IgE-expressing and IgE-secreting B cells from OVA-sensitized mice. On the other hand, the inhibitory effect of fucoidan on IgE production was proved due to preventing Cε germ line transcription and nuclear factor-kappa B (NF-κB) p52 translocation in B cells (Oomizu et al. 2006). However, the effect of fucoidan was not observed if B cells were prestimulated with IL-4 and anti-CD40 antibody before the administration of fucoidan. These observations suggested that fucoidan may not prevent a further increase of IgE in patients who have already developed allergic diseases and high levels of serum IgE. Conversely, Iwamoto et al. (2010) have determined that fucoidan effectively reduced IgE production in both peripheral blood mononuclear cells from atopic dermatitis patients and healthy donors. These findings indicated that fucoidan suppresses IgE induction by inhibiting immunoglobulin class-switching to IgE in human B cells, even after the onset of atopic dermatitis. Besides, porphyran, a sulfated polysaccharide isolated from red seaweeds, has been recognized to be effective against different allergic responses. According to Ishihara et al. (2005), porphyran of red algae *Porphyra tenera* and *Porphyra yezoensis* was capable of inhibiting the contact hypersensitivity reaction induced by 2,4,6-trinitrochlorobenzene through decreasing the serum levels of IgE and interferon gamma (IFN-γ) in BALB/c mice.

In addition, alginic acid, a naturally occurring hydrophilic colloidal polysaccharide obtained from the several species of brown seaweeds, exhibited different effects against hyaluronidase activity and histamine release from mast cells (Asada et al. 1997). In the in vivo conditions, alginic acid inhibited compound 48/80-induced systemic anaphylaxis with doses of 0.25–1 g/kg and significantly inhibited passive cutaneous anaphylaxis by 54.8% at 1 g/kg for 1 h pretreatment. Besides, alginic acid was found to have a maximum suppression rate (60.8%) on histamine release from rat peritoneal mast cells at concentration of 0.01 µg/mL. Furthermore, the antiallergic activities of alginic acid were also observed due to its suppressive effects on activity and expression of histidine decarboxylase, production of IL-1β and tumor necrosis factor-alpha (TNF-α), and protein level of NF-κB/*Rel A* in phorbol 12-myristate 13-acetate (PMA) plus A23187-stimulated HMC-1 cells (Jeong et al. 2006). Noticeably, alginic acid oligosaccharide (ALGO), a lyase lysate of alginic acid, has been revealed to be able to reduce IgE production in the serum of BALB/c mice immunized with beta-lactoglobulin (Uno et al. 2006). Moreover, antigen-induced Th2 development was blocked by ALGO treatment via enhancing the production of IFN-γ and IL-12 and downregulating IL-4 production in splenocytes of mice (Yoshida et al. 2004).

16.2.4 Anticoagulant Activity

Blood coagulation is processed by coagulation factors in order to stop the flow of blood through the injured vessel wall whenever an abnormal vascular condition and exposure to non-endothelial surfaces at sites of vascular injury occur. As endogenous or exogenous anticoagulants interfered with the coagulation factors, the blood coagulation can be stopped (Kim and Wijesekara 2010).

Heparin (a glycosaminoglycan extracted from porcine tissues) has been the most commonly used antithrombotic/anticoagulant drug. However, the use of heparin may be accompanied by side effects such as thrombocytopenia, hemorrhagic effect, ineffectiveness

TABLE 16.2

Marine Algae SP-Derived Anticoagulant Agents

Source	Major Sugar	References
Rhodophyceae (red algae)		
Grateloupia indica	Galactose	Sen et al. (1994)
Gigartina skottsbergii	Galactose	Carlucci et al. (1997)
Nothogenia fastigiata	Mannose	Kolender et al. (1997)
Schizymenia binderi	Galactose	Zuniga et al. (2006)
Lomentaria catenata	Galactose	Pushpamali et al. (2008)
Porphyra haitanensis	Galactose	Zhang et al. (2010)
Chlorophyceae (green algae)		
Monostroma nitidum	Rhamnose	Maeda et al. (1991)
Codium fragile	Arabinose	Hayakawa et al. (2000)
Codium pugniformis	Glucose	Matsubara et al. (2000)
Codium cylindricum	Galactose	Matsubara et al. (2001)
Ulva conglobata	Rhamnose	Mao et al. (2006)
Monostroma latissimum	Rhamnose	Mao et al. (2009)
Phaeophyceae (brown algae)		
Ecklonia kurome	Fucose	Nishino et al. (1991)
Ascophyllum nodosum	Fucose	Nardella et al. (1996)
Ecklonia cava	Fucose	Athukorala et al. (2006)
Lessonia vadosa	Fucose	Chandia and Matsuhiro (2008)
Laminaria japonica	Fucose	Wang et al. (2010)

in congenital or acquired antithrombin deficiencies, and incapacity to inhibit thrombin bound to fibrin (Costa et al. 2010). Due to several side effects of heparin, anticoagulant activity is among the most widely studied properties of SPs for alternative sources of heparinoid-active compounds as therapeutic agents. Therefore, various anticoagulant SPs from marine algae have been isolated and characterized (Table 16.2). Two types of SPs are identified with high anticoagulant activity including sulfated fucoidans from marine brown algae (Chevolot et al. 1999) and carrageenan from marine red algae (Carlucci et al. 1997). However, there are fewer reports of anticoagulant SPs reported from marine green algae compared to brown and red algae (Mao et al. 2006). Jurd et al. (1995) found that the anticoagulant-active SPs from *Codium fragile* subspecies *atlanticum* (Chlorophyceae) contain xyloarabinogalactans. A sulfated galactan with anticoagulant activity has also been reported from *Codium cylindricum* (Matsubara et al. 2001). In addition, Maeda et al. (1991) have revealed that the anticoagulant SPs from the green alga *Monostroma nitidum* yielded a sixfold higher activity than that of heparin. In comparison, marine brown algae extracts exhibit higher anticoagulant activity than red and green algae extracts (Chevolot et al. 1999).

The anticoagulant activity of the earlier SPs has been determined by prolongation of activated partial thromboplastin time (APTT), prothrombin time (PT), and thrombin time (TT) assays. Since a few studies reported the prolongation of PT by marine SPs, it suggests that marine SPs interfered a little or may not inhibit the extrinsic pathway of coagulation. The relationship between structure and anticoagulant activity of some SPs has been reported (Hayakawa et al. 2000). The presence of sulfate groups in SPs can increase both their specific and nonspecific binding to a wide range of biologically active proteins. Anticoagulant activity of sulfated galactans depends on the nature of the sugar residue, the sulfation position of the structure, and the sulfate content in the SPs (Silva et al. 2010). Moreover, the O-sulfated 3-linked α-galactans enhanced the inhibition of thrombin and factor Xa by antithrombin and/or heparin cofactor II in the intrinsic pathway of blood coagulation (Pereira et al. 2002). Furthermore, high molecular weight carrageenans with high sulfate content have shown higher anticoagulant activity than low molecular weight and low sulfate content SPs (Shanmugam and Mody 2000).

Low molecular weight heparins and unfractionated heparins are the only SPs currently used as anticoagulant drugs. Seaweed-derived SPs have been described to possess anticoagulant activity similar to or higher than heparin (Costa et al. 2010). Collectively, these evidences suggest that SPs derived from seaweeds have a promising potential to be used as anticoagulant nutraceuticals or medicinal food ingredients in the food industry.

16.2.5 Anticancer Activity

The formation of cancer cells in human body can be directly induced by free radicals and natural anticancer drugs as chemopreventive agents have gained a positive popularity in treatment of cancer. Hence, radical scavenging compounds such as SPs from seaweeds can be used indirectly to reduce cancer formation in human body. Recently, numerous studies reported that SPs inhibit tumor growth and metastatic process both by direct action on tumor cells and by the enhancement of immune response (Khotimchenko 2010). Yamamoto et al. (1986) reported that the oral administration of several seaweeds can cause a significant decrease in the incidence of carcinogenesis in vivo. SPs have antiproliferative activity in cancer cell lines in vitro as well as inhibitory property of tumor growth in mice (Rocha de Souza et al. 2007; Ye et al. 2008). In addition, they have antimetastatic activity by blocking the interactions between the cancer cells and the basement membrane (Rocha et al. 2005). Porphyran of red algae *P. yezoensis* can induce cancer cell death via apoptosis in a dose-dependent manner in vitro without affecting the growth of normal cells (Kwon and Nam 2006). According to recent study, the SPs from *Ecklonia cava* have potential antiproliferative effects on U-937 (human leukemic monocyte lymphoma), CT-26 (murine colon carcinoma), HL-60 (human promyelocytic leukemia), and B-16 (mouse melanoma) cell lines (Athukorala et al. 2009).

Antitumor activity of fucoidan from Korean brown seaweed *U. pinnatifida* in PC-3 (human prostate), Hela (human cervical), A549 (carcinomic human alveolar basal epithelial), and HepG2 (human hepatocellular liver carcinoma) cancer cell lines in a similar pattern to that of commercial fucoidan was reported (Synytsya et al. 2010). Fucoidan was found to inhibit proliferation and induce apoptosis in human lymphoma HS-Sultan cells accompanied by activation of caspase-3 and downregulation of ERK pathways (Aisa et al. 2004). Lee et al. (2008) discovered that the fucoidan from *Laminaria guryanovae* was effective in inhibiting cell transformation induced by epidermal growth factor in the mouse epidermal JB6 Cl41 cells. In addition, antitumor and antimetastatic activities of fucoidan isolated from brown alga *Fucus evanescens* were studied in C57Bl/6 mice with transplanted Lewis lung adenocarcinoma (Alekseyenko et al. 2007). *Cladosiphon okamuranus* TOKIDA is commercially cultured around the Okinawa Island, Japan. A fucoidan has been prepared on an industrial scale from the brown seaweed and used as an additive to health foods, drinks, and cosmetics in Japan. Fucoidan from *C. okamuranus* TOKIDA induced apoptosis of human T-cell leukemia virus type 1-infected T-cell lines and primary adult T-cell leukemia (ATL) cells (Heneji et al. 2005) and apoptosis of U937 cells via caspase-3 and caspase-7 activation-dependent pathways (Teruya et al. 2007). Their results suggested that fucoidan can be a potentially useful therapeutic agent for ALT patients.

Anticancer activity of fucoidans has been reported to be closely related to their sulfate content and molecular weight. When native fucoidans have hydrolyzed in boiling water with HCl acid for 5 min, it significantly increased anticancer activity. However, fucoidans hydrolyzed in a microwave oven showed little improvement of anticancer activity. This suggests that anticancer activity of fucoidans could be significantly enhanced by lowering their molecular weight only when they are depolymerized at mild conditions (Yang et al. 2008). Importantly, SPs from marine algae are known to be important free-radical scavengers and antioxidants for the prevention of oxidative damage, which is an important contributor in carcinogenesis. Therefore, these marine algae-derived SPs can be used as functional ingredients in pharmaceuticals or functional foods to reduce cancer formation in human body.

16.3 Concluding Remarks

Algal SPs are a source of numerous biological activities that may find therapeutic benefits. Furthermore, seaweed processing by-products with bioactive SPs can be easily utilized for producing functional ingredients. The possibilities of designing new functional foods and pharmaceuticals to support reducing or regulating the diet-related chronic malfunctions are promising. Therefore, it can be suggested that due to valuable biological functions with health beneficial effects, marine algae-derived SPs have much potential as active ingredients for preparation of nutraceutical products. Until now, most of the biological activities of marine-derived SPs have been observed in vitro or in mouse model systems. Therefore, further research studies are needed in order to investigate their activity in human subjects.

Acknowledgment

This study was supported by a grant from the Marine Bioprocess Research Center of the Marine Bio 21 Project funded by the Ministry of Land, Transport and Maritime, Republic of Korea.

References

Adhikari, U., C. G. Mateu, K. Chattopadhyay, C. A. Pujol, E. B. Damonte, and B. Ray. 2006. Structure and antiviral activity of sulfated fucans from *Stoechospermum marginatum*. *Phytochemistry* 67:2474–2482.

Aisa, Y., Y. Miyakawa, T. Nakazato, H. Shibata, K. Saito, Y. Ikeda, and M. Kizaki. 2004. Fucoidan induces apoptosis of human HS-Sultan cells accompanied by activation of caspase-3 and down-regulation of ERK pathways. *American Journal of Hematology* 78:7–14.

Alekseyenko, T. V., S. Y. Zhanayeva, A. A. Venediktova, T. N. Zvyagintseva, T. A. Kuznetsova, N. N. Besednova, and T. A. Korolenko. 2007. Antitumor and antimetastatic activity of fucoidan, a sulfated polysaccharide isolated from the Okhotsk sea *Fucus evanescens* brown alga. *Bulletin of Experimental Biology and Medicine* 143:730–732.

Asada, M., M. Sugie, M. Inoue, K. Nakagomi, S. Hongo, K. Murata, S. Irie, T. Takeuchi, N. Tomizuka, and S. Oka. 1997. Inhibitory effect of alginic acids on hyaluronidase and on histamine release from mast cells. *Bioscience, Biotechnology, and Biochemistry* 61:1030–1032.

Athukorala, Y., G. N. Ahn, Y. H. Jee, G. Y. Kim, S. H. Kim, J. H. Ha, J. S. Kang, K. W. Lee, and Y. J. Jeon. 2009. Antiproliferative activity of sulfated polysaccharide isolated from an enzymatic digest of *Ecklonia cava* on the U-937 cell line. *Journal of Applied Phycology* 21:307–314.

Athukorala, Y., W. K. Jung, T. Vasanthan, and Y. J. Jeon. 2006. An anticoagulative polysaccharide from an enzymatic hydrolysate of *Ecklonia cava*. *Carbohydrate Polymers* 66:184–191.

Bourgougnon, N., M. Lahaye, B. Quemener, J. C. Chermann, M. Rimbert, M. Cormaci, G. Furnari, and J. M. Komprobst. 1996. Annual variation in composition and in vitro anti-HIV-1 activity of the sulfated glucuronogalactan from *Schizymenia dubyi* (Rhodophyta, Gigartinales). *Journal of Applied Phycology* 8:155–161.

Carlucci, M. J., C. A. Pujol, M. Ciancia, M. D. Noseda, M. C. Matulewicz, E. B. Damonte, and S. A. Cerezo. 1997. Antiherpetic and anticoagulant properties of carrageenans from the red seaweed *Gigartina skottsbergii* and their cyclized derivatives: Correlation between structure and biological activity. *International Journal of Biological Macromolecules* 20:97–105.

Chandia, N. P. and B. Matsuhiro. 2008. Characterization of a fucoidan from *Lessonia vadosa* (Phaeophyta) and its anticoagulant and elicitor properties. *International Journal of Biological Macromolecules* 42:235–240.

Chattopadhyay, N., T. Ghosh, S. Sinha, K. Chattopadhyay, P. Karmakar, and B. Ray. 2010. Polysaccharides from *Turbinaria conoides*: Structural features and antioxidant capacity. *Food Chemistry* 118:823–829.

Chevolot, L., A. Foucault, F. Chaubet, N. Kervarec, C. Sinquin, A. M. Fisher, and C. Boisson-Vidal. 1999. Further data on the structure of brown seaweed fucans: Relationships with anticoagulant activity. *Carbohydrate Research* 319:154–165.

Costa, L. S., G. P. Fidelis, S. L. Cordeiro, R. M. Oliveira, D. A. Sabry, R. B. G. Câmara, L. T. D. B. Nobre et al. 2010. Biological activities of sulfated polysaccharides from tropical seaweeds. *Biomedicine Pharmacotherapy* 64:21–28.

Ghosh, P., U. Adhikari, P. K. Ghosal, C. A. Pujol, M. J. Carlucci, E. B. Damonte, and B. Ray. 2004. In vitro anti-herpetic activity of sulfated polysaccharide fractions from *Caulerpa racemosa*. *Phytochemistry* 65:3151–3157.

Ghosh, T., K. Chattopadhyay, M. Marschall, P. Karmakar, P. Mandal, and B. Ray. 2009. Focus on antivirally active sulfated polysaccharides: From structure–activity analysis to clinical evaluation. *Glycobiology* 19:2–15.

Hayakawa, Y., T. Hayashi, J. B. Lee, P. Srisomporn, M. Maeda, T. Ozawa, and N. Sakuragawa. 2000. Inhibition of thrombin by sulfated polysaccharides isolated from green algae. *Biochimica Biophysica Acta* 1543:86–94.

Heneji, K., T. Matsuda, M. Tomita, H. Kawakami, K. Ohshiro, J. N. Uchihara, M. Masuda et al. 2005. Fucoidan extracted from *Cladosiphon okamuranus* Tokida induces apoptosis of human T-cell leukemia virus type 1-infected T-cell lines and primary adult T-cell leukemia cells. *Nutrition and Cancer* 52:189–201.

Ishihara, K., C. Oyamada, R. Matsushima, M. Murata, and T. Muraoka. 2005. Inhibitory effect of porphyran, prepared from dried "Nori," on contact hypersensitivity in mice. *Bioscience, Biotechnology, and Biochemistry* 69:1824–1830.

Iwamoto, K., T. Hiragun, S. Takahagi, Y. Yanase, S. Morioke, S. Mihara, Y. Kameyoshi, and M. Hide. 2010. Fucoidan suppresses IgE production in peripheral blood mononuclear cells from patients with atopic dermatitis. *Archives of Dermatological Research* 303:425–431.

Jeong, H. J., S. A. Lee, P. D. Moon, H. J. Na, R. K. Park, J. Y. Um, H. M. Kim, and S. H. Hong. 2006. Alginic acid has anti-anaphylactic effects and inhibits inflammatory cytokine expression via suppression of nuclear factor-kappaB activation. *Clinical and Experimental Allergy* 36:785–794.

Jiao, G., G. Yu, J. Zhang, and H. S. Ewart. 2011. Chemical structures and bioactivities of sulfated polysaccharides from marine algae. *Marine Drugs* 9:196–223.

Jurd, K. M., D. J. Rogers, G. Blunden, and D. S. McLellan. 1995. Anticoagulant properties of sulphated polysaccharides and a proteoglycan from *Codium fragile* ssp. *atlanticum*. *Journal of Applied Phycology* 7:339–345.

Khotimchenko, Y. S. 2010. Antitumor properties of nonstarch polysaccharides: Fucoidans and chitosans. *Russian Journal of Marine Biology* 36:321–330.

Kim, S. H., D. S. Choi, Y. Athukorala, Y. J. Jeon, M. Senevirathne, and C. K. Rha. 2007. Antioxidant activity of sulfated polysaccharides isolated from *Sargassum fulvellum*. *Journal of Food Science and Nutrition* 12:65–73.

Kim, S. K. and I. Wijesekara. 2010. Development and biological activities of marine-derived bioactive peptides: A review. *Journal of Functional Foods* 2:1–9.

Kolender, A. A., C. A. Pujol, E. B. Damonte, M. C. Matulewicz, and A. S. Cerezo. 1997. The system of sulfated α-(1→3)-linked D-mannans from the red seaweed *Nothogenia fastigiata*: Structures, antiherpetic and anticoagulant properties. *Carbohydrate Research* 304:53–60.

Kwon, M. J. and T. J. Nam. 2006. Porphyran induces apoptosis related signal pathway in AGS gastric cancer cell lines. *Life Sciences* 79:1956–1962.

Lee, N. Y., S. P. Ermakova, T. N. Zvyagintseva, K. W. Kang, Z. Dong, and S. Choi. 2008. Inhibitory effects of fucoidan on activation of epidermal growth factor receptor and cell transformation in JB6 C141 cells. *Food and Chemical Toxicology* 46:1793–1800.

Liu, H., M. Geng, X. Xin, F. Li, Z. Zhang, J. Li, and J. Ding. 2005. Multiple and multivalent interactions of novel anti-AIDS drug candidates, sulfated polymannuronate (SPMG)-derived oligosaccharides, with gp120 and their anti-HIV activities. *Glycobiology* 15:501–510.

Maeda, M., T. Uehara, N. Harada, M. Sekiguchi, and A. Hiraoka. 1991. Heparinoid-active sulfated polysaccharides from *Monostroma nitidum* and their distribution in the Cholorophyta. *Phytochemistry* 30:3611–3614.

Mao, W., H. Li, Y. Li, H. Zhang, X. Qi, H. Sun, Y. Chen, and S. Guo. 2009. Chemical characteristics and anticoagulant activity of the sulfated polysaccharide isolated from *Monostroma latissimum* (Chlorophyta). *International Journal of Biological Macromolecules* 44:70–74.

Mao, W., X. Zhang, Y. Li, and H. Zhang. 2006. Sulfated polysaccharides from marine green algae *Ulva conglobata* and their anticoagulant activity. *Journal of Applied Phycology* 18:9–14.

Maruyama, H., H. Tamauchi, M. Hashimoto, and T. Nakano. 2005. Suppression of Th2 immune responses by Mekabu fucoidan from *Undaria pinnatifida Sporophylls*. *International Archives of Allergy and Immunology* 137:289–294.

Matsubara, K., Y. Matsuura, A. Bacic, M. L. Liao, K. Hori, and K. Miyazawa. 2001. Anticoagulant properties of a sulfated galactan preparation from a marine green alga, *Codium cylindricum*. *International Journal of Biological Macromolecules* 28:395–399.

Matsubara, K., Y. Matsuura, K. Hori, and K. Miyazawa. 2000. An anticoagulant proteoglycan from the marine green alga, *Codium pugniformis*. *Journal of Applied Phycology* 12:9–14.

Meiyu, G., L. Fuchuan, X. Xianliang, L. Jing, Y. Zuowei, and G. Huashi. 2003. The potential molecular targets of marine sulfated polymannuroguluronate interfering with HIV-1 entry. Interaction between SPMG and HIV-1 rgp120 and CD4 molecule. *Antiviral Research* 59:127–135.

Miao, B., J. Li, X. Fu, L. Gan, X. Xin, and M. Geng. 2005. Sulfated polymannuroguluronate, a novel anti-AIDS drug candidate, inhibits T cell apoptosis by combating oxidative damage of mitochondria. *Molecular Pharmacology* 68:1716–1727.

Nardella, A., F. Chaubet, C. Boisson-Vidal, C. Blondin, P. Durand, and J. Jozefonvicz. 1996. Anticoagulant low molecular weight fucans produced by radical process and ion exchange chromatography of high molecular weight fucans extracted from the brown seaweed *Ascophyllum nodosum*. *Carbohydrate Research* 289:201–208.

Nishino, T., Y. Aizu, and T. Nagumo. 1991. The influence of sulfate content and molecular weight of a fucan sulfate from the brown seaweed *Ecklonia kurome* on its antithrombin activity. *Thrombosis Research* 64:723–731.

Oomizu, S., Y. Yanase, H. Suzuki, Y. Kameyoshi, and M. Hide. 2006. Fucoidan prevents Cε germline transcription and NF-κB p52 translocation for IgE production in B cells. *Biochemical and Biophysical Research Communications* 350:501–507.

Pereira, M. S., F. R. Melo, and P. A. S. Mourao. 2002. Is there a correlation between structure and anticoagulant action of sulfated galactans and sulfated fucans? *Glycobiology* 12:573–580.

Pushpamali, W. A., C. Nikapitiya, M. De Zoysa, I. Whang, S. J. Kim, and J. Lee. 2008. Isolation and purification of an anticoagulant from fermented red seaweed *Lomentaria catenata*. *Carbohydrate Polymers* 73:274–279.

Qi, H., Q. Zhang, T. Zhao, R. Chen, H. Zhang, X. Niu, and Z. Li. 2005. Antioxidant activity of different sulfate content derivatives of polysaccharide extracted from *Ulva pertusa* (Chlorophyta) in vitro. *International Journal of Biological Macromolecules* 37:195–199.

Queiroz, K. C. S., V. P. Medeiros, L. S. Queiroz, L. R. D. Abreu, H. A. O. Rocha, C. V. Ferreira, M. B. Juca, H. Aoyama, and E. L. Leite. 2008. Inhibition of reverse transcriptase activity of HIV by polysaccharides of brown algae. *Biomedicine and Pharmacotherapy* 62:303–307.

Rocha, H. A., C. R. Franco, E. S. Trindade, S. S. Veiga, E. L. Leite, H. B. Nader, and C. P. Dietrich. 2005. Fucan inhibits Chinese hamster ovary cell (CHO) adhesion to fibronectin by binding to the extracellular matrix. *Planta Medica* 71:628–633.

Rocha de Souza, M. C., C. T. Marques, C. M. G. Dore, F. R. Ferreira da Silva, H. A. O. Rocha, and E. L. Leite. 2007. Antioxidant activities of sulphated polysaccharides from brown and red seaweeds. *Journal of Applied Phycology* 19:153–160.

Ruperez, P., O. Ahrazem, and J. A. Leal. 2002. Potential antioxidant capacity of sulfated polysaccharides from the edible marine brown seaweed *Fucus vesiculosus*. *Journal of Agricultural and Food Chemistry* 50:840–845.

Sen, A. K. Sr., A. K. Das, N. Banerji, A. K. Siddhanta, K. H. Mody, B. K. Ramavat, V. D. Chauhan, J. R. Vedasiromoni, and D. K. Ganguly. 1994. A new sulfated polysaccharide with potent blood anti-coagulant activity from the red seaweed *Grateloupia indica*. *International Journal of Biological Macromolecules* 16:279–280.

Shanmugam, M. and K. H. Mody. 2000. Heparinoid-active sulfated polysaccharides from marine algae as potential blood anticoagulant agents. *Current Science* 79:1672–1683.

Silva, F. R. F., C. M. P. G. Dore, C. T. Marques, M. S. Nascimento, N. M. B. Benevides, H. A. O. Rocha, S. F. Chavante, and E. L. Leite. 2010. Anticoagulant activity, paw edema and pleurisy induced carrageenan: Action of major types of commercial carrageenans. *Carbohydrate Polymers* 79:26–33.

Sun, L., C. Wang, Q. Shi, and C. Ma. 2009. Preparation of different molecular weight polysaccharides from *Porphyridium cruentum* and their antioxidant activities. *International Journal of Biological Macromolecules* 45:42–47.

Synytsya, A., W. J. Kim, S. M. Kim, R. Pohl, A. Synytsya, F. Kvasnicka, J. Copikova, and Y. I. Park. 2010. Structure and antitumor activity of fucoidan isolated from sporophyll of Korean seaweed *Undaria pinnatifida*. *Carbohydrate Polymers* 81:41–48.

Teruya, T., T. Konishi, S. Uechi, H. Tamaki, and M. Tako. 2007. Anti-proliferative activity of oversulfated fucoidan from commercially cultured *Cladosiphon okamuranus* TOKIDA in U937 cells. *International Journal of Biological Macromolecules* 41:221–226.

Trinchero, J., N. M. A. Ponce, O. L. Cordoba, M. L. Flores, S. Pampuro, C. A. Stortz, H. Salomon, and G. Turk. 2009. Antiretroviral activity of fucoidans extracted from the brown seaweed *Adenocystis utricularis*. *Phytotherapy Research* 23:707–712.

Uno, T., M. Hattori, and T. Yoshida. 2006. Oral administration of alginic acid oligosaccharide suppresses IgE production and inhibits the induction of oral tolerance. *Bioscience, Biotechnology, and Biochemistry* 70:3054–3057.

Vo, T. S. and S. K. Kim. 2010. Potential anti-HIV agents from marine resources: An overview. *Marine Drugs* 8:2871–2892.

Wang, S. C., S. W. A. Bligh, S. S. Shi, Z. T. Wang, Z. B. Hu, J. Crowder, C. Branford-White, and C. Vella. 2007. Structural features and anti-HIV-1 activity of novel polysaccharides from red algae *Grateloupia longifolia* and *Grateloupia filicina*. *International Journal of Biological Macromolecules* 41:369–375.

Wang, J., L. Liu, Q. Zhang, Z. Zhang, H. Qi, and P. Li. 2009. Synthesized oversulphated, acetylated and benzoylated derivatives of fucoidan extracted from *Laminaria japonica* and their potential antioxidant activity *in vitro*. *Food Chemistry* 114:1285–1290.

Wang, J., Q. Zhang, Z. Zhang, and Z. Li. 2008. Antioxidant activity of sulphated polysaccharide fractions extracted from *Laminaria japonica*. *International Journal of Biological Macromolecules* 42:127–132.

Wang, J., Q. Zhang, Z. Zhang, H. Song, and P. Li. 2010. Potential antioxidant and anticoagulant capacity of low molecular weight fucoidan fractions extracted from *Laminaria japonica*. *International Journal of Biological Macromolecules* 46:6–12.

Witvrouw, M. and E. De Clercq. 1997. Sulfated polysaccharides extracted from sea algae as potential antiviral drugs. *General Pharmacology* 29:497–511.

Xue, C., G. Yu, T. Hirata, J. Terao, and H. Lin. 1998. Antioxidative activities of several marine polysaccharides evaluated in a phosphatidylcholine-liposomal suspension and organic solvents. *Bioscience, Biotechnology and Biochemistry* 62:206–209.

Yamamoto, I., H. Maruyama, M. Takahashi, and K. Komiyama. 1986. The effect of dietary or intraperitoneally injected seaweed preparations on the growth of sarcoma-180 cells subcutaneously implanted into mice. *Cancer Letters* 30:125–131.

Yanase, Y., T. Hiragun, K. Uchida, K. Ishii, S. Oomizu, H. Suzuki, S. Mihara et al. 2009. Peritoneal injection of fucoidan suppresses the increase of plasma IgE induced by OVA-sensitization. *Biochemical and Biophysical Research Communications* 387:435–439.

Yang, C., D. Chung, I. S. Shin, H. Y. Lee, J. C. Kim, Y. J. Lee, and S. G. You. 2008. Effects of molecular weight and hydrolysis conditions on anticancer activity of fucoidans from sporophyll of *Undaria pinnatifida*. *International Journal of Biological Macromolecules* 43:433–437.

Ye, H., K. Wang, C. Zhou, J. Liu, and X. Zeng. 2008. Purification, antitumor and antioxidant activities in vitro of polysaccharides from the brown seaweed *Sargassum pallidum*. *Food Chemistry* 111:428–432.

Yoshida, T., A. Hirano, H. Wada, K. Takahashi, and M. Hattori. 2004. Alginic acid oligosaccharide suppresses Th2 development and IgE production by inducing IL-12 production. *International Archives of Allergy and Immunology* 133:239–247.

Zhang, Q., N. Li, G. Zhou, X. Lu, Z. Xu, and Z. Li. 2003. In vivo antioxidant activity of polysaccharide fraction from *Porphyra haitanensis* (Rhodophyta) in aging mice. *Pharmacological Research* 48:151–155.

Zhang, Z., Q. Zhang, J. Wang, H. Song, H. Zhang, and X. Niu. 2010. Regioselective syntheses of sulfated porphyrans from *Porphyra haitanensis* and their antioxidant and anticoagulant activities *in vitro*. *Carbohydrate Polymers* 79:1124–1129.

Zhao, X., C. Xue, Y. Cai, D. Wang, and Y. Fang. 2005. Study of antioxidant activities of fucoidan from *Laminaria japonica*. *High Technology Letters* 11:91–94.

Zuniga, E. A., B. Matsuhiro, and E. Mejias. 2006. Preparation of a low-molecular weight fraction by free radical depolymerization of the sulfated galactan from *Schizymenia binderi* (Gigartinales, Rhodophyta) and its anticoagulant activity. *Carbohydrate Polymers* 66:208–215.

17

Biological Activities and Potential Applications of Marine Biotoxins

Alberto Otero, María José Chapela, Jorge Lago, Juan M. Vieites, and Ana G. Cabado

CONTENTS

17.1 Nonneurotoxic Toxins

17.1.1 Lipophilic Toxins

17.1.1.1 Okadaic Acid-Group Toxins and Pectenotoxin-Group Toxins

17.1.1.1.1 Occurrence of Okadaic Acid-Group and Pectenotoxin-Group Toxins

In general terms, the occurrence of phycotoxins has increased dramatically in the last decades. The causes behind this expansion are debated, with possible explanations ranging from natural mechanisms of species dispersal to a host of human-related phenomena such as pollution, climatic shifts, increased scientific awareness and analytical capabilities, increased use of coastal water for aquaculture, and transport of algal species via ship ballast water. In addition to these factors, long-term increases of nutrient loading of coastal waters and unusual climatological conditions are believed to favor certain species and stimulate blooms (WHOI, 2007).

Diarrhetic shellfish poisoning (DSP) toxins belong to three different structural classes, okadaic acid (OA)-group toxins, pectenotoxin (PTX)-group toxins, and yessotoxin (YTX)-group toxins. The EU excluded the YTX-group from the DSP group, and nowadays, the present regulation considers these toxins as a separate group (European Parliament, 2004).

OA-group toxins are heat-stable lipophilic polyether compounds that include OA and dinophysistoxins (DTXs). OA was first isolated from the marine sponge *Halichondria okadai* in 1981 (Tachibana et al., 1981). In 1982, the structure of OA and DTX1 was elucidated and reported for the first time (Murata et al., 1982). Ten years later, DTX2 was isolated from mussels (Hu et al., 1992a,b). Reports of the parent toxins were followed by numerous studies of esterified derivatives from shellfish and algae. The causative organisms were identified as dinoflagellates belonging to the planktonic *Dinophysis* genus, such as *Dinophysis acuminate, Dinophysis acuta, Dinophysis rotundata,* and *Dinophysis novergica,* and the benthic *Prorocentrum* genus, such as *Prorocentrum lima, Prorocentrum belizeanum, Prorocentrum concavum,* and *Prorocentrum maculosum* (Yasumoto et al., 1985). DSP toxins accumulate in several bivalves, including mussels, scallops, cockles, oysters, and clams, which filter seawater, and in some crustaceans. Although they were first reported in the Netherlands in the 1960s (Kat, 1983a,b), similar outbreaks occurred in Japan in 1978 (Yasumoto et al., 1978). Since then, they were reported worldwide, and although Japan and Europe are the most affected areas, they also occur in North and South America, Australia, Indonesia, and New Zealand.

PTX-group toxins have been grouped together with DSP group because they always appear in shellfish contaminated with OA and derivatives; however, there is a great debate whether these toxins should be classified as DSP toxins or not because some research groups did not find evidence of its diarrheic effects (Burgess and Shaw, 2001).

PTXs are polyether macrolide toxins and include over 15 analogues. PTX1 and PTX2 were originally isolated from Japanese scallops, *Patinopecten yessoensis* (Yasumoto et al., 1985). In the same study, three other analogues were obtained (PTX3–5). Also, PTX6 and PTX7 were later isolated from Japanese scallops. *Dinophysis fortii* was initially identified as the real producer of these toxins. More recently PTX11 (Suzuki et al., 2003; Vale, 2004), PTX12 (Briggs et al., 2004; Miles et al., 2004), PTX13, and PTX14 (Miles et al., 2006) were found in *Dinophysis* spp., and PTX6 and PTX-2 seco acid (PTX2SA) were found in shellfish tissues (Suzuki et al., 1998, 2001a,b). To date many analogues of PTXs have been discovered, but only four (PTX2, PTX12, PTX11, and PTX13) have been identified as actual biosynthetic products of the algae. Other PTXs seem to be either product of the shellfish metabolism or artifacts (Blanco et al., 2007).

17.1.1.1.2 Okadaic Acid-Group and Pectenotoxin-Group Toxin Isolation

Reliable supplies of microalgal toxins are required for the development of assay methods, as standards for toxin analysis, and for biochemical and toxicological studies. The main methods used have been the isolation of toxins from microalgal cultures or from contaminated shellfish. DSP toxins and lipophilic toxins including PTXs are usually isolated from bivalves or algae harvested from natural blooms by acetone extraction, although aqueous methanol is sometimes used. Individual toxins are then isolated through a complex fractionation and purification procedure of raw extracts on the basis of a combination of chromatographic techniques.

These approaches require availability of suitable contaminated material, or cultures and facilities for growing microalgae on a large scale. Isolation of toxins from natural blooms of marine microalgae is possible but so far has been limited. However, a high proportion of toxins can be present in the water after filtration. This possibility has been evaluated by different research groups, but it needs to be improved to be used efficiently (Rundberget et al., 2007).

Several standards and reference materials of some of these toxin groups are available in the following:

- National Research Council (NRC Canada) offers OA, DTX1, DTX2, and PTX2.
- CIFGA (Lugo, Spain) offers OA, DTX1, DTX2, and PTX2.
- Wako Pure Chemical Industries, Ltd. (Osaka, Japan) offers OA and DTX1.
- Sigma-Aldrich Co. LLC. (St. Louis, MO) offers OA.
- World Ocean Solutions (Wilmington, NC) offers OA.

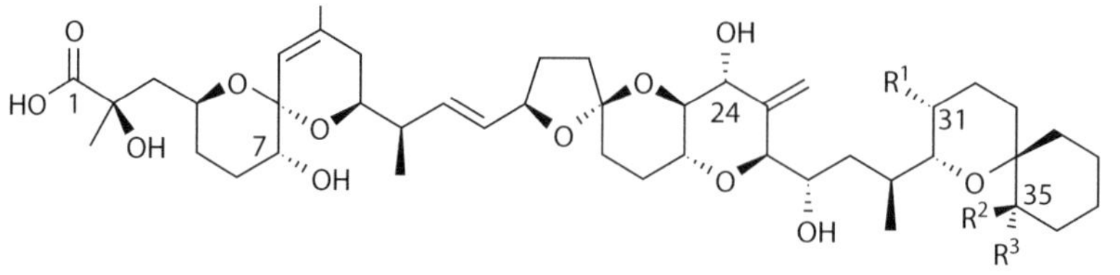

	R^1	R^2	R^3
1. Okadaic acid	CH_3	H	H
2. DTX-1	CH_3	CH_3	H
3. DTX-2	H	H	CH_3

FIGURE 17.1

Chemical structure of OA and DTX. (From Botana, L.M., *Seafood and Freshwater Toxins. Pharmacology, Physiology and Detection*, CRC Press/Taylor & Francis, Boca Raton, FL, 2008.)

17.1.1.1.3 Okadaic Acid-Group and Pectenotoxin-Group Toxin Chemical Characterization

OA and DTXs are polyketide compounds containing furan- and pyran-type ether rings and an alpha-hydrocarboxyl function, the difference between them being the number or position of the methyl groups (Dominguez et al., 2010) (Figure 17.1). Any of the parent OA analogues can be esterified at the 7-hydroxy position with a range of saturated and unsaturated fatty acids to form corresponding "acylated" derivatives known collectively as "DTX3" (EFSA, 2008b).

PTXs resemble OA in molecular weight and in having cyclic ethers and a carboxyl group in the molecule. Unlike OA, the carboxyl moiety in many PTXs is in the form of macrocyclic lactone (macrolide) (Suzuki, 2008).

17.1.1.1.4 Biological Activities and Potential Applications

OA was first identified as a potent inhibitor of Ser/Thr protein phosphatases about 35 years ago. These groups of enzymes perform the dephosphorylation of numerous proteins; this function is closely related to many essential metabolic processes in eukaryotic cells. To date, a myriad of studies have exploited the interaction of DSP toxins with phosphatases to examine the role of these proteins in cytoskeletal integrity. Nevertheless, very few of these reports have focused on the detailed study of the intracellular pathways involved in the reorganization of cytoskeletal components caused by DSP toxins. Recently, it was suggested that, in addition to protein phosphatases, other cellular targets could exist for OA (Leira et al., 2002; Cabado et al., 2004; Santaclara et al., 2005; Vale and Botana, 2008).

In addition, OA acts as a direct cytotoxic and genotoxic agent for human cells, but it is considered that its effect varies depending on the type of cell and the concentration employed (Valdiglesias et al., 2010). The toxin is known to act as a potent neurotoxin for cultured neurons, to induce apoptotic events in various cell lines, and to exert tumor-promoting activity in various organs. It induces DNA damages in the form of both strand breaks and oxidative damage; however, the mechanisms leading to the DNA damage are highly dependent on the cell type. This may be related to the antioxidant status of each cell type and capability of metabolizing OA among other reasons (Cabado et al., 2003; Lago et al., 2005; Franchini et al., 2010; Valdiglesias et al., 2011a–c).

The extent of the OA-induced injuries and the toxin organotrophicity are dose related and may be determined by the administration route. After intravenous administration, OA acts as a hepatotoxin with undetectable effects on the intestine but also has an impact on cytoskeletal elements at sublethal doses (Franchini et al., 2010).

Concerning PTXs, it is generally accepted that they are hepatotoxic compounds, but the mechanism of action has not been completely elucidated yet. Cytotoxicity in different human cancer cell lines (Lamas et al., 2006a,b) and induction of apoptosis in rat and salmon hepatocytes and also in p53-deficient cell lines are effects attributed to some PTXs (Espiña and Rubiolo, 2008).

In spite of the existence of early reports on PTX2 diarrheic toxicity, there have been more recent studies with pure PTXs that demonstrate that this group of toxins does not induce diarrhea or any other pathological signs by oral administration at doses considerably higher. The body distribution of PTX2 and 2SA was analyzed in mice after p.o. and i.p. administration. In vitro cytotoxicity assays have been the first step for the discovery of many drugs used in antitumor therapy (Vilarino and Espina, 2008). More information is needed about their toxicity to humans and their pharmacokinetics in order to make a better judgment about their usefulness in the management of human diseases.

17.1.1.2 Yessotoxins-Group Toxins

17.1.1.2.1 Origin and Occurrence of Yessotoxins

YTXs are polyether compounds produced by phytoplanktonic dinoflagellates *Protoceratium reticulatum* (=*Gonyaulax grinley*) and *Lingulodinium polyedrum* (=*Gonyaulax polyedra*), and *Gonyaulax spinifera* (Tubaro et al., 2010). Since its first isolation in Japan from the scallop *Patinopecten yessoensis* (Murata et al., 1987), YTXs have been described worldwide, in Asia (Korea) (Lee et al., 2011), America (Chile) (Alvarez et al., 2011), and Oceania (New Zealand) (Yasumoto and Takizawa, 1997). In Europe, it has been described in Norway, Adriatic Sea, and Spain (EFSA, 2008a; Custovic et al., 2009; de la Iglesia and Gago-Martinez, 2009).

17.1.1.2.2 Yessotoxins Isolation

Isolation from contaminated mollusks can be performed following the mouse bioassay methodology (EURLMB, 2009), which is based on an acetone extraction in a proportion 5:1 acetone:mollusk. After acetone evaporation, a liquid–liquid partitioning of the remaining extract is performed in a separatory funnel with a mixture 30:60 of dichloromethane:methanol 60% in water. Dichloromethane phase should be extracted twice with methanol 60% in water. YTXs will remain in the three aqueous methanol phase. Nevertheless, it has been stated that the less hydrophilic compounds, such as the desulfo derivatives, will be lost in the dichloromethane fraction (Ciminiello and Fattorusso, 2008).

Several separation methods have been proposed; usually, acetone extraction is the first step due to the lipophilic nature of YTXs and the ease of evaporating this solvent, but alternative extraction methods starting with 80% methanol or by mixing acetone extraction followed by methanol extraction have also been reported. Acetone extraction is then followed by partitioning with different solvents such as dichloromethane or hexane, in different proportions. These extracts can be further cleaned by means of filters, silica or alumina columns, or solid-phase extraction cartridges (Quilliam, 2003; Alfonso et al., 2007; Gerssen et al., 2009).

A second strategy for YTX purification is from microalgal culture (Loader et al., 2007). In this case, algal cultures were filtered and pumped through a column packed with resin. The resin was rinsed with water and drained dry, and then toxins were extracted with acetone, which was evaporated. The remaining aqueous solution was dried and then eluted in an alumina column with dichloromethane:methanol 1:1, methanol, and ammonium hydroxide 1%:methanol 1:1. The methanolic ammonia fraction was dried by rotary evaporation, suspended in water, washed with ethyl acetate, and extracted with butanol. Finally, the butanolic fraction was dried with anhydrous sodium sulfate, filtered, and evaporated in vacuo. The residue was subjected to further purification steps in flash column chromatography. Similar protocols with changes (solvents, type of columns among others) have been used by other authors (Miles et al., 2004, 2005).

A third strategy could be upscaling analytical chromatography to semipreparative or preparative chromatography. To our knowledge, none of the broad range of HPLC-based analytical methods for YTXs (Ciminiello and Fattorusso, 2008) have been upscaled, although preparative chromatography has been employed as last step after column chromatography (Miles et al., 2004, 2005).

Several standards and reference materials of some of these toxin groups are available in the following:

- National Research Council (NRC Canada) offers YTX.
- CIFGA (Lugo, Spain) offers YTX and homoYTX.

17.1.1.2.3 Chemical Characterization

YTXs are polyether compounds, consisting of 11 contiguously transfused ether rings, an unsaturated side chain, and two sulfate esters (EFSA, 2008a). YTX planar structure was determined in 1987 by NMR techniques (Murata et al., 1987), and later on the absolute configuration was reported (Satake et al., 1996; Takahashi et al., 1996). The parent compound, YTX, is shown in Figure 17.2. More than 90 YTX analogues have been described, but structures for most of them have not been determined and only 30 have been isolated (Miles et al., 2005; Paz et al., 2008). The group seems to be heat stable, since concentration procedures that use heat do not show a decrease in the amount (Alfonso et al., 2007).

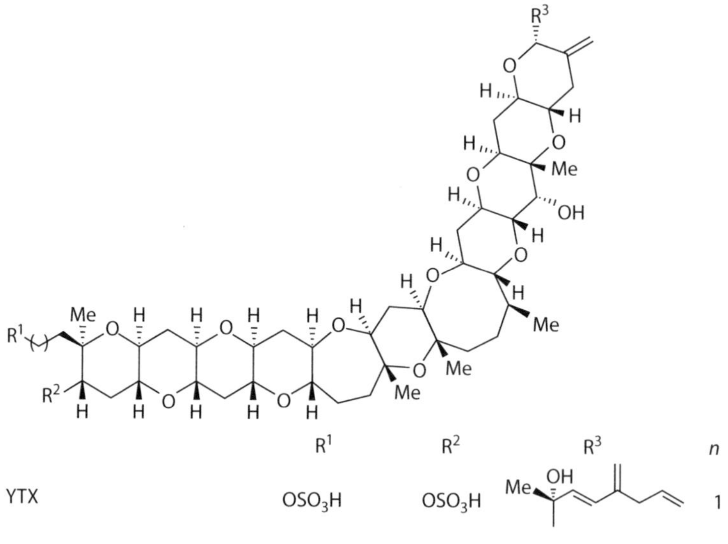

FIGURE 17.2
Structure of YTX, from Ciminello et al. (From Botana, L.M., *Seafood and Freshwater Toxins. Pharmacology, Physiology and Detection,* CRC Press/Taylor & Francis, Boca Raton, FL, 2008.)

17.1.1.2.4 Biological Activities and Potential Applications

The existence of this toxin group was discovered due to their high acute toxicity during mouse bioassay (intraperitoneal injection) for lipophilic toxin analysis of mollusks (Yasumoto et al., 1984; EURLMB, 2009). Symptomatology after injection includes dyspnea and, at high doses, nervous symptoms like cramps and jumping. Reported LD_{50} varies among authors, ranging from 80–100 to 750 µg/kg for YTX and 444 µg/kg for homoYTX, whereas di-desulfo-YTX was lethal at 301 µg/kg and 45-hydroxy-homoYTX was shown to be less toxic than YTX as it did not induce mice lethality or symptoms of toxicity at 750 mg/kg (Tubaro et al., 2010). With the discrepancies in LD_{50} of YTX, it is not easy to establish toxicity equivalence factor (TEF) of analogues; however, according to toxicological available data, the following TEFs have been proposed by EFSA Contaminants Panel: YTX = 1, 1a-homoYTX = 1, 45-hydroxyYTX = 1, and 45-hydroxy-1a homoYTX = 0.5 (EFSA, 2008a).

Oral administration has reported lower toxicity in mice. In fact, no lethality and no clinical symptoms were observed at doses up to 10 mg/kg body weight (b.w.) administered by gavage in single doses or repeated doses up to 5 m/kg b.w. given seven times. Regarding toxicity in humans, no reports about human intoxications caused by YTXs have been published so far. Indeed, no data regarding chronic exposure, carcinogenicity, or genotoxicity are available (EFSA, 2008a).

The target organ of YTXs seems to be the heart, since after i.p. injection, mice showed vacuolation in the cardiac muscle and intracellular edema, as examined by light microscopy (Aune et al., 2002). No pathological changes were seen in lung, thymus, liver, pancreas, kidney, adrenal gland, jejunum, colon, and spleen. Ultrastructural changes in cardiac muscle included swelling myocardial muscle cells in the wall of the left ventricle and separation of myofibrils and mitochondria, the latter organelles being rounded in appearance. These changes were more pronounced in the vicinity of capillaries. Other authors (Terao et al., 1990) have reported more severe microscopic alterations in cardiac muscle. The differences among these studies are not clear and it has been proposed to be due to differences in toxin purity and mice strains (EFSA, 2008a).

YTX increases cytosolic Ca^{2+} levels through Ca^{2+} influx channels in human lymphocytes and on rat cerebellar neurons. On the other hand, YTX shows an inhibitory effect on calcium entry induced by the calcium ATPase inhibitor thapsigargin or by incubation in a calcium-free medium (De la Rosa et al., 2001a,b; Perez-Gomez et al., 2006). Nevertheless, it has been proposed that YTX effect on cellular calcium homeostasis is quite modest and that it is not related to its cytotoxic effect (Tubaro et al., 2010).

YTXs did not induce any direct effect on sodium channels (Inoue et al., 2003).

On the other hand, YTX triggers a dose-dependent decrease of cAMP and cGMP levels after incubation. These effects are Ca^{2+} dependent and can be modified by specific phosphodiesterase (Alfonso and Alfonso, 2008). This decrease has been proposed to be due to an activation in the activity of phosphodiesterases, which hydrolyze these compounds (Alfonso et al., 2003).

Several cytotoxic effects of YTXs have been reported after in vitro experiments in different cellular models. Among them, YTX induces cell detachment from culture dishes (Ogino et al., 1997). It induced decreases in F-actin filaments in several cell models like cerebellar granule cells (CGCs), mouse fibroblast NIH3T3, rat L3, mouse BC3H1 myoblast cell lines, and MCF-7 human breast adenocarcinoma cells (Perez-Gomez et al., 2006; Tubaro et al., 2010). However, this seems not to be a universal effect, since no effects over F-actin levels were detected in M17 neuroblastoma cell line, in rabbit enterocytes, or in human Caco-2 cells (Leira et al., 2003; Ares et al., 2005). The cell adhesion protein E-cadherin degradation pathway is also affected by YTX at long incubation times and low concentrations. Since E-cadherin has been linked to tumor spreading and metastasis, it has been a concern if the disruption of E-cadherin by YTX could affect tumor expansion in YTX-contaminated mollusk consumers. Nevertheless, *in vivo* experiments demonstrated that although the resulting molecule of E-cadherin disruption had increased, YTXs did not induce any effect on E-cadherin system in *in vivo* experiments (Callegari et al., 2006).

YTX induced apoptotic events in different cellular lines, including cancer cells, primary cell cultures, and cell lines. There are reports related to YTX-induced apoptosis in rat hepatocytes, rat glioma cells, HeLa S$_3$ cells, BE(2) neuroblastoma cell line, rat cerebellar neurons, L6 myoblast cell line, BC3H1 myoblast cell line, mouse fibroblast NIH3T3 cell line, CaCo-2 cells, MCF-7 cancer cells, and HepG2 cell cultures reviewed in (Korsnes and Espenes, 2011), where the possibility of the use of YTX in therapeutic applications, for instance, as an antitumor drug, is discussed. In this line, the European patent application EP1875906 (Botana et al., 2008) considers to use YTX as an antitumor drug, and protoceratin I, the major compound with cytotoxic activity against human tumor cell lines isolated from *Protoceratium cf. reticulatum*, was proved to be identical to homoYTX (Ciminiello and Fattorusso, 2008).

17.1.1.3 Azaspiracid-Group Toxins

17.1.1.3.1 Origin and Occurrence of Azaspiracid throughout the World

Azaspiracids (AZAs) are a group of polyether marine biotoxins originated by several phytoplankton species that can accumulate in tissues of various phytoplankton-feeding shellfish species causing severe gastrointestinal human intoxications. The first documented episode of intoxication with AZA occurred in 1995 in the Netherlands and was associated with the ingestion of mussels originating from Killary Harbour, Ireland. Four additional events of intoxication with AZA-contaminated shellfish have been documented, all of them related to the intake of Irish mussels.

Since initial events focused on Irish waters, AZAs have been detected in shellfish, crustaceans, and other species from other localizations in European Atlantic coasts (Norway, England, Spain, France, Denmark, Portugal, and Sweden), North American Atlantic coasts (Canada), African Atlantic coasts (Morocco) (Twiner et al., 2008), Japan (Ueoka et al., 2009), and Chile (Alvarez et al., 2009; López-Rivera et al., 2009).

The identification of the AZA-producing organism has been a difficult task. James et al. detected the presence of AZAs 1, 2, and 3 in extracts from the heterotrophic dinoflagellate *Protoperidinium crassipes* (James et al., 2003). However, the heterotrophic nature of the species, together with the fact that the attempts to confirm its AZA production in laboratory cultures manipulating environmental variables were not successful, suggested that the real potential role of this organism is to act as a vector when feeding on the actual producer species rather than being a progenitor of these toxins. Finally, a small photosynthetic dinoflagellate designed as *Azadinium spinosum* was found to produce AZA1 and AZA2 and an AZA 2 isomer when cultured in pure culture, and it was also present in field samples rich in AZAs (Krock et al., 2009b; Tillmann et al., 2009). The role of this species in AZA contamination has been recently confirmed in experiments where 24 h feeding trial of blue mussels (*Mytilus edulis*) were performed using an algal suspension of *Az. spinosum* culture. It was demonstrated that *Az. spinosum* were filtered, consumed, and digested directly by mussels, and analysis showed that AZAs were accumulated in the shellfish hepatopancreas (Salas et al., 2011).

17.1.1.3.2 AZA Toxin Isolation

Complexity of the cellular effects and toxicology of AZA makes availability of pure AZA toxins or reference materials an important factor in their study. In addition, the recent change in EU legislation that improves the LC-MS/MS as reference method for the determination of AZA has increased the requirements of AZA reference materials for validation proposes.

Extraction and purification of AZA from contaminated mussel tissues can be summarized in three steps (Twiner et al., 2008):

1. Extraction with acetone or ethanol
2. Liquid–liquid partitions, first with ethyl acetate followed by a hexane partition step
3. Chromatographic separation steps including vacuum liquid chromatography in silica, size-exclusion chromatography, and reverse-phase chromatography on C8 or C18 columns

Following the schema above, Perez et al. (2010) described precisely the process of preparation of certified calibration solutions for AZAs 1, 2, and 3 from contaminated mussels. They achieved important amounts of calibration solutions of the three toxins in a concentration level suitable for its use in calibration of LC-MS/MS instrumentation, and the developed purification procedure yielded sufficient AZA recoveries for effective isolation.

Alfonso et al. (2008) described a complete procedure, slightly different of that described earlier, to obtain AZA analogues from mussels contaminated with DSP toxins and AZAs by means of three consecutive steps: an extraction procedure to remove toxins from shellfish, an solid phase extract (SPE) to clean the samples and separate DSP toxins and AZAs, and a preparative HPLC to isolate each analogue. They obtained large amounts of AZA1, AZA2, AZA3, AZA4, and AZA5 suitable for AZA toxicity studies or certified materials and standard production purposes. In all steps, LC-MS/MS was used to detect and quantify the toxins.

Several standards and reference materials of some of these toxin groups are available in the following:

- National Research Council (NRC Canada) offers AZA1, AZA 2, and AZA3.
- CIFGA (Lugo, Spain) offers AZA1, AZA 2, AZA 3, AZA 4, and AZA5.

17.1.1.3.3 Chemical Characterization

AZAs are nitrogen-containing polyether toxins comprising a unique spiral ring assembly containing a heterocyclic amine (piperidine) and an aliphatic carboxylic acid moiety (EFSA, 2008b).

Up to 28 different naturally occurring analogues of AZA1 have been identified as well as 4 methyl ester analogues that are artifacts of storage in methanolic solution (Rehmann et al., 2008). Only AZAs 1–3 (Figure 17.3) have been detected in water column or phytoplankton, suggesting that the other analogues isolated from shellfish are product of biotransformations once the former three analogues have been ingested by bivalves.

17.1.1.3.4 Biological Activities and Potential Applications

Although symptoms observed during episodes of AZA intoxication were similar to those typically observed in DSP intoxication, the administration to mice of AZA toxic materials

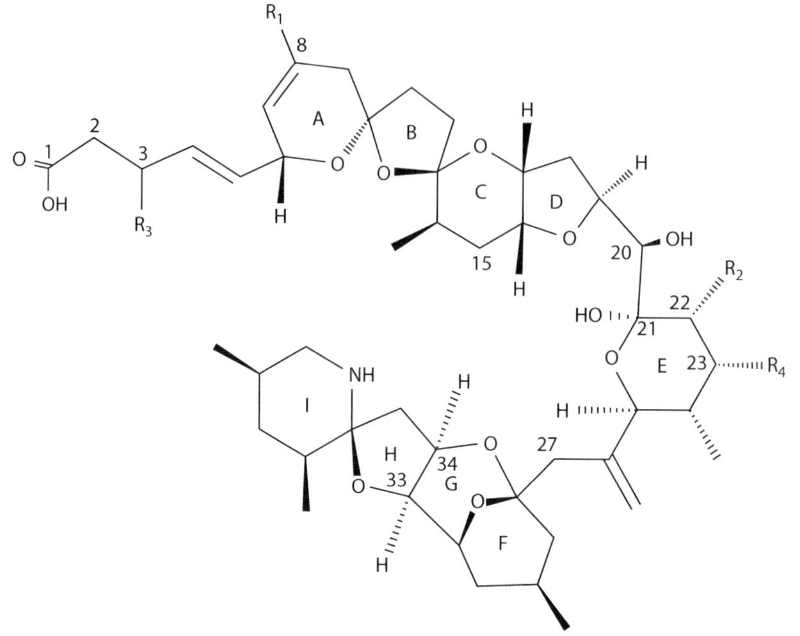

FIGURE 17.3
Molecular structure of azaspiracids. (From Botana, L.M., *Seafood and Freshwater Toxins. Pharmacology, Physiology and Detection,* CRC Press/Taylor & Francis, Boca Raton, FL, 2008.)

resulted in great differences from the symptomatology caused by DSP toxins. Mice injected with low doses of AZA did not suffer diarrhea (Ito et al., 2002), and in a few hours they develop slowly progressive paralysis, difficulties in breathing, and finally death (Satake et al., 1998). A 200 µg/kg dose seems to be the minimum lethal intraperitoneal dose in mice for AZA1, while AZA2 and AZA3 showed a higher toxicity (110 and 140 µg/kg, respectively) (Satake et al., 1998; Ofuji et al., 1999). Autopsy and histopathological analysis revealed damages in liver, pancreas, spleen, thymus, and stomach. After administration of sublethal doses of AZA by gavage, mice showed damage in small intestine, affecting epithelial cell in the fingerlike villi. The grade of tissue damage was progressively increasing from 4 to 24 h after administration (Ito et al., 1998, 2000).

In contrast to OA (main toxin of DSP toxin group), no inhibition effect of AZA has been found on protein phosphatase activity (PP1 and PP2A) (Flanagan et al., 1999, 2001).

The complexity of AZA *in vitro* effects, which seem to vary among different cell types together with the high diversity of proteins involved in cell volume regulation, makes it difficult to highlight only one specific target for AZA. AZA can cause cytotoxicity to a variety of cell types from various mammalian sources. Cytotoxicity was first observed by Flanagan et al. (2001) in hepatoblastoma cells and bladder carcinoma cells exposed to crude-contaminated mussel extract. Twiner et al. observed that AZA1 caused cytotoxicity to kidney, lung, and neuronal-, pituitary-, and immune-type cell cultures in a concentration- and time-dependent manner (Twiner et al., 2005). Curiously, the unique cell line that has not been observed to suffer AZA cytotoxicity is human colon adenocarcinoma (Caco-2) (Ronzitti et al., 2007; Vilariño et al., 2007). However, neurons seem to be especially sensible to AZAs, causing irreversible morphological changes with relatively short times of exposure and cytotoxicity with longer expositions to AZAs (Román et al., 2002;

Vilariño et al., 2006). Long exposure times were also required to achieve complete cyto-toxicity in primary cultures of CGCs (Vale et al., 2008). It is demonstrated that cytotoxicity effects of AZA include alterations in the cytoskeleton, but the difference in the concentration required to decrease F-actin content and that needed to decrease cell viability is high (>1000-fold), suggesting that F-actin is not a target for AZA (Furey et al., 2010). AZAs have also been observed to cause apoptotic activation, and this seems to be related to the activation of caspase activity (Vilariño et al., 2007; Cao et al., 2010).

AZAs appear to affect several membrane proteins involved in cell adhesion and tight junction, like claudins and cadherins. Caco-2 cells exposed to AZA1 demonstrated variations in fractions of claudin protein expression and upregulation of a fragment of E-cadherin (Hess et al., 2007; Ronzitti et al., 2007; Bellocci et al., 2010). AZAs also cause upregulation on gene expression and protein levels of low-density lipoprotein receptor, effect that seems to be a response to the decreased level in intracellular cholesterol caused by AZA1 (Twiner et al., 2008).

Cytosolic calcium is an important secondary messenger in several mammalian cell pathways. AZA1 was observed to cause increment in cytosolic calcium in human lymphocytes (Román et al., 2002). Similarly, AZA2 and AZA3 elevated both cytosolic calcium and cAMP (Román et al., 2004), whereas AZA4 and AZA5 did not affect calcium levels (Alfonso et al., 2005, 2006).

The effects of AZA on protein regulation in neuroblastoma cells were studied by Kellmann et al. They observed that the most highly upregulated proteins were involved in cellular energy metabolism, followed by cytoskeleton-regulating proteins. The majority of downregulated proteins were involved in transcription, translation, and protein modification. Another two proteins involved in the maintenance of the Golgi complex and vesicle transport were also downregulated (Kellmann et al., 2009).

17.2 Neurotoxic Toxins

17.2.1 Saxitoxin and Analogues (PSP)

17.2.1.1 Origin and Occurrence of Saxitoxin-Group Toxins throughout the World

Saxitoxin (STX)-group toxins include several naturally occurring neurotoxic alkaloids that induce the so-called paralytic shellfish poisoning (PSP) in humans. They are produced by a complex and unique biosynthetic pathway, identical for distantly related organisms, such as dinoflagellates and cyanobacteria (Kellmann et al., 2008). It was also reported that they can be produced by a bacterium, *Moraxella* sp., isolated from *Protogonyaulax tamarensis* (Kodama et al., 1990). Toxic dinoflagellates that belong to the genus *Alexandrium* (formerly *Gonyaulax*) are the main species responsible for PSP and for the worldwide outbreaks that impact human health. These toxic episodes induce poisonings and sometimes deaths as well as tremendous economical losses to the fishery products industry. Toxic microalgae synthesize a wide range of toxins that can be accumulated by shellfish along the food chain. Within the genus *Alexandrium*, great differences in toxin profiles (the presence and quantity of individual toxins) and allelochemical properties are well documented for the species *Alexandrium minutum* and *Alexandrium tamarense*. The "*Alexandrium tamarense/catenella/fundyense* species complex" (the "tamarensis complex") is defined by morphological attributes that reflect geographic distribution and the toxicity of populations

(Aguilera-Belmonte et al., 2011). In addition, the species *Alexandrium minutum, Alexandrium lusitanicum,* and *Alexandrium angustitabulatum* constitute the "minutum" species complex, although recently it was reported no distinction between *A. lusitanicum* and *A. minutum* (McCauley et al., 2009). Another toxic dinoflagellate, *Gymnodinium catenatum,* is one of the most widespread species that produces PSP toxins, and *Pyrodinium bahamense* also contributes to most PSP toxic episodes. Several reports of STX production by freshwater and brackish cyanobacteria, as well as calcareous red macroalgae, have also been published (Etheridge, 2010).

Phycotoxins show a nonhomogeneous distribution in terms of time and geographical location, and these data are confirmed for STX-group toxins. Several decades ago, relatively few countries appeared to be affected by PSP (Figure 17.4); however, in 2006, large geographic areas were threatened, many fishery resources were impacted, and higher economic losses occurred (WHOI, 2007; McCauley et al., 2009).

In addition to the places reported in this figure, the occurrence of these toxins has increased dramatically the last years. Recently, the first identification of PSP toxins in shellfish harvested from Icelandic waters was published (Burrel et al., 2011). Also, Ngy et al. have reported the first occurrence of STX, both in the indigenous puffer fish and in Cambodian marine waters (Ngy et al., 2008). Moreover, two species of *Alexandrium, Alexandrium catenella* and *Alexandrium tamarense,* were recently identified in the North Lake of Tunis (Armi et al., 2011).

The occurrence of high levels of STX-group toxins in mollusks usually is limited in time, even in the geographical areas that are affected by these toxins. Very high values were found in mussels and clams, but considering the p95, the highest levels were recorded for cockles and gastropods. Overall, the occurrence of these toxins appears to similarly affect all considered species, with somewhat higher presence in cockles. No final conclusions of crabs and gastropods contamination were drawn due to the low number of samples (EFSA, 2009).

17.2.1.2 STX-Group Toxin Isolation

Toxins can be isolated from the digestive gland of contaminated shellfish and quantified by NMR (Watanabe et al., 2010). Certified calibration solutions for PSP toxins are available from the Institute for Marine Biosciences (NRC-CNRC, 2011). Then, STX and derivatives are isolated, from large-scale laboratory culture of dinoflagellates, mainly from *A. tamarense* strains. The principal toxin in this source material is N-sulfocarbamoyl-gonyautoxin-3 that is extracted, purified, and then chemically converted to STX. Eventually, the final product is purified by preparative-scale chromatography. In other cases, where the principal toxins are C1 and C2, these are epimerized to an equilibrated ratio and then extracted and purified. Also, C2 can be extracted, purified, and chemically converted to dcSTX (Hall et al., 1990; Oshima, 1995).

To obtain GTX1, GTX4, and neoSTX, a large-scale laboratory culture of an *A. minutum* strain is normally used. GTX1, GTX4, and neoSTX are extracted and purified by preparative-scale chromatography. In contrast, to isolate dc-neoSTX, the alga *A. tamarense* is used to obtain neoSTX that is chemically converted to dc-neo STX and purified by preparative-scale chromatography (Laycock et al., 1994; Oshima, 1995).

Purity of these toxins is checked by several techniques including NMR spectroscopy, liquid chromatography with fluorescence detection (LC-FLD), capillary electrophoresis with UV detection (CE-UVD), and liquid chromatography with chemiluminescence nitrogen detection (LC-CLND) (Aversano et al., 2005).

• **PSP**

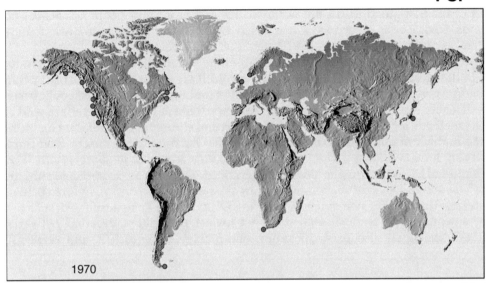

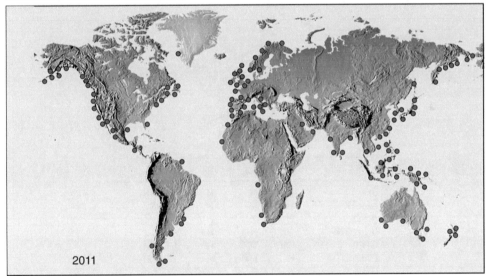

FIGURE 17.4
Global distribution of PSP toxins recorded in 1970 and comparison with 2011. (From WHOI, Harmful algae, Woods Hole Oceanographic Institution, http://www.whoi.edu/redtide/regions/world-distribution, accessed January 31, 2012, 2007.)

Several standards and reference materials of some of these toxin groups are available in the following:

- National Research Council (NRC Canada) offers C1-2, dcGTX2-3, dcNEO, dcSTX, GTX1–4, GTX2–3, GTX5, neoSTX, and STX.
- CIFGA (Lugo, Spain) offers C1-2, GTX1–4, and GTX2–3.
- Sigma-Aldrich Co. LLC. (St. Louis, MO) offers STX.

17.2.1.3 Chemical Characterization

Most of the STX-group toxins are water-soluble and heat-stable nonproteinaceous compounds whose basic structure is composed of a 3,4-propinoperhydropurine tricyclic system, as can be seen in Figure 17.5 (Wang, 2008; EFSA, 2009).

STX belongs to the large family of guanidinium-containing marine natural products, due to the presence of two guanidine groups, which are responsible for its high polarity. Structural diversity of STX-group toxins as well as the biosynthetic and metabolic basis for this diversity was recently characterized. An improvement in screening efforts and analytical methods for detection as well as the structural elucidation has referred an increase in the number of new PSP toxins reported in the literature. Each moiety then imparts a varying level of toxicity (Wiese et al., 2010). To date and since its discovery in 1957, 57 analogues of STX-group toxins have been described. They can be divided into subgroups based on substituent side chains such as carbamate, sulfate, hydroxyl, hydroxybenzoate, or acetate. They may be non-sulfated, such as STX and neoSTX; monosulfated, such as the gonyautoxins (GTX1–6); or disulfated (C1–C4 toxins). In addition, decarbamoyl variants of these analogues also exist, including decarbamoyl-STXs (dcSTX and dc-neoSTX),

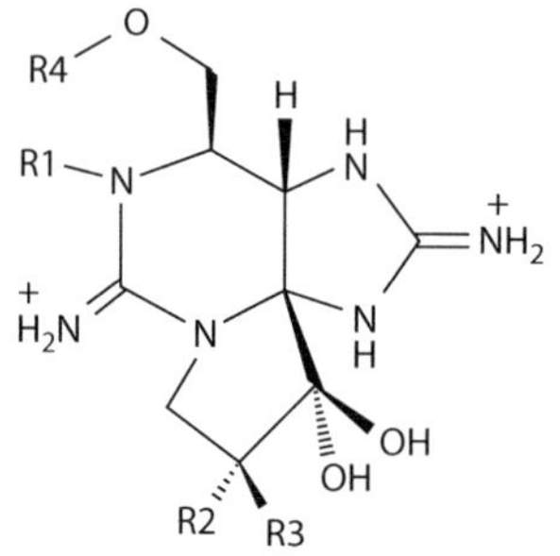

	R1	R2	R3	R4
STX	H	H	H	$CONH_2$
neoSTX	OH	H	H	$CONH_2$
dcSTX	H	H	H	H
dcneoSTX	OH	H	H	H
GTX1	OH	OSO_3^-	H	$CONH_2$
GTX2	H	OSO_3^-	H	$CONH_2$
GTX3	H	H	OSO_3^-	$CONH_2$
GTX4	OH	H	OSO_3^-	$CONH_2$
GTX5 B1	H	H	H	$CONHSO_3^-$
GTX6 B2	OH	H	H	$CONHSO_3^-$
dcGTX1	OH	OSO_3^-	H	H
dcGTX2	H	OSO_3^-	H	H
dcGTX3	H	H	OSO_3^-	H
dcGTX4	OH	H	OSO_3^-	H
C1	H	OSO_3^-	H	$CONHSO_3^-$
C2	H	H	OSO_3^-	$CONHSO_3^-$
C3	OH	OSO_3^-	H	$CONHSO_3^-$
C4	OH	H	OSO_3^-	$CONHSO_3^-$

FIGURE 17.5
Structures of STXs and its derivatives. (From Botana, L.M., *Seafood and Freshwater Toxins. Pharmacology, Physiology and Detection*, CRC Press/Taylor & Francis, Boca Raton, FL, 2008.)

decarbamoyl-GTX1-4, and 13-deoxy-decarbamoyl derivatives (do-STX, do-GTX2,3). Three structural families of STX are classified by the identity of the R4 side chain as either N-sulfocarbamoyl, decarbamoyl, or carbamoyl, each with increasing toxicity in mammalian bioassays (Wiese et al., 2010). Although STX analogues are recognized as hydrophilic compounds, a new subclass of STX-group toxins that contain a hydroxybenzoate moiety in place of the carbamoyl group (GC toxins: GC1–GC3) was discovered. GC toxins dominate the toxin profiles of many *Gymnodinium catenatum* strains and can contribute significantly to sample toxicity, yet these toxins may easily escape detection using conventional chromatography, resulting in significant underestimates of sample toxicity (Negri et al., 2007).

17.2.1.4 Toxicokinetics and Toxicity

STX-group toxins are very potent neurotoxins in humans, quickly absorbed and transported in the blood to other organs, including the brain. Paresthesia and numbness around the lips, tongue, and mouth, which appeared within minutes after eating toxic food, indicated local absorption of the toxin through the mouth mucous membranes (EFSA, 2009).

Concerning body distribution, biotransformation, and elimination, several studies related to STX detection show wide distribution in muscle, liver, kidney, small and large intestine, lung, heart, and spleen. Naturally occurring PSP toxins may be structurally modified by several biological factors. For instance, biotransformation in shellfish or by marine bacteria is well known. Less toxic PSP toxins may be converted into analogues with greater toxicity or vice versa. It has also been reported that STX-group toxins are metabolically transformed, and the urine is the main excretion route for these toxins in humans. The rapid onset of the symptoms suggests that STXs have a rapid excretion or metabolism, or both. In fact, if the intoxicated person survives the first 24 h, there is a very good chance for the patient to recover (EFSA, 2009; Wiese et al., 2010).

It has long been recognized that STX-group toxins act by interfering with voltage-gated sodium channel functioning. Sodium channels control several functions such as contraction of muscle, secretion of hormones, sensing on the environment, processing of information in the brain, and output from the brain to peripheral tissues (Catteral et al., 2007). The voltage-gated sodium channels are responsible for the rapid influx of sodium ions that underlies the rising phase of the action potential in nerve, muscle, and endocrine cells. They work by depolarizing themselves and repolarizing back by managing sodium and potassium ion flux through the channels: when the cell is depolarized, the sodium channel molecule undergoes a conformational change that opens up an aqueous path. This pathway allows extracellular sodium to move into the cell geared by the electrochemical driving forces. This stream of sodium getting into the cell is responsible for the rising phase of the action potential. The cell is repolarized back by the expulsion of potassium ions through the potassium channels, also present in the membrane and which are not affected by STX (FAO, 2004).

The voltage-gated sodium channels from mammalian brain have a common structural motif in a single protein complex that consists of two parts, a principal α-subunit of 220–260 kDa and two auxiliary β-subunits of 33–36 kDa. The toxins act from the exterior of the cells by getting access to the extracellular cavity of the channel and bind to receptor site 1 of the α-subunit in the sodium channel. Six receptor sites have been identified in the voltage-gated sodium channels and, STX and tetrodotoxin (TTX), other phycotoxins described elsewhere within this chapter, bind to the so-called site 1. STX forms hydrogen bonds and electrostatic interactions with the side chains of several amino acids, mostly the negatively charged dissociated groups of glutamic acid and aspartic acid, that participate in the ion selectivity filter of the channels. Then, when the sodium channels are blocked, the propagation of the action potential is slowed or abolished, representing the molecular basis of the toxic effects of STX. As a consequence of voltage-gated sodium channel blockade, a progressive loss of neuromuscular function ensues, leading to the reported neurotoxic or paralytic symptoms that can result in death by asphyxia. The structure of STX-group toxin molecules and the amino acid sequence in SS2 region of ion channels (encompassing site 1) determines the biological responses (Catteral et al., 2007).

Apparently, the channel blockade is specially associated with the 7,8,9-guanidine function, where the hydrated ketone C12-OH is very important and the carbamoyl side chain contributes but is not essential (FAO, 2004). An extensive study about the interaction of neoSTX with the sodium channels was made by Hu and Kao (1991).

The time that the channel remains open depends on the association constant and is reversibly correlated with the toxin concentration. This time does seem to depend not on the toxin concentration but on the dissociation velocity (FAO, 2004).

17.2.1.5 Pharmaceutical Potential

At present, marine alkaloids, including phycotoxins, constitute an extraordinary potential source of new bioactive compounds for pharmaceutical and medical uses. Their biological activities are harmful to the target organisms, since the function of the toxin is either to protect the toxic species from attack by a predator or to immobilize potential prey. Despite the damage in the target organism, toxins have a great potential for nontarget organisms, in particular for therapeutic purposes in humans. This apparent contradiction can be explained as a molecule that is toxic at one concentration and may be useful when delivered at a lower and more controlled dose or to a different receptor. In humans, the acute reference dose (ARfD) for STX and analogues established by EFSA is 0.5 mg STX equivalents/kg b.w. However, recently, based on daily intake estimations, EFSA's assessment is that there is a concern for the health of the consumer (EFSA, 2009; Paredes et al., 2011).

Sometimes the toxin components are directly used as drugs, although more often the toxic lead compound provides a design idea for the development of a drug molecule. Many drugs share some physicochemical considerations such as a molecular weight in the range of 300–500 and water–lipid partition coefficients (log P) that favor their bioavailability. Furthermore, they present potency and selectivity for target site/disease, low toxicity, limited side effects, easy and economical synthesis, and novelty, among others (Craik and Scanlon, 2000).

Marine toxins can potentially be used to develop modulatory drugs that inhibit or prolong ion channel functioning in specific channelopathies as well as interruption of neuropathic signaling (e.g., neuropathic pain).

Conotoxins, a group of toxins isolated from marine cone snails, target a broad range of ion channels and membrane receptors and are currently investigated for possible clinical trials (Halai and Craik, 2009). In 2004, a synthetic single conotoxin analogue, ϖ-conotoxin, MVIIA, also known as ziconotide (trade name Prialt®), was the first marine natural product to be approved for use by the U.S. FDA since 1976. Ziconotide acts by targeting N-type voltage-sensitive Ca^{+2} channels and is used for the treatment of chronic pain in spinal cord injury (Wiese et al., 2010).

STX also has a huge pharmaceutical potential for its ability to induce anesthesia through interaction with site 1 of the voltage-gated Na^+ channel. It has been suggested that site 1 blockers prolong the duration of anesthesia in a synergistic manner when it is combined with other local anesthetics. However, the use of STX to enter clinical trials has been hindered by its systematic toxicity. The use of STX as a slow-release, prolonged anesthetic was recently demonstrated using a novel controlled-release system in male Sprague–Dawley rats. Liposomal formulations of STX, either alone or in conjunction with dexamethasone and/or bupivacaine, were able to block the sciatic nerve within rats for long periods with no myotoxic, cytotoxic, or neurotoxic effects and little associated inflammation. Liposome formulations of STX for slow and site-directed release for prolonged anesthesia have been postulated as a putative treatment of localized pain and severe joint pain (Wiese et al., 2010).

Broadly speaking, sodium channel-modulating agents have potential applications in the treatment of several conditions, including epilepsy, stroke, and cardiac arrhythmias (Craik and Scanlon, 2000). Alterations of sodium channel may contribute to remodeling, ectopic action potentials, and ephaptic transmissions, resulting in spontaneous sensory disturbances, misperceptions of sensation, and neuropathically mediated pain (Watters, 2000).

GTX2–3 have clinical potential and have been used for the treatment of anal fissures by direct injection into both sides of the fissure. A success rate of 98% with remission after 15 and 28 days for acute and chronic conditions, respectively, was observed. A further study with an enhanced method improved time of healing of 7–14 days for chronic cases. Both studies identified GTX2–3 as safe and effective when compared to other treatments. GTX2–3 have also been used in the treatment of chronic tension-type headache, with 70% of patients responding to treatment. These studies recognize that other STX analogues have potential as future pharmaceutical leads. Their use in the past has also been limited mainly due to problems obtaining purified analogues.

Some authors pointed out that toxins are complex molecules that would be extremely expensive to synthesize on the large scale required for pharmaceutical production; often they have poor oral bioavailability and they may be toxic and/or immunogenic. However, toxins are potential candidates to be used as therapeutic agents or as a drug lead and deserve further investigation. The recent elucidation of the *sxt* gene clusters in cyanobacteria and the identification of novel STX analogues have provided many options for further STX-group toxin bioactivity studies (Craik and Scanlon, 2000).

This potential will increase as we continue to gain a better molecular understanding of the STX-group toxins, leading to future research of their use in combinatorial biosynthesis for the production of novel alkaloids with beneficial application. Bioactivity studies and molecular modeling of a range of these toxins could also lead to the design of unnatural analogues with improved pharmaceutical characteristics. For these reasons, toxins should be regarded as starting points for drug design rather than ends in themselves (Wiese et al., 2010).

17.2.2 Domoic Acid (ASP)

17.2.2.1 Occurrence of Domoic Acid

Domoic acid (DA) was first recognized as the causative toxin of the amnesic shellfish poisoning (ASP) accident that occurred in Canada in 1987 when over 143 people became ill and 4 died after consuming DA-contaminated mussels harvested from cultivation beds on the eastern coast of Prince Edward Island (Lefebvre and Robertson, 2010).

DA is a water-soluble, polar, nonprotein excitatory amino acid that is structurally related to kainic acid (Wright et al., 1989). It was first isolated from the rhodophyte *Chondria armata* following investigations on the anthelmintic and insecticidal activity of seaweed extracts. Although multiple macroalgal and diatom sources of DA have been identified (see Lefebvre and Robertson, 2010 for review), toxigenic diatoms pose the biggest threat to human health through the accumulation of DA in filter-feeding marine organisms. In the Canadian episode, marine diatoms of the genus *Pseudonitzschia* (*Pseudonitzschia pungens*) were found to be responsible for the production of DA (Perl et al., 1990a,b). Strains of *Pseudonitzschia* known to produce DA also include *Pseudonitzschia multiseries, Pseudonitzschia pseudodelicatissima*, and *Pseudonitzschia australis* (Jeffery et al., 2004). Levels of DA vary greatly with strain, geographical location, and environmental conditions like temperature (Mos, 2001). Shellfish such mussels, razor clams, scallops and also crustacea can accumulate DA either by direct filtration of the plankton or by feeding directly on contaminated organisms (Jeffery et al., 2004). DA also accumulates in certain fish, such as anchovies, sardines, mackerel, and albacore, though levels are usually lower than in shellfish. Toxic blooms of DA-producing diatoms are a global issue and appear to be increasing in frequency and toxicity, thereby presenting a continued threat to human health and seafood safety (Lefebvre et al., 2002).

17.2.2.2 Domoic Acid Isolation

DA is easily extracted from crude homogenates of shellfish or other biomaterials. The most common method is to drain the tissues to remove salt water and then to homogenize the pooled tissue in a blender. Tissue homogenates are suspended in water:methanol (1:1) followed by supernatant centrifugation and filtration and then used for analysis, or combined with a highly selective cleanup based on strong anion exchange (SAX). Although SPE has become the most common method for cleanup of shellfish samples, some authors concluded that an additional step with a SAX-SPE cartridge did not significantly improve the recovery of DA from sand crab samples (Powell et al., 2002).

Several standards and reference materials of some of these toxin groups are available in the following:

- National Research Council (NRC Canada) offers DA.
- CIFGA (Lugo, Spain) offers DA.
- Sigma-Aldrich Co. LLC. (St. Louis, MO) offers DA.

17.2.2.3 Domoic Acid Toxin Chemical Characterization

DA is a crystalline water-soluble potent neurotoxic amino acid, which has at least nine geometrical isomers (see Figure 17.6). Isodomoic acids A, B, and C and domoilactones, found in seaweed, have not been detected in extracts of plankton or shellfish tissue. However, isodomoic acids D, E, and F and the 50-epidomoic acid have been isolated from both plankton cells and shellfish tissue. Formation of these geometrical isomers can be achieved by brief exposure of dilute solutions of DA to UV light. In addition, heat can accelerate the conversion from DA to 50-epidomoic acid. Interestingly, pharmacological studies reported that these DA isomers are not as toxic as DA because they bind less strongly to the kainate receptor proteins than DA itself. However, 50-epidomoic acid and DA have the same or a similar toxicity (Wright and Quilliam, 1995; He et al., 2010).

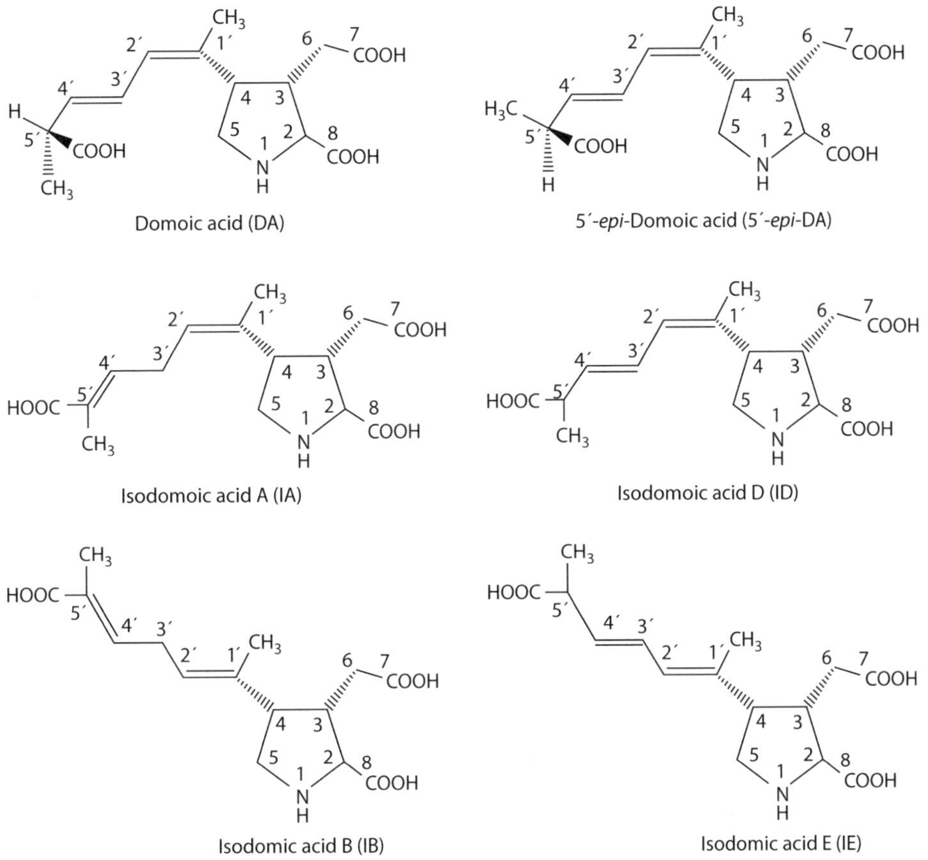

FIGURE 17.6
Chemical structures of DA and its isomers. (From Botana, L.M., *Seafood and Freshwater Toxins. Pharmacology, Physiology and Detection*, CRC Press/Taylor & Francis, Boca Raton, FL, 2008.)

17.2.2.4 Biological Activities and Potential Applications

DA is a potent excitotoxin and most studies on DA using experimental animals have focused on the mechanisms of neurotoxicity. Limited information is available on the intestinal absorption, distribution, metabolism, and excretion (ADME) of DA after ingestion. Truelove and Iverson (1994) investigated the pharmacokinetics of DA in monkeys and rats after intravenous dosing and reported the rapid excretion of DA: the plasma half-life for DA was 114.5 min in monkeys and 21.6 min in rats. Suzuki and Hierlihy (1993) investigated the excretion of DA in rats after intravenous dosing and reported that DA was completely recovered in the urine within 160 min. The absorption rate of DA, estimated from the urinary excretion of DA after oral administration, was trace in both monkeys (4%–7%) and rats (1.8%) (Truelove et al., 1996). Ross et al. (2000) investigated the effects of DA on the uptake of glutamic acid in rat astrocytes and reported that DA inhibited the uptake of glutamic acid in a dose-dependent manner. Some research groups reported that the uptake of glutamic acid across intestinal brush border membranes is predominantly mediated by a Na^+-dependent transport system. However, against expectations, DA transport appears not to share a transport system with glutamic acid. Subsequent studies conclude that absorption of DA is reduced in rodents compared to humans, but in adult rats, mice, monkeys, and humans, DA poorly penetrates the blood–brain barrier. In addition, DA has been shown to be very toxic not only to newborn but also to fetal mice in uterus where DA clearly induced hippocampal excitotoxicity (Mayer, 2000).

DA belongs to the kainoid class of compounds, which is a class of excitatory neurotransmitters. It can damage the neurons by activating R-amino-3-hydroxy-5-methyl-4-isoxazolepropionic acid (AMPA) and kainate receptors, causing an influx of calcium. In mammals, including humans, DA acts as a neurotoxin, causing short-term memory loss, brain damage, and, in severe cases, death. After the ingestion of bivalve mollusks or possibly fish contaminated with DA, gastrointestinal symptoms appear, including nausea, abdominal cramps, vomiting, diarrhea, and anorexia. The neurological symptoms (headaches, dizziness, ataxia, loss of memory) may occur after a delay of a few hours or up to 3 days according to the outbreak observed in 1987 (He et al., 2010).

17.3 Other Toxins

17.3.1 Brevetoxins

17.3.1.1 Origin and Occurrence of Brevetoxins

Brevetoxin (BTX)-group toxins are neurotoxic polyether toxins produced by the dinoflagellate *Karenia brevis* (formerly called *Gymnodinium breve* and *Ptychodiscus brevis*). Since its first identification in the Gulf of Mexico in 1947 (Gunter et al., 1947; Davis, 1948; EFSA, 2010), BTXs have been described in Florida, North Carolina, New Zealand, Australia, Japan, and Scotland (Van Dolah, 2000; FAO, 2004; Fleming et al., 2011). Some other algal species from the family *Raphidophyceae* (*Chattonella antiqua, Chattonella marina, Fibrocapsa japonica, Heterosigma akashiwo*) have also been reported to produce BTX-like toxins and, also, to produce BTXs. (Ramsdell, 2008). These species have been reported in the Pacific and Atlantic. *K. brevis* or *K. brevis*-like species have also been reported from Japan, New Zealand, West-Atlantic, Spain, Portugal, and Greece (FAO, 2004). Nevertheless, no intoxication outbreaks in humans or occurrence of BTX-group toxins in shellfish or fish have been reported in Europe (EFSA, 2010).

17.3.1.2 Brevetoxin Isolation

After identification in the Gulf of Mexico in 1947, bioactive principals were isolated from cultures and contaminated shellfish. McFarren et al. determined that BTXs cause neurological poisoning in mice, similar to ciguatera fish poisoning (CFP) (McFarren et al., 1965). Nevertheless, BTX isolation was a difficult task, yielding inconsistent results until the application of HPLC technology in 1979 (Risk et al., 1979).

Isolation of BTXs can be performed with diethyl ether from mussel homogenate, as it is done for the mouse bioassay, although it has been pointed out that those more polar BTX metabolites (e.g., cysteine conjugates) are poorly extracted with diethyl ether (Plakas and Dickey, 2010).

In order to perform isolation from cultures, cells can be separated by a dialysis method, and the toxins extracted with ethyl acetate. Consecutive steps of washing and fractioning with water first and then with acetone (Lekan and Tomas, 2010). Liquid–liquid partition with 1:1 hexane:methanol followed by chromatographic separation has been also suggested (Caillaud et al., 2009).

Several standards and reference materials of some of these toxin groups are available in the following:

- World Ocean Solutions (Wilmington, NC) offers BTX1, BTX2, BTX3, BTX6, BTX7, BTX9, BTX10, and BTX–COOH.
- Latoxan (France) offers BTX2 and BTX3.

17.3.1.3 Chemical Characterization

Several BTX-group toxins have been isolated and identified. These are grouped into two types (type A and B) based on their molecular backbone structures: BTX1 (or PbTx1)13 (type A) and BTX2 (or PbTx2)13 (type B) are considered to be the parent toxins from which other BTX-group toxins derive (see Figure 17.7). BTX A has a backbone of 10 fused cyclic ether rings; BTX B, which is reported to be the most abundant BTX-group toxin in *K. brevis*, has a backbone of 11 fused cyclic ether rings, BTX2 (Landsberg, 2002; Baden et al., 2005; Plakas and Dickey, 2010). It has been demonstrated that the family *Raphidophyceae*, besides the so-called BTX-like toxins, produce BTXs. Besides BTX-group toxins are metabolized in shellfish and fish, yielding several metabolites of BTX-group toxins. Hence, consumers of contaminated seafood are exposed to their metabolites rather than parental algal BTXs (Ramsdell, 2008; EFSA, 2010).

Brevetoxin A-type backbone

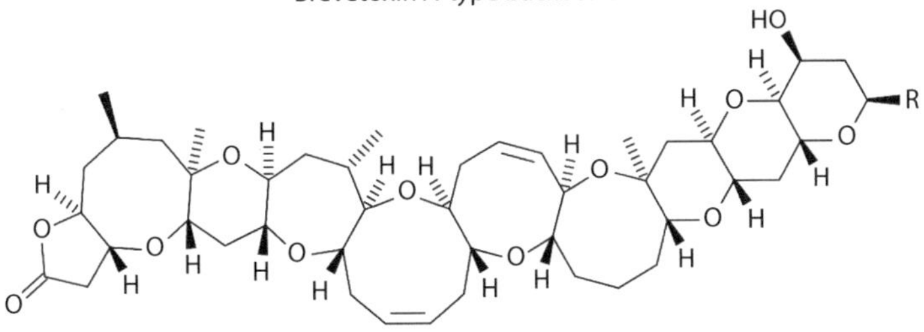

BTX1 R = –CH$_2$C(=CH$_2$)CHO
BTX7 R = –CH$_2$C(=CH$_2$)CH$_2$OH
BTX10 R = –CH$_2$CH(–CH$_3$)CH$_2$OH

Brevetoxin B-type backbone

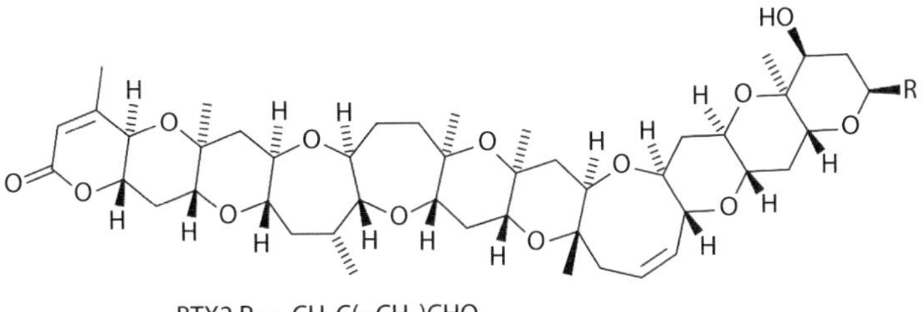

BTX2 R = –CH$_2$C(=CH$_2$)CHO
BTX3 R = –CH$_2$C(=CH$_2$)CH$_2$OH
BTX8 R = –CH$_2$COCH$_2$Cl
BTX9 R = –CH$_2$CH(CH$_3$)CH$_2$OH

FIGURE 17.7
Chemical structures of BTX-group toxins: A- and B-type backbone structures.

17.3.1.4 Biological Activities and Potential Applications

BTX-group toxins cause neurologic (neurotoxic) shellfish poisoning (NSP), which is characterized by mainly neurological and gastrointestinal effects. The symptoms and signs include, for example, nausea; vomiting; diarrhea; paresthesia; cramps; bronchoconstriction; paralysis; paresthesia of lips, face, and extremities; seizures; and coma. They typically occur within 30 min to 3 h after consuming contaminated shellfish and last for a few days. Reports of persistent symptoms or mortality have not been identified (FAO, 2004; EFSA, 2010).

Besides the consumption of contaminated seafood, inhalation of contaminated aerosols is another important route of intoxication. The inhalation of BTX-contaminated aerosols in coastal areas results in acute respiratory symptoms, which may persist, particularly, but not only, in persons with underlying lung disease such as asthma and include throat and nasal irritation, tightness of chest, wheezing, and shortness of breath (Ramsdell, 2008; Kirkpatrick et al., 2010; Fleming et al., 2011).

There is a mouse bioassay for detecting BTX-group toxins in shellfish based on shellfish extraction with diethyl ether. One mouse unit (MU) is approximately 0.2 mg/kg. BTX (BTX3) has a similar LD_{50} than the shellfish conjugates B1, B2, and B4 (200, 50, 306, and 100 µg/kg, respectively); the aldehyde and reduced BTX B present very similar LD_{50} (200 and 170 µg/kg, respectively), whereas there is no LD_{50} calculated for BTX A. LD_{50} of BTX B when administered orally is higher (6600 µg/kg) than by i.p. administration, and oral LD_{50} for BTX3 has been established in 520 µg/kg (Ramsdell, 2008).

Since BTX-producing blooms are accompanied by mortality of marine vertebrates (turtles, birds, mammals, and fish) (Gunter et al., 1947; Nam et al., 2010), bioassays based on fish lethality by bath exposure have been developed, with small fishes such as zebra fish (*Danio rerio*), mosquito fish (*Gambusia affinis*), and minnow (*Cyprinodon variegatus*).

BTXs target ion channels, binding with high affinity to receptor site 5 of the voltage-gated sodium channels in cell walls (Baden et al., 2005) leading to an uncontrolled Na^+ influx into cells and depolarization of neuronal and muscle cell membranes. BTXs interact in sodium homeostasis with other marine biotoxins, such as STX, TTX, and ciguatoxin (CTX) (Kulagina et al., 2004; Ramsdell, 2008). At the level of the sodium channel, BTX exerts at least four actions: shift of the voltage dependence, inhibition of inactivation, increase of mean open times, and multiple subconductance levels, all these actions leading to depolarization of excitable cell membranes. The global response to BTXs in different cells, organs, or in vivo models will be dependent on several factors, such as the existence of the different voltage-dependent sodium channel subtypes expressed. Also, BTXs have a reversal effect from excitatory to inhibitory. Within a few seconds, transient repetitive neuronal discharges are followed by action potential depression and eventually a complete blockade of neuronal excitability. In vivo, the interplay between autonomic pathways at the level of either the peripheral or central nervous systems will condition the final observed effect (Ramsdell, 2008).

Besides excitable cells, BTX has been shown to exert actions on nonexcitable cells, such as activation of mouse bone marrow–derived mast cell activation (Hilderbrand et al., 2010), trigger of inflammatory response in an alveolar macrophage cell line (Sas and Baatz, 2010), DNA damage, and apoptosis induction in Jurkat cells (Murrell and Gibson, 2009).

The use of BTX derivatives for enhancing neuronal growth and for the treatment of neurodegenerative diseases and neurological disorders and injuries, such as Alzheimer's disease, amyotrophic lateral sclerosis, cerebral strokes, traumatic brain, and spinal cord injuries, has been proposed (Taupin, 2009).

17.3.2 Ciguatoxins

17.3.2.1 *Origin and Occurrence of Ciguatoxin-Group Toxins throughout the World*

The causative toxins of CFP, an important human illness derived from consumption of seafood, are CTX-group toxins produced by the benthic dinoflagellate *Gambierdiscus* spp. Worldwide, between 50,000 and 500,000 human poisonings per year have been estimated (Litaker et al., 2009). Although *Gambierdiscus toxicus* was first identified as the producer of this global food-borne illness, nowadays it is known that this taxon is composed of genetically and morphologically distinct groups. Thus, *G. toxicus* is not a single cosmopolitan species; instead it is a species including several distantly related groups co-occurring across geography, and at present, the genus *Gambierdiscus* is undergoing taxonomic revision (Parsons et al., 2011). In fact, 10 *Gambierdiscus* species were documented by Litaker in the Atlantic and in the Pacific Region (Litaker et al., 2009, 2010), and new species of *Gambierdiscus* were detected in European Atlantic waters and in the Mediterranean Sea (Aligizaki and Nikolaidis, 2008). The presence of CFP in Africa and Europe including Canary Islands (Pérez-Arellano et al., 2005) and Madeira (Gouveia et al., 2009) was also reported. Furthermore, potential CTX producers were recorded in the Mediterranean Sea and in waters of the Canary Islands (Caillaud et al., 2010; EFSA, 2010). Another benthic dinoflagellate, *Ostreopsis* spp. that produces PlTX and derivatives, is a present threat outside of its purported role in ciguatera (it will be considered elsewhere within this chapter). Figure 17.8 illustrates *Ostreopsis'* and *Gambierdiscus'* worldwide distribution.

CTXs were mainly found in the Pacific (P), Caribbean (C), and Indian Ocean (I) regions, and they are classified as Pacific (P), Caribbean (C), and Indian Ocean (I) CTX-group toxins. However, as it was mentioned before, recently CTX-group toxins were identified for the first time in fish caught in Europe.

CFP is the most frequently reported seafood-toxin illness in the world producing gastrointestinal, neurologic, and/or cardiovascular symptoms that last days to even months. Humans acquire this illness by eating reef fish containing the naturally occurring toxins, CTXs.

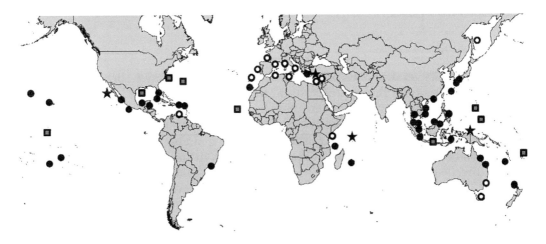

FIGURE 17.8
Global distribution of *Ostreopsis* and *Gambierdiscus* (April, 2011). The black circles indicate areas where both genera were reported. The open circles represent areas where only *Ostreopsis* was reported. The gray squares indicate where only *Gambierdiscus* was reported. The stars indicate places where fish has been caught that resulted in cases of CFP. (From Parsons, M.L. et al., *Harmful Algae*, 14, 107, 2011.)

17.3.2.2 Ciguatoxins Isolation

CTXs are lipophilic polyethers that can be isolated from fish and from *Gambierdiscus* spp. cell extracts, either wild samples or cultures.

To isolate and purify P-CTX1 standard from moray eels and blue-spotted groupers, reliable and sensitive methods were optimized by using LC-MS/MS coupled with accelerated solvent extraction (ASE) (Hamilton et al., 2002; Wu et al., 2011). The large, 3 nm in length, and complex molecular structure of CTXs had impeded chemists from completing their total synthesis. However, total chemical synthesis of CTX3C was outlined ensuring a practical supply of CTX for biological applications, and later the chemical structure of other analogues was also identified (Inoue et al., 2004; Hirama, 2005).

Several extraction and purification procedures of CTX-group toxins from fish or wild and cultured *Gambierdiscus* spp. cell pellets were compiled in a recent publication. In a first method and following a general protocol, these authors gathered different cleanup steps with Florisil SPE to increase the purity of the ether fractions. Other methods described are based on the use of successive solvent partitions, followed by various SPE cleanup procedures. Finally, a useful protocol when the flesh is limited was also reported in this chapter that includes the use of Sep-Pak cartridges (Caillaud et al., 2010).

17.3.2.3 Ciguatoxins-Group Toxin Chemical Characterization

CTXs are lipid-soluble polyether compounds, consisting of 13–14 rings fused by ether linkages into a rigid ladderlike structure and relatively heat stable, odorless, and tasteless.

To date, over 50 different chemical congeners of CTXs have been identified whose toxicity can vary significantly (Litaker et al., 2010). On the one hand, the chemical structures of more than 20 P-CTX analogues, main CTX-group toxins in Pacific areas, have been identified, and structural modifications are mainly seen in both termini of the toxin molecules, mostly by oxidation. On the other hand, the chemical structures of several Caribbean CTX-group toxins were also revealed. Some chemical structures are depicted in Figure 17.9; four Indian Ocean CTX-group toxins were also isolated although their structures were not reported yet (EFSA, 2010).

17.3.2.4 Toxicity

Based on toxicity studies following oral administration in mice, the absorption of CTX-group toxins from the gastrointestinal tract was reported. The biotransformation of CTX-group toxins in animals is indicated by the observation that 1 h after intraperitoneal injection of C-CTX, both nonpolar and polar CTX-group toxins were detected in blood. CTX-group toxins could be transferred from the mother to the fetus through the placenta and from the mother to her offspring through the milk (EFSA, 2010).

CTXs directly target the voltage-sensitive Na^+ channels binding to site 5 and forcing their opening. Then, an influx of Na^+ occurs, and as a result, the involved cells are depolarized, inducing action potentials. Secondary responses observed in cells exposed to CTX-group toxins include Ca^{2+} entry into the cell by reverse action of Na^+/Ca^{2+} exchangers eventually leading to muscular contraction and neurotransmitter release. Water entry into cells is another effect that follows sodium influx, leading to cell mitochondria swelling, blebbing, and cytotoxicity (EFSA, 2010).

P-CTX-4B (–4A)

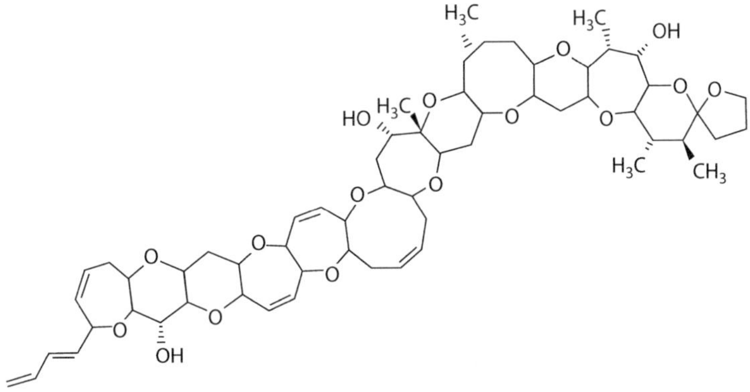

P-CTX-3C

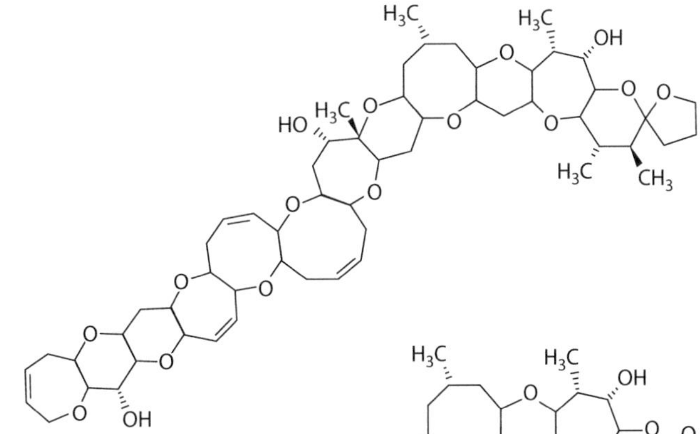

2,3-Dihydroxy P-CTX-3C

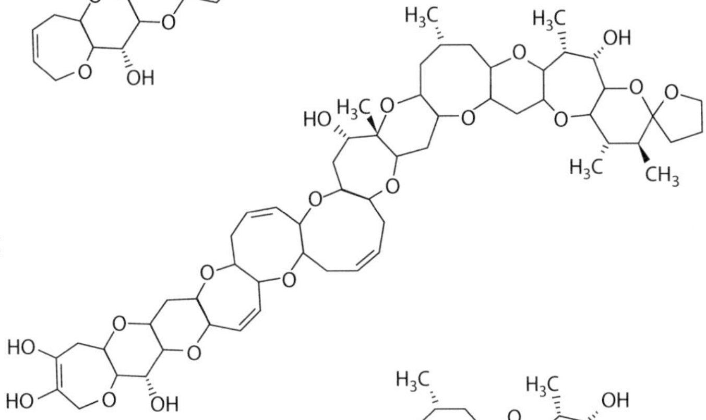

51-Hydroxy P-CTX-3C

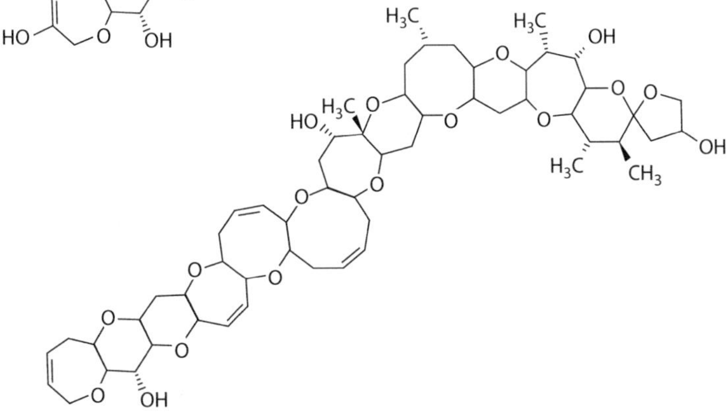

FIGURE 17.9
CTX structures from *Gambierdiscus* spp. (From Botana, L.M., *Seafood and Freshwater Toxins. Pharmacology, Physiology and Detection*, CRC Press/Taylor & Francis, Boca Raton, FL, 2008.)

17.3.2.5 Pharmaceutical Potential

CTXs are one of the most potent natural substances known. One of the CTXs poses a health risk at concentrations as low as 0.08–0.1 µg/kg, although CTX rarely accumulates in fish at levels that are lethal to humans.

CTX activates the voltage-gated sodium channels in cell membranes, which increases sodium ion permeability and depolarizes the nerve cell causing the array of neurological signs associated with CFP.

No pharmaceutical or medical use has been established or characterized for CTXs to date. However, many effects of these toxins in different cell types are thoroughly known. In vitro pharmacological studies have revealed that CTXs interfere in different intracellular pathways: activate Na^+ channels of excitable and nonexcitable cells, induce membrane depolarization and spontaneous and repetitive action potentials in excitable cells, and alter the Na^+ gradient driving the $Na^+–Ca^{2+}$ exchanger leading to an elevation in intracellular Ca^{2+} concentration. Also, they induce repetitive, synchronous, and asynchronous neurotransmitter release and transient increases and decreases in the quantal content of synaptic responses; cause spontaneous and titanic muscle contractions; impair synaptic vesicle recycling that exhausts neurotransmitters available for release; and cause swelling of axons, nerve terminals, and presynaptic Schwann cells (Lewis et al., 2000). Thus, all these effects drawing this scenario suggest that CTX-group toxins possess a big potential as new pharmacological tools.

17.3.3 Tetrodotoxin

17.3.3.1 Origin and Occurrence of Tetrodotoxin throughout the World

TTX is a neurotoxin that has been identified from taxonomically diverse marine organisms. Its name is derived from *Tetraodontidae*, the family of puffer fish from which it was first isolated. However, TTX has been found to occur in at least six phyla of organisms within the Animalia kingdom. Its presence was described in many sources including frogs, newts, nematodes, starfish, crabs, mollusks, and a lot more. It is not clear how or why TTX occurs in such a diverse range of phylogenetically unrelated organisms. The widespread occurrence of TTX suggests that symbiotic or commensal bacteria play a role in TTX biosynthesis, although this assertion is not completely proved (Chau et al., 2011). TTX-producing bacteria have been isolated from most but not all animals containing TTX. The debate into whether TTX is derived from bacteria or is endogenous to the host animals is ongoing, and the only published study into the substrates of TTX biosynthesis proved inconclusive. For instance, newts were unlikely to harbor TTX-producing bacteria, although the presence of TTX-producing bacteria in their gastrointestinal tract was later proved (Chau et al., 2011). It was also reported that some marine environment actinomycetes, mainly *Streptomyces*, produce TTX (Imada, 2005).

TTX-containing fish exists in tropical waters throughout the world, mainly Southeast Asia and more specifically Japan. Some areas include Taiwan, Thailand, Malaysia, Hong Kong, Singapore, Australia, Madagascar, China, Bangladesh, and the Philippines. Locally acquired TTX poisoning has been also reported in Mexico and the United States (Gessner and McLaughlin, 2008).

During the last years, there has been evidence of TTX being present in Europe for the first time, as, for example, in the lessepsian migrant puffer fish *Lagocephalus sceleratus*, in Greek waters (Bentur et al., 2008). The term "lessepsian migrant" refers to the Red Sea species that have passed through the Suez Canal and settled in the Eastern Mediterranean. Also, lately TTX has been found in a gastropod, the trumpet shell *Charonia lampas lampas* in Portugal (Rodriguez et al., 2008).

17.3.3.2 Tetrodotoxin Isolation

The amount of TTX isolated from laboratory cultures is usually quite small when compared to the high levels of TTX found in host animals supporting a bioaccumulation through the food chain.

TTX has a long history; both the ancient Egyptian and Chinese societies possessed knowledge of the toxic properties of the puffer fish. However, TTX was not isolated as a crystal until the early 1950s and also chromatographically in the 1960s. Despite its long knowledge regarding toxicity and pharmacology, neither the pathway to TTX nor even the biogenic origin of TTX is known.

TTX isolation and purification involves harvesting of puffer fish livers, but this procedure has a detrimental impact on aquatic life and is quite inefficient. Two TTXs were isolated, purified, and characterized from liver of puffer fish by thin-layer chromatography, and their structure was elucidated by means of NMR and mass spectroscopy (Hasan et al., 2007). Attempts at chemical synthesis of TTX have been successful although these generally involve complex, multistep reactions, are time consuming and expensive, and result in low yields (Chau et al., 2011). A reliable method to produce a constant source of TTX could be the use of biosynthesis genes. The knowledge related to the assembly of TTX together with genetic engineering in microbes by means of molecular technologies would facilitate the production of TTX in large quantities (Chau et al., 2011).

Several standards and reference materials of some of these toxin groups are available in the following:

- CIFGA (Lugo, Spain) offers TTX.
- Sigma-Aldrich Co. LLC. (St. Louis, MO) offers TTX.
- Abcam plc. (Cambridge, United Kingdom) offers TTX.

17.3.3.3 Tetrodotoxin Characterization

17.3.3.3.1 Chemical Characterization

Similar to STX, TTX is a heat-stable water-soluble heterocyclic guanidine. It has a highly unusual structure containing a single guanidinium moiety attached to a highly oxygenated carbon backbone that consists of a 2,4-dioxaadamantane structure with five hydroxyl groups. Figure 17.10 shows the chemical structure of TTX and derivatives (Chau et al., 2011).

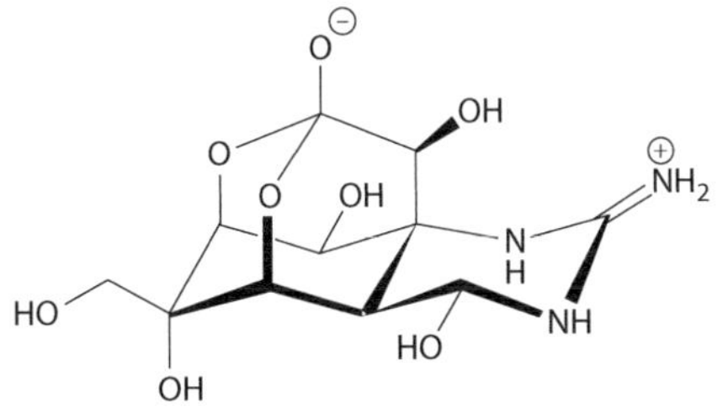

FIGURE 17.10
Tetrodotoxin (TTX) structure. (From Botana, L.M., *Seafood and Freshwater Toxins. Pharmacology, Physiology and Detection*, Marcel & Dekker, New York, 2000.)

17.3.3.4 Toxicity

TTXs share the STX mechanism of action. Both toxins block sodium channels by binding through site 1, in a selective way and with high affinity (Etheridge, 2010). TTX has different affinities for the variant sodium channel isoforms due to amino acid substitutions that confer TTX resistance to a variety of species (Lee and Ruben, 2008).

The toxicity of TTX relates to two factors: paralysis of skeletal muscle, including the diaphragm and intercostals muscles, leading to respiratory failure, and reduced blood pressure, predominantly due to vasodilatation. Early signs of this effect might include among others weakness, tingling of the lips, and dizziness (Berde et al., 2011).

The toxicity of TTX is much lower by oral or inhaled routes than by injection. TTX does not cause direct myocardial depression or arrhythmias because it does not bind significantly to Nav 1.5 sodium channels, the predominant channel subtype found in the heart. In addition, TTX crosses the blood–brain barrier poorly and does not generate seizures (Berde et al., 2011).

Concerning pharmacokinetics in puffer fish, it is known that TTX is absorbed into the systemic circulation from the gastrointestinal tract by saturable mechanism and finally accumulated in the liver (Matsumoto et al., 2008).

17.3.3.5 Pharmaceutical Potential

TTX selectively blocks voltage-gated sodium channels, and due to this selectivity, it has become an important chemical tool in neuroscience. The use of TTX in anesthesia and analgesia is being developed thus heightening its demand. This toxin, known as Tectin as brand name, is currently undergoing Phase III clinical trials in Canada as an injectable systemic analgesic for inadequately controlled pain due to advanced cancer, especially where the pain has neuropathic features (Berde et al., 2011).

The TTX formulation in these trials consists of 15 µg/mL of TTX (47 µM), in 2 mL ampules given by subcutaneous injection. Human subjects have tolerated doses of up to 90 µg daily, with mostly mild side effects observed at doses below 60 µg. It is important to mention that addition of either bupivacaine or epinephrine increases the LD_{50} of TTX in rats, that is, reduces systemic toxicity from TTX, and also increases its potency producing sensory blockade, thereby substantially improving the therapeutic index of TTX. The combination of bupivacaine, TTX, and epinephrine appears promising for prolonged duration of local anesthesia. Three-way combinations of TTX, bupivacaine, and epinephrine produce significant prolonged sciatic nerve blockade in rats, compared to bupivacaine plain or bupivacaine plus epinephrine. Neurobehavioral experiments support the inclusion of all three drugs in the mixture as an approach to prolong block durations while minimizing the systemic toxicity of either TTX or bupivacaine. This three-drug combination is likely to be especially important for clinical situations such as wound infiltration for a large open abdominal incision. For this application, very large injection volumes (e.g., 60–90 mL in adults) are required to provide blockade of afferents from multiple layers of the wound, and therefore, TTX concentrations must be low in order to keep the total systemic dose in a safe range. The three-drug combination is also likely to improve the reliability of blockade compared to formulations using TTX–epinephrine without bupivacaine (Berde et al., 2011). Then, peripheral nerve blockade and wound infiltration can provide useful contributions to multimodal approaches for postoperative recovery (Dahl and Moiniche, 2009).

In that study, Tectin appeared indistinguishable, in its neurobehavioral effects, from TTX supplied by Sigma, and Tectin and its placebo vehicle appeared benign in its histologic effects on rat sciatic nerves. Some authors believe that TTX can be a systemically safe drug over a particular dose range and point out that a convenient, flexible, and safe approach to clinical development would be to supply clinicians with a standard package containing two vials, a 2 mL ampule of TTX as Tectin along with a larger 30 mL vial of bupivacaine 2.5 mg/mL (0.25%) with epinephrine 5 µg/mL (1:200,000). This would permit the clinician to mix the vials immediately prior to use in several ratios for different clinical indications. However, it is necessary to provide preclinical data that confirm the contribution of each drug in the combination from the standpoint of both efficacy and safety (Berde et al., 2011).

Currently, a prolonged peripheral nerve blockade and wound analgesia can be supplied by indwelling catheters and infusion pumps. Catheters can become dislodged or can unintentionally preferentially block one trunk, cord, or division of a plexus. While portable elastomeric infusion pumps are convenient and can facilitate local anesthetic delivery at home, they are expensive, and delivery failures could occur (Remeral et al., 2008). An approach that could reliably prolong the duration of peripheral nerve blockade or infiltration analgesia by three- to fourfold would be very important for postoperative care. Since both the desirable effect (analgesia) and other effects (motor blockade) are greatly prolonged, in future clinical development, it will be important to restrict injections to body locations where motor effects are clinically unimportant.

Clinically relevant combinations of Tectin with commercially available bupivacaine 0.25% and epinephrine 5 µg/mL warrant further study for prolonged-duration local anesthesia. Then, a single-injection approach to prolonged local anesthesia will provide good pain relief as a component of multimodal analgesic regimens, will thereby reduce postoperative opioid requirements, and may improve the course of postoperative recovery and acute rehabilitation (Berde et al., 2011).

Also, TTX-sensitive subtypes of sodium channels play a role in the pathogenesis of chemotherapy-induced neuropathic pain. In this context, low doses of TTX can prevent and treat paclitaxel-induced neuropathic pain (Nieto et al., 2007).

Antineoplastic activities of TTX were reported on Ehrlich ascites carcinoma and on leukemia cell line (P388). TTX, by blocking Na^+ influx into the cells, prevents the carcinoma cells from getting sufficient Na^+ ions for the requirements of various intracellular functions and, above all, to maintain the normal charge distribution across the cell membrane, a process necessary to maintain cellular integrity. As a consequence, the proliferation and invasiveness of such cells are suppressed (Bragadeeswaran et al., 2010).

17.3.4 Palytoxin and Other Related Toxins

17.3.4.1 Occurrence of Palytoxin and Other Related Toxins

Palytoxin (PlTX) is one of the most poisonous nonprotein substances known to date, and it was first isolated and purified from *Palythoa toxica* (Moore and Scheuer, 1971).

The PlTX-group toxins are complex polyhydroxylated compounds with both lipophilic and hydrophilic areas. They are white, amorphous, hygroscopic solids, which have not yet been crystallized. They are insoluble in nonpolar solvents such as chloroform, ether, and acetone; are sparingly soluble in methanol and ethanol; and are soluble in pyridine, dimethyl sulfoxide, and water. At least eight different PlTX analogues are known: PlTX, ostreocin-D, ovatoxin-A, homopalytoxin, bishomopalytoxin, neopalytoxin, deoxypalytoxin, and 42-hydroxypalytoxin (Riobo and Franco, 2011).

The presence of PlTX and its derivatives has been well documented in invertebrates (Aligizaki and Nikolaidis, 2008) and in fish (Taniyama et al., 2003).

PlTX was also found in benthic dinoflagellates belonging to the genus *Ostreopsis*. Six of the nine currently recognized species are toxic and produce PlTX-related compounds. Ostreocin-D, an analogue of PlTX, was identified and isolated in *Ostreopsis siamensis* (Usami et al., 1995). In recent years, *Ostreopsis ovata* blooms in the Mediterranean region were found to cause respiratory illnesses due to inhalation of aerosols released during such blooms (Ciminiello et al., 2006a).

However, it is not demonstrated that the dinoflagellate is the primary producer, and it was suggested that bacteria might be the original producers of PlTX (Seemann et al., 2009).

This toxin and its analogues have become a global concern due to their effects on animals and especially on humans. In this sense, human intoxication arising from consumption of seafood suspected to be contaminated with PlTX or from dermal absorption has been reported in the Philippines, in Madagascar, in Hawaii, in Japan, in Germany, in the United States, and in Italy (Ramos and Vasconcelos, 2010).

17.3.4.2 Palytoxin and Other Related Toxin Isolation

Most of the extraction and purification processes for biological and chemical determinations of PlTXs follow a general procedure with slight modifications. Ethanol and methanol are the most common solvents used to extract PlTX, but the toxin is also quite soluble in water or other water-miscible solvents. The following steps include partitions with hexane and butanol and finally SPE cartridges or flash chromatography (Oku et al., 2004). Depending on the matrix, exhaustive extraction and purification processes may be required. In this sense, polyps, mollusks, crabs, and fish are the most complex ones. Extraction method can be simplified when dinoflagellate samples are obtained from cultures or seawater since the matrix is less complex and the amount of lipophilic compounds is smaller than in mollusks and fish. Thus, a simple extraction performed with methanol following a later partition with hexane is enough for their determination by HPLC-FLD or LC-MS/MS. PlTX dissolved in seawater has never been detected during *Ostreopsis* blooms. Extraction from this matrix is complicated due to the presence of low toxin levels in seawater and high concentration of salts (Riobo et al., 2011). Recently, extraction of PlTX from growth media of *O. ovata* cultures (945 mL) after removing *Ostreopsis* cells was performed using an equal volume of butanol for three times. The butanol layer was evaporated to dryness, then dissolved in 5 mL of methanol/water (1:1, v/v) and analyzed directly by LC-MS/MS (Guerrini et al., 2010). Likewise, the presence of PlTX in environmental aerosol samples has not yet been demonstrated despite respiratory intoxications reported (Riobo et al., 2011).

Several standards and reference materials of some of these toxin groups are available in the following:

- Wako Pure Chemical Industries, Ltd. (Osaka, Japan) offers PlTX.
- Sigma-Aldrich Co. LLC. (St. Louis, MO) offers PlTX.

17.3.4.3 Palytoxin and Other Related Toxin Chemical Characterizations

PlTX could be considered as one of the most complicated and largest molecules. The basic molecule consists of a long, partially unsaturated (with eight double bonds) aliphatic backbone with spaced cyclic ethers, 64 chiral centers, and 40–42 hydroxyl and 2 amide groups. The third nitrogen present as a primary amino group at C-115 end of the molecule accounts for the basicity of PlTX (Ramos et al., 2010).

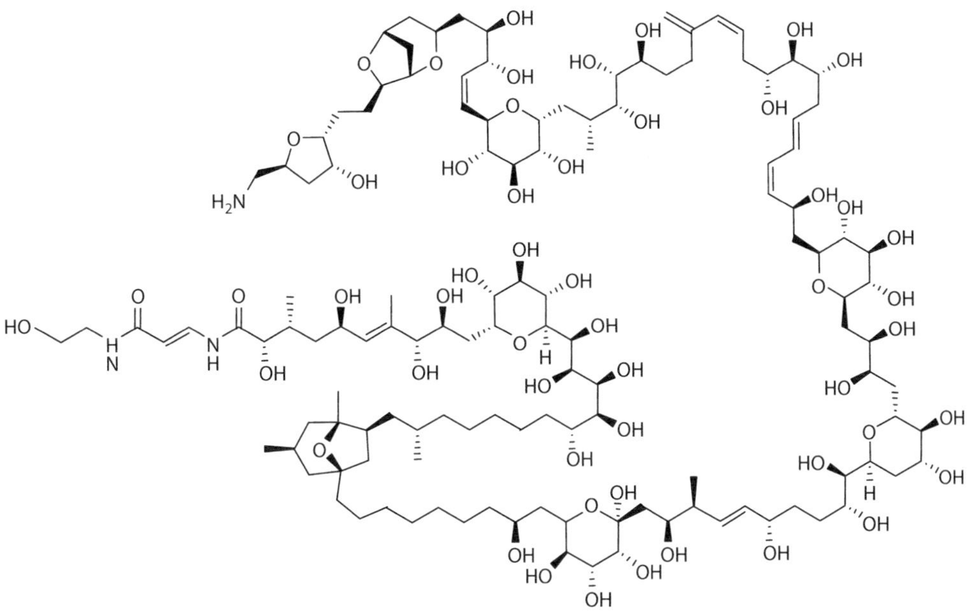

FIGURE 17.11
Structure of PlTX. (From Riobo, P. and Franco, J.M., *Toxicon*, 57(3), 368, 2011.)

The structure of PlTX (Figure 17.11) was elucidated by two independent groups, one led by Professor Hirata in Japan (Hirata and Uemura, 1985) and the other by Professor Moore at Honolulu in the United States (Moore and Bartolini, 1981). Chemical structure has only been characterized for PlTX (Cha et al., 1982), ostreocin-D (Ukena et al., 2001), and 42-hydroxypalytoxin (Ciminiello et al., 2009).

17.3.4.4 Biological Activities and Potential Applications

PlTX is one of the most potent natural nonprotein compounds exhibiting extreme toxicity in mammals. Lethal doses through intravenous administration in rats, mice, guinea pigs, rabbits, dogs, and monkeys ranged between 0.03 and 0.45 mg/kg (Wiles et al., 1974). By extrapolation, a toxic dose in humans would range between 2.3 and 31.5 mg (Uemura et al., 1991). Despite its high lethality in terrestrial animals, PlTX has also been detected in crabs, fishes, anemones, sponges, mussels, and soft corals without causing deleterious effects. PlTX shows remarkable biological activity even at very low concentration (Moore et al., 1971). For review, see Ramos and Vasconcelos (2010).

A broad range of studies indicates that the Na^+/K^+-ATPase is a high affinity cellular receptor for PlTX (Franchini et al., 2010). This enzyme plays a central role in regulation of ion fluxes and also functions as a signal transducer to relay messages from the plasma membrane to the intracellular organelles through several pathways (Louzao et al., 2011). PlTX is also a skin tumor promoter that stimulates a wide range of cellular responses such as arachidonic acid metabolism and the production of prostaglandins, modulation of the epidermal growth factor receptor, and modulation of mitogen-activated protein (MAP) kinase cascades (Wattenberg, 2007). The physiological role of MAP kinases is known for a multitude of cellular processes, including cytoskeleton rearrangement. Nevertheless how their regulation might be coupled to the interaction of PLT with the Na^+/K^+-ATPase remains to be determined. Similarly to ion channels, the Na^+/K^+-ATPase activity is regulated, in part, by cytoskeleton. Other studies were done to evaluate the cytotoxicity and cell death induced by PlTX in several cell lines (Valverde et al., 2008a,b). On the other hand, PlTX affects cytoskeleton dynamics by targeting microfilaments (Louzao et al., 2011).

17.3.5 Cyclic Imines

17.3.5.1 Origin and Occurrence of Cyclic Imine Toxins throughout the World

Cyclic imines (CIs) are a recently discovered group of marine biotoxins produced by dinoflagellates integrated by six described groups of toxins: spirolides (SPXs), gymnodimines (GYMs), pinnatoxins (PnTXs), pteriatoxins (PtTXs), prorocentrolides, and spiro-prorocentrimine. All of them are macrocyclic compounds with imine- (carbon–nitrogen double bond) and spiro-linked ether moieties. Their imino group is supposed to act as functioning pharmacophore (Krock et al., 2009a) causing similarities in their intraperitoneal toxicity in mice (EFSA, 2010; Otero et al., 2011).

SPXs were discovered in 1995 during routine monitoring of polar lipophilic toxic compound in mollusk extracts. An unusual toxicity was found during regular mouse bioassay testing of scallop (*Placopecten magellanicus*) and mussel (*M. edulis*) viscera harvested along the southeastern coast of Nova Scotia in Canada. These toxins are metabolites of the dinoflagellate *Alexandrium ostenfeldii* and *Alexandrium peruvianum* and are sometimes found in the presence of other toxins such as PSP toxins (Hu et al., 1995). Ten years after the first detection of the SPXs, two novel SPX derivatives were isolated and characterized from the culture of two clonal strains of *A. ostenfeldii* isolated from Limfjorden in Denmark (MacKinnon et al., 2006). Subsequently, SPXs were detected during analysis of blue mussel (*M. edulis*) digestive glands and algal biomass samples collected during a bloom at Sognefjord, Skjer in Norway (Aasen et al., 2006). Presence of amounts of SPX was revealed during the investigation of DSP toxin episode in Spain (Villar-Gonzalez et al., 2006), France (Amzil et al., 2007), and Chile (Alvarez et al., 2010). In 2007, investigation of a large culture of an Adriatic *A. ostenfeldii* strain allowed the isolation and structure elucidation of another congener of the SPX family (Ciminiello et al., 2007).

GYMs were first isolated from oysters (*Tiostrea chilensis*), collected at the Foveaux Strait, South Island of New Zealand (Seki et al., 1995). They are produced by the dinoflagellate *Karenia selliformis*. Besides the New Zealand coastal area, outbreaks of intoxication by GYM A have also been observed in Tunisia (Bire et al., 2002).

PnTXs were first discovered in extracts from the digestive glands of the pen shell *Pinna attenuata* after an outbreak of shellfish poisoning in China and Japan (Zheng et al., 1990). Selwood et al. isolated and structurally characterized three analogues of PnTXs from digestive glands of two bivalve species, Pacific oysters (*Crassostrea gigas*) and razor fish (*Pinna bicolor*), from the South Australian coast (Selwood et al., 2010). In 2010, PnTX presence (PnTXs G and A) has also been reported in shellfish from Norwegian waters (Miles et al., 2010). PtTXs were first described by Takada et al. (2001), who observed that a moray eel vomits the viscera of the Okinawan oyster *Pteria penguin*. These authors successfully isolated PtTXs A, B, and C as extremely toxic and minor components from *Pt. penguin* and reported the structural determination of these three compounds.

Prorocentrolide A has been isolated from *P. lima* for the first time in 1988 (Torigoe et al., 1988). The dinoflagellate was isolated at Sesoko Island, Okinawa, in 1985 and cultured in seawater enriched with ES-1 nutrient 3 at 25°C for 5 weeks. Hu et al. (1996)

isolated prorocentrolide B, a new toxin from *P. maculosum*, which causes the characteristic "fast-acting" symptoms. As the structural details began to emerge, it became apparent that the new compound was related to prorocentrolide A, previously isolated from a strain of *P. lima*. Spiro-prorocentrimine was isolated from a laboratory-cultured benthic *Prorocentrum* species of Taiwan by Lu et al. (2001).

17.3.5.2 Cyclic Imine Toxin Isolation

Isolation of all CI toxins can be summarized in three main steps including an initial extraction with intermediate polar organic solvents, such as aqueous methanol, aqueous ethanol, or acetone. This should be followed by a liquid–liquid partition, first against n-hexane and second with more polar solvents such as acetate, dichloromethane, or 1-butanol. Finally, a series of chromatographic separations on normal-phase, reverse-phase, size-exclusion gel, and/or ion-exchange resin chromatographic separation sholud be performed. This process was described by Cembella and Krock (Cembella and Krock, 2008).

Different organic solvents and chromatographic techniques could be employed depending on the toxin type and the matrix from where the toxin will be extracted (shellfish or phytoplankton).

Several standards and reference materials of some of these toxin groups are available in the following:

- National Research Council (NRC Canada) offers GYM and 13-desmethyl SPX C.
- CIFGA (Lugo, Spain) offers 13,19-didesmethyl SPX C and 13-desmethyl SPX C.

17.3.5.3 Chemical Characterization

The structure of the SPXs can be divided into two parts: the upper part containing a 6,7-bicyclic spiroimine unit, believed to be the pharmacophore, and the lower unit containing a spiroacetal or bis-spiroacetal moiety (Gueret and Brimble, 2010). To date, 14 members of the SPX family have been isolated all around the world (Ciminiello et al., 2006b, 2010a,b; Lassus et al., 2007; Touzet et al., 2008; Alvarez et al., 2010; Villar-Gonzalez et al., 2011). For review, see Otero et al. (2011). Structural variants and molecular weights of known SPXs are summarized in Figure 17.12.

GYM A was described as a complex pentacyclic derivative incorporating a C24 carboxylic acid and a fused azine (Seki et al., 1995). Its molecular mass is of 504.704 g/mol and the simple molecular formula is $C_{32}H_{45}NO_4$. The structure of GYM B is similar to that of GYM A but contains an exocyclic methylene at position C17 and allylic hydroxyl group at position C18, while GYM C is an oxidized isomer of GYM B at position C18 (Marrouchi et al., 2009) (Figure 17.13).

PnTXs and pteriatoxins are structurally and synthetically related to the better studied group of SPXs. PnTXs are amphoteric macrocyclic compounds possessing a common 27-membered carbocyclic backbone composed of a unique 6,7-azaspiro-linked imine fragment (AG ring), a bridged 5,6-bicycloketal (EF ring), and a 6,5,6-dispiroketal (BCD ring), as well as varying functional group substitutions at positions C21, C22, C28, and C33 (Beaumont et al., 2010). The chemical structures with the corresponding formula and molecular masses of the known PnTX analogues have been summarized in Figure 17.14.

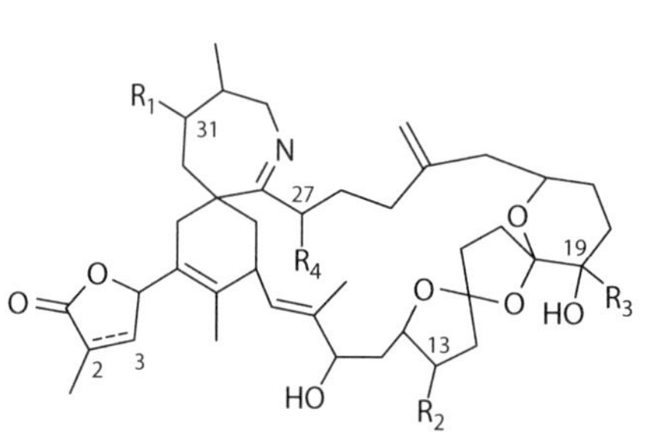

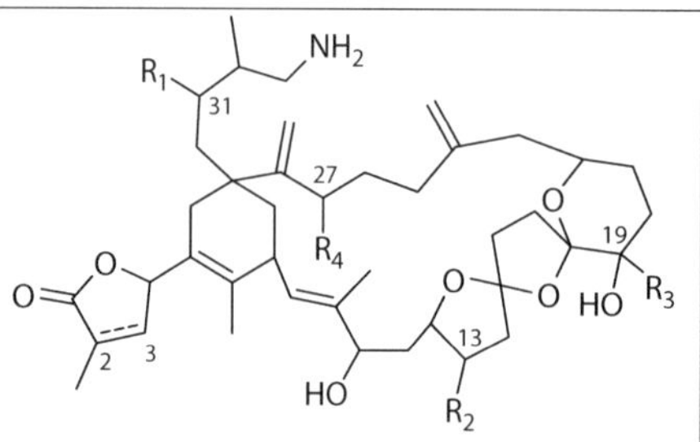

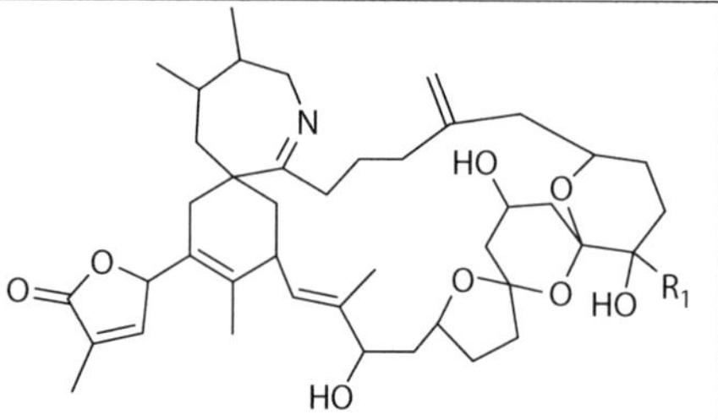

Spirolide	R_1	R_2	R_3	R_4	Δ	MW
A	H	CH_3	CH_3		$Δ^{2,3}$	691.5
B	H	CH_3	CH_3			693.5
C	CH_3	CH_3	CH_3		$Δ^{2,3}$	705.5
D	CH_3	CH_3	CH_3			707.7
13-desMeC	CH_3		CH_3		$Δ^{2,3}$	691.5
13,19-didesMeC	CH_3				$Δ^{2,3}$	677.5
13-desMeD	CH_3		CH_3			693.5
27-OH-13,19-didesMeC	CH_3			CH_3	$Δ^{2,3}$	691.5
E	H	CH_3	CH_3	H		709.5
F	H	CH_3	CH_3	H		711.5
G	H					691.5
20-MeG	CH_3					705.5

FIGURE 17.12
Structural variants and molecular weight (Mw) of known SPXs isolated from shellfish and plankton. (From Otero, A. et al., *Chem. Res. Toxicol.*, 24(11), 1817, 2011.)

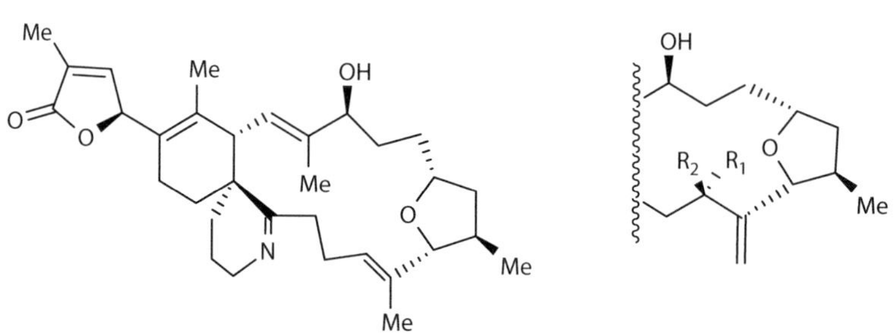

Gymnodimine A

Gymnodimine B: R_1 = OH, R_1 = H
Gymnodimine C: R_1 = H, R_2 = OH

FIGURE 17.13
2D Structures of known members of the GYM family. (From Otero, A. et al., *Chem. Res. Toxicol.*, 24(11), 1817, 2011.)

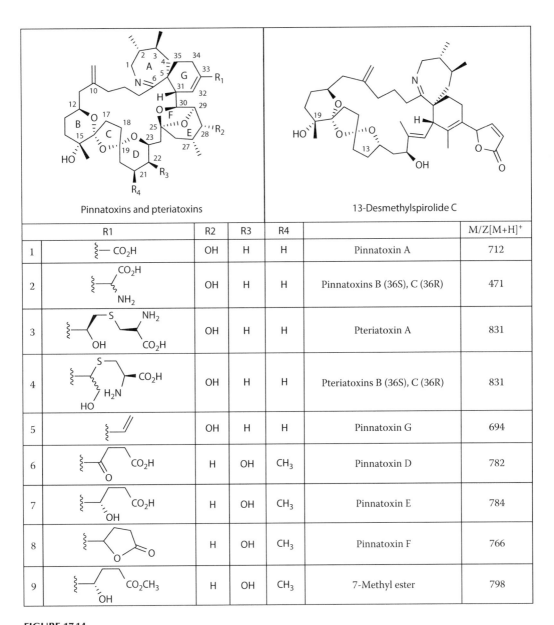

	R1	R2	R3	R4		M/Z[M+H]$^+$
1	$-$ CO$_2$H	OH	H	H	Pinnatoxin A	712
2	CO$_2$H / NH$_2$	OH	H	H	Pinnatoxins B (36S), C (36R)	471
3	S NH$_2$ / OH CO$_2$H	OH	H	H	Pteriatoxin A	831
4	S CO$_2$H / H$_2$N / HO	OH	H	H	Pteriatoxins B (36S), C (36R)	831
5		OH	H	H	Pinnatoxin G	694
6	CO$_2$H / O	H	OH	CH$_3$	Pinnatoxin D	782
7	CO$_2$H / OH	H	OH	CH$_3$	Pinnatoxin E	784
8	O / O	H	OH	CH$_3$	Pinnatoxin F	766
9	CO$_2$CH$_3$ / OH	H	OH	CH$_3$	7-Methyl ester	798

FIGURE 17.14

Chemical structural data of all known PnTX analogues to date and related 13-desmethyl SPX C and PtTX structures, shown for comparison. (From Otero, A. et al., *Chem. Res. Toxicol.*, 24(11), 1817, 2011.)

The molecular formula of PtTXs A, B, and C was determined to be C$_{45}$H$_{70}$N$_2$O$_{10}$S (A) and C$_{45}$H$_{70}$N$_2$O$_{10}$S (B and C). The position of duplicate signals in the 1H NMR spectrum suggested that PtTXs B (2) and C (3) are C34 epimers of each other (Figure 17.15). PtTXs A, B, and C have the same polyether macrocycles as in PnTX A, and they are considered PnTX analogues containing a cysteine moiety.

Planar structure of prorocentrolide A (Figure 17.16) was elucidated by Torigoe et al. (1988), and no stereochemical details have been reported.

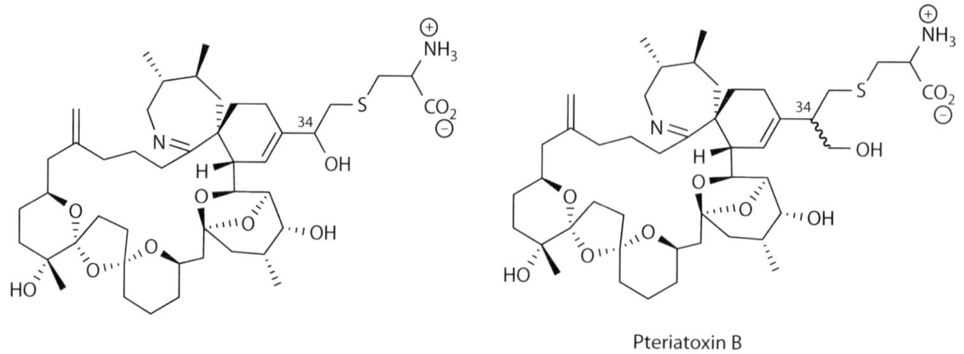

Pteriatoxin A

Pteriatoxin B
and C

FIGURE 17.15
1H NMR data for PtTXs A (1), B (2), and C (3) from Takada et al. (From Otero, A. et al., *Chem. Res. Toxicol.*, 24(11), 1817, 2011.)

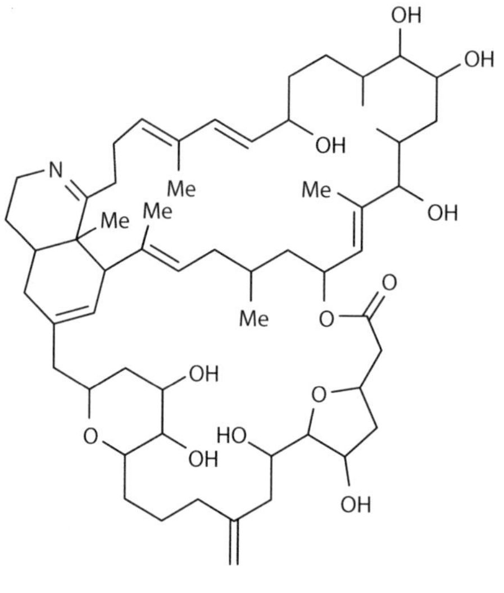

FIGURE 17.16
Prorocentrolide A structure from Torigoe et al. (From Otero, A. et al., *Chem. Res. Toxicol.*, 24(11), 1817, 2011.)

Details of the relative stereochemistry of prorocentrolide B are shown in Figure 17.17. However, the absolute stereochemistry of the rings and the relative configuration of one ring with respect to the others remain undetermined. The full distribution of this family of toxins is not well known, but it is reasonable to conclude from the structural data that prorocentrolide B from *P. maculosum* shares a common biosynthetic pathway with proro-centrolide A from *P. lima* (Hu et al., 1996).

Spiro-prorocentrimine, $C_{42}H_{69}NO_{13}S$, is a polar lipid-soluble toxin that was isolated from a laboratory-cultured benthic *Prorocentrum* species of Taiwan by Lu et al. (2001). X-ray diffraction analysis of the compound revealed a spiro-linked CI with the *ortho, para*-disubstituted 3%-cyclohexene in addition to its macrolide skeleton (Figure 17.18).

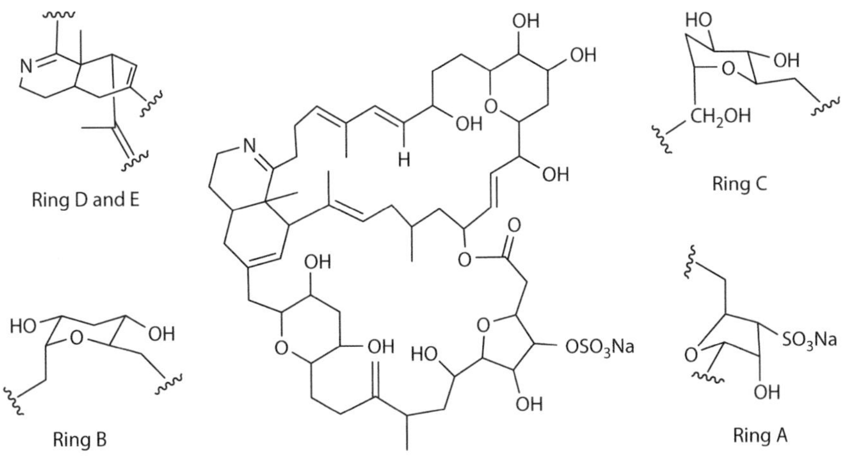

FIGURE 17.17
The relative stereochemistry of the five- and six-membered rings of prorocentrolide B from Hu et al. (1996). (From Otero, A. et al., *Chem. Res. Toxicol.*, 24(11), 1817, 2011.)

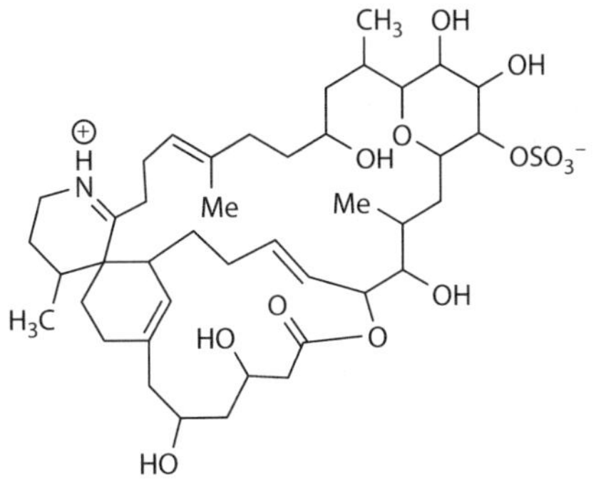

FIGURE 17.18
Structure of spiro-prorocentrimine from Lu (2001). (From Otero, A. et al., *Chem. Res. Toxicol.*, 24(11), 1817, 2011.)

17.3.5.4 Biological Activities and Potential Applications

Toxicological studies of different CIs have been a difficult task due to the lack of reference or toxic materials. Thus, only toxicity of GYMs and SPXs has been studied in depth.

Spiroimine moiety has been established as the common pharmacophore unit of CI group, although structural change in other parts of the molecules also can affect the toxicity (Gueret and Brimble, 2010).

Symptomatology after administration of a toxic dose is similar for all toxins of the group, including decreased activity and coordination, piloerection, moderated exophthalmia, marked abdominal muscle spasm, respiratory distress, tremor in the hind end limbs, opisthotonos, contraction of front legs, respiratory arrest, convulsion, and tremors involving the whole body. If animals survive after 20 min, they fully and quickly recover (Gill et al., 2003).

Initial studies on CIs' mechanism of action suggested that it could be related to the interference on transmission of nervous impulses at neuromuscular junction level. SPXs and GYMs have been demonstrated to act as potent antagonists of both nicotinic (nAChRs) and muscarinic (mAChRs) acetylcholine receptors, and probably, this antagonism on nAChRs is the main cause of the acute symptomatology observed during the mouse bioassay of samples containing these toxins (Kharrat et al., 2008; Bourne et al., 2010; Wandscheer et al., 2010).

Kharrat et al. demonstrated that GYM A broadly interferes in neuromuscular transmission by directly blocking muscle-type nAChRs, and this action could explain some of the acute toxic symptoms observed in mice following GYM A injection including paralysis of the hind legs and dyspnea. It was also concluded that GYM A interacts with a broad range of muscular and neuronal types of nAChRs, larger than other well-characterized toxins that also act on nicotinic receptors (Kharrat et al., 2008). Bourne et al. confirmed the interaction of SPX and GYM with several muscle and neuronal types of nAChRs by competition binding experiments against labeled α-bungarotoxin and epibatidine. They also performed functional analysis of both toxins using voltage-clamp recordings with oocytes expressing muscular and neuronal types of receptors. No agonist effect was observed with SPX or GYM, but both toxins showed a dose-dependent antagonism in muscle- and neuronal-type receptors. However, while GYM effect was reverted after washing with free-toxin solution, SPX antagonism was not abolished after 30–40 min of washout. It was concluded that SPX and GYM toxins display high affinity and potent antagonism but limited selectivity for the muscle type versus neuronal subtypes of nAChR (Bourne et al., 2010).

Wandscheer et al. studied the effect of SPXs on mAChRs in a human neuronal model known to have an acetylcholine-elicited calcium signal dependent on muscarinic AChR activation. They observed that 13-desmethyl SPX C caused a dose- and time-dependent inhibition on neuroblastoma cell response to acetylcholine extracellular stimulation. They demonstrated by competitive binding assays that the 13-desmethyl SPX is a competitive antagonist on mAChRs and also causes an internalization of the M3-type muscarinic receptor that might contribute to the inhibitory effect of the toxin on the calcium response to acetylcholine stimulation (Wandscheer et al., 2010).

17.3.6 Maitotoxin

17.3.6.1 Origin and Occurrence of Maitotoxin Toxins

Maitotoxins (MTX) are a group of water-soluble toxins produced by species of dinoflagellates of the genus *Gambierdiscus*, which grow on algae in tropical waters worldwide. This genus is known to produce both MTX and CTXs, which accumulate in the body of herbivorous fishes and then transmitted through the tropical food chain to carnivorous species. In contrast to CTX, MTX does not accumulate in the flesh but in the viscera of fish.

17.3.6.2 Maitotoxin Isolation

A general process for the isolation of MTX from *Gambierdiscus* sp. cells was described in 1988 by Yasumoto's group at Tohoku University (Yokoyama et al., 1988). They extracted the cells with methanol twice. Solvent was removed and the residue was liquid–liquid partitioned twice, first between 40% methanol and dichloromethane and then between water and butanol. MTX in the butanol fraction was chromatographed on a silica gel column.

Fraction containing the MTX was chromatographed on successive reverse-phase columns and finally purified on a Develosil TMS column with acetonitrile/water (35:65) to obtain the MTX that was eluted at around 33–35 min.

17.3.6.3 Chemical Characterization of Maitotoxins

MTX is a polyketide-derived polycyclic ether integrated by four rigid polyether ladders connected by mobile hydrocarbon chains. It has a molecular weight of 3422 Da and it is the largest non-biopolymeric natural toxin (Murata et al., 1994). See Figure 17.19.

17.3.6.4 Potential Pharmacological Application: Calcium-Dependent Mechanisms

MTX is a very potent toxin when administered intraperitoneally. Lethal dose to mice is 50 ng/kg depending on mice strain, sample source, and preparation procedure. Symptomatology includes reduced body temperature, piloerection, dyspnea, progressive paralysis, slight tremors to convulsions, and long death times. A high dose causes gaps, convulsions, and rapid death. In contrast, it has a very low oral toxicity (Trevino et al., 2008).

At cellular level, MTX causes an increase in the concentration of Ca^{2+} and Na^+ by means of the activation of Ca^{2+}-permeable nonselective cation channels, resulting in a potent cell membrane depolarization. This causes, in excitable cells, the opening of voltage-gated Ca^{2+} and Na^+ channels. This massive influx of ions could exceed buffering mechanisms of cells affecting cell viability. The activation of the Ca^{2+} seems to be intermediated by an intracellular second messenger, although the actual receptor for MTX remains unidentified (Trevino et al., 2008).

Due to its ability to activate Ca^{2+}-permeable nonselective cation channels, MTX is considered a powerful tool in the study of Ca^{2+}-dependent mechanisms, for example, the acrosome reaction, where MTX may be used as a substance to induce sperm capacitation to penetrate the outer egg envelope (Hamano et al., 2001; Trevino et al., 2006).

Another unusual effect of MTX is the formation of cytolytic/oncotic pores that finally conduce to cell membrane blebbing and oncotic cell death. The formation of cytolytic/oncotic pores is modulated by intracellular Ca^{2+} concentration (Schilling et al., 1999; Estacion and Schilling, 2001; Wisnoskey et al., 2004); then MTX results in a useful tool to understand oncotic/necrotic cell death mechanisms.

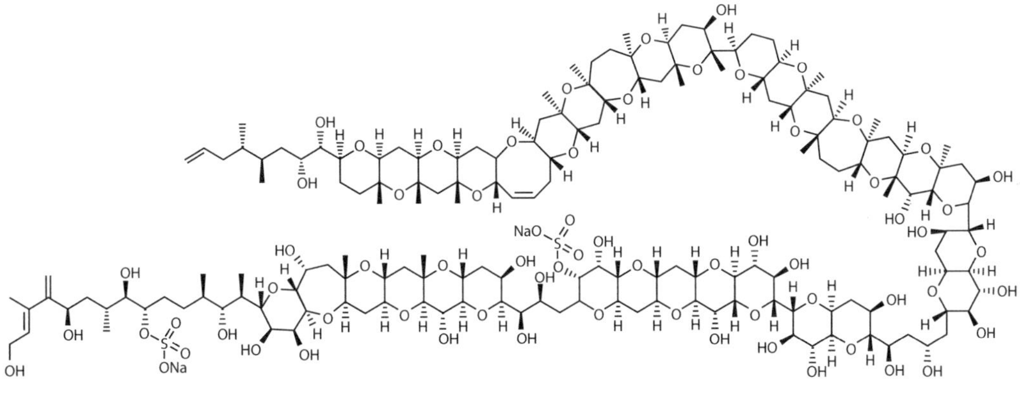

FIGURE 17.19
Structure of MTX.

Acknowledgments

This work was supported by the Ministry of Science and Innovation of Spain AGL2009-13581-C02-02, PHARMATLANTIC 2009-1/117.

References

Aasen, J.A.B., W. Hardstaff, T. Aune, and M.A. Quilliam. 2006. Discovery of fatty acid ester metabolites of spirolide toxins in mussels from Norway using liquid chromatography/tandem mass spectrometry. *Rapid Communications in Mass Spectrometry*, 20 (10): 1531–1537.

Aguilera-Belmonte, A., I. Inostroza, J. Franco, P. Riobo, and P.I. Gómez. 2011. The growth, toxicity and genetic characterization of seven strains of *Alexandrium catenella* (Whedon and Kofoid) Balech. 1985 (Dinophyceae) isolated during the 2009 summer outbreak in southern Chile. *Harmful Algae*, 12: 105–112.

Alfonso, A. and C. Alfonso. 2008. Yessotoxins, pharmacology and mechanism of action: Biological detection. In *Seafood and Freshwater Toxins. Pharmacology, Physiology and Detection*, ed. L.M. Botana, pp. 315–327. Boca Raton, FL: Taylor & Francis Group.

Alfonso, C., A. Alfonso, P. Otero et al. 2008. Purification of five azaspiracids from mussel samples contaminated with DSP toxins and azaspiracids. *Journal of Chromatography B*, 865 (1–2): 133–140.

Alfonso, C., A. Alfonso, M.J. Pazos et al. 2007. Extraction and cleaning methods to detect yessotoxins in contaminated mussels. *Analytical Biochemistry*, 363 (2): 228–328.

Alfonso, A., Y. Román, M.R. Vieytes et al. 2005. Azaspiracid-4 inhibits Ca^{2+} entry by stored operated channels in human T lymphocytes. *Biochemical Pharmacology*, 69 (11): 1627–1636.

Alfonso, A., L.A. de la Rosa, M.R. Vieytes, T. Yasumoto, and L.M. Botana. 2003. Yessotoxin a novel phycotoxin, activates phosphodiesterase activity. Effect of yessotoxin on cAMP levels in human lymphocytes. *Biochemical Pharmacology*, 65: 193–208.

Alfonso, A., M.R. Vieytes, K. Ofuji et al. 2006. Azaspiracids modulate intracellular pH levels in human lymphocytes. *Biochemical and Biophysical Research Communications*, 346 (3): 1091–1099.

Aligizaki, K. and G. Nikolaidis. 2008. Morphological identification of two tropical dinoflagellates of the genera *Gambierdiscus* and *Sinophysis* in the Mediterranean Sea. *Journal of Biological Research-Thessaloniki*, 9: 75–82.

Alvarez, G., E. Uribe, P. Avalos, C. Marino, and J. Blanco. 2010. First identification of azaspiracid and spirolides in *Mesodesma donacium* and *Mulinia edulis* from Northern Chile. *Toxicon*, 55 (2–3): 638–641.

Alvarez, G., E. Uribe, R. Diaz et al. 2011. Bloom of the Yessotoxin producing dinoflagellate *Protoceratium reticulatum* (Dinophyceae) in Northern Chile. *Journal of Sea Research*, 65 (4): 427–434.

Alvarez, G., E. Uribe, A. Vidal et al. 2009. Paralytic shellfish toxins in *Argopecten purpuratus* and *Semimytilus algosus* from northern Chile. *Aquatic Living Resources*, 22 (3): 341–347.

Amzil, Z., M. Sibat, F. Royer, N. Masson, and E. Abadie. 2007. Report on the first detection of pectenotoxin-2, spirolide-a and their derivatives in French shellfish. *Marine Drugs*, 5 (4): 168–179.

Ares, I.R., M.C. Louzao, M.R. Vieytes, T. Yasumoto, and L.M. Botana. 2005. Actin cytoskeleton of rabbit intestinal cells is a target for potent marine phycotoxins. *Journal of Experimental Biology*, 208 (Pt 22): 4345–4354.

Armi, Z., A. Milandri, S. Turki, and B. Hajjem. 2011. *Alexandrium catenella* and *Alexandrium tamarense* in the North Lake of Tunis: Bloom characteristics and the occurrence of Paralytic Shellfish Toxin. *African Journal of Aquatic Science*, 36 (1): 47–56.

Aune, T., R. Sorby, T. Yasumoto, H. Ramstad, and T. Landsverk. 2002. Comparison of oral and intraperitoneal toxicity of yessotoxin towards mice. *Toxicon*, 40 (1): 77–82.

Aversano, C.D., P. Hess, and M.A. Quilliam. 2005. Hydrophobic interaction liquid chromatography-mass spectrometry for the analysis of paralytic shellfish poisoning (PSP) toxins. *Journal of Chromatography A*, 1081: 190–201.

Baden, D.G., A.J. Bourdelais, H. Jacocks, S. Michelliza, and J. Naar. 2005. Natural and derivative brevetoxins: Historical background, multiplicity, and effects. *Environmental Health Perspectives*, 113 (5): 621–625.

Beaumont, S., E.A. Ilardi, N.D.C. Tappin, and A. Zakarian. 2010. Marine toxins with spiroimine rings: Total synthesis of pinnatoxin A. *European Journal of Organic Chemistry*, 2010 (30): 5743–5765.

Bellocci, M., G.L. Sala, F. Callegari, and G.P. Rossini. 2010. Azaspiracid-1 inhibits endocytosis of plasma membrane proteins in epithelial cells. *Toxicological Sciences*, 117 (1): 109–121.

Bentur, Y., J. Ashkar, Y. Lurie et al. 2008. Lessepsian migration and tetrodotoxin poisoning due to *Lagocephalus sceleratus* in the eastern Mediterranean. *Toxicon*, 52: 964–968.

Berde, C.B., U. Athiraman, B. Yahalom et al. 2011. Tetrodotoxin-bupivacaine-epinephrine combinations for prolonged local anesthesia. *Marine Drugs*, 9 (12): 2717–2728.

Bire, R., S. Krys, J.M. Fremy et al. 2002. First evidence on occurrence of gymnodimine in clams from Tunisia. *Journal of Natural Toxins*, 11 (4): 269–275.

Blanco, J., G. Alvarez, and E. Uribe. 2007. Identification of pectenotoxins in plankton, filter feeders, and isolated cells of a *Dinophysis acuminata* with an atypical toxin profile, from Chile. *Toxicon*, 49 (5): 710–716.

Botana, L.M. 2000. *Seafood and Freshwater Toxins. Pharmacology, Physiology and Detection.* New York: Marcel & Dekker.

Botana, L.M. 2008. *Seafood and Freshwater Toxins. Pharmacology, Physiology and Detection.* Boca Raton, FL: CRC Press/Taylor & Francis Group.

Botana, L.M., A. Alfonso, M.R. Vieytes, and M.I. Loza-García. 2008. Therapeutic use of yessotoxins as human tumor cell growth inhibitors, European Patent application EP1875906.

Bourne, Y., Z. Radic, R. Aráoz et al. 2010. Structural determinants in phycotoxins and AChBP conferring high affinity binding and nicotinic AChR antagonism. *Proceedings of the National Academy of Sciences*, 107 (13): 6076–6081.

Bragadeeswaran, S., D. Therasa, K. Prabhu, and K. Kathiresan. 2010. Biomedical and pharmacological potential of tetrodotoxin-producing bacteria isolated from marine pufferfish *Arothron hispidus* (Muller, 1841). *Journal of Venomous Animals and Toxins Including Tropical Diseases*, 16 (3): 421–431.

Briggs, L.R., C.O. Miles, J.M. Fitzgerald et al. 2004. Enzyme-linked immunosorbent assay for the detection of yessotoxin and its analogues. *Journal of Agricultural and Food Chemistry*, 52 (19): 5836–5842.

Burgess, V. and G. Shaw. 2001. Pectenotoxins—An issue for public health—A review of their comparative toxicology and metabolism. *Environment International*, 27 (4): 275–283.

Burrel, S., T. Gunnarsson, K. Gunnarsson, D. Clarke, and A. Turner. 2011. First report of paralytic shellfish poisoning toxins in blue mussels (*M. edulis*) from Breidafjord and Eyjafjord, Iceland. Poster in *Marine and freshwater toxins analyses: Second Joint Symposium and AOAC Task Force Meeting*, May 2011, Baiona, Spain.

Cabado, A.G., F. Leira, J.M. Vieites, M. Vieytes, and L.M. Botana. 2003. Caspase-8 activation initiates okadaic acid-induced apoptosis in neuroblastoma. In *Molluscan Shellfish Safety*, eds. A. Villalba, B. Reguera, J.L. Romalde, and R. Beiras, pp. 107–117. Santiago de Compostela, Spain: Consellería de Pesca e Asuntos Marítimos da Xunta de Galicia and Intergovernmental Oceanographic Commission of UNESCO.

Cabado, A.G., F. Leira, M. Vieytes, J.M. Vieites, and L.M. Botana. 2004. Cytoskeletal disruption is the key factor that triggers apoptosis in okadaic acid-treated neuroblastoma cells. *Archives of Toxicology*, 78: 74–85.

Caillaud, A., E. Canete, P. de la Iglesia, G. Gimenez, and J. Diogene. 2009. Cell-based assay coupled with chromatographic fractioning: A strategy for marine toxins detection in natural samples. *Toxicology in Vitro*, 23 (8): 1591–1596.

Caillaud, A., P. de la Iglesia, H.T. Darius et al. 2010. Update on methodologies available for ciguatoxin determination: Perspectives to confront the onset of Ciguatera fish poisoning in Europe. *Marine Drugs*, 8: 1838–1907.

Callegari, F., S. Sosa, S. Ferrari et al. 2006. Oral administration of yessotoxin stabilizes E-cadherin in mouse colon. *Toxicology*, 227: 145–155.

Cao, Z., K.T. LePage, M.O. Frederick, K.C. Nicolaou, and T.F. Murray. 2010. Involvement of caspase activation in azaspiracid-induced neurotoxicity in neocortical neurons. *Toxicological Sciences*, 114 (2): 323–334.

Catteral, W., S. Cestéle, V. Yarov-Yarovoy et al. 2007. Voltage-gated ion channels and gating modifier toxins. *Toxicon*, 49: 124–141.

Cembella, A. and B. Krock. 2008. Cyclic imine toxins: Chemistry, biogeography, biosynthesis and pharmacology. In *Seafood and Freshwaters Toxins: Pharmacology, Physiology and Detection*, ed. L.M. Botana, pp. 561–580. Boca Raton, FL: CRC Press/Taylor & Francis Group.

Ciminiello, P., C. Dell'Aversano, E. Dello Iacovo et al. 2009. Stereostructure and Biological activity of 42-hydroxy-palytoxin: A new palytoxin analogue from Hawaiian *Palythoa* subspecies. *Chemical Research in Toxicology*, 22 (11): 1851–1859.

Ciminiello, P., C. Dell'Aversano, E. Fattorusso et al. 2006a. The Genoa 2005 outbreak. Determination of putative palytoxin in Mediterranean *Ostreopsis ovata* by a new liquid chromatography tandem mass spectrometry method. *Analytical Chemistry*, 78 (17): 6153–6159.

Ciminiello, P., C. Dell'Aversano, E. Fattorusso et al. 2006b. Toxin profile of *Alexandrium ostenfeldii* (Dinophyceae) from the Northern Adriatic Sea revealed by liquid chromatography-mass spectrometry. *Toxicon*, 47 (5): 597–604.

Ciminiello, P., C. Dell'Aversano, E. Fattorusso et al. 2007. Spirolide toxin profile of Adriatic *Alexandrium ostenfeldii* cultures and structure elucidation of 27-hydroxy-13,19-didesmethyl spirolide C. *Journal of Natural Products*, 70 (12): 1878–1883.

Ciminiello, P., C. Dell'Aversano, E. Fattorusso et al. 2010a. Complex toxin profile of *Mytilus galloprovincialis* from the Adriatic sea revealed by LC-MS. *Toxicon*, 55 (2–3): 280–288.

Ciminiello, P., C. Dell'Aversano, E.D. Iacovo et al. 2010b. Characterization of 27-hydroxy-13-desmethyl spirolide C and 27-oxo-13,19-didesmethyl spirolide C. Further insights into the complex Adriatic *Alexandrium ostenfeldii* toxin profile. *Toxicon*, 56 (8): 1327–1333.

Ciminiello, P. and E. Fattorusso. 2008. Yessotoxins, chemistry, metabolism and chemical analysis. In *Seafood and Freshwater Toxins. Pharmacology, Physiology and Detection*, ed. L.M. Botana, pp. 287–314. Boca Raton, FL: CRC Press/Taylor & Francis Group.

Craik, D.J. and M.J. Scanlon. 2000. New toxins, new drugs. In: *Seafood and Freshwater Toxins. Pharmacology, Physiology and Detection*, ed. L.M. Botana, pp. 715–740. New York: Marcel Dekker, Inc.

Custovic, S., S. Orhanovic, Z. Nincevic-Gladan, T. Josipovic, and M. Pavela-Vrancic. 2009. Occurrence of yessotoxin (YTX) in the coastal waters of the eastern-mid Adriatic Sea (Croatia). *Fresenius Environmental Bulletin*, 18 (8): 1452–1455.

Cha, J.K., W.J. Christ, J.M. Finan et al. 1982. Stereochemistry of palytoxin.4. Complete structure. *Journal of the American Chemical Society*, 104 (25): 7369–7371.

Chau, R., J.A. Kalaitzis, and B.A. Neilan. 2011. On the origins and biosynthesis of tetrodotoxin. *Aquatic Toxicology*, 104 (1–2): 61–72.

Dahl, J. and S. Moiniche. 2009. Relief of postoperative pain by local anaesthetic infiltration: Efficacy for major abdominal and orthopedic surgery. *Pain*, 143: 7–11.

Davis, C.C. 1948. *Gymnodinium brevis* Sp Nov a cause of discolored water and animal mortality in the Gulf of Mexico. *Botanical Gazette*, 109 (3): 358–360.

De la Rosa, L.A., A. Alfonso, N. Vilariño et al. 2001a. Maitotoxin-induced calcium entry in human lymphocytes. Modulation by yessotoxin, Ca^{2+} channel blockers and kinases. *Cell Signal*, 13 (10): 711–716.

De la Rosa, L.A., A. Alfonso, N. Vilariño, M.R. Vieytes, and L.M. Botana. 2001b. Modulation of cytosolic calcium levels of human lymphocytes by yessotoxin, a novel marine phycotoxin. *Biochemical Pharmacology*, 61 (7): 827–833.

Dominguez, H.J., B. Paz, A.H. Daranas et al. 2010. Dinoflagellate polyether within the yessotoxin, pectenotoxin and okadaic acid toxin groups: Characterization, analysis and human health implications. *Toxicon*, 56 (2): 191–217.

EFSA. 2008a. Opinion of the Scientific Panel on Contaminants in the Food chain on a request from the European Commission on marine biotoxins in shellfish—Yessotoxin group. *The EFSA Journal*, 907: 1–62.

EFSA. 2008b. Opinion of the Scientific Panel on Contaminants in the Food chain on a request from the European Commission on marine biotoxins in shellfish—Azaspiracids. *The EFSA Journal*, 723: 1–52.

EFSA. 2010. Panel on Contaminants in the Food chain (CONTAM); Scientific opinion on marine biotoxins in shellfish—Emerging toxins: Brevetoxin group. *The EFSA Journal*, 8 (7): 1–29.

EFSA, E.F.S.A. 2009. Marine biotoxins in shellfish-Saxitoxin group. Scientific opinion of the Panel on Contaminants in the Food Chain. *The EFSA Journal*, 1019: 1–46.

Espiña, B. and J.A. Rubiolo. 2008. Marine toxins and the cytoskeleton: Pectenotoxins, unusual macrolides that disrupt actin. *FEBS Journal*, 275 (24): 6082–6088.

Estacion, M. and W.P. Schilling. 2001. Maitotoxin-induced membrane blebbing and cell death in bovine aortic endothelial cells. *BMC Physiology*, 1: 2.

Etheridge, S.M. 2010. Paralytic shellfish poisoning: Seafood safety and human health perspectives. *Toxicon*, 56: 108–122.

EURLMB. 2009. EU harmonised standard operating procedure for detection of lipophilic toxins by mouse bioassay, pp. 1–14. European Union Reference Laboratory for Marine Biotoxins, http://www.aesan.msssi.gob.es/CRLMB/docs/docs/metodos_analiticos_de_desarrollo/EU-Harmonised-SOP-MBA-Lipophilic-Version5-June2009.pdf

European Parliament. 2004. Regulation (EC) No 853/2004 of the European parliament and of the council of 29 April 2004 laying down specific hygiene rules for on the hygiene of foodstuffs. *Official Journal of the European Union*, L139: 55–205.

FAO. 2004. Marine biotoxins. Food and Nutrition Paper 80. Available from http://www.fao.org/docrep/007/y5486e/y5486e00.HTM

Flanagan, A.F., K.R. Callanan, J. Donlon et al. 2001. A cytotoxicity assay for the detection and differentiation of two families of shellfish toxins. *Toxicon*, 39 (7): 1021–1027.

Flanagan, A.F., M. Kane, J. Donlon, and R. Palmer. 1999. Azaspiracid, detection of a newly discovered phycotoxin in vitro. *Journal of Shellfish Research*, 18 (2): 716.

Fleming, L.E., B. Kirkpatrick, L.C. Backer et al. 2011. Review of Florida red tide and human health effects. *Harmful Algae*, 10: 224–233.

Franchini, A., D. Malagoli, and E. Ottaviani. 2010. Targets and effects of yessotoxin, okadaic acid and palytoxin: A differential review. *Marine Drugs*, 8 (3): 658–677.

Furey, A., S. O'Doherty, K. O'Callaghan, M. Lehane, and K.J. James. 2010. Azaspiracid poisoning (AZP) toxins in shellfish: Toxicological and health considerations. *Toxicon*, 56 (2): 173–190.

Gerssen, A., M.A. McElhinney, P.P.J. Mulder et al. 2009. Solid phase extraction for removal of matrix effects in lipophilic marine toxin analysis by liquid chromatography-tandem mass spectrometry. *Analytical and Bioanalytical Chemistry*, 394 (4): 1213–1226.

Gessner, B.D. and B. McLaughlin. 2008. Epidemiologic impact of toxic episodes: Neurotoxic toxins. In *Seafood and Freshwater Toxins. Pharmacology, Physiology and Detection*, ed. L.M. Botana, pp. 77–103. Boca Raton, FL: CRC Press/Taylor & Francis Group.

Gill, S., M. Murphy, J. Clausen et al. 2003. Neural injury biomarkers of novel shellfish toxins, Spirolides: A pilot study using immunochemical and transcriptional analysis. *Neurotoxicology*, 24 (4–5): 593–604.

Gouveia, N., J. Delgado, N. Gouveira, and P. Vale. 2009. Primeiro rexistro da ocorrência de episódios do tipo ciguatérico no arquipélago da Madeira. *Algas tóxicas e biotoxinas nas águas da Península Ibérica -2009: actas da X Reunião Ibérica Fitoplâncton Tóxico e Biotoxinas*, ed. P.R. Costa, M.J. Botelho, S.M. Rodrigues, A.S. Palma, M.T. Moita, pp. 152–157, IPIMAR, Lisboa, Portugal, May 12–15, 2009.

Gueret, S.M. and M.A. Brimble. 2010. Spiroimine shellfish poisoning (SSP) and the spirolide family of shellfish toxins: Isolation, structure, biological activity and synthesis. *Natural Product Reports*, 27 (9): 1350–1366.

Guerrini, F., L. Pezzolesi, A. Feller et al. 2010. Comparative growth and toxin profile of cultured *Ostreopsis ovata* from the Tyrrhenian and Adriatic Seas. *Toxicon*, 55: 211–220.

Gunter, G., F.G.W. Smith, and R.H. Williams. 1947. Mass mortality of marine animals on the lower west coast of Florida, November 1946–January 1947. *Science*, 105 (2723): 256–257.

Halai, R. and D.J. Craik. 2009. Conotoxins: Natural product drug leads. *Natural Products Report*, 26: 526–536.

Hall, S., G.R. Strichartz, E. Moczydlowski, A. Ravindran, and P.B. Reichardt. 1990. The saxitoxins: Sources, chemistry and pharmacology. In *Marine Toxins*, eds. S. Hall and G.R. Strichartz, pp. 29–65, ACS Symposium Series. Washington, DC: American Chemical Society.

Hamano, K., K. Sasaki, J. Masaki et al. 2001. Effect of maitotoxin on the acrosome reaction in bull spermatozoa. *Journal of Reproduction and Development*, 47 (5): 295–302.

Hamilton, B., M. Hurbungs, J.P. Vernoux, A. Jones, and R.J. Lewis. 2002. Isolation and characterisation of Indian Ocean ciguatoxin. *Toxicon*, 40 (6): 685–693.

Hasan, S., M.M. Rahman, T. Hossain et al. 2007. Purification, characterization and toxic profile of two toxins isolated from puffer fish *Tetraodon patoca*, available in Bangladesh. *Pakistan Journal of Biological Sciences*, 10 (5): 773–777.

He, Y., A. Fekete, G.N. Chen et al. 2010. Analytical approaches for an important shellfish poisoning agent: Domoic acid. *Journal of Agricultural and Food Chemistry*, 58 (22): 11525–11533.

Hess, P., T. McMahon, N. Rehmann et al. 2007. Isolation and purification of azaspiracids from naturally contaminated materials and evaluation of their toxicological effects. Final project report. Galway, Ireland: Marine Institute.

Hilderbrand, S.C., R.N. Murrell, J.E. Gibson, and J.M. Brown. 2010. Marine brevetoxin induces IgE-independent mast cell activation. *Archives of Toxicology*, 85 (2): 135–141.

Hirama, M. 2005. Total synthesis of ciguatoxin CTX3C: A venture into the problems of ciguatera seafood poisoning. *Chemical Record*, 5 (4): 240–250.

Hirata, Y. and D. Uemura. 1985. Toxic compounds of *Palythoa tuberculosa* (Coelenterata), palytoxin and its analogs. *Yakugaku Zasshi-Journal of the Pharmaceutical Society of Japan*, 105 (1): 1–10.

Hu, T.M., J.M. Curtis, Y. Oshima et al. 1995. Spirolide-B and Spirolide-D, two novel macrocycles isolated from the digestive glands of shellfish. *Journal of the Chemical Society-Chemical Communications*, (20): 2159–2161.

Hu, T.M., J. Doyle, D. Jackson et al. 1992a. Isolation of a new Diarrhetic shellfish poison from Irish mussels. *Journal of the Chemical Society-Chemical Communications*, 1: 39–41.

Hu, T.M., A.S.W. de Freitas, J.M. Curtis et al. 1996. Isolation and structure of prorocentrolide B, a fast-acting toxin from *Prorocentrum maculosum*. *Journal of Natural Products*, 59 (11): 1010–1014.

Hu, S. and C. Kao. 1991. Interactions of neosaxitoxin with the sodium-channel of the frog skeletal-muscle fiber. *Journal of General Physiology*, 97 (3): 561–578.

Hu, T.M., J. Marr, A.S.W. Defreitas et al. 1992b. New diol esters isolated from cultures of the dino-flagellates *Prorocentrum lima* and *Prorocentrum concavum*. *Journal of Natural Products*, 55 (11): 1631–1637.

de la Iglesia, P. and A. Gago-Martinez. 2009. Determination of yessotoxins and pectenotoxins in shellfish by capillary electrophoresis-electrospray ionization-mass spectrometry. *Food Additives and Contaminants: Part A Chemistry, Analysis, Control, Exposure, and Risk Assessment*, 26 (2): 221–228.

Imada, C. 2005. Enzyme inhibitors and other bioactive compounds from marine actinomycetes. *Antonie van Leeuwenhoek, International Journal of General and Molecular Microbiology*, 87 (1): 59–63.

Inoue, M., M. Hirama, M. Satake, K. Sugiyama, and T. Yasumoto. 2003. Inhibition of brevetoxins binding to the voltage-gated sodium channel by gambierol and gambieric acid-A. *Toxicon*, 41: 469–474.

Inoue, M., K. Miyazaki, H. Uehara, M. Maruyama, and M. Hirama. 2004. First- and second-generation total synthesis of ciguatoxin CTX3C. *Proceedings of the National Academy of Sciences of the United States of America*, 101 (33): 12013–12018.

Ito, A., M. Satake, K. Ofuji et al. 2000. Small intestine injuries in mice caused by a new toxin, azaspiracid, isolated from Irish mussels, pp. 395–398. *Ninth International Conference on Harmful Algal Blooms*, Hobart, Tasmania, Australia.

Ito, E., M. Satake, K. Ofuji et al. 2002. Chronic effects in mice caused by oral administration of sublethal doses of azaspiracid, a new marine toxin isolated from mussels. *Toxicon*, 40 (2): 193–203.

Ito, A., K. Terao, T. McMahon, J. Silke, and T. Yasumoto. 1998. Acute pathological changes in mice caused by crude extracts of novel toxins isolated from Irish mussels. In *Harmful Algae*, eds. B. Reguera, J. Blanco, M.L. Fernandez, and T. Wyatt, pp. 588–589. Santiago de Compostela, Spain: Xunta de Galicia and Intergovernmental Oceanographic Commission of UNESCO.

James, K.J., C. Moroney, C. Roden et al. 2003. Ubiquitous 'benign' alga emerges as the cause of shellfish contamination responsible for the human toxic syndrome, azaspiracid poisoning. *Toxicon*, 41: 145–151.

Jeffery, B., T. Barlow, K. Moizer, S. Paul, and C. Boyle. 2004. Amnesic shellfish poison. *Food and Chemical Toxicology*, 42 (4): 545–557.

Kat, M. 1983a. *Dinophysis acuminata* blooms in the Dutch coastal area related to diarrhetic mussel poisoning in the Dutch Waddensea. *Sarsia*, 68 (1): 81–84.

Kat, M. 1983b. Diarrhetic mussel poisoning in the Netherlands related to the dinoflagellate *Dinophysis acuminata*. *Antonie Van Leeuwenhoek. Journal of Microbiology*, 49 (4–5): 417–427.

Kellmann, R., T.K. Michali, and B.A. Neilan. 2008. Identification of a saxitoxin biosynthesis gene with a history of frequent horizontal gene transfers. *Journal of Molecular Evolution*, 67 (5): 526–538.

Kellmann, R., C.A.M. Schaffner, T.A. Gronset et al. 2009. Proteomic response of human neuroblastoma cells to azaspiracid-1. *Journal of Proteomics*, 72 (4): 695–707.

Kharrat, R., D. Servent, E. Girard et al. 2008. The marine phycotoxin gymnodimine targets muscular and neuronal nicotinic acetylcholine receptor subtypes with high affinity. *Journal of Neurochemistry*, 107 (4): 952–963.

Kirkpatrick, B., J.A. Bean, L.E. Fleming et al. 2010. Gastrointestinal emergency room admissions and Florida red tide blooms. *Harmful Algae*, 9 (1): 82–86.

Kodama, M., T. Ogata, S. Sakamoto et al. 1990. Production of paralytic shellfish toxins by a bacterium *Moraxella* sp. isolated from *Protogonyaulax tamarensis*. *Toxicon*, 28: 707–714.

Korsnes, M.S. and A. Espenes. 2011. Yessotoxin as an apoptotic inducer. *Toxicon*, 57 (7–8): 947–958.

Krock, B., C.G. Seguel, K. Valderrama, and U. Tillmann. 2009a. Pectenotoxins and yessotoxin from Arica Bay, North Chile as determined by tandem mass spectrometry. *Toxicon*, 54 (3): 364–367.

Krock, B., U. Tillmann, U. John, and A.D. Cembella. 2009b. Characterization of azaspiracids in plankton size-fractions and isolation of an azaspiracid-producing dinoflagellate from the North Sea. *Harmful Algae*, 8 (2): 254–263.

Kulagina, N.V., T.J. O'Shaughnessy, W. Ma, J.S. Ramsdell, and J.J. Pancrazio. 2004. Pharmacological effects of the marine toxins, brevetoxin and saxitoxin, on murine frontal cortex neuronal networks. *Toxicon*, 44 (6): 669–676.

Lago, J., F. Santaclara, J.M. Vieites, and A.G. Cabado. 2005. Collapse of mitochondrial membrane potential and caspases activation are early events in okadaic acid-treated Caco-2 cells. *Toxicon*, 46 (5): 579–586.

Lamas, C., I. Valverde, J. Lago, J.M. Vieites, and A.G. Cabado. 2006a. In vitro evaluation of apoptotic markers triggered by PTX-2 in Caco-2 and neuroblastoma cells. *Egyptian Journal of Natural Toxins*, 3: 17–33.

Lamas, C., I. Valverde, J. Lago, J.M. Vieites, and A.G. Cabado. 2006b. Comparison between cytotoxic effects induced by PTX-2 in vitro in two human cell lines. *Egyptian Journal of Natural Toxins*, 3: 1–16.

Landsberg, J.H. 2002. The effects of harmful algal blooms on aquatic organisms. *Reviews in Fisheries Science*, 10 (2): 113–390.

Lassus, P., Z. Amzil, R. Baron et al. 2007. Modelling the accumulation of PSP toxins in Thau Lagoon oysters (*Crassostrea gigas*) from trials using mixed cultures of *Alexandrium catenella* and *Thalassiosira weissflogii*. *Aquatic Living Resources*, 20 (1): 59–67.

Laycock, M.V., P. Thibault, S.W. Ayer, and J.A. Walter. 1994. Isolation and purification procedures for the preparation of paralytic shellfish poisoning toxin standards. *Natural Toxins*, 2: 175–183.

Lee, K.J., J.S. Mok, K.C. Song et al. 2011. Geographical and annual variation in lipophilic shellfish toxins from oysters and mussels along the south coast of Korea. *Journal of Food Protection*, 74 (12): 2127–2133.

Lee, C.H. and P.C. Ruben. 2008. Interaction between voltage-gated sodium channels and the neuro-toxin, tetrodotoxin. *Channels*, 2: 407–412.

Lefebvre, K.A., S. Bargu, T. Kieckhefer, and M.W. Silver. 2002. From sanddabs to blue whales: The pervasiveness of domoic acid. *Toxicon*, 40 (7): 971–977.

Lefebvre, K.A. and A. Robertson. 2010. Domoic acid and human exposure risks: A review. *Toxicon*, 56 (2): 218–230.

Leira, F., C. Alvarez, A.G. Cabado et al. 2003. Development of a F-actin-based live-cell fluorimetric microplate assay for diarrhetic shellfish toxins. *Analytical Biochemistry*, 317: 129–135.

Leira, F., C. Alvarez, J.M. Vieites, M.R. Vieytes, and L.M. Botana. 2002. Characterization of distinct apoptotic changes induced by okadaic acid and yessotoxin in the BE(2)-M17 neuroblastoma cell line. *Toxicology in Vitro*, 16 (1): 23–31.

Lekan, D.K. and C.R. Tomas. 2010. The brevetoxin and brevenal composition of three *Karenia brevis* clones at different salinities and nutrient conditions. *Harmful Algae*, 9 (1): 39–47.

Lewis, R.J., J. Molgó, and D.J. Adams. 2000. Ciguatera toxins: Pharmacology of toxins involved in ciguatera and related fish poisonings. In *Seafood and Freshwater Toxins. Pharmacology, Physiology and Detection*, ed. L.M. Botana, pp. 419–447. New York: Marcel Dekker.

Litaker, R.W., M.W. Vandersea, M.A. Faust et al. 2009. Taxonomy of Gambierdiscus including four new species, *Gambierdiscus caribaeus, Gambierdiscus carolinianus, Gambierdiscus carpenteri* and *Gambierdiscus ruetzleri* (Gonyaulacales, Dinophyceae). *Phycologia*, 48 (5): 344–390.

Litaker, R.W., M.W. Vandersea, M.A. Faust et al. 2010. Global distribution of ciguatera causing dino-flagellates in the genus *Gambierdiscus*. *Toxicon*, 56: 711–730.

Loader, J.I., A.D. Hawkes, V. Beuzenberg et al. 2007. Convenient large-scale purification of yesso-toxin from *Protoceratium reticulatum* culture and isolation of a novel furanoyessotoxin. *Journal of Agricultural and Food Chemistry*, 55 (26): 11093–11100.

López-Rivera, A., K. O'Callaghan, M. Moriarty et al. 2009. First evidence of azaspiracids (AZAs): A family of lipophilic polyether marine toxins in scallops (*Argopecten purpuratus*) and mussels (*Mytilus chilensis*) collected in two regions of Chile. *Toxicon*, 55 (4): 692–701.

Louzao, M.C., I.R. Ares, E. Cagide et al. 2011. Palytoxins and cytoskeleton: An overview. *Toxicon*, 57 (3): 460–469.

Lu, C.-K., G.-H. Lee, R. Huang, and H.-N. Chou. 2001. Spiro-prorocentrimine, a novel macrocyclic lactone from a benthic *Prorocentrum* sp. of Taiwan. *Tetrahedron Letters*, 42 (9): 1713–1716.

MacKinnon, S.L., J.A. Walter, M.A. Quilliam et al. 2006. Spirolides isolated from Danish strains of the toxigenic dinoflagellate *Alexandrium ostenfeldii*. *Journal of Natural Products*, 69 (7): 983–987.

Marrouchi, R., F. Dziri, N. Belayouni et al. 2009. Quantitative determination of gymnodimine-A by high performance liquid chromatography in contaminated clams from Tunisia Coastline. *Marine Biotechnology*, 12 (5): 579–585.

Matsumoto, T., Y. Nagashima, H. Kusuhara et al. 2008. Pharmacokinetics of tetrodotoxin in puffer fish *Takifugu rubripes* by a single administration technique. *Toxicon*, 51: 1051–1059.

Mayer, A.M.S. 2000. The marine toxin domoic acid may affect the developing brain by activation of neonatal brain microglia and subsequent neurotoxic mediator generation. *Medical Hypotheses*, 54 (5): 837–841.

McCauley, L.A.R., D.L. Erdner, S. Nagai, M.L. Richlen, and D.M. Anderson. 2009. Biogeographic analysis of the globally distributed harmful algal bloom species *Alexandrium minutum* (Dinophyceae) based on rRNA gene sequences and microsatellite markers. *Journal of Phycology*, 45 (2): 454–463.

McFarren, E.F., H. Tanabe, F. Silva et al. 1965. The occurrence of a ciguatera-like poison in oysters, clams, and *Gymnodinium breve* cultures. *Toxicon*, 3: 111.

Miles, C.O., T. Rundberget, M. Sandvik, J. Aasen, and A. Selwood. 2010. The presence of pinnatoxins in Norwegian mussels. *National Veterinary Institute's Report Series*, 07b: 1–9.

Miles, C.O., A.L. Wilkins, A.D. Hawkes et al. 2004. Isolation of a 1,3-enone isomer of heptanor-41-oxoyessotoxin from *Protoceratium reticulatum* cultures. *Toxicon*, 44 (3): 325–336.

Miles, C.O., A.L. Wilkins, A.D. Hawkes et al. 2005. Polyhydroxylated amide analogs of yessotoxin from *Protoceratium reticulatum*. *Toxicon*, 45 (1): 61–71.

Miles, C.O., A.L. Wilkins, A.D. Hawkes et al. 2006. Isolation and identification of pectenotoxins-13 and -14 from *Dinophysis acuta* in New Zealand. *Toxicon*, 48 (2): 152–159.

Moore, R.E. and G. Bartolini. 1981. Structure of palytoxin. *Journal of the American Chemical Society*, 103 (9): 2491–2494.

Moore, R.E. and P.J. Scheuer. 1971. Palytoxin—New marine toxin from a coelenterate. *Science*, 172 (3982): 495–498.

Mos, L. 2001. Domoic acid: A fascinating marine toxin. *Environmental Toxicology and Pharmacology*, 9 (3): 79–85.

Murata, M., M. Kumagai, J.S. Lee, and T. Yasumoto. 1987. Isolation and structure of yessotoxin, a novel polyether compound implicated in diarrhetic shellfish poisoning. *Tetrahedron Letters*, 28: 5869–5872.

Murata, M., H. Naoki, S. Matsunaga, M. Satake, and T. Yasumoto. 1994. Structure and partial stereochemical assignments for maitotoxin, the most toxic and largest natural non-biopolymer. *Journal of the American Chemical Society*, 116 (16): 7098–7107.

Murata, M., M. Shimatani, H. Sugitani, Y. Oshima, and T. Yasumoto. 1982. Isolation and structural elucidation of the causative toxin of the diarrhetic shellfish poisoning. *Bulletin of the Japanese Society of Scientific Fisheries*, 48 (4): 549–552.

Murrell, R.N. and J.E. Gibson. 2009. Brevetoxins 2, 3, 6, and 9 show variability in potency and cause significant induction of DNA damage and apoptosis in Jurkat E6–1 cells. *Archives of Toxicology*, 83 (11): 1009–1019.

Nam, D.H., D.H. Adams, L.J. Flewelling, and N. Basu. 2010. Neurochemical alterations in lemon shark (*Negaprion brevirostris*) brains in association with brevetoxin exposure. *Aquatic Toxicology*, 99 (3): 351–359.

Negri, A.P., C.J.S. Bolch, S. Geier et al. 2007. Widespread presence of hydrophobic paralytic shellfish toxins in *Gymnodinium catenatum*. *Harmful Algae*, 6 (6): 774–780.

Ngy, L., K. Tada, C.F. Yu, T. Takatani, and O. Arakawa. 2008. Occurrence of paralytic shellfish toxins in Cambodian Mekong pufferfish *Tetraodon turgidus*: Selective toxin accumulation in the skin. *Toxicon*, 51 (2): 280–288.

Nieto, F.R., J.M. Entrena, C.M. Cendana et al. 2007. Tetrodotoxin (TTX) inhibits the development and expression of neuropathic pain induced by paclitaxel in mice. *Pain*, 137: 520–531.

NRC-CNRC. 2011. Certified Reference Materials Program. National Research Council Canada. http://www.nrc-cnrc.gc.ca/eng/programs/imb/crmp.html (accessed January 31, 2012).

Ofuji, K., M. Satake, T. McMahon et al. 1999. Two analogs of azaspiracid isolated from mussels, *Mytilus edulis*, involved in human intoxication in Ireland. *Natural Toxins*, 7 (3): 99–102.

Ogino, H., M. Kumagai, and T. Yasumoto. 1997. Toxicological evaluation of yessotoxin. *Natural Toxins*, 5: 255–259.

Oku, N., N.U. Sata, S. Matsunaga, H. Uchida, and N. Fusetani. 2004. Identification of palytoxin as a principle which causes morphological changes in rat 3Y1 cells in the zoanthid *Palythoa aff. margaritae*. *Toxicon*, 43 (1): 21–25.

Oshima, Y. 1995. Postcolumn derivatization liquid chromatographic method for paralytic shellfish toxins. *Journal of AOAC International*, 78: 528–532.

Otero, A., M.J. Chapela, M. Atanassova, J.M. Vieites, and A.G. Cabado. 2011. Cyclic imines: Chemistry and mechanism of action: A review. *Chemical Research in Toxicology*, 24 (11): 1817–1829.

Paredes, I., I.M.C.M. Rietjens, J.M. Vieites, and A.G. Cabado. 2011. Update of risk assessments of main marine biotoxins in the European Union. *Toxicon*, 58: 336–354.

Parsons, M.L., K. Aligizaki, M.-Y. Dechraoui Bottein et al. 2011. *Gambierdiscus* and *Ostreopsis*: Reassessment of the state of knowledge of their taxonomy, geography, ecophysiology and toxicology. *Harmful Algae*, 14: 107–129.

Paz, B., A.H. Daranas, M. Norte et al. 2008. Yessotoxins, a group of marine polyether toxins: An overview. *Marine Drugs*, 6 (2): 73–102.

Perez, R., N. Rehmann, S. Crain et al. 2010. The preparation of certified calibration solutions for azaspiracid-1, -2, and -3, potent marine biotoxins found in shellfish. *Analytical and Bioanalytical Chemistry*, 398 (5): 2243–2252.

Perez-Gomez, A., A. Ferrero-Gutierrez, A. Novelli et al. 2006. Potent neurotoxic action of the shellfish biotoxin yessotoxin on cultured cerebellar neurons. *Toxicological Science*, 90 (1): 168–177.

Pérez-Arellano, J., O. Luzardo, A. Brito et al. 2005. Ciguatera fish poisoning, Canary Islands. *Emerging Infectious Diseases*, 11: 1981–1982.

Perl, T.M., L. Bedard, T. Kosatsky et al. 1990a. An outbreak of toxic encephalopathy caused by eating mussels contaminated with domoic acid. *New England Journal of Medicine*, 322 (25): 1775–1780.

Perl, T.M., J.C. Hockin, T. Kosatsky et al. 1990b. Neurologic sequelae after ingestion of mussels contaminated with domoic acid—Reply. *New England Journal of Medicine*, 323 (23): 1632–1632.

Plakas, S.M. and R.W. Dickey. 2010. Advances in monitoring and toxicity assessment of brevetoxins in molluscan shellfish. *Toxicon*, 56 (2): 137–149.

Powell, C.L., M.E. Ferdin, M. Busman, R.G. Kvitek, and G.J. Doucette. 2002. Development of a protocol for determination of domoic acid in the sand crab (*Emerita analoga*): A possible new indicator species. *Toxicon*, 40 (5): 485–492.

Quilliam, M. 2003. Chemical methods for lipophilic shellfish toxins. In *Manual on Harmful Marine Microalgae*, eds. G. Hallegraeff, D.M. Anderson, and A.D. Cembella, pp. 211–245. Paris, France: UNESCO.

Ramos, V. and V. Vasconcelos. 2010. Palytoxin and analogs: Biological and ecological effects. *Marine Drugs*, 8 (7): 2021–2037.

Ramsdell, J.S. 2008. The molecular and integrative basis to brevetoxin toxicity. In *Seafood and Freshwater Toxins. Pharmacology, Physiology and Detection*, ed. L.M. Botana, pp. 519–550. Boca Raton, FL: CRC Press/Taylor & Francis Group.

Rehmann, N., P. Hess, and M.A. Quilliam. 2008. Discovery of new analogs of the marine biotoxin azaspiracid in blue mussels (*Mytilus edulis*) by ultra-performance liquid chromatography/tandem mass spectrometry. *Rapid Communications in Mass Spectrometry*, 22 (4): 549–558.

Remeral, F., A.S. Vuitton, M. Palud et al. 2008. Elastomeric pump reliability in postoperative regional anesthesia: a survey of 430 consecutive devices. *Anesthesia and Analgesia*, 107: 2079–2084.

Riobo, P. and J.M. Franco. 2011. Palytoxins: Biological and chemical determination. *Toxicon*, 57 (3): 368–375.

Risk, M., Y.Y. Lin, V.M. Sadagoparamanujam et al. 1979. High-pressure liquid-chromatographic separation of 2 major toxic compounds from *Gymnodinium breve* (Davis). *Journal of Chromatographic Science*, 17 (7): 400–405.

Rodriguez, P., A. Alfonso, C. Vale et al. 2008. First toxicity report of tetrodotoxin and 5,6,11-trideoxyTTX in the trumpet shell *Charonia lampas lampas* in Europe. *Analytical Chemistry*, 80: 5622–5629.

Román, Y., A. Alfonso, M.C. Louzao et al. 2002. Azaspiracid-1, a potent, nonapoptotic new phycotoxin with several cell targets. *Cell Signalling*, 14: 703–716.

Román, Y., A. Alfonso, M.R. Vieytes et al. 2004. Effects of Azaspiracids 2 and 3 on intracellular cAMP, [Ca2+], and pH. *Chemical Research in Toxicology*, 17 (10): 1338–1349.

Ronzitti, G., P. Hess, N. Rehmann, and G.P. Rossini. 2007. Azaspiracid-1 Alters the E-cadherin pool in epithelial cells. *Toxicological Sciences*, 95 (2): 427–435.

Ross, I.A., W. Johnson, P.P. Sapienza, and C.S. Kim. 2000. Effects of the seafood toxin domoic acid on glutamate uptake by rat astrocytes. *Food and Chemical Toxicology*, 38 (11): 1005–1011.

Rundberget, T., M. Sandvik, K. Larsen et al. 2007. Extraction of microalgal toxins by large-scale pumping of seawater in Spain and Norway, and isolation of okadaic acid and dinophysistoxin-2. *Toxicon*, 50 (7): 960–970.

Salas, R., U. Tillmann, U. John et al. 2011. The role of *Azadinium spinosum* (Dinophyceae) in the production of azaspiracid shellfish poisoning in mussels. *Harmful Algae*, 10 (6): 774–783.

Santaclara, F., J. Lago, J.M. Vieites, and A.G. Cabado. 2005. Effect of okadaic acid on integrins and structural proteins in BE(2)-M17 cells. *Archives of Toxicology*, 79 (10): 582–586.

Sas, K.M. and J.E. Baatz. 2010. Brevetoxin-2 induces an inflammatory response in an alveolar macrophage cell line. *International Journal of Hygiene and Environmental Health*, 213 (5): 352–358.

Satake, M., K. Ofuji, H. Naoki et al. 1998. Azaspiracid, a new marine toxin having unique spiro ring assemblies, isolated from Irish mussels, *Mytilus edulis*. *Journal of the American Chemical Society*, 120 (38): 9967–9968.

Satake, M., K. Terasawa, Y. Kadowaki, and T. Yasumoto. 1996. Relative configuration of yessotoxin and isolation of two new analogs from toxic scallops. *Tetrahedron Letters*, 37 (33): 5955–5958.

Schilling, W.P., W.G. Sinkins, and M. Estacion. 1999. Maitotoxin activates a nonselective cation channel and a P2Z/P2X7-like cytolytic pore in human skin fibroblasts. *American Journal of Physiology—Cell Physiology*, 277 (4): C755–C765.

Seemann, P., C. Gernert, S. Schmitt, D. Mebs, and U. Hentschel. 2009. Detection of hemolytic bacteria from *Palythoa caribaeorum* (Cnidaria, Zoantharia) using a novel palytoxin-screening assay. *Antonie Van Leeuwenhoek International Journal of General and Molecular Microbiology*, 96 (4): 405–411.

Seki, T., M. Satake, L. Mackenzie, H.F. Kaspar, and T. Yasumoto. 1995. Gymnodimine, a new marine toxin of unprecedented structure isolated from New Zealand oysters and the dinoflagellate, *Gymnodinium* sp. *Tetrahedron Letters*, 36 (39): 7093–7096.

Selwood, A.I., C.O. Miles, A.L. Wilkins et al. 2010. Isolation, structural determination and acute toxicity of pinnatoxins E, F and G. *Journal of Agricultural and Food Chemistry*, 58 (10): 6532–6542.

Suzuki, T. 2008. Chemistry, metabolism and chemical detection methods of pectenotoxins. In *Seafood and Freshwater Toxins. Pharmacology, Physiology and Detection*, pp. 343–359. Boca Raton, FL: CRC Press/Taylor & Francis Group.

Suzuki, T., V. Beuzenberg, L. Mackenzie, and M.A. Quilliam. 2003. Liquid chromatography-mass spectrometry of spiroketal stereoisomers of pectenotoxins and the analysis of novel pectenotoxin isomers in the toxic dinoflagellate *Dinophysis acuta* from New Zealand. *Journal of Chromatography A*, 992 (1–2): 141–150.

Suzuki, C.A.M. and S.L. Hierlihy. 1993. Renal clearance of domoic acid in the rat. *Food and Chemical Toxicology*, 31 (10): 701–706.

Suzuki, T., L. Mackenzie, D. Stirling, and J. Adamson. 2001a. Conversion of pectenotoxin-2 to pectenotoxin-2 seco acid in the New Zealand scallop, *Pecten novaezelandiae*. *Fisheries Science*, 67 (3): 506–510.

Suzuki, T., L. Mackenzie, D. Stirling, and J. Adamson. 2001b. Pectenotoxin-2 seco acid: A toxin converted from pectenotoxin-2 by the New Zealand Greenshell mussel, *Perna canaliculus*. *Toxicon*, 39 (4): 507–514.

Suzuki, T., T. Mitsuya, H. Matsubara, and M. Yamasaki. 1998. Determination of pectenotoxin-2 after solid-phase extraction from seawater and from the dinoflagellate *Dinophysis fortii* by liquid chromatography with electrospray mass spectrometry and ultraviolet detection. Evidence of oxidation of pectenotoxin-2 to pectenotoxin-6 in scallops. *Journal of Chromatography A*, 815: 155–160.

Tachibana, K., P.J. Scheuer, Y. Tsukitani et al. 1981. Okadaic acid, a cyto-toxic polyether from 2 marine sponges of the genus *Halichondria*. *Journal of the American Chemical Society*, 103 (9): 2469–2471.

Takada, N., N. Umemura, K. Suenaga, and D. Uemura. 2001. Structural determination of pteriatoxins A, B and C, extremely potent toxins from the bivalve *Pteria penguin*. *Tetrahedron Letters*, 42 (20): 3495–3497.

Takahashi, H., T. Kusumi, Y. Kan, M. Satake, and T. Yasumoto. 1996. Determination of the absolute configuration of yessotoxin, a polyether compound implicated in diarrhetic shellfish poisoning, by NMR spectroscopic method using a chiral anisotropic reagent, methoxy-(2-naphthyl) acetic acid. *Tetrahedron Letters*, 37 (39): 7087–7090.

Taniyama, S., O. Arakawa, M. Terada et al. 2003. *Ostreopsis* spp., a possible origin of palytoxin (PTX) in parrotfish *Scarus ovifrons*. *Toxicon*, 42 (1): 29–33.

Taupin, P. 2009. Brevetoxin derivative compounds for stimulating neuronal growth. *Expert Opinion on Therapeutic Patents*, 19 (2): 269–274.

Terao, K., E. Ito, M. Oarada, M. Murata, and T. Yasumoto. 1990. Histopathological studies on experimental marine toxin poisoning—5. The effects in mice of yessotoxin isolated from Patinopecten yessoensis and of a desulfated derivative. *Toxicon*, 28: 1095–1104.

Tillmann, U., M. Elbrachter, B. Krock, U. John, and A. Cembella. 2009. *Azadinium spinosum* gen. et sp nov (*Dinophyceae*) identified as a primary producer of azaspiracid toxins. *European Journal of Phycology*, 44 (1): 63–79.

Torigoe, K., M. Murata, and T. Yasumoto. 1988. Prorocentrolide, a toxic nitrogenous macrocycle from a marine dinoflagellate, *Prorocentrum lima*. *Journal of the American Chemical Society*, 110: 7876–7877.

Touzet, N., J.M. Franco, and R. Raine. 2008. Morphogenetic diversity and biotoxin composition of *Alexandrium* (Dinophyceae) in Irish coastal waters. *Harmful Algae*, 7 (6): 782–797.

Trevino, C.L., J.L. De la Vega-Beltran, T. Nishigaki, R. Felix, and A. Darszon. 2006. Maitotoxin potently promotes Ca²⁺ influx in mouse spermatogenic cells and sperm, and induces the acrosome reaction. *Journal of Cell Physiology*, 206: 449–456.

Trevino, C.L., L. Escobar, L. Vaca et al. 2008. Maitotoxin: A unique pharmacological tool for elucidating Ca²⁺ dependent mechanisms. In *Seafood and Freshwater Toxins: Pharmacology, Physiology, and Detection*, ed. L.M. Botana, pp. 503–516. Boca Raton, FL: Taylor & Francis Group.

Truelove, J. and F. Iverson. 1994. Serum domoic acid clearance and clinical observations in the *Cynomolgus* monkey and Sprague-Dawley rat following a single iv-dose. *Bulletin of Environmental Contamination and Toxicology*, 52 (4): 479–486.

Truelove, J., R. Mueller, O. Pulido, and F. Iverson. 1996. Subchronic toxicity study of domoic acid in the rat. *Food and Chemical Toxicology*, 34 (6): 525–529.

Tubaro, A., V. Dell'ovo, S. Sosa, and C. Florio. 2010. Yessotoxins: A toxicological overview. *Toxicon*, 56 (2): 163–172.

Twiner, M.J., P. Hess, M.-Y. Bottein Dechraoui et al. 2005. Cytotoxic and cytoskeletal effects of azaspiracid-1 on mammalian cell lines. *Toxicon*, 45 (7): 891–900.

Twiner, M.J., N. Rehmann, P. Hess, and G.J. Doucette. 2008. Azaspiracid shellfish poisoning: A review on the chemistry, ecology, and toxicology with an emphasis on human health impacts. *Marine Drugs*, 6 (2): 39–72.

Uemura, Y., J.M. Miller, W.R. Matson, and M.F. Beal. 1991. Neurochemical analysis of focal Ischemia in rats. *Stroke*, 22 (12): 1548–1553.

Ueoka, R., A. Ito, M. Izumikawa et al. 2009. Isolation of Azaspiracid-2 from a marine sponge *Echinoclathria* sp. as a potent cytotoxin. *Toxicon*, 53 (6): 680–684.

Ukena, T., M. Satake, M. Usami et al. 2001. Structure elucidation of ostreocin D, a palytoxin analog isolated from the dinoflagellate *Ostreopsis siamensis*. *Bioscience Biotechnology and Biochemistry*, 65 (11): 2585–2588.

Usami, M., M. Satake, S. Ishida et al. 1995. Palytoxin analogs from the dinoflagellate *Ostreopsis siamensis*. *Journal of the American Chemical Society*, 117 (19): 5389–5390.

Valdiglesias, V., B. Laffon, E. Pasaro et al. 2011a. Induction of oxidative DNA damage by the marine toxin okadaic acid depends on human cell type. *Toxicon*, 57 (6): 882–888.

Valdiglesias, V., B. Laffon, E. Pasaro, and J. Mendez. 2011b. Evaluation of okadaic acid-induced genotoxicity in human cells using the micronucleus test and gamma H2AX analysis. *Journal of Toxicology and Environmental Health-Part A—Current Issues*, 74 (15–16): 980–992.

Valdiglesias, V., B. Laffon, E. Pasaro, and J. Mendez. 2011c. Okadaic acid induces morphological changes, apoptosis and cell cycle alterations in different human cell types. *Journal of Environmental Monitoring*, 13 (6): 1831–1840.

Valdiglesias, V., J. Mendez, E. Pasaro et al. 2010. Assessment of okadaic acid effects on cytotoxicity, DNA damage and DNA repair in human cells. *Mutation Research—Fundamental and Molecular Mechanisms of Mutagenesis*, 689 (1–2): 74–79.

Vale, P. 2004. Differential dynamics of dinophysistoxins and pectenotoxins between blue mussel and common cockle: A phenomenon originating from the complex toxin profile of *Dinophysis acuta*. *Toxicon*, 44: 123–134.

Vale, C. and L.M. Botana. 2008. Marine toxins and the cytoskeleton: Okadaic acid and dinophysistoxins. *FEBS Journal*, 275 (24): 6060–6066.

Vale, C., C. Wandscheer, K.C. Nicolaou et al. 2008. Cytotoxic effect of azaspiracid-2 and azaspiracid-2-methyl ester in cultured neurons: Involvement of the c-Jun N-terminal kinase. *Journal of Neuroscience Research*, 86 (13): 2952–2962.

Valverde, I., J. Lago, A. Reboreda, J.M. Vieites, and A.G. Cabado. 2008a. Characteristics of palytoxin-induced cytotoxicity in neuroblastoma cells. *Toxicology in Vitro*, 22 (6): 1432–1439.

Valverde, I., J. Lago, J.M. Vieites, and A.G. Cabado. 2008b. In vitro approaches to evaluate palytoxin-induced toxicity and cell death in intestinal cells. *Journal of Applied Toxicology*, 28 (3): 294–302.

Van Dolah, F. 2000. Marine algal toxins: Origins, health effects, and their increased occurrence. *Environmental Health Perspectives*, 108 (Supplement 1): 133–141.

Vilarino, N. and B. Espina. 2008. Pharmacology of pectenotoxins. In *Seafood and Freshwater Toxins. Pharmacology, Physiology and Detection*, ed. L.M. Botana, pp. 361–380. Boca Raton, FL: CRC Press/Taylor & Francis Group.

Vilariño, N., K.C. Nicolaou, M.O. Frederick et al. 2006. Cell growth inhibition and actin cytoskeleton disorganization induced by azaspiracid-1 structure-activity studies. *Chemical Research in Toxicology*, 19 (11): 1459–1466.

Vilariño, N., K.C. Nicolaou, M.O. Frederick, M.R. Vieytes, and L.M. Botana. 2007. Irreversible cytoskeletal disarrangement is independent of caspase activation during in vitro azaspiracid toxicity in human neuroblastoma cells. *Biochemical Pharmacology*, 74 (2): 327–335.

Villar-Gonzalez, A., M.L. Rodriguez-Velasco, B. Ben-Gigirey, and L.M. Botana. 2006. First evidence of spirolides in Spanish shellfish. *Toxicon*, 48 (8): 1068–1074.

Villar-Gonzalez, A., M.L. Rodriguez-Velasco, and A. Gago-Martinez. 2011. Determination of lipophilic toxins by LC/MS/MS: single-laboratory validation. *Journal of AOAC International*, 94 (3): 909–922.

Wandscheer, C.B., N. Vilariño, B. Espiña, M.C. Louzao, and L.M. Botana. 2010. Human muscarinic acetylcholine receptors are a target of the marine toxin 13-desmethyl C spirolide. *Chemical Research in Toxicology*, 23 (11): 1753–1761.

Wang, D.Z. 2008. Neurotoxins from marine dinoflagellates: A brief review. *Marine Drugs*, 6 (2): 349–371.

Watanabe, R., T. Suzuki, and Y. Oshima. 2010. Development of quantitative NMR method with internal standard for the standard solutions of paralytic shellfish toxins and characterisation of gonyautoxin-5 and gonyautoxin-6. *Toxicon*, 56: 589–595.

Wattenberg, E.V. 2007. Palytoxin: Exploiting a novel skin tumor promoter to explore signal transduction and carcinogenesis. *American Journal of Physiology—Cell Physiology*, 292 (1): C24–C32.

Watters, M.R. 2000. Toxins as a starting point to drugs. In *Seafood and Freshwater Toxins. Pharmacology, Physiology and Detection*, ed. L.M. Botana. New York: Taylor & Francis Group.

WHOI. 2007. Harmful algae. Woods Hole Oceanographic Institution. http://www.whoi.edu/redtide/page.do?pid=18103 (accessed January 31, 2012).

Wiese, M., P.M. D'Agostino, T.K. Mihali, M.C. Moffitt, and B.A. Neilan. 2010. Neurotoxic alkaloids: Saxitoxin and its analogs. *Marine Drugs*, 8 (7): 2185–2211.

Wiles, J.S., J.A. Vick, and M.K. Christen. 1974. Toxicological evaluation of Palytoxin in several animal species. *Toxicon*, 12 (4): 427–433.

Wisnoskey, B.J., M. Estacion, and W.P. Schilling. 2004. Maitotoxin-induced cell death cascade in bovine aortic endothelial cells: Divalent cation specificity and selectivity. *American Journal of Physiology—Cell Physiology*, 287 (2): C345–C356.

Wright, J.L.C., Boyd, K., de Freitas, A.S.W. et al. 1989. Identification of domoic acid, a neuroexcitatory amino acid, in toxic mussels from eastern Prince Edward Island. *Canadian Journal of Chemistry*, 67: 481–490.

Wright, J.L.C. and M.A. Quilliam. 1995. Methods for domoic acid, the amnesic shellfish poisoning (ASP) toxin. In *Manual on Harmful Marine Microalgae*, eds. G.M. Hallegraeff, D. Anderson, and A.D. Cembella, pp. 115–135. Paris, France: UNESCO.

Wu, J.J., Y.L. Mak, M.B. Murphy et al. 2011. Validation of an accelerated solvent extraction liquid chromatography-tandem mass spectrometry method for Pacific ciguatoxin-1 in fish flesh and comparison with the mouse neuroblastoma assay. *Analytical and Bioanalytical Chemistry*, 400: 3165–3175.

Yasumoto, T., M. Murata, Y. Oshima, G.K. Matsumoto, and J. Clardy. 1984. Diarrhetic shellfish poisoning. In *Seafood Toxins*, ed. E.P. Ragelis, pp. 207–214. Washington, DC: American Chemical Society.

Yasumoto, T., M. Murata, Y. Oshima et al. 1985. Diarrhetic shellfish toxins. *Tetrahedron*, 41 (6): 1019–1025.

Yasumoto, T., Y. Oshima, and M. Yamaguchi. 1978. Occurrence of a new type of shellfish poisoning in the Tohoku district. *Bulletin of the Japanese Society for the Science of Fish*, 44: 1249–1255.

Yasumoto, T. and A. Takizawa. 1997. Fluorometric measurement of yessotoxins in shellfish by high-pressure liquid chromatography. *Bioscience, Biotechnology, and Biochemistry*, 61 (10): 1775–1777.

Yokoyama, A., M. Murata, Y. Oshima, T. Iwashita, and T. Yasumoto. 1988. Some chemical properties of maitotoxin, a putative calcium channel agonist isolated from a marine dinoflagellate. *Journal of Biochemistry*, 104 (2): 184–187.

Zheng, S.Z., F.L. Huang, S.C. Chen et al. 1990. The isolation and bioactivities of pinnatoxin (in Chinese). *Chinese Journal of Marine Drugs*, 33 (9): 33–35.

18

Compounds from Marine Organisms with Antiviral Activity

Se-Kwon Kim, Fatih Karadeniz, and Mustafa Zafer Karagozlu

CONTENTS

18.1 HIV-1 and AIDS

High amounts of secondary metabolites produced by microorganisms, plants, and marine organisms have been of much attention as bioactive substances for disease treatment (Lam 2007). Among these diseases, acquired immunodeficiency syndrome (AIDS) stands as one of the most important diseases which needs urgent consideration worldwide with about 33.2 million people infected by human immunodeficiency virus type 1 (HIV-1) (UNAIDS 2010). HIV is a member of the lentivirus family for being an enveloped retrovirus. The structure of HIV is relatively complex with each virus expressing 160 kDa glycoproteins composed of gp120 and gp41 which are linked together by non-covalent bonds. The gp41 molecule is a transmembrane glycoprotein that crosses the membrane of the viral envelope. Infection of the host cell by HIV entrance occurs through the interaction of viral envelope protein, gp120, with a specific membrane glycoprotein called CD4 along a chemokine receptor (Kwong et al. 1998). Host cell membrane forms the viral envelope during infection process and within the envelope, viral core (nucleocapsid) that includes a layer of protein called p17, and an inner layer of protein called p24 is located. The HIV genome is composed of two identical single-stranded RNA (+), and some proteins are attached to the genome such as two molecules of reverse transcriptase, a protease, and an integrase.

In order to develop therapeutic agents and learn their mechanism of action, detailed knowledge of the viral replication of HIV-1 is strictly needed. Following infection of HIV and virus entry into cells, viral substances get into contact with the appropriate receptors and co-receptors. Next, formation of the viral double-stranded DNA genome is followed by the integration of proviral DNA into the host cell genome, creating a provirus.

Attachment of the virus occurs upon the binding of the gp120 on the viral envelope to the CD4+ host cell. Receptors on the host cells could be either one of the following major chemokine receptors, CXCR4 or CCR5. CXCR4 is found on naive T cells, whereas CCR5 is located on monocytes, macrophages, and activated or memory subset of T cells. Once in the cytoplasm, the viral RNA is converted to DNA by the action of a viral RNA-dependent DNA polymerase activity and a virus specified ribonuclease H activity found in the HIV-1 reverse transcriptase (RT) enzyme. Following several stages of integration through integrase enzyme activity, new virus particles are started to be synthesized by host cell genome. Forming new virus particles is followed by trimming the HIV protease inside the capsid. This process produces the functioning proteins such as reverse transcriptase, integrase, and protease enzymes. The newly released virions now have the capacity to infect new target cells, starting a new replication cycle as fully mature viruses.

AIDS is evidently caused by HIV-1 infection, and up to now there are significant advances in rational drug design and highly active compounds can be synthesized (De Clercq 2009). However, resistance of the virus to the drugs on the market, side effects of synthetic drugs, and the need for long-term antiviral treatment because of the longevity of the disease onset and progress urge the inevitable development of new anti-HIV agents, targets, and therapies (D'Aquila et al. 2003; Worm et al. 2010). In this regard, natural substances from both terrestrial and marine organisms are still known as the richest source of bioactive compounds. Among these sources, marine-derived substances promote excessive availability for discovering anti-HIV treatment, while they contain a massive amount of potential, being a consistent source for successful drug discovery. There are numerous marine-based natural products, which are reported to have bioactivities like antifungal, antimicrobial, and antiallergic effects. In addition, several natural products from marine organisms have been reported to express bioactivity against prevalent diseases worldwide which awake as much concern as AIDS such as cancer, diabetes, and obesity (Mayer et al. 2011). So far, high amounts of scientific evidences promote various compounds isolated from natural resources to show anti-HIV activity and to inhibit HIV-1 activity in almost every stage of the viral life cycle (Jiang et al. 2010). Several compounds of plant origin such as alkaloids, coumarins, carbohydrates, flavonoids, lignans, phenolics, quinines, phospholipids, terpenes, and tannins have been elucidated and reported to possess inhibitory activity against various targets in the viral life cycle of HIV such as crucial enzyme inhibition of reverse transcriptase and protease. Considering that the marine species comprise more than half of the total biodiversity of the earth, the sea holds considerably high potential of lead compounds for novel drugs. On this matter, among the terrestrial organism for compound isolation, the marine organisms present rich resources of diverse compounds with various crucial antiviral activities.

18.2 Compounds from Marine Algae with Anti-HIV Activity

18.2.1 Phlorotannins

Tannins are naturally occurring water-soluble polyphenolic compounds, and it has been considered that they possess anti-HIV activity by showing distinct inhibiting activities on polymerase and ribonuclease of HIV-1 life cycle. Phlorotannins are tannin derivatives which contain several phloroglucinol units linked to each other in different ways and formed by the polymerization of phloroglucinol (1,3,5-tryhydroxybenzene) monomer units and biosynthesized through the acetate–malonate pathway. So far, phlorotannins are mostly isolated from most of the terrestrial plants, however in marine environments mostly from red and brown alga. Numerous bioactivities of marine-derived phlorotannins have been reported up to date such as antioxidant, anti-inflammatory, antibacterial, and anti-MMP activities (Nagayama et al. 2002; Kim et al. 2006).

In early studies, seaweed extracts have been tested for their anti-HIV-1 activity in manners of inhibiting key viral life cycle enzymes such as RT, protease, and integrase of HIV-1 (Ahn et al. 2004). Following the referred study, two phlorotannins from brown alga *Ecklonia cava* KJELLMAN have been isolated and reported to inhibit the HIV-1 protease and reverse transcriptase. These phlorotannins, 8,8′-bieckol and 8,4‴-dieckol, which are dimers of eckol, were isolated from *E. cava* inhibited the RT and protease activity efficiently. In case of inhibition of HIV-1 RT, 8,8′-bieckol which has a biaryl linkage showed a 10-fold higher activity than that of 8,4‴-dieckol which has a diphenyl ether linkage with the IC_{50} values of 0.5 and 5.3 µM, respectively. This significant RT inhibitory activity of 8,8′-bieckol was favorable against its protease inhibition and comparable to the positive control nevirapine which has an IC_{50} value of 0.28 µM. In the light of recent reports, 8,8′-bieckol might be employed as a drug candidate for development of new-generation therapeutic agents against HIV. In addition to this results, in another report, 6,6′-bieckol from *E. cava* reduced the cytopathic effects of HIV-1 including HIV-1-induced syncytia formation and viral p24 antigen levels, as well as inhibited RT and HIV-1 entry activity (Artan et al. 2008). In this study, the lower cytotoxicity of 6,6′-bieckol compared to previous studied tannins raised the potential of this substance as a safe therapeutic agent. In detail, 6,6′-bieckol protected the 96% of the HIV-1 infected cells from infection-induced lytic effects and inhibited the syncytia formation up to 88% with an EC_{50} value of 1.72 µM. Moreover, 6,6′-bieckol inhibited the RT activity and p24 production with IC_{50} values of 1.07 and 1.26 µM, respectively. The performed studies also clearly showed that 6,6′-bieckol addition successfully prevented the HIV-1 entry dependent on the inhibition of production of specific proteins such as p55 and p41. These results were strengthened by coculture assays, which again show clear inhibitory effect against HIV-1 infection in vitro. This important anti-HIV activity in various stages of viral cycle including viral entry and RT activity, however excluding a sufficient protease inhibition, promotes 6,6′-bieckol as a significant lead for further drug design on the way to a fully inhibition of HIV-1 activity.

Another phlorotannin, diphlorethohydroxycarmalol, has been isolated from *Ishige okamurae* Yendo (Ahn et al. 2006) besides the brown alga *E. cava*. This phlorotannin was assayed for its inhibitory activity against HIV-1 RT, integrase, and protease, while any study for its HIV-1 activity in vitro has not been carried out. Diphlorethohydroxycarmalol inhibited the RT and protease activity with IC_{50} values of 9.1 and 25.2 µM, respectively; however, it failed to show any efficiency against HIV-1 protease. Although lacking of in vitro assessment of its potential as well as the failure to inhibit HIV-1 protease, this phlorotannin also can be regarded as an important compound for further anti-HIV drug design or present use in the nutraceutical and pharmaceutical industries for supplementary treatment.

18.2.2 Polysaccharides

Polysaccharides with bioactivities from different organisms have been characterized, assayed, and reported in many researches in past few decades. Activities such as anti-coagulant, anti-inflammatory, antitumor, and antiviral stand as the main bioactivities of polysaccharides from different natural sources. Expectedly, marine algae serve as a significant source of different type of polysaccharides with different bioactivities. The chemical structure, the amount of these polysaccharides, and therefore their bioactivity vary according to marine algae species and divisions such as Chlorophyta (green algae), Rhodophyta (red algae), and Phaeophyta (brown algae). In recent years, numerous saccharides isolated from marine algae have attracted quite attention in the fields of biochemistry and pharmacology due to their efficiency as anti-HIV-1, anti-adhesive, anticoagulant, anticancer, and anti-inflammatory agents (Schaeffer and Krylov 2000; Wijesekara et al. 2010). Moreover, polysaccharides have attracted much of attention as antiviral compounds since the inhibitory activities of algal polysaccharides against mumps and influenza virus were reported long time ago (Gerber et al. 1958). Further, a comparative study has been reported the inhibition of herpes simplex virus and other viruses by polysaccharide fractions from the extracts of ten red algae (Ehreshmann et al. 1977). It is proposed that polysaccharides are quite efficient in disrupting the viral peptide attachments which are supposed to be highly preserved in the drug-resistance mutation process. Therefore, polysaccharides are directed to affect these peptides as potential anti-HIV targets.

Fucans are sulfated polysaccharides of high molecular weight which can be found widely in various brown algae species. They have fucose as their main repeating unit; however, they can include other sugars as well such as glucose, mannose, galactose, and uronic acid. Several fucans from the seaweed species *Dictyota mertensii*, *Lobophora variegata*, *Spatoglossum schroederi*, and *Fucus vesiculosus* were reported to successfully inhibit the activity of HIV reverse transcriptase (RT) (Queiroz et al. 2008). An isolated galactofucan which is mainly formed by galactose-linked fucose and with lower sulfate content from *L. variegate* inhibited the 94% HIV-1 RT activity at a concentration of 1.0 μg/mL. Another isolated fucan with a higher sulfate content and contains mostly fucose units exerted a high inhibitory effect on RT as well. The same fucan from two different algae, *S. schroederi* and *D. mertensii*, showed similar inhibition ratio which is 99.03% and 99.30%, respectively, at 1.0 mg/mL concentration. However, a higher sulfate containing fucan from *S. schroederi* with the units of galactose and fucose could only show a 53.90% inhibitory against the RT activity at the same concentration. As a part of this comparative approach, a homofucan containing only sulfated fucose units have been isolated and surprisingly exhibited a strong RT inhibitory effect. At a concentration of 0.5 mg/mL, this fucan inhibited the 98.10% of the RT activity. Next, fucans were subjected to chemical modifications which help to understand the structure–activity relation in fucans' anti-HIV activity. Fucans which were modified by carboxyreduction and desulfation showed approximately fourfold lower inhibitory activities for RT under the same conditions. Reverse transcriptase inhibition of fucans are suggested to be dependent on both the ionic charges and the sugar rings regarding the comparison between structure and inhibitory activity. Sugar groups are supposed to orientate the ionic charges as well as recognize the enzyme and initiate enzyme-compound binding. These results suggest that the side chain of fucan, which was modified, was dominantly active during its efficiency against viral infection.

In a recent study, galactofucan fractions of brown algae *Adenocystis utricularis* possess in vitro anti-HIV-1 activity (Trinchero et al. 2009). Two fractions among five had strong inhibitory effects on HIV-1 replication with IC_{50} values of 0.6 and 0.9 μg/mL, respectively. Moreover, these fractions showed their activity against both wild type and drug-resistant viral strains which is a promising result against highly mutation-susceptible nature of HIV-1.

The glucoronogalactan from red algae *Schizymenia dubyi* was also reported to exhibit anti-HIV activity (Bourgougnon et al. 1996). Glucoronogalactan from *S. dubyi* successfully protected the MT4 cells from the cytopathic effects HIV-1 infection by means of reducing the syncytia formation almost to 1% of untreated infected control at a concentration of 5 µg/mL. In vitro studies on glucoronogalactan suggest that disturbing virus–host cell linkage and inhibiting early steps of HIV infection can be regarded as the possible action mechanism of this polysaccharide.

Two red alga *Grateloupia filicina* and *Grateloupia longifolia* are also sources for sulfated galactan fractions with promising antiviral effects (Wang et al. 2007). Two galactans named as GFP and GLP from *G. filicina* and *G. longifolia*, respectively, were confirmed to contain 25.7% and 18.5% sulfate of their whole chemical content. The sulfated galactan GFP has sulfate ester groups at carbon 2 and at carbon 2 and 6 for GLP. The anti-HIV activities of these polysaccharides have been tested on a primary isolate of HIV-1 and human peripheral blood mononuclear cells, and both GFP and GLP showed strong anti-HIV activity with low cytotoxicity. EC_{50} values for the HIV-1 infection protective effect of GFP and GLP addition were calculated as 0.010 and 0.003 µM, respectively.

Moreover, a variety of potential bioactive polysaccharides are also isolated from brown algae where some of them exhibit anti-HIV activity with different mechanism of action. Sulfated polymannuroguluronate (SPMG) is a novel member of polysaccharides extracted from brown algae (Meiyu et al. 2003; Miao et al. 2005). It has 8 kDa average molecular weight and rich in 1,4-linked β-D mannuronate with 1.5 sulfated and 1.0 carboxyl groups per sugar residue. Studies suggested a possible linkage between SPMG and gp120 of HIV-1. It has been reported that binding of SPMG to gp120 alone or gp120-CD4 complex occurred through V3 loop region of the protein. SPMG showed partial suppression of gp120 binding to CD4 when treated prior to infection. However, SPMG addition to pre-infected cells did not show any significant suppression of virus–host cell linkage. Therefore, it is suggested that SPMG either shares common binding sites on gp120 with CD4 or masks the docking sites of gp120 for CD4.

18.2.3 Lectins

Lectins can be found in lots of species ranging from prokaryotes to corals, algae, fungi, plants, invertebrates, and vertebrates and defined as carbohydrate-binding proteins. Owing to their distinct carbohydrate-binding properties, they are highly involved in crucial biological processes such as host–pathogen interaction, cell–cell communication, induction of intracellular signaling cascades, and cell targeting which are main targets for any viral life cycle starting from infection and followed by exit of newly formed virions. As expected in this regard, lectins are showed to have potential to block the interaction between HIV-1 and host cells, preventing the viral infection and dissemination as a result. Evidently, HIV-1 envelope glycoprotein gp120 is extensively glycosylated with numerous N-linked glycosylation sites. Glycans which are seated in these glycosylation sites are in rich of mannose and can easily serve as ligands for lectins. The importance of gp120 in viral infection of the target cell makes this protein suitable target for anti-HIV treatment or prophylaxis. In this manner, there are several types of lectins which were isolated from marine sources with potential anti-HIV activity (Sato and Hori 2009).

Red algae *Griffithsia* sp. is the source of a novel lectin identified as Griffithsin with a molecular weight of 12.7 kDa. This 121 amino acid protein is reported to display promising anti-HIV activity (Mori et al. 2005). Without any observable cysteine residues,

Griffithsin is completely novel and does not have any homology to any of the proteins or translated nucleotide sequences. Studies showed that Griffithsin potently prevented the T-lymphoblastic cells from the cytopathic effects of both laboratory strains and clinical primary isolates of HIV-1. It was also exhibited to be active against both T-cell-tropic and macrophage-tropic strains of HIV-1 at concentrations as low as 0.043 μM. More importantly, Griffithsin blocked cell–cell fusion between chronically infected and uninfected cells which is referred as syncytia and the crucial step toward cell death. Blockage of the formation of syncytia by Griffithsin occurred at sub-nanomolar concentrations without any cytotoxic effect. In connection with predicted mode of action, this lectin disturbed the binding of CD4 host cell membrane receptor to gp120 in a glycosylation-dependent manner and prevents HIV-1 infection. On the other hand, gp120–Griffithsin bond was inhibited by higher glucose and mannose but not by galactose, xylose, or sialic acid–containing glycoproteins. Unusual distinct activity of Griffithsin is credited to its linker sequences of Gly-Gly-Ser-Gly-Gly after a series of assays regarding structure–activity relationship.

In a recent study, a high-mannose binding lectin (BCA) is isolated from green alga *Boodlea coacta* with potent antiviral activity against HIV-1 and influenza viruses (Sato et al. 2011). Carbohydrate-binding specificity determination of BCA evidently showed that this lectin has strong specificity for α1–2-linked mannose at nonreducing terminal. The potent anti-HIV-1 activity of BCA was easily predicted from carbohydrate-binding propensity and similarity with formerly reported antiviral lectins. Studies showed that BCA inhibited the HIV-1 infection with EC_{50} value of 8.2 nM. Additionally, it has been reported that BCA's affinity to HIV-1 during its potent bioactivity is quite high, supporting its promising potential as an anti-HIV therapeutic agent.

18.2.4 Others

Screening of seaweed extracts as a part of series of experiments, 47 marine macroalgae extracts were tested for their ability to inhibit HIV-1 RT and integrase (Ahn et al. 2002). Results clearly showed that 1 of 4 Chlorophyta, 8 of 17 Phaeophyta, and 6 of 26 Rhodophyta species showed inhibitory activity against HIV-1 reverse transcriptase. Parallel to previous reports on algal compounds with antiviral activities, among these 47 algae extracts, five species (*E. cava, I. okamurae, Sargassum confusum, Sargassum hemiphyllum, Sargassum ringgoldianum*) were able to inhibit the activity of HIV-1 integrase. Moreover, in vitro studies confirmed that extracts of Bossiella sp. and Chondria crassicaulis successfully prevented the MT4 cells from HIV-1-induced cytopathic effects in case of non-cytotoxic concentrations. Following these screening results, a carmalol derivative, diphlorethohydroxycarmalol, was isolated from brown alga, *I. okamurae* (Ahn et al. 2006), as mentioned earlier, which urges the further isolation processes for elucidation of active compounds of these extracts.

Furthermore, two diterpenes, named (6R)-6-hydroxydichotoma-3,14-diene-1,17-dial (DT1) and (6R)-6-acetoxydichotoma-3,14-diene-1,17-dial (DT2), were isolated from the brown alga *D. menstrualis* (Pereira et al. 2004). It has been reported that DT1 and DT2 inhibited the virus replication with EC_{50} values of 40 and 70 μM, respectively, in addition to HIV-1 RT inhibitory activity with ICμ values of 10 and 35 μM. Another study reported a dolabellane diterpene, 8,10,18-trihydroxy-2,6-dolabelladiene from brown alga *Dictyota pfaffii* with a HIV-1 infection inhibitory effect with an EC_{50} of 8.4 and 1.7 μM in peripheral blood mononuclear cells and macrophages, respectively. Moreover, this diterpene inhibited the HIV-1 RT activity with an IC_{50} of 16.5 μM (Barbosa et al. 2004).

18.3 Conclusion

Taken together, studies in the past few decades evidently promoted highly promising results regarding potential treatment of viral infections with marine-derived substances. Several natural compounds have been put on stage to be a potential lead drug or a supplemental treatment. Most of them showed enough activity to be a drug candidate, nutraceutical, or a combination choice for antiviral cocktails. In reported studies, these natural compounds were able to reduce or regulate HIV-1 infection and related complications. Moreover, these promising results of agents from marine organisms with beneficial health effects and potential anti-HIV activity present quite valuable knowledge on the road to novel highly effective HIV-1 treatment.

References

Ahn, M. J., K. D. Yoon, C. Y. Kim, J. H. Kim, C. G. Shin, and J. Kim. 2006. Inhibitory activity on HIV-1 reverse transcriptase and integrase of a carmalol derivative from a brown alga, *Ishige okamurae*. *Phytotherapy Research* 20: 711–713.

Ahn, M. J., K. D. Yoon, C. Y. Kim, S. Y. Min, Y. U. Kim, J. H. Kim, C. G. Shin et al. 2002. Inhibition of HIV-1 reverse transcriptase and HIV-1 integrase and antiviral activity of Korean seaweed extracts. *Journal of Applied Phycology* 14: 325–329.

Ahn, M. J., K. D. Yoon, S. Y. Min, J. S. Lee, J. H. Kim, T. G. Kim, S. H. Kim et al. 2004. Inhibition of HIV-1 reverse transcriptase and protease by phlorotannins from the brown alga *Ecklonia cava*. *Biological and Pharmaceutical Bulletin* 27: 544–547.

Artan, M., Y. Li, F. Karadeniz, S. H. Lee, M. M. Kim, and S. K. Kim. 2008. Anti-HIV-1 activity of phloroglucinol derivative, 6,6'-bieckol, from *Ecklonia cava*. *Bioorganic and Medicinal Chemistry* 16: 7921–7926.

Barbosa, J. P., R. C. Pereira, J. L. Abrantes, C. C. Cirne Dos Santos, M. A. Rebello, and V. L. Texeira. 2004. In vitro antiviral diterpenes from the Brazilian brown alga *Dictyota pfaffii*. *Planta Medica* 70: 856–860.

Bourgougnon, N., M. Lahaye, B. Quemener, J. C. Chermann, M. Rimbert, M. Cormaci, G. Furnari, and J. M. Komprobst. 1996. Annual variation in composition and in vitro anti-HIV-1 activity of the sulfated glucuronogalactan from *Schizymenia dubyi* (Rhodophyta, Gigartinales). *Journal of Applied Phycology* 8: 155–161.

D'Aquila, R. T., F. Brun-Vézinet, B. Clotet, L. M. Demeter, R. M. Grant, J. M. Schapiro, and A. Telenti. 2002. Drug resistance mutations in HIV-1. *Topics in HIV Medicine* 10: 21–25.

De Clercq, E. 2009. Anti-HIV drugs: 25 compounds approved within 25 years after the discovery of HIV. *International Journal of Antimicrobial Agents* 33: 307–320.

Ehreshmann, D. W., E. F. Dieg, M. T. Hatch, L. H. DiSalvo, and N. A. Vedros. 1977. Antiviral substances from California marine algae. *Journal of Phycology* 13: 37–40.

Gerber, P., J. D. Dutcher, E. V. Adams, and J. H. Sherman. 1958. Inhibition of herpes virus replication by marine algae extracts. *Proceedings of the Society for Experimental Biology and Medicine* 99: 590–593.

Jiang, Y., T. B. Ng, C. R. Wang, D. Zhang, Z. H. Cheng, Z. K. Liu, W. T. Qiao, Y. Q. Geng, N. Li, and F. Liu. 2010. Inhibitors from natural products to HIV-1 reverse transcriptase, protease and integrase. *Mini-Reviews in Medicinal Chemistry* 10: 1331–1344.

Kim, M. M., Q. V. Ta, E. Mendis, N. Rajapakse, W. K. Jung, H. G. Byun, Y. J. Jeon, and S. K. Kim. 2006. Phlorotannins in *Ecklonia cava* extract inhibit matrix metalloproteinase activity. *Life Sciences* 79: 1436–1443.

Kwong, P. D., R. Wyatt, J. Robinson, R. W. Sweet, J. Sodroski, and W. A. Hendrickson. 1998. Structure of an HIV gp120 envelope glycoprotein in complex with the CD4 receptor and a neutralizing human antibody. *Nature* 393: 648–659.

Lam, K. S. 2007. New aspects of natural products in drug discovery. *Trends in Microbiology* 15: 279–289.

Mayer, A., A. Rodríguez, R. Berlinck, and N. Fusetani. 2011. Marine pharmacology in 2007–8: Marine compounds with antibacterial, anticoagulant, antifungal, anti-inflammatory, antimalarial, anti-protozoal, antituberculosis and antiviral activities; affecting the immune and nervous system and other miscellaneous mechanisms of action. *Comparative Biochemistry and Physiology—Part C: Toxicology and Pharmacology* 153: 191–222.

Meiyu, G., L. Fuchuan, X. Xianliang, L. Jing, Y. Zuowei, and G. Huashi. 2003. The potential molecular targets of marine sulfated polymannuroguluronate interfering with HIV-1 entry: Interaction between SPMG and HIV-1 rgp120 and CD4 molecule. *Antiviral Research* 59: 127–135.

Miao, B., J. Li, X. Fu, L. Gan, X. Xin, and M. Geng. 2005. Sulfated polymannuroguluronate, a novel anti-AIDS drug candidate, inhibits T cell apoptosis by combating oxidative damage of mito-chondria. *Molecular Pharmacology* 68: 1716–1727.

Mori, T., B. R. O'Keefe, R. C. Sowder, S. Bringans, R. Gardella, S. Berg, P. Cochran et al. 2005. Isolation and characterization of Griffithsin, a novel HIV-inactivating protein, from the red alga *Griffithsia* sp. *Journal of Biological Chemistry* 280: 9345–9353.

Nagayama, K., Y. Iwamura, T. Shibata, I. Hirayama, and T. Nakamura. 2002. Bactericidal activity of phlorotannins from the brown alga *Ecklonia kurome*. *Journal of Antimicrobial Chemotherapy* 50: 889–893.

Pereira, H. S., L. R. Leão-Ferreira, N. Moussatché, V. L. Teixeira, D. N. Cavalcanti, L. J. Costa, R. Diaz, and I. C. P. P. Frugulhetti. 2004. Antiviral activity of diterpenes isolated from the Brazilian marine alga *Dictyota menstrualis* against human immunodeficiency virus type 1 (HIV-1). *Antiviral Research* 64: 69–76.

Queiroz, K. C. S., V. P. Medeiros, L. S. Queiroz, L. R. D. Abreu, H. A. O. Rocha, C. Ferreira, M. B. Jucá, H. Aoyama, and E. L. Leite. 2008. Inhibition of reverse transcriptase activity of HIV by polysac-charides of brown algae. *Biomedicine and Pharmacotherapy* 62: 303–307.

Sato, Y., M. Hirayama, K. Morimoto, N. Yamamoto, S. Okuyama, and K. Hori. 2011. High mannose-binding lectin with preference for the cluster of α 1–2-mannose from the green alga *Boodlea coacta* is a potent entry inhibitor of HIV-1 and influenza viruses. *Journal of Biological Chemistry* 286: 19446–19458.

Sato, T. and K. Hori. 2009. Cloning, expression, and characterization of a novel anti-HIV lectin from the cultured cyanobacterium, *Oscillatoria agardhii*. *Fisheries Science (Tokyo, Japan)* 75: 743–753.

Schaeffer, D. J. and V. S. Krylov. 2000. Anti-HIV activity of extracts and compounds from algae and cyanobacteria. *Ecotoxicology and Environmental Safety* 45: 208–227.

Trinchero, J., N. M. A. Ponce, O. L. Córdoba, M. L. Flores, S. Pampuro, C. A. Stortz, H. Salomón, and G. Turk. 2009. Antiretroviral activity of fucoidans extracted from the brown seaweed *Adenocystis utricularis*. *Phytotherapy Research* 23: 707–712.

Unaids Global Report. 2010. UNAIDS report on the global AIDS epidemic 2010. *WHO Library Cataloguing* 2010: 1–3.

Wang, S. C., S. W. A. Bligh, S. S. Shi, Z. T. Wang, Z. B. Hu, J. Crowder, C. Branford-White, and C. Vella. 2007. Structural features and anti-HIV-1 activity of novel polysaccharides from red algae *Grateloupia longifolia* and *Grateloupia filicina*. *International Journal of Biological Macromolecules* 41: 369–375.

Wijesekara, I., R. Pangestuti, and S. K. Kim. 2010. Biological activities and potential health benefits of sulfated polysaccharides derived from marine algae. *Carbohydrate Polymers* 84: 14–21.

Worm, S. W., C. Sabin, R. Weber, P. Reiss, W. El-Sadr, F. Dabis, S. De Wit et al. 2010. Risk of myocardial infarction in patients with HIV infection exposed to specific individual antiretroviral drugs from the 3 major drug classes: The data collection on adverse events of anti-HIV drugs (D:A:D) study. *Journal of Infectious Diseases* 201: 318–330.

19

Biological Activities of Marine-Derived Bioactive Peptides

Chen Zhang, Yuanfeng Ruan, and Se-Kwon Kim

CONTENTS

19.1 Introduction

Marine organisms are rich sources of structurally diverse compounds with various biological activities. With marine species comprising approximately a half of the total global biodiversity, the sea offers an enormous resource for novel compounds (Barrow and Shahidi, 2008). Recently, a great deal of interest has been developed to study the structural, compositional, and sequential properties of concerning bioactive peptides. Marine bioactive peptides can be produced by either one of the three methods, namely, solvent extraction, enzymatic hydrolysis, and microbial fermentation of food proteins (Lahl and Braun, 1994). Depending on the amino acid sequence, they may be involved in various biological functions (Clare and Swaisgood, 2000). Marine-derived bioactive peptides have been shown to possess many physiological functions, including antihypertensive or angiotensin I–converting enzyme inhibition (Je et al., 2005b), antioxidant (Mendis et al., 2005b), anticoagulant (Jo et al., 2008), and antimicrobial (Stensvag et al., 2008) activities. Moreover, some of these bioactive peptides have been identified to possess nutraceutical potentials for human health promotion and disease risk reduction (Shahidi and Zhong, 2008), and recently, the possible roles of food-derived bioactive peptides in reducing the risk of cardiovascular disease have been demonstrated (Erdmann et al., 2008). Bioactive peptides derived from marine organisms as well as marine fish processing by-products have potential in the development of functional foods (Shahidi, 2007), and they can act as potential physiological modulators of metabolism after absorption.

19.2 Biological Activities of Marine Bioactive Peptides

19.2.1 Antihypertensive Activity

High blood pressure is one of the major independent risk factors for cardiovascular diseases (Kannel and Higgins, 1990). Angiotensin I–converting enzyme (EC 3.4.15.1; ACE) plays a crucial role in the regulation of blood pressure as it promotes the conversion of angiotensin I to the potent vasoconstrictor angiotensin II as well as inactivates the vasodilator bradykinin. This potent vasoconstrictor is also involved in the release of a sodium-retaining steroid, aldosterone from the adrenal cortex, which has a tendency to increase blood pressure (Li et al., 2003).

ACE is a multifunctional enzyme that also catalyzes the degradation of bradykinin, a blood pressure–lowering nonapeptide (Kumar et al., 1991; Sibony et al., 1993). Moreover, ACE has been shown to degrade neuropeptides including enkephalins, neurotensin, and substance P, which may interact with the cardiovascular system. Oshima et al. (1979) have reported the first ACE inhibitory peptides produced from food proteins by digestive proteases. Afterward, many other ACE inhibitory peptides have been discovered in enzymatic hydrolysates of different food proteins (Muruyama and Suzuki, 1982; Wu and Ding, 2001), including marine organisms (Lee et al., 2005; Sato et al., 2002), and they could be applied in the prevention of hypertension and in the initial treatment of mildly hypertensive individuals (Vercruysse et al., 2005).

Marine-derived antihypertensive peptides have shown potent ACE inhibition activities. The potency of these marine-derived peptides has expressed as an IC_{50} value, which the ACE inhibitor concentration leads to 50% inhibition of ACE activity. Moreover, the inhibition modes of ACE-catalyzed hydrolysis of these antihypertensive peptides have been determined by Lineweaver–Burk plots. Competitive ACE inhibitory peptides have most frequently been reported (Je et al., 2005c; Lee et al., 2010; Zhao et al., 2009). These inhibitors can bind to the active site to block it or to the inhibitor binding site that is remote from the active site to alter the enzyme conformation such that the substrate no longer binds to the active sites. In addition, a noncompetitive mechanism has also been observed in some peptides (Qian et al., 2007; Suetsuna and Nakano, 2000). Numerous in vivo studies of marine-derived antihypertensive peptides in spontaneously hypertensive rats have shown potent ACE inhibition activity (Lee et al., 2010; Qian et al., 2007; Zhao et al., 2009). Marine-derived bioactive peptides have potential for use as functional ingredients in nutraceuticals and pharmaceuticals due to their effectiveness in both prevention and treatment of hypertension. Moreover, cost-effective and safe drugs can be produced from marine bioactive peptides, and further studies are needed with clinical trials for these antihypertensive peptides.

19.2.2 Antioxidant Activity

Recently, a number of studies observed that peptides derived from different marine protein hydrolysates act as potential antioxidants, and they have been isolated from marine organisms such as jumbo squid (Mendis et al., 2005a; Rajapakse et al., 2005b), oyster (Qian et al., 2008), blue mussel (Jung et al., 2005), hoki (Je et al., 2005a; Kim et al., 2007; Mendis et al., 2005b), tuna (Je et al., 2007, 2008), Pacific hake (Samaranayaka and Li-Chan, 2008), capelin (Amarowicz and Shahidi, 1997), scad (Thiansilakul et al., 2007), mackerel (Wu et al., 2003), Alaska pollock (Cho et al., 2008; Je et al., 2005d), conger eel and yellow fin sole (Jun et al., 2004). The beneficial effects of antioxidant marine bioactive peptides are well known in scavenging free radicals and reactive oxygen species or in preventing oxidative damage by interrupting the radical chain reaction of lipid peroxidation (Mendis et al., 2005a; Qian et al., 2008; Rajapakse et al., 2005c). The inhibition of lipid peroxidation by marine bioactive peptide, isolated from jumbo squid, has been determined by a linoleic acid model system, and its activity was much higher than α-tocopherol and was close to highly active synthetic antioxidant, to that of BHT (Mendis et al., 2005a). It has been shown that this antioxidant potency is mostly due to the presence of hydrophobic amino acids in the peptide (Mendis et al., 2005a). Gelatin peptides contain mainly hydrophobic amino acids, and abundance of these amino acids favors higher emulsifying ability. Hence, marine gelatin–derived peptides are expected to exert higher antioxidant effects among other antioxidant peptide sequences (Mendis et al., 2005b). The challenge for food technologists will be to develop functional foods and nutraceuticals without the undesired side effects of the added peptides.

19.2.3 Anticoagulant Activity

The anticoagulant marine bioactive peptides have rarely been reported but have been isolated from marine organisms such as the marine echiuroid worm (Jo et al., 2008), starfish (Koyama et al., 1998), and blue mussel (Jung et al., 2009). Moreover, marine anticoagulant proteins have been purified from blood ark shell (Jung et al., 2001) and yellow fin sole (Rajapakse et al., 2005a). The anticoagulant activity of the earlier-mentioned peptides has been determined by prolongation of activated partial thromboplastin time (APTT), prothrombin time (PT), and thrombin time (TP) assays, and the activity was compared with heparin, the commercial anticoagulant. The anticoagulant peptide (amino acid sequence: GELTPESGPDLFVHFLDGNPSYSLYADAVPR) isolated from the marine echiuroid worm has potently prolonged the normal clotting time on APTT (32.3 ± 0.9 s) to 192.2 ± 2.1 s in a dose-dependent manner with IC_{50} being 42.6 µg mL^{-1} (Jo et al., 2008). In addition, a protein derived from blood ark shell has prolonged the APTT from a 32 s control clotting time to 325 s, and 2.8 µg mL^{-1} of heparin, a commercial anticoagulant, prolonged the APTT also more than 300 s on APTT, PT, and TT (Jung et al., 2001). However, these marine-derived anticoagulant peptides are non-cytotoxic and have potential to be used as functional ingredients in nutraceuticals or pharmaceuticals.

19.2.4 Antimicrobial Activity

Since the first discovery of antimicrobial peptides in insects, more than 700 molecules with this property have been isolated from a wide variety of insects, plants, and mammals (Reddy et al., 2004).

Marine-derived antimicrobial peptides have been well described in the hemolymph of the many marine invertebrates (Tincu and Taylor, 2004) including spider crab (Stensvag et al., 2008), oyster (Liu et al., 2008), American lobster (Battison et al., 2008), shrimp (Bartlett et al., 2002), and green sea urchin (Li et al., 2008). Antibacterial activity has been reported in the hemolymph of the blue crab, *Callinectes sapidus*, and it was highly inhibitory to gram-negative bacteria (Edward et al., 1996). Although there are several reports on antibacterial activity in seminal plasma, few antibacterial peptides have been reported in the mud crab, *Scylla serrata* (Jayasankar and Subramonium, 1999). The antimicrobial peptide derived from the American lobster (*Homarus americanus*) has shown bacteriostatic activity against some gram-negative bacteria, and both protozoastatic and protozoacidal activity against two scuticociliate parasites *Mesanophrys chesapeakensis* and *Anophryoides haemophila*; the latter is a significant of *H. americanus* (Battison et al., 2008). In addition, antimicrobial peptide, named arasin 1, derived from the spider crab (*Hyas araneus*) inhibited the growth of *Corynebacterium glutamicum* (Stensvag et al., 2008). Achour et al. (1997) found that oyster protein extract could enhance proliferation of immunocytes in human immunodeficiency virus (HIV-1).

The need to discover new antimicrobial substances is important due to progressive development of resistance by pathogenic microorganisms against the conventional antibiotics. Marine-derived antimicrobial peptides are considered as promising candidates with broad-spectrum antimicrobial activity. Therefore, it could be suggested that these antimicrobial peptides have potent capacities for new antibiotic development in the pharmaceutical industry as well as in food industry as novel antimicrobial or antifungal agents.

19.2.5 Other Biological Activities

Biologically active marine peptides are food-derived peptides that exert beyond their nutritional value a physiological, hormone-like effect, and their possible roles in reducing the risk of cardiovascular diseases by lowering plasma cholesterol level and anticancer activity by reducing cell proliferation on human breast cancer cell lines have been shown previously (Picot et al., 2006). Moreover, calcium-binding bioactive peptides derived from pepsin hydrolysates of marine fish species, Alaska pollock (*Theragra chalcogramma*) and hoki (*Johnius belengerii*) frame, can be introduced to oriental people with a lactose indigestion and intolerance and calcium-fortified supplements like fruit juices or calcium-rich foods as the alternative for dairy products (Jung and Kim, 2007; Jung et al., 2006). These calcium-binding peptides have shown high affinity to calcium and are also suitable for reducing the risk of osteoporosis. It has been proven that small peptides (di- and tripeptides) generated in the diet can be absorbed across the brush border membrane by a specific peptide transport system and thus produce diverse biological effects.

19.3 Conclusions

Recent studies have provided evidence that marine-derived bioactive peptides play a vital role in human health and nutrition. The possibilities of designing new functional foods and pharmaceuticals to support the reduction or regulation of diet-related chronic malfunctions are promising. Therefore, potential pharmaceuticals developed from marine bioactive peptides can be applied as oral administration instead of intravenous administration. Furthermore, fish processing by-products like food proteins can be easily utilized for producing bioactive peptides. These evidences suggest that due to valuable biological functions with health beneficial effects, marine-derived bioactive peptides have potential as active ingredients for preparation of various functional foods or nutraceutical and pharmaceutical products. Until now, most of the biological activities of marine-derived bioactive peptides have been observed in vitro or in mouse model systems. Therefore, further research studies are needed in order to investigate their activity in humans. However, marine-derived bioactive peptides are an optimistic present donated by the sea and have promising capabilities for the development of novel nutraceuticals and pharmaceuticals.

Acknowledgment

This study was supported by a grant from Marine Bioprocess Research Center of the Marine Bio 21 Project funded by the Ministry of Land, Transport and Maritime Affairs, Republic of Korea.

References

Achour, A., Lachgar, A., and Astgen, A. (1997). Potentialization of IL-2 effect on immune cells by oyster extract (JCOE) in normal and HIV-infected individuals. *Biomedicine and Pharmacotherapy*, 51, 427–429.

Amarowicz, R. and Shahidi, F. (1997). Antioxidant activity of peptide fractions of capelin protein hydrolysates. *Food Chemistry*, 58 (4), 355–359.

Barrow, C. and Shahidi, F. (2008). *Marine Nutraceuticals and Functional Foods*. CRC Press, Boca Raton, FL.

Bartlett, T. C., Cuthbertson, B. J., Shepard, E. F., Chapman, R. W., Grops, P. S., and Warr, G. W. (2002). Crustins, homologues of an 11.5-kDa antibacterial peptide, from two species of penaeid shrimp, *Litopenaeus vannamei* and *Litopenaeus setiferus*. *Marine Biotechnology*, 4, 278–293.

Battison, A. L., Summerfield, R., and Patrzykat, A. (2008). Isolation and characterization of two antimicrobial peptides from haemocytes of the American lobster *Homarus americanus*. *Fish and Shellfish Immunology*, 25, 181–187.

Cho, S. S., Lee, H. K., Yu, C. Y., Kim, M. J., Seong, E. S., Ghimire, B. K., Son, E. H., Choung, M. G., and Lim, J. D. (2008). Isolation and characterization of bioactive peptides from *Hwangtae* (yellowish dried Alaska pollack) protein hydrolysate. *Journal of Food Science and Nutrition*, 13, 196–203.

Clare, D. A. and Swaisgood, H. E. (2000). Bioactive milk peptides: A prospectus. *Journal of Dairy Science*, 83, 1187–1195.

Edward, N. J., Arroll, T. A., and Fan, Z. (1996). Specificity and some physicochemical characteristics of the antibacterial activity from blue crab *Callinectes sapidus*. *Fish and Shellfish Immunology*, 6, 403–413.

Erdmann, K., Cheung, B. W. Y., and Schroder, H. (2008). The possible roles of food-derived bioactive peptides in reducing the risk of cardiovascular disease. *Journal of Nutritional Biochemistry*, 19, 643–654.

Jayasankar, V. and Subramonium, T. (1999). Antibacterial activity of seminal plasma of the mud crab *Scylla serrata* (forskal). *Journal of Experimental Marine Biology and Ecology*, 236, 253–259.

Je, J. Y., Kim, S. Y., and Kim, S. K. (2005a). Preparation and antioxidative activity of hoki frame protein hydrolysate using ultrafiltration membranes. *European Food Research and Technology*, 221, 157–162.

Je, J. Y., Park, P. J., Byun, H. K., Jung, W. K., and Kim, S. K. (2005b). Angiotensin I converting enzyme (ACE) inhibitory peptide derived from the sauce of fermented blue mussel, *Mytilus edulis*. *Bioresource Technology*, 96, 1624–1629.

Je, J. Y., Park, J. Y., Jung, W. K., Park, P. J., and Kim, S. K. (2005c). Isolation of angiotensin I converting enzyme (ACE) inhibitor from fermented oyster sauce, *Crassostrea gigas*. *Food Chemistry*, 90, 809–814.

Je, J. Y., Park, P. J., and Kim, S. K. (2005d). Antioxidant activity of a peptide isolated from Alaska pollack (*Theragra chalcogramma*) frame protein hydrolysate. *Food Research International*, 38, 45–50.

Je, J. Y., Qian, Z. J., Byun, H. G., and Kim, S. K. (2007). Purification and characterization of an antioxidant peptide obtained from tuna backbone protein by enzymatic hydrolysis. *Process Biochemistry*, 42, 840–846.

Je, J. Y., Qian, Z. J., Lee, S. H., Byun, H. G., and Kim, S. K. (2008). Purification and antioxidant properties of bigeye tuna (*Thunnus obesus*) dark muscle peptide on free radical-mediated oxidation systems. *Journal of Medicinal Food*, 11(4), 629–637.

Jo, H. Y., Jung, W. K., and Kim, S. K. (2008). Purification and characterization of a novel anticoagulant peptide from marine echiuroid worm, *Urechis unicinctus*. *Process Biochemistry*, 43, 179–184.

Jun, S. Y., Park, P. J., Jung, W. K., and Kim, S. K. (2004). Purification and characterization of an antioxidative peptide from enzymatic hydrolysates of yellowfin sole (*Limanda aspera*) frame protein. *European Food Research and Technology*, 219, 20–26.

Jung, W. K., Je, J. Y., and Kim, S. K. (2001). A novel anticoagulant protein from *Scapharca broughtonii*. *Journal of Biochemistry and Molecular Biology*, 35, 199–205.

Jung, W. K., Karawita, R., Heo, S. J., Lee, B. J., Kim, S. K., and Jeon, Y. J. (2006). Recovery of a novel Ca-binding peptide from Alaska pollack (*Theragra chalcogramma*) backbone by pepsinolytic hydrolysis. *Process Biochemistry*, 41, 2097–2100.

Jung, W. K. and Kim, S. K. (2007). Calcium-binding peptide derived from pepsinolytic hydrolysates of hoki (*Johnius belengerii*) frame. *European Food Research and Technology*, 224, 763–767.

Jung, W. K., Rajapakse, N., and Kim, S. K. (2005). Antioxidative activity of a low molecular weight peptide derived from the sauce of fermented blue mussel, *Mytilus edulis*. *European Food Research and Technology*, 220, 535–539.

Kannel, W. B. and Higgins, M. (1990). Smoking and hypertension as predictors of cardiovascular risk in population studies. *Journal of Hypertension*, 8, S3–S8.

Kim, S. Y., Je, J. Y., and Kim, S. K. (2007). Purification and characterization of antioxidant peptide from hoki (*Johnius belengerii*) frame protein by gastrointestinal digestion. *Journal of Nutritional Biochemistry*, 18, 31–38.

Koyama, T., Noguchi, K., Aniya, Y., and Sakanashi, M. (1998). Analysis for sites of anticoagulant action of plancinin, a new anticoagulant peptide isolated from the starfish *Acanthaster planci*, in the blood coagulation cascade. *General Pharmacology*, 31, 277–282.

Kumar, R. S., Thekkumkara, T. J., and Sen, G. C. (1991). The mRNA encoding the two angiotensin-converting enzymes is transcribed from the same gene by a tissue-specific choice of alternative transcription initiation sites. *Journal of Biological Chemistry*, 266, 3854–3862.

Lahl, W. J. and Braun, S. D. (1994). Enzymatic production of protein by hydrolysates for food use. *Food Technology*, 48, 68–71.

Lee, S. H., Qian, Z. J., and Kim, S. K. (2010). A novel angiotensin I converting enzyme inhibitory peptide from tuna frame protein hydrolysate and its antihypertensive effect in spontaneously hypertensive rats. *Food Chemistry*, 118, 96–102.

Lee, T. G., Yeum, D. M., Kim, Y. S., Yeo, S. G., Lee, Y. W., Kim, J. S., Kim, I. S., and Kim, S. B. (2005). Peptide inhibitor for angiotensin converting enzyme from thermolysin hydrolysate of Manila clam protein. *Journal of Fisheries Science and Technology*, 8, 109–112.

Li, C., Haug, T., Styrvold, O. B., Jorgensen, T. O., and Stensvag, K. (2008). Strongylocins, novel antimicrobial peptides from the green sea urchin. *Developmental and Comparative Immunology*, 32, 1430–1440.

Li, G. H., Le, G. W., Shi, Y. H., and Shrestha, S. (2003). Angiotensin I—Converting enzyme inhibitory peptides derived from food proteins and their physiological and pharmacological effects. *Nutrition Research*, 24, 469–486.

Liu, Z., Dong, S., Xu, J., Zeng, M., Song, H., and Zhao, Y. (2008). Production of cysteine-rich antimicrobial peptide by digestion of oyster (*Crassostrea gigas*) with alcalase and bromelin. *Food Control*, 19, 231–235.

Mendis, E., Rajapakse, N., Byun, H. G., and Kim, S. K. (2005a). Investigation of jumbo squid (*Dosidicus gigas*) skin gelatin peptides for their in vitro antioxidant effects. *Life Sciences*, 77, 2166–2178.

Mendis, E., Rajapakse, N., and Kim, S. K. (2005b). Antioxidant properties of a radical-scavenging peptide purified from enzymatically prepared fish skin gelatin hydrolysate. *Journal of Agricultural Food Chemistry*, 53, 581–587.

Muruyama, S. and Suzuki, H. A. (1982). A peptide inhibitor of angiotensin I converting enzyme in the tryptic hydrolysate of casein. *Agricultural and Biological Chemistry*, 46, 1393–1394.

Oshima, G., Shimabukuro, H., and Nagasawa, K. (1979). Peptide inhibitors of angiotensin I-converting enzyme in digests of gelatin by bacterial collagenase. *Biochimica Biophysica Acta*, 566, 128–137.

Picot, L., Bordenave, S., Didelot, S., Fruitier-Arnaudin, I., Sannier, F., Thorkelsson, G., Berge, J. P., Guerard, F., Chabeaud, A. et al. (2006). Antiproliferative activity of fish protein hydrolysates on human breast cancer cell lines. *Process Biochemistry*, 41, 1217–1222.

Qian, Z. J., Je, J. Y., and Kim, S. K. (2007). Antihypertensive effect of angiotensin I converting enzyme-inhibitory peptide from hydrolysates of bigeye tuna dark muscle, *Thunnus obesus*. *Journal of Agricultural and Food Chemistry*, 55, 8398–8403.

Qian, Z. J., Jung, W. K., Byun, H. G., and Kim, S. K. (2008). Protective effect of an antioxidative peptide purified from gastrointestinal digests of oyster, *Crassostrea gigas* against free radical induced DNA damage. *Bioresource Technology*, 99, 3365–3371.

Rajapakse, N., Jung, W. K., Mendis, E., Moon, S. H., and Kim, S. K. (2005a). A novel anticoagulant purified from fish protein hydrolysate inhibits factor XIIa and platelet aggregation. *Life Sciences*, 76, 2607–2619.

Rajapakse, N., Mendis, E., Byun, H. G., and Kim, S. K. (2005b). Purification and in vitro antioxidative effects of giant squid muscle peptides on free radical-mediated oxidative systems. *Journal of Nutritional Biochemistry*, 16, 562–569.

Rajapakse, N., Mendis, E., Jung, W. K., Je, J. Y., and Kim, S. K. (2005c). Purification of a radical scavenging peptide from fermented mussel sauce and its antioxidant properties. *Food Research International*, 38, 175–182.

Reddy, K. V., Yedery, R. D., and Aranha, C. (2004). Antimicrobial peptides: Premises and promises. *International Journal of Antimicrobial Agents*, 24, 536–547.

Samaranayaka, A. G. P., and Li-Chan, C. Y. (2008). Autolysis-assisted production of fish protein hydrolysates with antioxidant properties from Pacific hake (*Merluccius productus*). *Food Chemistry*, 107, 768–776.

Sato, M., Hosokawa, T., Yamaguchi, T., Nakano, T., Muramoto, K., Kahara, T., Funayama, K., Kobayashi, A., and Nakano, T. (2002). Angiotensin I-converting enzyme inhibitory peptides derived from wakame (*Undaria pinnatifida*) and their antihypertensive effect in spontaneously hypertensive rats. *Journal of Agricultural and Food Chemistry*, 50, 6245–6252.

Shahidi, F. (2007). *Maximising the Value of Marine By-Products*. CRC Press, Boca Raton, FL.

Shahidi, F. and Zhong, Y. (2008). Bioactive peptides. *Journal of AOAC International*, 91, 914–931.

Sibony, M., Gasc, J. M., Soubrier, F., Alhenc-Gelas, F., and Corvol, P. (1993). Gene expression and tissue localization of the two isomers of ACE. *Hypertension*, 21, 827–835.

Stensvag, K., Haug, T., Sperstad, S. V., Rekdal, O., Indrevoll, B., and Styrvold, O. B. (2008). Arasin 1, a proline-arginine-rich antimicrobial peptide isolated from the spider crab, *Hyas araneus*. *Developmental & Comparative Immunology*, 32, 275–285.

Suetsuna, K., and Nakano, T. (2000). Identification of an antihypertensive peptide from peptic digest of wakame (*Undaria pinnatifida*). *Journal of Nutritional Biochemistry*, 11, 450–454.

Thiansilakul, Y., Benjakul, S., and Shahidi, F. (2007). Antioxidative activity of protein hydrolysate from round scad muscle using alcalase and flavourzyme. *Journal of Food Biochemistry*, 31, 266–287.

Tincu, J. A., and Taylor, S. W. (2004). Antimicrobial peptides from marine invertebrates. *Antimicrobial Agents and Chemotherapy*, 48, 3645–3654.

Vercruysse, L., Camp, J. V., and Smagghe, G. (2005). ACE inhibitory peptides derived from enzymatic hydrolysates of animal muscle protein: A review. *Journal of Agricultural and Food Chemistry*, 53, 8106–8115.

Wu, C. H., Chen, H. M., and Shiau, C. Y. (2003). Free amino acids and peptides as related to antioxidant properties in protein hydrolysates of mackerel (*Scomber austriasicus*). *Food Research International*, 36(9–10), 949–957.

Wu, J. and Ding, X. (2001). Hypotensive and physiological effect of angiotensin converting enzyme inhibitory peptides derived from soy protein on spontaneously hypertensive rats. *Journal of Agricultural and Food Chemistry*, 49, 501–506.

Zhao, Y., Bafang, L., Dong, S., Liu, Z., Zhao, X., Wang, J., and Zeng, M. (2009). A novel ACE inhibitory peptide isolated from *Acaudina molpadioidea* hydrolysate. *Peptides*, 30, 1028–1033.

20

Health Beneficial Effects of Docosahexaenoic Acid: A Marine Treasure

Na-Young Song and Young-Joon Surh

CONTENTS

20.1 Introduction

Polyunsaturated fatty acids (PUFAs) contain multiple double bonds in the backbone structures, which might be crucial for their biological actions. PUFAs include omega-3 (n-3) and omega-6 (n-6) essential fatty acids that contain the first double bond localized at the third and the sixth carbon from the omega end, respectively. The n-3 and n-6 "essential" fatty acids are required for biological processes, but not spontaneously synthesized in the body (Das, 2006). Thus, the n-3 and n-6 fatty acids must be provided by exogenous sources, principally daily diet.

Various plant oils provide the n-3 and n-6 PUFAs to our body as their precursor forms, α-linolenic acid and linoleic acid, respectively (Whelan and Rust, 2006). As illustrated

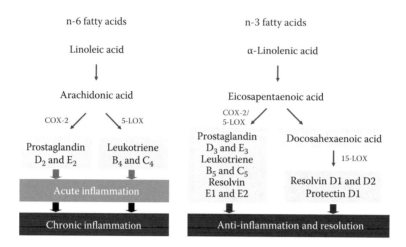

FIGURE 20.1

A general overview of synthesis of eicosanoids and lipid mediators from the n-3 and n-6 PUFAs. The precursor forms of the n-3 and n-6 PUFAs, α-linolenic acid (n-3) and linoleic acid (n-6), undergo metabolism to produce 20-carbon PUFAs, EPA (n-3), and arachidonic acid (n-6). COX and LOX can convert these 20-carbon PUFAs to various eicosanoids involved in cellular physiological processes.

in Figure 20.1, these precursors undergo desaturation and elongation mainly in the liver, producing the n-3 and n-6 PUFAs (Wall et al., 2010). Among the n-3 and n-6 fatty acids, 20-carbon PUFAs, eicosapentaenoic acid (EPA, n-3) and arachidonic acid (n-6), can be further metabolized by cyclooxygenase (COX) and lipoxygenase (LOX) to form a set of distinct eicosanoids involved in modulation of various cellular physiological processes. EPA also produces another representative n-3 PUFA docosahexaenoic acid (DHA) via serial elongation, desaturation, and β-oxidation. DHA is unable to yield eicosanoids. Instead, DHA can produce D series resolvins (RvDs) and protectins that also exert assorted physiological actions including resolution of inflammatory processes (Serhan and Petasis, 2011). Such n-3/n-6 PUFAs and their byproducts have been reported to confer diverse health beneficial effects. However, the n-6 PUFAs might offset the health benefits of the n-3 PUFAs due to adverse effects of arachidonic acid-derived eicosanoids (Calder, 2006). Therefore, the balanced ratio of n-3 to n-6 is important for health beneficial effects, and the higher ratio is preferable for reducing the risk of chronic diseases (Simopoulos, 2002).

As mentioned earlier, the enzymatic processes are required to obtain the n-3 fatty acids from natural dietary products such as plant seed, nut, and soy. However, DHA and EPA can be directly provided from the marine organisms, including salmon, herring, tuna, cod, and marine bacteria *Photobacterium* (Yano et al., 1994, Wall et al., 2010). Such marine organisms usually inhabit under low-temperature deep-sea environments where they have to store more lipids to survive (Wall et al., 2010). Thus, the marine organisms are the primary sources of the n-3 PUFAs, particularly DHA and EPA. As depicted in Figure 20.2, DHA is a carboxylic acid with 22 carbons and 6 *cis* double bonds, while EPA has 20 carbons and 5 *cis* double bonds. These two n-3 fatty acids have been reported to exert similar biological actions with slightly different potencies, due to the similar chemical structures (Deckelbaum and Torrejon, 2012, Mozaffarian and Wu, 2012). Generally, DHA is known to be more effective than EPA in terms of the health beneficial effects (Serini et al., 2011). Therefore, we will focus on the health beneficial effects of DHA herein.

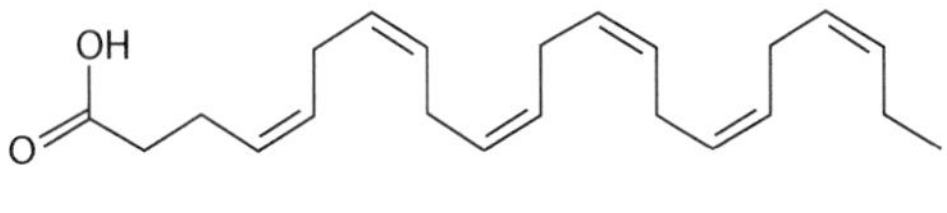

DHA (22:6n-3)

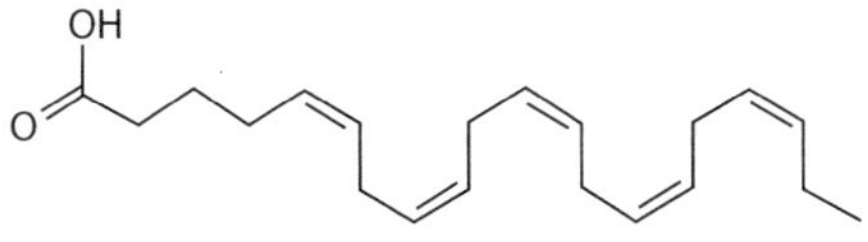

EPA (20:5n-3)

FIGURE 20.2
Chemical structures of DHA and EPA. DHA consists 22 carbons with 5 double bonds, whereas EPA has a 20-carbon chain and 6 double bonds.

20.2 DHA Modulates Inflammatory Processes

20.2.1 Inflammation and Lipid Mediators Derived from the n-3 and n-6 Fatty Acids

Inflammation is the main defense mechanism against infection and various deleterious insults. Once the acute inflammation is initiated, the pro-inflammatory cytokines, such as tumor necrosis factors (TNFs) and interleukins (ILs), are released to recruit neutrophils into the inflammatory site. Subsequently, monocytes and macrophages are further engaged for effective phagocytosis (Serhan and Petasis, 2011). During this process, a lipid mediator class switching occurs, from the initial pro-inflammatory mediators to the pro-resolving mediators in order to promote the resolution phase that returns the body to homeostasis (Serhan, 2007). If the acute inflammation is not completely resolved, the inflammatory responses might be prolonged and aggravated, leading to chronic inflammation. The unresolved chronic inflammation is the prime etiology of many human diseases, including rheumatoid arthritis, Crohn's disease, lupus, diabetes, asthma, obesity, cardiovascular diseases, neurodegenerative diseases, and cancer (Serhan et al., 2008).

The lipid mediators derived from n-3 and n-6 PUFAs play key roles in the overall inflammatory events. At the beginning of the inflammation, the n-6 arachidonic acid produces the pro-inflammatory eicosanoids, including prostaglandins (prostaglandin D_2 and E_2; PGD_2 and PGE_2) and leukotrienes (leukotriene B_4 and C_4) (see Figure 20.1; Calder, 2006). However, the n-3 fatty acid is known to take part in anti-inflammation. Cumulative evidence supports that fish oil supplementation abundant in the n-3 fatty acid remarkably reduces expression of the inflammatory markers and concomitantly induces the anti-inflammatory gene expression (Bouwens et al., 2009, Deike et al., 2012). A *fat-1* transgenic mouse rich in endogenous n-3 fatty acids was generated by knocking-in of *Caenorhabditis elegans fat-1* gene that encodes the n-3 fatty acid desaturase able to convert the n-6 into the n-3 PUFAs (Kang et al., 2004). Interestingly, this *fat-1* mouse exhibits low expression levels of the pro-inflammatory genes, such as COX-2, PGE_2, and ILs (Gravaghi et al., 2011). Moreover, the *fat-1* mice are less susceptible to dextran sodium sulfate (DSS)–induced colitis and cerulein-induced pancreatitis (Hudert et al., 2006, Weylandt et al., 2008). Based on these investigations, the n-3 fatty acids seem to be potential inhibitors of inflammation.

20.2.2 Anti-Inflammatory Effects of DHA

DHA is thought to be the prime ingredient responsible for the anti-inflammatory effect of the n-3 PUFAs. Oral administration of DHA (30 mg/kg/day) attenuates DSS-induced acute colitis in terms of symptomatic markers (colon length, stool consistency, and diarrhea), histopathological scores (inflammation score, crypt destruction, and infiltration of neutrophils), and myeloperoxidase activity (Cho et al., 2011). Furthermore, the microarray analysis shows downregulation of DSS-induced pro-inflammatory cytokines in DHA-fed mice (Cho et al., 2011). DHA-enriched diet also attenuated inflammatory edema in 2,4-dinitro-1-fluorobenzene-induced contact hypersensitivity in mice and carrageenan-induced rat paw edema (Nakamura et al., 1994, Tomobe et al., 2000). These findings suggest the immunosuppressive and anti-inflammatory effects of DHA.

The anti-inflammatory effects of DHA might be attributed to its direct influence on immune cells. DHA prevents adhesion of neutrophils to endothelial cells, the initial phase of inflammation, via downregulation of adhesion molecules, such as vascular adhesion molecule-1 and P-selectin (Wang et al., 2003, 2011b, Yates et al., 2011). Moreover, DHA intake at a dose of 36 mg/kg/day for 4 weeks reduced phagocytosis as well as chemotaxis in rat peritoneal macrophages (Bulbul et al., 2007). DHA also attenuates maturation and cytokine secretion of dendritic cells, the antigen presenting cells that link between innate and adaptive immunity (Kong et al., 2010, 2011). A study with human subjects reveals that supplementation with DHA suppresses activation of T lymphocytes (Kew et al., 2004).

The direct suppressive effect of DHA on the immune cells can extend to nonimmune cells and peripheral tissues in a paracrine manner. Activated immune cells produce various pro-inflammatory cytokines that circulate in the blood stream and provoke inflammatory responses in the peripheries. DHA inhibits LPS-induced secretion of IL-1β, IL-6, and TNF-α from THP-1 macrophages (Mullen et al., 2010). DHA also attenuates production of IL-12, a pro-inflammatory cytokine, in murine dendritic cells, while secretion of the anti-inflammatory cytokine IL-10 is enhanced (Draper et al., 2011). Moreover, deoxynivalenol-induced expression of IL-6 was found to be suppressed in peritoneal macrophages obtained from DHA-fed mice (Shi and Pestka, 2009). In addition to reduced secretion of the pro-inflammatory cytokines from the immune cells, DHA can attenuate inflammatory responses in nonimmune cells via suppression of pro-inflammatory proteins. COX-2 is one of the most well-known proteins induced in the inflammatory reactions (Morteau, 2000). Overexpression of COX-2 is implicated in numerous human diseases, including cancer (Ristimaki et al., 1997, Tucker et al., 1999, Warner and Mitchell, 2004). It has been reported that DHA inhibits IL-1α-induced expression as well as activity of COX-2 in human saphenous vein endothelial cells (Massaro et al., 2006). DHA also attenuates COX-2 expression induced by ultraviolet B (UVB) radiation in hairless mouse skin (Rahman et al., 2011). NADP(H) oxidases (NOXs) are involved in generation of reactive oxygen species (ROS), such as superoxide anion, leading to profound inflammation. DHA downregulates NOX4 in various types of cells, which might be suggested as an additional mechanism of the anti-inflammatory effect of DHA (Massaro et al., 2006, Richard et al., 2009, Rahman et al., 2011).

Multiple lines of evidence support that DHA also inhibits COX-2 expression in several types of human cancer cells, including hepatocellular carcinoma, cholangiocarcinoma, colon cancer, and breast cancer cells (Calviello et al., 2004, Horia and Watkins, 2007, Lim et al., 2008, 2009). The inhibition of COX-2 by DHA leads to reduced production of PGE$_2$, one of the COX-2-dependent metabolites that takes part in tumor promotion and progression (Calviello et al., 2004, Swamy et al., 2004, Horia and Watkins, 2007). Moreover, celecoxib, a well-known COX-2 inhibitor, potentiates DHA-induced growth arrest and apoptosis of cancer cells possibly via inhibition of nuclear factor-κB (NF-κB) activity (Swamy et al., 2004, Narayanan et al., 2005). These findings suggest that DHA may inhibit inflammation-associated tumorigenesis through downregulation of NF-κB-dependent COX-2 expression.

20.2.3 Molecular Mechanisms of DHA-Induced Anti-Inflammatory Effects

The primary molecular mechanism underlying the anti-inflammatory effects of DHA is inhibition of NF-κB, a key transcription factor responsible for expression of proteins mediating inflammation and immune responses, such as ILs and COX-2. NF-κB is normally present as a dimer, mainly composed of p50 and p65, and sequestered in the cytoplasm as an inactive complex with its negative regulator IκB proteins (Surh, 2003). When IκB is phosphorylated by IκB kinase (IKK), it undergoes proteasomal-dependent degradation, allowing NF-κB to translocate into the nucleus and transactivate target genes (Surh, 2003). DHA attenuates TNF-α-induced degradation of IκBα and nuclear accumulation of the p50 and p65 subunits in human aortic endothelial cells (Wang et al., 2011b). DHA shows the consistent effects on IκBα, p50, and p65 in LPS-treated THP-1 macrophages (Mullen et al., 2010). Furthermore, DHA inhibits NF-κB p65 DNA-binding activity provoked by LPS in THP1 macrophages and human kidney cells (Li et al., 2005, Martinez-Micaelo et al., 2012).

In addition to NF-κB, several transcription factors have been proposed as alternative molecular targets of DHA in its exerting anti-inflammatory responses. Peroxisome proliferator–activated receptors (PPARs) are transcription factors that regulate transcription of genes involved in metabolism and immunomodulation. It has been reported that DHA-induced PPARγ activation leads to inhibition of NF-κB as well as cytokine secretion (Li et al., 2005, Zapata-Gonzalez et al., 2008). Moreover, the n-3 fatty acid–enriched supplementation activates PPARα that subsequently interacts with the p65 subunit of NF-κB, interfering NF-κB-dependent transcription of the pro-inflammatory mediators (Zuniga et al., 2011). Suppression of activator protein 1 and cAMP response element-binding protein is responsible for the anti-inflammatory effect of DHA as well (Shi and Pestka, 2009, Wang et al., 2011b). Moreover, NF-E2-related factor 2 (Nrf2), a redox-sensitive transcription factor, mediates DHA suppression of COX-2, IL-1β, IL-6, and TNF-α, possibly by reducing the levels of ROS and nitric oxide (NO) (Wang et al., 2010b). DHA has been reported to block ROS and NO production in murine macrophages (Komatsu et al., 2003, Ambrozova et al., 2010). Thus, DHA exerts anti-inflammatory effects via multiple molecular mechanisms.

20.2.4 Pro-Resolving Properties of DHA

The lipid mediator class switching from anti-inflammatory to pro-resolving mediators occurs to better prepare the termination of the acute inflammation (Serhan, 2007). During the resolution phase, the pro-resolving mediators inhibit excessive recruitment of neutrophils and eliminate apoptotic cells and debris from inflamed sites in order to prevent the spread out of inflammation (Serhan et al., 2008). Resolvins and protectins are the representative pro-resolving lipid mediators. DHA is a crucial source for these two pro-resolving mediators, particularly D series of resolvins (RvD1 and RvD2) and protectin D1 (PD1) (Serhan and Petasis, 2011). RvD2 has been reported to reduce infiltration, adhesion, and emigration of leukocytes (Spite et al., 2009). Moreover, RvD1 switches macrophage polarization from inflammatory M1 to anti-inflammatory M2, resulting in stimulation of non-phlogistic macrophage phagocytosis (Titos et al., 2011). PD1 also increases macrophage phagocytosis of apoptotic polymorphonuclear neutrophils (PMNs), whereas it attenuates infiltration of PMNs (Serhan et al., 2006, Schwab et al., 2007). Thus, DHA-derived resolvins and protectins play crucial roles in orchestration of the resolution phase. When unresolved inflammation becomes chronic, it might cause various human diseases. In this regard, the anti-inflammatory and pro-resolving effects of DHA seem to be the fundamental feature for its health benefits.

20.3 DHA Retards, Prevents, and Suppresses Tumorigenesis

20.3.1 Lessons from fat-1 Mice: Chemopreventive Roles of the n-3 Fatty Acids

The *fat-1* transgenic mice display higher levels of the n-3 PUFAs due to expression of the *C. elegans* n-3 fatty acid *fat-1* desaturase, as mentioned in Section 20.2.1. When the *fat-1* mice are subcutaneously injected with murine B16 melanoma cells, growth rates and volumes of melanomas were remarkably reduced compared with wild-type mice (Xia et al., 2006). The *fat-1* mice are also resistant to diethylnitrosamine-induced hepatocarcinogenesis and colitis-induced colon carcinogenesis (Jia et al., 2008, Weylandt et al., 2011). Therefore, the knocking-in of *fat-1* gene can prevent tumor formation and also retard the tumor growth, which is attributable to enriched endogenous n-3 fatty acids, such as DHA. This chemopreventive effect of n-3 PUFAs accumulated in *fat-1* mice appears to be mediated by dampening of the NF-κB-dependent inflammatory signaling (Nowak et al., 2007, Griffitts et al., 2010).

20.3.2 DHA Inhibits Multistage Carcinogenesis

Carcinogenesis is generally described as a multistage process that can be divided into initiation, promotion, and progression. During the initiation stage of carcinogenesis, irreversible genetic changes occur. An intraperitoneal injection of DHA protected against 2,4,7,8-tetrachlorodibenzo-ρ-dioxin (TCDD)-induced DNA damage in rat liver (Turkez et al., 2011). Pretreatment with DHA also reduced formation of DNA adducts as well as aberrant crypt foci induced by 2-amino-1-methyl-6-phenylimidazo[4,5-b]pyridine (PhIP) in the rat colon (Takahashi et al., 1997). ROS play a crucial role in DNA damage (Ziech et al., 2011). A topical application of DHA onto mouse skin downregulates UVB-induced expression of NOX4, a key enzyme responsible for cellular ROS production (Rahman et al., 2011). DHA can also upregulate expression of diverse antioxidant enzymes and related proteins via activation of Nrf2 (Gao et al., 2007). Thus, DHA might prevent and retard the initial stage of carcinogenesis by hampering irreversible genetic alteration.

Once the cell has been mutated and transformed, its proliferation can be sped up during the promotion stage. DHA has been shown to suppress JB6 cell transformation on soft agar induced by the tumor promoter phorbol myristate acetate and epidermal growth factor (Liu et al., 2001). DHA has been shown to inhibit growth and proliferation of various types of cancer cells, such as breast, colon, liver, and pancreatic cancer cells (Wu et al., 2005, Kato et al., 2007, Lee et al., 2010, Song et al., 2011). DHA induces cell cycle arrest in the G1 to S phase as well as retardation of DNA synthesis, consequently delaying cell cycle progression in cancer cells (Khan et al., 2006, Kato et al., 2007, Lee et al., 2010). Furthermore, DHA induces apoptosis in several cancer cell lines through activation of caspases and repression of antiapoptotic proteins, such as Bcl-2 and Bcl-XL (Lim et al., 2008, Ghosh-Choudhury et al., 2009, Kang et al., 2010). Interestingly, DHA induces accumulation of ROS in MCF-7 human breast cancer cells, which seems crucial for DHA-induced apoptosis (Kang et al., 2010). This is contradictory to the investigation that DHA exerts an antioxidative effect. Leonardi et al. have shown that DHA has dual effects on the cellular redox status, anti- and pro-oxidative effects, depending on its dose and time, which might explain such a contradiction (Leonardi et al., 2007). In vivo data also support the inhibitory effect of DHA on tumor growth. DHA feeding reduced the growth of cancer cells transplanted in rodents (Rose et al., 1995, Calviello et al., 2004, Gleissman et al., 2011). The xenograft tumors of DHA-fed group displayed downregulation of a proliferation marker Ki67, while the tumors showed an increase in the percentage of apoptotic cells detected by the terminal deoxynucleotidyl transferase–mediated dUTP in situ nick-end labeling technique (Calviello et al., 2004).

Metastasis is the hallmark of poor prognosis for cancer treatment (Ruiter et al., 2001). DHA can inhibit tumor migration and invasion, the initial steps in metastasis. DHA reduces expression and activity of matrix metalloproteinases (MMPs), zinc-dependent endopeptidases that degrade extracellular matrix and thereby enable tumor cells to escape from the primary site (Connolly and Rose, 1993, Suzuki et al., 1997, Shinto et al., 2009, Wu et al., 2012). As a consequence, DHA inhibits cell migration and invasion in several cancer cell lines (McCabe et al., 2005, Isbilen et al., 2006, Horia and Watkins, 2007, D'Eliseo et al., 2011, Wu et al., 2012). Furthermore, DHA attenuates expression of vascular endothelial cell growth factor (VEGF), a major stimulator for angiogenesis, in human colon cancer cells and tumors obtained from HT-29 cells transplanted in nude mice (Calviello et al., 2004, 2007). In line with these observations, DHA-fed rats showed reduced vascularization in N-methylnitrosourea (NMU)-induced mammary tumors compared with a control group, which was assessed by the power Doppler sonography (Colas et al., 2006). The tube formation and mouse dorsal air sac assays also support an antiangiogenic effect of DHA in vitro and in vivo (Tsuzuki et al., 2007, Szymczak et al., 2008). The inhibitory effect of DHA on migration, invasion, and angiogenesis might be due to destabilization of hypoxia-inducible factor-1 α (HIF-1α), a transcription factor responsible for expression of genes required for rescue of hypoxic stress, such as MMPs and VEGF. Collectively, DHA has antimetastatic and antiangiogenic potential (Mandal et al., 2010).

In addition, DHA is suggested as an adjuvant agent in chemotherapy. The combination treatment with DHA potentiates growth arrest and apoptosis of cancer cells induced by chemotherapeutics, such as 5-fluorouracil and ectoposide (Calviello et al., 2005, Zhuo et al., 2009, Wang et al., 2011a). This might be attributable to inhibitory effects of DHA on expression and activity of multidrug-resistance protein 1 (Kuan et al., 2011). DHA increases uptake of vincristine, an anticancer drug, while reducing its efflux from the cancer cell (Das and Madhavi, 2011). Furthermore, DHA treatment depleted the intracellular glutathione in some cancer cells, thereby sensitizing apoptosis of cancer cells during the chemotherapy (Merendino et al., 2003, 2005).

20.4 DHA as a Brain Food

20.4.1 DHA Enhances the Brain Development

Hippocampal DHA accumulation occurs during brain development, implying that DHA plays a crucial role in brain functions (Green and Yavin, 1998). DHA promotes differentiation of neural stem cells into neurons (Kawakita et al., 2006). Moreover, DHA enhances neurite outgrowth and proliferation of neural cells (He et al., 2009). In hippocampal neuronal cultures, DHA supplementation induces synapsin puncta formation and synaptic activity, implying that DHA promotes synaptogenesis as well as functional maturation of synapses (Cao et al., 2009). However, depletion of DHA alters neurogenesis in the embryonic rat brain, which may lead to delay and/or inhibition of normal brain development (Coti Bertrand et al., 2006). Given these investigations, DHA might take part in the brain development, including neuronal differentiation, neurogenesis, neuritogenesis, and synaptogenesis.

20.4.2 DHA Improves the Learning Ability

DHA is involved in the learning ability as well. The *fat-1* transgenic mice rich in the n-3 PUFAs display about 220% higher levels of DHA in the brain cortex compared with wild-type littermates (Boudrault et al., 2010). In the Morris water maze, the *fat-1* mice spend less time reaching the hidden platform than wild-type counterparts (He et al., 2009). Moreover, the long-term oral administration of DHA over 10 weeks reduced reference and working memory errors in aged rats (Gamoh et al., 2001). Such improvement of learning and cognitive abilities by DHA supplementation might be due to induced expression of brain-derived neurotrophic factor (BNDF) responsible for memory functions in hippocampus tissues (Jiang et al., 2009). DHA deficiency in the brain, however, is associated with impaired spatial learning and memory abilities (Xiao et al., 2006). Taken together, these investigations suggest that DHA may improve the learning performance.

Attention-deficit hyperactivity disorder (ADHD) is characterized by hyperactivity, impulsivity, and inattention, which is likely to be associated with learning difficulty (Geissler and Lesch, 2011). Interestingly, children with ADHD show lower DHA levels in erythrocytes compared with control subjects (Stevens et al., 1995). Particularly, ADHD patients with learning disabilities have lower DHA levels than normal individuals, implying that DHA supplementation may improve learning difficulties related to ADHD (Milte et al., 2011). However, there is no significant correlation between DHA supplementation and alleviation of ADHD symptoms, although some reports show slight improvement by DHA (Hirayama et al., 2004, Transler et al., 2010). Thus, further investigation is required to fully understand the role of DHA in improvement of the learning ability in subjects with ADHD.

20.4.3 DHA Ameliorates Alzheimer Disease

Alzheimer disease (AD) is the most common neurodegenerative disorder in the elderly characterized by dementia. The main pathological hallmarks of AD are extracellular deposition of amyloid β (Aβ) and intracellular accumulation of hyperphosphorylated tau proteins (Jucker and Walker, 2011). It has been reported that a low serum level of DHA might be a pivotal risk factor for AD (Kyle et al., 1999). Notably, DHA-depleting diet results in poor acquisition performance and thigmotaxis deficit in mice, which is corrected by DHA supplementation (Calon et al., 2004). Multiple lines of evidence support DHA-induced amelioration of AD. Dietary supplementation of DHA mitigates impaired learning ability in Aβ-infused rats (Hashimoto et al., 2002, 2005a,b). DHA administration also improves the cognitive deficits in Tg2567 mice utilized as an animal model of AD due to deposition of Aβ in the brain (Calon et al., 2004).

The beneficial effect of DHA on AD might be closely related with reduction of Aβ. DHA-enriched diet lowered the level of Aβ as well as plaque burden in the brain cortex of Tg2536 mice (Lim et al., 2005). Moreover, DHA alters the processing module of amyloid precursor proteins from amyloidogenic status able to produce Aβ toward the non-amyloidogenic mode (Sahlin et al., 2007, Grimm et al., 2011). DHA also protects against Aβ-induced cell death in primary hippocampal cultures (Wang et al., 2010a). In addition, DHA influences tau pathology as well. The 3 × Tg-AD mouse model exhibits not only Aβ deposition but also tau pathology, another hallmark of AD (Oddo et al., 2003). Dietary DHA inhibits accumulation and phosphorylation of tau in 3 × Tg-AD mice (Green et al., 2007).

However, DHA-induced amelioration of AD is still controversial in clinical studies with human subjects. Morris et al. have demonstrated that dietary intake of DHA is associated with the reduced risk of AD in a prospective study conducted with total 815 normal subjects (Morris et al., 2003). In contrast, Quinn and colleagues have shown that DHA supplementation has no effect on improvement of cognitive decline in patients with mild to moderate AD (Quinn et al., 2010). It appears that DHA may reduce the incidence of AD, while it does not alleviate and/or treat the symptoms of AD in human subjects.

20.5 DHA and Metabolic Disorders

20.5.1 Antiobesity Effect of DHA

Obesity is the prime risk factor of developing metabolic disorders, such as diabetes, hypertension, and heart diseases (Grundy, 2004). It has been reported that obese subjects have a low plasma concentration of DHA compared with normal lean individuals (Micallef et al., 2009). Notably, DHA supplementation reduces body weight in obese KK mice (Arai et al., 2009). Furthermore, dietary DHA lowers the masses of retroperitoneal plus epididymal white fat pads in high-fat diet–fed rats (Oudart et al., 1997). A clinical study with human subjects also supports the antiobesity effect of DHA. Fish oil diet results in weight loss in overweight men (Thorsdottir et al., 2007). This might be due to an increase of the n-3 fatty acid accumulation, based on the report that fish consumption among overweight adults is positively correlated with the proportion of DHA plus EPA in erythrocyte phospholipids (Thorsdottir et al., 2009). Furthermore, an intervention study with 20 severely obese women shows that the n-3 PUFA supplement led to weight loss and the body mass index decrease, which was significantly correlated with the elevated DHA level in serum phospholipids (Kunesova et al., 2006). The antiobesity effect of DHA seems to be mainly attributed to regulation of energy balance and lipid metabolism. Chronic DHA intake induces expression of uncoupling protein 3 in mice, possibly facilitating energy expenditure (Cha et al., 2001). Moreover, DHA is involved in lipid metabolism, particularly inhibition of lipogenesis and induction of lipolysis. Taken all these findings together, DHA might be a useful nutraceutical for improvement of obesity.

20.5.2 DHA and Diabetes Mellitus

Diabetes mellitus is a metabolic disorder characterized by high blood sugar (hyperglycemia), mainly classified into type 1 (T1DM) and type 2 (T2DM) depending on insulin dependency. Whereas T1DM is an insulin-dependent disorder that can be treated by insulin injection, the insulin-independent T2DM results from insulin resistance, a situation of reduced insulin sensitivity (American Diabetes Association, 2011). Interestingly, the *fat-1* mice are resistant to streptozotocin-induced T1DM due to inhibition of inflammation and subsequent β-cell destruction (Bellenger et al., 2011). Moreover, the *fat-1* mice have improved glucose tolerance against high-carbohydrate diet challenge (Ji et al., 2009).

A clinical study also shows that fish oil intake ameliorates insulin resistance in overweight and obese human subjects (Ramel et al., 2008). Thus, the n-3 fatty acids may prevent and improve T1DM as well as T2DM. DHA alone exerts an antidiabetic effect as well. DHA supplementation lowered the incidence of T1DM and plasma glucose levels in the chemically induced T1DM rat model (Suresh and Das, 2003). Dietary intake of DHA prevented insulin sensitivity and improved insulin resistance in rodents (Shimura et al., 1997, Vemuri et al., 2007, Andersen et al., 2008). Furthermore, DHA-derived metabolites can potently activate PPARγ, like "glitazones" useful for T2DM treatment (Yamamoto et al., 2005). In this regard, chronic intake of DHA, both DHA alone and combination with other n-3 PUFAs, might be helpful to prevent and/or reverse type 1 and 2 diabetes mellitus.

20.5.3 DHA and Cardiovascular Diseases

Cardiovascular disease (CVD), one of the major metabolic disorders, is a collective term that refers to a class of diseases related to heart and blood vessels, such as hypertension, atherosclerosis, and coronary artery disease. The blood lipid profile is a predictable index of CVD. High serum levels of total cholesterol, low-density lipoprotein cholesterol (LDL-C), and triglycerides (TGs) as well as low plasma high-density lipoprotein cholesterol (HDL-C) are recognized as the primary risk parameters of CVD (Barter et al., 2007, Sarwar et al., 2007). Dietary supplementation with DHA lowers the TG concentration and increases the HDL-C level in normal subjects as well as patients with dyslipidemia, although DHA is unlikely to significantly affect the plasma level of LDL-C (Davidson et al., 1997, Grimsgaard et al., 1997, Maki et al., 2005). DHA intake also decreases serum levels of C-reactive protein and inflammatory cytokines, markers of systemic inflammation associated with high risk of CVD (Kelley et al., 2009, Makhoul et al., 2011). Consequently, DHA reduces the blood pressure and the heart rate, while increasing the coronary flow velocity (Mori et al., 1999, Theobald et al., 2007, Oe et al., 2008). Notably, a higher plasma DHA level is inversely related to progression of coronary atherosclerosis as well as the risk of sudden death from cardiac causes (Albert et al., 2002, Erkkila et al., 2006). DHA thus might lessen the risk of CVD, possibly due to improvement of the lipid profile and attenuation of systemic inflammation.

20.6 Concluding Remarks

The various health benefits of the n-3 PUFAs have been extensively investigated with substantial and convincing evidence (Das, 2006, Yashodhara et al., 2009). As illustrated in Table 20.1, the *fat-1* mice enriched with the n-3 fatty acids are less susceptible to inflammation, carcinogenesis, and some metabolic diseases, compared with the wild-type counterparts. DHA is the most prominent PUFA among the n-3. DHA possesses a wide spectrum of health beneficial effects, which have been confirmed in plenty of animal models and clinical studies as summarized in Tables 20.2 and 20.3, respectively. High dose and/or long-term intake of DHA are relatively safe without any deleterious effect, suggesting that DHA is suitable for controlling chronic diseases (Lien, 2009). In addition to DHA itself, its metabolites, such as RvDs and PD1, are emerging as important regulators of cellular physiology, especially resolution of acute inflammation, which merit further investigations.

TABLE 20.1

Attenuation of Tumorigenesis, Inflammation, and Other Related Events in the *fat-1* Mice

Treatment	Effects	References
Analysis of ratio of n-3/n-6 in organs	The n-3/n-6 ratio ranges from 0.7 to 5.7 in various organs of *fat-1* mice	Kang et al. (2004)
DSS-induced acute and chronic colitis models	↓ Levels of COX-2, PGE$_2$ and pro-inflammatory cytokines	Gravaghi et al. (2011)
DSS-induced colitis model	↓ Body weight loss and colon shortening ↓ Severity and thickness of the inflammatory infiltrate ↑ Levels of RvE1, RvD3, and PD1 ↓ NF-κB activity ↓ mRNA expression levels of TNF-α and IL-1β	Hudert et al. (2006)
Cerulein-induced acute and chronic pancreatitis model	↓ IL-1β, IL-6, myeloperoxidase activity, and pancreatic necrosis in acute pancreatitis ↓ IL-6, fibrosis, and pancreatic stellate cell activation in chronic pancreatitis	Weylandt et al. (2008)
B16 melanoma-implanted *fat-1* mice	↓ Tumor incidence, tumor volume, and growth of B16 melanoma xenograft	Xia et al. (2006)
Diethylnitrosamine-induced liver cancer model	↓ Number of tumors lager than 3-mm and largest tumor diameter ↓ Levels of TNF-α, COX-2, and alanine transaminase ↓ Liver fibrogenesis	Weylandt et al. (2011)
Azoxymethane-initiated and DSS-promoted colon cancer model	↓ Number of colonic adenocarcinomas ↓ Inflammation score ↑ Long-term resolution of inflammation ↓ Levels of PGD$_2$ and PGE$_2$ ↑ Level of PGE$_3$	Jia et al. (2008)
Azoxymethane-initiated and DSS-promoted colon cancer model	↓ Tumor incidence ↓ Severity of inflammation ↓ NF-κB activity	Nowak et al. (2007)
Comparison between mice with double mutations (*c-Myc/TGF-β*) and those with triple mutations (*c-Myc/TGF-β/fat-1*)	Delayed development of tumors in the triple mutation mice ↓ Tumor volume in the triple mutation mice ↓ NF-κB activity in the triple mutation mice	Griffitts et al. (2010)
Measurement of learning ability	↑ Hippocampal neurogenesis ↑ Performance in the Morris water maze	He et al. (2009)
Streptozotocin-induced diabetes model	Resistant to hyperglycemia, β-cell damage, and hyperinsulinemia ↓ Levels of TNF-α and IL-1β ↓ NF-κB activity	Bellenger et al. (2011)
High-carbohydrate diet	↑ Glucose tolerance ↓ Body weight	Ji et al. (2009)
Analysis of fatty acid composition and protein expression in the brain cortex	↑ Level of DHA ↓ Levels of the n-6 PUFAs and COX-2	Boudrault et al. (2010)

TABLE 20.2

Chemopreventive and Other Health Beneficial Effects of DHA in Animal Models

Animal	Route of Administration	Effects	References
DSS-induced colitis in BALB/c mice	Oral administration of 30 mg/kg/day DHA	↓ Weight loss and colon shortening ↓ Levels of IL-1β and MMPs ↓ Myeloperoxidase activity	Cho et al. (2011)
Contact hypersensitivity reaction mouse model	Diet containing 4.8% DHA ethyl ester (97% purity)	↓ Ear swelling ↓ Infiltration of CD4-positive T lymphocytes ↓ Levels of interferon γ, IL-1β, IL-2, and IL-6	Tomobe et al. (2000)
Carrageenan-induced paw edema rat model	DHA-rich diet	↓ Swelling of footpads	Nakamura et al. (1994)
Peritoneal macrophages of DHA-fed Wistar rats	Oral administration of 36 mg/kg/day DHA	↓ Phagocytic and chemotactic activities	Bulbul et al. (2007)
Hairless mice exposed to UVB radiation	Topical application of DHA (2.5 and 10 μmol)	↓ Levels of COX-2 and NOX 4 ↓ NF-κB activity	Rahman et al. (2011)
TCDD-injected Sprague-Dawley rats	Intraperitoneal injection of 250 mg/kg DHA	↑ Levels of DHA and antioxidant enzymes ↓ Number of micronucleated hepatocytes ↓ Parenchymal degeneration, sinusoidal dilatation, lymphocyte infiltration, and lipid accumulation	Turkez et al. (2011)
PhIP-treated F344 rats	Intragastrically administration of 1 mL/rat DHA	↓ Number of aberrant crypt foci in the colon ↓ PhIP-DNA adducts	Takahashi et al. (1997)
MDA-MB-435 human breast cancer cells–implanted nude mice	Diet containing 8% DHA	↓ Growth of mammary fat pad tumors ↓ Lung metastasis	Rose et al. (1995)
HT-29 human colon cancer cells–implanted nude mice	Oral administration of 1 g/kg DHA ethyl ester	↓ Tumor volume and weight ↓ Levels of VEGF, COX-2, and PGE$_2$ in tumors ↓ Proliferating cells in tumors ↑ Apoptotic cells in tumors	Calviello et al. (2004)
Neuroblastoma-implanted nude rats	Diet containing 16% DHA and oral administration of 0.5 and 1 g/kg DHA	↓ Tumor incidence in diet group ↓ Median tumor weight and volume in oral administration group	Gleissman et al. (2011)
NMU-treated Sprague-Dawley rats	Diet containing 8% DHA	↓ Power Doppler index of tumor vascularization	Colas et al. (2006)
ICR mice with a dorsal air sac containing a chamber ring filled with DLD-1 cells	Oral administration of 10 mg conjugated DHA and 50 mg DHA	↓ Vessel formation	Tsuzuki et al. (2007)
Aged Wistar rats	Oral administration of 300 mg/kg DHA	↓ Number of reference and working memory errors in eight-arm radial maze	Gamoh et al. (2001)

TABLE 20.2 (continued)

Chemopreventive and Other Health Beneficial Effects of DHA in Animal Models

Animal	Route of Administration	Effects	References
Aged Kunming-line mice	Oral administration of 50 and 100 mg/kg DHA	↓ Number of errors in the step-through test ↓ Number of errors in the passageway water maze ↑ Level of BNDF	Jiang et al. (2009)
Tg2576 mice	DHA-depleted 0.6% DHA-containing diets	↓ Acquisition performance and thigmotaxis in DHA-depleted diet group ↑ Acquisition performance and thigmotaxis in DHA-fed group	Calon et al. (2004)
Aβ-infused Wistar rats	Oral administration of 300 mg/kg DHA ethyl ester	↑ Number of avoidance responses in the escape/avoidance training	Hashimoto et al. (2002)
Aβ-infused Wistar rats	Oral administration of 300 mg/kg DHA ethyl ester	↓ Number of reference memory errors ↓ Level of cholesterol in detergent insoluble membrane fractions	Hashimoto et al. (2005a)
Aβ-infused Wistar rats	Oral administration of 300 mg/kg DHA ethyl ester	↓ Number of reference and working memory errors in eight-arm radial maze	Hashimoto et al. (2005b)
Tg2576 mice	Diet containing 0.6% DHA	↓ Total Aβ ↓ Plaque burden	Lim et al. (2005)
3 × Tg mice	DHA-enriched diet	↓ Intraneuronal accumulation of Aβ and tau	Green et al. (2007)
Obese KK mice	DHA-rich fish oil diet	↓ Body weight ↓ Liver weight ↓ Liver TG and total cholesterol levels ↓ Fat droplet accumulation ↓ Plasma insulin level	Arai et al. (2009)
High-fat diet–fed Wistar rats	DHA-rich diet	↓ Mass of retroperitoneal plus epididymal white fat pads ↓ Protein concentration and DNA content in brown adipose tissue	Oudart et al. (1997)
Aged C57BL/6NJcl mice	DHA-rich diet	↑ Level of uncoupling protein 3 in the gastrocnemius muscle	Cha et al. (2001)
Alloxan-treated Wistar rats	Oral administration of 500 μg/kg DHA	↓ Incidence of T1DM ↓ Plasma glucose level ↑ Plasma insulin level	Suresh and Das (2003)
Wistar rats	Oral administration of 500 mg/kg DHA methyl ester	↓ Fasting plasma levels of glucose and insulin ↓ Insulin resistance	Andersen et al. (2008)
Conjugated linoleic acid–treated C57BL/6N mice	Diet containing 1.5% DHA	↓ Insulin resistance ↓ Fatty liver ↑ Plasma levels of leptin and adiponectin	Vemuri et al. (2007)
Obese KK-Ay mice	Oral administration of 500 mg/kg DHA	↓ Plasma levels of glucose, TG, and free fatty acids	Shimura et al. (1997)

TABLE 20.3

Effects of DHA in Human Subjects

Subjects	Route of Administration	Effects	References
42 healthy adults	9 g/day DHA-enriched fish oil	↓ Activation of T lymphocytes	Kew et al. (2004)
40 ADHD children	Intake of 3.6 g/week DHA	No significant improvement	Hirayama et al. (2004)
A prospective study started with 815 residents aged 65–94		Inverse correlation between DHA intake and risk of AD	Morris et al. (2003)
402 individuals with mild AD	Intake of 2 g/day DHA	No significant effect	Quinn et al. (2010)
234 healthy nonsmoking men	Intake of 3.6 g/day DHA	↓ Plasma level of TG ↑ Plasma level of HDL-C	Grimsgaard et al. (1997)
Subjects with combined hyperlipidemia	Intake of 1.25 and 2.5 g/day DHA	↓ Plasma level of TG ↑ Plasma level of HDL-C	Davidson et al. (1997)
57 subjects aged 21–80	Intake of 1.52 g/day DHA	↓ Plasma level of LDL-C carried by small, dense particles	Maki et al. (2005)
17 hyperglyceridemic men aged 39–66	Intake of 3 g/day DHA	↓ Number of circulating neutrophils ↓ Levels of C-reactive proteins and IL-6 ↑ Level of anti-inflammatory MMP-2	Kelley et al. (2009)
59 overweight, mild hyperlipidemic men	Intake of 4 g/day DHA	↓ Ambulatory blood pressure ↓ Heart rate	Mori et al. (1999)
28 elderly Japanese individuals	Intake of 240 mg/day DHA	↑ Coronary flow velocity ↑ Coronary flow velocity reserve	Oe et al. (2008)
19 healthy adults aged 45–65	Intake of 0.7 g/day DHA	↓ Diastolic blood pressure ↓ Heart rate	Theobald et al. (2007)

   Notably, DHA is commonly referred to as the marine fatty acid, due to its primary source that includes algae and dark fish such as salmon and herring. DHA is also abundant in plants and seeds as its precursor form, α-linolenic acid (Das, 2006). Such plant sources, however, might be unable to provide a sufficient amount of DHA (Williams and Burdge, 2006). Thus, marine foods and ingredients, such as fish oils and marine bacteria, are more reliable and direct sources of DHA (Larsen et al., 2011). Taken together, DHA seems worthy to be referred to as a "marine treasure."

Acknowledgment

This work was supported by the Global Core Research Center (GCRC) grant (No. 2012-0001184) from the National Research Foundation (NRF), Ministry of Education, Science and Technology (MEST), Republic of Korea.

References

Albert, C. M., Campos, H., Stampfer, M. J., Ridker, P. M., Manson, J. E., Willett, W. C., and Ma, J. 2002. Blood levels of long-chain n-3 fatty acids and the risk of sudden death. *N Engl J Med*, 346, 1113–1118.

Ambrozova, G., Pekarova, M., and Lojek, A. 2010. Effect of polyunsaturated fatty acids on the reactive oxygen and nitrogen species production by raw 264.7 macrophages. *Eur J Nutr*, 49, 133–139.

American Diabetes Association. 2011. Standards of medical care in diabetes: 2011. *Diabetes Care*, 34 (Suppl 1), S11–S61.

Andersen, G., Harnack, K., Erbersdobler, H. F., and Somoza, V. 2008. Dietary eicosapentaenoic acid and docosahexaenoic acid are more effective than α-linolenic acid in improving insulin sensitivity in rats. *Ann Nutr Metab*, 52, 250–256.

Arai, T., Kim, H. J., Chiba, H., and Matsumoto, A. 2009. Anti-obesity effect of fish oil and fish oil-fenofibrate combination in female KK mice. *J Atheroscler Thromb*, 16, 674–683.

Barter, P., Gotto, A. M., Larosa, J. C., Maroni, J., Szarek, M., Grundy, S. M., Kastelein, J. J., Bittner, V., and Fruchart, J. C. 2007. HDL cholesterol, very low levels of LDL cholesterol, and cardiovascular events. *N Engl J Med*, 357, 1301–1310.

Bellenger, J., Bellenger, S., Bataille, A., Massey, K. A., Nicolaou, A., Rialland, M., Tessier, C., Kang, J. X., and Narce, M. 2011. High pancreatic n-3 fatty acids prevent STZ-induced diabetes in *fat-1* mice: Inflammatory pathway inhibition. *Diabetes*, 60, 1090–1099.

Boudrault, C., Bazinet, R. P., Kang, J. X., and Ma, D. W. 2010. Cyclooxygenase-2 and n-6 PUFA are lower and DHA is higher in the cortex of *fat-1* mice. *Neurochem Int*, 56, 585–589.

Bouwens, M., van de Rest, O., Dellschaft, N., Bromhaar, M. G., De Groot, L. C., Geleijnse, J. M., Muller, M., and Afman, L. A. 2009. Fish-oil supplementation induces antiinflammatory gene expression profiles in human blood mononuclear cells. *Am J Clin Nutr*, 90, 415–424.

Bulbul, M., Tan, R., Gemici, B., Hacioglu, G., Agar, A., and Izgut-Uysal, V. N. 2007. Effect of docosahexaenoic acid on macrophage functions of rats. *Immunobiology*, 212, 583–587.

Calder, P. C. 2006. Polyunsaturated fatty acids and inflammation. *Prostaglandins Leukot Essent Fatty Acids*, 75, 197–202.

Calon, F., Lim, G. P., Yang, F., Morihara, T., Teter, B., Ubeda, O., Rostaing, P. et al. 2004. Docosahexaenoic acid protects from dendritic pathology in an Alzheimer's disease mouse model. *Neuron*, 43, 633–645.

Calviello, G., Di Nicuolo, F., Gragnoli, S., Piccioni, E., Serini, S., Maggiano, N., Tringali, G., Navarra, P., Ranelletti, F. O. and Palozza, P. 2004. n-3 PUFAs reduce VEGF expression in human colon cancer cells modulating the COX-2/PGE$_2$ induced ERK-1 and -2 and HIF-1α induction pathway. *Carcinogenesis*, 25, 2303–2310.

Calviello, G., Di Nicuolo, F., Serini, S., Piccioni, E., Boninsegna, A., Maggiano, N., Ranelletti, F. O., and Palozza, P. 2005. Docosahexaenoic acid enhances the susceptibility of human colorectal cancer cells to 5-fluorouracil. *Cancer Chemother Pharmacol*, 55, 12–20.

Calviello, G., Resci, F., Serini, S., Piccioni, E., Toesca, A., Boninsegna, A., Monego, G., Ranelletti, F. O., and Palozza, P. 2007. Docosahexaenoic acid induces proteasome-dependent degradation of β-catenin, down-regulation of survivin and apoptosis in human colorectal cancer cells not expressing COX-2. *Carcinogenesis*, 28, 1202–1209.

Cao, D., Kevala, K., Kim, J., Moon, H. S., Jun, S. B., Lovinger, D., and Kim, H. Y. 2009. Docosahexaenoic acid promotes hippocampal neuronal development and synaptic function. *J Neurochem*, 111, 510–521.

Cha, S. H., Fukushima, A., Sakuma, K., and Kagawa, Y. 2001. Chronic docosahexaenoic acid intake enhances expression of the gene for uncoupling protein 3 and affects pleiotropic mRNA levels in skeletal muscle of aged C57BL/6NJcl mice. *J Nutr*, 131, 2636–2642.

Cho, J. Y., Chi, S. G., and Chun, H. S. 2011. Oral administration of docosahexaenoic acid attenuates colitis induced by dextran sulfate sodium in mice. *Mol Nutr Food Res*, 55, 239–246.

Colas, S., Maheo, K., Denis, F., Goupille, C., Hoinard, C., Champeroux, P., Tranquart, F., and Bougnoux, P. 2006. Sensitization by dietary docosahexaenoic acid of rat mammary carcinoma to anthracycline: A role for tumor vascularization. *Clin Cancer Res*, 12, 5879–5886.

Connolly, J. M. and Rose, D. P. 1993. Effects of fatty acids on invasion through reconstituted basement membrane ('Matrigel') by a human breast cancer cell line. *Cancer Lett*, 75, 137–142.

Coti Bertrand, P., O'Kusky, J. R., and Innis, S. M. 2006. Maternal dietary (n-3) fatty acid deficiency alters neurogenesis in the embryonic rat brain. *J Nutr*, 136, 1570–1575.

D'Eliseo, D., Manzi, L., Merendino, N., and Velotti, F. 2011. Docosahexaenoic acid inhibits invasion of human RT112 urinary bladder and PT45 pancreatic carcinoma cells via down-modulation of granzyme B expression. *J Nutr Biochem*, 35, 452–457.

Das, U. N. 2006. Essential fatty acids: Biochemistry, physiology and pathology. *Biotechnol J*, 1, 420–439.

Das, U. N. and Madhavi, N. 2011. Effect of polyunsaturated fatty acids on drug-sensitive and resistant tumor cells in vitro. *Lipids Health Dis*, 10, 159.

Davidson, M. H., Maki, K. C., Kalkowski, J., Schaefer, E. J., Torri, S. A., and Drennan, K. B. 1997. Effects of docosahexaenoic acid on serum lipoproteins in patients with combined hyperlipidemia: A randomized, double-blind, placebo-controlled trial. *J Am Coll Nutr*, 16, 236–243.

Deckelbaum, R. J. and Torrejon, C. 2012. The omega-3 Fatty Acid nutritional landscape: Health benefits and sources. *J Nutr*, 142, 587S–591S.

Deike, E., Bowden, R. G., Moreillon, J. J., Griggs, J. O., Wilson, R. L., Cooke, M., Shelmadine, B. D., and Beaujean, A. A. 2012. The effects of fish oil supplementation on markers of inflammation in chronic kidney disease patients. *J Ren Nutr*, 22, 572–577.

Draper, E., Reynolds, C. M., Canavan, M., Mills, K. H., Loscher, C. E., and Roche, H. M. 2011. Omega-3 fatty acids attenuate dendritic cell function via NF-kappaB independent of PPARgamma. *J Nutr Biochem*, 22, 784–790.

Erkkila, A. T., Matthan, N. R., Herrington, D. M., and Lichtenstein, A. H. 2006. Higher plasma docosahexaenoic acid is associated with reduced progression of coronary atherosclerosis in women with CAD. *J Lipid Res*, 47, 2814–2819.

Gamoh, S., Hashimoto, M., Hossain, S., and Masumura, S. 2001. Chronic administration of docosahexaenoic acid improves the performance of radial arm maze task in aged rats. *Clin Exp Pharmacol Physiol*, 28, 266–270.

Gao, L., Wang, J., Sekhar, K. R., Yin, H., Yared, N. F., Schneider, S. N., Sasi, S. et al. 2007. Novel n-3 fatty acid oxidation products activate Nrf2 by destabilizing the association between Keap1 and Cullin3. *J Biol Chem*, 282, 2529–2537.

Geissler, J. and Lesch, K. P. 2011. A lifetime of attention-deficit/hyperactivity disorder: Diagnostic challenges, treatment and neurobiological mechanisms. *Expert Rev Neurother*, 11, 1467–1484.

Ghosh-Choudhury, T., Mandal, C. C., Woodruff, K., St. Clair, P., Fernandes, G., Choudhury, G. G., and Ghosh-Choudhury, N. 2009. Fish oil targets PTEN to regulate NF-κB for downregulation of anti-apoptotic genes in breast tumor growth. *Breast Cancer Res Treat*, 118, 213–228.

Gleissman, H., Segerstrom, L., Hamberg, M., Ponthan, F., Lindskog, M., Johnsen, J. I., and Kogner, P. 2011. Omega-3 fatty acid supplementation delays the progression of neuroblastoma in vivo. *Int J Cancer*, 128, 1703–1711.

Gravaghi, C., La Perle, K. M., Ogrodwski, P., Kang, J. X., Quimby, F., Lipkin, M., and Lamprecht, S. A. 2011. Cox-2 expression, PGE_2 and cytokines production are inhibited by endogenously synthesized n-3 PUFAs in inflamed colon of *fat-1* mice. *J Nutr Biochem*, 22, 360–365.

Green, K. N., Martinez-Coria, H., Khashwji, H., Hall, E. B., Yurko-Mauro, K. A., Ellis, L., and Laferla, F. M. 2007. Dietary docosahexaenoic acid and docosapentaenoic acid ameliorate amyloid β and tau pathology via a mechanism involving presenilin 1 levels. *J Neurosci*, 27, 4385–4395.

Green, P. and Yavin, E. 1998. Mechanisms of docosahexaenoic acid accretion in the fetal brain. *J Neurosci Res*, 52, 129–136.

Griffitts, J., Saunders, D., Tesiram, Y. A., Reid, G. E., Salih, A., Liu, S., Lydic, T. A., Busik, J. V., Kang, J. X., and Towner, R. A. 2010. Non-mammalian *fat-1* gene prevents neoplasia when introduced to a mouse hepatocarcinogenesis model: Omega-3 fatty acids prevent liver neoplasia. *Biochim Biophys Acta*, 1801, 1133–1144.

Grimm, M. O., Kuchenbecker, J., Grosgen, S., Burg, V. K., Hundsdorfer, B., Rothhaar, T. L., Friess, P. et al. 2011. Docosahexaenoic acid reduces amyloid β production via multiple pleiotropic mechanisms. *J Biol Chem*, 286, 14028–14039.

Grimsgaard, S., Bonaa, K. H., Hansen, J. B., and Nordoy, A. 1997. Highly purified eicosapentaenoic acid and docosahexaenoic acid in humans have similar triacylglycerol-lowering effects but divergent effects on serum fatty acids. *Am J Clin Nutr*, 66, 649–659.

Grundy, S. M. 2004. Obesity, metabolic syndrome, and cardiovascular disease. *J Clin Endocrinol Metab*, 89, 2595–2600.

Hashimoto, M., Hossain, S., Agdul, H., and Shido, O. 2005a. Docosahexaenoic acid-induced amelioration on impairment of memory learning in amyloid β–infused rats relates to the decreases of amyloid β and cholesterol levels in detergent-insoluble membrane fractions. *Biochim Biophys Acta*, 1738, 91–98.

Hashimoto, M., Hossain, S., Shimada, T., Sugioka, K., Yamasaki, H., Fujii, Y., Ishibashi, Y., Oka, J., and Shido, O. 2002. Docosahexaenoic acid provides protection from impairment of learning ability in Alzheimer's disease model rats. *J Neurochem*, 81, 1084–1091.

Hashimoto, M., Tanabe, Y., Fujii, Y., Kikuta, T., Shibata, H., and Shido, O. 2005b. Chronic administration of docosahexaenoic acid ameliorates the impairment of spatial cognition learning ability in amyloid β-infused rats. *J Nutr*, 135, 549–555.

He, C., Qu, X., Cui, L., Wang, J., and Kang, J. X. 2009. Improved spatial learning performance of *fat-1* mice is associated with enhanced neurogenesis and neuritogenesis by docosahexaenoic acid. *Proc Natl Acad Sci USA*, 106, 11370–11375.

Hirayama, S., Hamazaki, T., and Terasawa, K. 2004. Effect of docosahexaenoic acid-containing food administration on symptoms of attention-deficit/hyperactivity disorder—A placebo-controlled double-blind study. *Eur J Clin Nutr*, 58, 467–473.

Horia, E. and Watkins, B. A. 2007. Complementary actions of docosahexaenoic acid and genistein on COX-2, PGE₂ and invasiveness in MDA-MB-231 breast cancer cells. *Carcinogenesis*, 28, 809–815.

Hudert, C. A., Weylandt, K. H., Lu, Y., Wang, J., Hong, S., Dignass, A., Serhan, C. N., and Kang, J. X. 2006. Transgenic mice rich in endogenous omega-3 fatty acids are protected from colitis. *Proc Natl Acad Sci USA*, 103, 11276–11281.

Isbilen, B., Fraser, S. P., and Djamgoz, M. B. 2006. Docosahexaenoic acid (omega-3) blocks voltage-gated sodium channel activity and migration of MDA-MB-231 human breast cancer cells. *Int J Biochem Cell Biol*, 38, 2173–2182.

Ji, S., Hardy, R. W., and Wood, P. A. 2009. Transgenic expression of n-3 fatty acid desaturase (fat-1) in C57/BL6 mice: Effects on glucose homeostasis and body weight. *J Cell Biochem*, 107, 809–817.

Jia, Q., Lupton, J. R., Smith, R., Weeks, B. R., Callaway, E., Davidson, L. A., Kim, W. et al. 2008. Reduced colitis-associated colon cancer in *Fat-1* (n-3 fatty acid desaturase) transgenic mice. *Cancer Res*, 68, 3985–3991.

Jiang, L. H., Shi, Y., Wang, L. S., and Yang, Z. R. 2009. The influence of orally administered docosahexaenoic acid on cognitive ability in aged mice. *J Nutr Biochem*, 20, 735–741.

Jucker, M. and Walker, L. C. 2011. Pathogenic protein seeding in Alzheimer disease and other neurodegenerative disorders. *Ann Neurol*, 70, 532–540.

Kang, J. X., Wang, J., Wu, L., and Kang, Z. B. 2004. Transgenic mice: Fat-1 mice convert n-6 to n-3 fatty acids. *Nature*, 427, 504.

Kang, K. S., Wang, P., Yamabe, N., Fukui, M., Jay, T., and Zhu, B. T. 2010. Docosahexaenoic acid induces apoptosis in MCF-7 cells in vitro and in vivo via reactive oxygen species formation and caspase 8 activation. *PLoS One*, 5, e10296.

Kato, T., Kolenic, N., and Pardini, R. S. 2007. Docosahexaenoic acid (DHA), a primary tumor suppressive omega-3 fatty acid, inhibits growth of colorectal cancer independent of p53 mutational status. *Nutr Cancer*, 58, 178–187.

Kawakita, E., Hashimoto, M., and Shido, O. 2006. Docosahexaenoic acid promotes neurogenesis in vitro and *in vivo*. *Neuroscience*, 139, 991–997.

Kelley, D. S., Siegel, D., Fedor, D. M., Adkins, Y., and Mackey, B. E. 2009. DHA supplementation decreases serum C-reactive protein and other markers of inflammation in hypertriglyceridemic men. *J Nutr*, 139, 495–501.

Kew, S., Mesa, M. D., Tricon, S., Buckley, R., Minihane, A. M., and Yaqoob, P. 2004. Effects of oils rich in eicosapentaenoic and docosahexaenoic acids on immune cell composition and function in healthy humans. *Am J Clin Nutr*, 79, 674–681.

Khan, N. A., Nishimura, K., Aires, V., Yamashita, T., Oaxaca-Castillo, D., Kashiwagi, K., and Igarashi, K. 2006. Docosahexaenoic acid inhibits cancer cell growth via p27Kip1, CDK2, ERK1/ERK2, and retinoblastoma phosphorylation. *J Lipid Res*, 47, 2306–2313.

Komatsu, W., Ishihara, K., Murata, M., Saito, H., and Shinohara, K. 2003. Docosahexaenoic acid suppresses nitric oxide production and inducible nitric oxide synthase expression in interferon-γ plus lipopolysaccharide-stimulated murine macrophages by inhibiting the oxidative stress. *Free Radic Biol Med*, 34, 1006–1016.

Kong, W., Yen, J. H., and Ganea, D. 2011. Docosahexaenoic acid prevents dendritic cell maturation, inhibits antigen-specific Th1/Th17 differentiation and suppresses experimental autoimmune encephalomyelitis. *Brain Behav Immun*, 25, 872–882.

Kong, W., Yen, J. H., Vassiliou, E., Adhikary, S., Toscano, M. G., and Ganea, D. 2010. Docosahexaenoic acid prevents dendritic cell maturation and in vitro and in vivo expression of the IL-12 cytokine family. *Lipids Health Dis*, 9, 12.

Kuan, C. Y., Walker, T. H., Luo, P. G., and Chen, C. F. 2011. Long-chain polyunsaturated fatty acids promote paclitaxel cytotoxicity via inhibition of the MDR1 gene in the human colon cancer Caco-2 cell line. *J Am Coll Nutr*, 30, 265–273.

Kundu, J. K. and Surh, Y. J. 2008. Inflammation: Gearing the journey to cancer. *Mutat Res*, 659, 15–30.

Kunesova, M., Braunerova, R., Hlavaty, P., Tvrzicka, E., Stankova, B., Skrha, J., Hilgertova, J. et al. 2006. The influence of n-3 polyunsaturated fatty acids and very low calorie diet during a short-term weight reducing regimen on weight loss and serum fatty acid composition in severely obese women. *Physiol Res*, 55, 63–72.

Kyle, D. J., Schaefer, E., Patton, G., and Beiser, A. 1999. Low serum docosahexaenoic acid is a significant risk factor for Alzheimer's dementia. *Lipids*, 34 (Suppl), S245.

Larsen, R., Eilertsen, K. E., and Elvevoll, E. O. 2011. Health benefits of marine foods and ingredients. *Biotechnol Adv*, 29, 508–518.

Lee, C. Y., Sit, W. H., Fan, S. T., Man, K., Jor, I. W., Wong, L. L., Wan, M. L., Tan-Un, K. C., and Wan, J. M. 2010. The cell cycle effects of docosahexaenoic acid on human metastatic hepatocellular carcinoma proliferation. *Int J Oncol*, 36, 991–998.

Leonardi, F., Attorri, L., Benedetto, R. D., Biase, A. D., Sanchez, M., Tregno, F. P., Nardini, M., and Salvati, S. 2007. Docosahexaenoic acid supplementation induces dose and time dependent oxidative changes in C6 glioma cells. *Free Radic Res*, 41, 748–756.

Li, H., Ruan, X. Z., Powis, S. H., Fernando, R., Mon, W. Y., Wheeler, D. C., Moorhead, J. F., and Varghese, Z. 2005. EPA and DHA reduce LPS-induced inflammation responses in HK-2 cells: Evidence for a PPARγ-dependent mechanism. *Kidney Int*, 67, 867–874.

Lien, E. L. 2009. Toxicology and safety of DHA. *Prostaglandins Leukot Essent Fatty Acids*, 81, 125–132.

Lim, G. P., Calon, F., Morihara, T., Yang, F., Teter, B., Ubeda, O., Salem, N., Jr., Frautschy, S. A., and Cole, G. M. 2005. A diet enriched with the omega-3 fatty acid docosahexaenoic acid reduces amyloid burden in an aged Alzheimer mouse model. *J Neurosci*, 25, 3032–3040.

Lim, K., Han, C., Dai, Y., Shen, M., and Wu, T. 2009. Omega-3 polyunsaturated fatty acids inhibit hepatocellular carcinoma cell growth through blocking β-catenin and cyclooxygenase-2. *Mol Cancer Ther*, 8, 3046–3055.

Lim, K., Han, C., Xu, L., Isse, K., Demetris, A. J., and Wu, T. 2008. Cyclooxygenase-2-derived prostaglandin E$_2$ activates beta-catenin in human cholangiocarcinoma cells: Evidence for inhibition of these signaling pathways by omega 3 polyunsaturated fatty acids. *Cancer Res*, 68, 553–560.

Liu, G., Bibus, D. M., Bode, A. M., Ma, W. Y., Holman, R. T., and Dong, Z. 2001. Omega 3 but not omega 6 fatty acids inhibit AP-1 activity and cell transformation in JB6 cells. *Proc Natl Acad Sci USA*, 98, 7510–7515.

Makhoul, Z., Kristal, A. R., Gulati, R., Luick, B., Bersamin, A., O'Brien, D., Hopkins, S. E., Stephensen, C. B., Stanhope, K. L., Havel, P. J., and Boyer, B. 2011. Associations of obesity with triglycerides and C-reactive protein are attenuated in adults with high red blood cell eicosapentaenoic and docosahexaenoic acids. *Eur J Clin Nutr*, 65, 808–817.

Maki, K. C., Van Elswyk, M. E., Mccarthy, D., Hess, S. P., Veith, P. E., Bell, M., Subbaiah, P., and Davidson, M. H. 2005. Lipid responses to a dietary docosahexaenoic acid supplement in men and women with below average levels of high density lipoprotein cholesterol. *J Am Coll Nutr*, 24, 189–199.

Mandal, C. C., Ghosh-Choudhury, T., Yoneda, T., Choudhury, G. G., and Ghosh-Choudhury, N. 2010. Fish oil prevents breast cancer cell metastasis to bone. *Biochem Biophys Res Commun*, 402, 602–607.

Martinez-Micaelo, N., Gonzalez-Abuin, N., Terra, X., Richart, C., Ardevol, A., Pinent, M., and Blay, M. 2012. Omega-3 docosahexaenoic acid and procyanidins inhibit cyclooxygenase activity and attenuate NF-κB activation through a p105/p50 regulatory mechanism in macrophage inflammation. *Biochem J*, 441, 653–663.

Massaro, M., Habib, A., Lubrano, L., Del Turco, S., Lazzerini, G., Bourcier, T., Weksler, B. B., and De Caterina, R. 2006. The omega-3 fatty acid docosahexaenoate attenuates endothelial cyclooxygenase-2 induction through both NADP(H) oxidase and PKC epsilon inhibition. *Proc Natl Acad Sci USA*, 103, 15184–15189.

McCabe, A. J., Wallace, J. M., Gilmore, W. S., Mcglynn, H., and Strain, S. J. 2005. Docosahexaenoic acid reduces in vitro invasion of renal cell carcinoma by elevated levels of tissue inhibitor of metalloproteinase-1. *J Nutr Biochem*, 16, 17–22.

Merendino, N., Loppi, B., D'Aquino, M., Molinari, R., Pessina, G., Romano, C., and Velotti, F. 2005. Docosahexaenoic acid induces apoptosis in the human PaCa-44 pancreatic cancer cell line by active reduced glutathione extrusion and lipid peroxidation. *Nutr Cancer*, 52, 225–233.

Merendino, N., Molinari, R., Loppi, B., Pessina, G., D'Aquino, M., Tomassi, G., and Velottia, F. 2003. Induction of apoptosis in human pancreatic cancer cells by docosahexaenoic acid. *Ann NY Acad Sci*, 1010, 361–364.

Micallef, M., Munro, I., Phang, M., and Garg, M. 2009. Plasma n-3 Polyunsaturated Fatty Acids are negatively associated with obesity. *Br J Nutr*, 102, 1370–1374.

Milte, C. M., Sinn, N., Buckley, J. D., Coates, A. M., Young, R. M., and Howe, P. R. 2011. Polyunsaturated fatty acids, cognition and literacy in children with ADHD with and without learning difficulties. *J Child Health Care*, 15, 299–311.

Mori, T. A., Bao, D. Q., Burke, V., Puddey, I. B., and Beilin, L. J. 1999. Docosahexaenoic acid but not eicosapentaenoic acid lowers ambulatory blood pressure and heart rate in humans. *Hypertension*, 34, 253–260.

Morris, M. C., Evans, D. A., Bienias, J. L., Tangney, C. C., Bennett, D. A., Wilson, R. S., Aggarwal, N., and Schneider, J. 2003. Consumption of fish and n-3 fatty acids and risk of incident Alzheimer disease. *Arch Neurol*, 60, 940–946.

Morteau, O. 2000. Prostaglandins and inflammation: The cyclooxygenase controversy. *Arch Immunol Ther Exp (Warsz)*, 48, 473–480.

Mozaffarian, D. and Wu, J. H. 2012. (n-3) Fatty acids and cardiovascular health: Are effects of EPA and DHA shared or complementary? *J Nutr*, 142, 614S–625S.

Mullen, A., Loscher, C. E., and Roche, H. M. 2010. Anti-inflammatory effects of EPA and DHA are dependent upon time and dose-response elements associated with LPS stimulation in THP-1-derived macrophages. *J Nutr Biochem*, 21, 444–450.

Nakamura, N., Hamazaki, T., Kobayashi, M., and Yazawa, K. 1994. The effect of oral administration of eicosapentaenoic and docosahexaenoic acids on acute inflammation and fatty acid composition in rats. *J Nutr Sci Vitaminol (Tokyo)*, 40, 161–170.

Narayanan, N. K., Narayanan, B. A., and Reddy, B. S. 2005. A combination of docosahexaenoic acid and celecoxib prevents prostate cancer cell growth in vitro and is associated with modulation of nuclear factor-kappaB, and steroid hormone receptors. *Int J Oncol*, 26, 785–792.

Nowak, J., Weylandt, K. H., Habbel, P., Wang, J., Dignass, A., Glickman, J. N., and Kang, J. X. 2007. Colitis-associated colon tumorigenesis is suppressed in transgenic mice rich in endogenous n-3 fatty acids. *Carcinogenesis*, 28, 1991–1995.

Oddo, S., Caccamo, A., Shepherd, J. D., Murphy, M. P., Golde, T. E., Kayed, R., Metherate, R., Mattson, M. P., Akbari, Y., and Laferla, F. M. 2003. Triple-transgenic model of Alzheimer's disease with plaques and tangles: Intracellular Aβ and synaptic dysfunction. *Neuron*, 39, 409–421.

Oe, H., Hozumi, T., Murata, E., Matsuura, H., Negishi, K., Matsumura, Y., Iwata, S. et al. 2008. Arachidonic acid and docosahexaenoic acid supplementation increases coronary flow velocity reserve in Japanese elderly individuals. *Heart*, 94, 316–321.

Oudart, H., Groscolas, R., Calgari, C., Nibbelink, M., Leray, C., Le Maho, Y., and Malan, A. 1997. Brown fat thermogenesis in rats fed high-fat diets enriched with n-3 polyunsaturated fatty acids. *Int J Obes Relat Metab Disord*, 21, 955–962.

Quinn, J. F., Raman, R., Thomas, R. G., Yurko-Mauro, K., Nelson, E. B., Van Dyck, C., Galvin, J. E. et al. 2010. Docosahexaenoic acid supplementation and cognitive decline in Alzheimer disease: A randomized trial. *JAMA*, 304, 1903–1911.

Rahman, M., Kundu, J. K., Shin, J. W., Na, H. K., and Surh, Y. J. 2011. Docosahexaenoic acid inhibits UVB-induced activation of NF-κB and expression of COX-2 and NOX-4 in HR-1 hairless mouse skin by blocking MSK1 signaling. *PLoS One*, 6, e28065.

Ramel, A., Martinez, A., Kiely, M., Morais, G., Bandarra, N. M., and Thorsdottir, I. 2008. Beneficial effects of long-chain n-3 fatty acids included in an energy-restricted diet on insulin resistance in overweight and obese European young adults. *Diabetologia*, 51, 1261–1268.

Richard, D., Wolf, C., Barbe, U., Kefi, K., Bausero, P., and Visioli, F. 2009. Docosahexaenoic acid down-regulates endothelial Nox 4 through a sPLA2 signalling pathway. *Biochem Biophys Res Commun*, 389, 516–522.

Ristimaki, A., Honkanen, N., Jankala, H., Sipponen, P., and Harkonen, M. 1997. Expression of cyclo-oxygenase-2 in human gastric carcinoma. *Cancer Res*, 57, 1276–1280.

Rose, D. P., Connolly, J. M., Rayburn, J., and Coleman, M. 1995. Influence of diets containing eicosa-pentaenoic or docosahexaenoic acid on growth and metastasis of breast cancer cells in nude mice. *J Natl Cancer Inst*, 87, 587–592.

Ruiter, D. J., Van Krieken, J. H., Van Muijen, G. N., and De Waal, R. M. 2001. Tumour metastasis: Is tissue an issue? *Lancet Oncol*, 2, 109–112.

Sahlin, C., Pettersson, F. E., Nilsson, L. N., Lannfelt, L., and Johansson, A. S. 2007. Docosahexaenoic acid stimulates non-amyloidogenic APP processing resulting in reduced Aβ levels in cellular models of Alzheimer's disease. *Eur J Neurosci*, 26, 882–889.

Sarwar, N., Danesh, J., Eiriksdottir, G., Sigurdsson, G., Wareham, N., Bingham, S., Boekholdt, S. M., Khaw, K. T., and Gudnason, V. 2007. Triglycerides and the risk of coronary heart disease: 10,158 incident cases among 262,525 participants in 29 Western prospective studies. *Circulation*, 115, 450–458.

Schwab, J. M., Chiang, N., Arita, M., and Serhan, C. N. 2007. Resolvin E1 and protectin D1 activate inflammation-resolution programmes. *Nature*, 447, 869–874.

Serhan, C. N. 2007. Resolution phase of inflammation: Novel endogenous anti-inflammatory and proresolving lipid mediators and pathways. *Annu Rev Immunol*, 25, 101–137.

Serhan, C. N., Chiang, N., and Van Dyke, T. E. 2008. Resolving inflammation: Dual anti-inflammatory and pro-resolution lipid mediators. *Nat Rev Immunol*, 8, 349–361.

Serhan, C. N., Gotlinger, K., Hong, S., Lu, Y., Siegelman, J., Baer, T., Yang, R., Colgan, S. P., and Petasis, N. A. 2006. Anti-inflammatory actions of neuroprotectin D1/protectin D1 and its natural stereoisomers: Assignments of dihydroxy-containing docosatrienes. *J Immunol*, 176, 1848–1859.

Serhan, C. N. and Petasis, N. A. 2011. Resolvins and protectins in inflammation resolution. *Chem Rev*, 111, 5922–5943.

Serini, S., Fasano, E., Piccioni, E., Cittadini, A. R., and Calviello, G. 2011. Differential anti-cancer effects of purified EPA and DHA and possible mechanisms involved. *Curr Med Chem*, 18, 4065–4075.

Shi, Y. and Pestka, J. J. 2009. Mechanisms for suppression of interleukin-6 expression in peritoneal macrophages from docosahexaenoic acid-fed mice. *J Nutr Biochem*, 20, 358–368.

Shimura, T., Miura, T., Usami, M., Ishihara, E., Tanigawa, K., Ishida, H., and Seino, Y. 1997. Docosahexanoic acid (DHA) improved glucose and lipid metabolism in KK-Ay mice with genetic non-insulin-dependent diabetes mellitus (NIDDM). *Biol Pharm Bull*, 20, 507–510.

Shinto, L., Marracci, G., Baldauf-Wagner, S., Strehlow, A., Yadav, V., Stuber, L., and Bourdette, D. 2009. Omega-3 fatty acid supplementation decreases matrix metalloproteinase-9 production in relapsing-remitting multiple sclerosis. *Prostaglandins Leukot Essent Fatty Acids*, 80, 131–136.

Simopoulos, A. P. 2002. The importance of the ratio of omega-6/omega-3 essential fatty acids. *Biomed Pharmacother*, 56, 365–379.

Song, K. S., Jing, K., Kim, J. S., Yun, E. J., Shin, S., Seo, K. S., Park, J. H. et al. 2011. Omega-3-polyunsaturated fatty acids suppress pancreatic cancer cell growth in vitro and in vivo via downregulation of Wnt/β-catenin signaling. *Pancreatology*, 11, 574–584.

Spite, M., Norling, L. V., Summers, L., Yang, R., Cooper, D., Petasis, N. A., Flower, R. J., Perretti, M., and Serhan, C. N. 2009. Resolvin D2 is a potent regulator of leukocytes and controls microbial sepsis. *Nature*, 461, 1287–1291.

Stevens, L. J., Zentall, S. S., Deck, J. L., Abate, M. L., Watkins, B. A., Lipp, S. R., and Burgess, J. R. 1995. Essential fatty acid metabolism in boys with attention-deficit hyperactivity disorder. *Am J Clin Nutr*, 62, 761–768.

Suresh, Y. and Das, U. N. 2003. Long-chain polyunsaturated fatty acids and chemically induced diabetes mellitus. Effect of omega-3 fatty acids. *Nutrition*, 19, 213–228.

Surh, Y. J. 2003. Cancer chemoprevention with dietary phytochemicals. *Nat Rev Cancer*, 3, 768–780.

Suzuki, I., Iigo, M., Ishikawa, C., Kuhara, T., Asamoto, M., Kunimoto, T., Moore, M. A., Yazawa, K., Araki, E., and Tsuda, H. 1997. Inhibitory effects of oleic and docosahexaenoic acids on lung metastasis by colon-carcinoma-26 cells are associated with reduced matrix metalloproteinase-2 and -9 activities. *Int J Cancer*, 73, 607–612.

Swamy, M. V., Cooma, I., Patlolla, J. M., Simi, B., Reddy, B. S., and Rao, C. V. 2004. Modulation of cyclooxygenase-2 activities by the combined action of celecoxib and decosahexaenoic acid: Novel strategies for colon cancer prevention and treatment. *Mol Cancer Ther*, 3, 215–221.

Szymczak, M., Murray, M., and Petrovic, N. 2008. Modulation of angiogenesis by omega-3 polyunsaturated fatty acids is mediated by cyclooxygenases. *Blood*, 111, 3514–3521.

Takahashi, M., Totsuka, Y., Masuda, M., Fukuda, K., Oguri, A., Yazawa, K., Sugimura, T., and Wakabayashi, K. 1997. Reduction in formation of 2-amino-1-methyl-6-phenylimidazo[4,5-b] pyridine (PhIP)-induced aberrant crypt foci in the rat colon by docosahexaenoic acid (DHA). *Carcinogenesis*, 18, 1937–1941.

Theobald, H. E., Goodall, A. H., Sattar, N., Talbot, D. C., Chowienczyk, P. J., and Sanders, T. A. 2007. Low-dose docosahexaenoic acid lowers diastolic blood pressure in middle-aged men and women. *J Nutr*, 137, 973–978.

Thorsdottir, I., Birgisdottir, B., Kiely, M., Martinez, J., and Bandarra, N. 2009. Fish consumption among young overweight European adults and compliance to varying seafood content in four weight loss intervention diets. *Public Health Nutr*, 12, 592–598.

Thorsdottir, I., Tomasson, H., Gunnarsdottir, I., Gisladottir, E., Kiely, M., Parra, M. D., Bandarra, N. M., Schaafsma, G., and Martinez, J. A. 2007. Randomized trial of weight-loss-diets for young adults varying in fish and fish oil content. *Int J Obes (Lond)*, 31, 1560–1566.

Titos, E., Rius, B., Gonzalez-Periz, A., Lopez-Vicario, C., Moran-Salvador, E., Martinez-Clemente, M., Arroyo, V., and Claria, J. 2011. Resolvin D1 and its precursor docosahexaenoic acid promote resolution of adipose tissue inflammation by eliciting macrophage polarization toward an M2-like phenotype. *J Immunol*, 187, 5408–5418.

Tomobe, Y. I., Morizawa, K., Tsuchida, M., Hibino, H., Nakano, Y., and Tanaka, Y. 2000. Dietary docosahexaenoic acid suppresses inflammation and immunoresponses in contact hypersensitivity reaction in mice. *Lipids*, 35, 61–69.

Transler, C., Eilander, A., Mitchell, S., and van de Meer, N. 2010. The impact of polyunsaturated fatty acids in reducing child attention deficit and hyperactivity disorders. *J Atten Disord*, 14, 232–246.

Tsuzuki, T., Shibata, A., Kawakami, Y., Nakagaya, K., and Miyazawa, T. 2007. Anti-angiogenic effects of conjugated docosahexaenoic acid in vitro and in vivo. *Biosci Biotechnol Biochem*, 71, 1902–1910.

Tucker, O. N., Dannenberg, A. J., Yang, E. K., Zhang, F., Teng, L., Daly, J. M., Soslow, R. A. et al. 1999. Cyclooxygenase-2 expression is up-regulated in human pancreatic cancer. *Cancer Res*, 59, 987–990.

Turkez, H., Geyikoglu, F., and Mokhtar, Y. 2011. Ameliorative effect of docosahexaenoic acid on 2,3,7,8-tetrachlorodibenzo-p-dioxin-induced histological changes, oxidative stress, and DNA damage in rat liver. *Toxicol Ind Health*, 28, 687–696.

Vemuri, M., Kelley, D. S., Mackey, B. E., Rasooly, R., and Bartolini, G. 2007. Docosahexaenoic acid (DHA) but not eicosapentaenoic acid (EPA) prevents trans-10, cis-12 conjugated linoleic acid (CLA)-induced insulin resistance in mice. *Metab Syndr Relat Disord*, 5, 315–322.

Wall, R., Ross, R. P., Fitzgerald, G. F., and Stanton, C. 2010. Fatty acids from fish: The anti-inflammatory potential of long-chain omega-3 fatty acids. *Nutr Rev*, 68, 280–289.

Wang, F., Bhat, K., Doucette, M., Zhou, S., Gu, Y., Law, B., Liu, X. et al. 2011a. Docosahexaenoic acid (DHA) sensitizes brain tumor cells to etoposide-induced apoptosis. *Curr Mol Med*, 11, 503–511.

Wang, T. M., Chen, C. J., Lee, T. S., Chao, H. Y., Wu, W. H., Hsieh, S. C., Sheu, H. H., and Chiang, A. N. 2011b. Docosahexaenoic acid attenuates VCAM-1 expression and NF-κB activation in TNF-α-treated human aortic endothelial cells. *J Nutr Biochem*, 22, 187–194.

Wang, P. Y., Chen, J. J., and Su, H. M. 2010a. Docosahexaenoic acid supplementation of primary rat hippocampal neurons attenuates the neurotoxicity induced by aggregated amyloid β protein(42) and up-regulates cytoskeletal protein expression. *J Nutr Biochem*, 21, 345–350.

Wang, H., Khor, T. O., Saw, C. L., Lin, W., Wu, T., Huang, Y., and Kong, A. N. 2010b. Role of Nrf2 in suppressing LPS-induced inflammation in mouse peritoneal macrophages by polyunsaturated fatty acids docosahexaenoic acid and eicosapentaenoic acid. *Mol Pharm*, 7, 2185–2193.

Wang, Y., Liu, Q., and Thorlacius, H. 2003. Docosahexaenoic acid inhibits cytokine-induced expression of P-selectin and neutrophil adhesion to endothelial cells. *Eur J Pharmacol*, 459, 269–273.

Warner, T. D. and Mitchell, J. A. 2004. Cyclooxygenases: New forms, new inhibitors, and lessons from the clinic. *FASEB J*, 18, 790–804.

Weylandt, K. H., Krause, L. F., Gomolka, B., Chiu, C. Y., Bilal, S., Nadolny, A., Waechter, S. F., Fischer, A., Rothe, M., and Kang, J. X. 2011. Suppressed liver tumorigenesis in *fat-1* mice with elevated omega-3 fatty acids is associated with increased omega-3 derived lipid mediators and reduced TNF-α. *Carcinogenesis*, 32, 897–903.

Weylandt, K. H., Nadolny, A., Kahlke, L., Kohnke, T., Schmocker, C., Wang, J., Lauwers, G. Y., Glickman, J. N., and Kang, J. X. 2008. Reduction of inflammation and chronic tissue damage by omega-3 fatty acids in *fat-1* transgenic mice with pancreatitis. *Biochim Biophys Acta*, 1782, 634–641.

Whelan, J. and Rust, C. 2006. Innovative dietary sources of n-3 fatty acids. *Annu Rev Nutr*, 26, 75–103.

Williams, C. M. and Burdge, G. 2006. Long-chain n-3 PUFA: Plant v. marine sources. *Proc Nutr Soc*, 65, 42–50.

Wolff, H., Saukkonen, K., Anttila, S., Karjalainen, A., Vainio, H., and Ristimaki, A. 1998. Expression of cyclooxygenase-2 in human lung carcinoma. *Cancer Res*, 58, 4997–5001.

Wu, M., Harvey, K. A., Ruzmetov, N., Welch, Z. R., Sech, L., Jackson, K., Stillwell, W., Zaloga, G. P., and Siddiqui, R. A. 2005. Omega-3 polyunsaturated fatty acids attenuate breast cancer growth through activation of a neutral sphingomyelinase-mediated pathway. *Int J Cancer*, 117, 340–348.

Wu, M. H., Tsai, Y. T., Hua, K. T., Chang, K. C., Kuo, M. L., and Lin, M. T. 2012. Eicosapentaenoic acid and docosahexaenoic acid inhibit macrophage-induced gastric cancer cell migration by attenuating the expression of matrix metalloproteinase 10. *J Nutr Biochem*, 23, 1434–1439.

Xia, S., Lu, Y., Wang, J., He, C., Hong, S., Serhan, C. N., and Kang, J. X. 2006. Melanoma growth is reduced in *fat-1* transgenic mice: Impact of omega-6/omega-3 essential fatty acids. *Proc Natl Acad Sci USA*, 103, 12499–12504.

Xiao, Y., Wang, L., Xu, R. J., and Chen, Z. Y. 2006. DHA depletion in rat brain is associated with impairment on spatial learning and memory. *Biomed Environ Sci*, 19, 474–480.

Yamamoto, K., Itoh, T., Abe, D., Shimizu, M., Kanda, T., Koyama, T., Nishikawa, M., Tamai, T., Ooizumi, H., and Yamada, S. 2005. Identification of putative metabolites of docosahexaenoic acid as potent PPARγ agonists and antidiabetic agents. *Bioorg Med Chem Lett*, 15, 517–522.

Yano, Y., Nakayama, A., Saito, H., and Ishihara, K. 1994. Production of docosahexaenoic acid by marine bacteria isolated from deep sea fish. *Lipids*, 29, 527–528.

Yashodhara, B. M., Umakanth, S., Pappachan, J. M., Bhat, S. K., Kamath, R., and Choo, B. H. 2009. Omega-3 fatty acids: A comprehensive review of their role in health and disease. *Postgrad Med J*, 85, 84–90.

Yates, C. M., Tull, S. P., Madden, J., Calder, P. C., Grimble, R. F., Nash, G. B., and Rainger, G. E. 2011. Docosahexaenoic acid inhibits the adhesion of flowing neutrophils to cytokine stimulated human umbilical vein endothelial cells. *J Nutr*, 141, 1331–1334.

Zapata-Gonzalez, F., Rueda, F., Petriz, J., Domingo, P., Villarroya, F., Diaz-Delfin, J., De Madariaga, M. A., and Domingo, J. C. 2008. Human dendritic cell activities are modulated by the omega-3 fatty acid, docosahexaenoic acid, mainly through PPARγ:RXR heterodimers: Comparison with other polyunsaturated fatty acids. *J Leukoc Biol*, 84, 1172–1182.

Zhuo, Z., Zhang, L., Mu, Q., Lou, Y., Gong, Z., Shi, Y., Ouyang, G., and Zhang, Y. 2009. The effect of combination treatment with docosahexaenoic acid and 5-fluorouracil on the mRNA expression of apoptosis-related genes, including the novel gene BCL2L12, in gastric cancer cells. *In Vitro Cell Dev Biol Anim*, 45, 69–74.

Ziech, D., Franco, R., Pappa, A., and Panayiotidis, M. I. 2011. Reactive oxygen species (ROS)-induced genetic and epigenetic alterations in human carcinogenesis. *Mutat Res*, 711, 167–173.

Zuniga, J., Cancino, M., Medina, F., Varela, P., Vargas, R., Tapia, G., Videla, L. A., and Fernandez, V. 2011. N-3 PUFA supplementation triggers PPARα activation and PPARα/NF-κB interaction: Anti-inflammatory implications in liver ischemia-reperfusion injury. *PLoS One*, 6, e28502.

21

Treatment of Obesity and Diabetes with Marine-Derived Biomaterials

Se-Kwon Kim, Fatih Karadeniz, and Mustafa Zafer Karagozlu

CONTENTS

21.1 Obesity and Diabetes

Obesity predisposes a person to a variety of pathological disorders and has become a serious public health problem. White adipose tissue (WAT) is a major energy reserve in higher eukaryotes, and storing triacylglycerol in intervals of energy excess and its mobilization during the energy requirement are its primary purposes. However, initiation and endurance of obesity occur pursuant to not only hypertrophy of adipose tissue but also differentiation of preadipocytes into adipocytes. This mechanism of adipogenesis is triggered by adipose tissue hypergenesis (Spiegelman and Flier 1996, 2001). Differentiated adipocytes secrete obesity-related factors called adipokines. Plasma leptin, tumor necrosis factor (TNF)-α, and nonesterified fatty acid levels are all elevated in obesity and play a role in causing insulin resistance. Therefore, obesity is closely correlated to the prevalence of diabetes as well as other crucial diseases such as cardiovascular disease, hypertension, and cancer (Langin 2006; Schwartz and Porte 2005).

Diabetes mellitus (DM) is a chronic metabolic disorder characterized by defects in both insulin secretion and insulin action, causing raised blood glucose levels, which in turn can damage many systems in the body, such as blood vessels and nerves. DM affects about 5% of the global population and is becoming the fifth leading cause of death, according to a recent survey of global mortality (Roglic et al. 2005). The disorder is still maintaining a surprising prevalence, and unfortunately, the current treatments are only limited to a weak control of disease to increase the life quality rather than a cure. DM can be classified into several types, while type I and type II are becoming the main and well-studied ones. The most common type is type II DM, which accounts for over 90% of all diabetes-diagnosed patients. It is well known that most of the diabetic complications and impaired cell function in type 2 diabetes are mediated by hyperglycemia (Ceriello 2005). Increasing levels of reducing sugars in the blood under hyperglycemic conditions trigger sets of reactions resulting in formation of reactive oxygen species (ROS), which promote oxidative-stress-induced tissue damage (Robertson and Harmon 2006). Glucose as a primary energy source and regulator of cell function especially induces such reactions. In type 2 diabetes, although patients can retain healthy pancreatic β-cells for many years after disease onset, chronic exposure to high glucose will impair β-cell function in later stages. Impaired β-cell function leads to cellular damage in type 2 diabetic patients (Robertson et al. 2003).

21.2 Antiobesity Activity of Marine-Derived Biomaterials

Obesity may be defined as an excessive accumulation of fat and causing an increased body weight (Kong et al. 2009). It is one of the challenging public health issues in the first half of this century. Moreover, obesity-related complications are shown to increase in many industrialized and developing countries, which cause a worrying health trend (Kelishadi 2007). In this context, the necessity of discovering alternative sources to overcome obesity-related problems has arisen along focused attention for safer products with activities against obesity. Therefore, marine sources especially macroalgae have been the center of attention for many researches with their potential to include diverse bioactive materials with lesser side effects.

A research group from Japan has isolated fucoxanthin from the seaweed *Undaria pinnatifida*. The experiments with this compound reported that oral treatment with fucoxanthin significantly reduced the amount of abdominal WAT of obese mice model, KKA[y] female mice, and normal mice fed with a high-fat diet (Maeda et al. 2005, 2007, 2008). Besides, no effect on normal mice fed with normal diet was observed. According to these results, fucoxanthin shows antiobesity effect by reducing the body weight specifically in obese conditions. WAT consists of adipocytes and is now recognized as an endocrine and active secretory organ through its production of biologically active mediators referred as adipokines secreted from mature adipocytes (Curat et al. 2006). Most studies reported that antiobesity effect of fucoxanthin was mainly mediated by the expression of uncoupling protein-1 (UCP-1) gene in visceral adipose tissues which lead to the induction of thermogenesis in adipose tissue and dissipating excess energy intake as heat to resist body weight gain (Mercader et al. 2010; Woo et al. 2009). Recent clinical study carried by Abidov et al. (2010) clearly showed antiobesity effect of Xanthigen™, an antiobesity supplement which consists of fucoxanthin and pomegranate seeds oil. In their study, they demonstrated that xanthigen promoted weight loss, reduced body and liver fat content, and improved liver function tests in obese nondiabetic women (Abidov et al. 2010).

Some reports have focused on the activities of alginate contained in several seaweeds. Sodium alginate isolated from the brown seaweed *Laminaria digitata* is recently exhibited as a weight-loss supplement; however, its side effects on gastric motor functions and satiation were of concern. Odunsi et al. (2010) clinically investigated and showed the effects of 10 days of treatment with alginate on gastric function, satiation, appetite, and gut hormones associated with satiety in obese adults. They found that treatment with alginate for 10 days resulted in no effect on aforementioned parameters. Therefore, these results point out that the daily intake of alginates may be safely effective to treat obesity.

Onset and longevity of obesity occur by not only hypertrophy of adipose tissue but also differentiation of preadipocytes into adipocytes. Suppression and regulation of obesity can be achieved by inhibiting adipocyte differentiation and forcing adipocytes to lipolysis to reduce accumulated WAT (Langin 2006). Thus, the increased control of the harmful effects on the accumulation of adipose tissue by adipocyte differentiation and its metabolism contribute to the search for a better understanding of the molecular mechanisms of obesity. Kim and Kong (2010) reported that dioxinodehydroeckol (DHE), isolated from *Ecklonia cava*, inhibited the differentiation of 3T3-L1 preadipocytes into adipocytes. It was shown that the presence of DHE significantly reduced lipid accumulation of preadipocytes. Additionally, DHE treatment downregulated the expression of peroxisome proliferator-activated receptor-γ (PPARγ), sterol regulatory element-binding protein 1 (SREBP1), and CCAAT/enhancer-binding protein (C/EBPα), which are key transcription factors for adipocyte differentiation. Moreover, DHE suppressed regulation of the adipocyte-specific gene promoters such as fatty acid binding protein (FABP4), fatty acid transport protein (FATP1), fatty acid synthase (FAS), lipoprotein lipase (LPL), acyl-CoA synthetase 1 (ACS1), leptin, and perilipin. The specific mechanism mediating the effects of DHE was confirmed by activation of phosphorylated AMP-activated protein kinase (pAMPK). Therefore, the results of Kong et al.'s study clearly demonstrated that DHE exerts anti-adipogenic, therefore, anti-obesity effect on adipocyte differentiation through the activation and modulation of the AMPK signaling pathway.

In several studies, similar anti-adipogenic effects of chitin-based derivative compounds have been reported in past decade. Chitin is mainly obtained from marine sources such as crustaceans (e.g., crabs, lobsters and shrimps) for these studies and derived to obtain more effective compounds. Karadeniz et al. (2011) reported the inhibitory activity of sulfated derivative of chitosan oligomers on adipogenesis. Sulfated chitosan could inhibit the mRNA expression of adipocyte-specific factors such as PPAR-γ, C/EBP-α, and SREBP-1. Correspondingly, sulfated chitosan decreased the stored triglyceride levels and facilitated lipolysis demonstrated by released glycerol content. In the light of these results, it can be easily suggested structural modification of chitin and chitosan by sulfation convincingly improved its antiobesity effect in the matter of inhibiting adipogenic differentiation of 3T3-L1 cells. In the same manner, it has been reported that treatment with carboxymethylated (CM)-chitin reduced triglyceride content and enhanced glycerol secretion resulting in less fat accumulation (Kong et al. 2011). CM-chitin induced the downregulation of adipogenesis-related transcriptional factors and adipocyte-specific gene promoters. Moreover, the specific mechanism by CM-chitin was confirmed by transcriptional activations of the phosphorylated adenosine monophosphate-activated protein kinase (AMPK) and aquaporin-7. These results suggest that CM-chitin exerts anti-adipogenic effect on lipid accumulation through modulations of AMPK and aquaporin-7 signal pathways.

Several researchers have demonstrated that chitosan tends to bond with the ingested dietary fat and carry it out in the stool while preventing their absorption through the gut (Kanauchi et al. 1995). Relevant researches about fat-lowering activity of chitosan also have shown that chitosan is capable of absorbing fat up to five times of its weight. Studies of chitosan and its fat-lowering activity have expressed that chitosan and its derivatives are highly effective hypocholesterolemic agents with the ability of decreasing blood cholesterol level up to as much as 50% (Jameela et al. 1994). In this context, blood cholesterol levels are also reported to be related with obesity and obesity-related complications especially in diabetic patients. Moreover, diabetic patient-based studies clearly showed that daily administration of chitosan could drop the blood cholesterol levels by 6% with an increased level of high-density lipoprotein. Additionally, chitosan oligosaccharides (COS) show high efficiency in regulation of blood cholesterol levels. Especially, studies reported that COS are capable of regulating cholesterol levels even in liver. COS prevent the development of fatty liver caused by the action of hepatotropic poisons. Although few studies were carried out for the action mechanism of COS in regulating the serum cholesterol level, several of them suggested possible mechanism of COS lowering the low-density lipoprotein levels. Remunan-Lopez et al. (1998) suggested ionic structure of COS binds bile salts and acid, which inhibit lipid digestion through micelle formation. However, Tanaka et al. (1997) suggested a different mechanism of chitosan and COS where lipids and fatty acids are directly bonded by chitosan.

21.3 Antidiabetes Activity of Marine-Derived Biomaterials

Diabetes mellitus (DM) is mainly characterized by hyperglycemia, and therefore, most of the complications are caused by high blood glucose levels. Expectedly, to prevent or treat diabetes, regulation of the blood glucose level and decreasing the level of postprandial hyperglycemia are known to be one of the most effective therapeutic approaches with fewer disadvantages than other approaches in the early period of DM. While the main absorption of blood glucose results from the intestinal reactions to digest the dietary carbohydrates, increasing efforts have been made to investigate and find potential inhibitors of α-glucosidase and α-amylase in natural resources (Naquvi et al. 2011). In the digestive process of dietary complex carbohydrates, α-glucosidase and α-amylase enzymes play a crucial role. Inhibition of either enzyme can reduce the digestion of oligosaccharides and disaccharides and delay glucose absorption as well as reduce glucose levels in plasma, finally resulting in suppression of postprandial hyperglycemia.

The edible marine brown alga *E. cava* has been reported to possess several bioactive materials with different bioactivities. It has been also reported that the phloroglucinol derivatives from *E. cava* show distinct inhibitory activities on α-glucosidase and α-amylase enzymes. Lee et al. (2009) reported that five phloroglucinal derivatives were isolated from *E. cava*: fucodiphloroethol G (1), dieckol (2), 6,6-bieckol (3), 7-phloroeckol (4), and phlorofucofuroeckol A (5). The antidiabetic activities of these derivatives were also assessed using an enzymatic inhibitory assay against rat intestinal α-glucosidase and porcine pancreatic α-amylase. Most of these phlorotannins showed significant inhibitory activities responding to both enzymes, especially compound 2, with the lowest IC_{50} values at $10.8\,\mu mol\,L^{-1}$ (α-glucosidase) and $124.9\,\mu mol\,L^{-1}$ (α-amylase), respectively. Further studies of compound 2 exerted a noncompetitive inhibitory activity against α-glucosidase. Therefore, *E. cava* is suggested to be an effective dietary supplement in order to prevent high blood glucose levels, especially in postprandial situations.

Effects of polysaccharides from marine seaweed extracts on post meal blood glucose and related insulin response have been examined in swine (Vaugelade et al. 2000). Three different algal fibers of different viscosities, extracted from *Palmaria palmata*, *Eucheuma cottonii*, or *L. digitata*, were used for the aforementioned examinations. The addition of *L. digitata* to the diet of swine resulted in a significantly reduced glucose absorption ratio, along an increased level of starch left in the digestive tract. This study demonstrated that highly viscous alginates from seaweeds could affect the intestinal absorption of glucose and responded insulin activity.

Jin et al. (2004) have reported the bioactivity of *Laminaria japonica* in respect to its possible antidiabetic effect. Administration of *L. japonica* aqueous extract to streptozotocin-induced diabetic rats at 100 mg/kg orally for 5 days significantly reduced blood glucose levels and hepatic lipid peroxidation due to the antioxidant activity of the extract. In a relative study,

Bu et al. (2010) investigated the a-glucosidase inhibitory effect of butyl-isobutyl-phthalate (BIP) from the rhizoid of *L. japonica*. BIP exhibited significant dose-dependent, noncompetitive inhibitory activity against α-glucosidase in vitro, with an IC_{50} of 38 µmol. Additionally, BIP had a significant effect in reducing hyperglycemic conditions of streptozotocin-induced diabetic mice in vivo. These results conclude that BIP could be considered an effective α-glucosidase inhibitor and may become a notable compound for diabetes treatment.

Protein tyrosine phosphatase 1B (PTP1B) is a negative regulator of insulin signaling, and PTP1B inhibition has been considered as a promising therapeutic target against type 2 diabetes. The natural compound hyrtiosal, from the marine sponge *Hyrtios erectus*, has been investigated for its ability to inhibit PTP1B (Sun et al. 2007). It has been reported that hyrtiosal showed extensive cellular effects on glucose transport as well as inhibition of the PTP1B activity. This compound was able to inhibit PTP1B activity with an IC_{50} of 42 µmol in a noncompetitive inhibition mode. Moreover, it was exerted that this identified PTP1B inhibitor could significantly enhance the membrane translocation of the important glucose transporter GLUT4 in PTP1B-overexpressed CHO cells. Additionally, PTP1B was found to regulate insulin-mediated inhibition of Smad2 activation, and hyrtiosal was also effective to facilitate insulin inhibition of Smad2 activation. The reported results of PTP1B inhibitor hyrtiosal have strongly suggested that this compound might serve as a potential lead compound for further research to treat diabetic complications.

A study by Zhu et al. (2010) reported that treatment with oligopeptides from marine salmon skin (OMSS) could regulate type 2 diabetes mellitus–related hyperglycemia, and β-cell deterioration in high-fat-diet-fed rats induced low doses of streptozotocin. Rats were fed with OMSS (3.0 g/kg/day) for 4 weeks, and therefore, their blood levels of fasting blood glucose (FBG) and insulin, serum superoxide dismutase (SOD), malondialdehyde (MDA), glutathione (GSH), tumor necrosis factor-alpha (TNFα), and interferon-gamma (IFNγ) were examined and measured as well as the adipocyte cell islets. Results clearly showed that the levels of FBG and amount of damaged pancreatic islet cells were significantly reduced in OMSS-treated rats. Lower levels of Fas expression were observed in the pancreatic islets of OMSS-treated rats. Significantly reduced levels of serum TNFα, IFNγ, and MDA, but increased levels of SOD and GSH, were detected in OMSS-treated rats. Taken together, treatment with OMSS significantly reduced diabetic conditions in diabetic rats and protected the pancreatic β-cells from apoptosis exhibiting a promising antidiabetic effect.

Chitosan is a functional and basic linear polysaccharide prepared by N-deacetylation of chitin which is a main compound of exoskeleton of crustaceans (e.g., crabs, lobsters, and shrimps), in the presence of alkaline. The industrial production and application fields of chitosan have been steadily increasing since 1970s. Early applications of chitosan were centered on the treatment of wastewater, heavy metal adsorption, food processing, immobilization of cells and enzymes, resin for chromatography, functional membrane in biotechnology, animal feed, and so on. The recent trend is toward producing highly valuable industrial products such as cosmetics, drug carriers, and pharmaceuticals. Chitin and chitosan are known to exhibit antitumor, antibacterial, hypocholesterolemia, and antihypertensive activity (Kim and Rajapakse 2005). The main motive for the development of new applications for chitosan lies in the fact that it is a very abundant polysaccharide, as well as nontoxic and biodegradable. In this respect, chitin, chitosan, and its derivatives with available large numbers of different chemical structures and bioactivities offer a great potential to recover and/or prevent obesity and diabetes.

In addition to fat-lowering mechanisms of chitosan and its derivatives, studies have also proven that chitosan administration can lead to the increase of insulin sensitivity of animal models (Neyrinck et al. 2009). It has been shown that 3 month administration of chitosan significantly increased insulin sensitivity in obese patients and expressed a highly notable decrease in body weight and triglyceride levels (Hernandez-Gonzalez et al. 2010).

Furthermore, chitosan and its oligosaccharides act as antidiabetic agents for treatment of diabetes for protecting pancreatic β-cells. In type two diabetes, although patients can retain healthy pancreatic β-cells for many years after the disease onset, chronic exposure to high glucose will impair β-cell function in later stages. Impaired β-cell functionality leads to cellular damage in type 2 diabetic patients. Therefore, the protection of beta cells is of quite importance for elevated insulin secretion as a part of diabetes treatment. Recent studies reported chitosan oligosaccharides as a protective agent for pancreatic beta cells against high glucose-dependent cell deterioration (Karadeniz et al. 2010). It is suggested that at the same time COS could effectively accelerate the proliferation of pancreatic islet cells with elevated insulin secretion in the aid of lowering blood glucose levels. Liu et al. (2007) reported that COS treatment could improve the general situation and diabetic symptoms of rats, decrease the blood glucose levels, and normalize the impaired insulin sensitivity. Moreover, COS were reported as a preventive agent in nonobese diabetic mice from developing type 1 diabetes, which might be related to several bioactivities of COS. These results supported the hypothesis that COS can prevent pancreatic beta cells of diabetic patients and normalize the crucial insulin secretion. The mechanism behind this protection is studied and suggested as related to immunopotentiation and antioxidation activity of COS.

Renal failure is one of the most common diseases caused by diabetes mellitus. The metal cross-linked complex of chitosan, chitosan–iron (III), has been recently reported to be highly active in reducing phosphorus serum levels to treat chronic renal failure (Schöninger et al. 2010). This relatively new derivative of chitosan is significantly capable of adsorbing serum phosphorus in alloxan diabetes-induced rats with symptoms of renal failure progression.

Moreover, recent studies indicate that diabetics may be at higher risk for blood coagulation than nondiabetics. This life-threatening condition needs to be treated urgently. Therefore, sulfated derivative of chitosan has been shown to possess anticoagulant potency (Vongchan et al. 2002). Furthermore, studies have reported that sulfated chitosan does not show antiplatelet activity unlike heparin, which is an effective anticoagulant agent. Collectively, results proved that sulfated chitosan is a more efficient agent than that of heparin, although heparin has been used for a long time for blood coagulation treatment.

In addition to COS, chitosan also reported to prevent the development and symptoms of non-insulin-dependent diabetes in rats as well as the complications of STZ inducement (Kondo et al. 2000). Briefly, reports suggest that chitosan products protect pancreatic cells and insulin secretion mechanism in diabetic conditions. Furthermore, these compounds can decrease the progression and complication rate of diabetes onset in animal models, demonstrating a great potential for chitosan products to be used as a nutraceutical for the treatment of diabetes.

21.4 Conclusion

High mortality and morbidity rates of diabetes make the diagnosis, prevention, and treatment more important as more and more patients are diagnosed with diabetes in the world in recent years. Besides diabetes, factors relating to diabetes such as obesity must be kept under control in order to prevent the diabetes onset. As a key inducing factor of type 2 diabetes with late onset, obesity urges researches to find a proper treatment to keep the increasing body weight and related complications of obesity. In this manner, natural agents from marine organisms possess various biological activities and have a remarkable potential to be used in several of therapeutic applications. Thus, many of the studies carried out to search antidiabetic activities of marine-derived compounds provide detailed acting mechanisms and activity for prevention and/or treatment of obesity as well as diabetic conditions. In addition, studies proved that structurally diverse compounds of marine origin could express better activity and understanding of the mechanism lying behind antidiabetic and antiobesity actions and efficiency. Therefore, future researches should be directed to enhance the effectiveness of marine-based substances in order to gain more active and fewer harmful agents. Collectively, in conclusion, this evidence suggests that marine natural agents are highly potent nutraceuticals for treatment and prevention of obesity, diabetes, and related complications.

References

Abidov, M., Z. Ramazanov, R. Seifulla, and S. Grachev. 2010. The effects of Xanthigen™ in the weight management of obese premenopausal women with non alcoholic fatty liver disease and normal liver fat. *Diabetes, Obesity and Metabolism* 12: 72–81.

Bu, T., M. Liu, L. Zheng, Y. Guo, and X. Lin. 2010. α-Glucosidase inhibition and the in vivo hypoglycemic effect of butyl-isobutyl-phthalate derived from the *Laminaria japonica* rhizoid. *Phytotherapy Research* 24: 1588–1591.

Ceriello, A. 2005. Postprandial hyperglycemia and diabetes complications: Is it time to treat? *Diabetes* 54: 1–7.

Curat, C., V. Wegner, C. Sengenes, A. Miranville, C. Tonus, R. Busse, and A. Bouloumie. 2006. Macrophages in human visceral adipose tissue: Increased accumulation in obesity and a source of resistin and visfatin. *Diabetologia* 49: 744–747.

Hernandez-Gonzalez, S. O., M. Gonzalez-Ortiz, E. Martinez-Abundis, and J. A. Robles-Cervantes. 2010. Chitosan improves insulin sensitivity as determined by the euglycemic-hyperinsulinemic clamp technique in obese subjects. *Nutrition Research* 30: 392–395.

Jameela, S. R., A. Misra, and A. Jayakrishnan. 1994. Cross-linked chitosan microspheres as carriers for prolonged delivery of macromolecular drugs. *Journal of Biomaterials Science, Polymer Edition* 6: 621–632.

Jin, D. Q., G. Li, J. S. Kim, C. S. Yong, J. A. Kim, and K. Huh. 2004. Preventive effects of *Laminaria japonica* aqueous extract on the oxidative stress and xanthine oxidase activity in streptozotocin-induced diabetic rat liver. *Biological and Pharmaceutical Bulletin* 27: 1037–1040.

Kanauchi, O., K. Deuchi, Y. Imasato, M. Shizukuishi, and E. Kobayashi. 1995. Mechanism for the inhibition of fat digestion by chitosan and for the synergistic effect of ascorbate. *Bioscience, Biotechnology, and Biochemistry* 59: 786–790.

Karadeniz, F., M. Artan, C. S. Kong, and S. K. Kim. 2010. Chitooligosaccharides protect pancreatic β-cells from hydrogen peroxide-induced deterioration. *Carbohydrate Polymers* 82: 143–147.

Karadeniz F., M. Z. Karagozlu, S. Y. Pyun, and S. K. Kim. 2011. Sulfation of chitosan oligomers enhances their anti-adipogenic effect in 3T3-L1 adipocytes. *Carbohydrate Polymers* 86 (2): 666–671.

Kelishadi, R. 2007. Childhood overweight, obesity, and the metabolic syndrome in developing countries. *Epidemiologic Reviews* 29: 62–76.

Kim, S. K. and C. S. Kong. 2010. Anti-adipogenic effect of dioxinodehydroeckol via AMPK activation in 3T3-L1 adipocytes. *Chemico-Biological Interactions* 186 (1): 24–29.

Kim, S. K. and N. Rajapakse. 2005. Enzymatic production and biological activities of chitosan oligosaccharides (COS): A review. *Carbohydrate Polymers* 62: 357–368.

Kondo, Y., A. Nakatani, K. Hayashi, and M. Ito. 2000. Low molecular weight chitosan prevents the progression of low dose streptozotocin-induced slowly progressive diabetes mellitus in mice. *Biological and Pharmaceutical Bulletin* 23: 1458–1464.

Kong, C. S., J. A. Kim, S. S. Bak, H. G. Byun, and S. K. Kim. 2011. Anti-obesity effect of carboxymethyl chitin by AMPK and aquaporin-7 pathways in 3T3-L1 adipocytes. *Journal of Nutritional Biochemistry* 22 (3): 276–281.

Kong, C. S., J. A. Kim, and S. K. Kim. 2009. Anti-obesity effect of sulfated glucosamine by AMPK signal pathway in 3T3-L1 adipocytes. *Food and Chemical Toxicology* 47: 2401–2406.

Langin, D. 2006. Adipose tissue lipolysis as a metabolic pathway to define pharmacological strategies against obesity and the metabolic syndrome. *Pharmacological Research* 53: 482–491.

Lee, S. H., Y. Li, F. Karadeniz, M. M. Kim, and S. K. Kim. 2009. α-Glucosidase and α-amylase inhibitory activities of phloroglucinal derivatives from edible marine brown alga, *Ecklonia cava*. *Journal of the Science of Food and Agriculture* 89: 1552–1558.

Liu, B., W. S. Liu, B. Q. Han, and Y. Y. Sun. 2007. Antidiabetic effects of chitooligosaccharides on pancreatic islet cells in streptozotocin-induced diabetic rats. *World Journal of Gastroenterology* 13: 725–731.

Maeda, H., M. Hosokawa, T. Sashima, K. Funayama, and K. Miyashita. 2005. Fucoxanthin from edible seaweed, *Undaria pinnatifida*, shows antiobesity effect through UCP1 expression in white adipose tissues. *Biochemical and Biophysical Research Communications* 332: 392–397.

Maeda, H., M. Hosokawa, T. Sashima, and K. Miyashita. 2007. Dietary combination of fucoxanthin and fish oil attenuates the weight gain of white adipose tissue and decreases blood glucose in obese/diabetic KKA^y mice. *Journal of Agricultural and Food Chemistry* 55: 7701–7706.

Maeda, H., M. Hosokawa, T. Sashima, and K. Miyashita. 2008. Antiobesity effect of fucoxanthin from edible seaweeds and its multibiological functions. In *Functional Food Health* eds. T. Shibamoto, K. Kanazawa, F. Shahidi, and C. T. Ho, pp. 376–388. Washington, DC: ACS Publications.

Mercader, J., A. Palou, and M. Luisa Bonet. 2010. Induction of uncoupling protein-1 in mouse embryonic fibroblast-derived adipocytes by retinoic acid. *Obesity* 18: 655–662.

Naquvi J. K., J. Ahamad, S. R. Mir, and A. Shuaib. 2011. Review on role of natural alpha-glucosidase inhibitors for management of diabetes mellitus. *Journal of Biomedical Research* 2 (6): 374–380.

Neyrinck, A. M., L. B. Bindels, F. De Backer, B. D. Pachikian, P. D. Cani, and N. M. Delzenne. 2009. Dietary supplementation with chitosan derived from mushrooms changes adipocytokine profile in diet-induced obese mice, a phenomenon linked to its lipid-lowering action. *International Immunopharmacology* 9: 767–773.

Odunsi, S. T., M. I. Vázquez-Roque, M. Camilleri, A. Papathanasopoulos, M. M. Clark, L. Wodrich, M. Lempke et al. 2010. Effect of alginate on satiation, appetite, gastric function, and selected gut satiety hormones in overweight and obesity. *Obesity (Silver Spring)* 18: 1579–1584.

Remunan-Lopez, C., A. Portero, J. L. Vila-Jato, and M. J. Alonso. 1998. Design and evaluation of chitosan/ethylcellulose mucoadhesive bilayered devices for buccal drug delivery. *Journal of Controlled Release* 55: 143–152.

Robertson, P. R. and J. S. Harmon. 2006. Diabetes, glucose toxicity, and oxidative stress: A case of double jeopardy for the pancreatic islet β cell. *Free Radical Biology & Medicine* 41: 177–184.

Robertson, P. R., J. Harmon, P. O. Tran, Y. Tanaka, and H. Takahashi. 2003. Glucose toxicity in β-cells: Type 2 diabetes, good radicals gone bad, and the glutathione connection. *Diabetes* 52: 581–587.

Roglic, G., N. Unwin, P. H. Bennett, C. Mathers, J. Tuomilehto, and S. Nag. 2005. The burden of mortality attributable to diabetes: Realistic estimates for the year 2000. *Diabetes Care* 28: 2130–2135.

Schöninger, L. M. R., R. C. Dall'Oglio, S. Sandri, C. A. Rodrigues, and C. Burger. 2010. Chitosan Iron(III) reduces phosphorus levels in alloxan diabetes-induced rats with signs of renal failure development. *Basic & Clinical Pharmacology & Toxicology* 106: 467–471.

Schwartz, M. and D. Porte Jr. 2005. Diabetes, obesity, and the brain. *Science* 307: 375–379.

Spiegelman, B. and J. Flier. 1996. Adipogenesis and obesity: Rounding out the big picture. *Cell* 87: 377–390.

Spiegelman, B. and J. Flier. 2001. Obesity and the regulation review of energy balance. *Cell* 104: 531–543.

Sun, T., Q. Wang, Z. Yu, Y. Zhang, Y. Guo, K. Chen, X. Shen, and H. Jiang. 2007. Hyrtiosal, a PTP1B inhibitor from the marine sponge *Hyrtios erectus*, shows extensive cellular effects on PI3K/AKT activation, glucose transport, and TGFbeta/Smad2 signaling. *ChemBioChem* 8 (2): 187–193.

Tanaka, Y., S. Tanioka, M. Tanaka, T. Tanigawa, Y. Kitamura, and S. Minami. 1997. Effects of chitin and chitosan particles on BALB/c mice by oral and parenteral administration. *Biomaterials* 18: 591–595.

Vaugelade, P., C. Hoebler, F. Bernard, F. Guillon, M. Lahaye, P. H. Duee, and B. Darcy-Vrillon. 2000. Non-starch polysaccharides extracted from seaweed can modulate intestinal absorption of glucose and insulin response in the pig. *Reproduction Nutrition Development* 40: 33–47.

Vongchan, P., W. Sajomsang, D. Subyen, and P. Kongtawelert. 2002. Anticoagulant activity of a sulfated chitosan. *Carbohydrate Research* 337: 1239–1242.

Woo, M. N., S. M. Jeon, Y. C. Shin, M. K. Lee, M. A. Kang, and M. S. Choi. 2009. Antiobese property of fucoxanthin is partly mediated by altering lipid-regulating enzymes and uncoupling proteins of visceral adipose tissue in mice. *Molecular Nutrition & Food Research* 53: 1603–1611.

Zhu, C. F., H. B. Peng, G. Q. Liu, F. Zhang, and Y. Li. 2010. Beneficial effects of oligopeptides from marine salmon skin in a rat model of type 2 diabetes. *Nutrition* 26 (10): 1014–1020.

22

Potential Anticoagulant Effect of Seaweed-Derived Biomaterials

Se-Kwon Kim and Quang Van Ta

CONTENTS

22.1 Introduction

As more than 70% of the world's surface is covered by oceans, the wide diversity of marine organisms offer a rich source of natural products, and the importance of marine organisms as a source of novel bioactive substances is growing rapidly. With marine species comprising approximately a half of the total global biodiversity, the sea offers an enormous resource for novel compounds (Aneiros and Garateix, 2004; Barrow and Shahidi, 2008). Moreover, a very different kind of substances has been obtained from marine organisms among other reasons because they are living in a very exigent, competitive, and aggressive surrounding, very different in many aspects from the terrestrial environment, a situation that demands the production of quite specific and potent active molecules. Marine environment contains a source of functional materials, including polyunsaturated fatty acids (PUFA), polysaccharides, essential minerals and vitamins, antioxidants, enzymes, and bioactive peptides (Kim and Wijesekara, 2010; Pomponi, 1999).

The blood coagulation system consists of intrinsic and extrinsic pathways, where a series of factors involve in the mechanism. Blood coagulation is preceded by coagulation factors in order to stop the flow of blood though the injured vessel walls whenever an abnormal vascular condition and exposure to nonendothelial surfaces at sites of vascular injury occurred. As endogenous or exogenous anticoagulants interfered with the coagulation factors by inactivation or restriction, the blood coagulation can be prolonged or stopped (Jung et al., 2001). These anticoagulants are used in therapeutic purposes, for example, as cure for hemophilia.

Heparin has been identified and used for more than 50 years as a commercial antico-agulant, and it is widely used for the prevention of venous thromboembolic disorders. However, several side effects of heparin have been reported such as development of thrombocytopenia, hemorrhagic effect, ineffectiveness in congenital or acquired anti-thrombin deficiencies, and incapacity to inhibit thrombin bound to fibrin (Pereira et al., 2002). Moreover, heparin is available in very low concentrations in pig intestine or bovine lungs from where it is primarily extracted. Therefore, the necessity of discovering alterna-tive sources of anticoagulants has been arisen with interesting demand for safer antico-agulant therapy. Therefore, marine organisms have gained much attention to find natural and safe anticoagulant agents.

Among marine organisms, marine algae are rich sources of structurally diverse bioac-tive materials with various biological activities. Recently, their importance as a source of novel bioactive substances is growing rapidly, and researchers have revealed that marine algae–originated compounds exhibit various biological activities with potential anticoagulant effect (Wijesekara and Kim, 2010; Wijesekara et al., 2010, 2011). Sulfated polysaccharides (SPs) and phlorotannins from marine algae have been shown to have potent anticoagulant effect, and according to most of studies, SPs are the main bioac-tive component for this anticoagulant effect. The anticoagulant activity of the SPs and phlorotannins from marine algae has been determined by prolongation of activated par-tial thromboplastin time (APTT), prothrombin time (PT), and thrombin time (TT) assays. Most of studies reported that the anticoagulant activity of marine SPs based on APTT and TT pathways. The prolongation of APTT suggests inhibition of the intrinsic factors and is the measure of the intrinsic pathway-dependent clotting time. The TT revealed the inhi-bition of thrombin activity or fibrin polymerization as thrombin inhibition-dependent clotting time. PT is the extrinsic pathway-dependent clotting time. This chapter focuses on anticoagulant agents derived from marine algae and presents an overview of their anticoagulant effect.

22.2 Anticoagulant Agents in Marine Algae

22.2.1 Sulfated Polysaccharides

Edible marine algae, sometimes referred as seaweeds, have attracted a special interest as good sources of nutrients, and one particular interesting feature is their richness in SPs, the uses of which span from food, cosmetic, and pharmaceutical industries to microbiol-ogy and biotechnology (Ren, 1997). Marine algae are the most important source of non-animal SPs, and the chemical structure of these polymers varies according to the algal species (Costa et al., 2010). The amount of SPs present is found to differ according to the three major divisions of marine algae, Chlorophyta (green algae), Rhodophyta (red algae), and Phaeophyta (brown algae). The major SPs (Figure 22.1) found in marine algae include fucoidan and laminarans of brown algae, carrageenan of red algae, and ulvan of green algae. Recently, various SPs from marine algae have attracted much attention in the fields of food, cosmetic, and pharmacology. For example, carrageenans from marine red algae are widely used as food additives, such as emulsifiers, stabilizers, or thickeners (Campo et al., 2009; Chen et al., 2007). Ulvan displays several physiochemical and biological features of

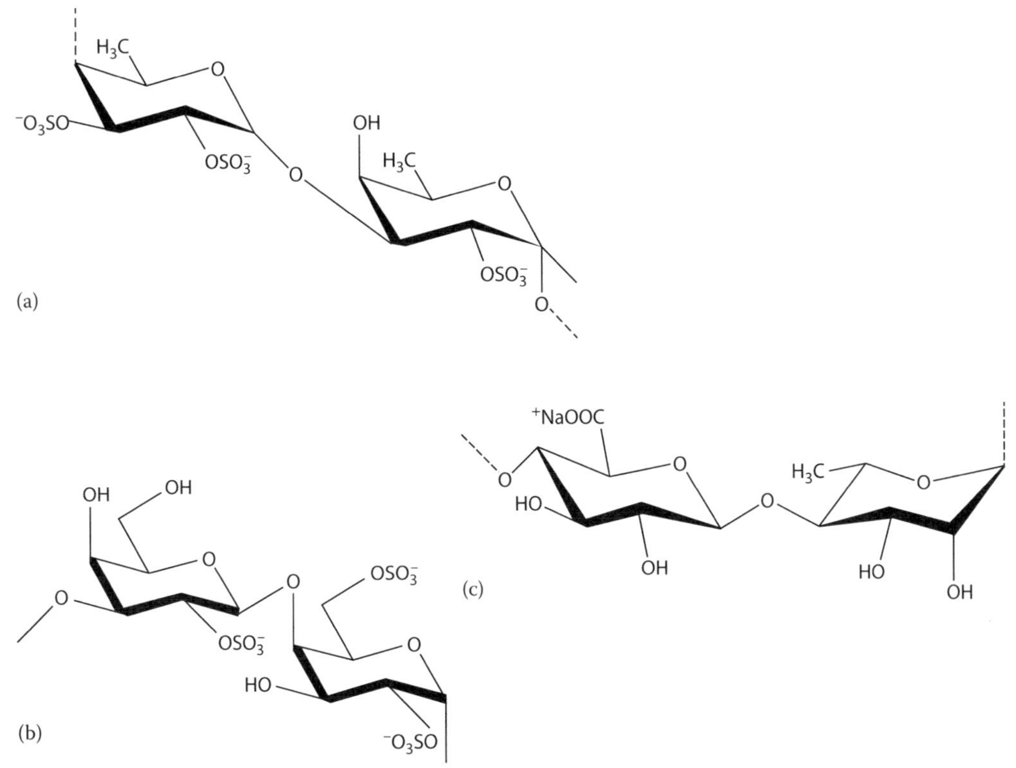

FIGURE 22.1
Anticoagulant SPs from marine algae (a) fucoidan, (b) carrageenan, and (c) ulvan.

potential interest for food, pharmaceutical, agricultural and chemical applications (Lahaye and Robic, 2007).

22.2.2 Phlorotannins

Marine brown algae accumulate a variety of phloroglucinol-based polyphenols, as phlorotannins of low, intermediate, and high molecular weight containing both phenyl and phenoxy units. Based on the means of linkage, phlorotannins can be classified into four subclasses such as fuhalols and phlorethols (phlorotannins with an ether linkage), fucols (with a phenyl linkage), fucophloroethols (with an ether and phenyl linkage), and eckols (with a dibenzodioxin linkage). The isolated and characterized phlorotannins from marine brown algae are compounds **1–7** (Figure 22.2), such as phloroglucinol (**1**), eckol (**2**), fucodiphloroethol G (**3**), phlorofucofuroeckol A (**4**), 7-phloroeckol (**5**), dieckol (**6**), and 6,6′-bieckol (**7**). In addition, triphloroethol A, 8,8′-bieckol and 8,4′-dieckol have been isolated. Among marine brown algae, *Ecklonia cava* is a rich source of phenolic compounds as phlorotannins than other brown algae (Wijesekara et al., 2010). However, other brown seaweeds also have been reported for various types of phlorotannins. These phlorotannins help to protect algae from stress conditions and herbivores. Due to the health beneficial various biological activities of phlorotannins, marine brown algae

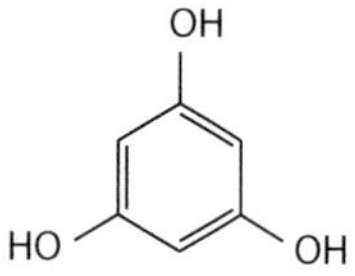

1

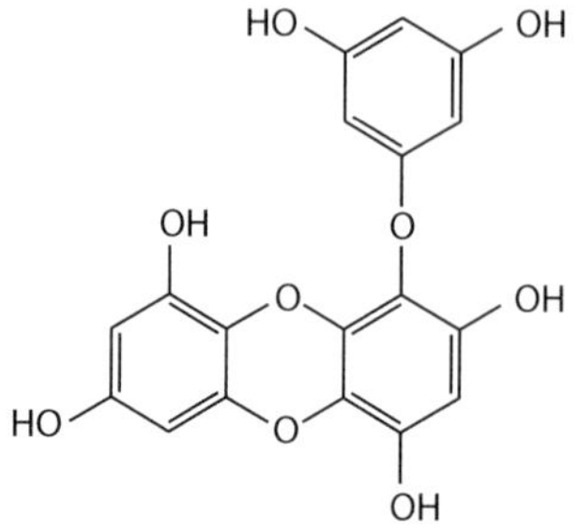

2

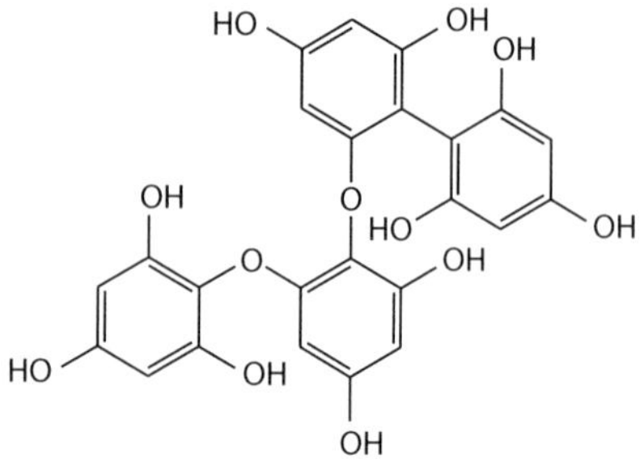

3

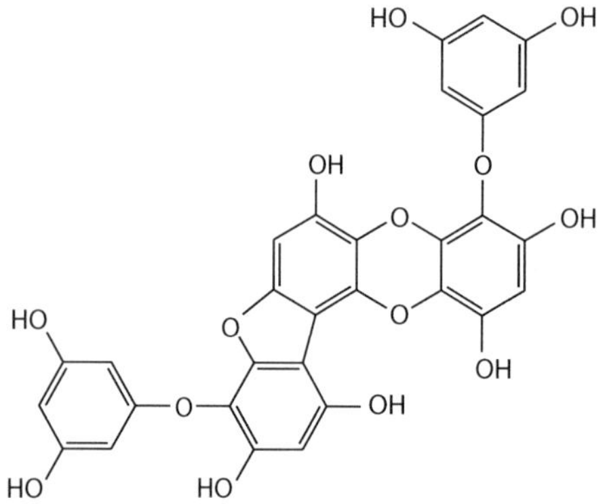

4

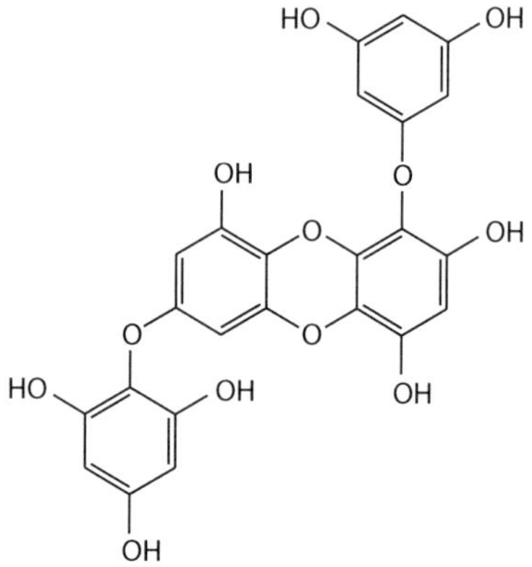

5

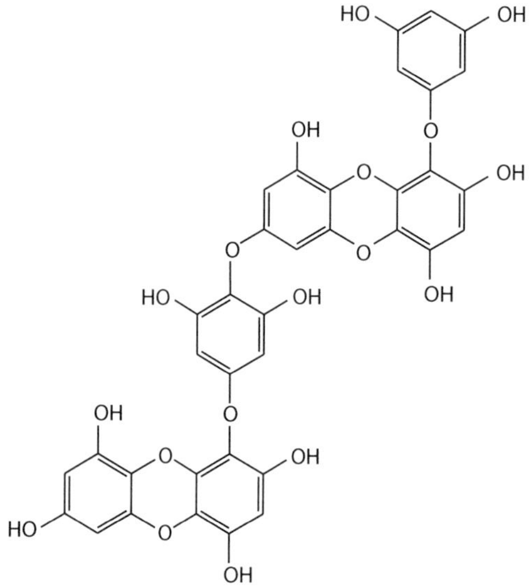

6

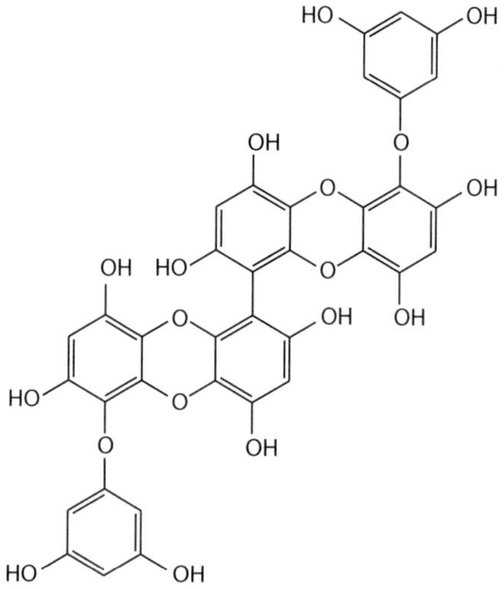

7

FIGURE 22.2
Phlorotannin derivatives from marine brown algae.

are known to be a rich source of healthy food. Among marine brown algae, *Ecklonia cava, E. stolonifera, E. kurome, Eisenia bicyclis, Ishige okamurae, Sargassum thunbergii, Hizikia fusiformis, Undaria pinnatifida,* and *Laminaria japonica* have been reported for phlorotannins with health beneficial biological activities.

22.3 Anticoagulant Activity of Marine Algae

After the investigation of blood anticoagulant properties from marine brown algae (Killing, 1913), it has been reported that SPs derived from marine algae are alternative sources for the manufacture of novel anticoagulant drugs (Church et al., 1989; Matsubara, 2004; Nishino et al., 2000). Anticoagulant activity is among the most widely studied properties of SPs, and anticoagulants from marine algae have previously been reviewed (McLellan and Jurd, 1992; Mestechkina and Shcherbukhin, 2010). Various anticoagulant SPs, from marine algae, have been isolated and characterized (Table 22.1). Two types of SPs are identified with high anticoagulant activity including sulfated galactans or also known as carrageenan from marine red algae (Carlucci et al., 1997; Kolender et al., 1997; Sen et al., 1994) and sulfated fucoidans from marine brown algae (Chevolot et al., 1999; Colliec et al., 1991; Dobashi et al., 1989). However, there are fewer reports of anticoagulant SPs reported from marine green algae compared to brown and red algae (Mao et al., 2009). Jurd et al. (1995) found that the

TABLE 22.1

Some Marine Algae with Anticoagulant SPs

Marine Algae with Anticoagulant SPs	References
Chlorophyta	
Monostroma latissimum	Mao et al. (2009)
Monostroma nitidum	Maeda et al. (1991)
Ulva conglobata	Mao et al. (2006)
Codium fragile	Hayakawa et al. (2000)
Codium pugniformis	Matsubara et al. (2000)
Codium cylindricum	Matsubara et al. (2001)
Phaeophyta	
Ecklonia cava	Athukorala et al. (2006)
Ecklonia kurome	Nishino et al. (1991)
Laminaria japonica	Wang et al. (2010)
Ascophyllum nodosum	Nardella et al. (1996)
Lessonia vadosa	Chandia and Matsuhiro (2008)
Rhodophyta	
Lomentaria catenata	Pushpamali et al. (2008)
Gigartina skottsbergii	Carlucci et al. (1997)
Schizymenia binderi	Zuniga et al. (2006)
Grateloupia indica	Sen et al. (1994)
Porphyra haitanensis	Zhang et al. (2010)
Nothogenia fastigiata	Kolender et al. (1997)

anticoagulant-active SPs from *Codium fragile* subspecies *atlanticum* (Chlorophyta) contain xyloarabinogalactans. A sulfated galactan with anticoagulant activity has also reported from *Codium cylindricum* (Matsubara et al., 2001). In addition, Maeda et al. (1991) have revealed that the anticoagulant SPs from *Monostroma nitidum* (Chlorophyceae) yielded a sixfold higher activity than that of heparin. In comparison, marine brown algae extracts exhibit higher anticoagulant activity than red and green algae extracts (Chevolot et al., 1999; Patanker et al., 1993).

Since a few studies reported the prolongation of PT by marine SPs, it suggests that marine SPs interfered a little or may not inhibit the extrinsic pathway of coagulation. The relationship between structure and anticoagulant activity of some SPs has been reported (Colliec et al., 1991; Hayakawa et al., 2000). The presence of sulfate groups in SPs can increase both their specific and nonspecific binding to a wide range of biologically active proteins. Anticoagulant activity of sulfated galactans depends on the nature of the sugar residue, the sulfation position of the structure, and the sulfate content in the SPs (Melo et al., 2004; Silva et al., 2010). Moreover, the O-sulfated 3-linked α-galactans enhanced the inhibition of thrombin and factor Xa by antithrombin and/or heparin cofactor II in the intrinsic pathway of blood coagulation (Pereira et al., 2002). Furthermore, high molecular weight carrageenans with high sulfate content have shown higher anticoagulant activity than low molecular weight and low sulfate content SPs (Shanmugam and Mody, 2000).

Unfractionated heparins and low molecular weight heparins are the only SPs currently used as anticoagulant drugs. Seaweed-derived SPs have been described to possess anticoagulant activity similar to or higher than heparin (Costa et al., 2010). Collectively, these evidences suggest that SPs derived from seaweeds have a promising potential to be used as anticoagulant agents in the pharmaceutical industry.

Phlorotannins from *Sargassum thunbergii* have been analyzed for their potential anticoagulant activity and suggested that phlorotannins are potential anticoagulants in vitro and in vivo (Li et al., 2007). According to their results, phlorotannins from *S. thunbergii* had a significant effect on the prolongation of APTT, PT, and TT especially at the concentration of 1 mg/mL. In addition, phloroglucinol can be developed as a novel anticoagulant in the pharmaceutical industry (Bae, 2011).

22.4 Conclusion

Recent studies have provided evidence that marine algal derived SPs and phlorotannins play a vital role in human health and nutrition. Furthermore, seaweed-processing by-products with bioactive SPs and phlorotannins can be easily utilized for producing functional ingredients. The possibilities of designing new pharmaceutical agents to support the reduction of blood clotting or regulation of the coagulant-related chronic malfunctions are promising. Therefore, it can be suggested that due to valuable biological functions with health beneficial effects, marine algae have much potential as active ingredients for preparation of nutraceutical and pharmaceutical products. Until now, most of researches of marine algal anticoagulant effect have been observed in vitro or in mouse model systems. Therefore, further research studies are needed in order to investigate their activity in human subjects.

References

Aneiros, A., Garateix, A. 2004. Bioactive peptides from marine sources: Pharmacological properties and isolation procedures. *J Chromatogr B* **803**:41–53.

Athukorala, Y., Jung, W.K., Vasanthan, T., Jeon, Y.J. 2006. An anticoagulative polysaccharide from an enzymatic hydrolysate of *Ecklonia cava*. *Carbohyd Polym* **66**:184–191.

Bae J.S. 2011. Antithrombotic and profibrinolytic activities of phloroglucinol. *Food Chem Toxicol* **49**:1572–1577.

Barrow, C., Shahidi, F. 2008. *Marine Nutraceuticals and Functional Foods*, CRC Press, New York.

Campo, V.L., Kawano, D.F., da Silva, D.B., Carvalho, I. 2009. Carrageenans: Biological properties, chemical modifications and structural analysis—A review. *Carbohyd Polym* **77**:167–180.

Carlucci, M.J., Pujol, C.A., Ciancia, M., Noseda, M.D., Matulewicz, M.C., Damonte, E.B. et al. 1997. Antiherpetic and anticoagulant properties of carrageenans from the red seaweed *Gigartina skottsbergii* and their cyclized derivatives: Correlation between structure and biological activity. *Int J Biol Macromol* **20**:97–105.

Chandia, N.P., Matsuhiro, B. 2008. Characterization of a fucoidan from *Lessonia vadosa* (Phaeophyta) and its anticoagulant and elicitor properties. *Int J Biol Macromol* **42**:235–240.

Chen, H., Yan, X., Lin, J., Wang, F., Xu, W. 2007. Depolymerized products of λ-carrageenan as a potent angiogenesis inhibitor. *J Agric Food Chem* **55**:6910–6917.

Chevolot, L., Foucault, A., Chaubet, F., Kervarec, N., Sinquin, C., Fisher, A.M. et al. 1999. Further data on the structure of brown seaweed fucans: Relationships with anticoagulant activity. *Carbohydr Res* **319**:154–165.

Church, F.C., Meade, J.B., Treanor, E.R., Whinna, H.C. 1989. Antithrombin activity of fucoidan. The interaction of fucoidan with heparin cofactor II, antithrombin III, and thrombin. *J Biol Chem* **264**:3618–3623.

Colliec, S., Fischer, A.M., Tapon-Bretaudiere, J., Boisson, C., Durand, P., Jozefonvicz, J. 1991. Anticoagulant properties of a fucoidan fraction. *Thromb Res* **64**:143–154.

Costa, L.S., Fidelis, G.P., Cordeiro, S.L., Oliveira, R.M., Sabry, D.A., Camara, R.B.G. et al. 2010. Biological activities of sulfated polysaccharides from tropical seaweeds. *Biomed Pharmacother* **64**:21–28.

Dobashi, K., Nishino, T., Fujihara, M., Nagumo, T. 1989. Isolation and preliminary characterization of fucose-containing sulfated polysaccharides with blood-anticoagulant activity from the brown seaweed *Hizikia fusiforme*. *Carbohydr Res* **194**:315–320.

Hayakawa, Y., Hayashi, T., Lee, J.B., Srisomporn, P., Maeda, M., Ozawa, T. et al. 2000. Inhibition of thrombin by sulfated polysaccharides isolated from green algae. *Biochim Biophys Acta* **1543**:86–94.

Jung, W.K., Je, J.Y., Kim, S.K. 2001. A novel anticoagulant protein from *Scapharca broughtonii*. *J Biochem Mol Biol* **35**:199–205.

Jurd, K.M., Rogers, D.J., Blunden, G., McLellan, D.S. 1995. Anticoagulant properties of sulphated polysaccharides and a proteoglycan from *Codium fragile ssp. atlanticum*. *J Appl Phycol* **7**:339–345.

Killing, H. 1913. Zur biochemie der meersalgen. *H-S Z Physiol Chem* **83**:171–197.

Kim, S.K., Wijesekara, I. 2010. Development and biological activities of marine-derived bioactive peptides: A review. *J Functional Foods* **2**:1–9.

Kolender, A.A., Pujol, C.A., Damonte, E.B., Matulewicz, M.C., Cerezo, A.S. 1997. The system of sulfated α-(1 → 3)-linked D-mannans from the red seaweed *Nothogenia fastigiata*: Structures, antiherpetic and anticoagulant properties. *Carbohydr Res* **304**:53–60.

Lahaye, M., Robic, A. 2007. Structure and functional properties of ulvan, a polysaccharide from green seaweeds. *Biomacromolecules* **8**:1765–1774.

Li, J., Wei, Y., Du, G., Hu, Y., Li, L. 2007. Anticoagulant activities of phlorotannins from *Sargassum thunbergii* Kuntz. *Trad Chinese Drug Res Clin Pharmacol* **18**:191–194.

Maeda, M., Uehara, T., Harada, N., Sekiguchi, M., Hiraoka, A. 1991. Heparinoid-active sulfated polysaccharides from *Monostroma nitidum* and their distribution in the Chlorophyta. *Phytochemistry* **30**:3611–3614.

Mao, W., Li, H., Li, Y., Zhang, H., Qi, X., Sun, H. et al. 2009. Chemical characteristics and anticoagulant activity of the sulfated polysaccharide isolated from *Monostroma latissimum* (Chlorophyta). *Int J Biol Macromol* **44**:70–74.

Mao, W., Zhang, X., Li, Y., Zhang, H. 2006. Sulfated polysaccharides from marine green algae *Ulva conglobata* and their anticoagulant activity. *J Appl Phycol* **18**:9–14.

Matsubara, K. 2004. Recent advances in marine algal anticoagulants. *Curr Med Chem* **2**:13–19.

Matsubara, K., Matsuura, Y., Bacic, A., Liao, M.L., Hori, K., Miyazawa, K. 2001. Anticoagulant properties of a sulfated galactan preparation from a marine green alga, *Codium cylindricum*. *Int J Biol Macromol* **28**:395–399.

Matsubara, K., Matsuura, Y., Hori, K., Miyazawa, K. 2000. An anticoagulant proteoglycan from the marine green alga, *Codium pugniformis*. *J Appl Phycol* **12**:9–14.

McLellan, D.S., Jurd, K.M. 1992. Anticoagulants from marine algae. *Blood Coagulation and Fibrinolysis* **3**:69–80.

Melo, F.R., Pereira, M.S., Foguel, D., Mourao, P.A.S. 2004. Antithrombin-mediated anticoagulant activity of sulfated polysaccharides. *J Biol Chem* **279**:20824–20835.

Mestechkina, N.M., Shcherbukhin, V.D. 2010. Sulfated polysaccharides and their anticoagulant activity: A review. *Appl Biochem Microbiol* **46**:267–273.

Nardella, A., Chaubet, F., Boisson-Vidal, C., Blondin, C., Durand, P., Jozefonvicz, J. 1996. Anticoagulant low molecular weight fucans produced by radical process and ion exchange chromatography of high molecular weight fucans extracted from the brown seaweed *Ascophyllum nodosum*. *Carbohydr Res* **289**:201–208.

Nishino, T., Aizu, Y., Nagumo, T. 1991. The influence of sulfate content and molecular weight of a fucan sulfate from the brown seaweed *Ecklonia kurome* on its antithrombin activity. *Thromb Res* **64**:723–731.

Nishino, T., Yamauchi, T., Horie, M., Nagumo, T., Suzuki, H. 2000. Effects of fucoidan on the activation of plasminogen by u-PA and t-PA. *Thromb Res* **99**:623–634.

Patankar, M.S., Oehninger, S., Barnett, T., Williams, R.L., Clerk, G.F. 1993. A revised structure for fucoidan may explain some of its biological activities. *J Biol Chem* **268**: 21770–21776.

Pereira, M.S., Melo, F.R., Mourao, P.A.S. 2002. Is there a correlation between structure and anticoagulant action of sulfated galactans and sulfated fucans? *Glycobiology* **12**:573–580.

Pomponi, S.A. 1999. The bioprocess-technological potential of the sea. *J Biotechnol* **70**:5–13.

Pushpamali, W.A., Nikapitiya, C., De Zoysa, M., Whang, I., Kim, S.J., Lee, J. 2008. Isolation and purification of an anticoagulant from fermented red seaweed *Lomentaria catenata*. *Carbohydr Polym* **73**:274–279.

Ren, D. 1997. Biotechnology and the red seaweed polysaccharide industry: Status, needs and prospects. *Trends Biotechnol* **15**:9–14.

Sen Sr, A.K., Das, A.K., Banerji, N., Siddhanta, A.K., Mody, K.H., Ramavat, B.K. et al. 1994. A new sulfated polysaccharide with potent blood anti-coagulant activity from the red seaweed *Grateloupia indica*. *Int J Biol Macromol* **16**:279–280.

Shanmugam, M., Mody, K.H. 2000. Heparinoid-active sulfated polysaccharides from marine algae as potential blood anticoagulant agents. *Curr Sci* **79**:1672–1683.

Silva, F.R.F., Dore, C.M.P.G., Marques, C.T., Nascimento, M.S., Benevides, N.M.B., Rocha, H.A.O. et al. 2010. Anticoagulant activity, paw edema and pleurisy induced carrageenan: Action of major types of commercial carrageenans. *Carbohydr Polym* **79**:26–33.

Wang, J., Zhang, Q., Zhang, Z., Song, H., Li, P. 2010. Potential antioxidant and anticoagulant capacity of low molecular weight fucoidan fractions extracted from *Laminaria japonica*. *Int J Biol Macromol* **46**:6–12.

Wijesekara, I., Kim, S.K. 2010. Angiotensin-I-converting enzyme (ACE) inhibitors from marine resources: Prospects in the pharmaceutical industry. *Mar Drugs* **8**:1080–1093.

Wijesekara, I., Pangestuti, R., Kim, S.K. 2011. Biological activities and potential health benefits of sulfated polysaccharides derived from marine algae. *Carbohydr Polym* **84**:14–21.

Wijesekara, I., Yoon, N.Y., Kim, S.K. 2010. Phlorotannins from *Ecklonia cava* (Phaeophyceae): Biological activities and potential health benefits. *Biofactors* **36**:408–414.

Zhang, Z., Zhang, Q., Wang, J., Song, H., Zhang, H., Niu, X. 2010. Regioselective syntheses of sulfated porpyrans from *Porphyra haitanensis* and their antioxidant and anticoagulant activities *in vitro*. *Carbohydr Polym* **79**:1124–1129.

Zuniga, E.A., Matsuhiro, B., Mejias, E. 2006. Preparation of a low-molecular weight fraction by free radical depolymerization of the sulfated galactan from *Schizymenia binderi* (Gigartinales, Rhodophyta) and its anticoagulant activity. *Carbohydr Polym* **66**:208–215.

23

Microbial Biomaterials and Their Applications

Se-Kwon Kim, Ira Bhatnagar, and Ramjee Pallela

CONTENTS

23.1 Introduction

Microbes have been long considered as producers of secondary metabolites with pharmaceutical applications. Avenues are now opening in the less explored potential of microorganisms in the field of probiotics and biomedical sciences including tissue engineering. However, most of the microbial species studies employed for such biomedical studies are terrestrial strains. Little attention is given to the microbial flora and fauna of the oceanic environments despite the fact that oceans have been a rich source of natural antioxidants, photoprotective (Pallela et al. 2010), anti-inflammatory (Himaya et al. 2010), anticancer (Bhatnagar and Kim 2010a), and antimicrobial or general pharmaceutical agents with varied actions (Bhatnagar and Kim 2010b).

Polyhydroxyalkanoates (PHAs) have the potential to replace petroleum-based plastics as biomedical materials for use in surgical pins, sutures, staples, blood vessel replacements, bone replacements and plates, medical implants, and drug delivery devices owing to their superior biodegradability and biocompatibility (Khanna and Srivastava 2005). Microbes are excellent producers of PHA and deserve to be studied further in this area. One of the present trends in implantable applications requires materials that are derived from nature. The impetus is twofold. First, such "natural" materials have been shown to better promote healing at a faster rate and are expected to exhibit greater compatibility with humans. Second, new concepts in implantable medical devices, especially in tissue engineering, derived from a combination of biomaterial onto which cells are seeded require the biomaterial to be biodegradable. Among the many other candidate biomaterials available from nature is chitin. Fungal cell wall is made up of chitin, and chitosan (CS) may be easily isolated from the fungal biomass. Yet, less attention is given in this field, and proper utilization of this fungal biomaterial is still not achieved.

With increasing environmental awareness and legal constraints being imposed on discharge of effluents, a need for cost-effective alternative technologies is essential. In this endeavor, microbial biomass has emerged as an option for developing economic and eco-friendly waste water treatment process. Biosorption is considered a potential instrument for the removal of metals from waste solutions and for precious metals recovery, an alternative to the conventional processes, such as those based on ion exchange or adsorption on activated carbon (Veglio and Beolchini 1997). This chapter would try to focus some of the aspects of these biomaterials and the use of microbial entities as a source for the same.

23.2 Microbial Biomaterials

23.2.1 Polyhydroxyalkanoates

Polyhydroxyalkanoates (PHAs) are biodegradable materials, which are accumulated to store carbon and energy in various microorganisms (Keshavarz and Roy 2010; Reddy et al. 2003). Certain nutritional factors, such as nutrient deficiency or the presence of excess carbon, limit their accumulation (Brandl et al. 1990; Reddy et al. 2003). Based on the number of carbon atoms in their monomers, PHAs are classified as "short-chain-length" PHAs, where the number of carbon atoms in the monomer is 3–5, such as polyhydroxybutyrate (PHB) and polyhydroxyvalerate, and "medium-chain-length" PHAs, with 6–16 carbons in the monomers. PHB is the most commonly used PHA, and the metabolic pathways of PHB have been elucidated in detail (Khanna and Srivastava 2005). The properties of PHB are similar to those of various synthetic thermoplastics such as polypropylene. Various microorganisms completely degrade PHB to water and carbon dioxide under aerobic conditions and to methane under anaerobic conditions.

In general, PHAs are polyesters that are synthesized by various microorganisms such as *Cupriavidus necator*, *Alcaligenes latus*, *Aeromonas hydrophila*, *Pseudomonas putida*, and *Bacillus* spp. Several halophilic microbes (including *Haloferax mediterranei*, *Vibrio* spp., *V. natriegens*, *V. nereis*, and *V. harveyi*) have been reported to produce PHB (Higgins and Sharp 1989; Sun et al. 1994; Weiner 1997). The identification of the gene that is involved in PHA synthesis, polyhydroxyalkanoic acid synthase, was verified using *V. parahaemolyticus* and *V. cholera*. The benefit of halophilic microbes in PHA production is that they produce PHA with high molecular weight, such as P(3HB-*co*-3HV). Therefore, they have potential industrial applications and may reduce the cost by some fermentation strategies, such as the immobilization of NaCl onto the walls of bioreactors. However, the disadvantage of halophilic microbes in PHA production is their low productivity (Chen et al. 2006; Don et al. 2006; Huang et al. 2006).

Few reports on marine PHA-producing microorganisms have been published in the recent past. A PHB-producing Gram-negative bacterium, identified as a *Vibrio* sp. BM-1 by the phylogenic analysis of its 16S rDNA, has been isolated from a marine environment in the north of Taiwan, which may be developed industrially for the production of PHB on a larger scale. Mineral salts such as Na_2HPO_4, KH_2PO_4, and $MgSO_4.7H_2O$ are believed to be important for supporting bacterial life and as critical elements for synthesizing metabolites (Ghanem et al. 2005; Mokhtari-Hosseini et al. 2009). The productivity of PHB may be enhanced by carefully studying the effects of mineral salts on PHB production and utilizing the modern biotechnological advancements.

23.2.2 Chitosan

Current tissue engineering strategies are focused on the restoration of pathologically altered tissue architecture by transplantation of cells in combination with supportive scaffolds and biomolecules. In recent years, considerable attention has been given to CS-based materials and their applications as wound-healing agent, bandage material, skin grafting template, hemostatic agent, hemodialysis membrane, dental implants, and drug delivery vehicle (Chandy and Sharma 1993; Hirano 1996; Muzzarelli et al. 1993; Patel and Amiji 1996; Vasudev et al. 1997). CS has been applied to conduct the extracellular matrix (ECM) formation in tissue regenerative therapy (Laurencin et al. 1996; Muzzarelli et al. 1994; Yaylaoglu et al. 1999).

Chitin, together with its variants, especially its deacetylated counterpart CS, has been shown to be useful as a wound dressing material, drug delivery vehicle, and increasingly a candidate for tissue engineering (Khor and Lim 2003). CS, a natural polymer obtained by alkaline deacetylation of chitin, is nontoxic, biocompatible, and biodegradable, and it has recently gained more interest due to its applications in food and pharmaceutics (Ramya et al. 2012). Interesting characteristics that render CS suitable for this purpose are a minimal foreign body reaction, an intrinsic antibacterial nature, and the ability to be molded in various geometries and forms such as porous structures, suitable for cell ingrowth, and osteoconduction. Due to its favorable gelling properties, CS can deliver morphogenic factors and pharmaceutical agents in a controlled fashion. Its cationic nature allows it to complex DNA molecules, making it an ideal candidate for gene delivery strategies (Figure 23.1). The ability to manipulate and reconstitute tissue structure and function using this material has tremendous clinical implications and is likely to play a key role in cell and gene therapies in coming years (Di Martino et al. 2005).

Much of the potential of CS as a biomaterial stems from its cationic nature and high charge density in solution. The charge density allows CS to form insoluble ionic complexes or complex coacervates with a wide variety of water-soluble anionic polymers (Francis Suh and Matthew 2000). One of CS's most promising features is its excellent ability to be processed into porous structures for use in cell transplantation and tissue regeneration. Porous CS structures can be formed by freezing and lyophilizing CS–acetic acid solutions in suitable molds (Madihally and Matthew 1999). CS/collagen composite scaffolds have also been made for skin tissue engineering (Ma et al. 2003).

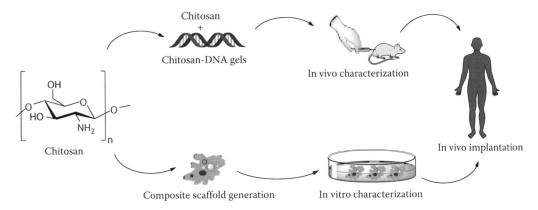

FIGURE 23.1
Schematic representation for application of CS in bone tissue engineering.

Venkatesan et al. (2010) have nicely reviewed the use of CS composite scaffolds in tissue engineering applications (Venkatesan and Kim 2010). Our group has further developed carbon nanotube-grafted CS and natural hydroxyapatite composite scaffolds for bone tissue engineering and achieved profound results (Venkatesan et al. 2011). Not only this, but CS–hydroxyapatite and marine collagen scaffolds have also been synthesized and characterized for bone tissue engineering usage (Pallela et al. 2012). Use of CS in cartilage tissue engineering has also been explored with studies on the feasibility of CS-based hyaluronic acid hybrid biomaterial scaffold generation (Yamane et al. 2005). A detailed review on the application of CS-based polysaccharide biomaterials in cartilage tissue engineering has been published by a leading research group of America in recent past (Francis Suh and Matthew 2000).

The direct use of in situ chitin with fungal mycelia from the fungus *Ganoderma tsugae* to produce wound-healing sacchachitin membranes has also been demonstrated (Su et al. 1997). A nonwoven mat obtained by first processing the mycelia to remove protein and pigment, followed by isolation of fibers in the 10–50 mm diameter range and final consolidation into a freeze-dried membrane under aseptic conditions, was used in a wound model study. The in vitro cell culture using rat fibroblasts and in vivo immunogenicity evaluations indicated no adverse responses (Hung et al. 2001). The wound healing of this fungal-based nonwoven mat as surmised from wound contraction measurements on two different animal model studies was favorable (Su et al. 1999). Fungal CS has also been reported to enhance disease resistance in case of fungal–pea interactions. CSs, (1) derived chemically from the chitin of fungal cell walls, (2) accumulated in *Fusarium solani*/pea interactions, or (3) released from chitinase and β-glucanase digestion of sporelings, were used to determine if these fungal polymers had the biological activity of the CS chemically derived from crustaceans. The biological activity of the cell wall chitin-derived CS from *F. solani* f. sp. *phaseoli* mimicked that of shrimp CS and was somewhat superior to that from f. sp. *pisi*. CSs derived from *F. solani* f. sp. *phaseoli* inhibited germination of *F. solani* macroconidia at concentrations as low as 8 μg mL^{-1} (Kendra et al. 1989). Apart from this, the food industry is also adopting the use of fungal CS for various processes including apple juice clarification. A study published a couple of years ago reported the use of fungal CS as a clarifying agent of apple juice. They reported that the clarity and color changes of the apple juice correlated closely for both fungal and shrimp CS treatment. However, the fungal CS proved highly effective in reducing the apple juice turbidity and gave lighter juices than the sample treated with shrimp CS (Rungsardthong et al. 2006). The use of fungal CS as a growth stimulator in orchid tissue culture has also been investigated and found to have profound effect on the growth of orchid plantlets (Nge et al. 2006). When examined for their antioxidant properties, fungal CS proved to be good antioxidant agents with an antioxidant activity of 61.6%–82.4% at 1 mg/mL concentration (Yen et al. 2007).

23.2.3 Biosorbents

Although the heavy metals occur in immobilized form in sediments and as ores in nature, a large deposition of heavy metals in terrestrial and aquatic environment may occur due to activities like ore mining and industrial processes disturbing the natural biogeochemical cycles. A proper predisposal treatment of these nonbiodegradable and persistent, detrimental heavy metals is mandatory as the release of these pollutants without proper treatment would pose a significant threat to both environment and public health. The phenomenon of biomagnification further deepens the threat where these heavy metals get accumulated in large numbers in food chains. Generally applied techniques for the treatment of heavy metal-contaminated water are reverse osmosis, electrodialysis, ultrafiltration, ion exchange, chemical precipitation, phytoremediation, etc. However, all these methods have disadvantages like incomplete metal removal, high reagent and energy requirements, and generation of toxic sludge or other waste products that require careful disposal (Ahalya et al. 2003).

An emerging cost-effective and eco-friendly technology to treat heavy metal-contaminated water seems to be that of biosorption. This technology employs various types of biomass as source to trap heavy metals in contaminated waters. The biosorbent is prepared by subjecting biomass to various processes like pretreatment, granulation, and immobilization, finally resulting in metal entrapped in bead-like structures. These beads are stripped of metal ions by desorption which can be recycled and reused for subsequent cycles (Figure 23.2). Biosorption can be defined as "a non-directed physicochemical interaction that may occur between metal/radionuclide species and microbial cells" (Alluri et al. 2007). It is a biological method of environmental control and can be an alternative to conventional contaminated water treatment facilities. It also offers several

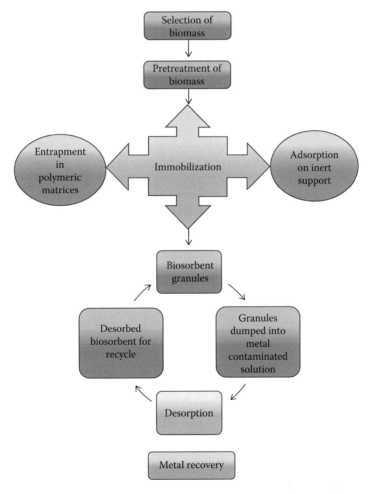

FIGURE 23.2
Utilization scheme for fungal and bacterial biomass for biosorption of metals.

advantages over conventional treatment methods including cost-effectiveness, efficiency, minimization of chemical/biological sludge, requirement of additional nutrients, and regeneration of biosorbent with possibility of metal recovery.

The unabated discharge of effluents by diverse industries constitutes one of the major causes of land and water pollution by chromium compounds and has become an obnoxious health hazard. Out of hexavalent and trivalent species of chromium which are prevalent in industrial waste solutions, the hexavalent form has been considered more hazardous to public health due to its mutagenic and carcinogenic properties. Cr(VI) causes severe diarrhea, ulcers, eye and skin irritation, kidney dysfunction, and probably lung carcinoma (Costa 2003). In reaching for these goals in pollution standards, many methods have been used for the removal of Cr(VI) from wastewaters including ion-exchange resins, filtration, and chemical treatment (Singh and Tiwari 1997). However, these methods are not completely satisfactory and have the following disadvantages: (1) generation of large amount of secondary waste products due to various reagents used in a series of treatments such as reduction of Cr(VI), neutralization of acidic solution and precipitation, and (2) the instability of ion-exchange resins due to serious oxidation by Cr(VI). Thus, there is a need for the development of new cost-effective methods that are more environmentally friendly (Park et al. 2005).

The removal of hexavalent chromium from aqueous solution was studied in batch experiments using dead biomass of three different species of marine *Aspergillus* after alkali treatment. All the cultures exhibited potential to remove Cr(VI), out of which, *Aspergillus niger* was found to be the most promising one. This culture was further studied by employing variation in pH, temperature, metal ion concentration, and biomass concentration with a view to understand the effect of these parameters on biosorption of Cr(VI). Higher biosorption percentage was evidenced at lower initial concentration of Cr(VI) ion, while the sorption capacity of the biomass increased with rising concentration of ions. Biomass as low as 0.8 g L^{-1} could biosorb 95% Cr(VI) ions within 2880 min from an aqueous solution of 400 mg L^{-1} Cr(VI) concentration. Optimum pH and temperature for Cr(VI) biosorption were 2.0°C and 50°C, respectively (Khambhaty et al. 2009).

Not only the dead fungal biomass of *Aspergillus* species but also other bacterial and fungal sp. has been employed for biosorption (Table 23.1). The removal of chromium from

TABLE 23.1

Microbial Species Used as Biomaterials in Heavy Metal Biosorption

Microbial Species	Heavy Metal	References
Phanerochaete chrysosporium	Ni(II), Pb(II)	Çeribasi and Yetis (2001)
Aspergillus niger	Cd	Barros Júnior et al. (2003)
Aspergillus fumigates	Ur(VI)	Bhainsa and D'Souza (1999)
Aspergillus terreus	Cu	Gulati et al. (2002)
Penicillium chrysogenum	Au	Niu and Volesky (1999)
Saccharomyces cerevisiae, Kluyveromyces fragilis	Cadmium	Hadi et al. (2003)
Saccharomyces cerevisiae	Methyl mercury and Hg(II)	Madrid et al. (1995)
Saccharomyces cerevisiae	Uranium	Volesky and May-Phillips (1995)
Bacillus polymyxa	Cu	Philip and Venkobachar (2001)
Bacillus coagulans	Cr(VI)	Alluri et al. (2007)
Escherichia coli	Hg	Bae et al. (2003)
Escherichia coli	Cu, Cr, Ni	Churchill and Churchill (1995)
Pseudomonas species	Cr(VI), Cu(II), Cd(II), Ni(II)	Muraleedharan et al. (1991)

aqueous solution was carried out in batch experiments using dead biomass of four fungal strains—*A. niger, Rhizopus oryzae, Saccharomyces cerevisiae,* and *Penicillium chrysogenum.* All of these dead fungal biomass completely removed Cr(VI) from aqueous solutions, that of *R. oryzae* being the most effective. The removal rate of Cr(VI) increased with a decrease in pH or with increases of Cr(VI) and biomass concentrations, thus supporting the mechanism that Cr(VI) is removed via a redox reaction. Park et al. have further concluded that from the practical view point, the abundant and inexpensive dead fungal biomass could be used for the conversion of toxic Cr(VI) into less toxic or nontoxic Cr(III) (Park et al. 2005).

23.3 Concluding Remarks

Microbial systems have long been proven to have a storehouse of potentialities in the health-care arena, and they form an inevitable component of many of the food processing industries. The promise for fungal chitin and CS as a biomaterial is vast and will continue to increase as the chemistry to extend its capabilities and new biomedical applications are investigated. The microbial biomaterials may be even further explored for tissue engineering applications as well. An extensive research for the use of PHB to manufacture biodegradable polymers using marine microorganisms is also a good area to look up to in terms of biomedical advances (Wei et al. 2011). Heavy metal contamination has also been a major area of concern among the environmentalists. Conventional technologies to clean up heavy metal ions from contaminated waters have been utilized, but these technologies are not all cost effective. An alternative to these technologies are the bioremediation methods which are inexpensive. Hence, microbial biosorbent systems could be envisaged as one of the promising solutions toward biodetoxification of heavy metal pollution.

In short, the microbial biomaterials should be given equal importance, and the marine microbial flora and fauna should be more deeply studied and discovered to get fruitful benefits from these unrevealed treasures of Mother Nature.

References

Ahalya, N., T.V. Ramachandra, and R.D. Kanamadi. 2003. Biosorption of heavy metals. *Research Journal of Chemistry and Environment* 7 (4):71–79.

Alluri, H.K., S.R. Ronda, V.S. Settalluri et al. 2007. Biosorption: An eco-friendly alternative for heavy metal removal. *African Journal of Biotechnology* 6 (25):2924–2931.

Bae, W., C.H. Wu, J. Kostal et al. 2003. Enhanced mercury biosorption by bacterial cells with surface-displayed MerR. *Applied and Environmental Microbiology* 69 (6):3176–3180.

Barros Júnior, L.M., G.R. Macedo, M.M.L. Duarte et al. 2003. Biosorption of cadmium using the fungus *Aspergillus niger. Brazilian Journal of Chemical Engineering* 20 (3):229–239.

Bhainsa, K.C. and S.F. D'Souza. 1999. Biosorption of uranium (VI) by *Aspergillus fumigatus. Biotechnology Techniques* 13 (10):695–699.

Bhatnagar, I. and S.K. Kim. 2010a. Marine antitumor drugs: Status, shortfalls and strategies. *Marine Drugs* 8 (10):2702–2720.

Bhatnagar, I. and S.K. Kim. 2010b. Immense essence of excellence: Marine microbial bioactive compounds. *Marine Drugs* 8 (10):2673–2701.

Brandl, H., R. Gross, R. Lenz et al. 1990. Plastics from bacteria and for bacteria: Poly (β-hydroxyalkanoates) as natural, biocompatible, and biodegradable polyesters. *Microbial Bioproducts* 41:77–93.

Çeribasi, I.H. and U. Yetis. 2001. Biosorption of Ni (II) and Pb (II) by *Phanerochaete chrysosporium* from a binary metal system-kinetics. *Water SA (Pretoria)* 27 (1):15–20.

Chandy, T. and C.P. Sharma. 1993. Chitosan matrix for oral sustained delivery of ampicillin. *Biomaterials* 14 (12):939–944.

Chen, C.W., T.M. Don, and H.F. Yen. 2006. Enzymatic extruded starch as a carbon source for the production of poly (3-hydroxybutyrate-co-3-hydroxyvalerate) by *Haloferax mediterranei*. *Process Biochemistry* 41 (11):2289–2296.

Churchill, S.A. and P.F. Churchill. 1995. Sorption of heavy metals by prepared bacterial cell surfaces. *Journal of Environmental Engineering* 121:706.

Costa, M. 2003. Potential hazards of hexavalent chromate in our drinking water. *Toxicology and Applied Pharmacology* 188 (1):1–5.

Di Martino, A., M. Sittinger, and M.V. Risbud. 2005. Chitosan: A versatile biopolymer for orthopaedic tissue-engineering. *Biomaterials* 26 (30):5983–5990.

Don, T.M., C.W. Chen, and T.H. Chan. 2006. Preparation and characterization of poly (hydroxyalkanoate) from the fermentation of *Haloferax mediterranei*. *Journal of Biomaterials Science, Polymer Edition* 17 (12):1425–1438.

Francis Suh, J.K. and H.W.T. Matthew. 2000. Application of chitosan-based polysaccharide biomaterials in cartilage tissue engineering: A review. *Biomaterials* 21 (24):2589–2598.

Ghanem, N.B., M.E.S. Mabrouk, S.A. Sabry et al. 2005. Degradation of polyesters by a novel marine *Nocardiopsis aegyptia* sp. nov.: Application of Plackett-Burman experimental design for the improvement of PHB depolymerase activity. *The Journal of General and Applied Microbiology* 51 (3):151–158.

Gulati, R., R.K. Saxena, and R. Gupta. 2002. Fermentation waste of *Aspergillus terreus*: A potential copper biosorbent. *World Journal of Microbiology and Biotechnology* 18 (5):397–401.

Hadi, B., A. Margaritis, F. Berruti et al. 2003. Kinetics and equilibrium of cadmium biosorption by yeast cells *S. cerevisiae* and *K. fragilis*. *International Journal of Chemical Reactor Engineering* 1 (1):47.

Higgins, D.G., and P.M. Sharp. 1989. Fast and sensitive multiple sequence alignments on a microcomputer. *Computer applications in the biosciences: CABIOS* 5 (2):151–153.

Himaya, S.W.A., B.M. Ryu, Z.J. Qian et al. 2010. Sea cucumber, *Stichopus japonicus* ethyl acetate fraction modulates the lipopolysaccharide induced iNOS and COX-2 via MAPK signaling pathway in murine macrophages. *Environmental Toxicology and Pharmacology* 30 (1):68–75.

Hirano, S. 1996. Chitin biotechnology applications. *Biotechnology Annual Review* 2:237–258.

Huang, T.Y., K.J. Duan, S.Y. Huang et al. 2006. Production of polyhydroxyalkanoates from inexpensive extruded rice bran and starch by *Haloferax mediterranei*. *Journal of Industrial Microbiology & Biotechnology* 33 (8):701–706.

Hung, W.S., C.L. Fang, C.H. Su et al. 2001. Cytotoxicity and immunogenicity of sacchachitin and its mechanism of action on skin wound healing. *Journal of Biomedical Materials Research* 56 (1):93–100.

Kendra, D.F., D. Christian, and L.A. Hadwiger. 1989. Chitosan oligomers from *Fusarium solani*/pea interactions, chitinase/β-glucanase digestion of sporelings and from fungal wall chitin actively inhibit fungal growth and enhance disease resistance. *Physiological and Molecular Plant Pathology* 35 (3):215–230.

Keshavarz, T. and I. Roy. 2010. Polyhydroxyalkanoates: Bioplastics with a green agenda. *Current Opinion in Microbiology* 13 (3):321–326.

Khambhaty, Y., K. Mody, S. Basha et al. 2009. Biosorption of Cr(VI) onto marine *Aspergillus niger*: Experimental studies and pseudo-second order kinetics. *World Journal of Microbiology and Biotechnology* 25 (8):1413–1421.

Khanna, S. and A.K. Srivastava. 2005. Recent advances in microbial polyhydroxyalkanoates. *Process Biochemistry* 40 (2):607–619.

Khor, E. and L.Y. Lim. 2003. Implantable applications of chitin and chitosan. *Biomaterials* 24 (13):2339–2349.

Laurencin, C.T., S.F. El-Amin, S.E. Ibim et al. 1996. A highly porous 3-dimensional polyphosphazene polymer matrix for skeletal tissue regeneration. *Journal of Biomedical Materials Research* 30 (2):133–138.

Ma, L., C. Gao, Z. Mao et al. 2003. Collagen/chitosan porous scaffolds with improved biostability for skin tissue engineering. *Biomaterials* 24 (26):4833–4841.

Madihally, S.V. and H.W.T. Matthew. 1999. Porous chitosan scaffolds for tissue engineering. *Biomaterials* 20 (12):1133–1142.

Madrid, Y., C. Cabrera, T. Perez-Corona et al. 1995. Speciation of methylmercury and Hg (II) using baker's yeast biomass (*Saccharomyces cerevisiae*). Determination by continuous flow mercury cold vapor generation atomic absorption spectrometry. *Analytical Chemistry* 67 (4):750–754.

Mokhtari-Hosseini, Z.B., E. Vasheghani-Farahani, A. Heidarzadeh-Vazifekhoran et al. 2009. Statistical media optimization for growth and PHB production from methanol by a methylotrophic bacterium. *Bioresource Technology* 100 (8):2436–2443.

Muraleedharan, T.R., L. Iyengar, and C. Venkobachar. 1991. Biosorption: An attractive alternative for metal removal and recovery. *Current Science* 61 (6):379–385.

Muzzarelli, R.A.A., G. Biagini, M. Bellardini et al. 1993. Osteoconduction exerted by methyl-pyrrolidinone chitosan used in dental surgery. *Biomaterials* 14 (1):39–43.

Muzzarelli, R.A.A., M. Mattioli-Belmonte, C. Tietz et al. 1994. Stimulatory effect on bone formation exerted by a modified chitosan. *Biomaterials* 15 (13):1075–1081.

Nge, K.L., N. Nwe, S. Chandrkrachang et al. 2006. Chitosan as a growth stimulator in orchid tissue culture. *Plant Science* 170 (6):1185–1190.

Niu, H. and B. Volesky. 1999. Characteristics of gold biosorption from cyanide solution. *Journal of Chemical Technology and Biotechnology* 74 (8):778–784.

Pallela, R., Y. Na-Young, and S.K. Kim. 2010. Anti-photoaging and photoprotective compounds derived from marine organisms. *Marine Drugs* 8 (4):1189–1202.

Pallela, R., J. Venkatesan, V.R. Janapala et al. 2012. Biophysicochemical evaluation of chitosan-hydroxyapatite-marine sponge collagen composite for bone tissue engineering. *Journal of Biomedical Materials Research Part A* 2:486–495.

Park, D., Y.-S. Yun, and J.M. Park. 2005. Use of dead fungal biomass for the detoxification of hexavalent chromium: Screening and kinetics. *Process Biochemistry* 40 (7):2559–2565.

Patel, V.R. and M.M. Amiji. 1996. Preparation and characterization of freeze-dried chitosan-poly (ethylene oxide) hydrogels for site-specific antibiotic delivery in the stomach. *Pharmaceutical Research* 13 (4):588–593.

Philip, L., and C. Venkobachar. 2001. An insight into the mechanism of biosorption of copper by *Bacillus polymyxa*. *International Journal of Environment and Pollution* 15 (4):448–460.

Ramya, R., J. Venkatesan, S.K. Kim et al. 2012. Biomedical applications of chitosan: An overview. *Journal of Biomaterials and Tissue Engineering* 2 (2):100–111.

Reddy, C.S.K., R. Ghai, and V.C. Kalia. 2003. Polyhydroxyalkanoates: An overview. *Bioresource Technology* 87 (2):137–146.

Rungsardthong, V., N. Wongvuttanakul, N. Kongpien et al. 2006. Application of fungal chitosan for clarification of apple juice. *Process Biochemistry* 41 (3):589–593.

Singh, V.K. and P.N. Tiwari. 1997. Removal and recovery of chromium (VI) from industrial waste water. *Journal of Chemical Technology and Biotechnology* 69 (3):376–382.

Su, C.H., C.S. Sun, S.W. Juan et al. 1997. Fungal mycelia as the source of chitin and polysaccharides and their applications as skin substitutes. *Biomaterials* 18 (17):1169–1174.

Su, C.H., C.S. Sun, S.W. Juan et al. 1999. Development of fungal mycelia as skin substitutes: Effects on wound healing and fibroblast. *Biomaterials* 20 (1):61–68.

Sun, W., J.G. Cao, K. Teng et al. 1994. Biosynthesis of poly-3-hydroxybutyrate in the luminescent bacterium, *Vibrio harveyi*, and regulation by the lux autoinducer, N-(3-hydroxybutanoyl) homoserine lactone. *Journal of Biological Chemistry* 269 (32):20785–20790.

Vasudev, S.C., T. Chandy, and C.P. Sharma. 1997. Development of chitosan/polyethylene vinyl acetate co-matrix: Controlled release of aspirin-heparin for preventing cardiovascular thrombosis. *Biomaterials* 18 (5):375–381.

Veglio, F. and F. Beolchini. 1997. Removal of metals by biosorption: A review. *Hydrometallurgy* 44 (3):301–316.

Venkatesan, J. and S.K. Kim. 2010. Chitosan composites for bone tissue engineering—An overview. *Marine Drugs* 8 (8):2252–2266.

Venkatesan, J., Z.J. Qian, B.M. Ryu et al. 2011. Preparation and characterization of carbon nanotube-grafted-chitosan-Natural hydroxyapatite composite for bone tissue engineering. *Carbohydrate Polymers* 83 (2):569–577.

Volesky, B. and H.A. May-Phillips. 1995. Biosorption of heavy metals by *Saccharomyces cerevisiae*. *Applied Microbiology and Biotechnology* 42 (5):797–806.

Wei, Y.-H., W.-C. Chen, H.-S. Wu et al. 2011. Biodegradable and biocompatible biomaterial, polyhydroxybutyrate, produced by an indigenous *Vibrio sp.* BM-1 isolated from marine environment. *Marine Drugs* 9 (4):615–624.

Weiner, R.M. 1997. Biopolymers from marine prokaryotes. *Trends in Biotechnology* 15 (10):390–394.

Yamane, S., N. Iwasaki, T. Majima et al. 2005. Feasibility of chitosan-based hyaluronic acid hybrid biomaterial for a novel scaffold in cartilage tissue engineering. *Biomaterials* 26 (6):611–619.

Yaylaoglu, M.B., P. Korkusuz, F. Korkusuz et al. 1999. Development of a calcium phosphate-gelatin composite as a bone substitute and its use in drug release. *Biomaterials* 20 (8):711–719.

Yen, M.T., Y.H. Tseng, R.C. Li et al. 2007. Antioxidant properties of fungal chitosan from shiitake stripes. *LWT-Food Science and Technology* 40 (2):255–261.

24

Marine Biomaterials for Antiallergic Therapeutics

Se-Kwon Kim, Thanh-Sang Vo, and Dai-Hung Ngo

CONTENTS

24.1 Introduction

The world's oceans, covering more than 70% of the earth's surface, represent an enormous resource for the discovery of promising therapeutic agents. Among 36 known living phyla, 34 of them are found in marine environments with more than 300,000+ known species of fauna and flora (Jirge and Chaudhari 2010). Although few marine natural products are currently on the market or in clinical trials, marine organisms have been known as the greatest unexploited source of potential pharmaceuticals. Due to the unusual diversity of chemical structures, marine organisms have received much attention in screening marine natural products for their biomedical potential (Haefner 2003; Newman and Cragg 2004; Molinski et al. 2009). During the last decades, marine organisms such as algae, tunicates, sponges, soft corals, bryozoans, sea slugs, mollusks, echinoderms, fishes, and microorganisms have been subjected to the isolation of numerous novel compounds. They have significant amounts of lipid, protein, peptide, acid amine, polysaccharides, chlorophyll, carotenoids, vitamins, minerals, and unique pigments (Faulkner 2001, 2002; Blunt et al. 2006). Notably, many of these compounds possess interesting biological activities and health benefit effects such as anticoagulant, antivirus, antioxidant, antiallergy, anticancer, anti-inflammation, and antiobesity (Blunden 2001; El Gamal 2010; Wijesekara et al. 2010; Gupta and Abu-Ghannam 2011; Mayer et al. 2011). Therefore, marine organisms are regarded as a huge source of novel biomaterials for the development of pharmaceutical and nutraceutical industries.

Allergy is a disorder of the immune system due to an exaggerated reaction of the immune system to harmless environmental substances, such as animal dander, house dust mites, foods, pollen, insects, and chemical agents (Milián and Díaz 2004). Allergic reaction is characterized by the excessive activation of mast cells and basophils by immunoglobulin E (IgE), resulting in an extreme inflammatory response (Galli et al. 2008). It can cause runny nose, sneezing, itching, rashes, swelling, or asthma (Kay 2000). It is noteworthy that the allergic diseases are among the commonest causes of chronic ill health. The prevalence, severity, and complexity of these diseases are rapidly rising and considerably adding to the burden of healthcare costs (Kay 2000). Currently, several classes of drugs, such as corticosteroids, antihistamines, and mast cell stabilizers, are used to treat the allergic disorders. All these therapeutics help to alleviate the symptoms, but, especially after long-term and high-dose medication, they can have quite substantial side effects (Baroody and Naclerio 2000; Rizzo and Sole 2006). Therefore, there is still a vital need for the development of new antiallergic drugs with satisfactory tolerability for long-term use. In this regard, natural bioactive compounds and their derivatives are great sources for the development of new generation antiallergic therapeutics which are more effective with fewer side effects.

24.2 Marine Biomaterials for Antiallergic Therapeutics

Acute allergic sensitization in individuals is involved in the generation of allergen-specific CD4+ Th2 cells. These cells secrete various cytokines, including IL-4, IL-5, IL-9, and IL-13, as well as chemokines such as thymus, leading to further Th2 cell recruitment and production of allergen-specific IgE by B cells. Subsequently, IgE circulates and binds surface receptors on mast cells and basophils. Further exposure to allergen results in cross-linking of IgE on mast cells and basophils causing cell degranulation, releasing histamine, proteases, chemokines, prostaglandins, leukotrienes, and a host of other mediators. This results in bronchoconstriction and recruitment of activated eosinophils, neutrophils, lymphocytes, and macrophages (Larche et al. 2003; Larche 2007). These allergic cascades are considered as a source of molecular targets for regulation of type I allergic reaction and management of allergic diseases. Recently, the role of marine organism-derived compounds as antiallergic agents has been determined in vitro and in vivo by many researchers. Simultaneously, numerous marine compounds have been found to be efficient for antiallergic therapeutics via suppression of allergic degranulation, inhibition of hyaluronidase enzyme, blockade of FcεRI activities, and modulation of allergic immune responses.

24.2.1 Phlorotannins

Brown algae have been recognized as a rich source of phlorotannins, which are formed by the polymerization of phloroglucinol (1,3,5-tryhydroxybenzene) monomer units and biosynthesized through the acetate–malonate pathway. The phlorotannins are highly hydrophilic components with a wide range of molecular sizes ranging between 126 Da and 650 kDa. Based on the means of linkage, phlorotannins can be classified into four subclasses, including fuhalols and phlorethols (phlorotannins with an ether linkage), fucols (with a phenyl linkage), fucophloroethols (with an ether and phenyl linkage), and eckols (with a dibenzodioxin linkage) (Vo and Kim 2010; Li et al. 2011). Notably, phlorotannins exhibited various beneficial bioactivities such as antioxidant, anticancer, antidiabetic, anti-HIV, matrix metalloproteinase enzyme inhibition, and antihypertensive activities (Wijesekara et al. 2010). In relation to antiallergic properties, many phlorotannins from brown algae have been known as potential natural inhibitors of allergic reactions. Several bioactive phloroglucinol derivatives, fucodiphloroethol G, eckol, dieckol, 6,6'-bieckol, phlorofucofuroeckol A, and 1-(3',5'-dihydroxyphenoxy)-7-(2",4",6-trihydroxyphenoxy)-2,4,9-trihydroxydibenzo-1,4-dioxin were isolated from *Ecklonia cava* and evidenced to be efficient against A23187 or FcɛRI-mediated histamine release from KU812 and RBL-2H3 cells (Li et al. 2008; Le et al. 2009). Especially, dieckol, 6,6'-bieckol, and fucodiphloroethol G exhibited a significantly inhibitory activity with IC_{50} range of 27.80–55.12 μM. The inhibitory mechanism of these compounds was determinedby blocking the binding activity between IgE and FcɛRI. In the same regard, Shim et al. (2009) have proved that phlorotannins of dioxinodehydroeckol and phlorofucofuroeckol A from *Ecklonia stolonifera* induced a suppression of the cell surface FcɛRI expression and total cellular protein and mRNA levels of the FcɛRI α chain in KU812 cells. Further, both of these compounds exerted inhibitory effects against intracellular calcium elevation and histamine release from anti-FcɛRI α chain antibody (CRA-1)-stimulated cells. Thus, these bioactive phloroglucinol derivatives were suggested as a promising candidate for the design of novel inhibitor of FcɛRI-mediated allergic reaction.

In addition, brown algae of *Eisenia bicyclis* and *Eisenia arborea* were also identified to contain many antiallergic phlorotannins, namely, phloroglucinol, phlorofucofuroeckol A, dieckol, and 8,8'-bieckol from *Eisenia bicyclis* considerably inhibited hyaluronidase enzyme with IC_{50} values of 280, 140, 120, and 40 μM, respectively (Shibata et al. 2002). The effect of these phlorotannins against hyaluronidase enzyme is stronger than well-known inhibitors such as catechins ($IC_{50} = 620$ μM) and sodium cromoglycate ($IC_{50} = 270$ μM). Notably, 8,8'-bieckol, the strongest hyaluronidase inhibitor among the tested phlorotannins, acted as a competitive inhibitor with an inhibition constant of 35 μM. Moreover, these phlorotannins caused the inactivation of enzyme secretory phospholipase A_2s, lipoxygenases, and cyclooxygenase. Herein, 8,8'-bieckol showed the pronouncedly inhibitory effects on soybean lipoxygenases and 5-lipoxygenases with IC_{50} values of 38 and 24 μM, respectively. Meanwhile, dieckol presented a significant inhibition of COX-1 with inhibition rate of 74.7% (Shibata et al. 2003). Likewise, several phlorotannins of eckol, 6,6'-bieckol, 6,8'-bieckol, 8,8'-bieckol, PFF-A, and PFF-B from *Eisenia arborea* were also confirmed as strong inhibitors of hyaluronidase, phospholipase A_2, cyclooxygenase, and lipoxygenases (Sugiura et al. 2008, 2009), which correlated to suppression in synthesis and release of leukotriene and prostaglandin from RBL cells (Sugiura et al. 2009). Among phlorotannins obtained from *Eisenia arborea*, PFF-B exposed the strongest activity against histamine and β-hexosaminidase release with IC_{50} value of 7.8 μM (Sugiura et al. 2006, 2007). Obviously, PFF-B had a 2.8–6.0 times greater inhibitory activity than those of epigallocatechin gallate ($IC_{50} = 22.0$ μM) or Tranilast ($IC_{50} = 46.6$ μM), a clinically used antiallergic drug (Matsubara et al. 2004).

24.2.2 Polysaccharides

Marine algae are the most important source of polysaccharides, and the chemical structure of polymers varies according to the alga species. In recent years, numerous polysaccharides isolated from marine algae have been used in many fields of food, cosmetic, and pharmacology due to their antiviral, anticoagulant, anticancer, and anti-inflammatory activities (Vo and Kim 2010). A role of polysaccharides from marine algae as antiallergic agents has been suggested. Alginic acid, a naturally occurring hydrophilic colloidal polysaccharide obtained from the several species of brown seaweeds, exhibited different effects against hyaluronidase activity and histamine release from mast cells (Asada et al. 1997). In the in vivo conditions, alginic acid inhibited compound 48/80-induced systemic anaphylaxis with doses of 0.25–1 g/kg and significantly inhibited passive cutaneous anaphylaxis by 54.8% at 1 g/kg for 1 h pretreatment (Jeong et al. 2006). Besides, alginic acid was found to have a maximum suppression rate (60.8%) on histamine release from rat peritoneal mast cells at concentration of 0.01 μg/mL. Furthermore, the antiallergic activities of alginic acid were also observed due to its suppressive effects on activity and expression of histidine decarboxylase, production of IL-1β and TNF-α, and protein level of nuclear factor (NF)-κB/*Rel A* in PMA plus A23187-stimulated HMC-1 cells (Jeong et al. 2006). Noticeably, alginic acid oligosaccharide (ALGO), a lyase–lysate of alginic acid, has been revealed to be able to reduce IgE production in the serum of BALB/c mice immunized with beta-lactoglobulin (Yoshida et al. 2004; Uno et al. 2006). Moreover, antigen-induced Th2 development was blocked by ALGO treatment via enhancing the production of IFN-γ and IL-12 and downregulating IL-4 production in splenocytes of mice (Yoshida et al. 2004).

Besides, Porphyran, a sulphated polysaccharide isolated from red seaweeds, has been recognized to be effective against different allergic responses. According to Ishihara et al. (2005), Porphyrans of red algae *Porphyra tenera* and *P. yezoensis* were capable to inhibit the contact hypersensitivity reaction induced by 2,4,6-trinitrochlorobenzene via decreasing the serum level of IgE in Balb/c mice. Meanwhile, fucoidan from *Undaria pinnatifida* reduced the concentrations of both IL-4 and IL-13 in bronchoalveolar lavage fluid and inhibited the increase of antigen-specific IgE in OVA-induced mouse airway hypersensitivity (Maruyama et al. 2005). In the recent study, Yanase et al. (2009) have reported that the peritoneal injection of fucoidan caused an alleviative effect of plasma IgE level by suppressing a number of IgE-expressing and IgE-secreting B cells from OVA-sensitized mice. On the other hand, the inhibitory effect of fucoidan on IgE production was determined by preventing Cε germ line transcription and NF-κB p52 translocation in B cells (Oomizu et al. 2006). Yet, the inhibitory activity of fucoidan would not be observed if B cells were prestimulated with IL-4 and anti-CD40 antibody before the administration of fucoidan. Thus, it suggested that fucoidan may not prevent a further increase of IgE in patients who have already developed allergic diseases and high levels of serum IgE. However, Iwamoto et al. (2011) have recently determined that fucoidan effectively reduced IgE production in both peripheral blood mononuclear cells from atopic dermatitis patients and healthy donors. These findings indicated that fucoidan suppresses IgE production by inhibiting immunoglobulin class switching to IgE in human B cells, even after the onset of atopic dermatitis.

24.2.3 Chitin, Chitosan, and Chitooligosaccharides

Chitin, a long-chain polymer of N-acetylglucosamine, is widely distributed as the principal component of living organisms such as insects, fungi, crustacean, and invertebrates. It is one of the most abundant polysaccharides and is usually prepared from the shells of crabs and shrimps. Chitosan, a partially deacetylated polymer of N-acetylglucosamine, is produced commercially by deacetylation of chitin (Dutta et al. 2004; Aranaz et al. 2009). During the past decades, chitosan has received considerable attention due to its biodegradable, nontoxic, and nonallergenic properties, which made it possible to be used in many fields including food, cosmetics, biomedicine, agriculture, and environmental protection (Shahidi et al. 1999; Kim and Rajapaksea 2005). Recent studies have focused on the conversion of chitosan to chitooligosaccharides (COS) since COS not only are water soluble (Yang et al. 2010) and possess higher oral absorption (Chae et al. 2005) but also have various biological effects, including antimicrobial, antitumor, anticancer, antioxidant, anti-inflammatory, and anti-angiotensin-I-converting enzyme activities (Kim and Rajapaksea 2005; Park and Kim 2010;

Xia et al. 2011). Especially, chitin and its derivatives have been determined to be therapeutic agents against allergic diseases (Catalli and Kulka 2010). For the early time, Shibata et al. (1997) have shown that intravenous administration of fractionated chitin particles (1–10 μm) into the mouse lung can activate alveolar macrophages to express cytokines such as IL-12 and IL-18, leading to INF-γ production mainly by NK cells. In a further study, Shibata et al. (2000) have demonstrated that orally given chitin downregulates allergen-induced IgE production and lung inflammation in a ragweed-immunized allergic animal model. Moreover, the production of Th2 cytokines including IL-4, IL-5, and IL-10 was inhibited by chitin treatment in the allergen-stimulated spleen cell culture. The inhibitory effects were found by enhancing the activity of NK cells and Th1 cells. Moreover, they have also shown that chitin is a strong Th1 adjuvant that upregulates Th1 immunity induced by heat-killed *Mycobacterium bovis* while downregulating Th2 immunity induced by mycobacterial protein (Shibata et al. 2001). On the other hand, Strong and colleagues have confirmed that intranasal application of chitin microparticles into the lung also significantly suppresses allergic response to *Dermatophagoides pteronyssinus* and *Aspergillus fumigatus* in a murine model of allergy (Strong et al. 2002). The suppressive effects were found by reducing the allergen-induced serum IgE levels, IL-4 production, peripheral eosinophilia, airway hyperresponsiveness, and lung inflammation. Similarly, intranasal application of water-soluble chitosan diminished mucus production and lung inflammation induced by *Dermatophagoides farina* (Chen et al. 2008). Furthermore, application of microgram quantities of chitin microparticles exhibited a beneficial effect in preventing and treating histopathologic changes in the airways of asthmatic mice (Ozdemir et al. 2006). Recently, Vo et al. (2011, 2012) have investigated the inhibitory effect of COS on mast cell activation induced by calcium ionophore A23187 or antigen. The pretreatment of COS causes significant inhibition on mast cell degranulation via reducing histamine and β-hexosaminidase release and intracellular Ca^{2+} elevation in RBL-2H3 mast cells. Moreover, the inhibitory effects of COS on expression as well as production of various cytokines such as TNF-α, IL-1β, IL-4, and IL-6 were also evidenced. Collectively, these results indicate that chitin and its derivatives can contribute to attenuation of allergic reactions and might be a promising candidate for novel inhibitor of allergic reaction.

24.2.4 Carotenoids

In the marine environment, algae serve as a reservoir of many secondary metabolites including carotenoids (Kay 1991; Spiller and Dewell 2003). So far, carotenoids have been known to possess many bioactivities, including anti-oxidative, anti-inflammatory, antiviral, and anticancer effect (Rao and Rao 2007). Moreover, dietary carotenoids have been associated with a decreased risk for certain types of immune diseases, such as asthma and atopic dermatitis. Indeed, feeding with both β-carotene and supplemental α-tocopherol enhances Th1 cell activity among splenocytes isolated from DO11.10 mice (Koizumi et al. 2006). Oral administration of β-carotene to OVA-immunized BALB/c mice led to a lowering of specific IgE and IgG_1 titer and caused inhibition of antigen-induced anaphylactic response by decreasing serum histamine level. In addition, Th1/Th2 balance was changed due to enhancement of Th1 cytokine production (IFN-γ, IL-12, and IL-2) and the downregulation of Th2 cytokine production (IL-4, IL-5, IL-6, and IL-10) in spleen cells from the mice fed β-carotene (Sato et al. 2004). A similar effect was observed from the OVA-sensitized B10A mice fed with high α- and β-carotene diets which are expected to inhibit oral sensitization to an antigen and prevent the development of food allergy (Sato et al. 2010). Recently, Sakai et al. (2009) have demonstrated the inhibitory effect of carotenoids on antigen-induced degranulation from rat basophilic leukemia 2H3 cells and mouse bone marrow-derived mast cells. Herein, fucoxanthin, astaxanthin, zeaxanthin, and β-carotene blocked the aggregation of FcεRI via inhibiting translocation of FcεRI to lipid rafts and caused the downregulation of FcεRI-mediated intracellular signaling, such as phosphorylation of Lyn kinase and Fyn kinase. Consequently, the downstream of intracellular signaling, especially β-hexosaminidase release, was suppressed in antigen-induced mast cells.

24.2.5 Polyunsaturated Fatty Acids

In general, polyunsaturated fatty acids are found in some vegetable oils, fish, and seafood. In addition, marine algae are also recognized to contain much more polyunsaturated fatty acids than terrestrial plants. Thus, marine algae are used as a source of essential fatty acids (Kay 1991; Khotimchenko 1993; Sanchez-Machado et al. 2002). Obviously, polyunsaturated fatty acids have attracted a great deal of attention because of their antioxidant, anti-atherosclerotic, anti-inflammatory, and immunoregulatory activities (Wojenski et al. 1991; Calder 1998; Kim et al. 2010). Especially, their potential inhibitory effects on allergic reactions have been evidenced recently. In particular, two polyunsaturated fatty acids of 18:4n-3 and 16:4n-3 purified from the marine algae *Undaria pinnatifida* and *Ulva pertusa* exhibited effective inhibition on the production of leukotriene B4, leukotriene C4, and 5-hydroxyeicosatetraenoic acid in MC/9 mouse mast cells (Ishihara et al. 1998). Moreover, α-linolenic acid (18:3 (n-3)) induced ameliorative changes in metabolism of omega-3/omega-6 polyunsaturated fatty acids, histamine content, and histamine release from RBL-2H3 cells. Namely, the concentration of α-linolenic acid and docosahexaenoic acid (DHA, 22:6 (n-3)) was increased, while linolenic acid (18:2 (n-6)) was slightly and arachidonic acid (20:4 (n-6)) was markedly decreased in mast cells (Kawasaki et al. 1994). Also, histamine content and release was remarkably lowered in the α-linolenic acid-treated RBL-2H3 cells. Likewise, PGE$_2$ production and histamine release were diminished in the canine mastocytoma cell line C2 treated with α-linolenic acid (Gueck et al. 2003), γ-linolenic acid, and docosahexaenoic acid (Gueck et al. 2004). Thus, the antiallergic effect of these polyunsaturated fatty acids was suggested either by the decrease in histamine content or by inhibition of the release of chemical mediator resulting from changes in the fatty acid composition.

24.2.6 Phycocyanins

Phycocyanin is one of the major pigment constituents of *Spirulina*, a microalgae used in many countries as dietary supplement (Romay et al. 2003; Liu et al. 2011). Recently, phycocyanin has been found to be an inhibitor of different allergic responses such as histamine release from rat peritoneal mast cells, ear swelling in mice induced by OVA, and skin reactions in rats caused by histamine and compound 48/80 (Remirez et al. 2002). Moreover, phycocyanin was shown to enhance biological defense activity against infectious diseases through suppressing antigen-specific IgE antibody and thus reducing allergic inflammation in mice (Nemoto-Kawamura et al. 2004). In the most recent study, Chang et al. (2011) have evaluated the therapeutic potential of R-phycocyanin (R-PC), a novel phycobiliprotein, against allergic airway inflammation. Interestingly, R-PC treatment resulted in a decrease of endocytosis and augmentation of IL-12 production in mouse BMDCs. Additionally, R-PC-treated dendritic cells promote CD4$^+$ T-cell stimulatory capacity and increase IFN-γ expression in CD4$^+$ T cells. Meanwhile, intraperitoneal administration of R-PC suppressed

OVA-induced airway hyperresponsiveness, serum levels of OVA-specific IgE, eosinophil infiltration, Th2 cytokine levels, and eotaxin in bronchoalveolar lavage fluid of mice. These findings implied that R-PC promoted activation and maturation of cultured dendritic cells and enhanced the immunological function toward Th1 activity. Taken together, *Spirulina* and its phycobiliprotein are expected to be a useful foodstuff for regulating allergic inflammatory responses.

24.3 Conclusion

Marine natural products have been a huge potential source for finding the safe and efficient alternative therapeutics in prevention and treatment of allergic diseases. Base on the specific assay system or screening approaches, a large number of antiallergic agents from marine organisms have been found to be effective against allergic reaction in vitro and in vivo. Therefore, marine biomaterials could be introduced for the preparation of novel functional ingredients in pharmaceuticals and functional foods for antiallergic therapeutics.

References

Aranaz, I., M. Mengíbar, R. Harris, I. Paños, B. Miralles, N. Acosta, G. Galed, and Á. Heras. 2009. Functional characterization of chitin and chitosan. *Current Chemical Biology* 3:203–230.

Asada, M., M. Sugie, M. Inoue, K. Nakagomi, S. Hongo, K. Murata, S. Irie, T. Takeuchi, N. Tomizuka, and S. Oka. 1997. Inhibitory effect of alginic acids on hyaluronidase and on histamine release from mast cells. *Bioscience, Biotechnology, and Biochemistry* 61:1030–1032.

Baroody, F. M. and R. M. Naclerio. 2000. Antiallergic effects of H1-receptor antagonists. *Allergy* 55:17–27.

Blunden, G. 2001. Biologically active compounds from marine organisms. *Phytotherapy Research* 15:89–94.

Blunt, J. W., B. R. Copp, M. H. G. Munro, P. T. Northcote, and M. R. Prinsep. 2006. Marine natural products. *Natural Product Reports* 23:26–78.

Calder, P. C. 1998. Immunoregulatory and anti-inflammatory effects of n-3 polyunsaturated fatty acids. *Brazilian Journal of Medicinal Biological Research* 31:467–490.

Catalli, A. and M. Kulka. 2010. Chitin and β-Glucan polysaccharides as immunomodulators of airway inflammation and atopic disease. *Recent Patents on Endocrine, Metabolic and Immune Drug Discovery* 4:175–189.

Chae, S. Y., M. K. Jang, and J. W. Nah. 2005. Influence of molecular weight on oral absorption of water soluble chitosans. *Journal of Controlled Release* 102:383–394.

Chang, C. J., Y. H. Yang, Y. C. Liang, C. J. Chiu, K. H. Chu, H. N. Chou, and B. L. Chiang. 2011. A novel phycobiliprotein alleviates allergic airway inflammation by modulating immune responses. *American Journal of Respiratory Critical Care Medicine* 183:15–25.

Chen, C. L., Y. M. Wang, C. F. Liu, and J. Y. Wang. 2008. The effect of water-soluble chitosan on macrophage activation and the attenuation of mite allergen-induced airway inflammation. *Biomaterials* 29:2173–2182.

Dutta, P. K., J. Dutta, and V. S. Tripathi. 2004. Chitin and chitosan: Chemistry, properties and applications. *Journal of Scientific and Industrial Research* 63:20–31.

El Gamal, A. A. 2010. Biological importance of marine algae. *Saudi Pharmaceutical Journal* 18:1–25.

Faulkner, D. J. 2001. Marine natural products. *Natural Product Reports* 18:1–49.

Faulkner, D. J. 2002. Marine natural products. *Natural Product Reports* 19:1–48.

Galli, S. J., M. Tsai, and A. M. Piliponsky. 2008. The development of allergic inflammation. *Nature* 454:445–454.

Gueck, T., A. Seidel, D. Baumann, A. Meister, and H. Fuhrmann. 2004. Alterations of mast cell mediator production and release by gamma-linolenic and docosahexaenoic acid. *Veterinary Dermatology* 15:309–314.

Gueck, T., A. Seidel, and H. Fuhrmann. 2003. Effects of essential fatty acids on mediators of mast cells in culture. *Prostaglandins, Leukotrienes and Essential Fatty Acids* 68:317–322.

Gupta, S. and N. Abu-Ghannam. 2011. Bioactive potential and possible health effects of edible brown seaweeds. *Trends in Food Science and Technology* 22:315–326.

Haefner, B. 2003. Drugs from the deep: Marine natural products as drug candidates. *Drug Discovery Today* 8:536–544.

Ishihara, K., M. Murata, M. Kaneniwa, H. Saito, K. Shinohara, and M. Maeda-Yamamoto. 1998. Inhibition of icosanoid production in MC/9 mouse mast cells by n-3 polyunsaturated fatty acids isolated from edible marine algae. *Bioscience, Biotechnology, and Biochemistry* 62:1412–1415.

Ishihara, K., C. Oyamada, R. Matsushima, M. Murata, and T. Muraoka. 2005. Inhibitory effect of porphyran, prepared from dried "Nori," on contact hypersensitivity in mice. *Bioscience, Biotechnology, and Biochemistry* 69:1824–1830.

Iwamoto, K., T. Hiragun, S. Takahagi, Y. Yanase, S. Morioke, S. Mihara, Y. Kameyoshi, and M. Hide. 2011. Fucoidan suppresses IgE production in peripheral blood mononuclear cells from patients with atopic dermatitis. *Archives of Dermatological Research* 303:425–431.

Jeong, H. J., S. A. Lee, P. D. Moon, H. J. Na, R. K. Park, J. Y. Um, H. M. Kim, and S. H. Hong. 2006. Alginic acid has anti-anaphylactic effects and inhibits inflammatory cytokine expression via suppression of nuclear factor-kappaB activation. *Clinical and Experimental Allergy* 36:785–794.

Jirge, S. and Y. Chaudhari. 2010. Marine: The ultimate source of bioactives and drug metabolites. *International Journal of Research in Ayurveda and Pharmacy* 1:55–62.

Kawasaki, M., M. Toyoda, R. Teshima, J. Sawada, and Y. Saito. 1994. Effect of alpha-linolenic acid on the metabolism of omega-3 and omega-6 polyunsaturated fatty acids and histamine release in RBL-2H3 cells. *Biological and Pharmaceutical Bulletin* 17:1321–1325.

Kay, R. A. 1991. Microalgae as food and supplement. *Critical Reviews in Food Science and Nutrition* 30:555–573.

Kay, A. B. 2000. Overview of 'Allergy and allergic diseases: With a view in the future'. *British Medical Bulletin* 56:843–864.

Khotimchenko, S. V. 1993. Fatty acids of green macrophytic algae from the sea of Japan. *Phytochemistry* 32:1203–1207.

Kim, J. A., C. S. Kong, and S. K. Kim. 2010. Effect of *Sargassum thunbergii* on ROS mediated oxidative damage and identification of polyunsaturated fatty acid components. *Food and Chemical Toxicology* 48:1243–1249.

Kim, S. K. and N. Rajapaksea. 2005. Enzymatic production and biological activities of chitosan oligosaccharides (COS): A review. *Carbohydrate Polymers* 62:357–368.

Koizumi, T., N. Bando, J. Terao, and R. Yamanishi. 2006. Feeding with both β-carotene and supplemental α-tocopherol enhances type 1 helper T cell activity among splenocytes isolated from DO11.10 mice. *Bioscience, Biotechnology, and Biochemistry* 70:3042–3045.

Larche, M. 2007. Regulatory T cells in allergy and asthma. *Chest* 132:1007–1014.

Larche, M., D. S. Robinson, and A. B. Kay. 2003. The role of T lymphocytes in the pathogenesis of asthma. *Journal of Allergy and Clinical Immunology* 111:450–463.

Le, Q. T., Y. Li, Z. J. Qian, M. M. Kim, and S. K. Kim. 2009. Inhibitory effects of polyphenols isolated from marine alga *Ecklonia cava* on histamine release. *Process Biochemistry* 44:168–176.

Li, Y., S. H. Lee, Q. T. Le, M. M. Kim, and S. K. Kim. 2008. Anti-allergic effects of phlorotannins on histamine release via binding inhibition between IgE and FcεRI. *Journal of Agricultural and Food Chemistry* 56:12073–12080.

Li, Y. X., I. Wijesekara, Y. Li, and S. K. Kim. 2011. Phlorotannins as bioactive agents from brown algae. *Process Biochemistry* 46:2219–2224.

Liu, J. G., C. W. Hou, S. Y. Lee, Y. Chuang, and C. C. Lin. 2011. Antioxidant effects and UVB protective activity of *Spirulina* (*Arthrospira platensis*) products fermented with lactic acid bacteria. *Process Biochemistry* 46:1405–1410.

Maruyama, H., H. Tamauchi, M. Hashimoto, and T. Nakano. 2005. Suppression of Th2 immune responses by Mekabu fucoidan from *Undaria pinnatifida Sporophylls*. *International Archives of Allergy and Immunology* 137:289–294.

Matsubara, M., S. Masaki, K. Ohmori, A. Karasawa, and K. Hasegawa. 2004. Differential regulation of IL-4 expression and degranulation by anti-allergic olopatadine in rat basophilic leukemia (RBL-2H3) cells. *Biochemical Pharmacology* 67:1315–1326.

Mayer, A. M. S., A. D. Rodriguez, R. Berlinck, and N. Fusetani. 2011. Marine pharmacology in 2007–8: Marine compounds with antibacterial, anticoagulant, antifungal, anti-inflammatory, antiprotozoal, antituberculosis and antiviral activities; affecting the immune and nervous system, and other miscellaneous mechanisms of action. *Comparative Biochemistry and Physiology—Part C* 153:191–222.

Milián, E. and A. M. Díaz. 2004. Allergy to house dust mites and asthma. *Puerto Rico Health Sciences Journal* 23:47–57.

Molinski, T. F., D. S. Dalisay, S. L. Lievens, and J. P. Saludes. 2009. Drug development from marine natural products. *Natural Reviews Drug Discovery* 8:69–85.

Nemoto-Kawamura, C., T. Hirahashi, T. Nagai, H. Yamada, T. Katoh, and O. Hayashi. 2004. Phycocyanin enhances secretary IgA antibody response and suppresses allergic IgE antibody response in mice immunized with antigen-entrapped biodegradable microparticles. *Journal of Nutritional Science and Vitaminology* 50:129–136.

Newman, D. J. and G. M. Cragg. 2004. Marine natural products and related compounds in clinical and advanced preclinical trials. *Journal of Natural Products* 67:1216–1238.

Oomizu, S., Y. Yanase, H. Suzuki, Y. Kameyoshi, and M. Hide. 2006. Fucoidan prevents Cε germline transcription and NF-κB p52 translocation for IgE production in B cells. *Biochemical and Biophysical Research Communications* 350:501–507.

Ozdemir, C., D. Yazi, M. Aydogan, T. Akkoc, N. N. Bahceciler, and P. Strong. 2006. Treatment with chitin microparticles is protective against lung histopathology in a murine asthma model. *Clinical and Experimental Allergy* 36:960–968.

Park, B. K. and M. M. Kim. 2010. Applications of chitin and its derivatives in biological medicine. *International Journal of Molecular Sciences* 11:5152–5164.

Rao, A. V. and L. G. Rao. 2007. Carotenoids and human health. *Pharmacological Research* 55:207–216.

Remirez, D., N. Ledón, and R. González. 2002. Role of histamine in the inhibitory effects of phycocyanin in experimental models of allergic inflammatory response. *Mediators of Inflammation* 11:81–85.

Rizzo, M. C. and D. Sole. 2006. Inhaled corticosteroids in the treatment of respiratory allergy: Safety vs. efficacy. *Journal of Pediatrics* 82:S198–S205.

Romay, C., R. González, N. Ledón, D. Remirez, and V. Rimbau. 2003. C-phycocyanin: A biliprotein with antioxidant, anti-inflammatory and neuroprotective effects. *Current Protein and Peptide Science* 4:207–216.

Sakai, S., T. Sugawara, K. Matsubara, and T. Hirata. 2009. Inhibitory effect of carotenoids on the degranulation of mast cells via suppression of antigen-induced aggregation of high affinity IgE receptors. *The Journal of Biological Chemistry* 284:28172–28179.

Sanchez-Machado, D. I., J. Lopez-Cervantes, J. Lopez-Hernandez, and P. Paseiro-Losada. 2002. Fatty acids, total lipid, protein and ash contents of processed edible seaweeds. *Food Chemistry* 85:439–444.

Sato, Y., H. Akiyama, H. Matsuoka, K. Sakata, R. Nakamura, S. Ishikawa, T. Inakuma et al. 2010. Dietary carotenoids inhibit oral sensitization and the development of food allergy. *Journal of Agricultural and Food Chemistry* 58:7180–7186.

Sato, Y., H. Akiyama, H. Suganuma, T. Watanabe, M. H. Nagaoka, T. Inakuma, Y. Goda, and T. Maitani. 2004. The feeding of β-carotene down-regulates serum IgE levels and inhibits the type I allergic response in mice. *Biological and Pharmaceutical Bulletin* 27:978–984.

Shahidi, F., J. K. V. Arachchi, and Y. J. Jeon. 1999. Food applications of chitin and chitosans. *Trends in Food Science and Technology* 10:37–51.

Shibata, Y., L. A. Foster, J. F. Bradfield, and Q. N. Myrvik. 2000. Oral administration of chitin down-regulates serum IgE levels and lung eosinophilia in the allergic mouse. *The Journal of Immunology* 164:1314–1321.

Shibata, Y., L. A. Foster, W. J. Metzger, and Q. N. Myrvik. 1997. Alveolar macrophage priming by intravenous administration of chitin particles, polymers of N-acetyl-D-glucosamine, in mice. *Infection and Immunity* 65:1734–1741.

Shibata, T., K. Fujimoto, K. Nagayama, K. Yamaguchi, and T. Nakamura. 2002. Inhibitory activity of brown algal phlorotannins against hyaluronidase. *International Journal of Food Science and Technology* 37:703–709.

Shibata, Y., I. Honda, J. P. Justice, M. R. Van Scott, R. M. Nakamura, and Q. N. Myrvik. 2001. Th1 adjuvant N-Acetyl-D-glucosamine polymer up-regulates Th1 immunity but down-regulates Th2 immunity against a mycobacterial protein (MPB-59) in interleukin-10-knockout and wild-type mice. *Infection and Immunity* 69:6123–6130.

Shibata, T., K. Nagayama, R. Tanaka, K. Yamaguchi, and T. Nakamura. 2003. Inhibitory effects of brown algal phlorotannins on phospholipase A2s, lipoxygenases and cyclooxygenases. *Journal of Applied Phycology* 15:61–66.

Shim, S. Y., J. S. Choi, and D. S. Byun. 2009. Inhibitory effects of phloroglucinol derivatives isolated from *Ecklonia stolonifera* on FcεRI expression. *Bioorganic and Medicinal Chemistry* 17:4734–4739.

Spiller, G. A. and A. Dewell. 2003. Safety of an astaxanthin-rich *Haematococcus pluvialis* algal extract: A randomized clinical trial. *Journal of Medicinal Food* 6:51–56.

Strong, P., H. Clark, and K. Reid. 2002. Intranasal application of chitin microparticles down-regulates symptoms of allergic hypersensitivity to *Dermatophagoides pteronyssinus* and *Aspergillus fumigatus* in murine models of allergy. *Clinical and Experimental Allergy* 32:1794–1800.

Sugiura, Y., K. Matsuda, T. Okamoto, Y. Yamada, K. Imai, T. Ito, M. Kakinuma, and H. Amano. 2009. The inhibitory effects of components from a brown alga, *Eisenia arborea*, on degranulation of mast cells and eicosanoid synthesis. *Journal of Functional Foods* 1:387–393.

Sugiura, Y., K. Matsuda, Y. Yamada, K. Imai, M. Kakinuma, and H. Amano. 2008. Radical scavenging and hyaluronidase inhibitory activities of phlorotannins from the edible brown alga *Eisenia arborea*. *Food Science and Technology Research* 14:595–598.

Sugiura, Y., K. Matsuda, Y. Yamada, M. Nishikawa, K. Shioya, H. Katsuzaki, K. Imai, and H. Amano. 2006. Isolation of a new anti-allergic phlorotannin, Phlorofucofuroeckol-B, from an edible brown alga, *Eisenia arborea*. *Bioscience, Biotechnology, and Biochemistry* 70:2807–2811.

Sugiura, Y., K. Matsuda, Y. Yamada, M. Nishikawa, K. Shioya, H. Katsuzaki, K. Imai, and H. Amano. 2007. Anti-allergic phlorotannins from the edible brown alga, *Eisenia arborea*. *Food Science and Technology Research* 13:54–60.

Uno, T., M. Hattori, and T. Yoshida. 2006. Oral administration of alginic acid oligosaccharide suppresses IgE production and inhibits the induction of oral tolerance. *Bioscience, Biotechnology, and Biochemistry* 70:3054–3057.

Vo, T. S. and S. K. Kim. 2010. Potential anti-HIV agents from marine resources: An overview. *Marine Drugs* 8:2871–2892.

Vo, T. S., J. A. Kim, D. H. Ngo, C. S. Kong, and S. K. Kim. 2012. Protective effect of chitosan oligosaccharides against FcεRI-mediated RBL-2H3 mast cell activation. *Process Biochemistry* 47:327–330.

Vo, T. S., C. S. Kong, and S. K. Kim. 2011. Inhibitory effects of chitooligosaccharides on degranulation and cytokine generation in rat basophilic leukemia RBL-2H3 cells. *Carbohydrate Polymers* 84:649–655.

Wijesekara, I., N. Y. Yoon, and S. K. Kim. 2010. Phlorotannins from *Ecklonia cava* (Phaeophyceae): Biological activities and potential health benefits. *Biofactors* 36:408–414.

Wojenski, C. M., M. J. Silver, and J. Waker. 1991. Eicosapentaenoic acid ethyl ester as an antithrombotic agent: Comparison to an extract of fish oil. *Biochimica et Biophysica Acta* 1081:33–38.

Xia, W., P. Liu, J. Zhang, and J. Chen. 2011. Biological activities of chitosan and chitooligosaccharides. *Food Hydrocolloids* 25:170–179.

Yanase, Y., T. Hiragun, K. Uchida, K. Ishii, S. Oomizu, H. Suzuki, S. Mihara et al. 2009. Peritoneal injection of fucoidan suppresses the increase of plasma IgE induced by OVA-sensitization. *Biochemical and Biophysical Research Communications* 387:435–439.

Yang, E. J., J. G. Kim, J. Y. Kim, S. C. Kim, N. H. Lee, and C. G. Hyun. 2010. Anti-inflammatory effect of chitosan oligosaccharides in RAW 264.7 cells. *Central European Journal of Biology* 5:95–102.

Yoshida, T., A. Hirano, H. Wada, K. Takahashi, and M. Hattori. 2004. Alginic acid oligosaccharide suppresses Th2 development and IgE production by inducing IL-12 production. *International Archives of Allergy and Immunology* 133:239–247.

Part III

Biomedical Applications of Marine Biomaterials

25

Biomedical Potential of Unchlorinated Briarane Diterpenes from Gorgonians and Sea Pens

Bruce F. Bowden and Ioana M. Vasilescu

CONTENTS

Coral reefs are generally comprised of a complex array of communities that may include many different types of coelenterates such as cnidarians (which include hard or stony corals, soft corals, sea whips and sea fans, sea pens, hydroids, zoanthids, and sea anemones) as well as ascidians (tunicates) and sponges. The corals are comprised of hexacorals (stony corals), where polyps have six or multiples of six tentacles, and octocorals, where polyps have eight tentacles. These sedentary coelenterates are generally not restricted to tropical coral reefs, and species are also found in subtropical, temperate, Arctic, and Antarctic waters.

Octocorals are members of the anthozoan subclass Octocorallia, which is comprised of the soft corals, gorgonians (sea fans, sea whips), sea pens, sea pansies, and blue coral. Octocorallia is estimated to include approximately 3000 species (Daly et al. 2007). Octocorals generally lack a hard calcium carbonate exoskeleton (notable exception: the blue coral, *Heliopora coerulea*), so many rely on chemical defense for survival. Octocoral chemical defenses are commonly (but not exclusively) terpenoid in nature and many octocorals are defended by diterpenes or sesquiterpenes. Among coral diterpenes, the most commonly encountered members are cembranoid diterpene that are based on a

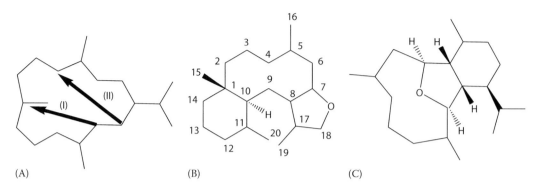

FIGURE 25.1
Structure A is the cembranoid diterpene carbon skeleton: arrows indicate cyclization positions that produce the carbon skeletons of (I) a briarane (structure B) and (II) a eunicellin (structure C). The conventional numbering system for briaranes is also indicated on structure B.

14-membered carbocyclic ring (Figure 25.1). In gorgonian and sea pen metabolites, the cembrane-derived diterpenes are often further cyclized and highly functionalized: two commonly encountered groups of such diterpenes that are found in both gorgonians and sea pens are the briarane and eunicellin skeletons (Figure 25.1).

Briarane diterpenes are a unique class of marine-derived secondary metabolites possessing a *trans*-fused bicyclo[8.4.0] skeleton that normally also features a fused γ-lactone (Joyner et al. 2011). All briaranes where the absolute stereochemistry has been determined have the same stereochemistry at most chiral centers, although descriptors (*R/S*) may vary. This is usually due to a change in substituent priorities rather than a change in the absolute arrangement at a center. To illustrate the point being made here, the absence or presence of an α-Cl substituent on C6 will change the descriptor for the stereochemical arrangements at C7 from *S* to *R* when the geometric arrangement at C7 remains unchanged; this effect may also result from a change in substituent on a more remote carbon (e.g., the C8 descriptor may also change with a change in the C6 substituent). The description of stereochemistry in briaranes has often been confused in the literature due to the solution conformation of the cyclodecane ring not matching the way in which the structure has been drawn. An α-oriented oxygen substituent on C9 with respect to the planar ring conformation depicted in structure B (Figure 25.1) for many briaranes is in fact located on the β-face of the briarane system in solution, but so is the C9 "β-oriented" proton due to an approximately 90° clockwise twist of the C9–C10 bond and nonplanarity of the cyclodecane ring. This results in the C5 double bond often being located below the (1,10)-ring junction. Despite literature structures that suggest the stereochemistry at C2 and C9 can vary, it is our belief that oxygen substituents on C2, C9, and C14 are always, respectively, β-, α-, and α-oriented relative to the conformation depicted in structure B. The normal stereochemical arrangements in briaranes are indicated in Figure 25.2 in terms of α or β substituent orientation to avoid confusion in *R/S* descriptors caused by priority changes.

This chapter is focused on the structural variations within unchlorinated briarane diterpenes that have been found in gorgonians (Gorgonacea), sea pens, and sea pansies (Pennatulacea); their reported biological activities and the potential to utilize the bioactivity as a lead for development of new pharmaceutical agents.

Despite the fact that a relatively small number of gorgonian and sea pen species have been chemically investigated, the briaranes isolated from those species number well in excess of 500 and their trivial nomenclature can be quite confusing and daunting for a

Carbon No.	1	2	3	4	5	6	7	8
Stereochem.	Always β-Me	Always β-O	Either α- or β-O	Either α- or β-O	Rarely chiral	Usually α-O/Cl	Usually β-H	Usually α-O
Carbon No.	9	10	11	12	13	14	17	
Stereochem.	Always α-O	Always α-H	β-H α- or β-O	Either α- or β-O	Either α- or β-O	Always α-O	α-Me when CH β-Me when CO	

FIGURE 25.2
More common stereochemical arrangements observed in briaranes when centers are chiral. Descriptors α and β relate to the planar conformation drawn in structure B of Figure 25.1.

newcomer to the area. For example, one species of gorgonian, *Briareum excavatum*, has been reported to afford a range of excavatolides (A–Z), excavatoids (A–P), briaexcavatolides (A–Z), briaexcavatins (A–Z), plus many other briarane diterpenes, while briaranolides reported from a *Briareum* species (Hoshino et al. 2005) have different structures from briarenolides (Su et al. 2007) and briareolides (Pordesimo et al. 1991, Mootoo et al. 1996) that also come from *Briareum* species, so beware of single-letter name differences!

Briarane diterpenes have been reviewed on a regular basis since 2005, but a large number of briaranes were reported prior to those survey reports that cover 262 briarane metabolites (Sung et al. 2005a, 2008e, 2011). A typical feature of briarane structures is the presence of numerous oxygen-containing functionalities such as alcohols, ketones, epoxides, other ethers, and esters. These corals are so prolific in their ability to oxidize and esterify carbon atoms that there are even quite a few examples where ester substituents are further esterified. Unlike most other coral metabolites where the esters are predominantly (or exclusively) acetates, known briaranes feature a variety of ester functions with acetate, hydroxyacetate, propanoate, butanoate, isobutanoate (=2-methylpropanoate), isovalerate (=3-methylbutanoate), hexanoate, and octanoate being some of the more commonly encountered ones. Among the known collection of briaranes, there are currently examples of oxygenation at every position of the carbobicyclic ring system except the ring junction carbons, the bridgehead methyl group (C15), and the methyl substituent on the lactone ring (C19).

There are almost as many chlorine-containing briaranes produced by gorgonians and sea pens as unchlorinated ones, but this chapter is focused only on the nonhalogenated briaranes. In chlorinated briaranes, chlorine generally occurs in allylic situations on either C6 (where it is normally α-oriented) or on C-16. These two substitution positions equate to a pair of allylic isomers. Halogens are rare in terpenoid metabolites of most other corals except *Clavularia*, a Stoloniferan octocoral that produces halogenated prostanoids (Watanabe 2003 and references therein).

Briaranes from sea pens demonstrate more diversity in the number and range of oxygen substituents found on the briarane ring system compared to those from gorgonians. Sea pens have afforded some of the simplest briaranes, but more commonly, the metabolites from sea pens display more oxygen functionality than those from gorgonians.

25.1 Briaranes That Lack the γ-Lactone Ring: Briareolate Esters

Although the defined structure for a briarane ring system includes a tetrahydrofuran ring with the oxygen bridging C7 and C18 (see, e.g., Ravi et al. 1980), a number of C18 methyl esters on a normal *trans*-fused bicyclo[8.4.0] briarane skeleton have been

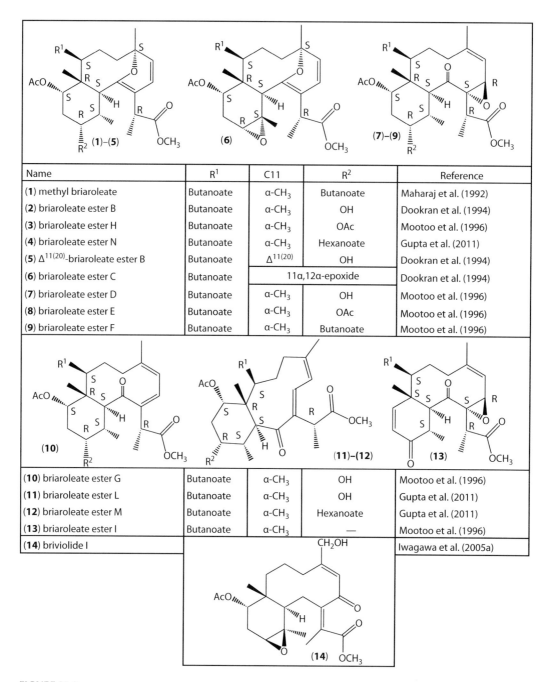

FIGURE 25.3
Methyl briareolate and related esters from *B. asbestinum* and *Briareum* sp.

reported from *Briareum asbestinum* (Figure 25.3), and these are included in this review for completeness.

The first of these was methyl briareolate (**1**) (Maharaj et al. 1992); further examples of 19-methyl esters were subsequently described that included five more 5,9-ethers: briareolate esters B (**2**) (Dookran et al. 1994), H (**3**) (Mootoo et al. 1996), N (**4**) (Gupta et al. 2011),

$\Delta^{11(20)}$-briareolate ester B (**5**), and briareolate ester C (**6**) (Dookran et al. 1994). Briareolate esters D to F (**7–9**) are Δ^5-7,8-epoxy-9-ones (Mootoo et al. 1996), while (Z,Z)-$\Delta^{5,7}$-9-one and (Z,E)-$\Delta^{5,7}$-9-one systems are respectively present in briareolate ester G (**10**) and in briareolate esters L (**11**) and M (**12**) (Gupta et al. 2011). Briareolate ester I (**13**) is a $\Delta^{5,13}$-7,8-epoxy-9,12-dione (Mootoo et al. 1996). The structure of methyl briareolate was confirmed by x-ray crystallography. Briviolide I (**14**) from a *Briareum* sp. (Iwagawa et al. 2005b) is a further example of a briarane with a methyl ester in place of the furan-based ring.

25.2 Rearranged Briarane Skeletons

This section is included to indicate the range of rearranged structures produced from the briarane system, so it is not a comprehensive list of rearranged briaranes and it includes chlorinated briaranes. Milolide F (**15**) (Figure 25.4) is currently the only metabolite with a *trans*-fused bicyclo[8.3.0] ring system (Kwak et al. 2001). It was isolated from *Briareum* (=*Solenopodium*) *stechei*. Although no other natural products with this ring system are known, a similar product was produced from stylatulide by reaction with BF_3 etherate (Wratten and Faulkner 1978).

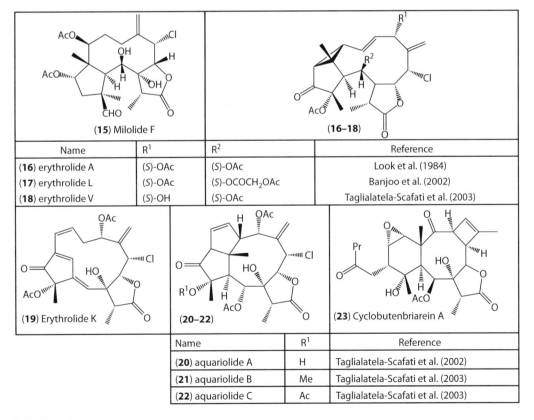

Name	R¹	R²	Reference
(**16**) erythrolide A	(S)-OAc	(S)-OAc	Look et al. (1984)
(**17**) erythrolide L	(S)-OAc	(S)-OCOCH₂OAc	Banjoo et al. (2002)
(**18**) erythrolide V	(S)-OH	(S)-OAc	Taglialatela-Scafati et al. (2003)

Name	R¹	Reference
(**20**) aquariolide A	H	Taglialatela-Scafati et al. (2002)
(**21**) aquariolide B	Me	Taglialatela-Scafati et al. (2003)
(**22**) aquariolide C	Ac	Taglialatela-Scafati et al. (2003)

FIGURE 25.4
Examples of rearranged briaranes.

Erythrolide A (**16**) from the Caribbean gorgonian *Erythropodium caribaeorum* was the first briarane-derived metabolite to display a 2-ketobicyclo[3.1.0]hexane fragment derived from a photochemical di-π-methane rearrangement (Look et al. 1984, Pordesimo et al. 1991).

Subsequently, the isolation of erythrolide L (**17**) (Banjoo et al. 2002) and erythrolide V (**18**) (Taglialatela-Scafati et al. 2003) that are also derived by a di-π-methane rearrangement from briaranes was reported (Figure 25.4). Erythrolide K (**19**) was isolated and its biogenetic origins from the rearranged briarane erythrolide A have also been discussed (Banjoo et al. 1998). A biogenetic proposal that links the carbon skeletons found in *E. caribaeorum* diterpenoids has been suggested to rationalize the biosynthesis of aquariolides A–C (**20–22**) (Taglialatela-Scafati et al. 2002, 2003). The final further cyclized briarane that has been included in this brief summary is cyclobutenbriarein A (**23**), the first diterpene reported with a tricyclo[8.4.0.0³,⁶]tetradec-4-ene ring system (Figure 25.4). It was isolated from the gorgonian *B. asbestinum* (González et al. 2002).

25.3 Briaranes with Substituted Furans

Briaranes with furan rings are among the simpler members of the briarane group with fewer oxygenated sites present (on average) than their γ-lactone counterparts; occurrence to date is limited to just three species. Two briarane furans (14-acetoxy-11,12-epoxy-3-oxo-briara-5,7,17-trien-2-yl 3-methylbutanoate ester (**24**) and 2, 14-diacetoxybriara-5,7,11,17-tetraen-3-one) (**25**), from the sea pen *Scytalium tentaculum*, that had been collected while trawling near Port Douglas in North Queensland were reported with semisystematic names based on the briarane ring system (Figure 25.5). Compound (**24**) affected heart rate and blood pressure in mice (Ravi et al. 1980).

Verecynarmins from the Mediterranean pennatulacean octocoral *Veretillum cynomorium* were isolated both from the coral and from a nudibranch, *Armina maculata*, that preys on the coral. The verecynarmins (Figure 25.5) are among the least functionalized briaranes known: verecynarmin A (**26**) (Guerriero et al. 1987) features a number of double bonds but just one ester group, an α-oriented acetate at C14. Verecynarmins B and C (**27–28**) (Guerriero et al. 1988) all feature a Δ^4 double bond rather than the more common Δ^5 unsaturation, which is observed in verecynarmins E–G (**29–31**) (Guerriero et al. 1990), and most other briaranes. 3,4-Dihydroverecynarmine A (**32**) and 4-O-acetylverecynarmine G (**33**) were reported from a *Pachyclavularia* species (Uchio et al. 1989). The taxonomy of *Pachyclavularia* has been a point of discussion, but many, including Dr. Phil Alderslade (a soft coral taxonomist), believe that *Pachyclavularia* belongs with *Briareum* in the Gorgonacea, with indistinguishable polyp morphology (and briarane chemistry).

25.4 $\Delta^{5,8(17)}$-Briaranes with γ-Lactones

Briarane lactones with double bonds at both C5, C8(17), and C11 include brianthein W (**34**), (Cardellina et al. 1984), anthoptilides A–E (**35–39**) (Pham et al. 2000), funicolides A and C (**40–41**) (Guerriero et al. 1995), briareolide J (**42**) (Mootoo et al. 1996), malayenolides

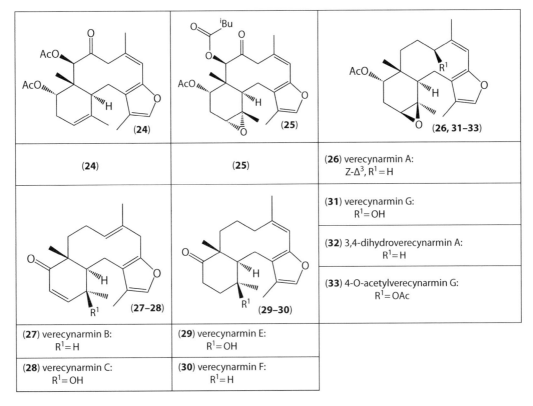

(24)	**(25)**	**(26)** verecynarmin A: Z-Δ³, R¹ = H
		(31) verecynarmin G: R¹ = OH
		(32) 3,4-dihydroverecynarmin A: R¹ = H
		(33) 4-O-acetylverecynarmin G: R¹ = OAc
(27) verecynarmin B: R¹ = H	**(29)** verecynarmin E: R¹ = OH	
(28) verecynarmin C: R¹ = OH	**(30)** verecynarmin F: R¹ = H	

FIGURE 25.5
Briaranes with a furan ring.

A and C (**43–44**) (Fu et al. 1999), briviolide J (**45**) (Iwagawa et al. 2005b), brianthein A (**46**) (Aoki et al. 2001), and excavatoid E (**47**) (Sung et al. 2009a). The lactone hemiketals, funicolides B and E (**48–49**), and 7-*Epi*-funicolide A (**50**) (Guerriero et al. 1995) have also been included here (Figure 25.6).

γ-Lactones or γ-lactone hemiketals with $\Delta^{5,8(17)}$ functionality, but with oxygenation instead of Δ^{11} unsaturation, are also well known. Examples feature alcohol, hydroperoxide, ester, or epoxide functionality (Figure 25.7). Briareolide G (**51**) (Pordesimo et al. 1991) and brianthein B (**52**) (Rodríguez et al. 1996, Aoki et al. 2001) have an OH or OOH, respectively, at C12, in addition to esters on C2 and C14 (briareolide G) or C2, C3, and C14 (brianthein B). Briviolide D (**53**), some of its naturally occurring derivatives (**54–56**), and briviolide E (**57**) all contain an 11,12-diol system, although C12 is acetylated in 12-O-acetylbriviolide D (**55**) (Iwagawa et al. 2005b).

Malayenolides B and D (**58** and **59**), from the sea pen *Veretillum malayense* (Fu et al. 1999), some briaranes from *Briareum* sp. that were given only semisystematic names (**60–64**) (Bowden et al. 1987, 1989); excavatolide S (**65**) from *B. excavatum* (Neve et al. 1999); and briviolides F and G (**66–67**) (Iwagawa et al. 2005b) all feature 11β,12β-epoxide functionality, while juncenolide K (**68**) (Wang et al. 2009) has an 11α,20-epoxy group. The hemiketal lactones (**69**) (Uchio et al. 1989) and "briarein (9)" (**70**) (Ospina et al. 2006), and the ketal lactone briviolide H (**71**) (Iwagawa et al. 2005b), have also been reported (Figure 25.7). Briviolide H is likely to be an artifact from MeOH/CH₂Cl₂ chromatography, formed from a similarly substituted hemiketal lactone.

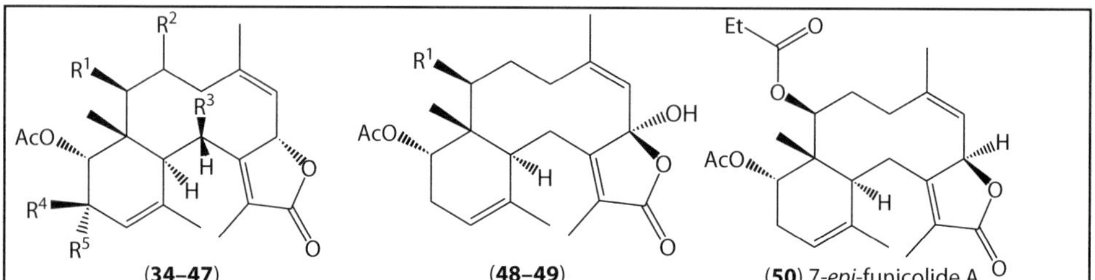

Name	R^1	R^2	R^3	R^4/R^5
(34) brianthein W	OAc	H	H	R^4=R^5=H
(35) anthoptilide A	tiglate	H	H	R^{4}R^5=O
(36) anthoptilide B	isobutanoate	H	H	R^{4}R^5=O
(37) anthoptilide C	propanoate	H	H	R^{4}R^5=O
(38) anthoptilide D	benzoate	H	H	R^{4}R^5=O
(39) anthoptilide E	propanoate	H	H	R^4=H; R^5=OH
(40) funicolide A	propanoate	H	H	R^4=R^5=H
(41) funicolide D	butanoate	H	H	R^4=R^5=H
(42) briareolide J	butanoate	H	OH	R^4=R^5=H
(43) malayenolide A	benzoate	H	H	R^4=R^5=H
(44) malayenolide C	3-methylpropenoate	H	H	R^4=R^5=H
(45) briviolide J	OAc	β-OAc	H	R^4=R^5=H
(46) brianthein A	OAc	α-OAc	H	R^4=R^5=H
(47) excavatoid E	OAc	α-butanoate	OH	R^4=R^5=H
(48) funicolide B	propanoate			
(49) funicolide E	OAc			

FIGURE 25.6
$\Delta^{5,8(17),11}$-briaranes with γ-lactones and lactone hemiketals.

25.5 Briaranes with an Oxygen Function at C8

The C8 oxygenated briaranes account for a large proportion of the terpenes found in the Gorgonacea and Pennatulacea and are the main metabolite group found in the genus *Briareum*.

Briaranes with an oxygen function at C8 include the following:

1. Briaranes with an 8α-hydroxyl group.
2. Briaranes with an ether linking C8 to either C2, C4, or C5, or alternately C9 to C5.
3. 8,17-Epoxybriaranes.
4. 8,17-Diols.

25.5.1 8-Hydroxybriaranes Where C19 Is a Secondary Methyl Group

Many Δ^5-briaranes have been reported with an 8α-OH. Shielding of the C19 methyl group due to steric compression (δ_C 7–8 ppm) is observed with an 8α-OH, so the upfield shift of the 19-Me ^{13}C signal is a diagnostic tool in elucidation of the stereochemistry.

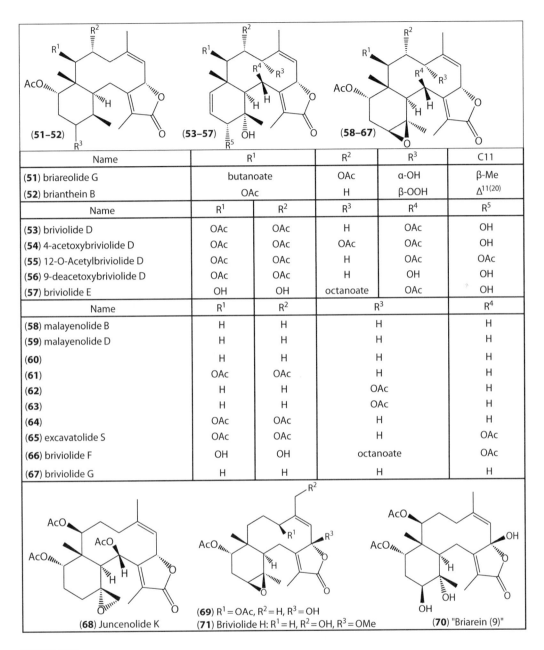

Name	R¹		R²	R³	C11
(51) briareolide G	butanoate		OAc	α-OH	β-Me
(52) brianthein B	OAc		H	β-OOH	Δ¹¹⁽²⁰⁾

Name	R¹	R²	R³	R⁴	R⁵
(53) briviolide D	OAc	OAc	H	OAc	OH
(54) 4-acetoxybriviolide D	OAc	OAc	OAc	OAc	OH
(55) 12-O-Acetylbriviolide D	OAc	OAc	H	OAc	OAc
(56) 9-deacetoxybriviolide D	OAc	OAc	H	OH	OH
(57) briviolide E	OH	OH	octanoate	OAc	OH

Name	R¹	R²	R³	R⁴
(58) malayenolide B	H	H	H	H
(59) malayenolide D	H	H	H	H
(60)	H	H	H	H
(61)	OAc	OAc	H	H
(62)	H	H	OAc	H
(63)	H	H	OAc	H
(64)	OAc	OAc	H	H
(65) excavatolide S	OAc	OAc	H	OAc
(66) briviolide F	OH	OH	octanoate	OAc
(67) briviolide G	H	H	H	H

(68) Juncenolide K
(69) R¹ = OAc, R² = H, R³ = OH
(71) Briviolide H: R¹ = H, R² = OH, R³ = OMe
(70) "Briarein (9)"

FIGURE 25.7
Δ⁵,⁸⁽¹⁷⁾-briaranes with γ-lactones, γ-lactone hemiketals, or γ-lactone ketals.

Briareolide K (**72**) and briarenolides A and B (**73–74**) are Δ⁵-8α-hydroxybriaranes that are among a small group of known 9-ketobriaranes (Figure 25.8). Briareolide K was presented with an 8β-hydroxyl group in a report that did not discuss C8 stereochemistry. The NMR data for the 19-methyl group (δ_H 1.13, δ_C 7.6 ppm) (Mootoo et al. 1996) matched those reported for briarenolide B in work that showed that the C8 hydroxyl and the 19-methyl group were both on the α-face of the briarane (Su et al. 2007). Briareolide K hence has an

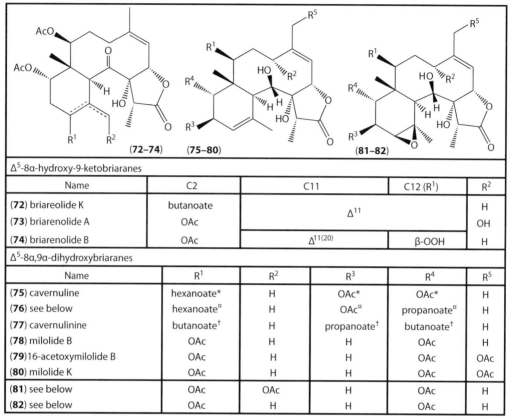

Δ^5-8α-hydroxy-9-ketobriaranes				
Name	C2	C11	C12 (R¹)	R²
(72) briareolide K	butanoate	Δ^{11}		H
(73) briarenolide A	OAc			OH
(74) briarenolide B	OAc	$\Delta^{11(20)}$	β-OOH	H

Δ^5-8α,9α-dihydroxybriaranes					
Name	R¹	R²	R³	R⁴	R⁵
(75) cavernuline	hexanoate*	H	OAc*	OAc*	H
(76) see below	hexanoate¤	H	OAc¤	propanoate¤	H
(77) cavernulinine	butanoate†	H	propanoate†	butanoate†	H
(78) milolide B	OAc	H	H	OAc	H
(79) 16-acetoxymilolide B	OAc	H	H	OAc	OAc
(80) milolide K	OAc	H	H	OAc	OAc
(81) see below	OAc	OAc	H	OAc	H
(82) see below	OAc	H	H	OAc	H

(76) O-deacetylpropionyl cavernuline　　　　　(81) 4β-acetoxy-9-deacetylstylatulide lactone

(82) 9-deacetylstylatulide lactone

*¤† Ester locations were not determined, so may be interchanged within these rows.

FIGURE 25.8
Δ^5-8α-hydroxy-9-keto and Δ^5-8α,9α-dihydroxybriaranes.

8α-hydroxyl group and that structure has been included here. Briarenolide A (73) was the first C20 hydroxymethyl briarane when its co-occurrence with the allylic hydroperoxide briarenolide B (74) was reported (Su et al. 2007). These two briaranes could potentially both be autoxidation artifacts.

The 8α,9α-dihydroxybriaranes in Figure 25.8 include cavernuline (75), O-deacetyl-propionyl cavernuline (76), and cavernulinine (77) from *Cavernulina grandiflora*, a pennatu-lacean octocoral (Clastres et al. 1984b). Structure determination of (75–77) was incomplete: the specific ester at each location (acetate, propanoate, butanoate, and hexanoate) was not determined. Milolide B (78), 16-acetoxymilolide B (79), milolide K (80) (all from *B. stechei*) (Kwak et al. 2001, 2002), 4β-acetoxy-9-deacetylstylatulide lactone (81), and 9-deacetylstylat-ulide lactone (82) (Sheu et al. 1996) (also from *Briareum* species) complete the list.

Together with 8α,9α-dihydroxybriaranes, 9α-acetoxy-8α-hydroxybriaranes represent about 25% of the known briarane metabolites. A large subgroup of these 9α-acetoxy-8α-hydroxybriaranes is a group that contains a $\Delta^{3,5}$-diene system. This functionality is also a commonly encountered structural feature among chlorinated briarane metabolites. The stereochemistry of the (Z)-Δ^3-alkene requires a different structural representation of the cyclodecadiene ring system from that used on preceding pages (Figure 25.9a and b). These briaranes contain some reported metabolites that feature a C15 methoxymethyl group; their natural occurrence should be regarded with skepticism until their metabolite status is verified. They are likely to be products of methanolysis from chloro, alcohol, or other labile groups during isolation.

Only three examples of $\Delta^{3,5,11}$-9α-acetoxy-8α-hydroxybriaranes, pachyclavulides B (**83**), C (**84**) (Iwasaki et al. 2006), and I (**85**) (Ito et al. 2007), have been reported, and all were isolated from *Pachyclavularia violacea* (Figure 25.9a). It is surprising that the only example of a $\Delta^{3,5,11(20)}$-9α-acetoxy-8α-hydroxy briarane that has been reported is robustolide C (**86**) from

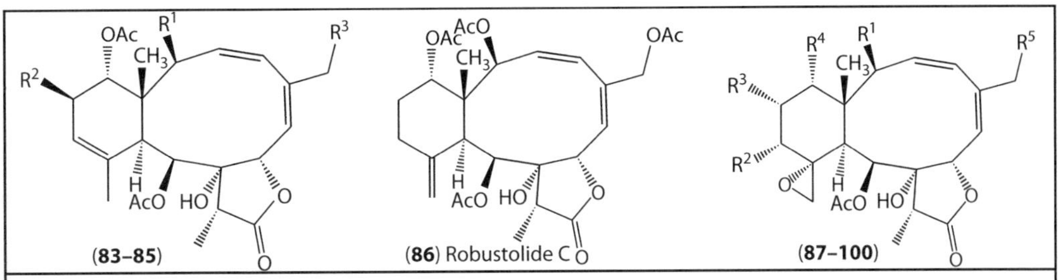

(83–85) (86) Robustolide C (87–100)

$\Delta^{3,5,11}$-9α-acetoxy-8α-hydroxybriaranes

Name	R^1	R^2	R^3
(**83**) pachyclavulide B	OAc	H	OH
(**84**) pachyclavulide C	OAc	H	OAc
(**85**) pachyclavulide I	OAc	β-OAc	OMe

$\Delta^{3,5,11(20)}$-9α-acetoxy-8α-hydroxybriaranes

(**86**) robustolide C			

$\Delta^{3,5}$-9α-acetoxy-11α,20-epoxy-8α-hydroxybriaranes

Name	R^1	R^2	R^3	R^4	R^5
(**87**) gemmacolide F	OH	OAc	OAc	OAc	OAc
(**88**) juncenolide B	OAc	H	OAc	OAc	OH
(**89**) juncenolide C	OAc	OAc	OAc	OAc	OH
(**90**) juncenolide D	OAc	OAc	OAc	OAc	OMe
(**91**) juncin U	OAc	OAc	R^1	OAc	OMe
(**92**) juncin Q	OAc	OH	OAc	OH	OH
(**93**) juncin V	OAc	OH	OAc	OH	OMe
(**94**) juncin W	OAc	OH	OAc	OH	OAc
(**95**) frajunolide D	OAc	OAc	H	OAc	OAc
(**96**) juncin I	OAc	OAc	R^2	OAc	OAc
(**97**) juncin J	OAc	R^2	R^2	OAc	OAc
(**98**) juncin K	OAc	R^2	H	R^2	OAc
(**99**) juncenolide E	R^2	H	OAc	OAc	OH
(**100**) juncin T	R^3	OAc	OAc	OAc	OH

R^1 = pentanoate R^2 = 3-methylbutanoate R^3 = 4-methylpentanoate ester of hydroxyacetate
(a)

FIGURE 25.9

(a) Briaranes that contain a $\Delta^{3,5}$-diene system.

(continued)

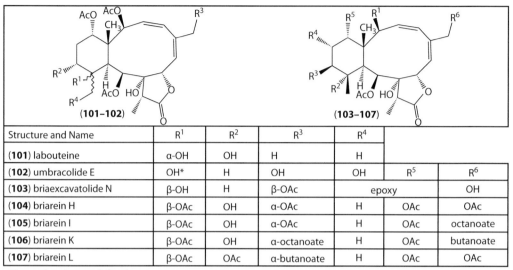

Structure and Name	R^1	R^2	R^3	R^4		
(**101**) labouteine	α-OH	OH	H	H		
(**102**) umbracolide E	OH*	H	OH	OH	R^5	R^6
(**103**) briaexcavatolide N	β-OH	H	β-OAc	epoxy		OH
(**104**) briarein H	β-OAc	OH	α-OAc	H	OAc	OAc
(**105**) briarein I	β-OAc	OH	α-OAc	H	OAc	octanoate
(**106**) briarein K	β-OAc	OH	α-octanoate	H	OAc	butanoate
(**107**) briarein L	β-OAc	OAc	α-butanoate	H	OAc	OAc

*Stereochemistry undefined

(b)

FIGURE 25.9 (continued)
(b) Other briaranes that contain a $\Delta^{3,5}$-diene system.

Ellisella robusta (Sung et al. 2007), because a significant number of 11α,20-epoxides have been isolated. These include gemmacolide F (**87**) (He and Faulkner 1991) from *Junceella gemmacea* as well as juncenolides B–D (**88–90**) (Shen et al. 2003) and juncins U (**91**), Q (**92**), V (**93**), and W (**94**) (Qi et al. 2006) from the gorgonian *Junceella juncea*. Juncenolide D and juncins U and V are all metabolites previously referred to as potential artifacts because of the presence of the C15 methoxymethyl group. Frajunolide D (**95**) from *J. fragilis* (Shen et al. 2007), together with juncins I–K (**96–98**) (Anjaneyulu et al. 2003), juncenolide E (**99**) (Wang et al. 2009), and juncin T (**100**) (Qi et al. 2006), all from *J. juncea,* completes the currently known members of this group (Figure 25.9a). Other briaranes that contain a $\Delta^{3,5}$-diene system (Figure 25.9b) are labouteine (**101**) from *Pteroides laboutei* (Clastres et al. 1984a), umbraculolide E (**102**) from *Gorgonella umbraculum* (Anjaneyulu et al. 2007), briaexcavatolide N (**103**) from *B. excavatum* (Sung et al. 2001), briareins H (**104**), I (**105**), K (**106**), and L (**107**) (Rodríguez et al. 1996). The structure of briaexcavatolide N is supported by an x-ray crystal structure. There are some interesting structural trends that begin to appear here and will be expanded upon later in this chapter as more examples are presented. The first observation is that when an 11α,20-epoxide group is present, the alcohol and acetate substituents on C12 are usually also α-oriented. The stereochemistry of C12 appears to correlate to the substituent and stereochemistry at C11.

The 9α-acetoxy-8α-hydroxybriarane group also includes the $\Delta^{5,11}$-9α-acetoxy-8α-hydroxybriaranes (Figure 25.10), the $\Delta^{5,11(20)}$-9α-acetoxy-8α-hydroxybriaranes (Figure 25.11), and their 11,12- and 11,20-epoxides (Figure 25.12), together with 11-hydroxybriaranes, 12-hydroxybriaranes, 11,12-dihydroxybriaranes, and their esters (Figure 25.13).

The $\Delta^{5,11}$-9α-acetoxy-8α-hydroxybriaranes (Figure 25.10) include pachyclavulide H (**108**) from *P. violacea* (Ito et al. 2007), its 2-butanoate analogue renillin C (**109**) from *Renilla reniformis* (Barsby and Kubanek 2005), and the 4α-hydroxy derivative, pachyclavulide H (**110**), also from *Pachyclavularia* (Ito et al. 2007). The isolation of milolide M (**111**), its 16-hydroxy (**112**) and 16-acetoxy (**113**) derivatives, milolide N (**114**) with 16-acetoxymilolide

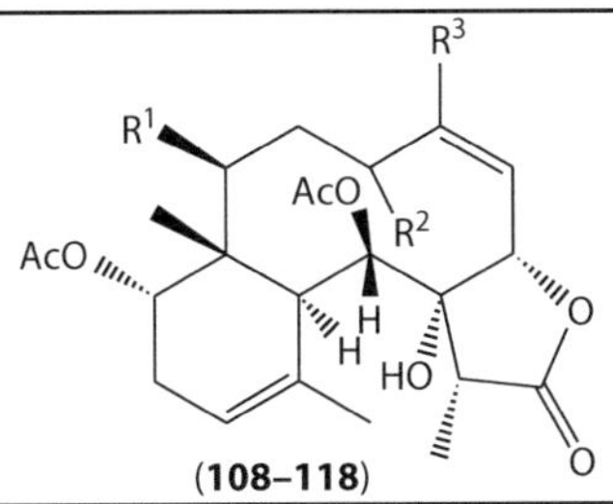

Compound	R^1	R^2	R^3
(108) pachyclavulide G	OAc	H	CH_2OAc
(109) renillin C	butanoate	H	CH_3
(110) pachyclavulide H	OAc	α-OH	CH_2OAc
(111) milolide M	OAc	β-OAc	CH_3
(112) 16-hydroxymilolide M	OAc	β-OAc	CH_2OH
(113) 16-hydroxymilolide M	OAc	β-OAc	CH_2OAc
(114) "compound 10"	OAc	β-OAc	COOMe
(115) milolide N	OAc	β-butanoate	CH_2OH
(116) 16-acetoxymilolide N	OAc	β-butanoate	CH_2OAc
(117) erythrolide M	OAc	β-3-acetoxybutanoate	CH_3
(118) erythrolide N	OAc	β-3-acetoxybutanoate	CH_2OH

The table header spanning reads: $\Delta^{5,11}$-9α-acetoxy-8α-hydroxybriaranes

FIGURE 25.10
$\Delta^{5,11}$-9α-acetoxy-8α-hydroxybriaranes.

N (115) (all from *B. stechei*) (Kwak et al. 2002), erythrolides M (116) and N (117) from *E. caribaeorum* (Banjoo et al. 2002), "compound 10" (118) from a sea pen, *Pteroeides* sp. (Tanaka et al. 2004), point to the wide range of gorgonian and sea pen/pansy genera where this metabolite group is found.

The $\Delta^{5,11(20)}$-9α-acetoxy-8α-hydroxybriaranes mainly come from the gorgonian genus *Junceella*. Frajunolides A, B, E, and J (119–122) (Shen et al. 2007, Liaw et al. 2008); junceellolide D (123) (Shin et al. 1989); junceellonoid B (124) (Zhang et al. 2004); junceellolide E (125) (Sung et al. 2000); and 4-deacetyljuncenolide D (126) (García et al. 1999) were all isolated from *J. fragilis*. Junceellolide D exhibited significant anti-inflammatory activity (Shin et al. 1989). Of the other compounds in this group derived from *J. fragilis* that have been screened, a number exhibited no significant cytotoxicity (Liaw et al. 2008), and several exhibited weak anti-inflammatory activity. The most active of these was junceellolide E, which suppressed the inflammatory response to the agonist FLMP/CB in human neutrophils with an approximate 40% inhibition of superoxide anion production and a 30% decrease in elastase release at a concentration of 10 μg/mL (Shen et al. 2007). Juncins Y and Z (127–128) (Qi et al. 2006), junceol A (129) (Sung et al. 2008d), and junceols D–H (130–134) (Sung et al. 2008c) were all isolated from *J. juncea*. "Compound 3," subsequently named umbraculolide A (135), however, was obtained from *G. umbraculum* (Subrahmanyam et al. 1998, 2001).

The known Δ^5-9α-acetoxy-8α-hydroxy-11,12-epoxybriaranes consist of both α- and β-oriented epoxides (Figure 25.12). In the milolide series of briaranes, milolide A (136), 16-hydroxymilolide A (137), and 16-acetoxymilolide A (138) from *B. stechei* all exhibit 11β,12β-epoxides (Kwak et al. 2001). Renillin D (139) from *R. reniformis* however contains an 11α,12α-epoxide (Barsby and Kubanek 2005). The situation with

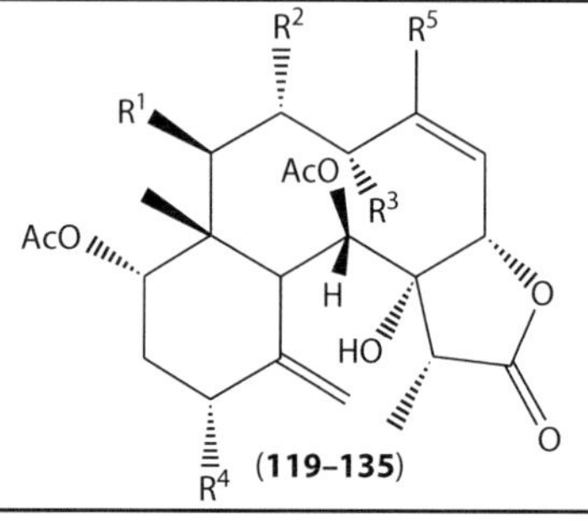

$\Delta^{5,11(20)}$-9α-acetoxy-8α-hydroxybriaranes

Compound	R^1	R^2	R^3	R^4	R^5
(**119**) frajunolide A	OAc	H	OAc	H	CH_3
(**120**) frajunolide B	OAc	H	OAc	OAc	CH_3
(**121**) frajunolide E	OAc	H	H	OAc	CH_3
(**122**) frajunolide J	OAc	H	R^a	H	CH_3
(**123**) junceellonoid B	OAc	H	H	H	CH_3
(**124**) junceellolide D	OAc	OAc	H	H	CH_3
(**125**) junceellolide E	R^a	H	H	H	CH_3
(**126**) 4-deacetyljunceellolide D	OAc	OH	H	H	CH_3
(**127**) juncin Y	OAc	OAc	H	H	CH_2OAc
(**128**) juncin Z	OAc	OAc	H	H	COOMe
(**129**) junceol A	OAc	R^c	H	H	CH_3
(**130**) junceol D	R^b	R^c	H	OAc	CH_3
(**131**) junceol E	R^b	OAc	H	H	CH_3
(**132**) junceol F	R^b	OAc	H	H	CH_3
(**133**) junceol G	R^b	H	H	OAc	CH_3
(**134**) junceol H	OAc	H	H	R^b	CH_3
(**135**) "Compound 3"	OAc	H	H	H	CH_3

"Compound 3" = Umbraculolide A
R^a = propanoate　R^b = 2-methylpropanoate　R^c = 3-methylbutanoate

FIGURE 25.11
$\Delta^{5,11(20)}$-9α-acetoxy-8α-hydroxybriaranes.

9α-acetoxy-8α-hydroxy-11,20-epoxybriaranes is similar, as both α- and β-arrangements have been reported at C11. They have normally been reported as either 11α,20α-epoxides or 11β,20β-epoxides, but the descriptor at C20 is meaningless given that three points define a plane (the epoxide ring) and the two groups attached to C20 (both Hs) are the same. It is therefore sufficient to describe these epoxides as either 11α,20-epoxides or 11β,20-epoxides. The known occurrence of these epoxides is restricted to the genus *Junceella*, with junceellolides F (**140**) (Sung et al. 2000) and K (**141**) (Sheu et al. 2006), 11α,20α-epoxyjunceellolide D (**142**), 11α,20α-epoxy-4-deacetyljunceellolide D (**143**), 11α,20α-epoxy-4-deacetoxyjunceellolide D (**144**) (García et al. 1999), and junceellolide J (**145**) and L (**146**) (Sheu et al. 2006), all isolated from *J. fragilis*. Juncin X (**147**) was from *J. juncea* (Qi et al. 2006).

The 8α,12-dihydroxy and 12-acetoxy-8α-hydroxybriaranes in Figure 25.12 are the *B. excavatum* metabolite briaexcavatin Z (**148**) (Sung et al. 2009b), pachyclavulide A (**149**) from *P. violacea* (Iwasaki et al. 2006), briviolide A (**150**) from *Briareum* sp. (Iwagawa et al. 2005b), the *B. stechei* metabolites milolide I (**151**) and G (**152**), 16-acetoxymilolide G (**153**) and J (**154**)

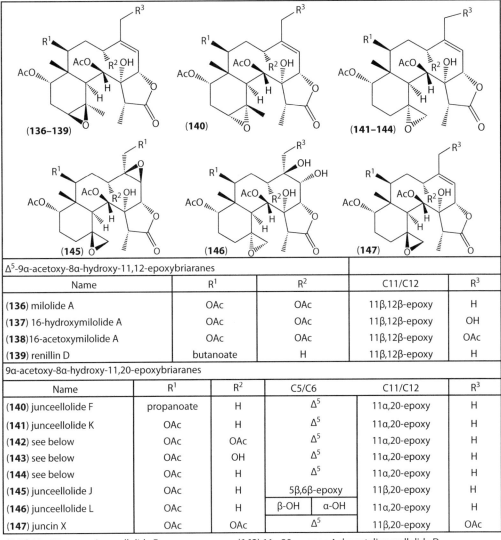

Δ⁵-9α-acetoxy-8α-hydroxy-11,12-epoxybriaranes				
Name	R¹	R²	C11/C12	R³
(**136**) milolide A	OAc	OAc	11β,12β-epoxy	H
(**137**) 16-hydroxymilolide A	OAc	OAc	11β,12β-epoxy	OH
(**138**)16-acetoxymilolide A	OAc	OAc	11β,12β-epoxy	OAc
(**139**) renillin D	butanoate	H	11β,12β-epoxy	H

9α-acetoxy-8α-hydroxy-11,20-epoxybriaranes						
Name	R¹	R²	C5/C6		C11/C12	R³
(**140**) junceellolide F	propanoate	H	Δ⁵		11α,20-epoxy	H
(**141**) junceellolide K	OAc	H	Δ⁵		11α,20-epoxy	H
(**142**) see below	OAc	OAc	Δ⁵		11α,20-epoxy	H
(**143**) see below	OAc	OH	Δ⁵		11α,20-epoxy	H
(**144**) see below	OAc	H	Δ⁵		11α,20-epoxy	H
(**145**) junceellolide J	OAc	H	5β,6β-epoxy		11β,20-epoxy	H
(**146**) junceellolide L	OAc	H	β-OH	α-OH	11α,20-epoxy	H
(**147**) juncin X	OAc	OAc	Δ⁵		11β,20-epoxy	OAc

(**142**) 11α,20α-epoxyjunceellolide D   (**143**) 11α,20α-epoxy-4-deacetyljunceellolide D

(**144**) 11α,20α-epoxy-4-deacetoxyjunceellolide D

FIGURE 25.12

Δ⁵-9α-acetoxy-11,12-epoxy-8α-hydroxybriaranes and Δ⁵-9α-acetoxy-11,20-epoxy-8α-hydroxybriaranes.

(Kwak et al. 2002); erythrolides O (**155**) (Banjoo et al. 2002), S (**156**) (Taglialatela-Scafati et al. 2003), and J (**157**) (Dookran et al. 1993) from *E. caribaeorum*, as well as milolide H (**158**) from *B. stechei* (Kwak et al. 2002) and excavatoid A (**159**) from cultured *B. excavatum* (Sung et al. 2009c). The remaining ungrouped briaranes are three from *J. fragilis* that all lack oxygen functionality at C12 and an 11-hydroxy-12-acetoxybriarane from *B. asbestinum*. The *J. fragilis* metabolites are 9-deacetylumbraculolide (**160**) (Sung and Fan 2003), junceellolides G (**161**) (Sung et al. 2000) and I (**162**) (Sung et al. 2004c), while briarein F (**163**) (Rodríguez et al. 1996) is from *B. asbestinum*. Although this is the only example of such functionality reported for 8-hydroxybriaranes, 11-hydroxy-12-alkoxybriaranes are commonly encountered when 8α,17α-epoxy functionality is present.

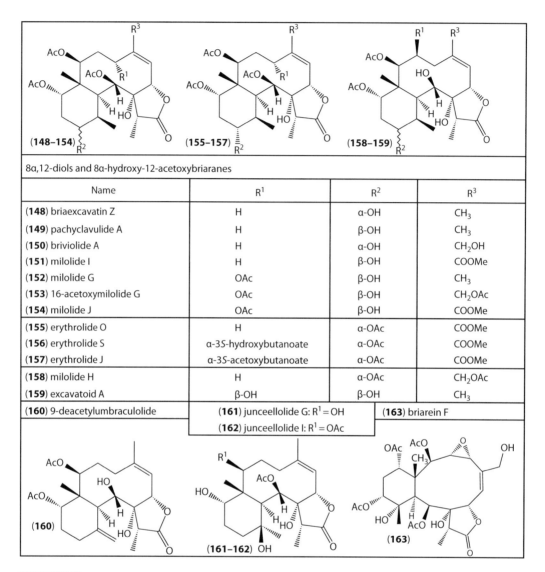

FIGURE 25.13
8α,12-dihydroxybriaranes, their C12 esters, and ungrouped 8α-hydroxybriaranes.

A stereochemical link between C11 and C12 substituents is observed among examples in Figure 25.11 and the metabolites (**149–159**) in Figure 25.13: in the presence of a Δ^{11(20)} double bond or β-methyl substituent on C11, ester substituents on C12 are usually α-oriented, while OH substituents more commonly have the opposite orientation. This observation also relies on other structural features, as observed for briaexcavatolide N (**103**), where Δ³ unsaturation and a 13α,14α-epoxide led to a 12β-OAc with the 11β-methyl substituent. Briaexcavatin Z (**148**) and briviolide A (**150**) are also exceptions to this general trend.

A small number of 8α-hydroxybriaranes with a Δ^{13}-12-one functionality are also known: they include renillafoulins A–C (**164–166**), three inhibitors of barnacle larval setting, that were isolated from the Atlantic sea pansy *R. reniformis* (Keifer et al. 1986) and erythrolide J (**167**) from *E. caribaeorum* (Banjoo et al. 1998). Renillafoulin A was also almost simultaneously reported under the name minabein 8 from a *Minabea* sp., an octocoral in the Alcyoniidae (Ksebati and Schmitz 1986); it has subsequently also been isolated from an *Eleutherobia* sp., another octocoral genus in the Alcyoniidae (Lievens et al. 2004). Erythrolide H (**168**) (Pordesimo et al. 1991) and 16-O-acetylerythrolide H (**169**) (Maharaj et al. 1999) are examples of Δ^{13}-8α-hydroxybriarane-12-ones that feature 2β,3α-epoxy functionality. There is also one example of a Δ^{13}-12α-acetate, solenolide F (**170**) that was isolated from a *Briareum* sp. (Groweiss et al. 1988).

25.5.2 Briaranes with Ether Functionality across the Cyclodecane Ring

The C5 to C9 ether linkage observed in some briareolate esters and the C2 to C8, C4 to C8, and C5 to C8 ethers that form a significant proportion of the known chlorinated briaranes have not been reported to date in unchlorinated briaranes. The sole example of an ether bridge in the cyclodecalin ring is the 4,7-dihydrofuran "compound 5" (**171**) (Figure 25.14), from *B. asbestinum* (Dookran et al. 1994). This ether probably arises through ketal formation from a briarane lactone hemiketal through OH displacement of a leaving group on C4.

25.5.3 Briaranes with 8,17-Epoxides

Briaranes that contain 8,17-epoxides invariably have the epoxide α-oriented. The simplest members of this group are those structures that maintain unsaturation at C5 and C11. The $\Delta^{5,11}$- and $\Delta^{5,11(20)}$-8α,17α-epoxybriaranes are shown in Figure 25.15. The C9 alcohols have been separated from the C9 acetates, and each group is tabulated in order of increasing substituent complexity from C2 then to C3 and C4. Junceellolide H (**172**) from *J. fragilis* (Sung et al. 2003) is a 2,9,14-triol, which lacks functionality at C3 and C4. "Compound 4" (**173**) from *J. gemmacea*

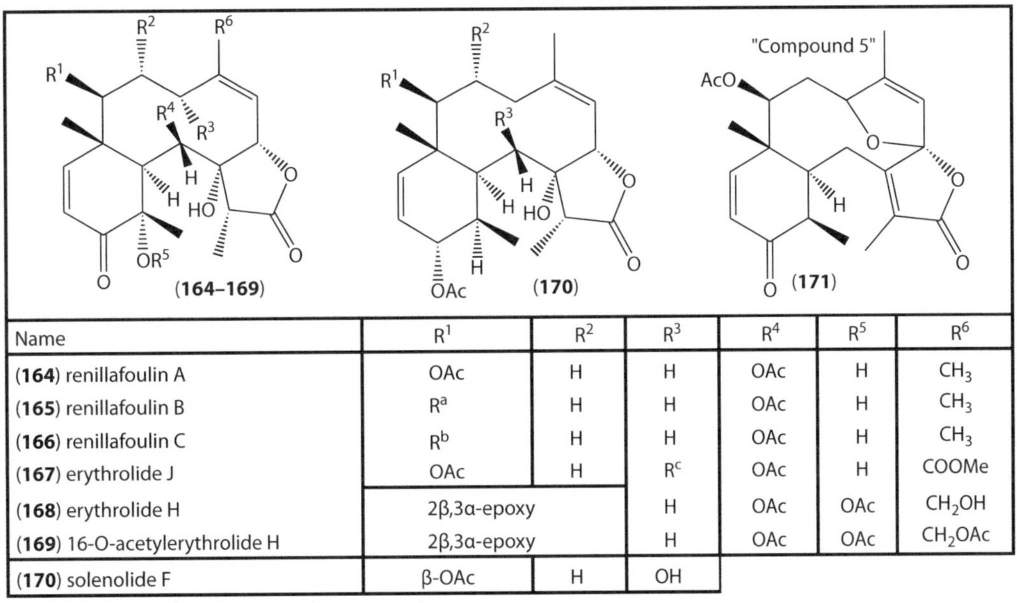

Name	R^1	R^2	R^3	R^4	R^5	R^6
(**164**) renillafoulin A	OAc	H	H	OAc	H	CH$_3$
(**165**) renillafoulin B	R^a	H	H	OAc	H	CH$_3$
(**166**) renillafoulin C	R^b	H	H	OAc	H	CH$_3$
(**167**) erythrolide J	OAc	H	R^c	OAc	H	COOMe
(**168**) erythrolide H	2β,3α-epoxy		H	OAc	OAc	CH$_2$OH
(**169**) 16-O-acetylerythrolide H	2β,3α-epoxy		H	OAc	OAc	CH$_2$OAc
(**170**) solenolide F	β-OAc	H	OH			

R^a = propanoate, R^b = butanoate, R^c = 3-acetoxybutanoate

FIGURE 25.14
Δ^{13}-12-ketobriaranes, a Δ^{13}-12-acetoxybriarane and an ether-bridged briaran-13-en-12-one.

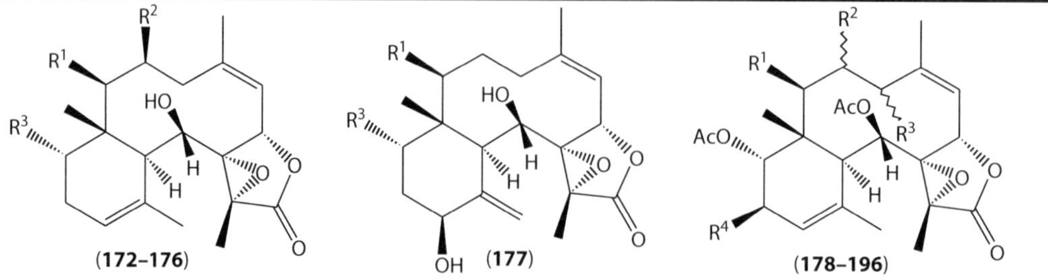

(172–176)   **(177)**   **(178–196)**

$\Delta^{5,11}$ and $\Delta^{5,11(20)}$-8α,17α-epoxybriaranes

Structure and Name	R^1	R^2	R^3	
(**172**) junceellolide H	OH	H	OH	
(**173**) compound 4	OAc	H	OAc	
(**174**) see below	butanoate	H	OAc	
(**175**) compound 12	OAc	OAc	OAc	
(**176**) compound 13	OAc	butanoate	OAc	
(**177**) compound 5	OAc	H	OAc	

Structure and Name	R^1	R^2	R^3	R^4
(**178**) briareolide H	OAc	H	H	H
(**179**) briarlide R	OH	α-OAc	H	H
(**180**) briaranolide G	OAc	β-OH	H	H
(**181**) briaranolide E	OAc	β-OAc	H	H
(**182**) briaranolide F	OAc	β-butanoate	H	H
(**183**) see below	OAc	α-OAc	H	H
(**184**) stecholide J	OAc	β-OAc	H	β-OH
(**185**) stecholide I	OAc	β-butanoate	H	β-OH
(**186**) briaranolide H	propanoate	α-propanoate	H	H
(**187**) see below	butanoate	H	α-OAc	H
(**188**) briaranolide I	OAc	Δ^3		H
(**189**) briarlide P	OAc	α-OH	α-OAc	H
(**190**) excavatolide O	OAc	α-OAc	α-OAc	H
(**191**) briaranolide A	OAc	β-OAc	β-OAc	H
(**192**) briaranolide D	OAc	β-OH	β-butanoate	H
(**193**) briaranolide B	OAc	β-OAc	β-butanoate	H
(**194**) briaranolide C	OAc	β-butanoate	β-butanoate	H
(**195**) briarlide O	OAc	α-OH	α-octanoate	H
(**196**) briarlide Q	OH	α-OAc	α-octanoate	H

(**174**) 11,12-deoxystecholide E   (**183**) 13-dehydroxystecholide J
(**187**) 11,12-Deoxystecholide A acetate

FIGURE 25.15
$\Delta^{5,11}$ and $\Delta^{5,11(20)}$-8α,17α-epoxy-9α-hydroxybriaranes and their 9α-acetates.

(Bowden et al. 1990) is the 2,14-diacetate of junceellolide H, while 11,12-deoxystecholide E (**174**) from *B. stechei* is the 14-acetate-2-butanoate diester of junceellolide H (Bloor et al. 1992). Compounds 12 (**175**) and 13 (**176**) from a *Briareum* sp. (Bowden et al. 1989) are esters at both C2 and C3. While stereochemistry at C2 is always the same, stereochemistry at C3 and C4 is variable and quite difficult to determine. The conformational flexibility of the cyclodecane ring system results in changes in conformational equilibria in solution when a substituent is altered, so homologous esters with the same stereochemistry at C3 and C4 (or the same esters at C3 and/or C4 with a structural change elsewhere in the molecule) do not necessarily exhibit consistency in either ^{1}H NMR shifts and couplings or ^{13}C NMR shifts. Some of these derivatives exhibit slow interconversion of conformers on the NMR timescale, so they give broad spectra. When conditions are altered to sharpen the spectra by heating, cooling, or changing the solvent, significant chemical shift changes may accompany sharpening of the spectrum, indicating that a shift in the equilibrium between the interconverting conformers has been caused by the change in conditions. It is conceivable that the stereochemistry for some of these substituents may have been incorrectly assigned. All stereochemistry presented here for C3 and C4 match those in the literature but have been redrawn in the same representation of the cyclodecane ring as has been used consistently for this chapter. This has, of course, resulted in multiple cases where substituents drawn with α- (or β-) orientation in the original literature are listed here with apparently the opposite orientation simply because of the change in representation of the ring conformation.

Compound 5 (**177**) from *J. gemmacea* (Bowden et al. 1990) is the only example of a $\Delta^{5,11(20)}$-8α,17α-epoxybriarane that has been reported to date.

Briareolide H (**178**) from a *Briareum* sp. (Pordesimo et al. 1991) is the triacetate of junceellolide H and is currently the only example of a $\Delta^{5,11}$-8α,17α-epoxy-9α-acetoxybriarane that lacks an oxygenated substituent at both C3 and C4. Briarlide R (**179**) (Iwagawa et al. 2005c); briaranolides G (**180**), E (**181**), and F (**182**) (Hoshino et al. 2005); 13-dehydroxystecholide J (**183**) (Bloor et al. 1992); stecholides J (**184**) and I (**185**) (Schmitz et al. 1993); and briaranolide H (**186**) (Hoshino et al. 2005) were all isolated from *Briareum* sp. and represent the known $\Delta^{5,11}$-8α,17α-epoxy-2,3-dihydroxybriarane mono- and diesters. These are all mono- or diesters of the 2β,3α- or 2β,3β-diols, where the esters are either acetate, propanoate, or butanoate, and they include two representatives (stecholides I and J) that also have a 13β-OH group. There is one representative of a 2,4-substitution pattern: 11,12-deoxystecholide A acetate (**187**), which was reported from *B. stechei* (Bloor et al. 1992). The remaining 9α-acetate derivatives in this group all present oxygen functionality at C2, C3, and C4; they include briaranolide I (**188**) (Hoshino et al. 2005); briarlide P (**189**) (Iwagawa et al. 2005c); excavatolide O (**190**) (Neve et al. 1999); briaranolides A (**191**), D (**192**), B (**193**), and C (**194**) (Hoshino et al. 2005); and briarlides O (**195**) and Q (**196**) (Iwagawa et al. 2005c). The briaranolides and briarlides were all isolated from *Briareum* sp., while excavatolide O was from the species *B. excavatum* (Figure 25.15).

Epoxidation at C11 is also prevalent among the 8α,17-epoxybriarane metabolites with 11β,12β-epoxides being the more commonly encountered isomer. The C9 alcohols and esters in this category are presented in Figure 25.16a. Among the C9-alcohols, 2β-acetoxy-2-(debutyryloxy)stecholide E (**197**) (Sheu et al. 1996) and stecholides F (**198**) and E (**199**) (Bloor et al. 1992), which were all isolated from *Briareum* sp., are the simplest, being the 2β-acetate, 2β-propanoate, and 2β-butanoate derivatives, respectively, with the only other unmentioned oxygen substituent being a 14α-acetate. Compounds 5 (**200**) and 6 (**201**) from a *Briareum* species (Bowden et al. 1989) are the 3α-acetate derivatives of (**197**) and (**199**), respectively. Compound 6 (Bowden et al. 1989) was also reported under the name 3-acetoxystecholide E (Bloor et al. 1992). Stecholide C (**202**), 16-hydroxystecholide C (**203**), and stecholides B (**204**) and A (**205**) (Bloor et al. 1992) complete the known 9α-alcohols in this structure group.

2β-Acetoxy-2-(debutyryloxy)stecholide E acetate (**206**) and stecholide E acetate (**207**) from *B. stechei* (Bloor et al. 1992) are the 9α-acetates of 2β-acetoxy-2-(debutyryloxy)stecholide E and stecholide E, respectively. The 2-acetate derivative of brianthein C (**208**) (Aoki et al. 2001)

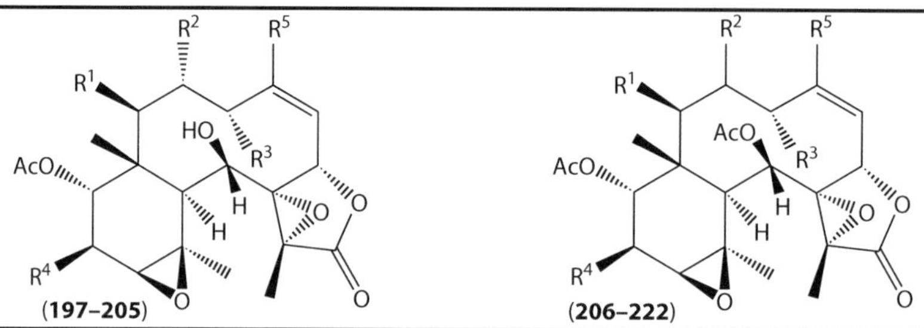

Structure and Name	R^1	R^2	R^3	R^4	R^5
(197) see below	OAc	H	H	H	Me
(198) stecholide F	propanoate	H	H	H	Me
(199) stecholide E	butanoate	H	H	H	Me
(200) compound 5	OAc	α-OAc	H	H	Me
(201) compound 6*	butanoate	α-OAc	H	H	Me
(202) stecholide C	OAc	H	α-OAc	H	Me
(203) 16-hydroxystecholide C	OAc	H	α-OAc	H	CH₂OH
(204) stecholide B	propanoate	H	α-OAc	H	Me
(205) stecholide A	butanoate	H	α-OAc	H	Me
(206) see below	OAc	H	H	H	Me
(207) stecholide E acetate	butanoate	H	H	H	Me
(208) brianthein C	OH	α-OAc	H	H	Me
(209) excavatolide P	OAc	α-OAc	H	H	Me
(210) stecholide L	OAc	β-OAc	H	β-OH	Me
(211) stecholide K	OAc	β-OAc	H	β-OAc	Me
(212) stecholide M	OAc	β-butanoate	H	β-OH	Me
(213) stecholide C acetate	OAc	H	α-OAc	H	Me
(214) see below	OAc	H	α-OAc	H	CH₂OH
(215) see below	OAc	H	α-OAc	H	CH₂OAc
(216) stecholide B acetate	propanoate	H	α-OAc	H	Me
(217) see below	propanoate	H	α-OAc	H	CH₂OAc
(218) stecholide D	butanoate	H	α-OH	H	Me
(219) stecholide A acetate	butanoate	H	α-OAc	H	Me
(220) see below	butanoate	H	α-OAc	H	CH₂OAc
(221) compound 12	butanoate	H	α-butanoate	H	Me
(222) excavatolide R	OAc	α-OAc	α-OAc	H	Me

* 3-Acetoxystecholide E (Bloor et al. 1992) = compound 6 (Bowden et al. 1989)

(197) 2β-acetoxy-2-(debutyryloxy)stecholide E **(206)** 2β-acetoxy-2-(debutyryloxy)stecholide E acetate

(214) 16-hydroxystecholide C acetate **(215)** 16-acetoxystecholide C acetate

(217) 16-acetoxystecholide B acetate **(220)** 16-acetoxystecholide A acetate

(a)

FIGURE 25.16

(a) Δ^5-8α,17α:11β,12β-bisepoxy-9α-hydroxy and 9α-acetoxybriaranes.

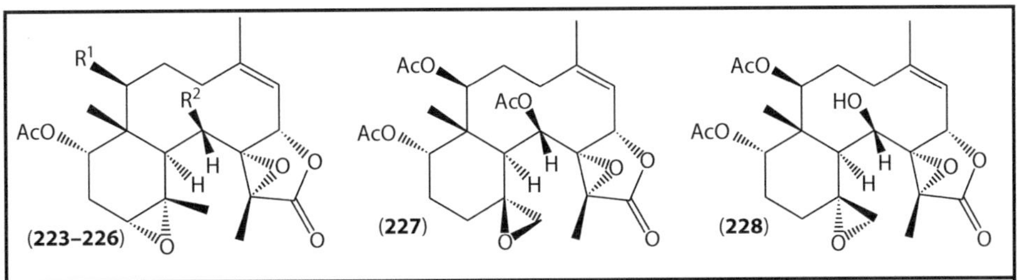

Structure and Name	R^1	C3	C4	R^1
(223) briareolide D	OAc	CH$_2$	CH$_2$	α-OAc
(224) briareolide C	butanoate	CH$_2$	CH$_2$	α-OAc
(225) briaranolide J	OAc	E-Δ^3		α-OAc
(226) briaexcavatin V	OAc	E-Δ^3		α-OH
(227) "compound 3"				
(228) umbraculolide B				

(b)

FIGURE 25.16 (continued)
(b) Δ^5-8α,17α:11α,12α-bisepoxy-9α-hydroxy and 9α-acetoxybriaranes and Δ^5-8α,17α:11,20-bisepoxy-9α-hydroxy and 9α-acetoxybriaranes.

is excavatolide P (**209**) (Neve et al. 1999); both were isolated from *B. excavatum*. Excavatolide P is also the 9α-acetate of compound 5 (Bowden et al. 1989) from a *Briareum* sp., while stecholide L (**210**) from *B. excavatum* (Schmitz et al. 1993) is the 3α-acetyl diastereomer of excavatolide P with a 13α-OH group added. Stecholide K (**211**) is the 13α-OAc ester of stecholide L, and stecholide M (**212**) is the 3β-butanoate homologue of stecholide L (Schmitz et al. 1993). Stecholide C acetate (**213**) (Bloor et al. 1992) was reported from *B. stechei*, while 16-hydroxystecholide C acetate (**214**) was found in *B. excavatum* (Schmitz et al. 1993). 16-Acetoxystecholide C acetate (**215**), stecholide B acetate (**216**), and its 16-acetoxy derivative (**217**) were all isolated from *B. stechei* (Bloor et al. 1992). A series of 2β-butanoates were also isolated from the same organism with the 4α-OH derivative named stecholide D (**218**), its 4α-OAc named stecholide A acetate (**219**), its 16-oxidized derivative 16-acetoxystecholide A acetate (**220**), and the 4α-butanoate of stecholide D (**221**) all reported. Excavatolide R (**222**), a 2β,3α,4α,9α-tetraacetate, was also reported from a Western Australian sample of *B. excavatum* (Neve et al. 1999).

A limited number of 11α,12α-epoxides and 11α,20-epoxides have also been reported, and these appear in Figure 25.16b. The four known 11α,12α-epoxides are briareolides D (**223**) and C (**224**) (Pordesimo et al. 1991), briaranolide J (**225**) (Hoshino et al. 2005), and briaexcavatin V (**226**) (Sung et al. 2009b). *Briareum* species were the source of these four briaranes. One 11β,20-epoxide, "compound 3" (**227**), a 9α-hydroxybriarane from *J. gemmacea* (Bowden et al. 1990), and one 11α,20-epoxide, umbraculolide B (**228**), a 9α-acetate from *G. umbraculum* (Subramanyam et al. 2000), have also been reported (Figure 25.16b).

Another large group of the 8α,17-epoxy briaranes contains either a Δ^{13}-12-one or the reduced Δ^{13}-12-hydroxybriarane. The stereochemistry of these alcohols is predominantly the 12α-isomer, although a few examples of 12-β isomers have been reported. The other usual structural features in the briaranes with these functional groups are either a β-oriented secondary methyl group (C20) on C11 or an α-oriented tertiary C20 methyl group if C11 carries an oxygen substituent. These Δ^{13}-12-ketones and the Δ^{13}-12-hydroxybriaranes are shown in Figure 25.17.

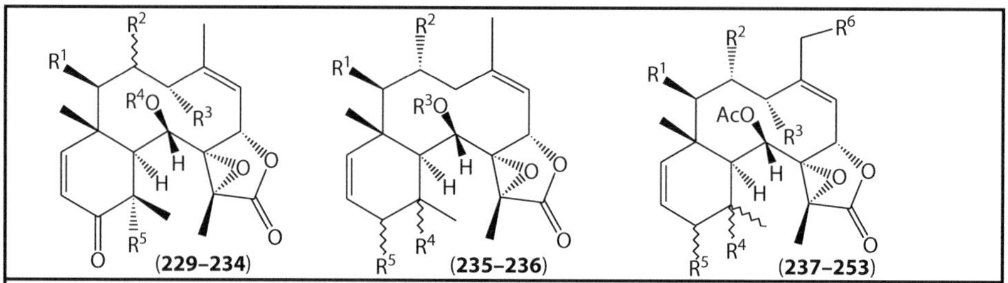

Structure and Name	R^1	R^2	R^3	R^4	R^5	
(229) briaexcavatolide D	OH	H	H	H	H	
(230) briaexcavatolide T	OAc	H	H	H	H	
(231) excavatolide Q	OAc	α-OAc	H	H	H	
(232) briareolide I	butanoate	H	H	Ac	H	
(233) briaexcavatolide A	OAc	β-OAc	H	Ac	H	
(234) briaexcavatin X	OAc	H	α-OH	Ac	α-OH	
(235) excavatolide N	OAc	OAc	H	α-H	α-OH	
(236) violide S	OAc	OAc	OAc	β-H	β-OH	

Structure and Name	R^1	R^2	R^3	R^4	R^5	R^6
(237) briarlide H	OH	OAc	H	α-OH	α-OH	H
(238) violide G	OAc	OAc	H	α-OH	α-OH	H
(239) violide H	OAc	H	octanoate	α-OH	α-OH	H
(240) compound 9	OAc	H	OAc	α-OH	α-OH	H
(241) violide I	OAc	H	hexanoate	α-OH	α-OH	H
(242) briarlide M	OAc	H	hexanoate	α-OH	α-OH	OH
(243) violide N	OAc	H	octanoate	α-OH	α-OH	OH
(244) violide F	OH	OH	octanoate	α-OH	α-OH	H
(245) briarlide J	OAc	OH	OAc	α-OH	α-OH	H
(246) violide E	OAc	OAc	butanoate	α-OH	α-OH	H
(247) violide D	OAc	OAc	hexanoate	α-OH	α-OH	H
(248) violide C	OAc	OAc	octanoate	α-OH	α-OH	H
(249) violide Q	OAc	octanoate	OH	α-OH	α-OH	H
(250) violide R	OAc	H	octanoate	β-OH	β-OH	H
(251) briaexcavatin W	OAc	H	H	β-OH	α-OH	H
(252) briaexcavatin K	OAc	H	OAc	β-OH	α-OH	H
(253) excavatoid B	OAc	H	β-butanoate	β-OH	α-OH	H

FIGURE 25.17
$\Delta^{5,13}$-9α-hydroxybriaradien-12-ones, 12-alcohols, and their 9α-acetates.

The Δ^{13}-12-ketones are the 9α-hydroxybriaranes, briaexcavatolides D (229) (Sheu et al. 1999a) and T (230) (Wu et al. 2003), and excavatolide Q (231) (Neve et al. 1999) plus the 9α-acetoxybriaranes, briareolide I (232) (Pordesimo et al. 1991), briaexcavatolide A (233) (Sheu et al. 1999a), and briaexcavatin X (234) (Sung et al. 2009b). All were from *B. excavatum* with the possible exception of briareolide I where the organism was only identified as a *Briareum* sp.; the first five structures all have an 11β-oriented secondary methyl group, while briaexcavatin X has an α-OH on C11.

Excavatolide N (235) from *B. excavatum* (Neve et al. 1999) and violide S (236) from a *Briareum* sp. (Iwagawa et al. 2005a) are Δ^{13}-9α,12α-dihydroxybriaranes with an 11β-secondary methyl group. Briarlide H (237) (Iwagawa et al. 2003), its 2β-acetate violide G (238), violide

H (**239**) (Iwagawa et al. 1999), compound 9 (**240**) (Bowden et al. 1989), violide I (**241**) (Iwagawa et al. 1999), briarlide M (**242**) (Iwagawa et al. 2005c), violides N (**243**) and F (**244**) (Iwagawa et al. 1999, 2000), briarlide J (**245**) (Iwagawa et al. 2005c), and violides E, D, C, and Q (**246–249**) (Iwagawa et al. 1999, 2005a) are all from *Briareum* sp. Violide R (**250**) (Iwagawa et al. 2005a) is an 11β,12β-diol,while briaexcavatins W (**251**) (Sung et al. 2009b) and K (**252**) (Sung et al. 2008b) and excavatoid B (**253**) (Sung et al. 2009c) are 11β,12α-diols.

Many C12 esters of these Δ^{13}-12-hydroxybriaranes have also been reported. Figure 25.18a depicts C12 esters of the 11α-hydroxy-$\Delta^{5,13}$-8α,17α-epoxybriarane structure. Compound 11 (**254**) (Bowden et al. 1989) and stecholide G (**255**) (Bloor et al. 1992), both from *Briareum* species, are 9α-hydroxybriaranes that feature an 11β-secondary methyl group with an α-acetate on C12. The remaining examples of C12-esters are 9α-acetoxybriaranes, and all have a hydroxyl group on C11. While examples with 11α-hydroxylation (Figure 25.18a) exceed those with an 11β-OH (Figure 25.18b), esters on C12 are predominantly α-oriented, with only two reported metabolites being 12β-esters. The 12-monoacetates of the 11α,12α-diols are represented by brianodin A (**256**) from a *Pachyclavularia* sp. (Ishiyama et al. 2008) and tubiporein (**257**), which was first reported (Natori et al. 1990) from the alcyonacean coral *Tubipora* sp. but subsequently re-reported under the name briarlide G when it was isolated from a *Briareum* sp. (Iwagawa et al. 2003). Brialaleptolide A (**258**) was isolated from a *Briareum* sp. (Joyner et al. 2007), and its 2-acetate, compound 10 (**259**) (Bowden et al. 1989), was renamed briarlide N in a subsequent reisolation (Iwagawa et al. 2005c). Brialaleptolides B (**260**) and C (**261**) (Joyner et al. 2007) and briarlides L (**262**), C (**263**), B (**264**), A (**265**), K (**266**), E (**267**), D (**268**), I (**269**), and F (**270**) (Iwagawa et al. 2003) were all reported from *Briareum* sp.

The 12-monoesters of 11β,12-diols (Figure 25.18b) are briaexcavatolides C (**271**) and B (**272**) (Sheu et al. 1999a) from *B. excavatum*; compound 8 (**273**) (Bowden et al. 1989) from a *Briareum* sp.; excavatolides X (**274**) and Y (**275**) (Sheu et al. 1999b), which all have 12α-esters; and briaexcavatolide S (**276**) (Wu et al. 2003), briaexcavatin N (**277**) (Sung et al. 2008a), and briaexcavatolide W (**278**) (Wu et al. 2004) that are 12β-esters from *B. excavatum*.

A small number of analogues of the 11,12-diols and 11-hydroxy-12-esters, all from *Briareum* species, have been reported that lack the Δ^{13} unsaturation present in the metabolites in Figures 25.17 and 25.18b: these are shown in Figure 2.19. Excavatolide Z (**279**) (Sheu et al. 1999b) has a 9α-OH and an ester on C12. Excavatoid F (**280**) (Sung et al. 2009a), briaexcavatin S (**281**), briaexcavatolides L (**282**) and U (**283**) (Wu et al. 2003), briaexcavatin L (**284**) (Sung et al. 2008b), and briareolide A (**285**) (Pordesimo et al. 1991), on the other hand, have a 9α-OAc and an alcohol on C12, while briareolide B (**286**) (Pordesimo et al. 1991) has acetates at both C9 and C12. These compounds can be envisaged as potential precursors for those with Δ^{13} unsaturation, which could result from elimination of the 14α-oxygen function. There are two examples of Δ^{12} briaranes: the 9α-alcohol, stecholide H (**287**) (Bloor et al. 1992), and the 9α-acetate, 2,9-diacetyl-2-debutyrylstecholide H (**288**) (Bloor et al. 1992).

A significant number of 11β-methyl-12-alcohols, esters, and ketones have also been reported predominantly from *B. excavatum*. These include the 9α-alcohols in Figure 25.20a—excavatolide E (**289**) (Sheu et al. 1998), L (**290**) (Sung et al. 1999), and W (**291**) (Sheu et al. 1999b); briaexcavatolide V (**292**) (Wu et al. 2003); excavatolide M (**293**) (Sung et al. 1999); and briarenol A (**294**) (Sung et al. 2005b), as well as 9α-acetates on the less common Δ^4-briarane: fragilide A (**295**) (Sung et al. 2004b) and excavatoids M and N (**296–297**) (Su et al. 2010).

The Δ^5-9α-acetoxybriaranes are well represented (Figure 25.20b). All unmentioned source organisms in the following discussion were identified samples of *B. excavatum*.

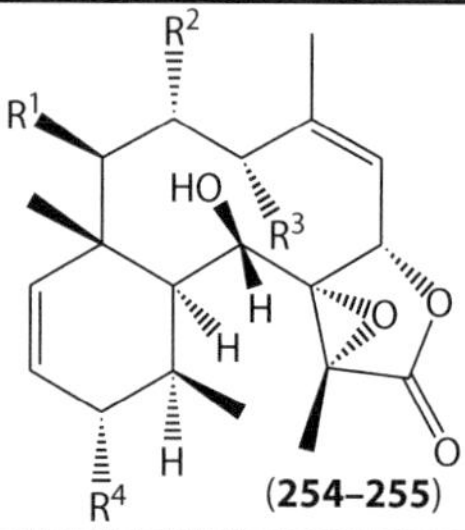

Structure and Name	R^1	R^2	R^3	R^4
(254) compound 11	OAc	H	H	α-OAc
(255) stecholide G	butanoate	H	H	α-OAc
(256) brianodin A	OH	OAc	H	α-OAc
(257) tubiporein*	OAc	OAc	H	α-OAc
(258) brialaleptolide A	OH	H	OAc	α-OAc
(259) compound 10[†]	OAc	H	OAc	α-OAc
(260) brialaleptolide B	OH	H	hexanoate	α-OAc
(261) brialaleptolide C	OH	H	octanoate	α-OAc
(262) briarlide L	OAc	H	octanoate	α-OAc
(263) briarlide C	OH	OH	OAc	α-OAc
(264) briarlide B	OAc	OH	OAc	α-OAc
(265) briarlide A	OAc	OAc	OAc	α-OAc
(266) briarlide K	OH	OH	octanoate	α-OAc
(267) briarlide E	OAc	OH	octanoate	α-OAc
(268) briarlide D	OAc	OH	octanoate	α-OAc
(269) briarlide I	OAc	OAc	octanoate	α-OAc
(270) briarlide F	OAc	octanoate	OH	α-OAc

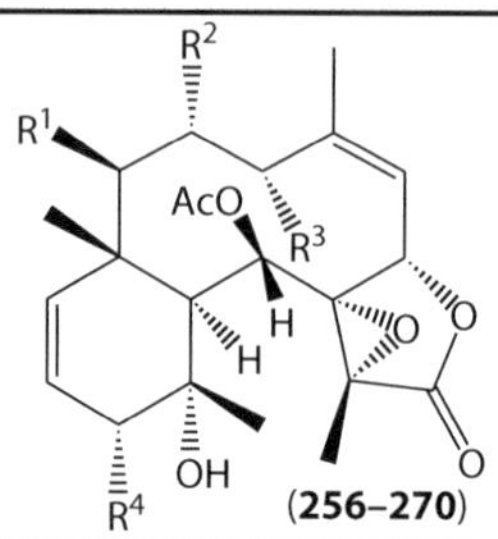

*Briarlide G (Iwagawa et al. 2003) = tubiporein (**257**) (Natori et al. 1990)
[†]Briarlide N (Iwagawa et al. 2005b) = compound 10 (**259**) (Bowden et al. 1989)

(a)

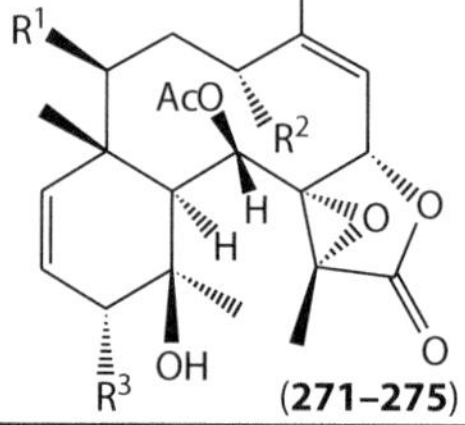

Structure and Name	R^1	R^2	R^3
(271) briaexcavatolide C	OAc	H	α-OAc
(272) briaexcavatolide B	OAc	H	α-butanoate
(273) compound 8	OAc	α-OAc	α-OAc
(274) excavatolide X	OAc	α-OAc	α-butanoate
(275) excavatolide Y	OAc	α-propanoate	α-OAc
(276) briaexcavatolide S	OH	α-OAc	β-OAc
(277) briaexcavatin N	OAc	β-OH	β-OAc
(278) briaexcavatolide W	OAc	OH	β-butanoate

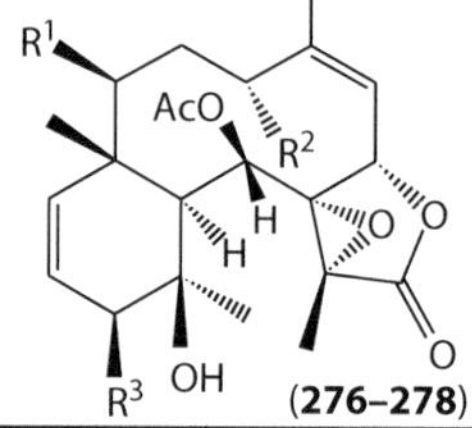

(b)

FIGURE 25.18

(a) C12 esters of the 11α-hydroxy-$\Delta^{5,13}$-8α,17α-epoxybriarane structure. (b) C12 esters of the 11β-hydroxy-$\Delta^{5,13}$-9α-acetoxy-8α,17α-epoxybriarane structure.

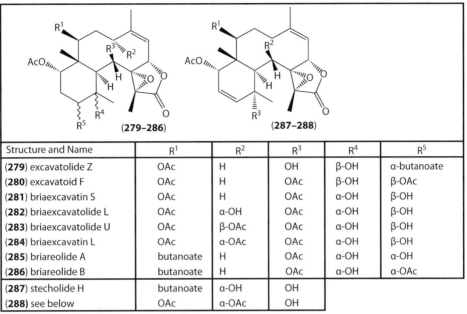

Structure and Name	R^1	R^2	R^3	R^4	R^5
(**279**) excavatolide Z	OAc	H	OH	β-OH	α-butanoate
(**280**) excavatoid F	OAc	H	OAc	β-OH	β-OAc
(**281**) briaexcavatin S	OAc	H	OAc	α-OH	β-OH
(**282**) briaexcavatolide L	OAc	α-OH	OAc	α-OH	β-OH
(**283**) briaexcavatolide U	OAc	β-OAc	OAc	α-OH	β-OH
(**284**) briaexcavatin L	OAc	α-OAc	OAc	α-OH	β-OH
(**285**) briareolide A	butanoate	H	OAc	α-OH	α-OH
(**286**) briareolide B	butanoate	H	OAc	α-OH	α-OAc
(**287**) stecholide H	butanoate	α-OH	OH		
(**288**) see below	OAc	α-OAc	OH		

(**288**) 2,9-diacetyl-2-debutyrylstecholide H

FIGURE 25.19
C11-alcohols that lack Δ^{13} unsaturation.

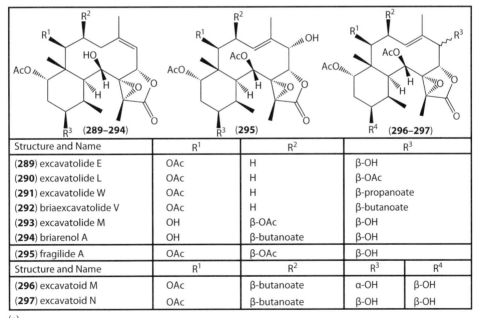

Structure and Name	R^1	R^2	R^3	
(**289**) excavatolide E	OAc	H	β-OH	
(**290**) excavatolide L	OAc	H	β-OAc	
(**291**) excavatolide W	OAc	H	β-propanoate	
(**292**) briaexcavatolide V	OAc	H	β-butanoate	
(**293**) excavatolide M	OH	β-OAc	β-OH	
(**294**) briarenol A	OH	β-butanoate	β-OH	
(**295**) fragilide A	OAc	β-OAc	β-OH	
Structure and Name	R^1	R^2	R^3	R^4
(**296**) excavatoid M	OAc	β-butanoate	α-OH	β-OH
(**297**) excavatoid N	OAc	β-butanoate	β-OH	β-OH

(a)

FIGURE 25.20
(a) 11β-methyl-12-alcohols and Δ^4-briaranes.

(*continued*)

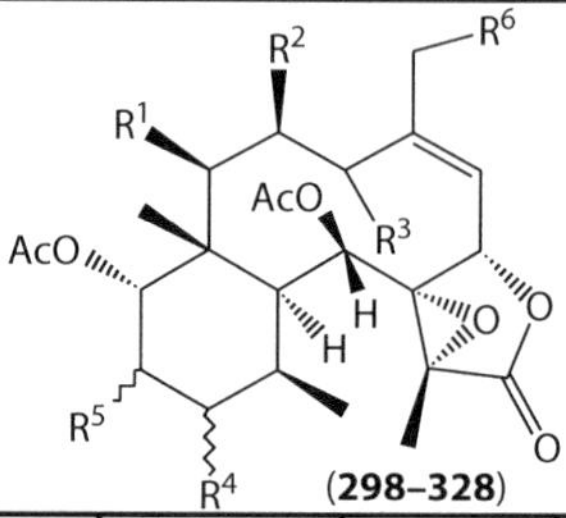

Structure and Name	R¹	R²	R³	R⁴	R⁵	R⁶
(**298**) briareolide F	OAc	H	H	α-OH	H	H
(**299**) briaexcavatin I	OAc	H	H	β-OH	H	H
(**300**) excavatolide G	OAc	H	H	β-OAc	H	H
(**301**) briareolide E	Rᵇ	H	H	α-OH	H	H
(**302**) see below	Rᵇ	H	H	β-OAc	H	H
(**303**) excavatoid L	OAc	OH	H	β-OH	H	H
(**304**) excavatolide C	OAc	OAc	H	β-OH	H	H
(**305**) stecholide N	OAc	OAc	H	β-OH	β-OH	H
(**306**) excavatolide D	OH	OAc	H	β-OH	H	H
(**307**) excavatolide B	OAc	OAc	H	β-OH	H	H
(**308**) briaexcavatin R	OAc	H	α-OH	β-OH	H	H
(**309**) briaexcavatin J	OAc	H	α-OH	β-OH	H	OAc
(**310**) briaexcavatin P	OAc	OAc	β-OAc	β-OH	H	H
(**311**) briaexcavatin O	OAc	Rᵇ	α-OAc	β-OH	H	H
(**312**) briaexcavatolide O	OH	OAc	Rᵇ	β-OH	H	H
(**313**) briaexcavatolide P	OAc	OH	Rᵇ	β-OH	H	H
(**314**) briaexcavatolide Q	OAc	OH	Rᵇ	β-OAc	H	H
(**315**) excavatolide K	OAc	OAc	H	β-OAc	H	H
(**316**) excavatolide I	OAc	Rᵇ	H	β-OAc	H	H
(**317**) excavatolide U	OAc	Rᵇ	H	Rᵃ	H	H
(**318**) excavatolide V	OAc	OAc	H	Rᵃ	H	H
(**319**) excavatolide F	OAc	Δ³		Rᵇ	H	H
(**320**) briaexcavatin M	OAc	Δ³		β-OH	H	H
(**321**) excavatolide H	OAc	Rᵇ	H	H	H	H
(**322**) excavatolide J	OAc	OAc	H	H	H	H
(**323**) briaexcavatin D	OAc	OAc	H	H	H	H
(**324**) briaexcavatin E	OAc	OAc	H	H	H	H
(**325**) briaexcavatin G	OAc	Rᵇ	H	Rᵈ	H	H
(**326**) briaexcavatin F	OAc	Rᵇ	H	Rᶜ	H	H
(**327**) briaexcavatolide R	OAc	Rᵇ	H	Rᵉ	H	H
(**328**) excavatolide T	OAc	OAc	H	=O	H	H

(**302**) 11,12-deoxy-11*H*-12-acetoxystecholide E acetate

Rᵃ = β-propanoate

Rᵇ = β-butanoate

Rᶜ = β-4-pentenoate

Rᵈ = β-3-methylbutanoate

Rᵉ = β-octanoate

(b)

FIGURE 25.20 (continued)

(b) 11β-methyl-12-esters and ketones.

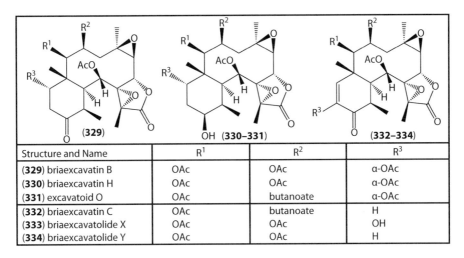

Structure and Name	R¹	R²	R³
(**329**) briaexcavatin B	OAc	OAc	α-OAc
(**330**) briaexcavatin H	OAc	OAc	α-OAc
(**331**) excavatoid O	OAc	butanoate	α-OAc
(**332**) briaexcavatin C	OAc	butanoate	H
(**333**) briaexcavatolide X	OAc	OAc	OH
(**334**) briaexcavatolide Y	OAc	OAc	H

FIGURE 25.21
5,6-epoxides.

The metabolites include briareolide F (**298**) from a *Briareum* sp. (Pordesimo et al. 1991); the *B. excavatum* metabolites briaexcavatin I (**299**) (Sung et al. 2008b); excavatolide G (**300**) (Sung et al. 1999); briareolide E (**301**) from *Briareum* (Pordesimo et al. 1991); 11,12-deoxy-11*H*-12-acetoxystecholide E acetate (**302**) from *B. stechei* (Bloor et al. 1992); excavatoid L (**303**) (Su et al. 2010); excavatolide C (**304**) (Sheu et al. 1998); stecholide N (**305**) (Schmitz et al. 1993); excavatolides D (**306**) and B (**307**) (Sheu et al. 1998); briaexcavatins R (**308**) (Hwang et al. 2008), J (**309**) (Sung et al. 2008b), P (**310**), and O (**311**) (Sung et al 2008a); briaexcavatolides O (**312**), P (**313**), and Q (**314**) (Wu et al. 2001); excavatolides K (**315**), I (**316**) (Sung et al. 1999), U (**317**), V (**318**) (Sheu et al. 1999b), and F (**319**) (Sung et al. 1999); briaexcavatin M (**320**) (Sung et al. 2008a); excavatolide H (**321**) and J (**322**) (Sung et al. 1999); briaexcavatins D (**323**), E (**324**) (Sung et al. 2006b), G (**325**) (Chen et al. 2006), and F (**326**) (Sung et al. 2006b); and briaexcavatolide R (**327**) (Wu et al. 2001). There is also one 12-ketone known in this grouping (Figure 25.20b): excavatolide T (**328**) (Neve et al. 1999).

The 5β,6α:8α,17α-bisepoxides include one C12-ketone, briaexcavatin B (**329**) (Sung et al. 2006a), two 12β-alcohols, briaexcavatin H (Chen et al. 2006) (**330**), and excavatoid O (**331**) (Sung et al. 2010), as well as three Δ¹³-12-ketones, briaexcavatin C (**332**) (Sung et al. 2006a), and briaexcavatolides X (**333**) and Y (**334**) (Sung et al. 2006b) all from *B. excavatum* (Figure 25.21). Originally published as 5,6-diols (Sung et al. 2004a), the structures of briaexcavatolides X and Y were subsequently revised, with structural changes in both the C5–C6 and C13–C14 regions.

25.5.4 8,17-Diols

A total of fourteen 8,17-diols (and two 8-hydroxy-17-esters) have been isolated (Figure 25.22), consisting of three briaexcavatolides and an excavatoid from *B. excavatum*, five violides, two unnamed diols and two unnamed monoesters from *Briareum* species, and three brianodins from *Pachyclavularia*. Briaexcavatolides Z (**335**) (Sung et al. 2004a), K (**336**), and L (**337**) (Sung et al. 2001); excavatoid D (**338**) (Sung et al. 2009c); and violide V (**339**) (Iwagawa et al. 2005a)

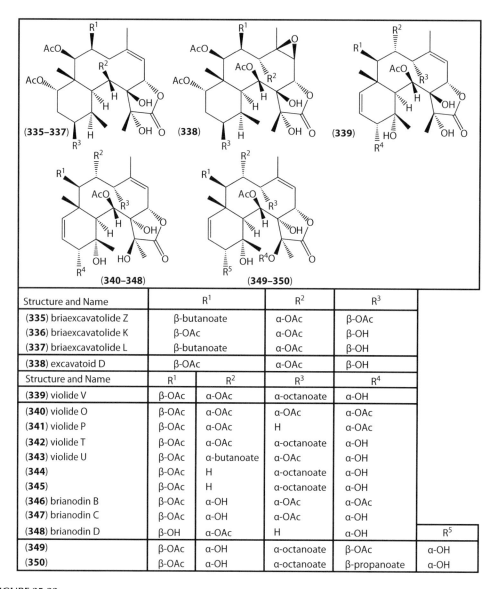

Structure and Name	R^1		R^2	R^3	
(335) briaexcavatolide Z	β-butanoate		α-OAc	β-OAc	
(336) briaexcavatolide K	β-OAc		α-OAc	β-OH	
(337) briaexcavatolide L	β-butanoate		α-OAc	β-OH	
(338) excavatoid D	β-OAc		α-OAc	β-OH	
Structure and Name	R^1	R^2	R^3	R^4	
(339) violide V	β-OAc	α-OAc	α-octanoate	α-OH	
(340) violide O	β-OAc	α-OAc	α-OAc	α-OAc	
(341) violide P	β-OAc	α-OAc	H	α-OAc	
(342) violide T	β-OAc	α-OAc	α-octanoate	α-OH	
(343) violide U	β-OAc	α-butanoate	α-OAc	α-OH	
(344)	β-OAc	H	α-octanoate	α-OH	
(345)	β-OAc	H	α-octanoate	α-OH	
(346) brianodin B	β-OAc	α-OH	α-OAc	α-OAc	
(347) brianodin C	β-OAc	α-OH	α-OAc	α-OH	
(348) brianodin D	β-OH	α-OAc	H	α-OH	R^5
(349)	β-OAc	α-OH	α-octanoate	β-OAc	α-OH
(350)	β-OAc	α-OH	α-octanoate	β-propanoate	α-OH

FIGURE 25.22
8,17-diols and their 17-monoesters.

are all 8β,17α-diols. Violides O (340), P (341) (Iwagawa et al. 2000), T (342), and U (343) as well as two unnamed diols (344 and 345) (Iwagawa et al. 2005a) and brianodins B (346), C (347), and D (348) (Ishiyama et al. 2008) are all 8α,17β-diols. Two unnamed 8α-hydroxy,17β-esters (349 and 350) have also been reported (Iwagawa et al. 2005a). The briaexcavatolides and the excavatoid have a β-secondary methyl group on C11 that distinguishes them from the violides and brianodins, which are comprised of five 11α,12α-diols and three 12α-acetoxy-11α-hydroxy compounds. The stereochemistry observed at C11/C12 is consistent with that of most other 11,12-diols and their monoesters (see Figures 25.17 through 25.19). The 8,17-diol system appears to be generated by nucleophilic attack by water on the 8α,17α-epoxide system from the β-face, as all isolated 8,17-diols here are *trans*-oriented on the lactone ring.

Both *trans* arrangements have however been isolated, indicative of epoxide ring opening by attack at either of the epoxide carbon atoms. Attack from the β-face is scarcely surprising, given the expected α-orientation of the precursor epoxide and steric constraints that block α-attack. The 8β,9α-diols are among a very limited number of naturally occurring unchlorinated briaranes known at this point in time that contain 8β-oxygen functionality.

25.6 Other Ungrouped Briaranes

A few ungrouped briaranes really don't fit into the classification system that has been used here: structure (**351**) (Figure 25.23) was proposed for briaexcavatin Y (Sung et al. 2009b). We consider structure (**352**) more likely in view of the fact that compound (**353**) was synthetically prepared from a 9α-hydroxy-8α,17α-briarane in DMSO-d_6 using the dimsyl anion (prepared by addition of NaH) as a base (Bowden et al. 1989). The difference between structures (**351**) and (**352**) is the stereochemistry at C8 and C9. Ring opening of the 8α,17α-epoxide would be expected to occur by an essentially S_N2 process at C8, leading to a *trans* rather than *cis* arrangement of the oxygen functions on C8 and C9, given that the 9α-OH (in the conformation that has been predominantly used throughout this chapter) is actually located on the β-face of the molecule, so S_N2 attack on the C8(17)-epoxide would be facilitated.

Briaexcavatin A (**354**) (Sung et al. 2006a) and excavatoid C (**355**) (Sung et al. 2009c) are briarane structures that have undergone Baeyer-Villiger-type oxidations in the 6-membered ring: briaexcavatin A has undergone C11–C12 bond cleavage, while the C12–C13 bond has been cleaved in excavatin C. These are at present the only examples of such oxidative ring cleavages that have been found from gorgonians and sea pens.

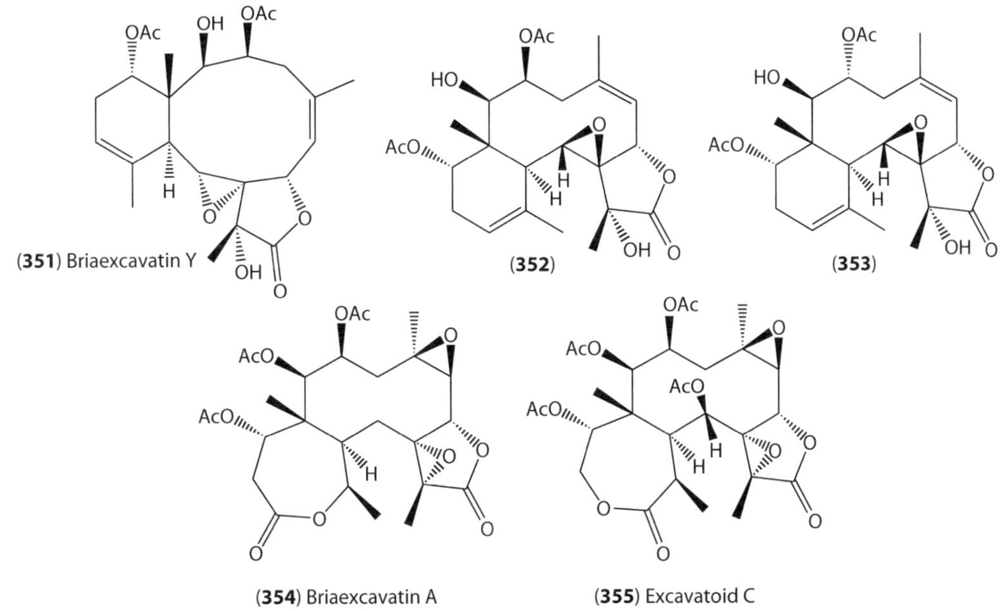

(**351**) Briaexcavatin Y   (**352**)   (**353**)

(**354**) Briaexcavatin A   (**355**) Excavatoid C

FIGURE 25.23
Briaranes that don't fit the structural categories previously presented.

25.7 Bioactivity and Structure

Over the years many different screening processes have been applied to marine natural products with some of the more common ones being investigations aimed at the following:

- Providing leads for cancer chemotherapy (cytostatic/cytotoxic activity)
- Modulation of the immune system (activation of the immune system for immuno-compromised patients, or suppression of the immune system for organ transplant therapy)
- Inhibition of inflammatory responses
- Discovery of new antimicrobial or antiviral agents
- Treatment of parasitic infections such as malaria and giardia

Other assays have also been used to look for insecticidal activity that might have application to agricultural production and to look for antifouling activity that might have industrial applications in the marine environment. An overview of the activities of briaranes in two of these areas (cytotoxicity and anti-inflammatory activity) follows:

25.8 Cytostatic Screening and Cytotoxicity Assays

The sophistication of assays used to indicate cytostatic or cytotoxic effects may vary

- Crude indicative assays (like brine shrimp lethality or inhibition of development of fertilized sea urchin eggs) may be used.
- *In vitro* assays using cell cultures of susceptible rapidly proliferating cells such as mouse leukemias are useful indicators of general cytotoxicity.
- *In vitro* assays involving multiple human cancer cell lines are capable of indicating cell-type specificity or the ability to act on multidrug-resistant (MDR) cancers.
- *In vivo* assays using animal models (typically mouse leukemias or nude mouse xenografts) are used to assess whether *in vitro* activity translates to activity in a living system.
- Cancer-specific biochemical enzyme assays can be used to specifically target the cancer cell and potentially induce apoptosis.

25.9 Briaranes that Disable the Multidrug-Resistant Pump in Cancer Cells

One strategy that can be utilized in the treatment of MDR cancers is to find molecules that effectively disable the MDR pump that results from overexpression of P-glycoprotein. Disabling the pump will improve the effectiveness of a chemotherapy treatment. A simple way to screen for molecules that disable the MDR pump is to grow cell cultures of MDR cancer cells in a medium with dye added. When the MDR pump is functioning, no dye gets into the cells, and when the MDR pump is disabled, the interior of the cell is colored. Another procedure compares the cytotoxicity of a drug such as colchicine against MDR cells in the absence and presence of the test material. These techniques have been used with a limited number of briaranes.

25.10 Cytotoxicity of Briaranes

The following discussion is an overview that utilizes specific examples to illustrate the views being expressed. It is in no manner meant to be a comprehensive literature review of reported briarane activities. In assays with briaranes, cytotoxicity methodologies have met with limited success; although many briaranes have been screened, as a general rule, the briarane system does not normally exhibit high cytotoxicity. Weak activity in a brine shrimp toxicity assay was, for example, reported for briareolate esters D (**7**), G (**10**), and I (**13**) (Mootoo et al. 1996), and moderate to weak cytostatic activity against two cancer cell lines has been reported for briareolate esters L (**11**) and M (**12**) (Gupta et al. 2011). Briaranes with 9-hydroxy groups initially appeared to be more cytotoxic than their esterified counterparts: three stecholides, stecholides A (**205**), B (**204**), and H (**287**) (of 20 stecholides that all contained 8,17-epoxy functionality that were screened), exhibited *in vitro* cytotoxic activity in the 5–10 µg/mL range against P388 murine leukemia. None of the 9-acetyl analogues of those three compounds exhibited significant cytotoxicity (Bloor et al. 1992). Since that report, many 9α-acetoxybriaranes have been reported to exhibit significant cytotoxic activity. Violide N (**243**) (which also has an 8,17-epoxide) was described as exhibiting cytotoxicity; however, it is a 9-acetoxybriarane (Iwagawa et al. 2000). Structurally, it is however a triol, with OH groups at C11, 12, and 20 that may compensate for the lack of a 9α-OH group. Another 9α-acetoxy-8,17-epoxide, briaexcavatolide P (**313**), exhibited cytotoxicity against P-388, A549, and HT-29 cancer cells with ED_{50} values of 0.9, 4.8, and 3.1 µg/mL, respectively (Wu et al. 2001). Although briaexcavatolide P lacks a C20-OH, it is still a diol with OH groups located on C3 and C12, so the presence or absence of a C20-OH would not appear to significantly influence binding for cytotoxicity. Juncenolide C (**89**), another 9α-acetoxy-20-hydroxybriarane (but with an 8α-OH instead of an 8α,17α-epoxide), also exhibited mild cytotoxicity in assays against human hepa adenocarcinoma (HEPA 59T/VGH) and oral epidermoid carcinoma (KB-16) cells at concentrations of 6.6 and 7.8 µg/mL, respectively (Shen et al. 2003). These observations support the premise that in order for briaranes to exhibit significant cytotoxicity, the presence of several binding groups such as hydroxyl or epoxide groups is required. As well as potentially playing a binding role (where location specificity would be a requirement), the presence of hydroxyl groups is probably an important factor for transport and absorption requirements: if the briarane is too lipophilic, aqueous solubility is likely to be an issue.

Recently, briareolate esters L (**11**) and M (**12**) were reported to contain a "springloaded (*E,Z*)-dienone Michael acceptor group that can form a reversible covalent bond to model sulfur-based nucleophiles" (Gupta et al. 2011). (The dienone system C5–C9 in fact has Z geometry for the C5 double bond and *E* for the C7 double bond; the *E*-geometry of C7 may well be a requirement for the reversible 1,4-Michael addition.) While the Z-C5 arrangement may well be important, its role has yet to be defined. Briareolate ester L exhibited EC_{50}

values in the 2–10 µM range against two cell lines, while M, which is more lipophilic, with a hexanoate ester replacing the α-OH on C12, was significantly less active. Activity was linked with the "*E,Z*-dienone" system and "reversible covalent bond formation to model sulfur nucleophiles." The authors concluded that the dienone with the correct geometry was required for the observed cytotoxicity, based on comparison with the assay result for briareolate N (**4**) that lacks the dienone system. This example would clearly provide cytotoxicity by an entirely different mechanism to previously discussed examples if the authors' conclusions are correct.

25.11 Anti-Inflammatory Activity of Briaranes

Three methods have been used to evaluate anti-inflammatory activity:

- Ability to inhibit mouse ear edema caused by application of an agonist
- Inhibition of elastase release and the generation of superoxide anion, in human neutrophils
- Suppression of COX-2 expression

Early work in this area (principally by Bob Jacobs at University of California, Santa Barbara, in collaboration with the Fenical and Faulkner groups) focused on alleviation of mouse ear edema. Junceellolide D (**124**) exhibited over 80% inhibition of inflammatory response in a mouse ear assay designed to assess topical efficacy (Shin et al. 1989). At a dose of 50 pg/ear, briareolides also displayed potential as anti-inflammatory agents with 71%, 55%, 75%, 85%, and 46% inhibition of inflammation, respectively, in the mouse ear assay for briareolides A–E (**285**, **286**, **224**, **223**, **301**) (Pordesimo et al. 1991).

Excavatolide C (**304**) (Sheu et al. 1998, Sung et al. 2008b), briaexcavatin E (**324**) (Sung et al. 2006b), frajunolides E (**121**) and J (**122**) (Liaw et al. 2008), and many other briaranes have been reported to exhibit weak inhibition of elastase release and superoxide anion generation at 10 µg/mL.

Excavatolide B (**307**) has been reported to significantly inhibit phorbol ester-induced vascular permeability in mice. This results in inhibition of edema formation by mechanisms that suppress COX-2, i-NOS, and MMP-9 expression in mouse skin. Excavatolide B was also shown to inhibit LPS-induced IL-6 and TNF-α expression in mouse bone marrow-derived dendritic cells. Structure–activity studies using the same assay indicated that acylation of the C12-OH group (to produce esters with 5–10 carbon atoms) resulted in reduced inhibitory bioactivity, with activity decreasing as the size of the 12-acyloxy substituent increased. Overall the SAR study led to conclusions that both the 8,17-epoxide and the 12-OH group were important in controlling the inflammatory response (Wei et al. 2011).

Brialaleptolides A–C (**258**, **260**, **261**) are further recent examples of 8,17-epoxybriaranes where screening that highlighted suppression of COX-2 expression, together with low-level cytotoxicity, suggested a possible application as leads for development of anticancer agents capable of inhibiting an inflammatory response (Joyner et al. 2011). Their structures are unexceptional in the realm of known briaranes, so the same activity may well be commonly observed for a larger number of briaranes when appropriate screening results become available.

25.12 Summary

The diverse range of unchlorinated briaranes that have been reported has been organized and is presented here in terms of chemical structural features. A brief overview of the biomedical potential of this group of metabolites is presented to highlight the potential that exists for developing this structure-based natural product library to identify lead structures for pharmaceutical research.

References

Anjaneyulu, A. S. R., V. L. Rao, V. G. Sastry, D. V. Rao, and H. Laatsch. 2007. Umbraculolide E, a new briarane diterpenoid from the Gorgonian *Gorgonella umbraculum*. *Nat. Prod. Commun.* 2:131–134.

Anjaneyulu, A. S. R., V. L. Rao, V. G. Sastry, M. J. R. V. Venugopal, and F. J. Schmitz. 2003. Juncins I-M, five new briarane diterpenoids from the Indian Ocean gorgonian *Junceella juncea* Pallas. *J. Nat. Prod.* 66(4):507–510.

Aoki, S., M. Okano, K. Matsui, T. Itoh, R. Satari, S. Akiyama, and M. Kobayashi. 2001. Brianthein A, a novel briarane-type diterpene reversing multidrug resistance in human carcinoma cell line, from the gorgonian *Briareum excavatum*. *Tetrahedron* 57(43):8951–8957.

Banjoo, D., A. R. Maxwell, B. S. Mootoo, A. J. Lough, S. McLean, and W. F. Reynolds. 1998. An unusual erythrolide containing a bicyclo [9.2.1] tetradecane skeleton. *Tetrahedron Lett.* 39:1469–1472.

Banjoo, D., B. S. Mootoo, R. S. Ramsewak, R. Sharma, A. J. Lough, S. McLean, and W. F. Reynolds. 2002. New erythrolides from the Caribbean gorgonian octocoral *Erythropodium caribaeorum*. *J. Nat. Prod.* 65(3):314–318.

Barsby, T. and J. Kubanek. 2005. Isolation and structure elucidation of feeding deterrent diterpenoids from the sea pansy, *Renilla reniformis*. *J. Nat. Prod.* 68(4):511–516.

Bloor, S. J., F. J. Schmitz, M. B. Hossain, and D. van der Helm. 1992. Diterpenoids from the gorgonian *Solenopodium stechei*. *J. Org. Chem.* 57(4):1205–1216.

Bowden, B. F., J. C. Coll, and G. M. König. 1990. Studies of Australian soft corals. XLVIII. New briaran diterpenoids from the gorgonian coral *Junceela gemmacea*. *Aust. J. Chem.* 43(1):151–159.

Bowden, B. F., J. C. Coll, W. Patalinghug, B. W. Skelton, I. Vasilescu, and A. H. White. 1987. Studies of Australian soft corals. XLII. Structure determination of new briaran derivatives from *Briareum stechei* (Coelenterata, Octocorallia, Gorgonacea). *Aust. J. Chem.* 40(12):2085–2096.

Bowden, B. F., J. C. Coll, and I. M. Vasilescu. 1989. Studies of Australian soft corals. XLVI. New diterpenes from a *Briareum* species (Anthozoa, Octocorallia, Gorgonacea). *Aust. J. Chem.* 42(10):1705–1726.

Cardellina, J. H., II, T. R., Jr., James, M. H. M. Chen, and J. Clardy. 1984. Structure of brianthein W, from the soft coral *Briareum polyanthes*. *J. Org. Chem.* 49(18):3398–3399.

Chen, Y.-P., S.-L. Wu, J.-H. Su, M.-R. Lin, W.-P. Hu, T.-L. Hwang, J.-H. Sheu, T.-Y. Fan, L.-S. Fang, and P.-J. Sung. 2006. Briaexcavatins G and H, Two new briaranes from the octocoral *Briareum excavatum*. *Bull. Chem. Soc. Jpn.* 79(12):1900–1905.

Clastres, A., A. Ahond, C. Poupat, P. Potier, and S. K. Kan. 1984a. Marine invertebrates of the New Caledonia lagoon. II. Structural study of three new diterpenes isolated from the sea pen *Pteroides laboutei*. *J. Nat. Prod.* 47(1):155–161.

Clastres, A., P. Laboute, A. Ahond, C. Poupat, and P. Potier. 1984b. Marine invertebrates of the New Caledonia lagoon. III. Structural study of three new diterpenes isolated from the sea pen *Cavernulina grandiflora*. *J. Nat. Prod.* 47(1):162–166.

Daly, M., M. R. Brugler, P. Cartwright, A. G. Collins, M. N. Dawson, D. G. Fautin, S. C. France et al. 2007. The phylum Cnidaria: A review of phylogenetic patterns and diversity 300 years after Linnaeus. *Zootaxa* 1668:127–182.

Dookran, R., D. Maharaj, B. S, Mootoo, R. Ramsewak, S. McLean, W. F. Reynolds, W. F. Tinto. 1993. Diterpenes from the gorgonian coral *Erythropodium caribaeorum* from the southern Caribbean. *J. Nat. Prod.* 56(7):1051–1056.

Dookran, R., D. Maharaj, B. S. Mootoo, R. Ramsewak, S. McLean, W. F. Reynolds, and W. F. Tinto. 1994. Briarane and asbestinane diterpenes from *Briareum asbestinum*. *Tetrahedron* 50(7):1983–1992.

Fu, X., F. J. Schmitz, and G. C. Williams. 1999. Malayenolides A-D, novel diterpenes from the Indonesian sea pen *Veretillum malayense*. *J. Nat. Prod.* 62(4):584–586.

García, M., J. Rodríguez, and C. Jiménez. 1999. Absolute structures of new briarane diterpenoids from *Junceella fragilis*. *J. Nat. Prod.* 62(2):257–260.

González, N., J. Rodríguez, R. G. Kerr, and C. Jiménez 2002. Cyclobutenbriarein A, the first diterpene with a tricyclo[8.4.0.03,6]tetradec-4-ene ring system isolated from the gorgonian *Briareum asbestinum*. *J. Org. Chem.* 67(15):5117–5123.

Groweiss, A., S. A. Look, and W. Fenical 1988. Solenolides, new antiinflammatory and antiviral diterpenoids from a marine octocoral of the genus *Solenopodium*. *J. Org. Chem.* 53(11):2401–2406.

Guerriero, A., M. D'Ambrosio, and F. Pietra. 1987. Verecynarmin A, a novel briarane diterpenoid isolated from both the Mediterranean nudibranch mollusk *Armina maculata* and its prey, the pennatulacean octocoral *Veretillum cynomorium*. *Helv. Chim. Acta* 70(4):984–991.

Guerriero, A., M. D'Ambrosio, and F. Pietra. 1988. Slowly interconverting conformers of the briarane diterpenoids Verecynarmin B, C, and D, isolated from the nudibranch mollusc *Armina maculata* and the pennatulacean octocoral *Veretillum cynomorium* of east Pyrenean waters. *Helv. Chim. Acta* 71:472–485.

Guerriero, A., M. D'Ambrosio, and F. Pietra. 1990. Isolation of the cembranoid preverecynarmin together with some briaranes, the verecynarmins, from both the nudibranch mollusk *Armina maculata* and its prey, the pennatulacean octocoral *Veretillum cynomorium* of east Pyrenean waters. *Helv. Chim. Acta* 73(2):277–283.

Guerriero, A., M. D'Ambrosio, and F. Pietra. 1995. 112. Bis-allylic reactivity of the funicolides, 5,8(17)-diunsaturated briarane diterpenes of the sea pen *Funiculina quadrangularis* from the Tuscan archipelago, leading to 16-nortaxane derivatives. *Helv. Chim. Acta* 78(6):1465–1478.

Gupta, P., U. Sharma, T. C. Schulz, E. S. Sherrer, A. B. McLean, A. J. Robins, and L. B. West, 2011. Bioactive diterpenoid containing a reversible "spring-loaded" (E,Z)-dieneone Michael acceptor. *Org. Lett.* 13(15):3920–3923.

He, H. Y. and D. J. Faulkner. 1991. New chlorinated diterpenes from the gorgonian *Junceella gemmacea*. *Tetrahedron* 47(20–21):3271–3280.

Hoshino, A., H. Mitome, S. Tamai, H. Takiyama, and H. Miyaoka. 2005. 8,17-Epoxybriarane diterpenoids, briaranolides A-J, from an Okinawan gorgonian *Briareum* sp. *J. Nat. Prod.* 68(9):1328–1335.

Hwang, T.-L., M.-R. Lin, W.-T. Tsai, H.-C. Yeh, W.-P. Hu, J.- H. Shen, and P.-J. Sung. 2008. New polyoxygenated briaranes from octocorals *Briareum excavatum* and *Ellisella robusta*. *Bull. Chem. Soc. Jpn.* 81(12):1638–1646.

Ishiyama, H., T. Okubo, T. Yasuda, Y. Takahashi, K. Iguchi, and J. Kobayashi. 2008. Brianodins A-D, briarane-type diterpenoids from soft coral *Pachyclavularia* sp. *J. Nat. Prod.* 71(4):633–636.

Ito, H., J. Iwasaki, Y. Sato, M. Aoyagi, K. Iguchi, and T. Yamori. 2007. Marine diterpenoids with a briarane skeleton from the Okinawan soft coral *Pachyclavularia violacea*. *Chem. Pharm. Bull.* 55(12):1671–1676.

Iwagawa, T., K. Babazono, M. Nakatani, M. Doe, Y. Mortmoto, and K. Takemura. 2005a. Briarane diterpenes from a gorgonian *Briareum* sp. *Heterocycles* 65(3):607–617.

Iwagawa, T., K. Babazono, H. Okamura, M. Nakatani, M. Doe, Y. Morimoto, M. Shiro, and K. Takamura. 2005b. Briviolides, new briarane diterpenes from a gorgonian *Briareum* sp. *Heterocycles* 65(9):2083–2093 [and Erratum *Heterocycles* 65(12):3093].

Iwagawa, T., T. Hirose, K. Takayama, H. Okamura, M. Nakatani, M. Doe, and K. Takemura. 2000. Violides N-P, New briarane diterpenes from a gorgonacean *Briareum* sp. *Heterocycles* 53(8):1789–1792.

Iwagawa, T., N. Nishitani, S. Kurosaki, H. Okamura, M. Nakatani, M. Doe, and K. Takemura. 2003. Briarlides, briarane diterpenes from a gorgonian *Briareum* sp. *J. Nat. Prod.* 66(11):1412–1415.

Iwagawa, T., N. Nishitani, M. Nakatani, M. Doe, Y. Morimoto, and K. Takemura. 2005c. Briarlides I-R, briarane diterpenes from a gorgonian *Briareum* sp. *J. Nat. Prod.* 68(1):31–35 [and Erratum *J. Nat. Prod.* 68(5):818].

Iwagawa, T., K. Takayama, H. Okamura, M. Nakatani, and M. Doe. 1999. New briarane diterpenes from a gorgonacean *Briareum* sp. *Heterocycles* 51(7):1653–1659 [and Erratum *Heterocycles* 53: 1237].

Iwasaki. J., H. Ito, M. Aoyagi, Y. Sato, and K. Iguchi. 2006. Briarane-type diterpenoids from the Okinawan soft coral *Pachyclavularia violacea*. *J. Nat. Prod.* 69(1):2–6.

Joyner, P. M., A. L, Waters, R. B, Williams, D. R. Powell, N. B. Janakiram, C. V. Rao, and R. H. Cichewicz. 2011. Briarane diterpenes diminish COX-2 expression in human colon adenocarcinoma cell. *J. Nat. Prod.* 74(4):857–861.

Keifer, P. A., K. L. Rinehart, Jr., and I. R. Hooper. 1986. Renillafoulins, antifouling diterpenes from the sea pansy *Renilla reniformis* (Octocorallia). *J. Org. Chem.* 51(23): 4450–4454.

Ksebati, M. B. and F. J. Schmitz. 1986. Diterpenes from a soft coral, *Minabea* sp., from Truk lagoon. *Bull. Soc. Chim. Belges* 95(9–10):835–851.

Kwak, J. H., F. J. Schmitz, and G. C. Williams. 2001. Milolides, new briarane diterpenoids from the Western Pacific octocoral *Briareum stechei*. *J. Nat. Prod.* 64(6):754–760.

Kwak, J. H., F. J. Schmitz, and G. C. Williams. 2002. Milolides G-N, new briarane diterpenoids from the western Pacific octocoral *Briareum stechei*. *J. Nat. Prod.* 65(5):704–708.

Liaw, C.-C., Y.-C. Shen, Y.-S. Lin, T.-L. Hwang, Y.-H. Kuo, and A. T. Khalil. 2008. Frajunolides E-K, briarane diterpenes from *Junceella fragilis*. *J. Nat. Prod.* 71(9):1551–1556.

Lievens, S. C., H. Hope, and T. F. Molinski. 2004. New 3-oxo-chol-4-en-24-oic acids from the marine soft coral *Eleutherobia* sp. *J. Nat. Prod.* 67(12):2130–2132.

Look, S. A., W. Fenical, D. van Engen, and J. Clardy. 1984. Erythrolides: Unique marine diterpenoids interrelated by a naturally-occurring di-π-methane rearrangement. *J. Am. Chem. Soc.* 106:5026–5027.

Maharaj, D., B. S. Mootoo, A. J. Lough, S. McLean, W. F. Reynolds, and W. F. Tinto. 1992. Methyl briareolate, the first briarein diterpene containing a C-19 methyl ester. *Tetrahedron Lett.* 33(50):7761–7764.

Maharaj, D., K. O. Pascoe, and W. F. Tinto. 1999. Briarane diterpenes from the gorgonian octocoral *Erythropodium caribaeorum* from the northern Caribbean. *J. Nat. Prod.* 62(2):313–314.

Mootoo, B. S., R. Ramsewak, R., R. Sharma, W. F. Tinto, A. J. Lough, S. McLean, W. F. Reynolds, J.-P. Yang, and M. Yu. 1996. Further briareolate esters and briareolides from the Caribbean gorgonian octocoral *Briareum asbestinum*. *Tetrahedron* 52(30):9953–9962.

Natori, T., H. Kawai, and N. Fusetani. 1990. Tubiporein, a novel diterpene from a Japanese soft coral *Tubipora* sp. *Tetrahedron Lett.* 31(5):689–690.

Neve, J. E., B. J. McCool, and B. F. Bowden. 1999. Excavatolides N-T, new briaran diterpenes from the Western Australian gorgonian *Briareum excavatum*. *Aust. J. Chem.* 52(5):359–366.

Ospina, C. A. and A. D. Rodriguez. 2006. Bioactive compounds from the gorgonian *Briareum polyanthes*. Correction of structures of four asbestinane-type diterpenes. *J. Nat. Prod.* 69(12):1721–1727.

Pham, N. B., M. S. Butler, P. C. Healy, and R. J. Quinn. 2000. Anthoptilides A-E, new briarane diterpenes from the Australian sea pen *Anthoptilum cf. Kukenthali*. *J. Nat. Prod.* 63(3):318–321.

Pordesimo, E. O., F. J. Schmitz, L. S. Ciereszko, M. B. Hossain, and D. Van der Helm 1991. New briarein diterpenes from the Caribbean gorgonians *Erythropodium caribaeorum* and *Briareum* sp. *J. Org. Chem.* 56(7):2344–2357.

Qi, S.-H., S. Zhang, P.-Y. Qian, Z.-H. Xiao, and M.-Y. Li. 2006. Ten new antifouling briarane diterpenoids from the South China sea gorgonian *Junceella juncea*. *Tetrahedron* 62(39):9123–9130.

Ravi, B. N., J.F. Marwood, and R. J. Wells. 1980. Three new diterpenes from the sea pen *Scytalium tentaculatum*. *Aust. J. Chem.* 33(10):2307–2316.

Rodríguez, A. D., C. Ramírez, and O. M. Cóbar. 1996. Briareins C-L, 10 new briarane diterpenoids from the common Caribbean gorgonian *Briareum asbestinum*. *J. Nat. Prod.* 59(1):15–22.

Schmitz, F. J., M. M. Schultz, J. Siripitayananon, M. B. Hossain, and D. van der Helm. 1993. New diterpenes from the gorgonian *Solenopodium excavatum*. *J. Nat. Prod.* 56(8):1339–1349.

Shen, Y.-C., Y.-H. Chen, T.-L. Hwang, J.-H. Guh, and A. T. Khalila. 2007. Four new briarane diterpenoids from the gorgonian coral *Junceella fragilis*. *Helv. Chim. Acta* 90(7):1391–1398.

Shen, Y.-C., Y.-C. Lin, C.-L. Ko, and L.-T. Wang. 2003. New briaranes from the Taiwanese gorgonian *Junceella juncea*. *J. Nat. Prod.* 66:302–305.

Sheu, J.-H., Y.-P. Chen, T.-L. Hwang, M. Y. Chiang, L.-S. Fang, and P.-J. Sung. 2006. Junceellolides J-L, 11,20-epoxybriaranes from the gorgonian coral *Junceella fragilis*. *J. Nat. Prod.* 69(2):269–273.

Sheu, J.-H., P.-J. Sung, M.-C. Cheng, H.-Y. Liu, L.-S. Fang, C.-Y. Duh, and M. Y. Chiang. 1998. Novel cytotoxic diterpenes, excavatolides A-E, isolated from the Formosan gorgonian *Briareum excavatum*. *J. Nat. Prod.* 61(5):602–608.

Sheu, J.-H., P.-J. Sung, L.-H. Huang, S.-F. Lee, T. Wu, B.-Y. Chang, C.-Y. Duh, L.-S. Fang, K. Soong, and T.-J. Lee. 1996. New cytotoxic briarane diterpenes from the Formosan gorgonian *Briareum* sp. *J. Nat. Prod.* 59(10):935–938.

Sheu, J.-H., P.-J. Sung, J.-H. Su, H.-Y. Liu, C.-Y. Duh, and M. Y. Chiang. 1999a. Briaexcavatolides A-J, new diterpenes from the gorgonian *Briareum excavatum*. *Tetrahedron* 55(51):14555–14564.

Sheu, J. H., P.-J. Sung, J.-H. Su, G.-H. Wang, C.-Y. Duh, Y. C. Shen, M. Y. Chiang, and I. T. Chen. 1999b. Excavatolides U–Z, New briarane diterpenes from the gorgonian *Briareum excavatum*. *J. Nat. Prod.* 62(10):1415–1420.

Shin, J., M. Park, and W. Fenical. 1989. The junceellolides, new anti-inflammatory diterpenoids of the briarane class from the Chinese gorgonian *Junceella fragilis*. *Tetrahedron* 45(6):1633–1638.

Su, J.-H., B.-Y. Chen, T.-L. Hwang, Y.-H. Chen, I.-C. Huang, M.-R. Lin, J.-J. Chen et al. 2010. Excavatoids L-N, new 12-hydroxybriaranes from the cultured octocoral *Briareum excavatum* (Briareidae). *Chem. Pharm. Bull.* 58(5):662–665.

Su, J.-H., P.-J. Sung, Y,-H. Kuo, C.-H. Hsu, and J.-H. Sheu. 2007. Briarenolides A-C, briarane diterpenoids from the gorgonian coral *Briareum* sp. *Tetrahedron* 63(34):8282–8285.

Subrahmanyam, C., R. Kulatheeswaran, and R.S. Ward. 1998. Briarane diterpenes from the Indian Ocean gorgonian *Gorgonella umbraculum*. *J. Nat. Prod.* 61(9):1120–1122.

Subrahmanyam, C., R. Sreekantha, and R. S. Ward. 2000. Umbraculolides B-D, further briarane diterpenes from the gorgonian *Gorgonella umbraculum Tetrahedron* 56(26):4585–4588.

Sung, P.-J., P.-C. Chang, L.-S. Fang, J.-H. Sheu, W.-C. Chen, Y.-P. Chen, and M.-R. Lin. 2005a. Survey of briarane-related diterpenoids-Part II. *Heterocycles* 65(1):195–204.

Sung, P.-J., C.-H. Chao, Y.-P. Chen, J.-H. Su, W.-P. Hu, and J.-H. Sheu. 2006a. Briaexcavatins A and B, novel briaranes from the octocoral *Briareum excavatum*. *Tetrahedron Lett.* 47(2):167–170.

Sung, P.-J., Y.-P. Chen, S.-L. Hwang, W.-P. Hu, L.-S. Fang, Y.-C. Wu, J.-J. Li, and J.-H. Sheu. 2006b. Briaexcavatins C-F, four new briarane-related diterpenoids from the Formosan octocoral *Briareum excavatum* (Briareidae). *Tetrahedron* 62(24):5686–5691.

Sung, P.-J., B.-Y. Chen, M.-R. Lin, T.-L. Hwang, W.-H. Wang, J.-H. Sheu, and Y.-C. Wu. 2009a. Excavatoids E and F: discovery of two new briaranes from the cultured octocoral *Briareum excavatum*. *Mar. Drugs* 7(3):472–482.

Sung, P.-J. and T.-Y. Fan. 2003. 9-O-Deacetylumbraculolide A, a new diterpenoid from the gorgonian *Junceella fragilis*. *Heterocycles* 60(5):1199–1202.

Sung, P.-J., T.-Y. Fan, L.-S. Fang, S.-L. Wu, J.-J. Li, M.-C. Chen, Y.-M. Cheng, and G.-H. Wang. 2003. Briarane derivatives from the gorgonian coral *Junceella fragilis*. *Chem. Pharm. Bull.* 51(12):1429–1431.

Sung, P.-J., W.-P. Hu, L.-S. Fang, T.-Y. Fan, and J.-J. Wang. 2005b. Briarenol A, a new diterpenoid from a gorgonian *Briareum* sp. (Briareidae). *Nat. Prod. Res.* 19(7):689–694.

Sung, P.-J., W.-P. Hu, S.-L. Wu, J.-H. Su, L.-S. Fang, J.-J. Wang, and J.-H. Sheu. 2004a. Briaexcavatolides X–Z, three new briarane-related derivatives from the gorgonian coral *Briareum excavatum*. *Tetrahedron* 60(40):8975–8979.

Sung, P.-J., G.-Y. Li, Y.-D. Su, M.-R. Lin, Y.-C. Chang, T.-H. Kung, C.-S. Lin et al. 2010. Excavatoids O and P, new 12-hydroxybriaranes from the octocoral *Briareum excavatum*. *Mar. Drugs* 8(10):2639–2646.

Sung, P.-J., M.-R. Lin, W.-C. Chen, L.-S. Fang, C.-K. Lu, and J.-H. Sheu. 2004b. Fragilide A, a novel diterpenoid from *Junceella fragilis*. *Bull. Chem. Soc. Jpn.* 77(6):1229–1230.

Sung, P.-J., M.-R. Lin, M.Y. Chiang, and T.-L. Hwang. 2009b. Briaexcavatins V–Z, discovery of new briaranes from a cultured octocoral *Briareum excavatum*. *Bull. Chem. Soc. Jpn.* 82(8):987–996.

Sung, P.-J., M.-R. Lin, and L.-S. Fang. 2004c. Briarane diterpenoids from the Formosan gorgonian coral *Junceella fragilis*. *Chem. Pharm. Bull.* 52(12):1504–1506.

Sung, P.-J., M.-R. Lin, T.-L. Hwang, T.-Y. Fan, W.-C. Su, C.-C. Ho, L.-S. Fang, and W.-H. Wang. 2008a. Briaexcavatins M-P, four new briarane-related diterpenoids from cultured octocoral *Briareum excavatum* (Briareidae). *Chem. Pharm. Bull.* 56(7):930–935.

Sung, P.-J., M.-R. Lin, Y.-D. Su, M. Y. Chiang, W.-P. Hu, J.-H. Su, M.-C. Cheng, T.-L. Hwang, and J.-H. Sheu. 2008b. New briaranes from the octocorals *Briareum excavatum* (Briareidae) and *Junceella fragilis* (Ellisellidae). *Tetrahedron* 64:2596–2604.

Sung, P.-J., C.-H. Pai, T.-L. Hwang, T.-Y. Fan, J.-H. Su, J.-J. Chen, L.-S. Fang, W.-H. Wang, and J.-H. Sheu. 2008c. Junceols D-H, new polyoxygenated briaranes from sea whip gorgonian coral *Junceella juncea* (Ellisellidae) *Chem. Pharm. Bull.* 56(9):1276–1281.

Sung, P.-J., C.-H. Pai, Y.-D. Su, T.-L. Hwang, F.-W. Kuo, T.-Y. Fan, and J.-J. Li. 2008d. New 8-hydroxybriarane diterpenoids from the gorgonians *Junceella juncea* and *Junceella fragilis* (Ellisellidae). *Tetrahedron* 64(19):4224–4232.

Sung, P.-J., J.-H. Sheu, W.-H. Wang, L.-S. Fang, H.-M. Chung, C.-H. Pai, Y.-D. Su et al. 2008e. Survey of briarane-related diterpenoids-Part III. *Heterocycles* 75(11):2627–2648.

Sung, P.-J., J.-H. Su, C.-Y. Duh, M. Y. Chiang, and J.-H. Sheu. 2001. Briaexcavatolides K-N, new briarane diterpenes from the gorgonian *Briareum excavatum*. *J. Nat. Prod.* 64(3):318–323.

Sung, P.-J., Y.-D. Su, G.-Y. Li, M. Y. Chiang, M.-R. Lin, I.-C. Huang, J.-J. Li, L.-S. Fang, and W.-H. Wang. 2009c. Excavatoids A–D, new polyoxygenated briaranes from the octocoral *Briareum excavatum*. *Tetrahedron* 65(34):6918–6924.

Sung, P.-J., J.-H. Su, G.-H. Wang, S.-F. Lin, C.-Y. Duh, and J. H. Sheu. 1999. Excavatolides F-M, new briarane diterpenes from the gorgonian *Briareum excavatum*. *J. Nat. Prod.* 62(3):457–463.

Sung, P.-J., J.-H. Su, W.-H. Wang, J.-H. Sheu, L.-S. Fang, Y.-C. Wu, Y.-H. Chen, H.-M. Chung, Y.-D. Su, and Y.-C. Chang. 2011. Survey of briarane-related diterpenoids-Part IV. *Heterocycles* 83(6):1241–1258.

Sung, P.-J., W.-T. Tsai, M. Y. Chiang, Y.-M. Su, and J. Kuo. 2007. Robustolides A–C, three new briarane-type diterpenoids from the female gorgonian coral *Ellisella robusta* (Ellisellidae). *Tetrahedron* 63(32):7582–7588.

Sung, P.-J., S.-L. Wu, H.-J. Fang, M. Y. Chiang, J.-Y. Wu, L.-S. Fang, and J.-H. Sheu. 2000. Junceellolides E-G, new briarane diterpenes from the west Pacific ocean gorgonian *Junceella fragilis*. *J. Nat. Prod.* 63(11):1483–1487.

Taglialatela-Scafati, O., K. S. Craig, D. Rebérioux, M. Roberge, and R. J. Andersen. 2003. Briarane, erythrane, and aquariane diterpenoids from the Caribbean gorgonian *Erythropodium caribaeorum*. *Eur. J. Org. Chem.* 2003:3515–3523.

Taglialatela-Scafati, O., U. Deo-Jangra, M. Campbell, M. Roberge, and R. J. Andersen. 2002. Diterpenoids from cultured *Erythropodium caribaeorum*. *Org. Lett.* 4(23):4085–4088.

Tanaka, C., Y. Yamamoto, M. Otsuka, J. Tanaka, T. Ichiba, G. Marriott, R. Rachmat, and T. Higa. 2004. Briarane diterpenes from two species of octocorals, *Ellisella* sp. and *Pteroeides* sp. *J. Nat. Prod.* 67(8):1368–1373.

Uchio, Y., Y. Fukazawa, B. F. Bowden, and J. C. Coll. 1989. New diterpenes from an Australian *Pachyclavularia* species (Coelenterata, Anthozoa, Octocorallia). *Tennen Yuki Kagobutsu Toronkai Koen Yoshishu* 31:548–553.

Wang, S.-S., Y.-H. Chen, J.-Y. Chang, T.-L. Hwang, C.-H. Chen, A. T. Khalil, and Y.-C. Shen. 2009. Juncenolides H– K, new briarane diterpenoids from *Junceella juncea*. *Helv. Chim. Acta* 92(10):2092–2100.

Watanabe, K., M. Sekine, and K. Iguchi. 2003. Isolation and structures of new halogenated prostanoids from the Okinawan soft coral *Clavularia viridis*. *J. Nat. Prod.* 66(11):1434–1440.

Wei, W.-C., S.-Y. Lin, Y.-J. Chen, C.-C. Wen, C.-Y. Huang, A. Palanisamy, N.-S. Yang, and J.-H. Sheu. 2011. Topical application of marine briarane-type diterpenes effectively inhibits 12-O-tetradecanoylphorbol-13-acetate-induced inflammation and dermatitis in murine skin. *J. Biomed. Sci.* 18:94–106.

Wratten, S. J. and D. J. Faulkner. 1978. Some diterpenes from the sea pen *Stylatula* sp. *Tetrahedron* 35(16):1907–1912.

Wu, S.-L., P.-J. Sung, M. Y. Chiang, J.-Y. Wu, and J.-H. Sheu. 2001. New polyoxygenated briarane diterpenoids, briaexcavatolides O–R, from the gorgonian *Briareum excavatum*. *J. Nat. Prod.* 64(11):1415–1420.

Wu, S.-L., P.-J. Sung, J.-H. Su, and J.-H. Sheu. 2003. Briaexcavatolides S-V, four new briaranes from a Formosan gorgonian *Briareum excavatum*. *J. Nat. Prod.* 66(9):1252–1256.

Wu, S.-L., P.-J. Sung, J.-H. Su, G.-H. Wang, and J.-H. Sheu. 2004. Briaexcavatolide W, a new diterpenoid from *Briareum excavatum*. *Heterocycles* 63(4):895–898.

Zhang, W., Y.-W. Guo, E. Mollo, and G. Cimino. 2004. Junceellonoids A and B, two new briarane diterpenoids from the Chinese gorgonian *Junceella fragilis*. *Helv. Chim. Acta* 84(9):2341–2345.

26

Application of Marine Collagen–Based Scaffolds in Bone Tissue Engineering

Ramjee Pallela, Jayachandran Venkatesan, Ira Bhatnagar,
Yoon-Bo Shim, and Se-Kwon Kim

CONTENTS

26.1 Introduction

Collagen is one of the important extracellular matrix (ECM) biomacromolecules that have been under extensive exploration for the past several decades. Besides its characteristic mechanical, hemostatic, and cell-binding properties, collagen has good biological compatibility toward the physiobiological systems and can be degraded into physiologically tolerable compounds (Song et al. 2006). Numerous innovations occurred in the field of collagen-based biomaterials ranging from injectable collagen solutions to bone regeneration scaffolds. Multiple cross-linking patterns within the collagens as well as with other biopolymers were explored in order to improve the generation of tissue and its function. The easy availability and high versatility, compatibility, and degradability are advantageous factors for utilizing collagens in the preparation of biomimetic scaffolds for tissue engineering applications (Parenteau-Bareil et al. 2010). The properties of collagen to be used in scaffold preparation further include osteocompatibility; minimal potential for antigenicity after removal of telopeptides; adhesiveness and cohesiveness; being fibrous but nonfriable; fibers appear to become incorporated into the new tissue matrix; suturable; high porosity gives space for neohistogenesis; can be combined with other materials; medium can be perfused; and fluid pressure can be transduced (Glowacki and Mizuno 2008).

Numerous collagen-dependent scaffolds have been developed by the utilization of various naturally derived collagens; being for example, bovine and porcine sources are traditionally been used in the preparation and application of collagen scaffolds in biology and medicine (Rodrigues et al. 2003). However, marine-derived collagens are gaining tremendous importance as they are proved to be less immunogenic and can avoid secondary complications occurring within the human body (Rao et al. 2011;

Pallela et al. 2012). The importance of these marine-derived, collagen-based biomaterials is, however, not put forward toward the clinical application in biomedical engineering. Hence, it is very necessary to understand the biophysicochemical properties as well as the physiofunctional role of these novel tissue engineering materials. Moreover, the biomedical implications of marine-derived collagen scaffolds in bone tissue engineering are to be well focused to meet the current-day necessities of human beings. A brief introduction of the collagen and their marine sources, and application of marine-derived collagen scaffolds in bone tissue engineering along with the recent advancements are presented in the chapter.

26.2 Collagen

Collagen belongs to a family of highly characteristic fibrous proteins present in multicellular animals and is the most abundant protein found in mammals (Scheibel 2005; Rao et al. 2011). Collagen serves as the structural backbone or scaffolding of animals and plays a crucial role in maintaining structural integrity as well as a regulating role in developing tissues. It is the common protein (about 30% of the human body) that provides texture, resiliency, and shape and is found in most of the animal connective tissues, namely, dermis, bones, tendons, cartilage (hyaline), ligaments, blood vessels, teeth, cornea, intervertebral disks, vitreous bodies, and placenta (fetal) (Prockop 1998). Although the function of the recently discovered collagen is still unknown, there are around 29 different types of collagen that are discovered and classified under several groups, based on their primary structures or forms of supramolecular organization and function (Rao et al. 2011). The diverse structural and functional properties of collagen make them occupy a significant level in tissue engineering and biomedical engineering fields. The current-day healthcare demands of human beings depend more on the collagen-based food, cosmeceutical, pharmaceutical, and biomedical products to combat not only the aging complications but also the emergency medical needs, for example, in the case of skin- and bone-damaged patients due to various accidents.

26.2.1 Properties of Collagen as Bone Tissue Engineering Scaffold

Collagen has unique applications in drug delivery systems, for example, collagen shields in ophthalmology, sponges for burns/wounds, minipellets and tablets for protein delivery, gel formulation in combination with liposomes for sustained drug delivery, as controlling material for transdermal delivery, and nanoparticles for gene delivery and basic matrices for various cell culture systems (Lee et al. 2001). Although the applications vary depending on the type and occurrence of disease in the human body, the properties of collagen are almost the same in each physiofunctional significance of various collagens.

The networking and porosity formation of collagen has been considered to be of greater advantage, because the mechanoelastic and tensile behavior of the collagen in 2D and 3D scaffold systems is very unique and suitable for various biomedical applications (Bonebreak 2005). These postulations are well supported by Boyce and Arruda, who narrated that the hyperelastic materials such as collagen produce a nonlinear stress–strain curve characterized by two regions. At small strains, the material exhibits low stiffness as the collagen fibers unkink and align themselves parallel to the stretch direction (Boyce and Arruda 2000). At higher strains, the collagen fibers have been sufficiently aligned and begin to stretch, resulting in a higher stiffness region. Unlike materials that exhibit a linear stress–strain relationship, the nonlinear behavior of hyperelastic materials in tension is not as easily defined. A constitutive model derived from the mechanical behavior of long-chain molecules such as those found in fibrous collagen networks can predict the mechanical response of scaffolds in tension. According to the Arruda–Boyce model of a scaffold, the stress–strain behavior of a collagen fiber network is primarily governed by the changes in entropy as the randomly oriented network becomes more organized with stretching. The elastic behavior of the network depends on two parameters: the number of rigid links N and the collagen fiber density n, which is most directly associated with the initial stiffness of the scaffold.

Biologically speaking, collagen and collagen porous scaffolds possess the excellent quality of biocompatibility and controllable biodegradability that signifies its role in tissue engineering of cartilage and bone where they serve as support and template for cell infiltration, proliferation, and differentiation (Ma et al. 2004). Moreover, with a combination of biomimetic bone materials like hydroxyapatite (HAp) and chitosan, a multicomponent scaffold system is well suitable for bone tissue engineering applications (Pallela et al. 2012). Hence, the mechanobiological properties of the collagen scaffolds are very important to consider them as potential biomedical materials/devises in bone tissue engineering.

26.2.2 Various Marine Sources of Collagen

The diversity in marine environment signifies the development and application of novel chemicobiological molecules used in various biomedical fields. The importance of these molecules is increasing day by day because of the increased need of these molecules to combat various health problems. Despite the chemical molecules, protein molecules like collagen from marine origin are gaining their potentiality toward the development of various pharmaceutical, cosmeceutical, and biomedical materials. Collagen is found to be ubiquitous in many marine organisms, namely, sponges (Porifera), jellyfish (Cnidaria), octopus and squid (Mollusca), and fish (Pisces) (Melnick 1958; Kuo et al. 1991; Trotter et al. 1994; Sivakumar and Chandrakasan 1998; Mizuta et al. 2003a,b; Sadowska et al. 2003; Kim and Park 2004; Song et al. 2006; In Jeong et al. 2007).

Sponge species belonging to the class Demospongiae (Porifera) structurally consist of a skeleton made up of siliceous spicules or spongin/collagen fibers or both. In the latter case, the spongin or collagen fibers provide a matrix in which the spicules are embedded. The abundance of silica as well as calcium and carbonate ions in the ancient marine environments, on the one hand, and the existence of chitin and collagen primary scaffolds, on the other hand, make them suitable for several biomimetic applications (Ehrlich 2010).

Scyphozoan jellyfish species have been proved to have collagens, where the mesoglea supports the attachment, spreading, and migration of anthozoan cells *in vitro* (Frank and Rinkevich 1999). In the later studies, the presence and role of collagens in various species have been well recognized for their biomedical applications (Song et al. 2006).

The elastic extensibility of proximal byssus in mussel is extraordinarily due to the construction of collagen-like filaments formed as byssal threads (Coyne et al. 1997; Qin and Waite 1998). Recent studies revealed that the main components of byssal threads include a set of various collagen-like structural proteins (preCols) consisting of a collagenous core sequence flanked by globular domains (Hagenau et al. 2011).

Several animals of the phylum Mollusca possess unique muscular arrangement made up of collagen and collagen-like proteins that are involved in various functional mechanisms of the animals like mussel, squid, cuttlefish, and octopus (Gosline and

Shadwick 1983; Kier 1988). The sucker musculature is enclosed on its inner and outer surface by sheets of connective tissue fibers forming an inner and outer connective tissue capsule. The fibers of the capsules are highly birefringent and show staining characteristics typical of collagen (Kier and Smith 2002).

On the other hand, certain species of echinoderms also possess collagen fibrils to fulfill their functional purpose. Echinoderms have collagenous tissues that are similar to vertebrate collagens; however, they can be manipulated to easily relinquish their collagen fibrils, which provides an excellent opportunity for the exploration of the native fibrillar structure (Szulgit 2007). The tissues of these animals have the unique capacity to rapidly and reversibly alter their mechanical properties, resembling the collagenous tissues of other phyla consisting of collagen fibrils in a nonfibrillar matrix (Trotter et al. 1994). According to these studies, sea cucumber collagens are of the same length as those from vertebrate collagen fibrils, and they assemble into fibrils with the repeated band periodicity similar to that of vertebrate collagen fibrils.

Not only the marine invertebrate collagen sources, but also marine vertebrate sources are huge and enormous and show much similarity to the human collagens. Fish would be the richest source of collagens in terms of its production and application in various bioprocess and biomedical engineering. Several species of fish are well investigated for their tissue collagen and gelatin toward various applications in functional foods, nutraceuticals, and important food ingredients of medical and biomedical importance (Hayashi et al. 2012). Other marine mammals (e.g., baleen whales, sea otters, and walruses) have significant mean bone collagen that is well explored for various biophysicochemical analyses (Schoeninger and DeNiro 1984). Few of the marine collagen sources with species names are given in Table 26.1.

26.2.3 Marine-Based Collagen Scaffolds in Bone Tissue Engineering

Skeletal bones mainly comprise collagen (predominantly type I) and carbonate-substituted HAp; both are osteoconductive components. Thus, an implant developed from such components is likely to mimic and use more than a monolithic device (Wahl and Czernuszka 2006). Collagen along with HAp and other natural and synthetic macromolecules was found to enhance the osteoblast differentiation, thereby accelerating osteogenesis in their combined form. However, the selection of a suitable scaffold matrix is critical and crucial for cell-based bone tissue engineering studies (Lin et al. 2011). Current strategies for bone repair have limitations for synthetic graft materials or for the scaffolds that support *ex vivo* bone tissue engineering. Hence, biomimetic strategies have been considered to be more important for the investigation of naturally occurring porous structures toward their use as templates for bone growth (Clarke et al. 2011).

Marine organisms like corals, algae (diatoms), and sponges are rich in mineralized porous structures, some of which are currently being used as bone graft materials (Biocoral, Pro Osteon 200R, Pro Osteon 500R, Algipore, etc.) and others are in their early stage of development. Despite these structural mineralized materials, collagen from marine organisms has also been considered as functionally important bone grafting material. Isolation, characterization, and design of collagen and its composite scaffolds for their *in vitro* and *in vivo* application as biomedical materials for bone tissue engineering is a continuous process of searching from marine sources (Rao et al. 2011). The structure and chemical composition of marine sponges, possessing calcareous or siliceous spicules and/or collagen/spongin, mimic the cancellous architecture of bone tissue and the complex canal system to create a porous biomimetic environment that is ideal for cellular integration within the bone matrix and promotes osteogenesis *in vitro* (Green et al. 2003; Lin et al. 2011).

TABLE 26.1

List of a Few Marine Animals Explored for Collagen and Collagen-Like Proteins

Name of the Animal[a]	Classification (Class: Phylum)	References
Sponges		
Chondrosia reniformis	Demospongiae: Porifera	Swatschek et al. (2002)
Several species of the genus *Ircinia* (e.g., *I. fusca*)	Demospongiae: Porifera	Pallela et al. (2011, 2012)
Suberites domuncula	Demospongiae: Porifera	Krasko et al. (2000)
Spongia sp.	Demospongiae: Porifera	Green et al. (2003)
Coelenterates		
Rhizostoma pulmo	Scyphozoa: Cnidaria	Addad et al. (2011)
Aurelia aurita	Scyphozoa: Cnidaria	
Cotylorhiza tuberculata	Scyphozoa: Cnidaria	
Pelagia noctiluca	Scyphozoa: Cnidaria	
Rhopilema asamushi	Scyphozoa: Cnidaria	Nagai et al. (2000)
Rhopilema esculentum	Scyphozoa: Cnidaria	
Stomolophus meleagris	Scyphozoa: Cnidaria	Nagai et al. (1999); Song et al. (2006)
Stomolophus nomurai	Scyphozoa: Cnidaria	Kimura et al. (1983); Miura and Kimura (1985)
Aurelia coerulea	Scyphozoa: Cnidaria	Kimura et al. (1983)
Nemopilema nomurai	Scyphozoa: Cnidaria	Sugahara et al. (2006)
Metridium dianthus	Anthozoa: Cnidaria	Katzman and Kang (1972)
Annelids		
Neanthes japonica	Polychaeta: Annelida	Kimura and Tanzer (1977)
Nereis virens	Polychaeta: Annelida	
Heterodrilus paucifascis, H. pentcheffi, H. flexuosus, H. minisetosus	Clitellata: Annelida	Sjölin and Gustavsson (2008)
Molluscs		
Mytilus galloprovincialis	Bivalvia: Mollusca	Hagenau et al. (2011)
Crassostrea gigas	Bivalvia: Mollusca	Mizuta et al. (2005)
Loliolus japonicus	Cephalopoda: Mollusca	Fu et al. (2008)
Doryteuthis gahi	Cephalopoda: Mollusca	Sadowska and Sikorski (1987)
Illex argentinus	Cephalopoda: Mollusca	
Octopus bimaculoides	Cephalopoda: Mollusca	Kier and Smith (2002)
Thysanoteuthis rhombus	Cephalopoda: Mollusca	Nagai (2004)
Callistoctopus ornatus	Cephalopoda: Mollusca	Nagai et al. (2002)
Todarodes pacificus	Cephalopoda: Mollusca	Nam et al. (2008)
Echinoderms		
Eucidaris tribuloides	Echinoidea: Echinodermata	Trotter et al. (1994)
Cucumaria frondosa	Holothuroidea: Echinodermata	
Apostichopus japonicus	Holothuroidea: Echinodermata	Saito et al. (2002)
Asterias amurensis	Asteroidea: Echinodermata	Kimura et al. (1993)
Heliocidaris crassispina	Echinoidea: Echinodermata	Nagai and Suzuki (2000a)
Asthenosoma ijimai	Echinoidea: Echinodermata	Omura et al. (1996)
Holothuria forskali	Holothuroidea: Echinodermata	Bailey et al. (1982)

(continued)

TABLE 26.1 (continued)

List of a Few Marine Animals Explored for Collagen and Collagen-Like Proteins

Name of the Animal[a]	Classification (Class: Phylum)	References
Fish		
Okamejei kenojei	Elasmobranchii: Chordata	Mizuta et al. (2003b)
Heterodontus japonicus	Elasmobranchii: Chordata	Nagai and Suzuki (2000b)
Katsuwonus pelamis	Actinopterygii: Chordata	
Lateolabrax japonicus	Actinopterygii: Chordata	
Plecoglossus altivelis	Actinopterygii: Chordata	
Evynnis tumifrons	Actinopterygii: Chordata	
Scomber japonicus	Actinopterygii: Chordata	
Trachurus japonicus	Actinopterygii: Chordata	
Merluccius merluccius, Oncorhynchus mykiss	Actinopterygii: Chordata	Wang et al. (2007)
Arius maculates	Actinopterygii: Chordata	Bama et al. (2010)
Ictalurus punctatus	Actinopterygii: Chordata	Liu et al. (2007)
Megalaspis cordyla	Actinopterygii: Chordata	Sampath Kumar et al. (2012)
Otolithes rubber	Actinopterygii: Chordata	
Priacanthus macracanthus	Actinopterygii: Chordata	Jongjareonrak et al. (2005)
Priacanthus tayenus	Actinopterygii: Chordata	Kittiphattanabawon et al. (2005)
Mammals		
Balaenoptera acutorostrata	Mammalia: Chordata	Ishikawa et al. (1999)

[a] According to the latest nomenclature adopted from World Register of Marine Species (WoRMS).

Marine sponge collagen/spongin is well proved to be comparable to vertebrate collagen and, as such, has been extracted for use as a functional additive to composite biomaterials. Previously, *Chondrosia reniformis*-derived collagen was used in conjunction with silica templating to produce hydrogels that supported attachment and growth and differentiation of human mesenchymal cells (hMSCs) into osteoblast-like cells (Heinemann et al. 2007). Recent studies on collagen scaffolds from marine sponge species that belong to Callyspongiidae were proved to serve as potent bone tissue engineering scaffolds (Lin et al. 2011).

When compared to the individual monocomponent bone substitutes, bi-, tri-, and multicomponent composite scaffolds are gaining much significance in terms of retaining biophysicochemical and physiofunctional properties of the biomimetic matrix. HAp and collagen composites (Col) have the potential in mimicking and replacing skeletal bones and prove to be beneficial for bone tissue engineering due to their resemblance to a natural bone (Sionkowska and Kozłowska 2010). Moreover, a tricomponent system of marine sponge collagen, HAp, and chitosan became a promising bioscaffold for the assessment of bone tissue engineering applications (Pallela et al. 2012).

Jellyfish collagen scaffolds are gaining much importance as there is not much impurity in their body parts. Hence, the extraction of jellyfish collagen from their umbrella or arms has been very interesting for application in biomedical sciences. Although the integration of these collagens with other bio-macromolecules is at the budding stage, few attempts are made to generate the bone tissue engineering scaffolds or devises. Previously, porous jellyfish collagen-based scaffolds were prepared by freeze-drying and cross-linking with 1-ethyl-(3-3-dimethylaminopropyl) carbodiimide hydrochloride (EDC) and N-hydroxysuccinimide (NHS) to be used in tissue engineering applications

(Song et al. 2006). Application of these scaffolds can be further extended to use in bone tissue engineering with combination of other bone augmentation materials like HAp and chitosan. Moreover, the osteogenic differentiation of mesenchymal stem cells (MSCs) can be investigated in jellyfish collagen, by making the observations based on bone marker expression and calcium accumulation.

Marine fish collagens are tremendously used for various biomedical applications (Hayashi et al. 2011). Just recently, salmon skin collagen/HAp composite scaffolds have been elucidated for their potential application in bone tissue engineering, based on the biomimetic mineralization principle (Hoyer et al. 2012). The developed scaffolds are highly resorbable with interconnecting porosity, sufficiently stable under cyclic compression, and show elastic mechanical properties. Further, it is observed that hMSCs were able to adhere and proliferate on these scaffolds, thereby promoting a well-demonstrated osteogenic differentiation. In other studies, biomimetic bioabsorbable composites of HAp and collagen (HA-C) powder were designed utilizing salmon bone and skin by a dissolution–precipitation method (Akazawa et al. 2012). When HA-C powders were implanted into the subcutaneous tissue at the dorsal region in rats, collagen was completely bioabsorbed and body fluid permeated into large agglomerated particles, and bioabsorption through the multigiant cell infiltration was noticeable around the surface layers of HAp particles.

26.3 Conclusion

Marine environment proved to be a good source of not only chemical molecules but also of several protein molecules like collagen. The implications of several marine-derived collagens in biology and biomedicine are noteworthy although the applications of these marine-based composite scaffolds in bone tissue engineering are still in the budding stage. The current chapter covered the basic knowledge of several marine sources of collagen and their possible and prospective implications in bone tissue engineering through the development of bone mimicking marine collagen composite materials or scaffolds. The cumulative information given in the chapter is hoped to serve the new marine researchers, who are interested in biomedicine, especially bone tissue engineering.

References

Addad, S., J.Y. Exposito, C. Faye et al. 2011. Isolation, characterization and biological evaluation of jellyfish collagen for use in biomedical applications. *Marine Drugs* 9(6):967–983.

Akazawa, T., M. Murata, M. Ito et al. 2012. Characterization of bio-absorbable and biomimetic apatite/collagen composite powders derived from fish bone and skin by the dissolution-precipitation method. *Key Engineering Materials* 493:114–119.

Bailey, A.J., L.J. Gathercole, J. Dlugosz et al. 1982. Proposed resolution of the paradox of extensive crosslinking and low tensile strength of cuvierian tubule collagen from the sea cucumber *Holothuria forskali*. *International Journal of Biological Macromolecules* 4(6):329–334.

Bama, P., M. Vijayalakshimi, R. Jayasimman et al. 2010. Extraction of collagen from cat fish (*Tachysurus maculatus*) by pepsin digestion and preparation and characterization of collagen chitosan sheet. *International Journal of Pharmacy and Pharmaceutical Sciences* 2(4):133–137.

Bonebreak, C.M. 2005. Biomechanical properties of engineered collagen scaffolds. Thesis (S.B.), Department of Mechanical Engineering, Massachusetts Institute of Technology, Cambridge, MA, http://hdl.handle.net/1721.1/32876.

Boyce, M.C. and E.M. Arruda. 2000. Constitutive models of rubber elasticity: A review. *Rubber Chemistry and Technology* 73:504–523.

Clarke, S.A., P. Walsh, C.A. Maggs et al. 2011. Designs from the deep: Marine organisms for bone tissue engineering. *Biotechnology Advances* 29(6):610–617.

Coyne, K.J., X.X. Qin, and J.H. Waite. 1997. Extensible collagen in mussel byssus: A natural block copolymer. *Science* 277(5333):1827–1830.

Ehrlich, H. 2010. *Biological Materials of Marine Origin.* Vol. 1, Springer Verlag, New York, p. 569.

Frank, U. and B. Rinkevich. 1999. Scyphozoan jellyfish's mesoglea supports attachment, spreading and migration of anthozoans' cells *in vitro. Cell Biology International* 23(4):307–311.

Fu, X., C. Xue, L. Jiang et al. 2008. Structural changes in squid (*Loligo japonica*) collagen after modification by formaldehyde. *Journal of the Science of Food and Agriculture* 88(15):2663–2668.

Glowacki, J. and S. Mizuno. 2008. Collagen scaffolds for tissue engineering. *Biopolymers* 89(5):338–344.

Gosline, J.M. and R.E. Shadwick. 1983. Molluscan collagen and its mechanical organization in squid mantle. In: *The Mollusca, Vol. 1, Metabolic Biochemistry and Molecular Biomechanics.* Hochachka, P.W. (ed.), Academic Press, New York, pp. 371–398.

Green, D., D. Howard, X. Yang et al. 2003. Natural marine sponge fiber skeleton: A biomimetic scaffold for human osteoprogenitor cell attachment, growth, and differentiation. *Tissue Engineering* 9(6):1159–1166.

Hagenau, A., P. Papadopoulos, F. Kremer et al. 2011. Mussel collagen molecules with silk-like domains as load-bearing elements in distal byssal threads. *Journal of Structural Biology* 175(3):339–347.

Hayashi, Y., Y. Shizuka, K.Y. Guchi et al. 2012. Chitosan and fish collagen as biomaterials for regenerative medicine. In: *Advances in Food and Nutrition Research.* Kim, S.-K. (ed.), Academic Press, New York, pp.105–120.

Hayashi, Y., Y. Shizuka, I. Takeshi et al. 2011. Fish collagen and tissue Repair. In: *Marine Cosmeceuticals: Trends and Prospects.* Kim, S.-K. (ed.), CRC-Taylor & Francis Group, Boca Raton, FL, pp. 133–141

Heinemann, S., C. Heinemann, H. Ehrlich et al. 2007. A novel biomimetic hybrid material made of silicified collagen: Perspectives for bone replacement. *Advanced Engineering Materials* 9(12):1061–1068.

Hoyer, B., A. Bernhardt, S. Heinemann et al. 2012. Biomimetically mineralized salmon collagen scaffolds for application in bone tissue engineering. *Biomacromolecules* 13(4):1059–1066.

Ishikawa, H., H. Amasaki, H. Dohguchi et al. 1999. Immunohistological distributions of fibronectin, tenascin, type I, III and IV collagens, and laminin during tooth development and degeneration in fetuses of minke whale, *Balaenoptera acutorostrata. The Journal of Veterinary Medical Science* 61(3):227–232.

Jeong, S., S.Y. Kim, S.K. Cho et al. 2007. Tissue-engineered vascular grafts composed of marine collagen and PLGA fibers using pulsatile perfusion bioreactors. *Biomaterials* 28(6):1115–1122.

Jongjareonrak, A., S. Benjakul, W. Visessanguan et al. 2005. Isolation and characterization of collagen from bigeye snapper (*Priacanthus macracanthus*) skin. *Journal of the Science of Food and Agriculture* 85(7):1203–1210.

Katzman, R.L. and A.H. Kang. 1972. The presence of fucose, mannose, and glucosamine-containing heteropolysaccharide in collagen from the sea anemone *Metridium dianthus. Journal of Biological Chemistry* 247(17):5486–5489.

Kier, W.M. 1988. The arrangement and function of molluscan muscle. *The Mollusca, Form and Function* 11:211–252.

Kier, W.M. and A.M. Smith. 2002. The structure and adhesive mechanism of octopus suckers. *Integrative and Comparative Biology* 42(6):1146–1153.

Kim, J.S. and J.W. Park. 2004. Characterization of acid-soluble collagen from pacific whiting surimi processing byproducts. *Journal of Food Science* 69(8):C637–C642.

Kimura, S., S. Miura, and Y. H. Park. 1983. Collagen as the major edible component of jellyfish (*Stomolophus nomurai*). *Journal of Food Science* 48(6):1758–1760.

Kimura, S., Y. Omura, M. Ishida et al. 1993. Molecular characterization of fibrillar collagen from the body wall of starfish *Asterias amurensis*. *Comparative Biochemistry and Physiology Part B: Comparative Biochemistry* 104(4):663–668.

Kimura, S. and M.L. Tanzer. 1977. Nereis cuticle collagen: Isolation and characterization of two distinct subunits. *Biochemistry* 16(11):2554–2560.

Kittiphattanabawon, P., S. Benjakul, W. Visessanguan et al. 2005. Characterisation of acid-soluble collagen from skin and bone of bigeye snapper (*Priacanthus tayenus*). *Food Chemistry* 89(3):363–372.

Krasko, A., B. Lorenz, R. Batel et al. 2000. Expression of silicatein and collagen genes in the marine sponge *Suberites domuncula* is controlled by silicate and myotrophin. *European Journal of Biochemistry* 267(15):4878–4887.

Kuo, J.D., H.O. Hultin, M.T. Atallah et al. 1991. Role of collagen and contractile elements in ultimate tensile strength of squid mantle. *Journal of Agricultural and Food Chemistry* 39(6):1149–1154.

Lee, C.H., A. Singla, and Y. Lee. 2001. Biomedical applications of collagen. *International Journal of Pharmaceutics* 221(1):1–22.

Lin, Z., K.L. Solomon, X. Zhang et al. 2011. In vitro evaluation of natural marine sponge collagen as a scaffold for bone tissue engineering. *International Journal of Biological Sciences* 7(7):968–977.

Liu, H.Y., D. Li, and S. Guo. 2007. Studies on collagen from the skin of channel catfish (*Ictalurus punctatus*). *Food Chemistry* 101(2):621–625.

Ma, L., C. Gao, Z. Mao et al. 2004. Enhanced biological stability of collagen porous scaffolds by using amino acids as novel cross-linking bridges. *Biomaterials* 25(15):2997–3004.

Melnick, S.C. 1958. Occurrence of collagen in the phylum Mollusca. *Nature*, 181:1483.

Miura, S. and S. Kimura. 1985. Jellyfish mesogloea collagen. Characterization of molecules as $\alpha 1 \alpha 2 \alpha 3$ heterotrimers. *Journal of Biological Chemistry* 260(28):15352–15356.

Mizuta, S., J.H. Hwang, and R. Yoshinaka. 2003b. Molecular species of collagen in pectoral fin cartilage of skate (*Raja kenojei*). *Food Chemistry* 80(1):1–7.

Mizuta, S., T. Miyagi, and R. Yoshinaka. 2005. Characterization of the quantitatively major collagen in the mantle of oyster *Crassostrea gigas*. *Fisheries Science* 71(1):229–235.

Mizuta, S., T. Tanaka, and R. Yoshinaka. 2003a. Comparison of collagen types of arm and mantle muscles of the common octopus (*Octopus vulgaris*). *Food Chemistry* 81(4):527–532.

Nagai, T. 2004. Collagen from diamondback squid (*Thysanoteuthis rhombus*) outer skin. *Zeitschrift Fur Naturforschung C* 59 (3/4):271–275.

Nagai, T., K. Nagamori, E. Yamashita et al. 2002. Collagen of octopus *Callistoctopus arakawai* arm. *International Journal of Food Science and Technology* 37(3):285–289.

Nagai, T. and N. Suzuki. 2000a. Partial characterization of collagen from purple sea urchin (*Anthocidaris crassispina*) test. *International Journal of Food Science and Technology* 35(5):497–501.

Nagai, T. and N. Suzuki. 2000b. Isolation of collagen from fish waste material—Skin, bone and fins. *Food Chemistry* 68(3):277–281.

Nagai, T., O. Tomoe, N. Takashi et al. 1999. Collagen of edible jellyfish exumbrella. *Journal of the Science of Food and Agriculture* 79(6):855–858.

Nagai, T., W. Wanchai, S. Nobutaka et al. 2000. Isolation and characterization of collagen from rhizostomous jellyfish (*Rhopilema asamushi*). *Food Chemistry* 70(2):205–208.

Nam, K.A., S.G. You, and S.M. Kim. 2008. Molecular and physical characteristics of squid (*Todarodes pacificus*) skin collagens and biological properties of their enzymatic hydrolysates. *Journal of Food Science* 73(4):C249–C255.

Omura, Y., U. Naoto, and S. Kimura. 1996. Occurrence of fibrillar collagen with structure of $(\alpha 1)2\alpha 2$ in the test of sea urchin *Asthenosoma ijimai*. *Comparative Biochemistry and Physiology Part B: Biochemistry and Molecular Biology* 115(1):63–68.

Pallela, R., S. Bojja, and V. R. Janapala. 2011. Biochemical and biophysical characterization of collagens of marine sponge, *Ircinia fusca* (Porifera: Demospongiae: Irciniidae). *International Journal of Biological Macromolecules* 49(1):85–92.

Pallela, R., J. Venkatesan, V.R. Janapala et al. 2012. Biophysicochemical evaluation of chitosan-hydroxyapatite-marine sponge collagen composite for bone tissue engineering. *Journal of Biomedical Materials Research Part A* 100A(2):486–495.

Parenteau-Bareil, R., R. Gauvin, and F. Berthod. 2010. Collagen-based biomaterials for tissue engineering applications. *Materials* 3(3):1863–1887.

Prockop, D.J. 1998. What holds us together? Why do some of us fall apart? What can we do about it? *Matrix Biology* 16(9):519–528.

Qin, X.X. and J.H. Waite. 1998. A potential mediator of collagenous block copolymer gradients in mussel byssal threads. *Proceedings of the National Academy of Sciences of the United States of America* 95(18):10517–10522.

Rao, J.V., R. Pallela, and G.V.S.B. Prakash. 2011. Prospects of marine sponge collagen and its applications in cosmetology. In: *Marine Cosmeceuticals: Trends and Prospects*. Kim, S. K. (ed.), CRC-Taylor & Francis Group, pp. 77–103.

Rodrigues, C.V.M., P. Serricella, A.B.R. Linhares et al. 2003. Characterization of a bovine collagen–hydroxyapatite composite scaffold for bone tissue engineering. *Biomaterials* 24(27):4987–4997.

Sadowska, M., I. Kolodziejska, and C. Niecikowska. 2003. Isolation of collagen from the skins of Baltic cod (*Gadus morhua*). *Food Chemistry* 81(2):257–262.

Sadowska, M. and Z.E. Sikorski. 1987. Collagen in the tissues of squid *Illex argentinus* and *Loligo patagonica*-contents and solubility. *Journal of Food Biochemistry* 11(2):109–120.

Saito, M., N. Kunisaki, N. Urano et al. 2002. Collagen as the major edible component of Sea cucumber (*Stichopus japonicus*). *Journal of Food Science* 67(4):1319–1322.

Sampath Kumar, N.S., R.A. Nazeer, and R. Jaiganesh. 2012. Wound healing properties of collagen from the bone of two marine fishes. *International Journal of Peptide Research and Therapeutics* 18(3):185–192.

Scheibel, T. 2005. Protein fibers as performance proteins: New technologies and applications. *Current Opinion in Biotechnology* 16(4):427–433.

Schoeninger, M.J. and M.J. DeNiro. 1984. Nitrogen and carbon isotopic composition of bone collagen from marine and terrestrial animals. *Geochimica et Cosmochimica Acta* 48(4):625–639.

Sionkowska, A. and J. Kozłowska. 2010. Characterization of collagen/hydroxyapatite composite sponges as a potential bone substitute. *International Journal of Biological Macromolecules* 47(4):483–487.

Sivakumar, P. and G. Chandrakasan. 1998. Occurrence of a novel collagen with three distinct chains in the cranial cartilage of the squid *Sepia officinalis*: Comparison with shark cartilage collagen. *Biochimica et Biophysica Acta (BBA)—General Subjects* 1381(2):161–169.

Sjölin, E. and L.M. Gustavsson. 2008. An ultrastructural study of the cuticle in the marine annelid *Heterodrilus* (Tubificidae, Clitellata). *Journal of Morphology* 269(1):45–53.

Song, E., S. Yeon Kim, T. Chun et al. 2006. Collagen scaffolds derived from a marine source and their biocompatibility. *Biomaterials* 27(15):2951–2961.

Sugahara, T., M. Ueno, Y. Goto et al. 2006. Immunostimulation effect of the jellyfish collagen. *Bioscience Biotechnology and Biochemistry* 70(9):2131–2137.

Swatschek, D., W. Schatton, J. Kellermann et al. 2002. Marine sponge collagen: Isolation, characterization and effects on the skin parameters surface-pH, moisture and sebum. *European Journal of Pharmaceutics and Biopharmaceutics* 53(1):107–113.

Szulgit, G. 2007. The echinoderm collagen fibril: A hero in the connective tissue research of the 1990s. *BioEssays* 29(7):645–653.

Trotter, J.A., F.A. Thurmond, and T.J. Koob. 1994. Molecular structure and functional morphology of echinoderm collagen fibrils. *Cell and Tissue Research* 275(3):451–458.

Wahl, D.A. and J.T. Czernuszka. 2006. Collagen-hydroxyapatite composites for hard tissue repair. *European Cells and Materials* 11:43–56.

Wang, L., X. An, Z. Xin et al. 2007. Isolation and characterization of collagen from the skin of deep-sea redfish (*Sebastes mentella*). *Journal of Food Science* 72(8):E450–E455.

27

Biocomposites Containing Chitosan for Bone Tissue Engineering

Sekaran Saravanan, Mohita Trivedi, Ambigapathi Moorthi, and Nagarajan Selvamurugan

CONTENTS

27.1 Introduction

Bone is a complex living connective tissue, which plays a vital role in providing structural framework, mechanical support, and flexibility to the body. In addition to these, bone is also involved in mineral storage and homeostasis especially calcium and blood pH regulation and possesses other secondary functions (Harold and Shim 1963). Bone is traumatized under various circumstances such as accidents, and growth defect and primary tumor resection, which lead to bone defect. The traditional treatment strategies such as grafting (auto-, allo-, and xenografting) and metallic implants are followed to treat bone loss or bone defect. Implementation of these procedures is limited due to donor site morbidity, tissue availability, inflammation, and the risk of transmission of bacterial infection. Bone tissue engineering, considerably a new field, has emerged that uses the principles of bone biology and engineering discipline in generating various artificial synthetics as well as natural biodegradable substitutes known as scaffolds to treat bone loss.

Scaffolds are temporary structures that provide adhesive matrix for cell infiltration and growth. Porous architecture, biodegradability, biocompatibility, surface characteristics, and mechanical strength are some vital features for a successful scaffold to be used as an implant for bone tissue engineering. Various metals have been used in addition to the polymeric and ceramic biomaterials to enhance the properties such as antibacterial activity, low toxicity, chemical stability, long-lasting action period, and thermal resistance. Doping with metals such as copper, zinc, and silver has effectively improved for possessing the antimicrobial properties (Sahiti et al. 2010, Saravanan et al. 2011, Swetha et al. 2012).

27.2 Choice of Biomaterials

Biomaterials, when compared to the conventional materials, offer better results in terms of cell adhesion, spreading, proliferation, and differentiation. Various biomaterials are in use with regard to their nature, origin, and site of application. In our laboratory, we mostly use biomaterials such as chitosan to form the base of the scaffolds. The criteria behind the selection of this material are as follows: firstly, it is biocompatible and nontoxic. Secondly, the degradation of chitosan is initiated by lysozyme, and the degraded products are incorporated into various metabolic pathways and eliminated from the system.

Chitosan is a linear polysaccharide, obtained from the deacetylation of chitin, the primary structural polymer of the exoskeleton of crustaceans, and cuticles of insects, and cell wall of fungi is composed of randomly distributed α-(1–4)-linked D-glucosamine (deacetylated unit) and N-acetyl-D-glucosamine (acetylated unit). Partial deacetylation of chitin leads to the formation of chitosan, and chemical modifications yield various chitosan derivatives (Muzzarelli and Peter 1997), which may have more potential applications. Chitosan is a biocompatible, biodegradable polycationic polymer, which has minimum immunogenicity and low cytotoxicity (Sarasam et al. 2008). Its derivatives have been tested for their ability of gene transfer (Saranya et al. 2011). To bring additional features necessary for bone tissue engineering, we also include bioactive glasses and hydroxyapatite (HA) materials as other biocomposite components in the scaffolds. Bioactive glasses are osteoconductive and biodegradable biomaterials used for bone repair (Roman et al. 2003). They can also bond to hard and soft tissues. Hydroxyapatite, $Ca_{10} [PO_4]_5 (OH)_2$, a crystallochemical analogue of the mineral component of bone, has been used as a chief inorganic component of synthetic materials in orthopedics for decades (Elliot 2002). HA can promote the formation of bone-like apatite on its surface (Sabokbar et al. 2001). Composites of HA promote various properties including osteoblast adhesion, migration, proliferation, and differentiation (Eserelcin et al. 1998). The structural aspects of HA play a vital role in cell attachment and viability. Protein adsorption and cell adhesion to the scaffolds containing nanosized HA particles (nHAp) have been improved. The inclusion of nHAp also improved the mechanical and biological properties of the scaffolds (Kim et al. 2005, Peter et al. 2010b).

27.3 Biomaterial Synthesis and Scaffold Fabrication

Biomaterials used in the tissue engineering should possess great commercialization aspect with low production cost. Fine modifications to the biomaterials yield optimized or modified products, which possess improved properties than original or parent biomaterial.

In a study aimed at imparting antibacterial properties to the HA, we synthesized copper- and zinc-substituted nanohydroxyapatite (Zn-nHAp, Cu-nHAp) through solgel synthesis (Sahithi et al. 2010, Swetha et al. 2012). The synthesized compounds showed enhanced antibacterial activity when compared with native nHAp.

Engineered scaffold biomaterial provides and enhances the functionalities for cell adhesion, tissue ingrowths by providing large surface area, and porous structure for harboring large number of cells. The pores are also required for the nutrient transportation to the interior of the scaffolds and, subsequently, elimination of the metabolic wastes (Wang et al. 2000). Approaches in scaffold design must be able to create hierarchical porous structures to attain desired mechanical function and transport properties and to design accordingly to various anatomical or structural shapes. Therefore, a 3D architecture is required, and this could involve different scaffold fabrication methods. Freeze-drying is one of the methods employed in our laboratory to fabricate scaffolds. It is based on the phase separation strategy. Scaffolds with various biocomposite materials are fabricated by this technique. The direct sublimation of solvent ice crystals to vapor state yields porous structures that result from the space originally occupied by the water molecule resulting in spongy scaffolds (Freyman et al. 2001). This is easy and reliable compared with other fabrication methods. Electrospinning is also used in our laboratory and is a versatile fabrication method for scaffolds. This method utilizes electrostatic charges for producing thin matrix of polymer fibers with both micron and nanosized diameters (Subbiah et al. 2005). By tailoring the experimental parameters, scaffolds of varied fiber diameters and thickness can be fabricated. We developed a nanofibrous carboxymethyl chitin (CMC)/poly(vinyl alcohol) (PVA) blend scaffold with the property of apatite deposition, cell support, and adhesion suitable for tissue engineering applications (Shalumon et al. 2009). With electrospinning technique, we also prepared the nanostructured and microstructured scaffolds using synthetic biopolymer, polycaprolactone (PCL) for cell attachment, proliferation, and differentiation (Binulal et al. 2010). Other methods of scaffold fabrication include leaching, microsphere, phase separation, and printing and prototyping method.

27.4 Scaffold Characterization

27.4.1 Surface Morphology

The implanted scaffolds should possess surface roughness for strong interlocking with host tissue. This rough topography is also required for better cell adhesion and spreading. Cell spreading in the form of lamelipodia may be influenced by surface roughness, and that could result in promotion of cell proliferation. The grooved surfaces are also considered better than the rough surfaces (Jayaraman et al. 2004). Nanostructures obtained by controlling the reaction parameters on the titanium surfaces exhibited increased protein adsorption compared with polished titania surfaces, as this serves as a prerequisite for proper cell attachment and proliferation (Divya Rani et al. 2009). This kind of roughness greatly affects the properties of cell seeded on the scaffolds. In addition to the surface roughness, the sizes of biomaterials play an important role for cell adhesion and spreading. As we mentioned earlier, electrospinning, a newly developed technique for scaffold fabrication, is used to generate fibers of the polymers for bone tissue engineering. This technique yields fibrillar woven matrix with porous architecture. The diameter of the fiber can be varied from micron to nanoscale by tuning the experimental parameters.

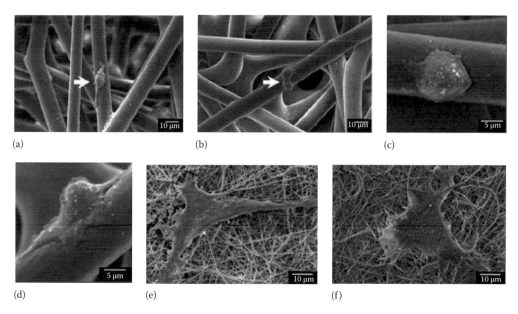

FIGURE 27.1
Human mesenchymal stem cell (hMSC) adhesion and spreading delayed on microfibrous scaffolds. Scanning electron micrographs of hMSCs on microfibrous structure after 12 h of incubation showed more or less round morphology with or without slight elongation along the axis of the fiber (a,b) (white arrows). Images under higher magnification clearly showed lack of spreading (c,d). Scanning electron micrographs of hMSCs on nanofibrous scaffolds at the same incubation time showed well-spread morphology (e,f). (From Binulal, N.S. et al., *Tissue Eng. A*, 16(2), 393, 2010.)

We developed PCL fibers through electrospinning, and the diameter of the fibers were adjusted and sized to both micro- and nanolevels. The micro- and nanostructured fibers were used for determining cell adhesion and spreading (Figure 27.1). Scanning electron microscopic studies revealed that cell adhesion and spreading onto nanofibrous PCL scaffolds were greater when compared to microfibrous scaffolds (Binulal et al. 2010). Thus, the nanosized architecture influences the properties of cell adhesion and spreading.

27.4.2 Pore Distribution

The scaffolds should possess porous architecture with interconnectivity so that they can act as template and they can guide cell for proliferation, differentiation, and tissue growth. Scaffolds may also act as controlled release devices to deliver various bioactive molecules according to the tissues' physiological need (Langer 1990). Pores greater than 20–100 μm favor cell penetration, but pores above 100 μm provide large space for neovascularization (Freyman et al. 2001). When the porosity is greater, the mechanical strength of the scaffolds will become reduced. A biocomposite scaffold containing chitosan, nanohydroxyapatite, and nanocopper–zinc alloy (CS/nHAp/nCu–Zn) exhibited interconnecting pores (Figure 27.2), and this architecture is indispensable to support cell migration, proliferation, and vascularization deep inside the scaffold (Tripathi et al. 2012).

27.4.3 Protein Adsorption

The adsorption of proteins onto the scaffolds is important as this will influence cell adhesion. The adsorbed proteins not only serve as a structural support but also promote

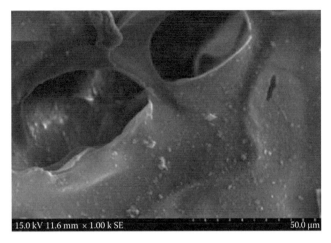

FIGURE 27.2
Scanning electron microscopic image of CS/nHAp/nCu–Zn scaffold indicating the interconnecting porous architecture. (From Tripathi, A. et al., *Int. J. Biol. Macromol.*, 50(1), 294, 2012.)

various chemical cues or signaling, thereby regulating cell activities (Silva and Menezes 2004, Wilson et al. 2005, Kennedy et al. 2006). More proteins are adsorbed onto nanosized particles due to the extended or more surface area (Binulal et al. 2010), thus generating more focal adhesion points for the cells (Divya Rani et al. 2009). On considering this property, we aimed fabricating scaffolds having increased protein adsorption. The addition of Cu–Zn alloy nanoparticles increased the surface area and hydrophilicity of the scaffolds, and hence more protein adsorption was seen (Tripathi et al. 2012). Increased protein adsorption of the scaffolds would lead to have better cell matrix interaction, adhesion, and spreading on the scaffolds. We showed that the biomaterials at nanoscale adsorb more proteins like fibronectin or vitronectin (Binulal et al. 2010), which could influence cell matrix interaction. The matrix or the scaffold material greatly affects the extent of cell adhesion, thereby modulating the cell proliferation (Bissell 2007). Integrins are the primary cell surface receptors that mediate cell matrix adhesion. Initial binding of integrins generally results in the clustering of additional adhesive proteins that leads to local remodeling of cytoskeletal arrangements in the cell (Berrier and Yamada 2007). These cytoskeletal rearrangement factors provide signals promoting the activation of various cytoplasmic proteins to control a number of key cellular processes including differentiation, cell polarity, gene regulation, apoptosis, actin organization, proliferation, and cell migration (Mooney et al. 1992, Cukierman et al. 2001, van der Flier and Sonnenberg 2001, Schwartz 2001). Wettability is another feature of the scaffolds, which greatly affects cell attachment. In our laboratory, we prepared and characterized a biocomposite scaffold containing chitosan/nanosilica/nanozirconia (CS/Si/Zr) scaffold, which showed increased wettability and in turn increased protein adsorption of the scaffold (Pattnaik et al. 2011) (Figure 27.3). The increased wettability would be preferred for improvement of the attachment of osteoblasts on the surface of the biocomposite materials.

27.4.4 Swelling Studies

After implantation of the scaffold under in vivo conditions, the scaffolds absorb fluids from the surrounding tissue and swells; this property is known as the swelling ability.

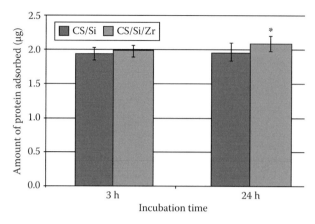

FIGURE 27.3
Protein adsorption studies of CS/Si/Zr scaffolds compared with chitosan/silica scaffolds. The CS/Si/Zr scaffolds exhibited a significant increase in the amount adsorbed on 24 h incubation when compared with CS/Si scaffolds. (From Pattnaik, S. et al., *Int. J. Biol. Macromol.*, 49(5), 1167, 2011.)

The absorption of tissue fluid results in the change in architecture of the scaffolds. As the pore size increases, the mechanical strength starts decreasing due to the weakening of the structural bonds. Increase in pore size leads to more cell penetration, and easy diffusion of ions and nutrients occurs (Chapekar 2000, LeBaron and Athanasiou 2000). Higher swelling ability may cause increased loss in structural integrity and strain to the surrounding tissues. Hence, the swelling property of the scaffolds is critical because that also determines the mechanical strength of the scaffolds. The swelling study in vitro is usually carried out by immersing the scaffolds in phosphate buffered saline (PBS) and measuring the weights at different time intervals. The biomaterials of their size and hydrophilic properties could have impact on the swelling properties of scaffolds. We investigated whether the addition of nanoparticles had any significant effect on the swelling behavior to various biocomposite scaffolds. When zirconia nanoparticles (nZr) were added to the chitosan–silicon dioxide matrix (CS/Si), the swelling ratio was decreased (Pattnaik et al. 2011). Similar effect was seen on addition of nBGC particles to chitosan–gelatin (CG) matrix (Peter et al. 2010a) (Figure 27.4.). In contrast, addition of nCu–Zn alloy to CS/nHAp matrix resulted in increased water uptake potential (Tripathi et al. 2012). The increased water uptake might result in increased pore size, thus leading to infiltration of cells and diffusion of ions with ease.

27.4.5 In Vitro Biodegradation Studies

The term biodegradation defines the chemical process of gradual breakdown of materials in a biological system (Williams and Zhong 1994). The implanted scaffolds interact with so many active substances and components present in the physiological environment that involves degrading the biomaterials. It involves breaking of scission of the chemical bonds in the biopolymers. Another phenomenon of degradation is by erosion. It usually takes place in devices that are fabricated from soluble polymers. The implanted scaffold erodes as water is absorbed into the systems. This could cause the polymer chain hydration leading to swelling, disentanglement of the scaffold, and ultimately dissolved away. Hydrolysis, degradation at the cross-links, and hydrolysis of liable bonds lead to the erosion of the polymeric implants (Heller 1980). Hydrolysis reactions may be catalyzed

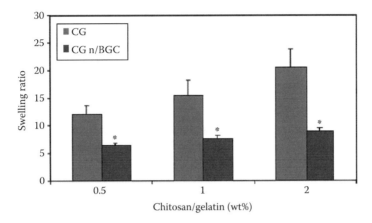

FIGURE 27.4
Swelling ratio of CG scaffolds and CGnBGC scaffolds prepared at different wt%. The swelling ratio significantly decreased with addition of nBGC particles. (From Peter, M. et al., *Chem. Eng. J.*, 158(2), 353, 2010a.)

by acids, bases, salts, or enzymes (Williams and Zhong 1994). Controlled biodegradation is essential so as to keep bone formation and degradation of the scaffold biomaterials in synchrony. The nature of biomaterials determines the degradation characteristics since the degradation is important for the release of bioactive ingredients. The degradation can be controlled or altered by the use of cross-linkers and tailored by tuning the concentration of cross-linkers and by chemical modifications (Nordtveit et al. 1996, Tomihata and Ikada 1997, Mi et al. 2001). The inclusion of nanomaterials could influence degradation properties. In our laboratory, we developed scaffolds with chitosan as the base material, and the in vitro degradation of the scaffolds was studied by the enzymatic action of lysozyme, which targets the glycosidic linkages in the chitosan structure. Incorporation of components like nanosilver into CS/nHAp scaffolds reduced the biodegradation to a great extent (Saravanan et al. 2011). Similarly, the incorporation of nCu–Zn alloy into CS/nHAp scaffolds decreased the biodegradation compared to CS/nHAp scaffolds (Figure 27.5) (Tripathi et al. 2012). Understanding the degradation mechanisms of biomaterials is vital in the selection of

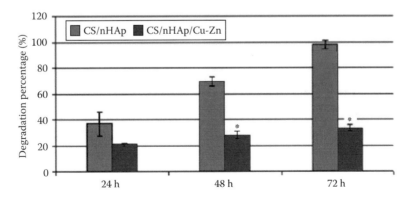

FIGURE 27.5
In vitro biodegradation of CS/nHAp scaffolds was found to be significantly decreased on addition of nCu–Zn alloy particles when compared to parent scaffolds. (From Tripathi, A. et al., *Int. J. Biol. Macromol.*, 50(1), 294, 2012.)

biomaterials for specific tissue engineering applications, because the degradation of the scaffold materials may affect various events such as cell growth, tissue regeneration, host response, and the material function.

27.4.6 In Vitro Biomineralization

Biomineralization refers to the deposition of ions and minerals present in the surrounding body fluid onto the implanted scaffolds. The deposition of calcium and phosphate enhances the attachment of osteoblasts and their activity (Grégoire et al. 1990). The biomineralization can be studied under laboratory conditions as in vitro. The in vitro biomineralization is carried out by immersing the scaffold in a solution called as simulated body fluid (SBF), which contains the ions and minerals at a concentration similar to the concentration present in the human plasma. The nanoparticles are expected to possess greater surface area and more nucleation sites leading to higher mineral deposition. The biocomposite scaffolds containing CS/Si and nZr were fabricated and compared with CS/SiO$_2$ scaffolds for the in vitro biomineralization capacity (Figure 27.6). The results proved that the incorporation of nZr into the CS/Si enhanced the biomineralization and bioactivity of scaffolds (Pattnaik et al. 2011). We also showed in another work that the addition of nHAp to CG scaffolds enhanced nucleation sites, thus leading to more efficient apatite formation (Peter et al. 2010b).

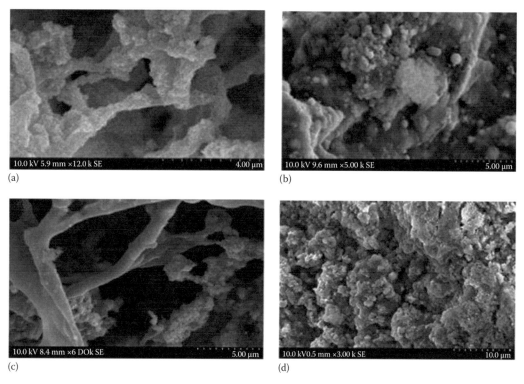

FIGURE 27.6
SEM images of the in vitro biomineralization of the CS/Si scaffolds after 7 days (a) and 14 days (b); SEM images of the in vitro mineralization of the CS/Si/Zr scaffolds after 7 days (c) and 14 days (d). The biomineralization was increased on addition of nZr particles to CS/Si matrix, and it was increased with the incubation time. (From Pattnaik, S. et al., *Int. J. Biol. Macromol.*, 49(5), 1167, 2011.)

27.4.7 Antibacterial Property

Infection is often defined as loss of homeostatic balance between the host tissue and the number of microorganism at a concentration exceeding 10^5/g of tissue (Zilberman and Elsner 2008). Reconstructive surgery-associated infections are very common and limit the tissue healing and regeneration capacity, ultimately leading to implant loosening and failure (Suci et al. 1998). Postsurgical administration of antibiotics is required to minimize the risk of infection. The loss of site-specific action and decrease in bioavailability lead to a new strategy of developing scaffolds incorporated with either antibacterial drugs and/or metal ions for local action against the pathogens. With this principle behind, the biocomposite scaffolds with antibacterial properties have been developed for bone tissue engineering. Copper- and zinc-doped nHAp were synthesized with greater antibacterial action compared with native nHAp (Sahiti et al. 2010, Swetha et al. 2012). Silver ions were also introduced onto the chitosan–nHAp scaffolds, and they showed enhanced antibacterial activity (Saravanan et al. 2011). nCu–Zn alloy at nanoscale was used in fabricating the CS/nHAp/Cu–Zn biocomposite scaffolds, and the results showed that these biocomposite scaffolds had enhanced antibacterial activity than CS/nHAp scaffolds (Tripathi et al. 2012).

27.4.8 Biocompatibility

The biomaterials and fabricated scaffolds should be biocompatible for their use in in vivo conditions. The scaffolds are tested for their biocompatibility by in vitro assessment through indirect cytotoxicity assay (Tripathi et al. 2012). Cytotoxicity assessment is therefore an important criterion for the fabricated scaffolds, and it can be carried out using the MTT (3-(4,5-dimethylthiazol-2-yl)-2,5-diphenyltetrazolium bromide) reagent. The MTT assay is based on the colorimetric analysis of the colored formazan crystal products formed by the conversion of MTT by mitochondrial succinate dehydrogenase enzyme inside the cell (Wataha et al. 1991).Cells are directly cultured with the scaffolds, or the conditioned media can be used for testing cytotoxicity. Several biocomposite scaffolds prepared in our laboratory were tested whether they are toxic or not using rat osteoprogenitor cells, osteoblastic cells, or mesenchymal stem cells, and these scaffolds were found to be nontoxic and cell friendly (Binulal et al. 2010, Peter et al. 2010a,b, Sahiti et al. 2010, Pattnaik et al. 2011, Saravanan et al. 2011, Swetha et al. 2012, Tripathi et al. 2012).

27.5 Conclusions

This chapter reviewed and highlighted several biocomposite materials/scaffolds prepared and characterized in our laboratory for bone tissue engineering applications. Most importantly, the characteristic features required for bone tissue engineering are discussed. Although conventional methods are in great implications, the advanced approach is highly encouraged especially utilization of the biomaterials at nanoscale. The structural and content modifications of biomaterials especially at nanoscale could contribute a great deal toward cell adhesion, spreading, proliferation, and differentiation. This would prove that there is a great scope of further research in this field for better applications.

Acknowledgment

This work was initiated by the financial support provided by SRM University. This work was also supported, in part, by Indian Council for Medical Research, India (Grant Nos. 5/13/2009-NCD-III; 80/10/2010-BMS to N.S.).

References

Berrier, A. L. and K. M. Yamada. 2007. Cell–matrix adhesion. *Journal of Cellular Physiology* 213(3):565–573.

Binulal, N. S., M. Deepthy, N. Selvamurugan, K. T. Shalumon, S. Suja, U. Mony, R. Jayakumar, and S. V. Nair. 2010. Role of nanofibrous poly (caprolactone) scaffolds in human mesenchymal stem cell attachment and spreading for in vitro bone tissue engineering—Response to osteogenic regulators. *Tissue Engineering Part A* 16(2):393–404.

Bissell, M. J. 2007. Modeling molecular mechanisms of breast cancer and invasion: Lessons from the normal gland. *Biochemical Society Transactions* 35(1):18–22.

Chapekar, M. S. 2000. Tissue engineering: Challenges and opportunities. *Journal of Biomedical Materials Research* 53(6):617–620.

Cukierman, E., R. Pankov, D. R. Stevens, and K. M. Yamada. 2001. Taking cell–matrix adhesions to the third dimension. *Science* 294(5547):1708–1712.

Divya Rani, V. V., K. Manzoor, D. Menon, N. Selvamurugan, and S. V. Nair. 2009. The design of novel nanostructures on titanium by solution chemistry for an improved osteoblast response. *Nanotechnology* 20(19):195101.

Elliott, J. C. 2002. Calcium phosphate biominerals. In *Phosphates: Geochemical, Geobiological and Material Importance*, M. J. Kohn, J. Rakovan, and J. M. Hughes (eds.), pp. 427–454. Reviews in Mineralogy and Geochemistry, Mineralogical Society of America, Washington, DC.

EserElçin, A., Y. M. Elçin, and G. D. Pappas. 1998. Neural tissue engineering: Adrenal chromaffin cell attachment and viability on chitosan scaffolds. *Neurological Research* 20(7):648–654.

van der Flier, A. and A. Sonnenberg. 2001. Function and interactions of integrins. *Cell and Tissue Research* 305(3):285–298.

Freyman, T. M., I. V. Yannas, and L. J. Gibson. 2001. Cellular materials as porous scaffolds for tissue engineering. *Progress in Materials Science* 46(3–4):273–282.

Grégoire, M., I. Orly, and J. Menanteau. 1990. The influence of calcium phosphate biomaterials on human bone cell activities-An in vitro approach. *Journal of Biomedical Materials Research* 24(2):165–177.

Harold Copp, D. and S. S. Shim. 1963. The homeostatic function of bone as a mineral reservoir. *Oral Surgery, Oral Medicine, and Oral Pathology* 16(6):738–744.

Heller, J. 1980. Controlled release of biologically active compounds from bioerodible polymers. *Biomaterials* 1(1):51–57.

Jayaraman, M., U. Meyer, M. Bühner, U. Joos, and H. P. Wiesmann. 2004. Influence of titanium surfaces on attachment of osteoblast-like cells *in vitro*. *Biomaterials* 25(24):625–631.

Kennedy, S. B., N. R. Washburn, C. G. Simon, and E. J. Amis. 2006. Combinatorial screen of the effect of surface energy on fibronectin-mediated osteoblast adhesion, spreading and proliferation. *Biomaterials* 27(20):3817–3824.

Kim, H. W., J. C. Knowles, and H. E. Kim. 2005. Hydroxyapatite and gelatin composite foams processed via novel freeze-drying and crosslinking for use as temporary hard tissue scaffolds. *Journal of Biomedical Materials Research A* 72(2):136–145.

Langer, R. 1990. New methods of drug delivery. *Science* 249:1527–1533.

LeBaron, R. G. and K. A. Athanasiou. 2000. *Ex-vivo* synthesis of articular cartilage. *Biomaterials* 21(24):2575–2587.

Mooney, D., L. Hansen, J. Vacanti, R. Langer, S. Farmer, and D. Ingber. 1992. Switching from differentiation to growth in hepatocytes: Control by extracellular-matrix. *Journal of Cellular Physiology* 151(3):497–505.

Mi, F. L., Y. C. Tan, H. C. Liang, R. N. Huang, and H. W. Sung. 2001. In vitro evaluation of a chitosan membrane cross-linked with genipin. *Journal of Biomaterials Science. Polymer Edition* 12(8):835–850.

Muzzarelli, R. A. A. and M. G. Peter. 1997. *Chitin Handbook*, European Chitin Society, Atec, Grottammare, Italy.

Nordtveit, R. J., K. M. Vårum, and O. Smidsrød. 1996. Degradation of partially N-acetylated chitosans with hen egg white and human lysozyme. *Carbohydrate Polymers* 29(2):163–167.

Pattnaik, S., S. Nethala, A. Tripathi, S. Saravanan, A. Moorthi, and N. Selvamurugan. 2011. Chitosan scaffolds containing silicon dioxide and zirconia nano particles for bone tissue engineering. *International Journal of Biological Macromolecules* 49(5):1167–1172.

Peter, M., N. S. Binulal, S. V. Nair, N. Selvamurugan, H. Tamura, and R. Jayakumar. 2010a. Novel biodegradable chitosan/gelatin/nano-bioactive glass ceramic composite scaffolds for alveolar bone tissue engineering. *Chemical Engineering Journal* 158(2):353–361.

Peter, M., N. Ganesh, N. Selvamurugan, S. V. Nair, T. Furuike, H. Tamura, and R. Jayakumar. 2010b. Preparation and characterization of chitosan–gelatin/nanohydroxyapatite composite scaffolds for tissue engineering applications. *Carbohydrate Polymers* 80(3):687–694.

Roman, J., S. Padilla, and M. Vallet-Regý. 2003. Sol-gel glasses as precursors of bioactive glass ceramics. *Chemical Materials* 15(3):798–806.

Sabokbar, A., R. Pandey, J. Díaz, J. M. Quinn, D. W. Murray, and N. A. Athanasou. 2001. Hydroxyapatite particles are capable of inducing osteoclast formation. *Journal of Materials Science. Materials in Medicine* 12(8):659–664.

Sahithi, K., M. Swetha, M. Prabaharan, A. Moorthi, N. Saranya, K. Ramasamy, N. Srinivasan, N. C. Partridge, and N. Selvamurugan. 2010. Synthesis and characterization of nanoscale-hydroxyapatite-copper for antimicrobial activity towards bone tissue engineering applications. *Journal of Biomedical Nanotechnology* 6(4):333–339.

Saranya, N., A. Moorthi, S. Saravanan, M. Pandima Devi, and N. Selvamurugan. 2011. Chitosan and its derivatives for gene delivery. *International Journal of Biological Macromolecules* 48(2):234–238.

Sarasam, A. R., P. Brown, S. S. Khajotia, J. J. Dmytryk, and S. V. Madihally. 2008. Antibacterial activity of chitosan-based matrices on oral pathogens. *Journal of Materials Science. Materials in Medicine* 19(3):1083–1090.

Saravanan, S., S. Nethala, S. Pattnaik, A. Tripathi, A. Moorthi, and N. Selvamurugan. 2011. Preparation, characterization and antimicrobial activity of a bio-composite scaffold containing chitosan/nano-hydroxyapatite/nano-silver for bone tissue engineering. *International Journal of Biological Macromolecules* 49(2):188–193.

Schwartz, M. A. 2001. Integrin signaling revisited. *Trends in Cell Biology* 11(12):466–470.

Shalumon, K. T., N. S. Binulal, N. Selvamurugan, S. V. Nair, M. Deepthy, T. Furuike, H. Tamura, and R. Jayakumar. 2009. Electrospinning of carboxymethyl chitin/poly(vinyl alcohol) nanofibrous scaffolds for tissue engineering applications. *Carbohydrate Polymers* 77(4):863–869.

Silva, F. C. and G. C. Menezes. 2004. Osteoblasts attachment and adhesion: How bone cells fit fibronectin-coated surfaces. *Materials Science and Engineering C-Biomimetic and Supramolecular Systems* 24(5):637–641.

Subbiah, T., G. S. Bhat, R. W. Tock, S. Pararneswaran, and S. S. Ramkumar. 2005. Electrospinning of nanofibers. *Journal of Applied Polymer Science* 96(2):557–569.

Suci, P. A., J. D. Vrany, and M. W. Mittelman. 1998. Investigation of interactions between antimicrobial agents and bacterial biofilms using attenuated total reflection Fourier transform infrared spectroscopy. *Biomaterials* 19(4–5):27–339.

Swetha, M., K. Sahithi, A. Moorthi, N. Saranya, S. Saravanan, K. Ramasamy, N. Srinivasan, and N. Selvamurugan. 2012. Synthesis, characterization, and antimicrobial activity of nano-hydroxyapatite-zinc for bone tissue engineering applications. *Journal of Nanoscience and Nanotechnology* 12(1):167–172.

Tomihata, K. and Y. Ikada. 1997. In vitro and in vivo degradation of films of chitin and its deacetylated derivatives. *Biomaterials* 18(7):567–575.

Tripathi, A., S. Saravanan, S. Pattnaik, A. Moorthi, N. C. Partridge, and N. Selvamurugan 2012. Bio-composite scaffolds containing chitosan/nano-hydroxyapatite/nano-copper-zinc for bone tissue engineering. *International Journal of Biological Macromolecules* 50(1):294–299.

Wang, J. H. C., E. S. Grood, J. Florer, and R. Wenstrup. 2000. Alignment and proliferation of MC3T3-E1 osteoblasts in microgrooved silicone substrata subjected to cyclic stretching. *Journal of Biomechanics* 33(6):729–735.

Wataha, J. C., C. T. Hanks, and R. G. Craig. 1991. The in vitro effects of metal cations on eukaryotic cell metabolism. *Journal of Biomedical Materials Research* 25(9):1133–1149.

Williams, D. F. and S. P. Zhong. 1994. Biodeterioration/biodegradation of polymeric medical devices *in situ*. *International Biodeterioration and Biodegradation* 34(2):95–130.

Wilson, C. J., R. E. Clegg, D. I. Leavesley, and M. J. Pearcy. 2005. Mediation of biomaterial-cell interactions by adsorbed proteins: A review. *Tissue Engineering* 11(1–2):1–18.

Zilberman, M. and J. J. Elsner. 2008. Antibiotic-eluting medical devices for various applications. *Journal of Controlled Release* 130(3):202–215.

28

Marine Plants and Algae as Promising 3D Scaffolds for Tissue Engineering

M. López-Álvarez, J. Serra, J.M. Sánchez, A. de Carlos, and P. González

CONTENTS

28.1 Introduction

Recent market studies estimate a globally and dramatic annual growth for the biomaterials sector due, mainly, to the aging of the population and to higher social welfare requirements. The pressing need to provide solutions for the replacement, repair, and regeneration of tissues and organs brings new challenges and opportunities for expansion to the field of biomaterials. Thus, new disciplines such as tissue engineering and regenerative medicine emerged in this way. In the case of bone tissue regeneration, one of the solutions proposed is the design of 3D scaffolds, based on porous biomaterials, with the specific morphology needed by the patient, to be cultured in the laboratory with cells taken from the sufferer. Later, the specific grown tissue will be implanted. This solution is thought to avoid the current implant rejections and to improve the quality of life of the patients.

Ideal scaffolds should have an internal structure designed with a predetermined density, pore shape, and size, with appropriate interconnection pathways. High porosity levels are necessary to support migration and proliferation of osteoblasts and mesenchymal cells, bone tissue ingrowth, vascular invasion, nutrient delivery, and matrix deposition in empty spaces. In fact, the main critical factor affecting bone formation is the presence of a combined macro- and microporosity, since macropores (size >100 µm) have a critical impact on osteogenic outcomes, promotion of vascularization, and mass transportation of nutrients and waste products (Wang et al. 2000), while micropores (size around 10 µm) favor capillary formation. Currently, it is commonly accepted that 3D scaffolds should also contain nanoporosity to allow the diffusion of molecules for nutrition and signaling (Ratner 2004). Pore interconnection also plays a key role in the overall biological system, since it provides the channel for cell distribution and migration, allowing efficient in vivo blood vessel formation. Furthermore, pore wall roughness contributes to increase the surface area, protein adsorption, and ion exchange (Bettinger et al. 2008; Yang et al. 2008).

The biodiversity that characterizes the marine environment represents an enormous potential for the acquisition of new microstructures that do in many cases display a complex and hierarchical organization similar to the ones present or required in the human organism. This approach represents a new way of understanding nature as a source of inspiration, the result of a need to find more efficient solutions with a less expensive processing. The use of biostructures derived from the marine environment for their application as biomaterials is very recent. For instance, several authors have proposed, in the last years, the use of different marine species like coral skeletons, sea urchins, and sponges as 3D biomatrices (Abramovitch-Gottlib et al. 2006; Green 2008; Cunningham et al. 2010). The results have confirmed that the 3D topography and the surface parameters of these materials influence positively the cell differentiation. Topography and composition of the material have been proven to affect cellular functions, such as adhesion, growth, motility, secretion, and apoptosis.

It is in this context that the main objective of this chapter is framed, in which the procurement of porous 3D biomatrices, obtained from marine plant and algae precursors, and their application in the biomedical field are proposed. The purpose is to obtain interesting bioinspired scaffolds of biocompatible materials that preserve the original microstructure of their natural precursors, with the aim of providing solutions to the development of medical devices and specific applications in tissue engineering and regenerative medicine. Highly porous scaffolds with appropriate pore size and interconnected pores will promote the invasion of blood vessels in vivo and neotissue ingrowth into the scaffold.

This chapter describes the process of the selection of the marine species, where the seaweed *Laminaria ochroleuca* and the marine plants *Zostera marina* and *Juncus maritimus* were the selected ones. The production of bioinspired ceramic scaffolds, the physicochemical characterization, in terms of porosity and chemical composition, and some biocompatibility in vitro tests are presented.

28.2 Selection of Marine Precursors

The selection of the precursors was based both on the requirements needed to fulfill by the final scaffold to be obtained and on the demands of the production process to transform the marine samples into the chosen materials: pyrolytic carbon (C) and biomorphic silicon carbide (SiC) ceramics, both already proven as biocompatible materials. All of them include as a common prerequisite the presence in the precursors of an interconnected porosity, which, in the case of the plant species, is closely linked to the presence of a developed vascular system. Another limiting characteristic, defined by the production process, is the composition of the precursors and, more specifically, their content in C with structural function: polysaccharides as cellulose, hemicelluloses, and lignin in the walls of the pores (Varela-Feria et al. 2008; González et al. 2009). These structural composites are present in the structure between the different cells and in the cell walls as a glue to give them rigidity. Therefore, two basic criteria were taken into account to select the marine species: consistent pores delimited by walls able to support the original structure until the end of the bioceramization process, and interconnectivity between those pores. These two requirements will help to obtain uniform and compact 3D scaffolds that will let the human cells to grow inside their pores giving a major integration of the biological tissue with the material.

In the case of marine plants and regarding the selection criteria based on pores delimited by consistent walls and the interconnectivity of these pores, the plant vascular system constitutes a developed distribution system extended throughout the whole body of the plant, from the root to the leafs. Going into more detail, this system of interconnected channels is composed of two different conduction tissues: the xylem and the phloem. The former transports water and dissolved substances from the root to the entire plant by means of two kinds of elongated tubular cells with lignified walls, without content of cytoplasm when they are mature, called tracheae and tracheids; the latter spreads the photosynthesized organic substances throughout the plant by vascular elements called sieve tubes and sieve cells (Paniagua et al. 1994).

In relation with the consistency of that tubular interconnected structure, the main composition of the cell walls varies with the type of plant considered. Thus, the Plantae kingdom is divided into four divisions (after Dawes 1998): nonvascular plants (bryophytes), seedless vascular plants (ferns), the naked seed vascular plants (gymnosperms), and the seed vascular flowering plants (angiosperms). The species of plants that can meet the requirements of porosity and consistency and have their habitat in the marine environment belong to the flowering plants (angiosperms). Their cell walls consist of cellulose (a long-chain polysaccharide whose unit is glucose that is added in the form of aligned microfibers), hemicelluloses (polysaccharides of lower molecular weight than cellulose and shorter chains that interconnect the microfibers to obtain a matrix for the cellulose superstructure), and lignin (an amorphous matrix of the conglomerate, which is located between different cells as a glue and in the cell walls to give them rigidity) (see Figure 28.1). The three components are distributed in layers, varying their proportion. Moreover, this proportion also varies depending on the type of plant, since obviously there is not the same proportion of lignin, for example, in a eucalyptus tree than in any marsh plant. The variation in the proportions will determine whether the selected precursors will be able to resist the fabrication process: the pyrolysis, in order to obtain C scaffolds that will maintain the interconnected tubular structure, and the reactive infiltration with molten silicon. This will be necessary to produce SiC scaffolds, with the appropriate consistency and porosity, avoiding the clogging of pores by the molten silicon flow (De Arellano et al. 2004; Borrajo 2006).

Going into detail with the techniques of processing selected to obtain the C and SiC ceramics, the marine algae and plants were subjected to the method described previously (Varela-Feria et al. 2008) after optimizing the parameters for these precursors (Figure 28.2). The first step consisted on removing the water from the marine structures, what was carried out by air-drying or lyophilization (depending on the precursor). Then they were introduced into a pyrolysis furnace to obtain the C scaffold. The latter is obtained by the thermal decomposition of the plant precursor with a gradual increase of temperature at a rate of 2°C/min up to 500°C, the maintenance of that temperature for 10 min, followed by a gradual decrease of 20°C/min down to room temperature. To obtain the SiC scaffold, the C scaffolds were covered by an optimized amount of pure silicon powder and infiltrated, under vacuum conditions, at 1550°C for 30 min, exceeding the melting point of silicon (1410°C) so that it flows through the interconnected pores reacting with the C. This temperature is achieved by following a gradual heating ramp of 10°C/min up to 1200°C and of 5°C/min from 1200°C to 1550°C. After the 30 min of permanence, the furnace temperature was decreased by a well-controlled ramp of 10°C/min to room temperature (López-Álvarez et al. 2011, 2012).

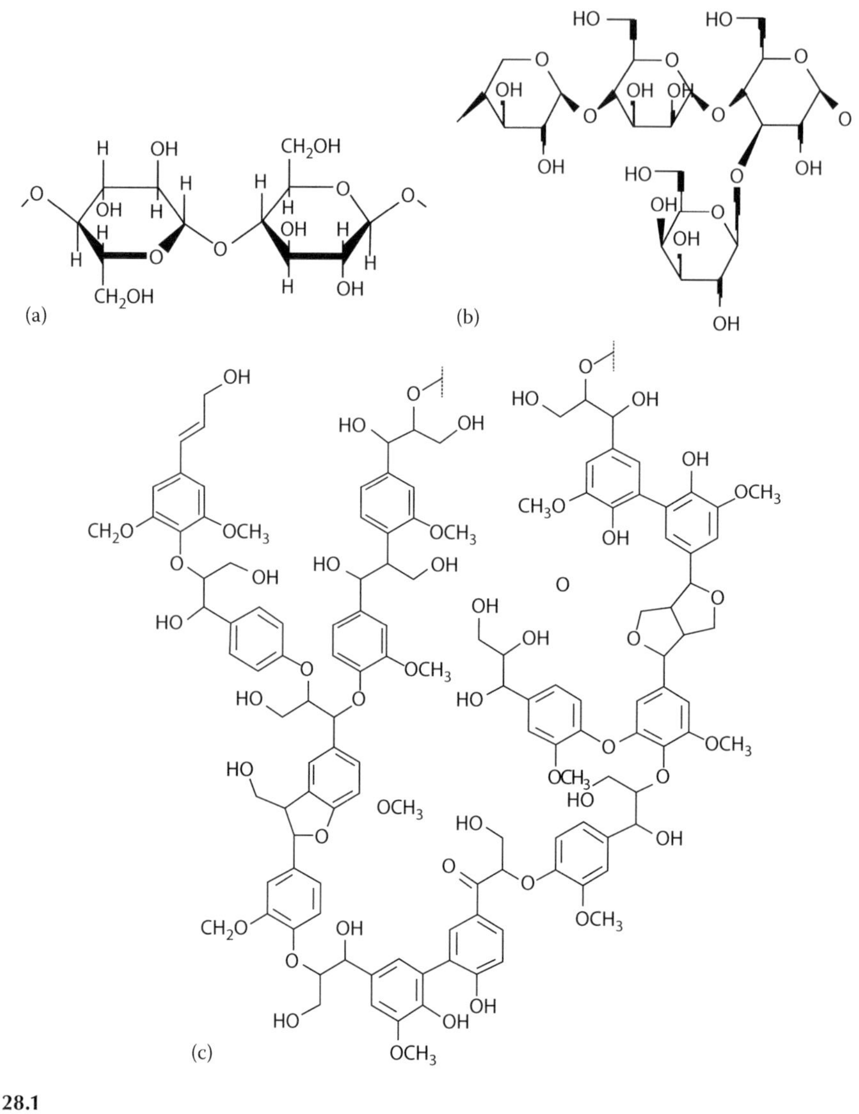

FIGURE 28.1
Cellulose (a), hemicelluloses (b), and lignin (c) partial molecules structure.

The marine plants finally selected were *J. maritimus* L. and *Z. marina* L. (Figure 28.3a and b), respectively. Both of them are angiosperms or flowering plants, the former integrated in salt marsh plant communities and the latter in seagrass meadows that can be the dominant vegetation type in many shallow water regions (Dawes 1998). Regarding the porosity and interconnectivity requirements established for the selection, when dealing with plants, a developed vascular system is ensured in principle; however, it should be mentioned that in the case of marine angiosperms, the exact function of the sieve elements must still be demonstrated. In addition, it is well known that, in aquatic plants, the xylem is reduced, which is interpreted as a result of the loss of a functional need (conductive and mechanical) in such plants with a constant supply of water and mechanically supported by the higher

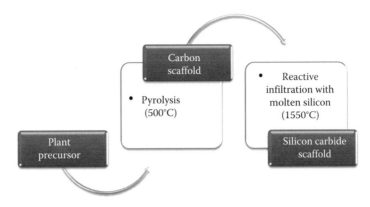

FIGURE 28.2
Diagram of the fabrication process of the two different scaffolds.

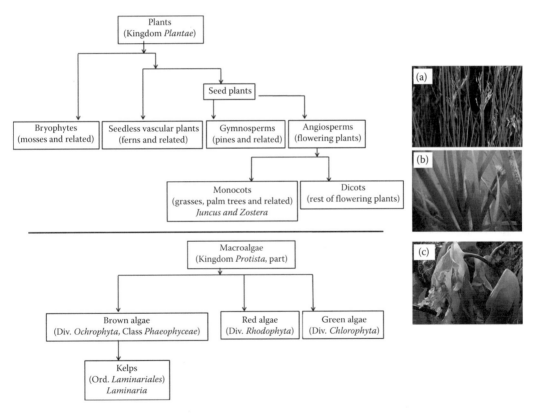

FIGURE 28.3
Taxonomic classification of the marine plants *J. maritimus* (a) and *Z. marina* (b) within the kingdom Plantae (Modified from Judd, W.S. et al., *Plant Systematics: A Phylogenetic Approach*, 2nd edn., Sinauer Associates, Inc., Sunderland, MA, 2002.) and the macroalgae *L. ochroleuca* (c) within the kingdom Protista. (Modified from Graham, L.E. and Wilcox, L.W., *Algae*, Prentice Hall, Upper Saddle River, NJ, 2000.)

density of the aquatic environment (Larkum et al. 2006). Within the angiosperms, both selected plants belong to the monocotyledons group. The choice of monocots is based on that, in addition of being the major components in many marine plant communities, the vascular bundles in monocots are scattered throughout the section of the stem, and not concentrated only in the central section as in dicotyledons (Murray 2005).

In regard to the selection of the seaweed species that meet the requirements set for the selection, and considering the definition of algae as *nonvascular autotrophic photosynthetic that contains chlorophyll a and a simple reproductive structure* (Dawes 1998), the difficulty to find species of algae with a developed vascular system is evident. In fact, this does not exist in algae, probably because their completely immersed way of life avoids the necessity to present a system to conduct the water from one side to the other of the seaweed body. However, the solutes originated in the photosynthetic cells must be distributed to the parts of the thallus situated far from the light, or more immature; this is the case of certain species of algae characterized by their large size and complexity. In them, a very primitive vascular system can be still found. It is formed by the sieve tubes and sieve cells (Graham and Wilcox 2000). Therefore, taking into account the selection criteria (defined by walls consisting of pores and interconnectivity of these pores), these species of macroalgae meet the porosity requirements. According to the taxonomic classification of the algae (Graham and Wilcox 2000), they are not included in the kingdom Plantae but in the Protista (Figure 28.3c). Within this kingdom, there are three different divisions containing macroalgae: Rhodophyta (red algae), Chlorophyta (green algae), and Ochrophyta, which includes the class Phaeophyceae (brown algae). The selected seaweed belongs to the order Laminariales of that class. The choice is due to its relatively large size and because they are among the most developed and complex seaweeds, with a rudimentary vascular system (sieve elements).

Regarding the consistency of the pore walls in the case of brown algae, the cell wall usually contains three compounds: cellulose that provides structural support; sodium, potassium, magnesium, and calcium alginates; and sulfated polysaccharides. Cellulose is usually the smallest constituent of the three (between 1% and 10% of thallus dry weight) and consists of microfibers generated at the cell surface by terminal complexes embedded in the cell membrane that are thought to include cellulose-synthesizing enzymes. The cells may regulate the presence and density of the cellulose-synthesizing complexes. Alginates are located within the intercellular matrix where they give flexibility to the thallus, helping it to prevent desiccation when emerged and where they play a role in the ion exchange. They represent between 20% and 40% of thallus dry weight (Graham and Wilcox 2000).

28.3 Marine Scaffolds: Physicochemical and Biological Characterization

28.3.1 Laminaria Ochroleuca Bachelot de La Pylaie

Laminaria ochroleuca is one of the largest and most complex brown seaweeds in the European coasts that dominate the low intertidal and the subtidal environment from temperate to Arctic latitudes (Dawes 1998). It can reach 2.5 m in length, and its attachment to the substrate is made possible by the presence of coarse holdfasts. It is also composed by the stipe, which is cylindrical and thick (from 2 to 6 cm in diameter). At the top, a blade or frond is located, which has a large heart-shaped part at the base, divided into multiple lacinia (Dawes 1998). Within the stipe and the frond, the tissue specialization occurs such

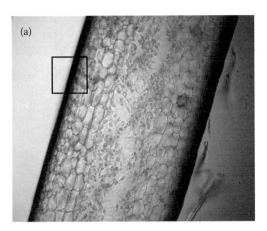
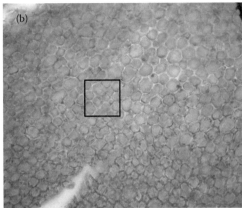
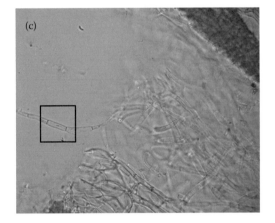

FIGURE 28.4
Tissue specialization of the cross section (a) of the frond of *L. ochroleuca* where pigmented cells (black square), colorless cells that constitute the cortex (also in b), and, in the innermost part, elongated cells specialized for the conduction of solutes (also in c) can be observed.

that the meristoderm is the outermost layer of pigmented cells (Figure 28.4a). Below this layer, colorless cells that constitute the cortex appear (Figure 28.4b), and in the innermost part of the cortex, the medulla cells, which are specialized in the conduction of solutes synthesized in the photosynthetic cells and that compose a vascular system similar to the plants, are found (Figure 28.4c). These driving elements (sieve elements) are elongated cells with perforated end walls (sieve plates) arranged in rows in order to form long continuous tubes. This system is disposed throughout the whole thallus of the macroalga except at the rhizoidal base (Graham and Wilcox 2000). Solutes transported through the vascular system include mannitol, free amino acids, and inorganic ions, which originated in the photosynthetic cells of the meristodermis and in the outermost cortex. This transport occurs in both daylight and darkness that is an advantage when the light levels are insufficient to permit photosynthesis, and it allows the algae to balance the respiration in the deeper portions of the thallus (Graham and Wilcox 2000).

The stipe of the selected algae was subjected to the scaffold's fabrication due to the amazing resemblance existing between its structure and the human trabecular bone.

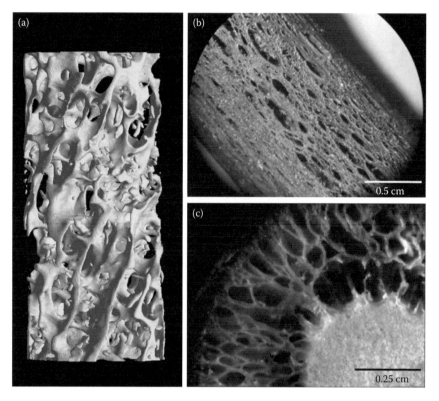

FIGURE 28.5
Resemblance between the porous structure of the human trabecular bone (a) (micro-CT image) and the stipe of *L. ochroleuca* (external appearance (b) and cross section (c)) (optical microscope images).

Figure 28.5 shows a micro-CT image of human trabecular bone (Figure 28.5a) and two images of the stipe (Figure 28.5b external appearance and Figure 28.5c cross section) obtained by optical microscopy (Nikon SMZ 10A). The hierarchical and interconnected porosity is evident in both images.

The C scaffold obtained (Figure 28.6a and c) presents a uniform pore distribution throughout the cross section where the large cavities (>1 mm) (shown in the unprocessed algae in Figure 28.5c) are still present. Between and inside of them, there are pores of around 40–50 μm of diameter distributed throughout the scaffold in a very generous and homogeneous distribution. The SiC scaffold (Figure 28.6b and d) maintained the large cavities that are still connected to each other by a porous structure (Figure 28.6b). At higher magnification (Figure 28.6d), it can be seen that these pores of around 50 μm were not clogged by the flow of molten silicon during the processing. Both C and SiC scaffolds presented apparently the high porosity levels needed to support the bone tissue ingrowth, vascular invasion, nutrient delivery, and matrix deposition in empty spaces.

The distribution of the porosity, studied by mercury porosimetry, confirmed these high levels of porosity in both scaffolds (Figure 28.7). The C scaffold was found to present macropores of 150 μm and mesopores of 40 and 25 μm, with a smaller contribution of pores of 5 μm in diameter. The average pore diameter was estimated at 48.05 μm and the total porosity of 39%. SiC scaffolds presented the same porosity range but with a peak at 10 μm instead of the peak at 5 μm. This can be explained by the possible rupture of the cell walls

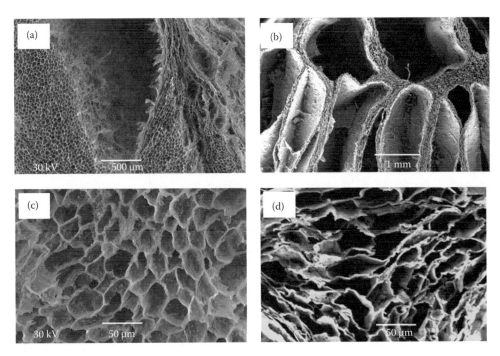

FIGURE 28.6
SEM images in cross section of the C scaffold (a) and (c) and of the SiC scaffold (b) and (d) obtained from the stipe of *L. ochroleuca*.

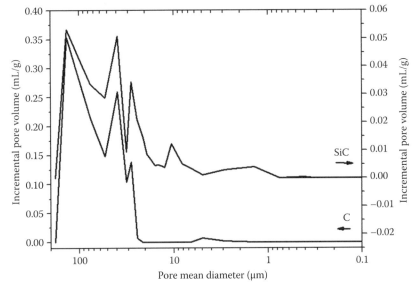

FIGURE 28.7
Pore size distribution obtained by mercury porosimetry of C and SiC scaffolds.

during the reactive infiltration causing the binding of several pores. At the same time, in the SiC scaffolds, pores of about 1.5 µm were also detected. The average pore size was set to 19.91 µm, and the value of total porosity detected was 45%. The considerable reduction at the mean pore size, compared to C, is probably due to the formation of SiC crystals inside and around the pores. It is important for understanding the total percentage of porosities to take into account that the large cavities present in both scaffolds are not detected as pores by this technique. However, in the case of the SiC, some of them could have been considered due to the fact of their decreased size as result of the formation of SiC crystals inside of them and, therefore, be counted as pores.

As previously mentioned, scaffolds for bone tissue regeneration should be porous to promote the integration of the new tissue with cell ingrowth and permit its vascularization. Moreover, the main critical factor affecting bone formation is the combination of macro and microporosity, where macropores with a size above 100 µm have a critical impact on osteogenic outcomes, promotion of vascularization, and mass transportation of nutrients and waste products, while micropores (size around 10 µm) favor capillary formation (Wang et al. 2000). Pore interconnection plays also a key role in the overall biological system, since it provides the channel for cell distribution and migration, allowing efficient in vivo blood vessel formation. According to Karageorgiou and Kaplan (2005), the total percentage of pores per volume of the human femoral trabecular bone varies between 50% and 90%. A review of the literature focused on scaffolds for bone regeneration showed a wide range of total porosity and pore sizes. In the case of ceramic materials, hydroxyapatite has been successfully tested as scaffolds with interconnected porosities varying from 36% to 80% and with pore size values between 150 and 600 µm (Kuboki et al. 1998; Nishiguchi et al. 2001; Chen et al. 2002; More et al. 2004). The same variability is observed in metal implants such as titanium and titanium alloys with a porosity between 50% and 60% and a pore size between 200 and 400 µm (Pilliar 1998; Nishiguchi et al. 2001) and in polymers with values of porosity found between 62% and 99% and pore sizes between 2 and 465 µm (Park et al. 2002; Li and Shi 2007). In the case of the C and SiC scaffold obtained from *L. ochroleuca*, the percentages of porosity that could be taken into account by this technique, unable to detect the cavities of more than 1 mm and, therefore, underestimating them, were 39% and 45% with pore diameters between 1.5 and 150 µm, plus the cavities (>1 mm). These values satisfied, for both materials (C and SiC), the general requirements to guarantee their success as scaffolds in terms of porosity.

Apart from porosity, the chemical composition of both C and SiC is essential for an adequate biocompatibility. Table 28.1 presents the elemental composition in atomic percentage of both materials compared to the composition of the natural algae analyzed by the x-ray fluorescence (XRF) technique. The results confirmed a major content of C (93.9%) in the C scaffold and a percentage of 67.5% in silicon and of 28.9% in C in the SiC composition. The remaining of 6.1% and 3.6%, respectively, corresponded in both scaffolds to oxygen, sodium, potassium,

TABLE 28.1

Elemental Composition in Atomic Percentage of the Natural Algae (Nat) and Both Scaffolds of the C and the SiC Measured by XRF

%	C	H	O	N	Cl	K	Na	Si	Al	S	Ca	P	Mg	I	F
Nat	24.9	2.1	36	29	2.3	1.6	0.8	0.3	1	0.5	0.2	0.2	0.3	0.1	0.4
C	93.9		2.3		0.2	0.4	0.9			0.4	0.7	0.4	0.8		
SiC	28.9		1.4		0.5	0.1	0.3	67.5	1.1	0.1	0.1	0.1			

calcium, magnesium, phosphorus, sulfur, and chlorine. The presence of those elements is explained by the marine origin of the precursor, which implies marine salts and also other nutrients in its composition. The main marine salts NaCl and KCl have even persisted after the high temperatures of the reactive infiltration process, in SiC, whose maximum temperature (1550°C) exceeds the salt temperature of evaporation (1413°C for NaCl and 1420°C for KCl). The reason for this can be that once their respective melting temperature is achieved, the molten marine salts flowed to the inside of the porous structure, which acted as a protection and prevented them from evaporating. In the case of SiC, the presence of aluminum was also detected due probably to the incorporation during the infiltration process from the melting pot (made of alumina), where the piece was placed inside the furnace.

As potential biomaterials, both the C and the SiC were subjected to a first basic cytotoxicity test, formally described by the ISO 10993-5 standard. It consists of immersing the scaffolds in cellular growth medium to evaluate their potential release of cytotoxic particles. The extracted solvents were then diluted with fresh cellular growth medium to obtain dilutions of 0%, 20%, 30%, 50%, and 100% of the extract. The same procedure was followed with phenol solution at 6.4 g/L and with supplemented growth medium as positive and negative controls, respectively. Finally, different dilutions, including controls, were incubated for 24 h with monolayers of the preosteoblastic cell line MC3T3-E1 (ECACC, United Kingdom), and cellular viability was evaluated by means of the Cell Proliferation Kit I from Roche Molecular Biochemicals (an MTT assay). Figure 28.8 presents a plot of the optical density, which is proportional to the cell viability, against the different dilutions of the extracts obtained from both materials and controls. It was observed that when a 20% of cytotoxic extract was added to the cells, the optical density in the positive control of cytotoxicity presented values close to zero, value that was maintained for the rest of the dilutions of the cytotoxic control. When a 20% of C and SiC extracts were added the optical density presented close values to the negative control of cytotoxicity (cell growth medium), to even achieve the highest values of viability when cells were incubated with the

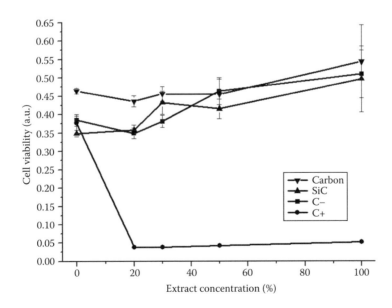

FIGURE 28.8
Relative cellular viability obtained from the solvents extracted from *L. ochroleuca*. A diluted phenol solution was used as positive control of cytotoxicity and cell growth medium as negative control.

undiluted extract. This figure clearly demonstrated the complete absence of cytotoxicity of the extracts obtained from C and SiC from *L. ochroleuca*, where no detrimental effects on the MC3T3-E1 preosteoblast viability were observed at any dilution tested.

28.3.2 *Zostera marina* L.

Zostera marina is a perennial plant, common in tropical, subtropical, and temperate climates, prostrated when exposed during the low tide in the muddy soil of the external marsh, only emerging during the low tide of the most intense tides. It is therefore one of the species that constitute the so-called sea grasses, adapted to live underwater (hydrophilic), forming beds in the shallow subtidal areas (Dawes 1998). It presents a well-developed rhizome with long internodes below the surface of the substrate. It also has numerous unbranched roots and a leaf at each node. Leaves are flat, ribbon shaped, and also flexible, so they can endure the movement of water remaining upright (Dawes 1998). The cell walls are mainly composed of polysaccharides and proteins with little cellulose and never lignified (Larkum et al. 2006). The mesophyll tissue is characterized by cells with thin cell walls surrounding cavities (air lacunae) regularly distributed so that every three or five of these cavities are interspersed between longitudinal vascular bundles (see Figure 28.9). This aerenchyma is developed to increase the internal gas space of aquatic plants that grow in oxygen-poor substrates (Larkum et al. 2006). *Zostera marina* has three or more parallel longitudinal vascular bundles, which are interconnected by transverse channels at regular intervals, and its vascular system is similar in structure and composition to the vascular land plants, so it has sieve elements, xylem, and parenchyma vascular cells (Larkum et al. 2006).

This plant has an interesting porous microstructure never used before from nature, with many possibilities in the field of the trabecular bone regeneration, especially oriented toward the tissue engineering application instead of the traditional implants. The hierarchical disposition of its abundant porosity, shown in Figure 28.9 with vascular bundles of around 20 μm of diameter and air cavities of around 200 μm, together with the own shape of the plant shoot, in sheets that can be overlapped to generate even a greater porosity (between sheets), constitutes the main advantages offered by this plant. At the same time, it is easily manipulated (favored by its laminar structure) with the possibility to

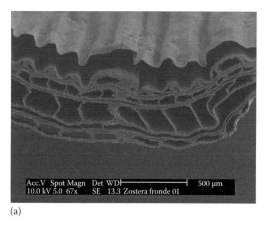

(a)

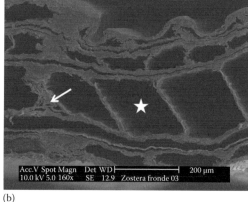

(b)

FIGURE 28.9
SEM images in cross section of a leaf of *Z. marina* in two different magnifications where white star indicates the air lacunae, and white arrow the vascular bundles.

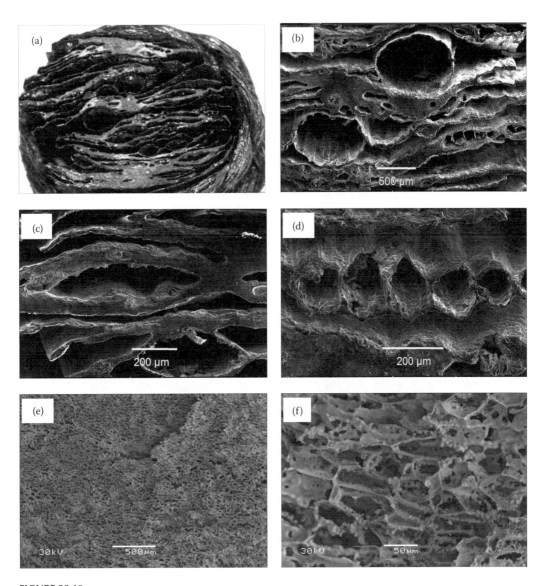

FIGURE 28.10
Optical microscopy (a) and SEM images (b–d) of the SiC scaffold obtained after overlapping several shoots of *Z. marina* in different magnifications. Longitudinal section of one of the sheets of *Z. marina* in SEM images in two magnifications are also presented (e, f).

give the final scaffold the specific dimensions and morphology needed to repair the bone defect in each patient. Figure 28.10 presents the morphology of a SiC scaffold obtained after overlapping several shoots of the plant. Great cavities (>500 μm diameter) that were generated as a consequence of the overlapping of several sheets can be perfectly observed (Figure 28.10a–c). The porosity retained from the air lacunae of the natural plant can be also perfectly observed (Figure 28.10d) with a diameter of around 100 μm. Finally, the porosity in longitudinal section of one of the sheets of this marine plant can be observed in two magnifications (Figure 28.10e–f) with the predominance of elongated macropores of around 70 μm in length.

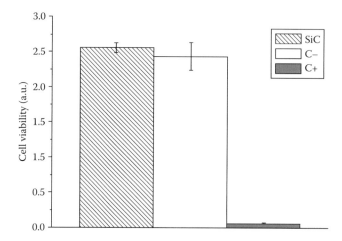

FIGURE 28.11
Relative cellular viability obtained from the solvents extracted from *Z. marina*. Phenol solution as positive control of cytotoxicity and cellular growth medium as negative control.

The absence of cytotoxicity exhibited by this ceramic, evaluated with the solvent extraction test, was demonstrated. Figure 28.11 presents the optical density, as a measure of the cell viability (in this case fibroblast L929) plotted, against the undiluted of extract obtained from the SiC of this marine plant and from both negative and positive controls of cytotoxicity (cell growth medium and latex, respectively). The result obtained, validated by the close to zero values in cellular viability in the case of the positive control of cytotoxicity, gave great values in cell viability in both the SiC and the negative control. Once again, the absence of cytotoxicity was clearly demonstrated.

28.3.3 *Juncus maritimus* L.

Juncus maritimus is a salt marsh plant able to grow in environments of intense water stress (xerophytes). It is distributed in temperate latitudes from middle to upper intertidal zone where tidal currents and wave action will not cause erosion and where the plants are not always submerged (Dawes 1998). It is a shallow rooted plant with rhizomes extended just below the soil surface and roots that are buried up to almost 100 cm. It presents interesting anatomical adaptations such as a considerable content in lignin, a high degree of epidermal development, an endodermic layer, and, finally, the modification of the leaf structure with a thick and continuous cuticle. This plant presents cylindrical leaves with a well-developed spongy parenchyma in the central region with numerous longitudinal air channels. The vascular bundles (Figure 28.12a) are distributed throughout the whole leaf where the phloem is constituted by pores of around 5 μm and the xylem is surrounding the phloem with pores between 20 and 25 μm. The outer region of the leaf, the mesophyll area, is characterized by a large number of bands of sclerenchyma or fiber bundles. The stomata, oval-shaped pores of around 30 μm used by the plant to regulate gas exchanges and water loss, are aligned in rows and sunk along the epidermis (Figure 28.12b) (Dawes 1998).

From the point of view of the potential biostructures to be used in the field of biomaterials, the sea rush *J. maritimus* has a vascular system uniformly distributed throughout its section that provides a hierarchical interconnected porosity along the entire plant, and, as an added value, this plant presents a double surface patterning in the upper

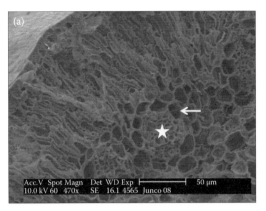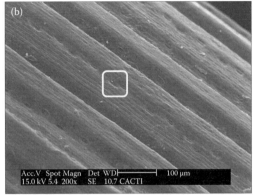

FIGURE 28.12

SEM images of *J. maritimus*. Micrograph (a) presents the unprocessed plant in cross section where white star indicates the vascular bundles corresponding to phloem and a white arrow the xylem. Micrograph (b) shows the surface of the plant constituted by fiber bundles and stomata (white square).

epidermal layers, with dimensions within the ranges previously tested and aligned in the direction of the plant's growth (Dawes 1998). This patterning presents grooves/ridges at the macroscale of approximately 100 μm width, oriented longitudinally, and within each of them, micropatterns of about 7 μm width oriented in the same direction. Arranged in rows on both sides of the macropattern, there are stomata, with a size of around 30 μm in diameter. This pattern could be used as a physical mold to promote the aligned growth of certain cell lines. In bone tissue, this aligned growth is of interest in long bones, where the calcium phosphate crystals present an aligned orientation. An oriented growth of osteoblasts will provide a bridge for bone regeneration in disrupted areas, in order to correct defects in this type of bones, and will improve the distribution of forces in load-bearing implants by guiding the growth of bone tissue in certain areas and in certain directions (Wiemann et al. 2007; Wise et al. 2008). The ingrowth of the aligned tissue into the stomata will promote a better fixation to the scaffold (Karageorgiou and Kaplan 2005).

Both C and SiC scaffolds were produced (Figure 28.13), and the surface morphology is analyzed by SEM and interferometric profilometry. The double macro- and microscaled patterning appeared perfectly preserved or even enhanced once the organic matter had been removed from the C scaffolds (Figure 28.13a and b). In the case of SiC scaffolds (Figure 28.13c and d), the preservation of the macropatterning is especially highlighted, and, due to the formation of the SiC crystals on the surface, the roughness has increased considerably along the channels mitigating the topography of microchannels (Figure 28.13c and d). It is important to note the conservation of the pores in both scaffolds. The interferometric profiles (Figure 28.13b and d), where the lower regions of the profile are represented in blue and the higher ones in red, revealed the distance between the highest point of a ridge and the lowest at the depressed areas (grooves) in the C scaffold (mean profile deviation value) of around 90 μm, being of 60 μm in the SiC. At the same time, the values obtained for the arithmetic average of the roughness profile (Ra), calculated with measures of the scaffolds taken in the perpendicular direction of the patterning structure (Ra perpendicular) and along one of the macroprojections (Ra along channel), were 10.9 and 1.6 μm in the case of the C scaffold and 7.7 and 3.5 μm for SiC. The decrease of roughness across the patterning in the SiC scaffold can be possibly attributed to the formation of SiC crystals in the lowest zones of the profile combined with the deposition of a higher volume of molten silicon in

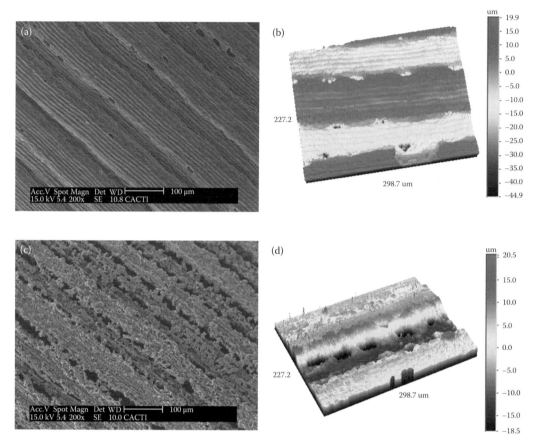

FIGURE 28.13
Surface patterning of the C (a, b) and the SiC scaffolds (c, d) obtained from *J. maritimus* by SEM micrographs (a, c) and interferometric profilometry (b, d) are represented.

the lowest regions during the processing. The increase in roughness along the channels in the ceramic scaffolds can be attributed again to the SiC crystals formed on their surface. Stomata pores can be perfectly distinguished in both profiles.

The C and SiC patterned scaffolds were incubated with the preosteoblastic cell line MC3T3-E1 in order to check if the double patterning of the surface promoted the alignment of these cells and also if cells differentiate to osteoblasts on both materials after induction with 2P-L-ascorbic acid, 2P-glicerol, and melatonin (Sigma). Figure 28.14 presents the cell morphology on the surface of the C scaffold after 24 h of incubation (Figure 28.14a) and after 28 days (Figure 28.14b). In both cases, cells remain aligned. After 24 h, the cells clearly proliferated by extending their filopodia following the orientation marked by the micropatterning of about 7 μm in width. After 28 days of incubation, the surface appeared completely covered by a thick layer of cells, and, what is more interesting, they still maintained the orientation marked by the patterned surface, despite the fact that they were growing on a thick layer of cells and not directly on the patterning. At the same time, the cell showed in image (Figure 28.14b) appears within a complex network of filaments and premineralized extracellular matrix that suggests its differentiation to osteoblast (for detailed information, see M. López-Álvarez 2011, 2012).

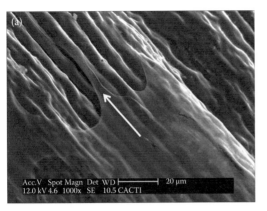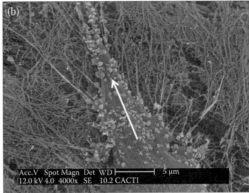

FIGURE 28.14
SEM images of MC3T3-E1 preosteoblasts incubated for 24 h (a) and 28 days (b) on the patterned surface of the C scaffold obtained from *J. maritimus*. (White arrows indicate the cell alignment.)

The mechanism by which the cells align is unclear, but one possible cause is believed to be the mechanical restraint imposed by the walls of the microchannels during the formation of the actin filaments from the cytoskeleton, which are involved in locomotion and cell expansion. In addition, the cell alignment on the microchannels also affects focal adhesions, and it is believed that microtubules also play an important role, since they are the first cellular structures to align (Wang et al. 2000; Li and Shi 2007; Wiemann et al. 2007; Wise et al. 2008; Regan et al. 2010). This marine plant offers great possibilities in the field of tissue engineering due to its great porosity, a patterning that promotes the cell alignment and, finally, demonstrated favorable behavior in terms of cell differentiation.

28.4 Conclusion

This chapter discussed the potentiality of three marine species, the plants *J. maritimus* and *Z. marina* and the macroalgae *L. ochroleuca*, as 3D scaffolds for bone tissue engineering in the form of porous C and SiC ceramics. Porosity, morphology, composition, and biocompatibility have been evaluated for each of the proposed precursors. Three marine-origin biomatrices in two different materials (C and SiC) have been proposed with great perspectives in terms of porosity, composition, and biocompatibility.

Acknowledgments

This work was partially financed by POCTEP 0330IBEROMARE1P project, Xunta de Galicia 2010/83, and Ministerio de Ciencia e Innovación (MAT 2010-18281). The technical staff of CACTI (University of Vigo), Dr. Mariana Landín (University of Santiago de Compostela), and TRABECULAE® Limited Society are gratefully acknowledged.

References

Abramovitch-Gottlib, L., S. Geresh, and R. Vago. 2006. Biofabricated marine hydrozoans: A bioactive crystalline material promoting ossification of mesenchymal stem cells. *Tissue Engineering* 12(4):729–739.

Bettinger, C.J., J.T. Borenstein, and R. Langer. 2008. Microfabrication techniques in scaffold development. In: *Nanotechnology and Tissue Engineering. The Scaffold*, Laurencin, C.T. and L.S. Nair (eds.), pp. 87–113. Boca Raton, FL: CRC Press.

Borrajo, J.P. 2006. Cerámicas biomórficas de carburo de silicio recubiertas con materiales bioactivos para aplicaciones biomédicas. PhD thesis, Universidade de Vigo, Vigo, Spain.

Chen, F., T. Mao, K. Tao, S. Chen, G. Ding, and X. Gu. 2002. Bone graft in the shape of human mandibular condyle reconstruction via seeding marrow-derived osteoblasts into porous coral in a nude mice model. *Journal of Oral and Maxillofacial Surgery* 60:1155–1159.

Cunningham, E., N. Dunne, G. Walker, C. Maggs, R. Wilcox, and F. Buchanan. 2010. Hydroxyapatite bone substitutes developed via replication of natural marine sponges. *Journal of Material Science: Materials in Medicine* 21(8):2255–2261.

Dawes, J.C. 1998. *Marine Botany*. New York: John Wiley & Sons, Inc.

De Arellano-López, A.R., J. Martínez-Fernández, P. González, C. Domínguez, V. Fernández-Quero, and M. Singh. 2004. Biomorphic SiC: A new engineering ceramic material. *International Journal of Applied Ceramic Technology* 1(1):1–12.

González, P., J.P. Borrajo, J. Serra et al. 2009. A new generation of bio-derived ceramic materials for medical applications. *Journal of Biomedical Materials Research (A)* 88(3):807–813.

Graham, L.E. and L.W. Wilcox. 2000. *Algae*. Upper Saddle River, NJ: Prentice Hall.

Green, D.W. 2008. Tissue bionics: Examples in biomimetic tissue engineering. *Biomedical Materials* 3:1–11.

Judd, W.S., C.S. Campbell, E.A. Kellogg, P.F. Stevens, and M.J. Donoghue. 2002. *Plant Systematics: A Phylogenetic Approach*, 2nd edn. Sunderland, MA: Sinauer Associates, Inc.

Karageorgiou, V. and D. Kaplan. 2005. Porosity of 3D biomaterial scaffolds and osteogenesis. *Biomaterials* 26:5374–5491.

Kuboki, Y. H., Takita, D. Kobayashi et al. 1998. BMP-induced osteogenesis on the surface of hydroxyapatite with geometrically feasible and non feasible structures: Topology of osteogenesis. *Journal of Biomedical Materials Research* 39:190–199.

Larkum, W.D., R.J. Orth, and C.M. Duarte. 2006. *Seagrasses: Biology, Ecology and Conservation*. Dordrecht, the Netherlands: Springer.

Li, J. and R. Shi. 2007. Fabrication of patterned multi-walled poly-L-lactic acid conduits for nerve regeneration. *Journal of Neuroscience Methods* 165:257–264.

López-Álvarez, M., I. Pereiro, J. Serra, A. de Carlos, and P. González. 2011. Osteoblast-like cell response to macro and micro-patterned carbon scaffolds obtained from the sea rush Juncus maritimus. *Biomedical Materials* 6(4):045012.

López-Álvarez, M., I. Pereiro, J. Serra, A. de Carlos, and P. González. 2012. Porous silicon carbide scaffolds with patterned surfaces from the sea rush *Juncus maritimus* for tissue engineering applications. *International Journal of Applied Ceramics Technology* 9(3):486–496.

More, R.B., A.D. Haubold, and J.C. Bokros. 2004. Pyrolytic carbon for long-term medical implants. In: *Biomaterials Science: An Introduction to Materials in Medicine*, Ratner, por B.D., A.S. Hoffmann, and F.J. Schoen (eds.), pp. 170–181. London, U.K.: Elsevier Academic Press.

Murray, W.N. 2005. *Introducción a la botánica*. Madrid, Spain: Ed. Pearson/Addison Wesley.

Nishiguchi, S., H. Kato, M. Neo et al. 2001. Alkali and heat treated porous titanium for orthopedic implants. *Journal of Biomedical Materials Research* 54:198–208.

Paniagua, R., M. Nistal, M. Álvarez-Uría, and B. Fraile. 1994. *Citología e Histología Vegetal y Animal*. Madrid, Spain: McGraw-Hill-Interamericana de España.

Park, S.N., J.C. Park, H.O. Kim, M.J. Song, and H. Suh. 2002. Characterization of porous collagen/ hyaluronic acid scaffold modified by 1-ethyl-3-(3-dimethylaminopropyl) carbodiimide cross-linking. *Biomaterials* 23:1205–1212.

Pilliar, R.M. 1998. Overview of surface variability of metallic endosseous dental implants: Textured and porous surface-structured designs. *Implant Dentistry* 7:305–314.

Ratner, B.D. 2004. A history of biomaterials. In: *Biomaterials Science: An Introduction to Materials in Medicine*, Ratner, B.D., A.S. Hoffmann, and F.J. Schoen (eds.), pp. 10–19. London, U.K.: Elsevier Academic Press.

Regan, E.M., J.B. Uney, A.D. Dick et al. 2010. Differential patterning of neuronal, glial and neural progenitor cells on phosphorus-doped and UV irradiated diamond-like carbon. *Biomaterials* 31:207–215.

Varela-Feria, F.M., J. Ramírez-Rico, A.R. de Arellano-López, J. Martínez-Fernández, and M. Singh. 2008. Reaction-formation mechanisms and microstructure evolution of biomorphic SiC. *Journal of Materials Science* 43(3):933–941.

Wang, J.H.C., E.S. Grood, J. Florer, and R. Wenstrup. 2000. Alignment and proliferation of MC3T3-E1 osteoblasts in microgrooved silicone substrata subjected to cyclic stretching. *Journal of Biomechanics* 33:729–735.

Wiemann, M., D. Bingmann, S. Franzka, N. Hartmann, H. Urch, and M. Epple. 2007. Oriented growth of osteoblast-like cells on two-dimensionally structured films of functionalized calcium phosphate nanoparticles on a silicon substrate. *Advanced Engineering Materials* 9(12):1077–1081.

Wise, J.K., M. Cho, E. Zussman, C.M. Megaridis, and A.L. Yarin. 2008. Electrospinning techniques to control deposition and structural alignment of nanofibrous scaffolds for cellular orientation and cytoskeletal reorganization. In: *Nanotechnology and Tissue Engineering. The Scaffold*, Laurencin, C.T. and L.S. Nair (eds.), pp. 243–260. Boca Raton, FL: CRC Press.

Yang, F., W.L. Neeley, M.J. Moore, J.M. Darp, A. Shukla, and R. Langer. 2008. Tissue engineering: The therapeutic strategy of the twenty-first century. In: *Nanotechnology and Tissue Engineering. The Scaffold*, Laurencin, C.T. and L.S. Nair (eds.), pp. 3–33. Boca Raton, FL: CRC Press.

29

Application of Marine Biomaterials in Orthopedic and Soft Tissue Surgical Challenges

Samit Kumar Nandi, Uttam Datta, and Subhasish Biswas

CONTENTS

29.1 Introduction

Life-saving organ transplantation and reconstruction surgery have made considerable dimension as routine procedures in advanced medical treatment but sometimes are associated with limitations. These procedures need either organ donation from a donor or tissue transplantation from a second surgical site from the individual under treatment. In the earlier one, there is an acute scarcity of donor organs, while the latter is connected with pain and morbidity of the sufferer. As a result, attempts have been initiated in tissue engineering to develop organs, tissues, and synthetic materials ex situ for future transplant use (Bell 1993; Langer and Vacanti 1993; Lauffenburger 1994; Peppas and Langer, 1994; Lanza et al. 1997; Healy et al. 1999; Service 2000).

Bone and joint problems are the major concern for millions of people worldwide. Indeed, they account for half of all chronic diseases in people over 50 years of age in developed countries. Additionally, it is predicted that the percentage of similar problems of the same age group would be doubled by 2020 (Kon et al. 2000). These diseases often necessitate surgery, including total joint replacement in cases of deterioration of the natural joint. Moreover, numerous bone fractures, low back pain, osteoporosis, scoliosis, and other musculoskeletal problems need to be solved by using permanent, temporary, or biodegradable devices.

From the inception till today, the search for an effective protocol for treatment of simple defect and management of segmental bone loss is only to understand that many miles are yet to be traversed for harnessing the effective remedial steps to win over these complications.

Bone is the second most frequently transplanted tissue (second only to transfused blood) (Kelly 2000). In human orthopedics, bone is used annually in more than 2.2 million graft procedures worldwide to repair defects created upon removal of infected tissue, bone cysts, tumor, and fracture nonunion; traumatic and pathological fractures; joint and spinal fusion; revision arthroplasty; and plastic surgery (Vaccaro 2002).

Bone grafting has also become a vital part of orthopedic surgery during the past two decades. It is mainly used to promote fracture healing, to fill gaps in the fracture site, or to replace missing bone fragments (Kelly 2000). Bone grafts are named according to their source histocompatibility or their structure–composition. Based on the source histocompatibility, an autograft (autogenous graft) is tissue that is transferred from one site to another in the same individual. An allograft is tissue transplanted from one individual to another of the same species. Xenograft is tissue transplanted between individuals of different species. The most desirable form of bone substitute is the autologous bone graft for their superior osteoconduction, ease of incorporation, and lack of immunological reactions (Naber et al. 1972; Marciani et al., 1977). Besides, it contains noncollagenous bone matrix proteins that stimulate osteoinduction and incorporates progenitor stem cells for osteogenesis. However, massive replacements of bone are not easily achieved by bone autografts (Mankin et al., 1976) as autogenous bone is limited in availability and may result in the donor-site morbidity. Furthermore, harvesting the autograft requires an additional surgery at the donor site that can result in its own complications, such as increased patient recovery time, inflammation, risk of extensive blood loss, infection, structural damage to donor bone disability, and chronic pain. In a retrospective study of 214 human patients with iliac crest bone grafting, the percentage of severe procurement complications (infection, severe blood loss, neurological damage) was only 2%, but about 24% of the patients showed chronic donor-site pain, and pain that was severe enough to interfere with daily activity at a mean follow-up of more than 4 years was significantly high (15%) (Skaggs et al. 2000). Another limitation of the efficacy of autogenous graft is damage of most viable cells taken from the harvest site when they are separated from their blood supply and processed in the surgical suite even with appropriated handling (McLaughlin and Roush 1998; Betz 2002). Allograft material is readily available, without the requirement of a secondary surgical site. They provide a source of type I collagen, which is the sole organic component of bone. However, they do not produce the inorganic calcium or scaffolding necessary for bone regeneration. Besides, the possible immune response and disease transmission may be detrimental for the recipient (Gazdag et al. 1995; Chapman et al. 1997). In addition, the efficacy of allograft material is inconsistent. The processing of allograft tissue to lower contamination risk can also significantly degrade the biologic and mechanical properties initially present in the donated tissue. Moreover, an abundant supply is not guaranteed; processed and banked donor bone is not always available at the time of surgery (Betz 2002). Based on the second criteria, structure–composition, bone grafts can be classified as cancellous (prepared from a bone trabeculae network collected mainly from the metaphyseal areas of long bones), cortical (prepared from a tubular segment of compact bone), corticocancellous (having both cortical and cancellous bone, e.g., rib graft), and osteochondral (prepared from articular cartilage and bone tissue, e.g., distal radius from bone bank to limb-sparing procedures).

Bone grafts can tender therapeutic benefits in terms of mechanical support and/or enhancing fracture healing. In large bony defects, cortical or osteochondral autogenous or allogeneic grafts are generally used and rigid internal fixation must be used to ensure the stability of the graft within the recipient site. In general, the ideal properties of grafts to stimulate bone healing should have one or several of the following properties: osteogenesis, osteoinduction, or osteoconduction. Osteogenesis is the formation of new bone in the recipient site by donor cells such as osteoblasts and undifferentiated mesenchymal cells that survive the transfer, in short, provides stem cells with osteogenic potential, which directly lays down new bone. Osteoinduction is the differentiation of undifferentiated mesenchymal cells of the fracture site into osteogenic cells (osteoblasts; chondroblast) by the action of different factors present in the graft such as bone morphogenic proteins (BMP; BMP-2), transforming growth factor-β (TGF-β), insulin-like growth factor (IGF), platelet-derived growth factor (PDGF), and cytokines, in short, induces a differentiation of stem cells into osteogenic cells. Osteoconduction is a 3D process of ingrowths of capillaries, perivascular tissue, and mesenchymal cells from the recipient bed into the structure of the graft, which provides scaffolding for this new bone formation, in short, provides a passive porous scaffold to support direct bone formation.

In order to get rid of the need for autograft collection and avoid potential complications related with allografts, various substances have been investigated as synthetic bone graft substitutes in human and animals (Elkins and Jones 1998; Sandhu and Grewal 1999; Moore et al. 2001; Galois et al. 2002; Dorea et al. 2005); however, none are ideal to satisfy all three requisite properties of osteoinduction, osteogenesis, and osteoconduction present in fresh cancellous bone autografts. Gradually, advances in bone grafting have stimulated the science through tissue, cellular, and molecular levels with the use of osteoblast cell cultures, demineralized bone matrix (DBM), bone marrow aspirates, recombinant bone morphogenetic protein (rhBMP-2), osteogenic protein (OP-1) as growth factors, etc. However, their high cost and logistics needed noticeably restrict their use in orthopedics application.

Calcium phosphate (CP) ceramics (β-tricalcium phosphate [β-TCP], hydroxyapatite [HAp]) have also been developed and used as a synthetic osteoconductive scaffold for three decades with successful research and clinical application (Elkins and Jones 1988; Szpalski and Gunzburg 2002), in human orthopedics and dental applications with excellent results (Anker et al. 2005; Arts et al. 2005). In order to promise a good osteoconductive effect, porosity of the ceramic structure is a key determinant of the amount of surface area exposed to the biological setting (Galois et al. 2002). Interconnected porosity and pore sizes in the range of 150–500 μm are optimal for interface activity, cellular migration, and bone ingrowth (Galois et al. 2002) throughout the ceramic implant because it more closely resembles the trabecular structure of cancellous bone (Elkins and Jones 1988).

Apart from the tremendous role of biomaterials in bone healing, several biomaterials are also using a wound enhancer. Wound healing is a complicated and well-orchestrated process involving multiple biological pathways and signaling and is of major importance especially in chemotherapeutic wound and chronic diabetic wounds and to the survival and clinical outcome of burn patients irrespective of man and animals. Clinically, the current treatment in topical wound management includes debridement, topical antibiotics, and a state-of-the-art topical dressing, which are a multilayer system that can include a collagen cellulose substrate, neonatal foreskin fibroblasts, growth factor-containing cream, and a silicone sheet covering for moisture control. Wound healing time can be up to 20 weeks. Although topical application of different drugs and/or agents has shown to favor healing, the subject is still controversial. Extensive research in this aspect has been conducted for the treatment of open wounds and revealed that topical medicaments either do not affect wound healing or inhibit rather than trigger it. Scanty information is available for proper guideline for treatment of wounds especially diabetic and chemotherapeutic in animal and human subject.

During the last decade, a variety of materials, such as metals, metal alloys, collagen, carbon-based materials, polymers, ceramics, and composites of the previously mentioned materials with growth factors and stem cells, have been recommended to fill and reconstruct bone defects with varying success. Irrespective of soft and hard tissue healing, angiogenesis plays the most vital role that remains a significant challenge in regenerative medicine applications. Whether the goal is to induce vascular growth in ischemic tissue or scale up tissue-engineered constructs, the ability to induce the growth of patent, stable vasculature is a critical obstacle. At present, a large focus of clinical and preclinical work is centered on local delivery strategy/vehicle of angiogenetic agents either in orthopedic or wound areas in a controlled microenvironment.

Marine environment has been recognized as an important and alternate source of bioactive biomaterials having medicinal potential. Apart from human medicines, the research on marine natural product in the last three decades has also brought forth the discovery of many chemically and biologically interesting molecules. The development of marine compound as therapeutic agent is still in its infancy due to lack of an analogous ethnomedical history as compared with terrestrial habitats, together with the relative technical difficulties in collecting marine organisms. The marine environment is rich in mineralizing organisms with porous structures, some of which are currently being used as bone graft materials and others that are in early stages of development (Clarke et al. 2011). Chitosan, a natural product derived from the polysaccharide chitin (aminopolysaccharide; combination of sugar and protein), an abundantly available natural biopolymer found in the exoskeletons of crustacean like shrimp, crabs, lobster, and other shellfish, would be an effective material to repair bone defects due to its biocompatibility. Coral exoskeleton, a marine product derived from *Porites* sp., acts as a scaffold because of its interconnected porous architecture, high compressive breaking stress, good biocompatibility, and resorbability. This chapter focuses on the application of different marine biomaterials for wound and orthopedic surgical challenges.

29.2 Coral as Bone Graft Substitute

For many years, resorbable porous ceramics derived from chemically converted corals have been used successfully as bone graft substitutes in both orthopedic and maxillo-cranio-facial surgery. This natural material is now extensively replaced by synthetic biomaterials like HAp or bioglasses with various mineral composition and porosity. Coral is mainly composed of calcium carbonate in the form of aragonite that was quickly absorbed by the body, which didn't allow for enough time for new bone to grow on the coralline scaffolding. Coral has optimal strength and structural characteristics due to its natural origin. The converted corals afford a 3D porous architecture that resembles cancellous bone with a pore diameter of 200–700 μm and lead to vascular ingrowth, differentiation of osteoprogenitor cells, remodeling, and graft resorption together with host bone ingrowth into the porous microstructure during resorption (Dee and Bizios 1996; Hu et al. 2000). It has been suggested that this natural biomaterial might be used as subchondral graft to support resurfacing of articular cartilage (Shahgaldi 1998) and hard tissue healing (Vago et al. 2002). Bamboo coral internodes exhibit bone-like mechanical and biochemical properties; structural and biochemical analyses of these natural biomineral composites and separation of proteinaceous components were carried out. Because of its high potential for colonization with both human osteoblasts and osteoclasts, the organic matrix, composed of an acidic fibrillar protein framework, proved to be a very successful model for possible applications in tissue engineering especially in orthopedic surgery and as "living bone implants" (Ehrlich et al. 2006).

Coralline ceramics have the benefit of being completely biocompatible, accepted by the patient's body as so similar to bone that they do not cause a negative immune reaction. Pore interconnection sizes are of paramount importance to achieve excellent mechanical bond when hard and soft tissue is involved. Biomaterials with interconnective pores are considered to be superior as compared to dead-end pores, because a spatial continuous connection of the pore system has an important meaning for the ingrowth of new bone (Osborn and Newesely 1980) especially in long-term tissue interface maintenance (Lemons 1996). It has been observed that implants with average pore sizes of 260–500 μm is of utmost necessity for ingrowth of osteoblasts and 200 μm for coralline HAp (Kuhne et al. 1994). Hydrothermal conversion of coral preserves the interconnected structure while altering the chemical structure from aragonite to HAp (Roy and Linnehan 1974; Holmes et al. 1984; White and Shors 1986). Depending on the coral species used, HAp and TCP can be produced with varying porosities. Coralline HAp surpassed cancellous bone strength after 6 months due to infiltration of bone and provides early structural support (Elsinger and Lear 1996). In a serial study up to 52 weeks involving calcium carbonate–HAp coral in animal bone defect model, it has been observed based on radiography, torsional testing, and quantitative histomorphometry using backscattering scanning electron microscopy that implants were nearly completely resorbed by 52 weeks with only a few percent of implant remaining (Chapman-Sheath et al. 2003). Based on the measurements of hardness, compressive strength, bulk density, and apparent porosity, marine coral could be an alternative xenograft due to its mechanical properties, osteoconductive nature (Alvarez et al. 2002), and micromechanical elastic properties (Nomura et al. 2005).

Coral implant as bone graft substitute should be used mainly as support in non-load-bearing situations. If it is necessary to use the material in load-bearing areas, the implant should be directionally oriented to obtain maximum strength, and maximum surface area should be in the direction of load (Hu et al. 2000). Based on the conversion process in commercial coralline HAp, the dissolution rate is very high as the structure possesses nanopores within the interpore trabeculae and ultimately reduces durability and strength. To overcome these limitations, two-stage application routes involving complete conversion of coral to pure HAp is achieved followed by solgel-derived HAp nano-coating applied to cover the micro- and nanopores within the intrapore material without hampering the large pores. This newer material can be applied in load-bearing situations (Ben-Nissan et al. 2004). The resorption rate of the coral can be controlled by partial conversion to provide a HAp layer via thermal modification. To increase the mechanical properties and to overcome the lower mechanical properties of HAp, fluorine-doped HAp from Indian coast corals and zirconia composites using coralline HAp and coralline fluorapatite has been developed for biomedical application (Sivakumar and Manjubala 2001).

In clinical setting, autogenous bone grafting has been the standard approach to reconstruction of trauma-induced metatarsal defects but having well-known disadvantages related to the harvesting, size, shape, and availability of autografts. Synthetic HAp bone graft substitute manufactured from a marine coral has been successfully used in a large, posttraumatic first metatarsal defect with effective outcome (Nesheiwat et al. 1998).

29.2.1 Coral in Maxillofacial, Dentistry, and Ear Application

Coral grafts have been successfully applied in maxillofacial surgery since 1992 and observed that in clinical cases they are well tolerated and are simultaneously partially ossified as the calcified skeleton is resorbed. Clinical cases show that use of this material has been successful (Soost 1996; Soost et al. 1998). Coralline HAp is a highly biocompatible material, which exhibited abundant ingrowth when in contact with host bone and good soft tissue ingrowth and fibrous tissue fixation within the middle ear and against the tympanic membrane. In animal model (canine) for middle ear and mastoid reconstruction, porous (coralline) HAp showed excellent results as otologic graft material (Jahn 1992). Successful outcome of an implant in the grafted maxillary sinus is dependent on the formation of new vital autogenous bone and its mineral density. Marine algae HAp graft material with autogenous bone has been used in the sinus augmentation procedure to support dental implants under occlusal loads that permits early loading of implants in the grafted maxillary sinus (Lee et al. 2011). Biocoral has also been successfully used in dentistry (Figueiredo et al. 2010).

29.2.2 Coral as Drug Delivery System

Coralline hydroxyapatite (CHA) can also be used as an efficient carrier system for the local delivery of growth factors to enhance osteointegration and implant fixation into peri-implant osseous tissue (Damien and Revell 2004).

29.3 Marine Sponge Skeleton as Bone Graft Substitute

Marine sponges are aquatic, sessile, filter-feeding metazoans of collagen origin (Simpson 1984). The Western Australia coast is the rich and diverse range of sources of marine sponges (Fromont et al. 2006). Marine sponges have been used as commercial bath sponges since early Greek civilization and, of late, as potential sources of therapeutic drugs and antibiotic substances (Hooper and Van Soest 2002; Shim et al. 2003). The abundance and structural diversity of natural marine sponge skeletons and their potential as multifunctional, cell conductive and inductive frameworks along with collagenous composition of the fiber indicate a promising new source of scaffold for tissue regeneration (Lin et al. 2011). Collagen-based marine sponge skeletons indicate that the collagenous fiber skeleton of marine sponges provides a suitable bioscaffold for bone regeneration, as it supports the adhesion, migration, and proliferation of osteoblasts in vitro (Zheng et al. 2007). The complex canal system within sponges creates a porous environment, which is ideal for cellular integration when combined with cells for tissue engineering. The possession of open interconnected channels created by a porous structured network in sponge is capable to induce osteoblast attachment, proliferation, migration, and differentiation in vitro, signifying its potential as a bioscaffold for bone tissue engineering (Green et al. 2003). The sponge–cell constructs help osteogenesis as observed by alkaline phosphatase expression, an early marker of osteoblast differentiation, mineral deposition, and the expression of osteogenic markers such as osteocalcin and osteopontin.

Spongin as a component of fibrous skeleton, pseudokeratin, neurokeratin, horny protein, and collagen-like protein in sponges can be used in several biomedical applications including osteoarthritis (OA). Spongin derived from *Hymeniacidon sinapium* can help bone mineralization of osteoblast-like MG-63 cells, increased ALP activity, collagen synthesis, and osteocalcin secretion in addition to bone mineralization in osteoblastic cells in vitro (Kim et al. 2009).

Silicatein-mediated "biosilica" formation in marine sponges, the involvement of further molecules in silica metabolism, and their potential application have been studied in biomedicine especially in bone replacement material and in the treatment of osteoporosis (Wang et al. 2011).

29.4 Chitosan as Bone Graft Substitute

During the past 25 years, chitosan has been recognized as a biomaterial for tissue engineering applications. Chitin, the source material for chitosan, is one of the most abundant organic materials, being second only to cellulose in the amount produced annually by biosynthesis. Chitosan is produced from chitin, which is a natural polysaccharide found in exoskeleton of crab, shrimp, lobster, coral, jellyfish, butterfly, ladybug, mushroom, and fungi. Nevertheless, marine crustacean shells are extensively used as primary sources for the production of chitosan (Madhavan and Nair 1974; Shahidi and Abuzaytoun 2005). Chitosan is a linear polysaccharide, composed of glucosamine and N-acetyl glucosamine units linked by β (1–4) glycosidic bonds. The chemical nature of chitosan in turn provides many potential for covalent and ionic modifications, which allow extensive adjustment of mechanical and biological properties.

A number of natural and synthetic polymers have been considered for overcoming the limitations as bone substitutes. In particular, chitosan has been extensively used in bone reconstruction due to its capacity to promote growth, biocompatibility, biodegradability, and biological and chemical similarities to natural tissues, and it can be molded into porous structures (Barbara 2005; Di Martino et al. 2005). In addition, the biological, physical, and chemical properties of chitosan can be tailored under mild conditions (Barbara 2005) and can be implanted into human body safely (Chenite et al. 2000). In the present times, most of the chitosan-based research is designed on 3D composite scaffolds as permanent implant in human body (Dhiman et al. 2005; Rezwan et al. 2006).

Varieties of composites on chitosan–CPs especially with β-TCP and HAp have been used in bone tissue engineering. CP bioceramic implanted with chitosan sponge has been used to enhance mechanical property of the ceramic phase via matrix reinforcement and preserving the osteoblast phenotype (Zhang and Zhang 2002; Zhang et al. 2003). The in vivo effect of HAp/chitosan materials through its application on the surface of the tibia after periosteum removal has been carried out with evidence of new bone after 1 week (Kawakami et al. 1992). Zhao et al. (2002) developed HAp/chitosan–gelatin network composites in the form of 3D porous scaffolds with the characteristics of improved adhesion, proliferation, and expression of rat calvarium osteoblasts on these highly porous scaffolds. HAp–chitin composite material exhibited rapid degradation and neovascularization in vivo during a 3-month period (Ge et al. 2004). In a study, it has been observed that chitosan may act as an adjuvant to improve injectability of the cement while keeping the physicochemical properties suitable for surgical application: setting time suitable for surgery, minimum disintegration of the cement in biological fluids, and mechanical properties suited to the kind of operation (Leroux et al. 1999). The said composites may be helpful for the regeneration of larger, non-load-bearing bone defects although in vivo evaluation of the composites is still under progress (Gutowska et al. 2001). For creation of macropores in injectable, bioabsorbable calcium phosphate ceramic (CPC) scaffold, chitosan has been used without compromising the strength and provided strength and elasticity for the implantation during tissue regeneration (Xu et al. 2004). Apart from this CPC, composites of chitosan with polymethyl-methacrylate (PMMA) have been developed as osteoconductive material for bone healing (Kim et al. 2004). The pore size of this composite material increased with the passage of time due to biodegradation of the chitosan. In addition, chitosan has been used to modify the surface properties of prosthetic materials for the attachment of osteoblasts (Lee et al. 2002a,b). Titanium (Ti) surface coated with chitosan via silane–glutaraldehyde chemistry exhibited increased osteoblast attachment and proliferation (Bumgardner et al. 2003). In wrapping up, chitosan is a promising candidate scaffold material in clinical practice particularly in orthopedic surgery due to the novel ability to bind anionic molecules such as growth factors, even though it needs to improve their mechanical properties for bone tissue engineering.

29.5 Marine Biomaterials in Bone Tissue Engineering

Tissue engineering as termed "regenerative medicine" is regarded as a finally ideal medical treatment for diseases that have been too intricate to be cured by existing approaches. This biomedical engineering is designed to repair injured body parts and restore their functions by using laboratory-grown tissues, materials, and artificial implants.

Bone tissue engineering aims to mimic the natural process of bone formation by delivering a source of cells and/or growth factors in a scaffold matrix, which can induce cellular attachment, migration, proliferation, and osteoblastic differentiation (Bruder and Fox 1999; Goldstein et al. 1999). Despite the rapid development in the area and having significant regenerative capacity of bone, bone tissue engineering plays a vital role in different serious clinical conditions like pathological and nonunion fracture, spinal arthrodesis, and management of maxillofacial fractures (Bruder and Fox 1999; Gittens and Uludag 2001).

Bone tissue engineering involves the use of scaffold matrices through which bone marrow stromal cells can be delivered to the defect site using different vehicles. A number of scaffold materials are available, but the ideal one should have biocompatibility and osteoconductive and osteoinductive properties together with a structure that mimics the trabecular network of bone tissue (Bruder and Fox 1999). Both natural and synthetic materials are being used in bone tissue engineering, but natural materials are superior because they are more biocompatible and tender a better biointeractive surface for cell attachment and growth (Sharma and Elisseeff 2004). Moreover, natural scaffolds derived from biological tissues exhibit highly optimized structures and comprise extracellular matrix components that offer a basis for cell attachment, migration, and proliferation (Green et al. 2002a). One of the satisfactory approaches is using biodegradable coral, and engineered bone from osteogenically induced bone marrow mesenchymal stromal cells (BMSCs) achieved satisfactory biomechanical properties at 32 weeks post-operation and can successfully repair the critical-sized segmental mandibular defects in canines, and the seeding cells could be used for bony restoration (Yuan et al. 2010). In another study, spontaneous induction of bone formation by coral-derived calcium carbonate-based macroporous constructs is initiated by secreted BMPs/OP-1 (Ripamonti et al. 2010). It is well established that human bone marrow (hBM) is an excellent source of mesenchymal stem cells (MSCs), which may differentiate into different cell phenotypes such as osteoblasts, chondrocytes, adipocytes, myocytes, cardiomyocytes, and neurons. Biomaterial, such as corals as osteoconductive material has been used to home human derived stem cells and is able to differentiate into osteoblasts that can be applied for clinical regenerative purposes (Tran et al. 2011).

The application for tissue-engineered bone of fiber skeleton of natural marine sponge was first reported by Green et al. (2003). Porosity within the marine sponge skeleton is formed by a system of pores (ostia), channels, and chambers throughout the sponge body that afford the living sponge with nutrition and gas exchange from the surrounding water. The open porosity of this scaffold enables maximal invasion of cells and bone tissue that is necessary for bone reconstruction while minimizing the volume of space taken up by the biomaterial (Gibson and Ashby 1988). The pore dimension of the scaffold plays a vital role for osteoblast integration into bone tissue. In general, optimum pore dimensions for bone tissue regeneration in synthetic scaffolds are between 100 and 250 μm (Karande et al. 2004). The pore dimension of the sponge, ranging from 100 to 300 μm, was equivalent to the pore size in human compact bone, indicating an ideal scaffold for tissue-engineered bone (Bilezikian et al. 2002).

The osteoinductive potential of coral, sea sponge, and nacre and the capacity of these materials to support human osteoprogenitor cell attachment, migration, growth, and differentiation were investigated (Green et al. 2002b). A novel tricomponent scaffold comprising of natural marine materials like chitosan, HAp derived from *Thunnus obesus* bone, and marine sponge (*Ircinia fusca*) collagen (MSCol) has been developed using freeze-drying and lyophilization method that paved the way for bone augmentation (Pallela et al. 2011).

29.6 Marine Biomaterials for Wound Healing

Irrespective of animal or human being, wound healing is a complicated and well-orchestrated process involving multiple biological pathways and signaling. Various kinds of intracellular and intercellular mechanisms encompassing the immune system, blood coagulation cascade, and pro-inflammatory signaling are intricately associated with the healing and repair process (Deodhar and Rana 1997; Nguyen et al. 2009). Healing in major organs cannot regenerate the functional and structural integrity of original tissues for which better scientific understanding is necessary to accelerate the healing process as well as to regenerate the original tissue architecture as it happens during prenatal development. Marine biomaterials can be an untapped gold mine for this purpose.

The wounds in acute and chronic cases, particularly more extensive wounds, need skin substitutes to repair. The aim of skin tissue engineering is to produce a construct that offers the complete regeneration of functional skin and allow the skin to fulfill normal functions like barrier formation, pigmentory defense against UV irradiation, thermoregulation, and mechanical and aesthetic functions (Metcalfe and Ferguson 2007). Among all the functions, some can be managed with existing skin substitutes, but in many situations, skin substitutes are mandatory. Previously, many skin substitutes such as xenograft, allografts, and autografts have been used for wound healing. However, several disadvantages like antigenicity or the limitation of donor sites restrict their widespread use as skin substitutes (Yanas and Burke 1980; Bell et al. 1981; Schul et al. 2000; Ma et al. 2003). Skin substitutes promote wound healing by simulating the host to produce various cytokines, which in turn play an important role not only in preventing dehydration and increasing inflammation but also in promoting the formation of granulation tissue in wound healing processes.

Chitosan as a skin substitute material has many advantages for wound healing such as hemostasis, enhancing the tissue regeneration and stimulating the fibroblast synthesis of collagen (Taravel and Domard 1995, 1996; Ma et al. 2001). Chitosan in the form of chitosan cotton triggers the wound healing by promoting infiltration of polymorpho-nuclear (PMN) cells at the wound site that is an indispensable event in rapid wound healing (Ueno et al. 1999). Recent studies indicate that incorporation of basic fibroblast growth factor (bFGF) in chitosan accelerated the rate of wound healing (Mizuno et al. 2003). Chitosan in combination with alginate as polyelectrolyte complex (PEC) membranes showed greater stability to pH changes and hence more rapid healing (Yan et al. 2000). Porous chitosan/collagen scaffold by their cross-linking with glutaraldehyde and freeze-drying improves and provides biostability and good biocompatibility and could successfully induce the fibroblast infiltration from the surrounding tissue of wound (Ma et al. 2003).

29.7 Conclusion

Marine biomaterials possess enormous future potentiality for bone repairing/regeneration as well as for wound healing over the conventional methods of treatment. The unique properties of marine biomaterials will pave the way for new directions of treatment and to combat many diseases that are yet to be solved.

References

Alvarez, K., S. Camero, M.E. Alarcón, A. Rivas, and G. González. 2002. Physical and mechanical properties evaluation of *Acropora palmata* coralline species for bone substitution applications. *J Mater Sci Mater Med* 13(5):509–515.

Anker, C.J., S.P. Holdridge, B. Baird, H. Cohen, and T.A. Damron. 2005. Ultraporous beta-tricalcium phosphate is well incorporated in small cavitary defects. *Clin Orthop Relat Res* 434:251–257.

Arts, J.J., J.W. Gardeniers, M.L. Welten, N. Verdonschot, B.W. Schreurs, and P. Buma. 2005. No negative effects of bone impaction grafting with bone and ceramic mixtures. *Clin Orthop Relat Res* 438:239–247.

Barbara, K. 2005. Membrane-based processes performed with use of chitin/chitosan materials. *Sep Purif Technol* 41(3):305–312.

Bell, E. 1993. *Tissue Engineering: Current Perspectives*. Boston, MA: Birkhauser.

Bell, E., H.P. Ehrlich, D.J. Battle, and T. Nakatsuji. 1981. Living tissue formed in vitro and accepted as skin-equivalent tissue of full thickness. *Science* 211:1052–1054.

Ben-Nissan, B., A. Milev, and R. Vago. 2004. Morphology of sol-gel derived nano-coated coralline hydroxyapatite. *Biomaterials* 25(20):4971–4975.

Betz, R.R. 2002. Limitations of autograft and allograft: New synthetic solutions. *Orthopedics* 25(5):561–570.

Bilezikian, J.P., G.A. Rodan, and L.G. Raisz. 2002. *Principles of Bone Biology*, 2nd edn. San Diego, CA: Academic Press.

Bruder, S.P. and B.S. Fox. 1999. Tissue engineering of bone. Cell based strategies. *Clin Orthop Relat Res* 367:S68–S83.

Bumgardner, J.D., R. Wiser, P.D. Gerard, P. Bergin, B. Chestnutt, M. Marin et al. 2003. Chitosan: Potential use as a bioactive coating for orthopaedic and craniofacial/dental implants. *J Biomater Sci Polym Ed* 14:423–438.

Chapman, M.W., R., Bucholz, and C. Cornell. 1997. Treatment of acute fracture with collagen-calcium phosphate graft material. *J Bone and Joint Surg* 79-A:143–147.

Chapman-Sheath, P., S. Cain, J. Debes, M. Svehla, W. Bruce, Y. Yu, and W.R. Walsh. 2003. In vivo response of coral biomaterials. *J Bone Joint Surg Br* 85-B:1–2.

Chenite, A., C. Chaput, D. Wang, C. Combes, M.D. Buschmann, C.D. Hoemann, J.C. Leroux, B.L. Atkinson, F. Binette, and A. Selmani. 2000. Novel injectable neutral solutions of chitosan form biodegradable gels in situ. *Biomaterials* 21(21):2155–2161.

Clarke, S.A., P. Walsh, C.A. Maggs, and F. Buchanan. 2011. Designs from the deep: Marine organisms for bone tissue engineering. *Biotechnol Adv* 29(6):610–617.

Damien, E. and P.A. Revell. 2004. Coralline hydroxyapatite bone graft substitute: A review of experimental studies and biomedical applications. *J Appl Biomater Biomech* 2(2):65–73.

Dee, K.C. and R. Bizios. 1996. Proactive biomaterials and bone tissue engineering. *Biotechnol Bioeng* 50:438–442.

Deodhar, A.K. and R.E. Rana. 1997. Surgical physiology of wound healing: A review. *J Postgrade Med* 43:52–56.

Dhiman, H.K., A.R. Ray, and A.K. Panda. 2005. Three-dimensional chitosan scaffold-based MCF-7 cell culture for the determination of the cytotoxicity of tamoxifen. *Biomaterials* 26(9):979–986.

Di Martino, A., M. Sittinger, and M.V. Risbud. 2005. Chitosan: A versatile biopolymer for orthopaedic tissue engineering. *Biomaterials* 26(30):5983–5990.

Dorea, H.C., R.M. McLaughlin, H.D. Cantwell, R. Read, L. Armbrust, R. Pool, J.K. Roush, and C. Boyle. 2005. Evaluation of healing in feline femoral defects filled cancellous autograft, cancellous allograft or bioglass. *Vet Comp Orthop Traumatol* 18:157–168.

Ehrlich, H., P. Etnoyer, S.D. Litvinov, M.M. Olennikova, H. Domaschke, T. Hanke, R. Born, H. Meissner, and H. Worch. 2006. Biomaterial structure in deep-sea bamboo coral (Anthozoa: Gorgonacea: Isididae): Perspectives for the development of bone implants and templates for tissue engineering. *Material wissenschaft und Werkstofftechnik* 37(6):552–557.

Elkins, A.D. and L.P. Jones. 1988. The effects of plaster of Paris and autogenous cancellous bone on the healing of cortical defects in the femurs of dogs. *Vet Surg* 17(2):71–76.

Elsinger, E.C. and L. Lear. 1996. Coralline hydroxyapatite bone graft substitutes. *J Foot Ankle Surg* 30:396.

Figueiredo, M., J. Henriques, G. Martins, F. Guerra, F. Judas, and H. Figueiredo. 2010. Physicochemical characterization of biomaterials commonly used in dentistry as bone substitutes—Comparison with human bone. *J Biomed Mater Res B Appl Biomater* 92(2):409–419.

Fromont, J., M. Vanderklift, and G. Kendrick. 2006. Marine sponges of the Dampier Archipelago, Western Australia: Patterns of species distributions, abundance and diversity. *Biodivers Conserv* 15:3731–3750.

Galois, L., D. Mainard, and J.P. Delagoutte. 2002. Beta-tricalcium phosphate ceramic as a bone substitute in orthopaedic surgery. *Int Orthop* 26(2):109–115.

Gazdag, A.R., J.M. Lane, D. Glaser, and R.A. Forster. 1995. Alternatives to autogenous bone graft: Efficacy and indications. *J Am Acad Orthop Surg* 3:1–8.

Ge, Z., S. Baguenard, L.Y. Lim, A. Wee, and E. Khor. 2004. Hydroxyapatite–chitin materials as potential tissue engineered bone substitutes. *Biomaterials* 25:1049–1058.

Gibson, L.J. and M.F. Ashby. 1988. *Cellular Solids: Structures and Properties*. London, U.K.: Pergamon Press.

Gittens, S.A. and H. Uludag. 2001. Growth factor delivery for bone tissue engineering. *J Drug Target* 9:407–429.

Goldstein, S.A., P.V. Patil, and M.R. Moalli. 1999. Perspectives on tissue engineering of bone. *Clin Orthop Relat Res* 367:S419–S423.

Green, D., D. Howard, X. Yang, M. Kelly, and R.O. Oreffo. 2003. Natural marine sponge fiber skeleton: A biomimetic scaffold for human osteoprogenitor cell attachment, growth, and differentiation. *Tissue Eng* 9:1159–1166.

Green, D., D. Howard, X. Yang, K. Partridge, N.M.P. Clarke, and R.O.C. Oreffo. 2002a. Marine invertebrate skeletons: Promising tissue engineering scaffolds particularly for orthopaedic applications. *Third Smith and Nephew International Symposium—Translating Tissue Engineering into Products*, p. 80.

Green, D., D. Walsh, S. Mann, and R.O. Oreffo. 2002b. The potential of biomimesis in bone tissue engineering: Lessons from the design and synthesis of invertebrate skeletons. *Bone* 30:810–815.

Gutowska, A., B. Jeong, and M. Jasionowski. 2001. Injectable gels for tissue engineering. *Anat Rec* 263:342–349.

Healy, K.E., A. Rezania, and R.A. Stile. 1999. Designing biomaterials to direct biological responses. *Annals NY Acad Sci* 875:24–35.

Holmes, R., V. Mooney, R. Bulcholz, and A. Tencer. 1984. A coralline hydroxyapatite bone graft substitute. *Clin Orthop Relat Res* 188:252–262.

Hooper, J.N.A. and R.W. Van Soest. 2002. *Systema Porifera: A Guide to the Classification of Sponges*, Vol. 1. New York: Kluwer Academic Plenum.

Hu, J., R. Fraser, J.J. Russell, and B. Ben-Nissan. 2000. Australian coral as a biomaterial: Characteristics. *J Mater Sci Technol* 16(6):591–595.

Jahn, A.F. 1992. Experimental applications of porous (coralline) hydroxylapatite in middle ear and mastoid reconstruction. *Laryngoscope* 102(3):289–299.

Karande, T.S., J.L. Ong, and C.M. Agrawal. 2004. Diffusion in musculoskeletal tissue engineering scaffolds: Design issues related to porosity, permeability, architecture, and nutrient mixing. *Ann Biomed Eng* 32:1728–1743.

Kawakami, T., M. Antoh, H. Hasegawa, T. Yamagishi, M. Ito, and S. Eda. 1992. Experimental study on osteoconductive properties of a chitosan bonded hydroxyapatite self-hardening paste. *Biomaterials* 13:759–763.

Kelly, E.B. 2000. New frontiers in bone grafting. *Orthop Technol Rev* 2(9):28–35.

Kim, S.B., Y.J. Kim, T.L. Yoon, S.A. Park, I.H. Cho, E.J. Kim et al. 2004. The characteristics of a hydroxyapatite–chitosan–PMMA bone cement. *Biomaterials* 25:5715–5723.

Kim, M.M., E. Mendis, N. Rajapakse, S.H. Lee, and S.K. Kim. 2009. Effect of spongin derived from *Hymeniacidon sinapium* on bone mineralization. *J Biomed Mater Res B Appl Biomater* 90(2):540–546.

Kon, E., A. Muraglia, A. Corsi, P. Bianco, M. Marcacci, I. Martin et al. 2000. Autologous bone marrow stromal cells loaded onto porous hydroxyapatite ceramic accelerate bone repair in critical-size defects of sheep long bones. *J Biomed Mater Res* 49:328–337.

Kuhne, J.H., R. Bartl, B. Frisch, C. Hammer, V. Jansson, and M. Zimmer. 1994. Bone formation in coralline hydroxyapatite. Effects of pore size studied in rabbits. *Acta Orthop Scand* 65(3):246.

Langer, R. and J.P. Vacanti. 1993. Tissue engineering. *Science* 260:920–926.

Lanza, R., R. Langer, and J.P. Vacanti. 1997. *Principles of Tissue Engineering*. Austin, TX: R.G. Landes Company and Academic Press Inc.

Lauffenburger, D.A. 1994. Cell engineering. In: *The Biomedical Engineering Handbook*, J.D. Bronzine (ed.). Boca Raton, FL: CRC Press.

Lee, B.H., Y.M. Lee, Y.S. Sohn, and S.C. Song. 2002a. Thermosensitive poly (organophosphazene) gel. *Macromolecules* 35(10):3876–3879.

Lee, J.Y., S.H. Nam, S.Y. Im, Y.J. Park, Y.M. Lee, Y.J. Seol et al. 2002b. Enhanced bone formation by controlled growth factor delivery from chitosan-based biomaterials. *J Control Release* 78:187–197.

Lee, C.Y.S., H.S. Prasad, J.B Suzuki, J.D Stover, and M.D. Rohrer. 2011. The correlation of bone mineral density and histologic data in the early grafted maxillary sinus: A preliminary report. *Implant Dent* 20(3):202–214.

Lemons, J.E. 1996. Ceramics: Past, present, and future. *Bone* 19:121S–128S.

Leroux, L., Z. Hatim, M. Freche, and J.L. Lacout. 1999. Effects of various adjuvants (lactic acid, glycerol, and chitosan) on the injectability of a calcium phosphate cement. *Bone* 25(Suppl 2):31S–34S.

Lin, Z., K.L. Solomon, X. Zhang, N.J. Pavlos, T. Abel, C. Willers, K. Dai, J. Xu, Q. Zheng, and M. Zheng. 2011. In vitro evaluation of natural marine sponge collagen as a scaffold for bone tissue engineering. *Int J Biol Sci* 7(7):968–977.

Ma, L., C. Gao, Z. Mao, J. Zhou, J. Shen, X. Hu et al. 2003. Collagen/chitosan porous scaffolds with improved biostability for skin tissue engineering. *Biomaterials* 24:4833–4841.

Ma, J., H. Wang, B. He, and J. Chen. 2001. A preliminary in vitro study on the fabrication and tissue engineering applications of a novel chitosan bilayer material as a scaffold of human fetal dermal fibroblasts. *Biomaterials* 22:331–336.

Madhavan, P. and K. Nair. 1974. Utilization of prawn waste: Isolation of chitin and its conversion to chitosan. *Fish Technol* 11:50–53.

Mankin, H.J., F.S. Fogelson, Z.A. Thrasher, and F. Jaffer. 1976. Massive resection and allograft transplantation in the treatment of malignant bone tumours. *N Engl J Med* 294:1247–1250.

Marciani, R.D., A.A. Gonty, J.S. Giansanti, and J. Avila. 1977. Autogenous cancellous marrow bone graft in irradiated (i) long mandibles. *Oral Surg* 43:365–368.

McLaughlin, R.M. and J.K. Roush. 1998. Autogenous cancellous and cortico-cancellous bone grafting. *Vet Med* 93(12):1071–1074.

Metcalfe, A.D. and M.W. Ferguson. 2007. Tissue engineering of replacement skin: The crossroads of biomaterials, wound healing, embryonic development, stem cells and regeneration. *J R Soc Interface* 4(14):413–437.

Mizuno, K., K. Yamamura, K. Yano, T. Osada, S. Saeki, N. Takimoto et al. 2003. Effect of chitosan film containing basic fibroblast growth factor on wound healing in genetically diabetic mice. *J Biomed Mater Res* 64:177–181

Moore, W.R., S.E. Graves, and G.I. Bain. 2001. Synthetic bone graft substitutes. *Anz J Surg* 71:354–361.

Naber, C.L., O.M. Reid, and J.E. Hammer III. 1972. Gross and histologic evaluation of an autogenous bone graft 57th month post operatively. *J Periodontal* 43:702.

Nesheiwat, F., W.M. Brown, and K.M. Healey. 1998. Post-traumatic first metatarsal reconstruction using coralline hydroxyapatite. *J Am Podiatr Med Assoc* 88(3):130–134.

Nguyen, D.T., D.P. Orgill, and G.F. Murphy. 2009. The pathophysiologic basis for wound healing and cutaneous regeneration. In: *Biomaterials for Treating Skin Loss* Orgill, D. and C. Blanco (eds.), Boca Raton, FL: CRC Press, Chapter 4, pp. 25–57.

Nomura, T., J.L. Katz, M.P. Powers, and C. Saito. 2005. Evaluation of the micromechanical elastic properties of potential bone-grafting materials. *J Biomed Mater Res B Appl Biomater* 73(1):29–34.

Osborn, J.F. and H. Newesely. 1980. The material science of calcium phosphate ceramics. *Biomaterials* 1:108–111.

Pallela, R., J. Venkatesan, V.R. Janapala, and S.K. Kim. 2011. Biophysicochemical evaluation of chitosan-hydroxyapatite-marine sponge collagen composite for bone tissue engineering. *Biomed Mater Res A* 100:486–495, doi: 10.1002/jbm.a.33292.

Peppas, N.A. and R. Langer. 1994. New challenges in biomaterials. *Science* 263:1715–1720.

Rezwan, K., Q.Z. Chen, J.J. Blaker, and A.R. Boccaccini. 2006. Biodegradable and bioactive porous polymer/inorganic composite scaffolds for bone tissue engineering. *Biomaterials* 27(18):3413–3431.

Ripamonti, U., R.M. Klar, L.F. Renton, and C. Ferretti. 2010. Synergistic induction of bone formation by hOP-1, hTGF-beta3 and inhibition by zoledronate in macroporous coral-derived hydroxyapatites. *Biomaterials* 31(25):6400–6410.

Roy, D.M. and S.K. Linnehan. 1974. Hydroxyapatite formed from coral skeletal carbonate by hydrothermal exchange. *Nature* 247:220–222.

Sandhu, H.S. and H.S. Grewal. 1999. The use of allograft bone in lumbar spine. *Orthop Clin North Am* 30(4):685–698.

Schulz, J.T., R.G. Tompkins, and J.F. Burke. 2000. Artificial skin. *Annual Review of Medicine* 51:231–244.

Service, R.F. 2000. Tissue engineers build new bone. *Science* 289:1498–1500.

Shahgaldi, B.F. 1998. Coral graft restoration of osteochondral defects. *Biomaterials* 19:205–213.

Shahidi, F. and R. Abuzaytoun. 2005. Chitin, chitosan, and co products: Chemistry, production, applications, and health effects. *Adv Food Nutr Res* 49:93–135.

Sharma, B. and J.H. Elisseeff. 2004. Engineering structurally organized cartilage and bone tissues. *Ann Biomed Eng* 32:148–159.

Shim, J.S., H.S. Lee, J. Shin, H.J. Kwon, and A. Psammaplin. 2003. A marine natural product inhibits aminopeptidase N and suppresses angiogenesis in vitro. *Cancer Lett* 203:163–169.

Simpson, T.L. 1984. *The Cell Biology of Sponges*. New York: Springer-Verlag.

Sivakumar, M. and I. Manjubala. 2001. Preparation of hydroxyapatite/fluoroapatite-zirconia composites using Indian corals for biomedical applications. *Mater Lett* 50(4):199–205.

Skaggs, D.L., M.A. Samuelson, J.M. Hale, R.M. Kay, and V.T. Tolo. 2000. Complications of posterior iliac crest bone grafting in spine surgery in children. *Spine* 25:2400–2402.

Soost, F. 1996. Biocoral—An alternative bone substitute. *Chirurg* 67(11):1193–1196.

Soost, F., B. Reisshauer, A. Herrmann, and H.J. Neumann. 1998. Natural coral calcium carbonate as alternative substitute in bone defects of the skull. *Mund Kiefer Gesichtschir* 2(2):96–100.

Szpalski, M. and R. Gunzburg. 2002. Applications of calcium phosphate–based cancellous bone void fillers in trauma surgery. *Orthopedics* 25(5 Suppl):601–612.

Taravel, M.N. and A. Domard. 1995. Collagen and its interaction with chitosan II. Influence of the physicochemical characteristics of collagen. *Biomaterials* 16:865–871.

Taravel, M.N. and A. Domard. 1996. Collagen and its interaction with chitosan III. Some biological and mechanical properties. *Biomaterials* 17:451–455.

Tran, C.T., C. Gargiulo, H.D. Thao, H.M. Tuan, L. Filgueira, and D. Michael Strong. 2011. Culture and differentiation of osteoblasts on coral scaffold from human bone marrow mesenchymal stem cells. *Cell Tissue Bank* 12(4):247–261.

Ueno, H., H. Yamada, I. Tanaka, N. Kaba, M. Matsuura, M. Okumura et al. 1999. Accelerating effects of chitosan for healing at early phase of experimental open wound in dogs. *Biomaterials* 20:1407–1414.

Vaccaro, A.R. 2002. The role of the osteoconductive scaffold in synthetic bone graft. *Orthopedics* 25(5 Suppl):571–578.

Vago, R., D. Plotquin, A. Bunin, I. Sinelnikov, D. Atar, and D. Itzhak. 2002. Hard tissue remodeling using biofabricated coralline biomaterials. *J Biochem Biophys Methods* 50(2–3):253–259.

Wang, S.F., X.H. Wang, and L. Gan. 2011. Biosilica-glass formation using enzymes from sponges [silicatein]: Basic aspects and application in biomedicine [bone reconstitution material and osteoporosis]. *Front Mater Sci* 5(3):266–281.

White, E. and E.C. Shors. 1986. Biomaterial aspects of Interpore-200 porous hydroxyapatite. *Dent Clin N Am* 30(1):49–67.

Xu, H.H., J.B. Quinn, S. Takagi, and L.C. Chow. 2004. Synergistic reinforcement of in situ hardening calcium phosphate composite scaffold for bone tissue engineering. *Biomaterials* 25:1029–1037.

Yan, X., E. Khor, and L.Y. Lim. 2000. PEC films prepared from Chitosan-Alginate coacervates. *Chem Pharm Bull* 48(7):941–946.

Yanas, I.V. and J.F. Burke. 1980. Design of an artificial skin I. Basic design principles. *J Biomed Mater Res* 14(4):65–81.

Yuan, J., W.J. Zhang, G. Liu, M. Wei, Z.L. Qi, W. Liu, L. Cui, and Y.L. Cao. 2010. Repair of canine mandibular bone defects with bone marrow stromal cells and coral. *Tissue Eng Part A* 16(4):1385–1394.

Zhang, Y., M. Ni, M. Zhang, and B. Ratner. 2003. Calcium phosphate chitosan composite scaffolds for bone tissue engineering. *Tissue Eng* 9:337–345.

Zhang, Y. and M. Zhang. 2002. Calcium phosphate/chitosan composite scaffolds for controlled in vitro antibiotic drug release. *J Biomed Mater Res* 62:378–786.

Zhao, F., Y. Yin, W.W. Lu, J.C. Leong, W. Zhang, J. Zhang et al. 2002. Preparation and histological evaluation of biomimetic three-dimensional hydroxyapatite/chitosan–gelatin network composite scaffolds. *Biomaterials* 23:3227–3234.

Zheng, M.H., K. Hinterkeuser, K. Solomon, V. Kunert, N.J. Pavlos, and Xu, J. 2007. Collagen-derived biomaterials in bone and cartilage repair. *Macromol Symp* 253:179–185.

30

Marine Materials in Drug Delivery and Tissue Engineering: From Natural Role Models to Bone Regeneration and Repair and Slow Delivery of Therapeutic Drugs, Proteins, and Genes

Besim Ben-Nissan and David W. Green

CONTENTS

30.1 Introduction

Marine structures like any other natural living structures are made with immaculate resource and energy efficiency using common, readily available materials through self-assembly into highly organized hierarchies. All functional structures optimized to their environment are produced in this way. This gives us the opportunity to produce structures with intricate shapes and architectures that are tailored to their functions. Biomimetic approaches using marine structures have yield promising outcomes for application in the tissue engineering of skeletal tissues (Weiner 1986, 2008). One such approach involves conjuring material environments at the molecular and macromolecular scales that try to mimic native extracellular matrix (ECM) (Huebsch and Mooney 2009). The aim has been to further extend this ongoing research toward the design of clinically relevant scaffolds for regenerative medicine using a unique set of self-organizing hierarchical structures designed and synthesized according to biological principles of design. A number of researchers have started to investigate marine structures by harnessing as nature does with enormous precision and control inorganic molecules and nanoparticles to construct advanced functional bioceramics with application in tissue engineering and newly pharmaceutical drug and gene delivery.

A common characteristic of natural biomaterials such as bone, nacre, sea urchin tooth, and other tough hybrid materials in nature is the strong nanoscale interaction between the inorganic and the organic phases. This characteristic allows the organic phase to act as a plastic energy-dissipating network, forming stretching (bridging) ligaments across the faces of a propagating crack in a nanoscale level (Dunlop et al. 2011). Such complexity has led to the common perception that to mimic natural designs, in situ synthesis techniques should be adopted.

Chemically derived hybrid materials lie at the interface of organic–inorganic and biological realms. Main advantages in the use of these hybrids result from their high versatility offering a wide range of possibilities to elaborate tailor-made materials in terms of chemical and physical properties, and shaping. Moreover, these hybrid nanocomposites present the paramount advantage to facilitate integration, miniaturization, and multifunctionalization of the devices, opening a new range of opportunities for many bioengineering applications.

Bone and joint degeneration is a fast-growing healthcare problem in the world. The best way of tackling the root causes of this tissue loss is by growing fresh tissue— literally in a petri dish—from the patient's own healthy bone and stem cells. So far, only small volumes of tissue can be produced in this way because vast numbers of starting bone cells—taken from a biopsy sample—must be used and getting nutrition to the growing mass of tissue is problematic. Surgeons have large amounts of tissues to treat bone diseases and trauma injuries with pinpoint clinical effectiveness. The potential of stem cells to make larger volumes of tissues more rapidly is very high, and they must be properly used for this goal.

In the light of these difficulties, bioengineers are developing templates—made from a variety of different materials—which support the growth of new tissues as if they were in the body.

The standard bone replacement materials conduct the growth of new bone through their well-defined pores and channels rather slowly, which is clinically ineffective. Regenerative growth has to be rapid, highly organized, and invested with blood supply. So the material has to stimulate and induce bone regeneration within its structure. However, there is a paucity of materials and structures with the right combination of structure and bone stimulation properties and possessing the right type of environments for stem cell productivity. Internationally the leading-edge researchers are devising synthetic materials that assemble themselves in the test-tube, with increasing elements that mimic natural bone. However, a clinically useful bone-like material made in this way is probably a decade away. Simpler approaches have been explored using natural templates such as ready-made marine structures.

There is prolific ongoing diversification of pharmaceutical and therapeutic proteins, carbohydrates, and lipids to treat degenerative diseases and trauma (Elliott et al. 2003; Carter 2006; Akinc et al. 2009; Ernst and Magnani 2009). This has been promoted by accumulating knowledge of molecular events in health and disease of tissues and organs. However, their clinical effectiveness and patient safety needs to be improved. For example, potent drugs produce unwanted and potentially damaging side effects and toxicity in otherwise healthy tissues and organs. Excessive concentration of any therapeutic biomolecule distributed to the incorrect, disease-free location can also degrade normal physiological function. Accurate targeting of proteins into elected cells and tissues may only eliminate such problems. This is most effectively achieved by conveying the protein cargo inside small highly mobile transplantation modules with equivalent mobility and targeting efficiency, as lentivirus-mediated gene-to-cell transfer. One of the most universally effective units for targeted delivery is a spherical capsule—a boundary-limited 3D volume with dimensions between 100 nm and 10 μm. Spheres compared with any other 3D shape possess the largest surface areas for their given volume meaning that release is maximized in all surrounding space. A sphere also is the most effect shape that can be carried in a physiological fluid and best suited to uninterrupted flow inside tubes and vessels (Zufferey et al. 1997; Sukhorukov et al. 2005; Yan et al. 2010).

Biomimicry to be applied as a method of innovation is not altogether straightforward. For many years biomimicry projects were empirical in nature. Certain systematic methods have been devised to make the transition from natural innovation into technology easier. Methods such as biomimicry facilitate the accession of functional adaptations—which have evolved by natural selection—randomly devised to solve the contradictions, trade-offs, and problems of survival so that it can be reused to solve analogous problems under investigation (Vincent et al. 2007). The first and most difficult step in this process is discovering the best biological analogue for the problem under investigation and associating it with usable technological functions (Bhushan 2009).

The essence of better-performing natural materials compared to their man-made counterparts is more attention given to detailed design, ability to be self-assembled, use of organic–inorganic mixtures, and optimization both in assembly and usage (Fratzl 2007). This is exemplified by the biological effectiveness of marine structures and sponges to support self-sustaining musculoskeletal tissues and the promotion of bone formation by extracts of skeletal proteins such as *spongin* and proteins from the organic matrix of *nacre seashell* (*Haliotis laevigata*) (abalone) nacre protein (Weiss et al. 2001). Molecules pivotal to the regulation and guidance of bone morphogenesis and particularly the events in mineral metabolism and deposition similarly exist in the earliest marine organisms because they represent the first molecular components established for calcification, morphogenesis, and wound healing. It emerges that bone morphogenic protein (BMP) molecules—the major bone growth factors in human bone morphogenesis—are secreted by endodermal cells into the developing skeleton (Zoccola et al. 2000). And signaling proteins, TGF-β and Wnt—targets for therapeutic bone regeneration—are present in early marine sponge development.

In human biology, a study of matrix vesicles will teach us valuable lessons on how proteins are captured and coated and how the vesicle is able to dock and fuse with their target. A second role model for biomimicry is the use of an existing template, for example, a filtering marine microskeleton of *Foraminifera* (Figure 30.1). Later in this chapter, we will describe significant technological trends aimed at producing delivery vehicles using natural-origin soft and hard organized matter, fabricated into capsules and cell-delineated assemblies. We will then outline new selected strategies for the engineering of new bone, based on biomimicry themes using calcium phosphate bioceramics as building blocks.

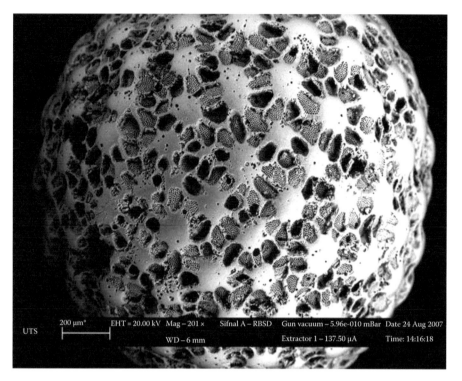

FIGURE 30.1
SEM image of a *Foraminifera (B. sphaerulata) macrosphere.*

30.2 Using Biomimicry for Tissue Engineering

30.2.1 Musculoskeletal Tissues

Tissue engineering is a multidisciplinary venture aimed at reproducing healthy, living human tissue and organs in the laboratory. Within this controlled laboratory environment, tissues are ready-made for each and every patient. Engineering natural tissue requires scaffolding to anchor and support it in precise anatomical arrangements. Growth factors, remodeling enzymes, and signaling molecules are also essential to control and regulate the dynamics of tissue morphogenesis housed within the frameworks during cultivation and following transplantation. Growth factors are key elements in bone healing. They are released during osteoclastic remodeling, from blood clots and damaged bone stimulating osteoblast activity at the periosteum and endosteum. They are also important in recruiting and stimulating exogenous cells and structures. As an example, VEGF is vital to signaling blood vessel invasion and stimulating network formation (Seipel et al. 2004). The most potent and universally accepted group of bone growth factors are the BMPs (types 1–8) discovered in the bone matrix by Urist (1965), Urist and Strates (1971), Wozney et al. (1988), Lind (1996), and Reddi (1998).

BMPs are widely used in experimental musculoskeletal tissue engineering and in orthopedic surgery to promote bone and cartilage tissue formation and gene expression profiles leading to bone formation and restoration of skeletal architecture. BMP's efficacy has undergone multiple in vitro, in vivo, and clinical trials with BMP-2/7 showing increased osteogenesis compared with autograft. It is clear though that bone healing and morphogenesis occur through the activity of multiple factors. Alternative biological factors with unique cellular functions and activities are sought to establish more precise control of the regenerative response and provide completeness and permanency of the final tissue. Until recently there has been a paucity of scaffolding to support tissue morphogenesis faithful to native bone. The key to this problem is engineering a high degree of bioresponsiveness necessary to generate normal tissues. It is possible to provide mechanically strong bone by properly integrating cultivated bone tissue within a framework that can directly elicit regenerative responses say through sets of functional groups, receptor molecules, mineral ion enrichment, and nanotopographic cues (Ehrbar et al. 2011). The current trend in framework design is to generate structures that mimic the structures and cellular functions of native tissue extracellular matrices (Liao et al. 2006; Dahlin et al. 2011).

As a result, frameworks are now constructed with native structural biopolymers (such as collagen) and decorated with receptors, cross-linkers, and functional groups. Biomimicry approaches are also at the forefront of material synthesis into ECM-like structures. This has led to tailored engineering of molecular building blocks and engineering at the nanoscale facilitating precision control of physical and chemical properties in the natural macrostructure. This can be achieved in synthetic chemical environments or through use of microbes (Hartgerink et al. 2001; Zhang 2003; Lutolf and Hubbell 2005; Harrington et al. 2006; Smith et al. 2008; Kyle et al. 2009; Sengupta and Heilshorn 2010).

These intricate structures are designed to better match naturally occurring ones. For example, electrospun materials offer broad range of constructs with dimensions analogous to native extracellular matrices and thus provide equivalent physical and chemical properties. The fibers can be tailored with specific surface chemistries alike to native ECM, to encourage cell adhesion (Li et al. 2002; Xu et al. 2004; Chew et al. 2006; Teo et al. 2006; Grafahrend et al. 2011).

In order to control cellular activities, the physical and chemical surroundings play a pivotal role in the quality of tissue organization, formation, and quantity, hence the focus on materials design and synthesis. Studies of the way natural materials are built into organized functioning units and the way they adapt to their environment will enable the future tissue engineer to produce an exciting array of self-responsive structures and materials for regenerative medicine and structural applications in biomedicine. Regeneration of calcified tissues has benefited greatly from the principles and concepts offered by biomimetic material chemistry (Mann 1988, 2001; Mann and Ozin 1996). Thus, to succeed with biomimetic approach, there must be a detailed blueprint of the anatomy and physiology of the tissue under observation.

30.2.2 Natural Templates

The natural templates of choice are the skeletons of three individual marine animals such as corals, shells, and sponges (Weiner 1986, 2008; Vago et al. 2002; Ben-Nissan 2003; Green et al. 2003, 2012; Heinemann et al. 2007; Green and Ben-Nissan 2008). Many of them possess exquisite architectures—down to the nanoscale that mimics human bone and chemical compositions that are identical to bone. The use of natural skeletons directly for bone surgery is not new and neither is the use of animal skeletons to grow bone tissue from stem cells (Ben-Nissan 2003). But what is emerging from early studies into the composition

TABLE 30.1

List of Marine Sponges and Corals with Utility for Regenerative Medicine

Marine Sponges	*Spongia ceylonensis*	*Verongid Ianthella basta*	*S. ceylonensis*	*Calcarea*	*Callyspongia ramosa*
Protein product	Skeletal proteins ECM proteins	Skeletal proteins ECM proteins	Skeletal proteins ECM proteins	Skeletal proteins (organic matrix)	3D framework
Corals	*Porites porites*	*Porites cylindrica*			
Protein product	3D framework Organic matrix proteins	3D framework Organic matrix proteins			

of natural skeletons is the unique qualities of the organic matrix for providing framework materials, promoting regeneration of mineralized tissues, and stimulating bone cells into bone formation and healing. This has not been properly investigated (Heinemann et al. 2007; Ehrlich et al. 2010, 2011). List of marine sponges and corals with utility for regenerative medicine is given in Table 30.1.

Currently in clinics and hospitals, there are two general bone graft replacement procedures: the first that is regarded as the gold standard for bone replacement procedures is the use of autograft (incorporating patients bone), which involves a secondary procedure during surgery and possible pain, and the second is the synthetic bone graft (allograft) techniques that are based on cadaver or animal bone that is demineralized and used as synthetic bone grafts and has been somehow controversial. This group also involves a range of ceramic and polymeric scaffolds.

Replacement autograft of musculoskeletal tissues is not available in the clinic because the volumes needed cannot be routinely obtained or cultivated. In addition, the anatomical organization of any cultivated tissues does not sufficiently replicate native tissues. Frameworks that are engineered to simulate the ECM will provide the ideal 3D architecture and anchorage to orchestrate proper tissue architecture, blood supply invasion, and organization with supply of tissue-promotive factors and developmental signals (Lutolf and Hubbell 2005). Therefore, science in regenerative medicine is fundamentally about biomimicry, simulating development of tissues in the laboratory by closely emulating biological processes and mechanisms using synergetic collectives of cells and biological molecules. Biomimicry does not have to be used to copy every element of the natural model. Simplified versions or copies of key elements may only be needed to achieve clinically acceptable outcomes at least until true mimics of the ECM can be generated in the laboratory (Lutolf and Hubbell 2005).

30.2.3 Coral as Bone Graft Material

It is highly advantageous to transform natural coral into a stronger form of mineral so that it is able to support higher loads. There are several methods in which to do this. Roy and Linnehan (1974) were first to develop a method to convert coral by hydrothermal exchange at high temperatures and pressures (Roy and Linnehan 1974). White and Shors applied the technique commercially by converting only partially, hence controlling the solubility rate of coral in vivo (White and Shors 1986). Hu et al. (2000) produced a highly crystalline complete hydroxyapatite (HA) structure that originated from Australian *Porites*, with uniform properties for long bone applications by a hydrothermal method that had additional processing steps. HA thus synthesized allows quick tissue ingrowth and fixation of the natural bone leading to good strength and chemical attachments. Many other natural marine structures have been converted into strengthened HA candidates for bone replacement applications including conch and clam sea shells. Conversion of sea urchin spines to resorbable Mg-substituted tricalcium phosphate by hydrothermal reaction at relatively low temperatures and AB-type carbonated nanopowder of HA prepared by hydrothermal transformation of milled oyster shell powders was also investigated. Hydroxyapatite (HAp) structures for tissue engineering by hydrothermal treatment of aragonite in the form of cuttlefish bone were covered by Ivankovic et al. (2009).

Although the first pioneering clinical work on TCP was carried out by two surgeons, Albee and Morrison, in 1920, the main theoretical work on bone chemistry and structure that is calcium phosphate (substituted carbonate HAp) was not adequately coved until LeGeros and her coworkers work in 1967 (LeGeros et al. 1967). Some of the current commercial bone graft materials are mainly produced from coralline HAp. By design and to keep the dissolution rate fast, their coral product is only partially converted and so retains a calcium carbonate core. Under certain conditions, dissolution rate is accelerated and this reduces durability and strength, respectively, and is not utilized where high structural strength—such as in long bones—is required. To overcome these limitations, a new double-stage conversion technique was developed by Ben-Nissan and coworkers (Ben-Nissan et al. 2000, 2004, 2011; Hu et al. 2000, 2001; Ben Nissan 2003, 2004; Novak et al. 2009; Chou et al. 2011).

This improved technique involves a two-stage application route whereby, in the first stage, complete conversion of coral to pure HAp is achieved. While in the second stage, a sol–gel-derived HAp nanocoating is directly applied to cover the meso- *and* nanopores within the intrapore material while maintaining the large pores for appropriate bone growth (Figure 30.2).

Compression and biaxial strengths, fracture toughness, and Young's modulus were improved due to this unique double treatment. Application of this treatment method results in enhanced bioactivity due to the nanograin size and hence large surface area that increases the reactivity of the nanocoating. It is anticipated that this new material can be applied to load-bearing bone graft applications where high strength requirements are pertinent.

The coral (*Porites*) was obtained from the Australian Great Barrier Reef and contained micropores of 150–400 µm size. The coral was shaped in the form of a block and was treated with 5% NaClO solution. Hydrothermal conversion was carried out in a Parr reactor (Parr Instrument Company, Moline, IL) with a Teflon liner at 250°C and 3.8 MPa pressure with excess $(NH_4)_2HPO_4$. Total conversion to single-phase HAp was achieved. By controlling the chemistry and treatment conditions, other types of calcium phosphates were easily produced.

Mechanical testing involved a standard four-point bend test according to ASTM C1161 to measure the flexural strength and flexural modulus of the natural coral. Comparative compression and biaxial strength tests were also carried out. Fracture surfaces were then viewed using scanning electron microscope (SEM), which was performed on a LEO-Supra55VP. Samples were analyzed by x-ray diffraction with a Siemens D-5000 (Karlsruhe, Germany). The XRD scan was carried out from 20.0 to 60.0 in 0.020 steps at a step time of 2.0 s. Thermogravimetric analyses (TGA/DTA) were performed on a TA Instrument SDT 2960, at a heating rate of 10°C/min. Characterization studies of the natural and converted corals using XRD, SEM, DTA/TGA, NMR, and Raman spectroscopy were

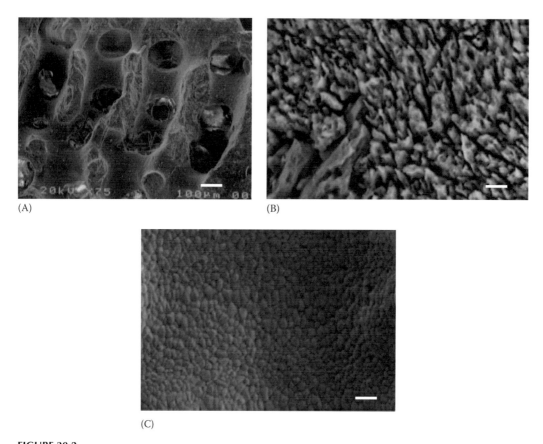

FIGURE 30.2
Nanocoating layer over the coralline structure. (A) Coral macrostructure (scale bar 100 μm), (B) interpore area showing nano- and mesopores (scale bar 300 nm), and (C) hydroxyapatite nanocoated region (scale bar 300 nm).

reported in previous publications. These results showed a large increase in all mechanical properties, specifically the compression strength, and bioactivity due to the application of hydrothermal conversion and nanocoating methods.

30.3 Drug Delivery

Bringing accumulations of therapeutic biomolecules to a destination inside the body needing immediate corrective treatment in physiologically relevant dosages over time spanning hours, days to months, and even years has evaded even the best engineered designs (Langer 1990, 1998). This arises because there are many layers of functional simplicity (protection, mobility, targeting, programmed release, environment responsiveness, intracellular transport), which have yet to be purposefully integrated into a single working device. In the future, biomedical engineers must develop better solutions to the exacting conflicts between the variety of competing physical (viscosity and surface tension at small scales) and chemical (bond energies, steric hindrance) constraints on functions (such as punctuated off-loading of proteins) and actions (such as mobility). To illustrate this, drug particles must be biodegradable but not dissolve away too rapidly and release the drug in a single bolus. Typically, drugs are delivered into the body by injection (directly into the eye or blood vessels) or by ingestion. They may however also be delivered in a solution across the tear film into ocular blood vessels, into nasal cavities as an aerosol and absorbed through skin where blood vessels are close to the skin surface. They must also be permeable but simultaneously immobilize the drug for set times. The size of the device will differ depending on how it is delivered to the patient. Ingested particles should be below 1 mm, particles for injection must be below 200 μm, and inhaled particles ideally should be 100 μm (LaVan et al. 2003). However, dosages are set by their biological effect and maximum possible function. For example, antibiotics are usually given in volumes of 1 g/day, whereas 300 μg of epinephrine is administered for anaphylactic shock (LaVan et al. 2003). Arguably, the two most essential functions are targeting to a cell and controlled delivery into the cell. This would ensure that less volumes are needed than currently set by standard, existing dosage regimes based on systemic administration (LaVan et al. 2003).

Most pharmaceutical drugs and therapeutic proteins have short residence periods inside the body because they are rapidly assimilated and metabolized, while genes have considerably more lengthy sustained activities once they are incorporated into the genetic machinery of the cell (Saltzman 1999; Luo and Saltzman 2000). Gene therapy is at a more advanced position than protein and cell therapy. For example, small RNAs damaging mRNA molecules and silencing gene action have shown efficacy in multiple clinical trials particularly with modified viral vectors. These biological vehicles produce stronger, more sustained expression than synthetic oligonucleotides (Fire et al. 1998).

However, oligonucleotides only need to enter the cytoplasm to have a potent biological effect. Yet delivering them to the right locations has proven equally as difficult as it has for proteins (Baker et al. 2010). Encapsulation strategies for siRNAs have been very varied and exploit nanotechnology (Davis et al. 2010). Small RNAs are modified to protect them against degradation by nucleases and increase knockdown potency.

Drug molecules introduced into the body are quickly assaulted and degraded by enzymes and so need protection. The protection must be also effective to evade interrogation by the patient's host immune system. However, the most important task to be tackled remains at targeting specific cells, tissues, and intracellular compartments and engineering the release of one drug or multiple drugs in tandem or in one single, continuous burst. By release we mean diffusion and desorption from the wall or the enclosed interior of the drug delivery device.

The rate of release and the quantity released must also be programmed in advance and anticipate the host responses in synchrony.

30.3.1 Microsphere Delivery Devices

The sphere is the indivisible and discrete unit of drug delivery. At any selected scale, the sphere is an ideal device for targeted delivery. A sphere possesses the highest volumes possible within the lowest possible surface area, which generates 3D structures with high encapsulation and packing efficiencies. These drug-loaded particles must be delivered to the patient by injection at an intramuscular site or into the blood stream so that they can be passively and speedily carried anywhere in the body to proceed to their exact localization and final destination. Therapeutic biomolecules can be delivered inside more diffuse packaging made from biomimicking dendritic polymers and liquid crystal dispersions—a common organizing substrate in nature used to process biomaterials (Esfand and Tomalia 2001; Patri et al. 2005; Guo et al. 2010; Rizwan et al. 2010). The most technologically promising polymer contributions are a new generation of peptidomimetic (Jabbari 2009), "guest" molecule-imprinted (Venkatesh et al. 2008) stimuli-responsive and self-actuating hydrogels, which are all attempts at simulating biology (Stayton et al. 2005; Swann and Ryan 2009). Natural hydrogels use the chemical energy from their environment to produce a variety of mechanical adaptations needed to influence their local environment. So the development of synthetic polymers that do the same will lead to better actively responsive emulates. Other bioengineers are contemplating fabrication of machines with moving parts. Small mechanical machines such as the nanovalve may be able to operate inside the body. Stimuli-responsive silica-based nanovalves open only when pH changes, as is the case in diseased tissue, so that they release their contents in the correct location to treat disease (Saha et al. 2007). With every delivery vehicle, there are added financial costs, lengthy testing procedures, and stringent regulation protocols that must be tackled. Hence, the pursuit of other strategies where the deliverable molecule is itself augmented with molecular components for targeting (Baker et al. 2010).

A drug delivery device is made to reside in the body at a particular location for prolonged time to achieve function throughout that lifetime. Characteristic patterns of engineered release with time would include continuous, oscillatory, declining, and periodic pulsation "release on–release off." This most closely matches the way hormones are regulated in the body. The aspiration is to control the release rate of proteins, genes, and polysaccharides accurately and sustain the desired drug concentration within set limits, reproducibly and predictably. Maintaining a biological effect for extended times is vital. Fundamentally, the ideal device must of its own "built-in" accord relocate to an elected destination, maintain its position there, release its contents at one place, remain under control, or have autonomous control of drug release. Having this remote sensing capability is an ultimate aim for any designer of drug delivery devices to maximize targeting efficiency.

30.3.2 Targeting and Delivering Biomolecules to Where They Are Needed

A first approach to targeting of an active drug into a region of tissue requiring therapeutic treatment has been to adsorb the drug onto the external and/or internal surfaces of an implant. Control of delivery is limited using this strategy because the drug dissociates from its template too transiently to produce long-lasting biological effects. However, studies have indicated the effectiveness of this strategy for localized gene and growth factor delivery (Chen and Mooney 2003; Silva et al. 2009; Salvay et al. 2010). In one study, delivery of DNA plasmid by resorbing polymer 3D scaffolds resulted in significantly better transfection efficiencies than by direct injection into an identical area of tissue (Shea et al. 1999). Combining the individual DNA molecules with a chaperone increased their entry into the cell (Jang et al. 2006). This can be achieved by infusing growth factors into the monomer mixture before it is synthesized into a polymer. As the polymer is resorbed, the proteins enter into the immediate surroundings. It is significantly more biologically realistic to have multiple drugs and their adjuvants released at the same time since drug effects sometimes require an agonist to function optimally. This results in a more complete biological effect and a permanent one as well (Richardson et al. 2001; Simmons et al. 2004). In one notable example, dual release of two growth factors that produce a complimentary outcome, from polymer scaffolds, has been demonstrated most effectively by including polymeric spheres within a 3D polymer scaffold (Richardson et al. 2001). New ways of administering drugs through the skin are producing promising biological and preclinical results. For instance, the Nanopatch is a bandage covered with nanometric needles on one side. The nanoneedles are each coated with vaccine. When the patch is taped onto the skin, it brings the vaccine into the exact area where there are high densities of resident antigen-presenting cells (Prow et al. 2010; Raphael et al. 2010).

Reduction in surgical invasiveness is crucial to the well-being of the patient and has led to development of a rich diversity of small (micron to nanometer) carriers. Some are even proposing that nanometric self-powered machines and computer-controlled robots could fulfill this role (Freitas 2006).

A significant number of biomaterials have been examined for drug delivery and new micrometric and nanometric platforms that couple drugs to sensors and implants (LaVan et al. 2003). Cylindrical nanotubes and nanowires offer new levels of sensory behavior and delivery options. Drug targeting directly into tumors is a highly significant prolific research effort. Alternate approaches have adopted the use of carbon nanotubes studded with quantum dots and cell-binding antibodies and peptides for targeting (De la Zerda and Gambhir 2007). Other fundamental approaches include developing a microdimensional chemical synthesizer and co-opting programmed cells to make the compound on-site. Further engineering challenges remain to be figured out and tackled. For example, it is important that there is capacity to encapsulate precise volumes of each candidate drug, ranging between microliter to nanoliter. The encapsulation medium must be also engineered to allow the freedom to immobilize insoluble and unstable drug compounds (LaVan et al. 2003). It seems likely that there will not be one single universal design for every demonstrable application. As the Nanopatch strategy demonstrates, a well-designed delivery device for a specific purpose tends to be the most effective and purposeful.

Another way forward has been consensually to use small-scale fabrication to produce highly detailed structures resolved at submicron and nanometric scales using micro-machining and lithography techniques adopted and adapted from the microelectronics industry. These platforms present many compartmentalized chambers as a way of controlling and regulating elution and effective dosage (Tao and Desai 2003). Diffusion chambers enclosed spaces that have the advantage of a narrative of clinical success, in the inner ear, the spinal cord, and the eye, but they do require highly invasive surgery particularly at deeply embedded tissue locations. Nanoparticles possess significant advantages for administering drugs and proteins in that they are highly stable, penetrate tissue linings, evade the immune system, and are ingested into the cell with high efficiencies. Unlike diffusion chambers and microchips, they do not need to be directly implanted. Owing to overall gains in functioning efficiency, a reduction in the quantity of encapsulates is possible.

30.3.3 Delivery Vehicles Designed with Nature's Input

If we were to ask questions of nature for likely inventions that correspond to current difficulties in drug delivery, then we will find many useful solutions evolved by millions of years of natural selection. Evolution has been highly successful at arriving at the most optimal solutions to the problems of survival and producing flawless high-quality materials (Vincent et al. 2006). Biologically inspired innovative design makes use of design analogies as the source of new technological inventions (Helms et al. 2009). They may not be the obvious ones, which is why it is important to study nature for ideas and inspiration (Jones 2006; Vincent et al. 2006). Nature can show us how to painlessly inject fluids through the skin by looking at the design of mosquito mouthparts. A study of the mechanics of mosquito fascicle mouthpart has provided important insight for the future design of painless, miniaturized hypodermic needles (Ramasubramanian et al. 2008). It can show us new ways by which cells in the body move themselves by examining how white blood cells roll along blood vessel walls with surface proteins called selectins (Eniola et al. 2002; Pennisi 2002). The adhesive ligands from leukocytes have been isolated and added onto polymer microspheres to provide them with this rolling capacity along cell linings (Eniola et al. 2002). Important lessons can be learned of the mechanisms of cell infection by bacterial and viral pathogens (Pizarro-Cerda and Cossart 2006) and leukocytes (Ranney 2000). The direct use of modified viral particles (e.g., attenuated lentiviruses) is not a new tactic as they are highly successful vehicles to transfer genes into animal and human cells with long-term expression potency (Zufferey et al. 1997; Wiznerowicz and Trono 2003). One suggested area of future study is the self-deployment structures in nature particularly in the plant kingdom (Kobayashi et al. 2000, 2003; Kobayashi and Horikawa 2009). One example is to understand the way seeds are dispersed from their capsules (Attenborough 1995) and the way pollen folds itself into 3D spherical capsules (Katifori et al. 2010). Much can be learned from natural history and natural history collections. Drug delivery can be informed by a rational study of biological molecule transport to the cell, into the cell, and inside the cell (Ranney 2000).

Traditionally biomimetic approaches have been empirical, wholly based on observation of natural phenomena and their history. There are more sophisticated ways of approaching nature for new ideas that are based on systematic organization into classification tables such as BioTriz and AskNature taxonomies (www.asknature.org). BioTriz is a method of extracting inventive solutions to the problems of existence and transferring them into technologies (Vincent 2003; Vincent et al. 2006).

In this review, we highlight the strategy of marine structures and biomimicry (copying significant elements of a natural role model for reuse in technology) for (a) drug delivery and (b) transplantation of therapeutic proteins and cells. Bioinspired design may have significant impact on future drug and protein delivery developments. It is hoped that this may offer better clinical outcomes than conventional strategies because it is based on nature's wisdom over millions of years of optimization, conservation of energy, and resolution of conflicting functions. The most obvious biomimicry model available is the virus capsule (Hoffman et al. 2001). The most significant lesson viruses have taught bioengineers is how to overcome the barriers to entry into the cell cytoplasm and into the nucleus. Viruses possess special protein coats that transfer their contents of DNA and proteins into endosomes and the cytoplasm where they produce their biological effect. As the pH drops inside the endosome, the conformation of the viral protein is altered so that it binds onto the membrane and punctures pores through it (Hoffman et al. 2001).

We confine ourselves to our own selected examples that harness natural-origin substrates and our own biomimetic approaches. Calcium minerals, lipids, polysaccharides, and proteins are common substrates used to manufacture micrometric and nanometric 3D spheres for drug delivery. Specifically, glycosaminoglycans (GAGs) (Yip et al. 2006), heparin, collagen, fibrin, elastin, silk fibroin (Wenk et al. 2008; Wu et al. 2008; Willerth et al. 2009), and artificial proteins (Silva et al. 2008) have all been tested as candidates for universal drug delivery substrates. How they are used to build structures for this role is one part of this review. The second is to focus upon structural design for targeting and programmed release. We envisage that by studying the appropriate biological analogues, we will discover inventive principles of design that can be transferred into fabrication of new drug delivery devices. This can be best defined as abstracting good design from nature or biomimicry (Parker and Townley 2007). We will then highlight spheres and capsules aimed at delivering packages of proteins and cells for tissue modulation and repair. We will also mention an example whereby we hope to use living cells to help fabricate biomaterial frameworks. Our search begins with the vesicles, ubiquitous semipermeable lipid bilayer delineating sacs that store, segregate, and transport biological substances from cell to cell and within the cell. Vesicles include vacuoles, lysozymes, transport vesicles, and secretory vesicles. Natural phospholipids and polymer amphiphiles are used to create engineered versions. Liposomes can also be chemically modulated with functional molecules to direct their attachment to designated cell and tissue addresses such as the calcium phosphate of bone (Anada et al. 2009). This highlights the limit of those structural solutions evolved by natural selection, which operate on a different time frame and set of constraints than man-made versions possibly can at present. For example, man-made versions allow for investment of more energy for their fabrication because they are not constrained by getting energy from the environment and selectively partitioning it (Vincent 2003). Organisms are constrained by path dependency, historical legacy, and trade-offs and then give rise to imperfections. A study of these can aid the design of improved versions of natural counterparts, which can function in situations (e.g., certain debilitating pathologies) not selected for.

30.3.4 Bioceramic-Based Delivery Vehicles

Bioceramics are a significant group of biomaterials tailored to the tissue engineering of bone teeth and cartilage. Despite their innate crystallographic structure, biominerals can be remodeled into a richly diverse collection of curved shapes and intricate 3D morphologies through specialized biological controls and regulation of mineral deposition on organic membranes and within and between cells (Addadi and Weiner 1992; Mann 1995, 2001). Many of the morphologies that are produced by biology are more architecturally elaborate than mineral crystals formed, which can produce rotated, twisted, and even spherical 3D structures by screw dislocations and the addition of impurities. For example, spheroidal graphite can be formed with addition of minute magnesium that generates twist boundaries, hence microspheres (Lux and Minkoff 1974). However, in geology, silica typically precipitates as spherical colloidal particles, whereas unicellular organisms can shape silica minerals into "lacelike" structures. With defined macromolecular organization and macroscopic form, there arises specific function. Hard mineralized materials and their built structures are appropriate for calcified bone and joint tissues owing to their complementarity, biocompatibility, and bioresorption properties. For bone replacement surgery, biphasic calcium phosphate bone substitutes derived from mixed HAp and β-tricalcium phosphate (β-TCP) are one the most promising materials for bone drug delivery systems in calcified tissues. Efforts are under way to increase the biological activity by a number of methods. Chemical and biological properties are intertwined with nanoscale dimensions of the mineral (Palazzo et al. 2007, 2009). Natural bone as stated earlier is comprised of nanometric carbonated HA nanocrystals. An increasingly important and necessary element of a biomimetic drug delivery device for bone repair and reconstruction is release of multiple therapeutic drugs and biological molecules from the same device (Green and Ben-Nissan 2008). Take, for example, the strategy to treat osteoarthritis. Current opinion is to bring a cooperative balance of bone-promoting and bone-resorbing drugs alongside antibiotics because of the constant and recurrent threat from bacterial infection due to the highly invasive nature of bone surgery (Chou et al. 2011). This principle was similarly used to develop biomimetic nanoapatite crystals tailored for dual release of alendronate and anticancer/ antimetastatic drugs by controlled desorption onto the crystal surface (Palazzo et al. 2007). The release rates were defined by using either needle-shaped or plate-shaped crystals with different surface charge and surface areas.

30.3.5 Calcium Phosphate- and Carbonate-Based Delivery Vehicles

The rich taxonomic diversity of intricate calcium carbonate structures throughout the lower orders of the animal kingdom provides a highly accessible library of structural designs. Many will offer functions for which they had not originally evolved but, which by chance, are predisposed to suit another function. An example of this is the reticulated filtration system, which fortuitously makes an ideal structure for drug entrapment and delivery. Although much is known about how they are synthesized at a molecular level and how these intricate structures are constructed, natural invertebrate skeletons are however almost impossible, at present, to copy by artificial means. Instead chemistry that emulates simple organizing steps in the morphogenesis of shell structures has produced materials and structures with similarly detailed morphology and function. Structures that mimic the morphology of calcium carbonate shells of microscopic planktons having been synthesized in an analogous process have been shown to accelerate the differentiation of osteoprogenitors into osteoid and cartilage tissues when cultivated together (Figure 30.3). Moreover, it was found that growth factors could be entrapped between and within the crystal plates during microsphere assembly. As the calcium carbonate slowly dissolves, these growth factors are released into the surrounding environment (Green 2004; Green and Ben-Nissan 2010).

Mature mineralized bone and neocartilage was regenerated in vivo by mixing these bone-conductive microporous spheres with human allograft and human bone marrow stromal cells—the precursors to osteoblasts (Figure 30.4).

Similarly naturally occurring *Foraminifera* shells possess a network of submicron and nanoscale interconnected pores and channels (Figure 30.1), which provide an added network of fluid flow routes that potentially increases their capacity for the uptake of growth medium, metabolites, and waste products. The specific arrangement of structural elements (pores, struts, and channels) introduces biotemplates for the organization and aggregation of different cell types into coherent and anatomically correct functional tissues. For example, the estimated 70,000 species of corals provide enough structural diversity to correspond with the varied textures present in human bone. Selected elements of tropical coral sand, as shown in Figures 30.1 and 30.5, have evolved a kaleidoscope of unique filtration architectures. These are comprised of macropores, micropores, and nanopores that can be completely converted to a range of soluble calcium phosphates. These small pores, which can control loaded drug release, are very difficult if not impossible to synthetically produce and hence make an important and novel slow drug delivery device. The future promise of these structures is that other tissue engineering components including BMP, stem cells, and antibiotics can be integrated within them. It must be noted that we are not confined by the structural designs enforced by environment, competition, genes, and evolution. The unicellular organisms that produce these micrometric shells could conceivably be cultured inside fermentation vats with high precision and reproducibly. Judicious regulation of their culturing conditions can direct growth patterns and ultimately the structures that they synthesize as previously illustrated by Townley et al. (2007, 2008). Nature has highly efficient manufacturing techniques that can be harnessed in this way for human technologies (Parker and Townley 2007).

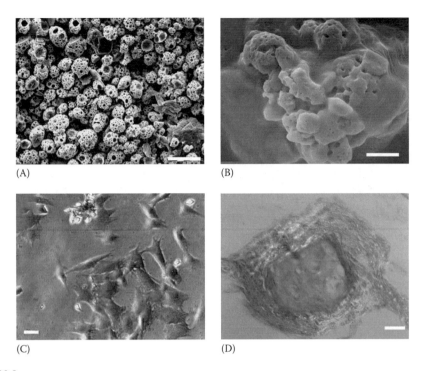

FIGURE 30.3
Synthetic microporous vaterite spheres (10 μm) that mirror the structure and morphology of natural plankton shells (A). SEM image of hBMS cells integrated with an aggregation of microporous vaterite spheres in pellet culture at 7 days in serum-supplemented media (B). Demonstrated functional release of an adsorbed osteoinductive factor (BMP 1,3,5,7 "retentate") as shown by positive alkaline phosphatase red staining in myoblast cells (C). These structures also provide a seeding template for osteoid (immature bone) formation into a distinct nodule in pellet culture at 14 days in serum-supplemented media (D).

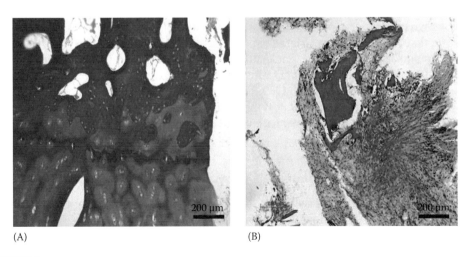

FIGURE 30.4
Histological sections of maturing bone and cartilage (intermediary) tissues produced from human mesenchymal stromal cells (hMSC) supported within vaterite microspheres admixed with allograft after implantation into severe combined immunodeficiency mouse for 4 weeks. Mature cartilage and bone regeneration exclusive to microsphere, hBMSC, and allograft combinations as shown in (A) contrasted with histological section of allograft and hBMS cells alone (B) (scale bar 200 μm).

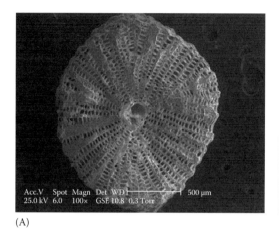
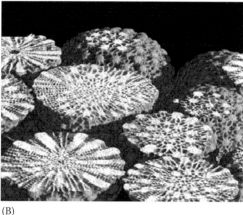

(A)   (B)

FIGURE 30.5

SEM image (A) and micro–computer tomography (CT) scan image (B) of coral sand *Foraminifera, floresianus,* and *B. sphaerulata* showing the cross-sectional area and unique natural filtration system of interconnected micropores and channels.

In our research, *Foraminifera, floresianus,* and *Baculogypsina sphaerulata,* which have unique filtration structures, were converted to solubility-controllable calcium phosphates and were loaded with a range of drugs and biological materials for targeted delivery, slow dissolution, and ultimately tissue regeneration and repair (Chou et al. 2011) (Figures 30.1 and 30.5).

Crab shell *chitosan* and seaweed-derived *alginate* polysaccharides are one of the most prolific substrates in use for biomedicine ranging from tissue engineering to drug and gene delivery (Kumar et al. 2004; Muzzarelli et al. 2007, 2009a,b). However, chemical and physical alterations are necessary to maximize its function inside the body. *Chitosan* nanoparticles, by far the most useful size for therapeutic intracellular delivery, are classed as smart delivery vehicles because chitosan is highly responsive to changes in environmental pH, within a restricted range, and temperature (Rinaudo 2006). Alginates are equally versatile vehicles for encapsulation and sustained delivery of proteins and genes by virtue of their chemical versatility (e.g., gelling can be caused by pH change or ionic substitution) (Martinsen et al. 1989; Thu et al. 1996a,b; Rowley et al. 1999; Orive et al. 2006). Once again physical and chemical modulation of alginates is being hotly pursued to tailor their properties with greater specificity for cell, gene, and protein delivery (Tonnesen and Karlsen 2002).

30.3.6 Transportation of Antibiotics

The development of microbial biofilms and their importance in medical implant infections have been extensively investigated over recent years. The development of a biofilm is initiated when bacterial cells attach to a surface and begin to excrete glue-like substances, which serve to anchor the cells. The environment created by the biofilm therefore enhances antimicrobial resistance. Microbial cells floating in surrounding fluids shed off new planktonic cells. This dynamic explains the relapsing nature of biofilm infections and the need for lengthy, controlled antibiotic delivery (Schroeder et al. 2010).

The current problem in the use of antibiotics for the treatment of osteomyelitis (bone degeneration) is the need for frequent dosage in order to gain maximum therapeutic effect due to their short residence times and low stability. This can in turn lead to toxicity and antibiotic resistance (Gao et al. 2011). Antibiotics must be maintained at levels above the minimum inhibitory concentration (MIC) for the shortest time necessary to effectively kill bacterial populations. Since direct intravenous delivery of antibiotics to the infected bone in sufficiently high concentrations results in systemic toxic effects, local administration using such procedures as closed irrigation and suction, local injection, and implantable pumps is widely used. However, these approaches are clinically inconvenient (O'Gara and Humphreys 2001).

As stated earlier, gentamicin sulfate is a potent antibiotic, widely used by clinicians to treat *Staphylococcus aureus* bacterial infections arising from orthopedic surgery and osteomyelitis. Antibiotics are poorly localized and can accumulate with toxic effects on the body. Achieving better targeted release and controlled dissolution has been an ongoing tissue engineering challenge.

Converted *Foraminifera*, β-TCP macrospheres were produced by a previously described method (Ben-Nissan 2003). It was demonstrated that calcium phosphate-converted *Foraminifera* micro- and macrospheres aided the slow release of encapsulated drug agents. Principally, this arises owing to their unique architecture of pores, struts, and channels, which amplifies physiological degradation and calcium phosphate dissolution to release attached drugs in a controlled manner. In a recent study, Chou et al. provided a focused evaluation of the antibiotic potential of these β-TCP macrospheres to eradicate *S. aureus* and maintaining osteoblast biocompatibility (Chou et al. 2011). They demonstrated that gentamicin coats these spheres entirely and that osteoblasts attach and grow onto the spheres. It was shown that gentamicin is quickly released and fast acting and finally that *S. aureus* do not attach to the spheres. Furthermore, gentamicin release is continued with no reemergence of bacteria in the presence of antibacterial micro- and macrospheres. In the light of these results, marine structure-based β-TCP macrospheres show promise as potential bone void filler particles with antibacterial effects. They have further reported that these unique structures could be used in regenerative orthopedics to treat osteomyelitis caused by *S. aureus* owing to their morphology, excellent drug retention, and release properties (Figure 30.6).

In the experimental work, the converted *Foraminifera* macrospheres were loaded with gentamicin (100 mg of gentamicin sulfate, Sigma Aldrich) (Figure 30.4 inset). The actual amount of gentamicin loaded into each β-TCP microsphere was calculated by taking the difference between the weight of the microsphere before and after soaking in gentamicin solution. All measurements were performed with a sample number of six (n = 6).

In this study, it was shown that the macrospheres can be stably loaded with sufficient quantities of the antibiotic gentamicin to kill *S. aureus* bacteria grown in the same culture within 30 min, with no evidence of bacterial growth within 24 h after adding macrospheres, while conversely, bacterial growth occurred in the presence of macrospheres not loaded with gentamicin (Figure 30.6).

It is important for bone regeneration that bone cells are unaffected by antibiotic treatment. In tests combining gentamicin macrospheres and cultured human osteoblasts, the in vitro cell growth was found to be normal and the cells were seen to adhere and spread onto the surface of all macrospheres. This is promising by indicating biocompatibility of the macrospheres. Furthermore, the β-TCP macrospheres, in addition to supplying calcium and phosphate ions during dissolution, possess properties for fast-acting drug release (Chou et al. 2011). In this study, antibiotic action of the gentamicin-loaded β-TCP macrospheres has been demonstrated, which when combined with their physical scaffolding support for contacting osteoblasts provides scope for their use as novel therapeutic bone void fillers.

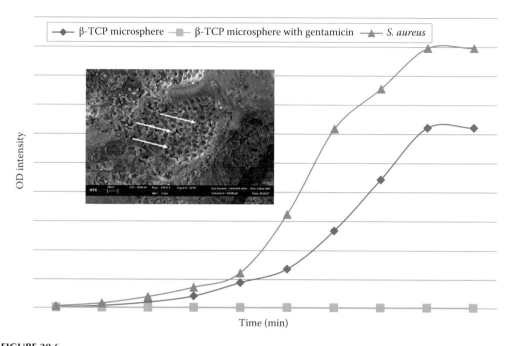

FIGURE 30.6
Cumulative effect of gentamicin release from macrospheres on *S. aureus* coculture. Inset image: a SEM to show trapped and adherent gentamicin particles on a β-TCP macrosphere outer surface.

30.4 Stem Cells and Tissue Engineering

Therapeutic stem cells require environments conducive to their propagation and continued survival. The simulation of similar or identical environments using biomaterials is being pursued to nurture stem cells in the laboratory. Those same attributes of porosity and biological responsiveness that made coral suited to bone invasion and morphosynthesis were thought equally useful for stem cell-based bone formation (Tohma et al. 2008).

Coral skeletons did show promotion of stem cell specialization and mature bone formation when implanted an in vivo segmental defect. Nanometric surface structure and crystallinity are increasingly being viewed as important elements in influencing MSC behavior and also supporting neural network formation. The internal environment—of geometrical spaces, nanotopography, and surface features—of coral skeletons could prove sufficient to expand added stem cell populations into the estimated numbers needed to be therapeutically relevant and this prior to implantation (Green et al. 2012). This propensity has been indicated by pilot studies to support the anchorage and proliferation of stem cells on the outer surfaces of *Foraminifera* (*B. sphaerulata*, floresianus) macrospheres (Figure 30.7). In a separate study, adipogenic cells could be transdifferentiated into osteoblast phenotype by growing on particular crystalline biomatrix. The promotive effect of crystallinity, mineral type, and ion composition on human cell populations was demonstrated within cultured crystalline aragonite hydrozoan corals (*Millepora dichotoma*). In this study, mesenchymal stem cells cultured on cloned *M. dichotoma* induced their differentiation into bone cell phenotype (Abramovitch-Gottlib et al. 2005).

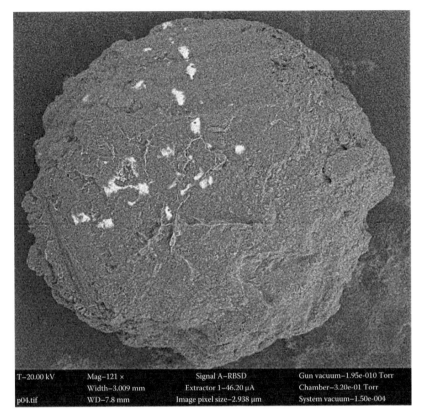

FIGURE 30.7
The potential of macrospheres to anchor and transport adherent stem cells fit for transplantation. SEM image of β-TCP macrosphere coated in adipocyte-derived stem cells in 3D pellet culture.

To emphasize the possible importance of surface nanoarchitecture, in pilot studies, coral skeletons transformed into calcium phosphate and coated with sol–gel HAp nanocoating were rapidly colonized by mesenchymal stem cells, whereas converted corals were less rapidly colonized by MSC. The chemical composition of skeletal biomatrix is also a significant factor that can induce the differentiation of attached cells (Green et al. 2012).

So it was demonstrated that spongin from the marine sponge, *Hymeniacidon sinapium*, was shown to promote bone mineralization of human preosteoblastic cells. Spongin also inhibited production of inflammatory cytokines, TNF-alpha, IL-1, and PGE, by macrophages adding to its credentials as a potential future osteoinductive scaffold material.

In the light of these and other examples, the potential for skeletal proteins—such as growth factors—to influence and control human cell proliferation and differentiation is being investigated. Growth factors common to humans and marine invertebrates are shown in Table 30.2. It is envisaged that by combining the innovative osteoaccelerant potential of skeletal proteins, the already established potential of bone-mimicking marine skeletons with regenerative potency of mesenchymal stem cells' self-sustaining living bone composites can be generated. Anticipated role and the rationale of the proteins, mesenchymal stem cells, and new biomaterial structures that can be used with marine skeletons for regenerative medicine are given in Table 30.3.

TABLE 30.2

Growth Factors Common to Humans and Marine Invertebrates

Growth Factors Active in Bone	Marine Organism with Growth Factor Analogue
BMP	Corals: *Turbinaria reniformis*, *Acropora* sp., *Pavona cactus*, *Galaxea fascicularis*, *Hydnophora pilosa*, *Stylophora pistillata*, *Lobophyllia* sp. (Zoccola et al. 2000; Lelong et al. 2001)
Transforming growth factor (TGF)	Marine sponge, Mollusca: *Planorbarius corneus*, *Viviparus ater*, *Viviparus contectus*, *Lymnaea stagnalis*, *Mytilus galloprovincialis* (Nichols et al. 2006; Adamski et al. 2011)
Vascular endothelial growth factor (VEGF)	Cnidaria: *Podocoryne carnea* (Seipel et al. 2004)
Fibroblast growth factor (FGF)	Cnidaria: *Nematostella vectensis* (Ornitz et al. 2002; Matus et al. 2007)
Insulin-like growth factor (IGF)	Mollusk nacre seashell: *H. laevigata* (Weiss et al. 2001)
Tissue necrosis factor (TNF)	Mollusk TNF-alpha present in *Mytilus edulis* (Hughes et al. 1992)
Epithelium growth factor (EGF)	Marine sponge: *Lubomirski baicalensis* (Gerber et al. 2000)
Platelet-derived growth factor (PDGF)	Mollusca P. corneus, V. ater, V. contectus, L. stagnalis, My. galloprovincialis (Franchini et al. 2000)

TABLE 30.3

Anticipated Role and the Rationale of the Proteins, Mesenchymal Stem Cells, and New Biomaterial Structures That Can Be Used with Marine Skeletons for Regenerative Medicine

Anticipated Role	Rationale
Stem cell microenvironment	Promotion of proliferation and differentiation
Alternative source of structural biomaterials	Structural biomaterials with new and enhanced properties
New source of regenerative proteins and sugars	Command and control of proliferation and differentiation

30.5 Concluding Remarks

Drug therapy works in tandem with tissue regeneration. It has been argued that the drug compound can be replaced by harnessing specific cells, genetically engineered to oversecrete therapeutic proteins in tempo with the local physiology. It may also be possible to harness a functional unit of cells to undertake the same role. We are using capsules to support cells that produce the desired proteins. In our laboratories, we are integrating the capsule with specific cells. Cellular assemblies are functional modules ringed with ordered arrangement of cells of different cell types with a discrete role in rebuilding tissues. It would be highly advantageous to be able to produce the basic units of tissue and then assembled into multiple layers and hierarchies in the laboratory. In other words, establish environments in which co-opted cells build their own structures from synthetic building blocks.

The formation of mineralized tissues is controlled by a number of factors based on human biology, biomechanics, and partition chemistry that directs the construction into defined spaces. The molecular functions of these compartments include control of size, shape, and organization of mineral; control of ion diffusion, solution concentrations, and pacifying minerals; accumulation of products; nucleation; transportation; and functional loadings. Cells of mineralized tissue are intrinsically involved in these processes. They themselves are assembled and confined within boundaries composed of impervious substrates to enclose mineralization and to control the structure and chemistry of the fluid-filled environment (Mann 1995; Mann and Ozin 1996). Inside the bone during the mineralization process, cells arrange themselves into groups. In one theory of bone growth, it has been suggested that osteoblasts come together and generate a fluid-filled compartment isolated from blood and other mineralized tissue.

Allowing human progenitor cells to reassemble their matrix environment using tailored synthetic biomaterial "building blocks" (multicomponent segments) is an evolving concept. Novel biomaterials generated by modular self-assembly are already well advanced. The cell-mediated approach promises a new class of biomaterials designed and constructed by biology in real time. This will allow any cell-engineered biomaterial to be precisely tailored with optimized properties. Tissue engineers are presently developing prefabricated scaffolds with built-in biorecognition motifs (ligands) that are modulated by the naturally occurring activities and responses of progenitor cells that proceed during early development and regeneration in adults. It is an attempt to simulate the complex time-dependent interactions between cells and between cells and its matrix. The change is styled to give rise to matrix events that reinforce regeneration processes. While among other researchers, the strategy has been to develop cell-independent self-assembling biomaterial structures, which increasingly simulate their natural counterparts. The promise of both approaches is to maximize biological responses and increase the speed and quality of tissue regeneration. In previous experiments, calcium carbonate microsponges at or below the dimension of a single cell were manipulated (by individual cells) and preferentially arranged into aggregates by cocultured human bone marrow stromal cells in monolayer culture at a range of cell densities (Green 2004; Green and Ben-Nissan 2008).

Bringing the correct dosage of regenerative factors to the treatable site, in a temporal sequence, has proven somewhat elusive. This arises out of the technical difficulty of coordinating release in synergy with host physiology and the variety of biological responses that can occur (Mooney et al. 2005). Proteins degrade too rapidly and possess limited stability. Gene correction strategies are aimed at increasing the effectiveness and potency of protein synthesis and secretion from the cell compared to direct delivery of proteins to the cell (Hoffman et al. 2001; Bianco et al. 2006). Cell-mediated gene therapy using nonviral transduction agents depends on synthetic biomaterials, lipids, and physical disruption of the cell membrane to allow entry of influential new genes and transcription factors. In all of these procedures, there are unproductive inefficiencies in gene targeting, gene expression levels, and inappropriate gene integration.

It is imperative that added bioactive factors are released in well-defined sequences at cell-instructive doses and for specific time periods in synchronization with the body's own biochemistry. Such actions will ensure that the added biological factors provide their maximum effect and potency. One of the main problems is releasing each factor in a slow and sustained manner for long periods of time to permanently restore tissue function. There are two ways that the release of encapsulates can be regulated. The first is to modify the composition and thickness of the capsule shell and, by doing so, slow down release of the contents by diffusion. This has been shown effective at delaying the release of plasmid deoxyribose nucleic acid. Alternatively it is possible to create nested arrangements of beads—one inside another (Green et al. 2003). The host–guest arrangement of capsules is seemingly an effective system for the temporal control of encapsulate release into the outside medium. Experimentally tyrosinase-containing capsules (containing identical volumes of tyrosinase) were inserted into a vacant host capsule, repeated twice. The repeated nesting increases the mass the enzyme must diffuse through and so slows its release to the outside environment.

Biomedical engineers are continually striving to improve and update therapeutic medical treatments to reduce pain, inflammation, surgery time, and invasiveness of surgery using drug and protein delivery vehicles. However, current devices are deficient in two crucial ways. They are not well targeted and delivery is not sufficiently well regulated. As a result, there is an ongoing, prolific research and discovery of new more clinically acceptable technologies that can remotely arrive at a tissue destination to deliver drugs, growth factors, and genes continuously in any elected spatial and temporal patterns. Spheres at a small scale can be put to effective use to carry these biological molecules and protect them from physiological degradation. Spheres conform to the shape of the cell during transportation (rounded up), possess the highest surface area to volume ratio of any 3D shape, have high packing efficiencies, and are smoothly carried away within fluids efficiently. We have selectively highlighted biomimicry approaches using marine structures to produce new devices that may potentially deliver drugs and genes to their intended destination in the correct dosages. Biomimicry in our terms involves selecting an appropriate analogy from nature that solves similar problems to the one under examination. We believe these approaches best repay study because nature provides us with highly refined solutions to conflicts that characterize problems. Often we find that non–human biology provides simpler and more convenient solutions. We showed how bioceramic macrospheres were made from marine structures synthetically using biomimicry chemistry for packaging and delivering growth factors to osteoprogenitors. Perhaps more advantageous of all is the direct use of natural skeletons appropriated to deliver bone-promoting drugs and antibiotics in tandem. Cells may also have a role in delivery of beneficial therapeutic proteins. In all probability, this might be the best way forward because cells can be genetically programmed to secrete proteins in synchrony with the host. Packaging cells into collective units and modules within these structures is necessary to properly protect cells transplanted into the host. Future work may also encompass ways of detecting the status and position of integrated devices.

We have highlighted our different approach to developing new drug delivery devices using nature throughout evolution as a philosopher and guide and hope this stimulates further investigation and clinical use.

References

Abramovitch-Gottlib, L., T. Gross, D. Naveh, S. Geresh, S. Rosenwaks, I. Bar, and R. Vago. 2005. Low level laser irradiation stimulates osteogenic phenotype of mesenchymal stem cells seeded on a three-dimensional biomatrix. *Lasers Med Sci*, 20(3–4), 138–146.

Addadi, L. and S. Weiner. 1992. Control and design principles in biological mineralization. *Ange Chem Int*, 31(2), 153–169.

Akinc, A. et al. 2009. Development of lipidoid-siRNA formulations for systemic delivery to the liver. *Mol Ther*, 17, 872–879.

Albee, F.H. and H.F. Morrison. 1920. Studies in bone growth. *Ann Surg*, 71, 32.

Anada, T. et al. 2009. Synthesis of calcium phosphate-binding liposome for drug delivery. *Bioorg Med Chem Lett*, 19(15), 4148–4150.

Attenborough, D. 1995. *Private Life of Plants: A Natural History of Plant Behaviour*. BBC Books, London.

Baker, M. 2010. Homing in on delivery. *Nature*, 464(7292), 1225–1230.

Ben-Nissan, B. 2003. Natural bioceramics: From coral to bone and beyond. *Curr Opin Solid State Mater Sci*, 7(4–5), 283–288.

Ben-Nissan, B. 2004. Biomimetics and bioceramics, in *Learning from Nature How to Design New Implantable Biomaterials*, NATO Science Series, Vol. 171 (Eds) Reis, R.L. and S. Weiner, Kluwer Academic Publishers, Dordrecht, the Netherlands, pp. 89–103, ISBN 1-4020-2647-7.

Ben-Nissan, B., A.H. Choi, D.W. Green, B.A. Latella, J. Chou, and A. Bendavid. 2011. Synthesis of hydroxyapatite nanocoatings by sol-gel A. Method for clinical applications, in *Biological and Biomedical Coatings Handbook, Vol. 1, Processing and Characterisation*, (Ed) Zhang, S., Taylor & Francis Group, Boca Raton, FL, Chapter 2, pp. 37–79, ISBN 9781439849958.

Ben-Nissan, B., A. Milev, and R. Vago. 2004. Morphology of sol-gel derived nano-coated coralline hydroxyapatite, *Biomaterials*, 25, 4971–4976.

Ben-Nissan, B., J.J. Russell, J. Hu, A. Milev, D. Green, R. Vago, W. Walsh, and R.M. Conway. 2000. Comparison of surface morphology in sol-gel treated coralline hydroxyapatite structures for implant purposes, in *Bioceramics, Vol. 13, Key Engineering Materials*, pp. 959–962, Trans Tech Publications, Zurich, Switzerland.

Bhushan, B. 2009. Biomimetics: Lessons from nature—An overview. *Philos Trans A Math Phys Eng Sci*, 367, 1445–1486.

Bianco, P. et al. 2006. Postnatal skeletal stem cells. *Adult Stem Cells*, 419, 117–148.

Carter, P.J. 2006. Potent antibody therapeutics by design. *Nat Rev Immunol*, 6, 343–357.

Chen, R.R. and D.J. Mooney. 2003. Polymeric growth factor delivery strategies for tissue engineering. *Pharmaceut Res*, 20(8), 1103–1112.

Chew, S.Y., Y. Wen, Y. Dzenis, and K.W. Leong. 2006. The role of electrospinning in the emerging field of nanomedicine. *Curr Pharm Des*, 12(36), 4751–4770.

Chou, J., B. Ben-Nissan, D.W. Green, S.M. Valenzuela, and L. Kohan. 2011. Targeting and dissolution characteristics of bone forming and antibacterial drugs by harnessing the structure of microspherical shells from coral beach sand. *Adv Eng Mater*, 13(1–2), 93–99.

Dahlin, R.L., F.K. Kasper, and A.G. Mikos. 2011. Polymeric nanofibers in tissue engineering. *Tissue Eng Part B Rev*, 17(5), 349–364.

Davis, M.E. et al. 2010. Evidence of RNAi in humans from systemically administered siRNA via targeted nanoparticles. *Nature*, 464(7291), 1067–1070.

De la Zerda, A. and S.S. Gambhir. 2007. Drug delivery: Keeping tabs on nanocarriers. *Nat Nanotechnol*, 2(12), 745–746.

Dunlop, J.W.C., R. Weinkamer, and P. Fratzl. 2011. Artful interfaces within biological materials. *Mater Today*, 14(3), 70–78.

Ehrbar, M. et al. 2011. Elucidating the role of matrix stiffness in 3D cell migration and remodeling. *Biophys Journal*, 100(2), 284–293.

Ehrlich, H. et al. 2010. Three-dimensional chitin-based scaffolds from *Verongida sponges* (Demospongiae: Porifera). Part I. Isolation and identification of chitin. *Int J Biol Macromol*, 47(2), 132–140.

Ehrlich, H. et al. 2011. Simple method for preparation of nanostructurally organized spines of sand dollar *Scaphechinus mirabilis* (Agassiz, 1863). *Mar Biotechnol (NY)*, 13(3), 402–410.

Elliott, S. et al. 2003. Enhancement of therapeutic protein in vivo activities through glycoengineering. *Nat Biotechnol*, 21(4), 414–421.

Eniola, A.O., S.D. Rodgers, and D.A. Hammer. 2002. Characterization of biodegradable drug delivery vehicles with the adhesive properties of leukocytes. *Biomaterials*, 23(10), 2167–2177.

Ernst, B. and Magnani, J.L. 2009. From carbohydrate leads to glycomimetic drugs. *Nat Rev Drug Discov*, 8(8), 661–677.

Esfand, R. and D.A. Tomalia. 2001. Poly(amidoamine) (PAMAM) dendrimers: From biomimicry to drug delivery and biomedical applications. *Drug Discov Today*, 6(8), 427–436.

Fire, A. et al. 1998. Potent and specific genetic interference by double-stranded RNA in *Caenorhabditis elegans*. *Nature*, 391(6669), 806–811.

Fratzl, P. 2007. Biomimetic materials research: What can we really learn from nature's structural materials? *J R Soc Interface*, 4(15), 637–642.

Freitas, R.A. 2006. Pharmacytes: An ideal vehicle for targeted drug delivery. *J Nanosci Nanotechnol* 6(9–10), 2769–2775.

Gao, P., X. Nie, M. Zou, Y. Shi, and G. Cheng. 2011. Recent advances in materials for extended-release antibiotic delivery system. *J Antibiot (Tokyo)*, 64(9):625–634.

Grafahrend, D., K.H. Heffels, M.V. Beer, P. Gasteier, M. Möller, G. Boehm, P.D. Dalton, and J. Groll. 2011. Degradable polyester scaffolds with controlled surface chemistry combining minimal protein adsorption with specific bioactivation. *Nat Mater*, 10(1), 67–73.

Green, D. 2004. Stimulation of human bone marrow stromal cells using growth factor encapsulated calcium carbonate porous microspheres. *J Mater Chem*, 14(14), 2206–2212.

Green, D.W. and B. Ben-Nissan. 2008. Bio-inspired engineering of human tissue scaffolding for regenerative medicine. Chapter 23, in *Biomaterials in Asia*, (Ed) Tateishi, T., World Scientific Publishing Co. Pte. Ltd. Singapore, pp. 364–385.

Green, D.W. and B. Ben-Nissan. 2010. Biomimetic applications in regenerative medicine: Scaffolds, transplantation modules and tissue homing devices, Chapter 21, in *Handbook of Materials for Nanomedicine*. (Eds) Torchilin, V.P. and M.M. Amiji, Pan Stanford Publishing, Pte. Ltd., Singapore, pp. 821–850.

Green, D.W., D. Howard, X.B. Yang, and M. Kelly. 2003. Oreffo ROC. Natural marine sponge fibre skeleton: A biomimetic scaffold for human osteoprogenitor cell attachment, growth and differentiation. *Tissue Eng*, 9(6), 1159–1166.

Green, D.W., G. Li, B. Milthorpe, and B. Ben-Nissan. 2012. Adult stem cell coatings using biomaterials for regenerative medicine. *Mater Today*, 15(1–2), 60–66.

Guo, C., J. Wang, F. Cao, R.J. Lee, and G. Zhai. 2010. Lyotropic liquid crystal systems in drug delivery. *Drug Discov Today*, 15, 1032–1040.

Harrington, D.A., E.Y. Cheng, M.O. Guler, L.K. Lee, J.L. Donovan, R.C. Claussen, and S.I. Stupp. 2006. Branched peptide-amphiphiles as self-assembling coatings for tissue engineering scaffolds. *J Biomed Mater Res A*, 78(1), 157–167.

Hartgerink, J.D., E. Beniash, and S.I. Stupp. 2001. Self-assembly and mineralization of peptide-amphiphile nanofibers. *Science*, 23(5547), 1684–1688.

Heinemann, S., H. Ehrlich, T. Douglas, C. Heinemann, H. Worch, W. Schatton, and T. Hanke. 2007. Ultrastructural studies on the collagen of the marine sponge *Chondrosia reniformis Nardo*. *Biomacromolecules*, 8(11), 3452–3457.

Helms, M., S.S. Vattam, and A.K. Goel. 2009. Biologically inspired design: Process and products. *Des. Stud*, 30(5), 606–622.

Hoffman, A. et al. 2001. Bioinspired polymers that control intracellular drug delivery. *Biotechnol Bioprocess Eng*, 6(4), 205–212.

Hu, J., R. Fraser, J.J. Russell, R. Vago, and B. Ben-Nissan. 2000. Australian coral as a biomaterial: Characteristics. *J Mater Sci Technol*, 16(6), 591–595.

Hu, J., J.J. Russell, B. Ben-Nissan, and R. Vago. 2001. Production and of hydroxyapatite from Australian corals via hydrothermal analysis process. *J Mater Sci Lett*, 20(1), 85–87.

Huebsch, N. and D.J. Mooney. 2009. Inspiration and application in the evolution of biomaterials. *Nature*, 462(7272), 426–432.

Ivankovic, H. et al. 2009. Preparation of highly porous hydroxyapatite from cuttlefish bone. *J Mater Sci Mater Med* 20(5), 1039–1046.

Jabbari, E. 2009. Engineering bone formation with peptidomimetic hybrid biomaterials. *Conf Proc IEEE Eng Med Biol Soc*, 2009, 1172–1175.

Jang, J.H. et al. 2006. Surface adsorption of DNA to tissue engineering scaffolds for efficient gene delivery. *J Biomed Mater Res A*, 77(1), 50–58.

Jones, R. 2006. What can biology teach us? *Nat Nanotechnol*, 1(2), 85–86.

Katifori, E. et al. 2010. Foldable structures and the natural design of pollen grains. *Proc Natl Acad Sci USA*, 107(17), 7635–7639.

Kobayashi, H., M. Daimaruya, and H. Fujita. 2003. Unfolding of morning glory flower as a deployable structure. *IUTAM Symposium on Dynamics of Advanced Materials and Smart Structures*, Yonezawa, Japan, Vol. 106, pp. 207–216.

Kobayashi, H., M. Daimaruya, and J.F.V. Vincent. 2000. Folding/unfolding manner of tree leaves as a deployable structure. *IUTAM-IASS Symposium on Deployable Structures: Theory and Applications*, Yonezawa, Japan, Vol. 80, pp. 211–220.

Kobayashi, H. and K. Horikawa. 2009. Deployable structures in plants. *Min Smart Nat*, 58, 31–40.

Kumar, M.N.V.R. et al. 2004. Chitosan chemistry and pharmaceutical perspectives. *Chem Rev*, 104(12), 6017–6084.

Kyle, S., A. Aggeli, E. Ingham, and M.J. McPherson. 2009. Production of self-assembling biomaterials for tissue engineering. *Trends Biotechnol*, 27(7) 423–433.

Langer, R. 1990. New methods of drug delivery. *Science*, 249(4976), 1527–1533.

Langer, R. 1998. Drug delivery and targeting. *Nature*, 392(Suppl 6679), 5–10.

LaVan, D.A., T. McGuire, and R. Langer. 2003. Small-scale systems for in vivo drug delivery. *Nat Biotechnol*, 21(10), 1184–1191.

LeGeros, R.Z., O.R. Trautz, J.P. Legeros, E. Klein, and W.P. Shirra. 1967. Apatite crystallites: Effects of carbonate on morphology. *Science*, 155(3768), 1409–1411.

Li, W.J., C.T. Laurencin, E.J. Caterson, R.S. Tuan, and F.K. Ko. 2002. Electrospun nanofibrous structure: A novel scaffold for tissue engineering. *J Biomed Mater Res*, 60(4), 613–621.

Liao, S., B. Li, Z. Ma, H. Wei, C. Chan, and S. Ramakrishna. 2006. Biomimetic electrospun nanofibers for tissue regeneration. *Biomed Mater*, 1(3), R45–R53.

Lind, M. 1996. Growth factors: Possible new clinical tools. *Acta Orthop Scand*, 67, 407.

Luo, D. and W.M. Saltzman. 2000. Synthetic DNA delivery systems. *Nat Biotechnol*, 18(1), 33–37.

Lutolf, M.P. and J.A. Hubbell. 2005. Synthetic biomaterials as instructive extracellular microenvironments for morphogenesis in tissue engineering. *Nat Biotechnol*, 23(1), 47–55.

Lux, B. and I. Minkoff. 1974. In *The Metallurgy of Cast Iron* (Eds) Lux, B., I. Minkoff, and F. Mollard, Georgi Publishing Co., St. Saphorin, Switzerland, pp. 495–508.

Mann, S. 1988. Molecular recognition in biomineralization. *Nature*, 332(6160), 119–124.

Mann, S. 1995. Biomineralization and biomimetic materials chemistry. *J Mater Chem*, 5(7), 935–946.

Mann, S. 2001. *Biomineralization: Principles and Concepts in Biomimetic Materials Chemistry*. Oxford.

Mann, S. and G.A. Ozin. 1996. Synthesis of inorganic materials with complex form. *Nature*, 382(6589), 313–318.

Martinsen, A., G. Skjakbraek, and O. Smidsrod. 1989. Alginate as immobilization material.1. Correlation between chemical and physical-properties of alginate gel beads. *Biotechnol Bioeng*, 33(1), 79–89.

Mooney, D.J. et al. 2005. Actively regulating bioengineered tissue and organ formation. *Orthod Craniofac Res*, 8(3), 141–144.

Muzzarelli, R.A.A. 2009a. Chitins and chitosans for the repair of wounded skin, nerve, cartilage and bone. *Carbohydr Polym*, 76(2), 167–182.

Muzzarelli, R.A.A. 2009b. Genipin-crosslinked chitosan hydrogels as biomedical and pharmaceutical aids. *Carbohydr Polym*, 77(1), 1–9.

Muzzarelli, R.A.A. et al. 2007. Chitin nanofibrils/chitosan glycolate composites as wound medicaments. *Carbohydr Polym*, 70, 274–284.

Nowak, D. et al. 2009. Morphology and the chemical make-up of the inorganic components of black corals. *Mater Sci Eng C*, 29(3), 1029–1038.

O'Gara, J.P. and H. Humphreys. 2001. *Staphylococcus epidermidis* biofilms: Importance and implications. *J Med Microbiol*, 50, 582–587.

Orive, G. et al. 2006. Biocompatibility of alginate-poly-L-lysine microcapsules for cell therapy. *Biomaterials*, 27(20), 3691–3700.

Palazzo, B. et al. 2007. Biomimetic hydroxyapatite drug nanocrystals as potential bone substitutes with antitumor drug delivery properties. *Adv Funct Mater*, 17(13), 2180–2188.

Palazzo, B. et al. 2009. Amino acid synergetic effect on structure, morphology and surface properties of biomimetic apatite nanocrystals. *Acta Biomater*, 5(4), 1241–1452.

Parker, A.R. and Townley, H.E. 2007. Biomimetics of photonic nanostructures. *Nat Nanotechnol*, 2(6), 347–353.

Patri, A.K., J.F. Kukowska-Latallo, and J.R. Baker. 2005. Targeted drug delivery with dendrimers: Comparison of the release kinetics of covalently conjugated drug and non-covalent drug inclusion complex. *Adv Drug Delivery Rev*, 57(15), 2203–2214.

Pennisi, E. 2002. Materials science. Biology reveals new ways to hold on tight. *Science*, 296(5566), 250–251.

Pizarro-Cerda, J. and P. Cossart. 2006. Bacterial adhesion and entry into host cells. *Cell*, 124(4), 715–727.

Prow, T.W. et al. 2010. Nanopatch-targeted skin vaccination against West Nile virus and Chikungunya virus in mice. *Small*, 6(16), 1776–1784.

Ramasubramanian, M.K., O.M. Barham, and V. Swaminathan. 2008. Mechanics of a mosquito bite with applications to microneedle design. *Bioinspir Biomim*, 3(4), 046001.

Ranney, D.F. 2000. Biomimetic transport and rational drug delivery. *Biochem Pharmacol*, 59(2), 105–114.

Raphael, A.P. et al. 2010. Targeted, needle-free vaccinations in skin using multilayered, densely-packed dissolving microprojection arrays. *Small*, 6(16), 1785–1793.

Reddi, A.H. 1998. Role of morphogenetic proteins in skeletal tissue engineering and regeneration. *Nat Biotechnol*, 16(3), 247–252.

Richardson, T.P. et al. 2001. Polymeric system for dual growth factor delivery. *Nat Biotechnol*, 19(11), 1029–1034.

Rinaudo, M. 2006. Chitin and chitosan: Properties and applications. *Prog Polym Sci*, 31(7), 603–632.

Rizwan, S.B. et al. 2010. Bicontinuous cubic liquid crystals as sustained delivery systems for peptides and proteins. *Expert Opin Drug Delivery*, 7(10), 1133–1144.

Rowley, J.A., G. Madlambayan, and D.J. Mooney. 1999. Alginate hydrogels as synthetic extracellular matrix materials. *Biomaterials*, 20(1), 45–53.

Roy, D.M. and S.K. Linnehan. 1974. Hydroxyapatite formed from coral skeletal carbonate by hydrothermal exchange. *Nature*, 247, 220–222.

Saha, S. et al. 2007. Nanovalves. *Adv Funct Mater*, 17(5), 685–693.

Saltzman, W.M. 1999. Delivering tissue regeneration. *Nat Biotechnol*, 17(6), 534–535.

Salvay, D.M., M. Zelivyanskaya, and L.D. Shea. 2010. Gene delivery by surface immobilization of plasmid to tissue-engineering scaffolds. *Gene Ther*, 17(9), 1134–1141.

Schroeder, A. et al. 2010. Using liposomes to target infection and inflammation induced by foreign body injuries or medical implants. *Expert Opin Drug Delivery*, 7(10), 1175–1189.

Seipel, K., M. Eberhardt, P. Muller, E. Pescia, N. Yanze, and V. Schmid. 2004. Homologs of vascular endothelial growth factor and receptor, VEGF and VEGF-R, in the jellyfish *Podocoryne carnea*. *Dev Dynam*, 231, 303.

Sengupta, D. and S.C. Heilshorn. 2010. Protein-engineered biomaterials: Highly tunable tissue engineering scaffolds. *Tissue Eng Part B Rev*, 16(3), 285–293.

Shea, L.D. et al. 1999. DNA delivery from polymer matrices for tissue engineering. *Nat Biotechnol*, 17(6), 551–554.

Silva, E.A. et al. 2008. Material-based deployment enhances efficacy of endothelial progenitor cells. *Proc Natl Acad Sci USA*, 105(38), 14347–14352.

Silva, A.K. et al. 2009. Growth factor delivery approaches in hydrogels. *Biomacromolecules*, 10(1), 9–18.

Simmons, C.A. et al. 2004. Dual growth factor delivery and controlled scaffold degradation enhance in vivo bone formation by transplanted bone marrow stromal cells. *Bone*, 35(2), 562–569.

Smith, L.A., X. Liu, and P.X. Ma. 2008. Tissue engineering with nano-fibrous scaffolds. *Soft Matter*, 4(11), 2144–2149.

Stayton, P.S. et al. 2005. Intelligent biohybrid materials for therapeutic and imaging agent delivery. *Proc IEEE*, 93(4), 726–736.

Sukhorukov, G.B. et al. 2005. Nanoengineered polymer capsules: Tools for detection, controlled delivery, and site-specific manipulation. *Small*, 1, 194–200.

Swann, J.M. and A.J. Ryan. 2009. Chemical actuation in responsive hydrogels. *Polym Int*, 58(3), 285–289.

Tao, S.L. and T.A. Desai. 2003. Microfabricated drug delivery systems: From particles to pores. *Adv Drug Delivery Rev*, 55(3), 315–328.

Teo, W.E., W. He, and S. Ramakrishna. 2006. Ramakrishna, electrospun scaffold tailored for tissue-specific extracellular matrix. *Biotechnol J*, 1(9), 918–929.

Thu, B. et al. 1996a. Alginate polycation microcapsules. 1. Interaction between alginate and polycation. *Biomaterials*, 17(10), 1031–1040.

Thu, B., P. Bruheim, T. Espevik, O. Smidsrød, P. Soon-Shiong, and G. Skjåk-Braek. 1996b. Alginate polycation microcapsules. 2. Some functional properties. *Biomaterials*, 17(11), 1069–1079.

Tohma, Y., H. Ohgushi, T. Morishita, Y. Dohi, M. Tadokoro, Y. Tanaka, and Y. Takakura. 2008. Bone marrow-derived mesenchymal cells can rescue osteogenic capacity of devitalized autologous bone. *J Tissue Eng Regen Med*, 2(1), 61–68.

Tonnesen, H.H. and Karlsen, J. 2002. Alginate in drug delivery systems. *Drug Dev Ind Pharm*, 28(6), 621–630.

Townley, H.E. et al. 2007. Modification of the physical and optical properties of the frustule of the diatom *Coscinodiscus wailesii* by nickel sulfate. *Nanotechnology*, 18(29), 295101.

Townley, H.E., A.R. Parker, and H. White-Cooper. 2008. Exploitation of diatom frustules for nanotechnology: Tethering active biomolecules. *Adv Funct Mater*, 18(2), 369–374.

Urist, M.R. 1965. Bone: Formation by autoinduction. *Science*, 150(3698), 893–899.

Urist, M.R. and B.S. Strates. 1971. Bone morphogenetic protein. *J. Dent Res*, 50(6), 1392–1406.

Vago, R., D. Plotquin, A. Bunin, I. Sinelnikov, D. Atar, and D. Itzhak. 2002. Hard tissue remodeling using biofabricated coralline biomaterials. *J Biochem Biophys Methods*, 50(2–3), 253–259.

Venkatesh, S. et al. 2008. Transport and structural analysis for controlled of molecular imprinted hydrogels drug delivery. *Eur J Pharm Biopharm*, 69(3), 852–860.

Vincent, J.F.V. 2003. Biomimetic modelling. *Philos Trans R Soc London [Biol]*, 358(1437), 1597–1603.

Vincent, J.F. et al. 2006. Biomimetics: Its practice and theory. *J R Soc Interface*, 3(9), 471–482.

Vincent, J., O. Bogatyreva, and N. Bogatyrev. 2007. Towards a theory of biomimetics. *Comp Biochem Physiol A—Mol Integr Physiol*, 146(4), S129.

Weiner, S. 1986. Organization of extracellularly mineralized tissues—A comparative-study of biological crystal-growth. *CRC Crit Rev Biochem*, 20(4), 365–408.

Weiner, S. 2008. Biomineralization: A structural perspective. *J Struct Biol*, 163(3), 229–234.

Weiss, I.M., W. Göhring, M. Fritz, K. Mann, 2001. Perlustrin, a *Haliotis laevigata* (Abalone) Nacre protein, is homologous to the insulin-like growth factor binding protein N-terminal module of vertebrates. *Biochem Biophys Res Commun*, 285(2), 244.

Wenk, E. et al. 2008. Silk fibroin spheres as a platform for controlled drug delivery. *J Controlled Release*, 132(1), 26–34.

White, E. and E.C. Shors. 1986. Biomaterial aspects of Interpore-200 porous hydroxyapatite. *Dent Clin North Am*, 30(1), 49–67.

Willerth, S.M., A. Rader, and S.E. Sakiyama-Elbert. 2009. The effect of controlled growth factor delivery on embryonic stem cell differentiation inside fibrin scaffolds. *Stem Cell Res* 2(3), 231–236.

Wiznerowicz, M. and D. Trono. 2003. Conditional suppression of cellular genes: Lentivirus vector-mediated drug-inducible RNA interference. *J Virol*, 77(16), 8957–8961.

Wozney, J.M. et al. 1988. Novel regulators of bone formation: Molecular clones and activities. *Science*, 242(4885), 1528–1534.

Wu, Y. et al. 2008. Fabrication of elastin-like polypeptide nanoparticles for drug delivery by electrospraying. *Biomacromolecules*, 10(1), 19–24.

Xu, C., R. Inai, M. Kotaki, and S. Ramakrishna. 2004. Electrospun nanofiber fabrication as synthetic extracellular matrix and its potential for vascular tissue engineering. *Tissue Eng*, 10, 1160–1168.

Yan, M. et al. 2010. A novel intracellular protein delivery platform based on single-protein nanocapsules. *Nat Nanotechnol*, 5, 48–53.

Yip, G.W., M. Smollich, and M. Gotte 2006. Therapeutic value of glycosaminoglycans in cancer. *Mol Cancer Ther*, 5(9), 2139–2148.

Zhang, S.G. 2003. Fabrication of novel biomaterials through molecular self-assembly. *Nat Biotechnol*, 21(10), 1171–1178.

Zoccola, D., A. Moya, G.E. Beranger, E. Tambutte, D. Allemand, G.F. Carle, and S. Tambutte. 2000. Specific expression of BMP2/4 ortholog in biomineralizing tissues of corals and action on mouse BMP receptor. *Mar Biotechnol*, 11, 260.

Zufferey, R. et al. 1997. Multiply attenuated lentiviral vector achieves efficient gene delivery in vivo. *Nat Biotechnol*, 15(9), 871–875.

31

Polysaccharides from Seaweeds: Modification and Potential Application in Drug Delivery

Héctor J. Prado, María C. Matulewicz, Pablo R. Bonelli, and Ana L. Cukierman

CONTENTS

31.1 Introduction

Carrageenans, agarans, and alginates are the most abundant seaweed polysaccharides. All of them have been extensively employed as excipients in pharmaceutical tablet dosage forms for various decades (Bhardwaj et al., 2000; Laurienzo, 2010).

Carrageenans and agarans are obtained from red seaweeds. They are linear-chain galactans constituted by alternating 3-linked β-galactopyranose residues (unit A) and 4-linked α-galactopyranose residues (unit B). The A units always belong to the D series, whereas the B units can present D or L configuration; occasionally, the B unit appears as 3,6-anhydrogalactopyranose. The structural variability is given by the substitution of the different hydroxyl groups by sulfate esters and, to a lower extent, by pyruvic acid ketals, methyl ethers, or different types of branching. Sulfation confers negative charges to the polysaccharide at most pH values. These galactans are classified as carrageenans when the B unit belongs to the B series and as agarans when the configuration is L. As a result of the aforementioned variations, carrageenans are divided into different families such as kappa (κ), lambda (λ), beta (β), or omega (ω). Agarans, however, do not have a comparable classification to that of carrageenans; the best known member of this group is agarose formed by a regular sequence of 3-linked β-D-galactopyranose and 4-linked 3,6-anhydro-α-L-galactopyranose without any sulfate groups. Depending on what galactan they biosynthesize, seaweeds are known as carrageenophytes or agarophytes. It is important to point out that the term agar or agar-agar, known from ancient times, usually refers to gelling polysaccharides extracted from an agarophyte (Stortz and Cerezo, 2000; Estévez et al., 2003; Usov, 2011).

Carrageenans have been incorporated in tablet matrices with various drugs and other excipients to alter release profiles. They have shown to be suitable tableting excipients for controlled-release applications (Bonferoni et al., 1993, 1994, 1998; Hariharan et al., 1997; Picker, 1999a,b; Gupta et al., 2001; Bani-Jaber et al., 2005; Gursoy and Cevik, 2008; Rowe et al., 2009). Besides, formulation of tablets with potassium chloride and kappa- or iota-carrageenans creates a microenvironment for gelation occurrence, which further controls drug release (Picker, 1999b). The elastic moduli of kappa-carrageenan (KC) gels depend on the type of cation and follow the Hofmeister series: $Cs^+ > Rb^+ > K^+ \gg Na^+ > Li^+$ (Ofner and Klech-Gelotte, 2007).

Agar has been investigated as a sustained-release agent in tablets, among several other pharmaceutical applications (Boraie and Naggar, 1984; Bhardwaj et al., 2000). Agarans have been reported to act as disintegrants in tablets (Fassihi, 1989). Agar has been used in floating controlled-release tablets; the buoyancy has been in part attributed to air entrapped in the agar gel network (Desai and Bolton, 1993; Rowe et al., 2009). Agarose gels are based on a double-helix structure (Arnot et al., 1974; Haggett et al., 1997).

Alginic acid, extracted from brown seaweeds, is a linear polymer composed of 4-linked β-D-mannuronic acid residues and 4-linked α-L-guluronic acid residues, both in the pyranose form. The monomers can appear in homopolymeric blocks of consecutive mannuronic residues (M-blocks), consecutive guluronic residues (G-blocks), or alternating M- and G-residues (MG-blocks). The mannuronic to guluronic ratio varies in the different species of alginophytes. As in alginic acids, the ionic groups are carboxylic acids, and their ionization is dependent on pH. The salts of alginic acids are called alginates (sodium and calcium alginates are the most used). Alginic acid or its salts are also known as algin (Aspinall, 1985).

Alginic acid and alginates are used in tablet formulation both as binders and as disintegrating agents at concentrations of 1%–5% w/w (Shotton and Leonard, 1976;

Esezobo, 1989; Rowe et al., 2009). Alginic acid has been patented as a stabilizing agent of levosimendan in tablets (Larma and Harjula, 1999). The influence of pH and drug solubility on the release kinetics of matrix tablets of sodium alginate has been evaluated (Hodsdon et al., 1995). Therapeutically, alginic acid has been used as an antacid (Vatier et al., 1996) and in the management of gastroesophageal reflux (Stanciu and Bennett, 1974). Alginate forms gels at pH > 6 by ionotropic gelation with divalent cations as Ca^{2+}, Ba^{2+}, or Zn^{2+}; at low pH, hydration of alginic acid leads to the formation of a high-viscosity "acid gel" (Russo et al., 2007; Laurienzo, 2010). Calcium alginate gels have been described mainly by the "eggbox" model (Grant et al., 1973; Morris et al., 1978; Ofner and Klech-Gelotte, 2007), although some other possible structures have been proposed (Li et al., 2007).

An innovative alternative for matrix systems for controlled drug release involves the use of interpolyelectrolyte complexes (IPECs), particularly those based on seaweed polysaccharides. IPECs are generally insoluble complexes formed by ionic association of the repeating units (RUs) of polymers with opposite charges (Lowman, 2000). Most IPECs are hydrogels, extensively investigated for controlled release (Peppas et al., 2000; Satish et al., 2006; Laurienzo, 2010). In recent years, research interest has been directed toward physically cross-linked hydrogels in order to avoid the use of chemical cross-linking agents. Chemical cross-linkers can affect the integrity of the substances to be entrapped and they are often bi- or multifunctional toxic compounds, which have to be removed from the hydrogels before they can be applied. As mentioned earlier, cross-linking in IPECs is achieved through ionic interactions (Hennink and Van Nostrum, 2002).

Differences between gels and hydrogels should be taken into account. As polymeric networks, both might be similar from a chemical viewpoint, but they are physically different. Gels are semisolid materials comprising small amounts of solid, dispersed in relatively large amounts of liquid yet possessing more solid-like than liquid-like character. Instead, hydrogels are cross-linked networks of hydrophilic polymers. They possess the ability to absorb large amounts of water and swell while maintaining their 3D structure. Gels are polymeric networks already swollen to equilibrium, and further addition of fluids results only in dilution of the polymeric network. Although some gels are rigid enough to maintain their structure under a small stress after exceeding the yield value, gel fluidity is observed with loss of polymer structure. A hydrogel exhibits swelling in aqueous media for the same reasons that an analogous linear polymer dissolves in water to form an ordinary polymer solution. Thus, the central feature to the functioning of a hydrogel is its inherent cross-linking. Although conventional gels can also develop small levels of cross-links, as a result of a gain in energy under the influence of shear forces, they are reversible because of the involvement of weak physical forces (Gupta et al., 2001)

In general, preparation of IPECs involves mixing aqueous solutions of the two constituting polymers at a pH for which both present opposite charges. To reach certain pH values, buffer systems may be required. The interaction of both polymers usually leads to precipitation. The solid is separated from the aqueous phase by filtration or centrifugation, followed by a washing stage to remove the salts and the subsequent removal of solvent. As final steps, grinding and sieving of solid may be carried out if necessary (Prado et al., 2008b, 2009). Drug loading may be conducted during IPEC formation (de la Torre et al., 2003), by imbibition of the already formed IPEC with the drug solution (Rodríguez et al., 2003), or by solid physical mixing of the drug and the IPEC, and further tableting (Prado et al., 2008b, 2009). The latter option would allow using the IPEC as a solid excipient in order to obtain controlled-release matrix systems by the direct compression technique.

Since carrageenans, agarans, and alginates present negative charges, they can constitute the anionic components of IPECs. Besides, by appropriate chemical modification of seaweed polysaccharides, cationic derivatives can be synthesized and used as the cationic polyelectrolyte components in the formation of IPECs. Among research studies on the use of IPECs in monolithic matrix systems for controlled release of drugs, only a few have employed seaweed polysaccharides, previous to our research, and should be highlighted. They include Eudragit E (EE)–sodium alginate (Moustafine et al., 2005b, 2009), chitosan–alginate, and chitosan–carrageenan (Tapia et al., 2002, 2004).

Within this context, this chapter deals with the preparation and characterization of different IPECs based on seaweed polysaccharides and their application as monolithic matrix systems for the controlled release of drugs. The systems initially prepared and characterized were IPECs formed between EE and KC and between a cationic corn starch (MS, $DS = 0.04$) and KC. These raw materials were of commercial origin. Then, IPECs between EE and polysaccharides of the red seaweed *Polysiphonia nigrescens* (PN) were prepared (Prado et al., 2012). Finally, IPECs between cationized agaroses (CAGs) obtained by organic synthesis and the polysaccharides of PN were also prepared (Prado et al., 2011, 2012). To the best of our knowledge, IPEC CAG-PN is the first reported one completely based on seaweed polysaccharides, both in the cationic and the anionic components.

Some of the starting materials, such as EE and KC, are excipients codified in pharmacopeias. Polysaccharides from PN could be purified in the same way as commercial agars to reach a pharmacopeial quality. The cationized starch (MS) employed in this chapter is for personal care use. However, since modified starch is codified in the U.S. Pharmacopeia, it may be used for medical purposes, after being adequately processed. CAGs are new compounds and should meet all regulatory requirements applicable to other excipients. However, the fact that agar is codified and the low toxicity history of other polysaccharides cationized with the same group such as cellulose, ethylcellulose, and starch (Annon, 1988; Krentz et al., 2006; Song et al., 2008), or of IPECs formed by cationized polysaccharides (Ito et al., 1986a,b), makes their study promising.

Ibuprofen (IBF), namely, (±)-α-methyl-4-(2-methylpropyl)benzeneacetic acid, was employed as model drug for the release tests in the present study. It is a nonsteroidal anti-inflammatory agent belonging to the group of propionic acid derivatives (apparent pK_a of 5.2) and presents a plasmatic half-life of 1.8–2.0 h. As a result, it has to be administered three to six times a day, making this drug a suitable candidate for controlled-release formulations (Chiao and Robinson, 1998).

Several of the numerous factors affecting the performance of IPECs in controlled drug release are examined in this chapter for some of the investigated IPECs. For the IPEC system between EE and KC (IPEC EE-KC), three different relationships of IBF:IPEC matrix composing the tablets were evaluated. In the case of the IPEC between MS and KC (IPEC MS-KC), two IBF:IPEC relationships were tested. In the IPECs between EE and the polysaccharides of PN, two different extracts of PN, which differed mainly in their molecular weight (M_n), were employed, thus obtaining IPEC EE-PNRT1 and IPEC EE-PN702. PNRT1 was extracted at room temperature ($M_n = 7.0$ kDa) and PN702 at 70°C ($M_n = 25.1$ kDa). These IPECs were used to prepare tablets with different IBF:IPEC relationships. In the IPECs between CAG and the polysaccharides of PN (IPEC CAG-PN), the degree of substitution (DS_{EA}) of the cationic component and its molecular weight were varied (CAG19 with $DS_{EA} = 0.19$ and $M_n = 134.5$ kDa and CAG77 with $DS_{EA} = 0.77$ and $M_n = 196.6$ KDa) as well as the molecular weight of the polysaccharides of PN (PNRT1 and PN702). In this way, four different IPECs were obtained: IPEC CAG19-PNRT1, IPEC CAG77-PNRT1, IPEC CAG19-PN702, and IPEC CAG77-PN702. In the preparation of tablets, the IBF:IPEC relationship was also changed.

31.2 Experimental

31.2.1 Materials

Basic butylated methacrylate copolymer, commercialized with the trademark Eudragit® E PO, maize (*Zea mays* L.) starch modified with cationic groups marketed under the name Farmal MS 5960® (MS), and KC Gelcarin® GP911 were kindly provided by Etilfarma SA/ Evonik Degussa Argentina SA, Corn Products SA/Corn Products Int., Buenos Aires, Argentina, and Productos Destilados/FMC Biopolymer Corp., respectively. The MS is a starch modified by the manufacturer by etherification with 2-hydroxy-3-(N, N, N-trimethylammonium)propyl. It has a *DS* of 0.04 and an amylose:amylopectin ratio of 27:73.

PN was collected in Cabo Corrientes (38° 03′ S, 57° 31′ W, Mar del Plata, Province of Buenos Aires, Argentina), dried in the open air, carefully hand sorted, and identified according to the literature. A voucher specimen (BAc 46.664) was deposited in the herbarium of the Museo de Ciencias Naturales Bernardino Rivadavia (Buenos Aires, Argentina). The seaweed was milled and sequentially extracted with water at room temperature, 70°C, and 90°C (×3 at each temperature). In the present work, the first extract at room temperature (PNRT1) and the second extract at 70°C (PN702) were employed. They were the two major extracts obtained (Prado et al., 2008a).

CAGs were obtained by chemical synthesis employing Agar Bacteriological (Agar No. 1, Oxoid Ltd.) and the cationizing reagent 3-chloro-2-hydroxypropyl trimethylammonium chloride (60% w/w aqueous solution, Sigma-Aldrich, Inc.), in an alkaline aqueous media. The synthetic procedure has been described in detail elsewhere (Prado et al., 2011). During the cationization of native agarose, alkaline modification is also produced through the cyclization of L-galactose 6-sulfate units to 3,6-anhydrogalactose (LA) and elimination of the few sulfate groups present in the natural polysaccharide (elemental S composition decreased from 0.41% w/w to 0.00% w/w). Briefly, as a result of this one-pot synthetic process, a minimally anionic polysaccharide turns into a cationic one with a controlled *DS*. For the preparation of IPECs, CAG19 (*DS* determined by elemental analysis of nitrogen or DS_{EA} = 0.19, M_n = 134.5, M_w = 242.0) and CAG77 (DS_{EA} = 0.77, M_n = 196.6, M_w = 354.0) were used. The acronym CAG followed by the *DS* of the product is applied to denote the CAGs (i.e., CAG19 denotes a CAG with DS_{EA} of 0.19).

All reagents used were of analytical grade. IBF was purchased from Droguería Todofarma SA (Buenos Aires, Argentina) and met USP requirements.

31.2.2 Repeating Unit Calculation

Concentration of the polymer solutions was calculated according to the RUs of each polyelectrolyte (Figure 31.1). As a result, values of 278, 4205, and 408 Da were used for EE, MS, and KC, respectively. For CAGs, the *RU* was calculated applying Equation 31.1:

$$RU = \frac{153 + (DS_{EA} \times 152) - DS_{EA}}{DS_{EA}} \tag{31.1}$$

where
   153 is the molecular weight of the mean unit of agarose $(162 + 144)/2 = 153$
   152 is the molecular weight of the cationic substituting group
   DS_{EA}, the experimental *DS* determined by elemental analysis of nitrogen (Prado et al., 2011).
      In this way, values of 956 and 350 Da were calculated for CAG19 and CAG77, respectively.

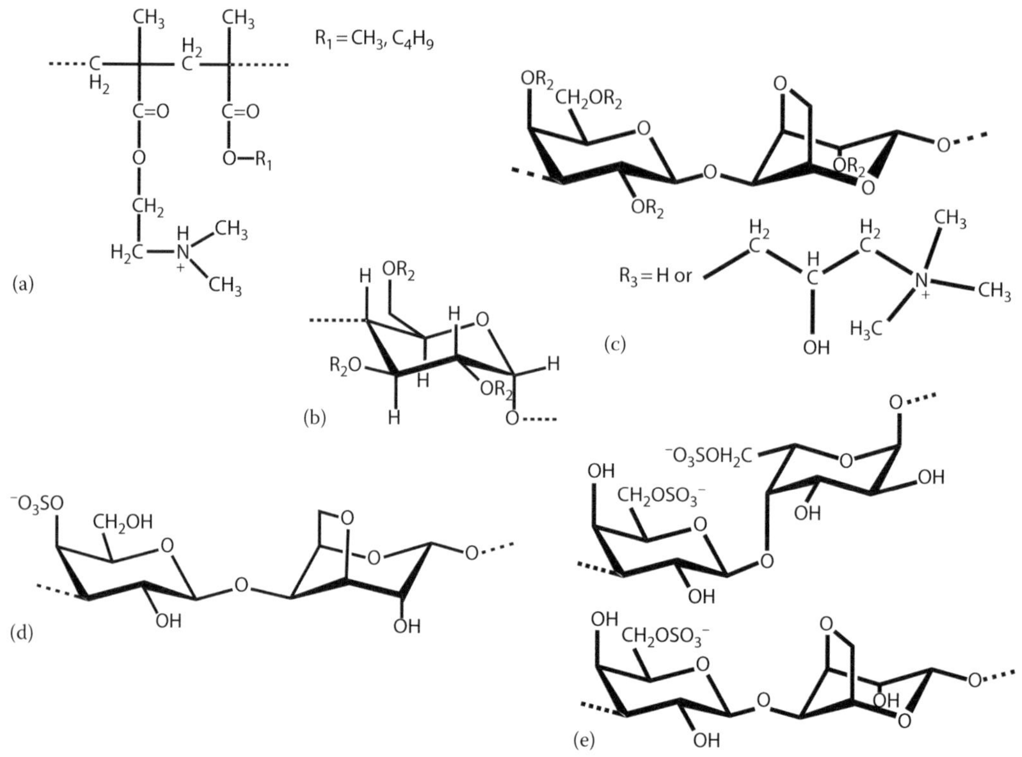

FIGURE 31.1
RUs of basic butylated methacrylate copolymer (EE) (a), cationized starch (MS) (b), cationized agaroses (CAGs) (c), kappa-carrageenan (KC) (d), and dyads present in the polysaccharides of PN (e).

For the polysaccharides of PN, the *RU*s were calculated applying Equation 31.2:

$$RU = \frac{(G \times 162) + (AG \times 144) + (SO_3Na \times 103) - SO_3Na}{SO_3Na} \tag{31.2}$$

where
   G is the relative composition of galactose (equal to 1, as the results are expressed with regard to agarose) (Prado et al., 2008a, 2012)
   162 is the molecular weight of the anhydrous galactose unit
   AG is the relative composition of anhydrogalactose
   144 is the molecular weight of the anhydrous anhydrogalactose unit
   SO_3Na is the relative sulfate composition
   103 is the molecular weight of SO_3Na

Applying Equation 31.2, values of 395 and 336 Da were calculated for PNRT1 and PN702, respectively.

31.2.3 Turbidimetry Measurements

Polymer solutions were separately dissolved in a final volume of 100 mL. IPEC EE-KC and IPEC EE-PN were prepared dissolving the components in pH 5.0 acetic acid/sodium acetate buffer. IPEC MS-KC and IPEC CAG-PN were prepared dissolving the components in distilled water. All the solutions were 0.5 mM of *RUs*, except those for IPEC MS-KC, where a concentration of 0.25 mM was employed for both components due to the high viscosity of MS.

For all the IPECs, the same procedure was applied: different volumes of the cationic polymer solution were added to volumes of the anionic polymer solution, for different values of molar mixing ratio in the range of 1:9 (0.11) to 9:1 (9.00), with a constant final volume. The molar mixing ratios are molar ratios of *RUs* of the cationic polymer to the ones of the anionic polymer. The process was repeated for all the mixtures but reversing the order of addition of the polymers. The system was allowed to stand for 1 h and then it was shaken vigorously. The relative turbidity was calculated as the ratio of the absorbance of a certain mixture at 600 nm to the maximum absorbance of each curve at 600 nm, multiplied by 100.

31.2.4 Preparation of Solid IPECs

Polymer solutions were separately dissolved in a final volume of 1 L. IPEC EE-KC and IPEC EE-PN were prepared dissolving the components in pH 5.0 acetic acid/sodium acetate buffer. IPEC MS-KC and CAG-PN were prepared dissolving the components in distilled water. All the solutions were 5 mM of RUs, except those for IPEC MS-KC, where a concentration of 2.5 mM was employed for both components.

Solutions of the corresponding cationic and anionic polymers were poured simultaneously in a vessel fitted with magnetic stirring. The agitation was maintained for 1 h and the system was allowed to stand for another hour. After isolation by centrifugation for 10 min (13,000 G), the precipitate was washed with distilled water. The centrifugation and washing process was repeated twice. IPEC suspensions were lyophilized. The dried products were sieved and the particle size fraction less than 250 μm (60 mesh Tyler) was used.

31.2.5 Elemental Analysis

The composition of IPECs and raw materials was investigated by elemental analysis, using a Carlo Erba EA 1108 CHNS elemental analyzer (Carlo Erba, Milan, Italy).

31.2.6 Fourier Transform Infrared Spectroscopy Analysis

Fourier transform infrared (FTIR) spectra of the raw materials, the IPECs, and the physical mixtures were determined with a 510P Nicolet FTIR spectrophotometer (Thermo Fisher Scientific Inc., Waltham, MA) in the range 4000–5000 cm^{-1}. The KBr transmission disk method was employed, and 32–64 scans were taken with a resolution of 2–4 cm^{-1}.

31.2.7 Scanning Electronic Microscopy Characterization

Scanning electronic microscopy (SEM) images of the surface of the raw materials, the IPECs, and the physical mixtures were obtained, without prior metallization. A Zeiss DSM 982 Gemini electronic microscope (Carl Zeiss, Oberkochen, Germany), equipped with a field emission gun (FEG) and an in-lens secondary electron detector, was employed. Acceleration voltages were 2–4 kV. The magnifications used were in the range ×200–×50,000.

31.2.8 Optical Microscopy

Particle size determination was performed using a Primo Star (Carl Zeiss, Oberkochen, Germany) microscope equipped with a graduated ocular, previously calibrated with a Zeiss graduated object micrometer. The accuracy of this system is ±1 μm. For each sample, 625 particles at random were chosen and their Feret diameters (Lieberman and Lachman, 1980) were measured. Preliminary observations of the particles' shape were also performed.

From the Feret diameter, the mean volume surface diameter (d_{vs}) was calculated; d_{vs} is defined by the following equation:

$$d_{vs} = \frac{\sum n_i X_i^3}{\sum n_i X_i^2} \tag{31.3}$$

where
  n_i is the number of particles in each size interval (sizes between 0 and 250 μm were taken, with intervals of 10 μm)
  X_i is the arithmetical mean of each size interval employed

31.2.9 Determination of Specific Surface Areas

Samples were degassed overnight at 310 K at a final pressure of 1.33×10^{-4} Pa (10^{-6} mm Hg). N_2 adsorption isotherms (77 K) were determined for IPECs by the volumetric technique. The conventional Brunauer, Emmett, and Teller (BET) procedure was applied to evaluate the specific surface areas of the samples (Rouquerol et al., 1999). A Gemini 2360 sorption instrument (Micromeritics Instrument Corp., Norcross, Georgia) was used.

31.2.10 Flowability

The flow properties of the IPECs were evaluated semiquantitatively by measuring the static angle of repose (Lieberman and Lachman, 1980; USP 30/NF 25, 2007). A funnel filled with the IPEC was maintained 2 cm above a graduated surface; the funnel was emptied and the angle of repose was calculated measuring the diameter of the cone formed.

31.2.11 Preparation of Tablets

For the swelling and erosion tests of the different IPECs, round flat tablets were prepared (total weight 100 ± 1 mg, 7.0 ± 0.1 mm of diameter) by compressing the solid IPEC or the physical mixture. A hydraulic press (W.A. Whitney, Rockford, IL) was employed. A compression force of 500 kiloponds (kp) was applied to the tablets. To determine the compactibility profile, tablets of the same characteristics were prepared by applying compression forces in the range 300–1000 kp.

For the release tests, IPEC and IBF were manually mixed and tablets were prepared (100 ± 1 mg or 150 ± 1 mg) by compressing 50 mg IPEC and 50 mg IBF or 100 mg IPEC and 50 mg IBF, respectively. In the case of IPEC EE-KC, tablets containing 75 mg IPEC and 50 mg IBF were also prepared. For comparative purposes, tablets containing 100 mg of the physical mixture and 50 mg IBF were additionally obtained. The compression force applied was 500 kp.

31.2.12 Compactibility Profile

Tablets were prepared by applying different compression forces (300–1000 kp), and their hardness was measured with an automatic durometer (Vanderkamp VK200, VanKel Technologies, Inc, NJ). The mean of three determinations is reported.

31.2.13 Degree of Swelling of Tablets

The degree of swelling (S%) of tablets of the IPECs and the physical mixtures was investigated, simulating the physiological conditions of the gastrointestinal tract (Moustafine et al., 2005a, 2006). For this purpose, tablets were placed in a preweighed basket of the dissolution tester and immersed for 2 h in 30 mL of 0.1 M HCl, then 10 mL of 0.20 M Na_3PO_4 were added to obtain a pH of 6.8 ± 0.05 and the test was allowed to continue for another 22 h. The temperature of the medium was $37.0°C \pm 0.5°C$. Measurements consisted in removing the basket from the medium, drying with filter paper, and weighing in an analytical balance. Weight differences were measured at 15 min and from 0.5 to 8 h every 30 min; an equilibrium value of swelling was determined after 24 h, as evaluated by further determinations.

The S% at each time was calculated by means of the following equation:

$$S\% = \frac{m_2 - m_1}{m_1} \times 100 \tag{31.4}$$

where
   m_1 is the initial weight of the tablet (dry)
   m_2 is the weight of the swollen tablet at different times

The results reported are the mean of three determinations.

31.2.14 Degree of Erosion of Tablets

The degree of erosion (E%) of the IPECs and the corresponding physical mixtures was determined by lyophilizing the tablets after reaching the equilibrium swelling values (24 h) and was calculated by

$$E\% = \frac{m_1 - m_3}{m_1} \times 100 \tag{31.5}$$

where
   m_1 is the weight of the initial (dry) tablet
   m_3 is the weight of the lyophilized tablet after erosion

The reported results are the mean of three determinations.

31.2.15 Ibuprofen Release Tests

The release profile of IBF was determined employing a dissolution equipment (Alycar Instruments, Argentina) that meets USP requirements for Apparatus 1 (basket). A rotating speed of 100 rpm was used and the temperature of the medium was $37.0°C \pm 0.5°C$. The dissolution medium employed was 750 mL of 0.1 M HCl for the first 2 h, then 250 mL of 0.20 M Na_3PO_4 solution were added to reach a pH of 6.8 ± 0.05 (if necessary, pH was rapidly adjusted with 2 M HCl or 2 M NaOH); the test was allowed to continue for six more hours (total release time evaluated 8 h) (Moustafine et al., 2005a, 2006; USP 30/NF 25, 2007). Tablets containing 50 mg IPEC and 50 mg IBF, 100 mg IPEC and 50 mg IBF, and 100 mg of physical mixtures and 50 mg IBF were tested. In the case of IPEC EE-KC, tablets containing 75 mg IPEC and 50 mg IBF were also evaluated.

Aliquots of 3 mL were taken every 30 min and were filtered immediately through 0.45 μm PVDF membranes. The reduction of volume was taken into account for the calculations. The amount of IBF released was determined spectrophotometrically at 221 nm (Cary 1E, Varian Inc., Palo Alto, CA). The results reported for each tablet formulation are the mean of three determinations. Previous studies indicated that IPECs or physical mixtures did not interfere with the determination of the model drug.

31.3 Results and Discussion

31.3.1 Preparation and Characterization of the Different IPEC Systems

Figure 31.1 shows the structures of the cationic and anionic components employed for IPEC formation. Among the cationic components, only EE is a synthetic polymer, whereas MS and CAG are natural polysaccharides modified with 2-hydroxy-3-(N,N,N-trimethylammonium)propyl groups. Besides, among all the cationic components employed, EE is the only one that presents tertiary amino groups whose protonation depends on the pH. According to the manufacturer, EE is soluble in acidic medium up to pH 6.0 due to the hydration of protonated dimethylamine groups. As a result, IPECs in which EE intervened as cationic components were independently prepared dissolving both polymer solutions in acetic acid/sodium acetate buffer of pH 5.0. More acidic pH were avoided in order to protect KC, PNRT1, and PN702 from eventual degradations. Unlike EE, MS and CAG possess quaternary ammonium groups that remain cationic in the whole range of pH. Due to the difficulty in achieving dissolution in the case of MS, IPEC MS-KC was prepared by heating both components at 80°C for 20 min and more diluted starting solutions were employed (2.5 mM instead of 5.0 mM).

The two CAGs (CAG19 and CAG77) employed in this work differ mainly in their DS (0.19 and 0.77, respectively) (Prado et al., 2011). The structure of MS presented in Figure 31.1b corresponds to cationized amylose: linear chains of α-1,4 glucose units, cationized or not. Besides, MS is also composed by cationized amylopectin (branched polysaccharide), formed by α-(1→4) and α-(1→6) glucose units, cationized or not.

In Figure 31.1, the structures of the anionic polysaccharides employed, KC, and the main dyads in the agarans of PN are also shown. The negative charge of the sulfate groups in KC and PN is also independent of pH. The polysaccharides of PN employed presented different molecular weights (PNRT1 $M_n = 7.0$ KDa and PN702 $M_n = 25.1$ KDa) (Prado et al., 2008a).

The IPECs are labeled by using the word IPEC, followed by the name of the cationic and the anionic components; both components are separated by a hyphen.

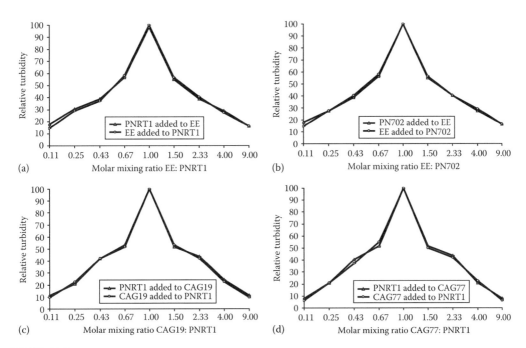

FIGURE 31.2
Relative turbidity of different IPEC systems as a function of the molar mixing ratio: IPEC EE-PNRT1 (a), IPEC EE-PN702 (b), IPEC CAG19-PNRT1 (c), and IPEC CAG77-PNRT1 (d).

31.3.2 Turbidimetry Results

IPEC formation was initially examined by turbidity measurements. Figure 31.2 shows, as an example, the results corresponding to IPEC EE-PNRT1, IPEC EE-PN702, IPEC CAG19-PNRT1, and IPEC CAG77-PNRT1. Similar curves were obtained for the other IPECs. As may be appreciated in Figure 31.2, maximum turbidity was achieved for a molar ratio of mixture of 1. Likewise, the results show that when the experiments were performed inverting the order of addition of the polymer solutions, the curves were similar, indicating that IPEC composition is independent of the mixing order.

31.3.3 Elemental Analysis

In order to confirm the stoichiometry of each component in the different solid IPECs, elemental analysis was performed. Table 31.1 shows experimental values and those calculated considering a 1:1 interaction of the RUs. The experimental N:S molar ratio is also presented. A good correlation between experimental and calculated values was found. A slight increase in the N:S molar ratio above the value expected (equal to 1) was detected for the IPECs containing polysaccharides from PN as the anionic components. This may be attributed to the presence of small quantities of seaweed proteins as impurities in the PN extracts. Elemental analyses of PNRT1 and PN702 indicated N contents of 0.89% w/w and 1.35% w/w, respectively. No elemental S was found in EE, MS, and CAG. Accordingly, all the sulfur in the IPECs arises from the anionic components (KC PNRT1 or PN702). On the other hand, no elemental N was found in KC; in this case, all the N content in IPEC EE-KC and MS-KC arises from the cationic polyelectrolytes, EE and MS, respectively.

TABLE 31.1

Elemental Analyses of the IPECs

IPEC	Experimental Value (% w/w)				Calculated Value (% w/w)				Experimental N:S
	C	H	N	S	C	H	N	S	Molar Ratio
EE-KC	46.07	6.66	1.98	4.77	47.92	6.60	2.11	4.83	0.95
MS-KC	43.74	6.24	0.32	0.72	44.31	6.20	0.31	0.70	1.02
EE-PNRT1	47.69	6.88	2.33	4.88	47.25	6.76	2.15	4.92	1.16
EE-PN702	47.46	6.85	2.63	5.45	47.63	6.80	2.36	5.41	1.10
CAG19-PNRT1	44.99	6.15	1.19	2.46	45.28	6.08	1.08	2.48	1.11
CAG77-PNRT1	43.06	6.26	2.27	4.64	43.56	6.22	2.04	4.66	1.12
CAG19-PN702	45.40	6.18	1.26	2.64	45.28	6.07	1.13	2.60	1.09
CAG77-PN702	43.18	6.21	2.52	5.14	43.57	6.21	2.23	5.10	1.12

31.3.4 Infrared Spectroscopy Results

In the FTIR spectra of IPEC EE-PNRT1 (Figure 31.3a) and IPEC EE-PN702, the disappearance of the absorption bands at 2770 and 2824 cm^{-1} of EE was detected. Those signals were present in the spectra of the raw materials and the physical mixtures (obtained by dry mixing the powders of the raw materials). This is due to the formation of the corresponding quaternary ammonium. Also, the appearance of the band at 2550 cm^{-1} was observed and assigned to the interaction of the quaternary ammonium with the polyelectrolyte of opposite charge (Moustafine et al., 2005a,b, 2006). On the other hand, the band at 822 cm^{-1} of PNRT1 and PN702 assigned to the sulfate group in the primary hydroxyl (C-6) of the galactose was shifted to 809 and 811 cm^{-1}, respectively, in the IPECs. There were differences in the fingerprint region between the spectra of the IPEC EE-PN and the corresponding components and physical mixtures.

Figure 31.3b shows the spectra of IPECs based on CAG and PNRT1 and individual polymer components. The band at 822 cm^{-1} (sulfate on C-6) of PNRT1 and PN702 was not observed in IPEC CAG19-PNRT1 and IPEC CAG19-PN702, whereas a weak band shift to 812 cm^{-1} was found in IPEC CAG77-PNRT1 and IPEC CAG77-PN702. The band at 1482 cm^{-1} (C–N bond stretching) of the cationic substituent of CAG shifted to 1469–1473 cm^{-1} in the IPECs. For the physical mixtures, the bands at 822 and 1482 cm^{-1} remained in the same position as in the raw materials. The IPECs also showed differences in the fingerprint regions with regard to the respective physical mixtures.

Similarly to the results for the IPEC EE-PN, in the FTIR spectra of IPEC EE-KC, a considerable reduction of the absorption bands at 2770 and 2824 cm^{-1}, corresponding to the non-ionized dimethylamino groups in EE spectrum, was detected. It indicates the formation of an ammonium salt. A wide and weak band at 2550 cm^{-1} was also detected in the IPEC spectra. There were also differences in the fingerprint region between the spectra of the IPEC EE-KC and the corresponding components and physical mixtures.

The FTIR spectra of the MS-KC physical mixture and of the IPEC were very similar to those corresponding to MS (not shown). This result is consistent with the composition of the physical mixture and the IPEC as they are constituted by 91% w/w of MS. The important difference in the proportion of the components, expressed as % w/w, is due to the different degrees of substitution of the IPEC constituents. KC has a *DS* of 0.5, and MS has a *DS* of 0.04. As a result, for a molar ratio of 1, IPEC MS-KC is mostly composed by MS. The spectrum of this IPEC, however, presented small differences when compared with

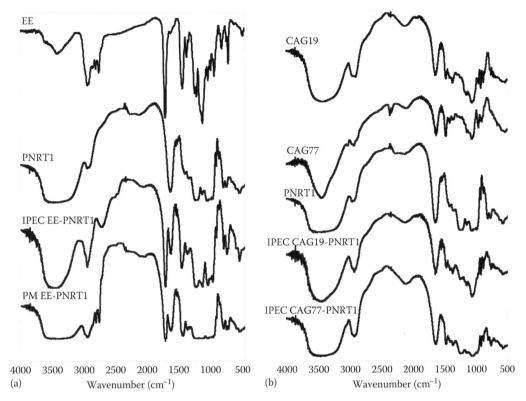

FIGURE 31.3
Fourier transform infrared spectra of EE, PNRT1, IPEC EE-PNRT1, and the physical mixtures PM EE-PNRT1 (a), CAGs CAG19 (DS_{EA} = 0.19), CAG77 (DS_{EA} = 0.77), PNRT1, IPEC CAG19-PNRT1, and IPEC CAG77-PNRT1 (b).

that corresponding to the physical mixture. The band at 850 cm^{-1} assigned to the sulfate group of KC (Anderson et al., 1968) shifted to 835 cm^{-1}, while the band at 1491 cm^{-1} assigned to the C–N bond of MS (Zhang et al., 2007) shifted to 1480 cm^{-1}. These displacements could be due to ionic interactions between the sulfate groups and the quaternary ammonium groups in the IPEC. There were also very small differences in the fingerprint region.

31.3.5 Scanning Electronic Microscopy Characterization

SEM was used for the characterization of raw materials, physical mixtures, and IPEC particles in solid state, providing information of shape, particle size, surface, and presence of pores. Some SEM images are displayed in Figure 31.4. For the physical mixtures, they indicated that the individual particles of the components retain its original characteristics in these mixtures. For example, EE appeared as particles of irregular shape, whereas PN presented fibrillar structures, of larger size; in the physical mixture PM EE-KC, KC particles surrounded by many EE particles may be easily identified. In contrast, all the IPECs studied presented very different characteristics when compared with the raw materials; these characteristics were inherent to each IPEC in particular.

IPEC EE-KC presented irregular-shaped particles of bigger size than its raw materials. At higher magnifications, a 3D reticular structure was revealed, showing pore diameters in the range 100–300 nm that resembles the structure of a "sponge" (Figure 31.4a and b).

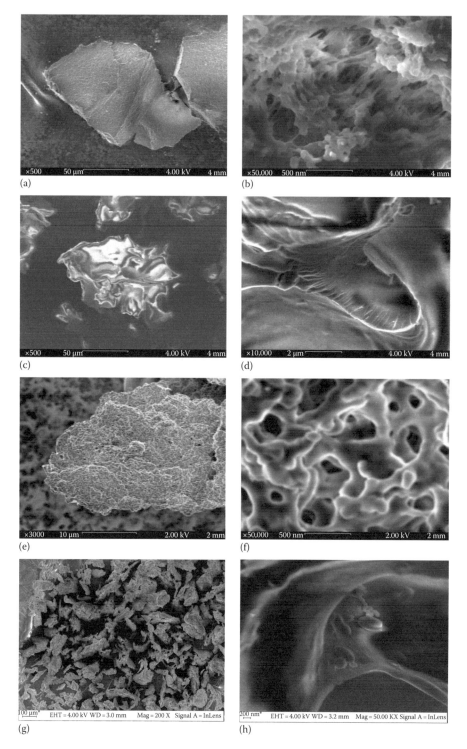

FIGURE 31.4
Scanning electron micrographs of IPEC EE-KC ×500 (a), ×50,000 (b), IPEC MS-KC ×500 (c), ×10,000 (d), IPEC EE-PN702 ×3,000 (e), ×50,000 (f), IPEC CAG19-PNRT1 ×200 (g), and IPEC CAG77-PN702 ×50,000 (h).

The appearance of MS particles was very similar to the native starch (not shown); this indicates that cationization of the starch was carried out by the manufacturer employing a heterogeneous-phase method that preserves the structure of granules. IPEC MS-KC (Figure 31.4c and d) presented irregular smooth particles, different to the IPEC EE-KC.

The samples of PNRT1 and PN702 presented fibrous characteristics, very similar to each other. The IPECs formed with these agarans and EE:IPEC EE-PNRT1 and IPEC EE-PN702 were in turn very similar to each other, presenting irregular shapes with a reticular 3D structure (similar to IPEC EE-KC). However, in this case, pore diameters were in the range 250–600 nm (Figure 31.4e and f).

Finally, the particles of the four IPEC CAG-PN (Figure 31.4g and h) showed shapes of irregular characteristics, with smooth surfaces. No differences were identified among the IPEC CAG-PN. Images of CAG19 and CAG77 have been earlier published elsewhere (Prado et al., 2011).

From the images, it can be inferred that IPECs based on EE (IPEC EE-KC and EE-PN) presented porous structures, whereas IPEC MS-KC and IPEC CAG-PN were nonporous (Prado et al., 2008b, 2009). Unfortunately, no SEM results have been reported in the literature for other IPEC systems in order to perform comparisons.

31.3.6 Optical Microscopy Results

This technique was applied in order to determine the Feret diameter of particles and to calculate, from this parameter, the mean volume surface diameter (d_{vs}) of each IPEC (Lieberman and Lachman, 1980). The results are presented in Table 31.2. Optical microscopy was also useful to perform preliminary observations on the shape of the particles. These observations were in agreement with those obtained by SEM.

31.3.7 Specific Surface Area

In Table 31.2, values of BET surface area of the different IPECs are reported. The theoretical areas of nonporous monodispersed spheres of the same diameter to that determined for each sample (considering a density of 1 g cm^{-3}) (Lieberman and Lachman, 1980) are included in the last column of the table, for comparative purposes. The BET area of IPEC EE-KC (3.012 m^2 g^{-1}) was 2 orders of magnitude higher than the theoretical one for a sample with a volume surface diameter (d_{vs}) of 171 μm. This result points to a porous structure, in agreement with SEM observations. Similar considerations apply to the BET areas of IPEC

TABLE 31.2

Mean Volume Surface Diameter (d_{vs}), BET Area, and Theoretical Area for the IPECs

IPEC	d_{vs} (μm)	BET Area (m^2 g^{-1})	Theoretical Area (m^2 g^{-1})
EE-KC	171	3.012	0.035
MS-KC	91	0.058	0.066
EE-PNRT1	86	0.985	0.070
EE-PN702	89	0.990	0.067
CAG19-PNRT1	189	0.050	0.032
CAG77-PNRT1	195	0.054	0.031
CAG19-PN702	190	0.045	0.032
CAG77-PN702	178	0.048	0.034

TABLE 31.3

Static Angles of Repose for IPECs

IPEC	Static Angle of Repose (°)	Flow Properties
EE-KC	27	Excellent
MS-KC	38	Fair—aid not needed
EE-PNRT1	31	Good
EE-PN702	32	Good
CAG19-PNRT1	37	Fair—aid not needed
CAG77-PNRT1	38	Fair—aid not needed
CAG19-PN702	37	Fair—aid not needed
CAG77-PN702	37	Fair—aid not needed

EE-PNRT1 and IPEC EE-PN702 (0.985 and 0.990 $m^2\ g^{-1}$), being one order of magnitude higher than the theoretical values for samples with d_{vs} of 86 and 89 μm, respectively. IPEC MS-KC and the four IPEC CAG-PN presented BET areas consistent with theoretical values and with SEM observations, where they appeared as nonporous materials.

31.3.8 Static Angle of Repose Results

The static angles of repose for each IPEC are shown in Table 31.3. Flow properties (USP 30/NF 25, 2007) are also included in the same table. IPEC EE-KC was the sample that presented the best flow properties among those evaluated in this chapter. It was followed in decreasing sequence by IPEC EE-PN, IPEC MS-KC, and IPEC CAG-PN. There was almost no difference between the two IPECs obtained from EE and PN, or among the four IPEC CAG-PN. Although in all cases the flowability of the IPECs could allow its use for industrial purposes, it is probable that flowability could be limited by the irregular shape of IPEC particles. This could be improved by applying spray drying after IPEC formation by the conventional method, since this method is known to lead to more spherical particles with better flow properties (Singh and Naini, 2007).

31.3.9 Compactibility Profiles

In Figure 31.5, the compactibility profiles of IPECs are shown. The mean of three determinations is reported with a confidence interval of 95%. As may be observed in the figure, the hardness follows the order IPEC MS-KC > IPEC CAG-PN > IPEC EE-PN > IPEC EE-KC. The differences between IPEC EE-PN (IPEC EE-PNRT1 and IPEC EE-PN702) were not important. In the same way, the four IPEC CAG-PN (IPEC CAG19-PNRT1, IPEC CAG77-PNRT1, IPEC CAG19-PN702, and IPEC CAG77-PN702) presented similar compactibility profiles. The slopes of the curves for all the IPECs tested were alike. In general, all the IPECs exhibited good compactibility properties, achieving appropriate hardness values when low compression forces were applied.

31.3.10 Degree of Swelling and Erosion of Tablets

The swelling profile of the different IPEC systems is illustrated in Figure 31.6. For IPEC EE-KC (Figure 31.6a), swelling reached a value of 103% after 1.5 h in the first stage of the experiment (acid medium of pH 1.0). At time = 2 h, the buffer stage started (pH 6.8) and

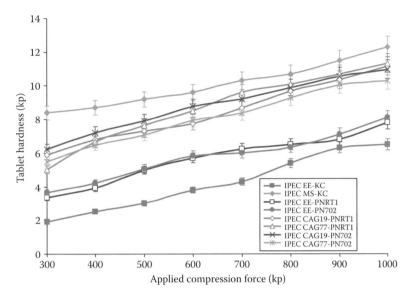

FIGURE 31.5
Compactibility profiles of tablets containing 100 mg of IPECs.

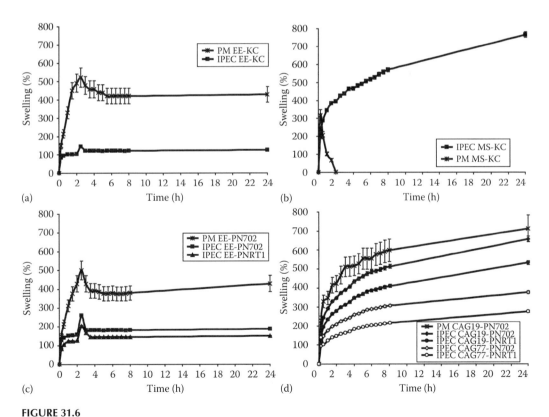

FIGURE 31.6
Swelling profiles of tablets containing 100 mg of IPECs or 100 mg of physical mixtures: (a) EE-KC, (b) MS-KC, (c) EE-PN, and (d) CAG-PN.

swelling increased to a maximum of 145% half an hour later. This behavior could be due to the gradual neutralization of the protonated dimethylamino groups, causing reduction in the interaction between both polymers and subsequent relaxation of the matrix. Moreover, these free dimethylamino groups could intervene as acceptors in hydrogen bond with the hydroxyl groups of KC, and the rearrangement would lead to the equilibrium swelling value of 125% at time = 24 h. The physical mixture PM EE-KC presented higher values of swelling than IPEC EE-KC (Figure 31.6a). The maximum achieved in the acid stage was 450%, and swelling continued growing during the buffer stage up to a value of 522% at time = 2.5 h; at equilibrium (time = 24 h), swelling was 429%. This behavior could be attributed to negligible interactions between both polymers, acting independently in the physical mixture. Final erosion of IPEC EE-KC tablets and of the physical mixture tablets was 5.1% and 7.3%, respectively.

During the swelling test of IPEC MS-KC (Figure 31.6b), tablets retained their integrity in agreement with a hydrogel structure. In the first stage of the experiment (acid medium), a rapid swelling was detected during the first hour. Then, swelling increased more slowly and reached a value of 380% at the end of that stage. At time = 2 h, the buffer stage began and the *S*% continuously increased, at a rate similar to that corresponding to the two last determinations of the acid stage. An equilibrium value of swelling of 742% was observed at time = 24 h. The erosion of tablets of IPEC MS-KC was 4.2%. The *DS* of the two polymers used to prepare the IPEC is very different: MS presents a *DS* of 0.04 (confirmed by elemental analysis), which means that 1 of 25 units of glucose is modified with a cationic group. KC, however, has a *DS* of 0.5 (1 of 2 units of galactose is substituted with a sulfate group). This could allow MS to eventually form long hydrophilic loops of glucose protected from disentanglement by means of the physical cross-linking with KC. The described structure is consistent with the high swelling observed. The association between stronger mismatching of the charge distances of the components and higher degrees of swelling has been previously reported for other IPECs (Philipp et al., 1989; Dautzenberg et al., 1994). Besides, the similar rate of swelling in the acid and buffer stages could be attributed to the fact that both polymers involved in the IPEC present ionic groups (quaternary ammonium and sulfate) whose ionization is pH independent.

The swelling/erosion behavior of the MS-KC physical mixture tablets was completely different. Swelling reached a maximum of 317% at time = 0.5 h. Extensive turbidity of the medium observed since the initial minutes of the experiments provided evidence of erosion. At time = 2 h, the tablet was completely disintegrated. Starch constitutes an important class of tablet disintegrant (Zhang et al., 2007). Moreover, in 0.1 M hydrochloric acid solution, both polysaccharides acting independently are also known to suffer dissolution and a certain degree of hydrolysis in the case of KC (Capron et al., 1996). Native starches poor in amylose reportedly reach a higher *S*% (Li and Yeh, 2001).

IPEC EE-PNRT1 and IPEC EE-PN702 presented swelling profiles that resembled those of IPEC EE-KC, reaching values of 126% and 158%, respectively, at the end of the acid stage (2 h) (Figure 31.6c). When the pH was changed to pH 6.8 (buffer stage), swelling values sharply rose to 204% and 261%, respectively. Equilibrium values of 150% and 188% were determined after 24 h, at the end of the buffer stage. An increase in the molecular weight of the anionic component was related to a higher experimental swelling value. The sharp increase in swelling followed by a reduction, after an increase of the pH, seems to be a typical behavior of IPECs composed of EE as the cationic component; this is the case of IPEC EE100–Eudragit L100 (Moustafine et al., 2005a, 2006), IPEC EE–alginate (Moustafine et al., 2009), and the aforementioned IPEC EE-KC (Prado et al., 2008b).

The physical mixture PM EE-PN exhibited higher values of swelling than the corresponding IPEC, due to similar considerations to those discussed in the case of the EE-KC system. The erosion after 24 h for IPEC EE-PN702, IPEC EE-PNRT1, and the physical mixture was 2.7%, 3.4%, and 6.7%, respectively.

IPEC CAG-PN presented a similar behavior to IPEC MS-KC. It is consistent with the fact that both IPECs shared the same cationic and anionic groups (2-hidroxy-3-(N,N,N-trimethylammonium)propyl and sulfate, respectively). IPEC CAG-PN showed a more gradual increase in swelling after pH change (Figure 31.6d), likely because the ionization of their ionic groups was independent of the pH. Swelling values followed the order IPEC CAG19-PN702 > IPEC CAG19-PNRT1 > IPEC CAG77-PN702 > IPEC CAG77-PNRT1, reaching maximum values of 347%, 278%, 208%, and 146% for the acid stage, with equilibrium values (24 h) of 658%, 532%, 377%, and 276% in the buffer stage at pH 6.8, respectively. An increase in swelling was related to an increase in the molecular weight of the anionic component, and to a decrease in the *DS* of the cationic component. For IPEC chitosan—Eudragit L100 and IPEC chitosan—Eudragit L100-55, a higher swelling has been reported when chitosan of higher molecular weight was employed (Moustafine et al., 2008).

Besides, physical mixture PM CAG19-PN702 showed a gradual increase in swelling, with a value of 423% at the end of the acid stage and of 713% after 24 h.

The values of erosion after 24 h for the different IPECs were as follows: 2.2% for IPEC CAG19-PN702, 2.7% for IPEC CAG19-PNRT1, 2.4% for IPEC CAG77-PN702, 3.5% for IPEC CAG77-PNRT1, and 6.7% for the physical mixture PM CAG19-PN702. From the values of erosion for all the investigated IPECs, it can be concluded that this phenomenon is less important than swelling, at least, for the experimental conditions employed in the present study.

31.3.11 Ibuprofen Release Profiles

IBF release profiles from tablets containing 50 or 100 mg of the different IPECs and 50 mg of IBF are shown in Figure 31.7. In the case of IPEC EE-KC, results of a formulation with 75 mg IPEC and 50 mg IBF are also presented. For comparative purposes, drug release profiles of tablets containing the physical mixtures and IBF are also shown in the same figure.

The profiles in the Figure 31.7a through d show two distinguished regions: acid stage and buffer stage. Comparison of the release values during the first 30 min (first experimental point) with those corresponding to equivalent successive intervals allowed to detect the presence or the lack of a "burst release" effect (Huang and Brazel, 2001) for each IPEC system; this effect is difficult to predict a priori. IPECs based on EE, IPEC EE-KC and IPEC EE-PN, presented a small degree of burst release (Prado et al., 2008b). On the contrary, IPEC MS-KC and IPEC CAG-PN showed release values in the first interval similar to those in the next ones, not exhibiting that effect. Burst release is frequently considered as undesirable, but it can be deleterious or beneficial, depending on the therapeutic goal. On the other hand, it is a fact inherently undesirable, if the burst release varies from one therapeutic unit to another (in the case of IPEC EE-KC and IPEC EE-PN, the magnitude of this effect was constant). Among the many causes that have been attributed to burst release, the more likely one for the monolithic hydrophilic matrices formed by the IPECs studied in this chapter is the fact that some drug may be trapped on the surface of the matrix during compression, especially in the case of high drug loads such as those used herein. When the dissolution medium contacts the tablet, this fraction is released immediately. The burst release would then occur in the IPECs that are less efficient in quickly generating a layer of hydrogel, capable of controlling the release of the drug on the surface. Nevertheless,

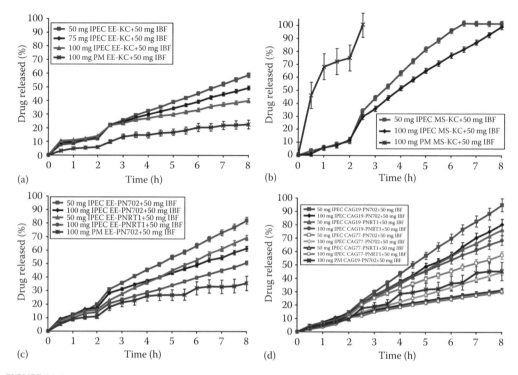

FIGURE 31.7
Release of IBF from tablets containing 50, 75, or 100 mg of IPECs (plus 50 mg IBF), or 100 mg of the physical mixtures (plus 50 mg IBF): (a) EE-KC, (b) MS-KC, (c) EE-PN, and (d) CAG-PN.

the existence of heterogeneity in the IPEC matrix that gives rise to different microdomains should not be neglected (Huang and Brazel, 2001).

During the acid stage, release values were low for the systems based on IPEC EE-KC (12.0%–13.9%), IPEC MS-KC (10.9%–12.9%), IPEC EE-PN (11.0%–20.0%), and IPEC CAG-PN (11.0%–14.7%). This could be mainly attributed to the action of the matrix and to the low solubility of IBF in the acid medium. The sharp change in pH from the acid to the buffer stage generated a relative increase in the amount of drug released for most IPEC systems. The pH change affected release not only because of variations in matrix swelling (in the case of IPEC EE-KC and EE-PN) but also because the carboxylic group of IBF ionized in the buffer stage, turning the drug more soluble in that condition. The solubility of IBF at pH 1.0 is 0.027 mg mL^{-1} and it increases to 10.1 mg mL^{-1} at pH 7.0, namely, 374 times higher (Higgins et al., 2001).

The IPEC systems examined in this chapter led to obtain a variety of release profiles with near zero-order kinetics in the buffer stage. The higher release was obtained for IPEC MS-KC; the formulation with 50 mg of this IPEC achieved a release of 100% after 6 h, and the formulation with 100 mg achieved complete release after 8 h (Figure 31.7b). For IPEC EE-KC, release values of 40.1%, 49.4%, and 58.7% were obtained after 8 h of test, employing 100, 75, and 50 mg of IPEC in the formulation, respectively. For IPEC EE-PN, the molecular weight of the anionic component (7.0 kDa for PNRT1 and 25.1 kDa for PN702) and the amount of the IPEC in the tablets formulation were varied. 100 mg IPEC EE-PNRT1 and 50 mg IPEC EE-PNRT1 formulations (plus 50 mg IBF in each case) achieved releases of 50.7% and 69.4%, respectively, after 8 h of test (Figure 31.7c).

Instead, 100 mg EE-PN702 and 50 mg EE-PN702 formulations attained values of 61.4% and 82.0%, respectively, for the same period. It follows that increasing the molecular weight of the anionic component increased drug release. For IPEC CAG-PN, in addition to the variation in the molecular weight of the anionic component (PN) and the amount of IPEC in the tablets, the *DS* of the cationic component (CAG) was also modified. In this way, final release values ranging from 30.5% for 100 mg IPEC CAG77-PNRT1 formulation to 95.0% for 50 mg IPEC CAG19-PN702 formulation were achieved (Figure 31.7d). With regard to the variation in the molecular weight of PN, similar conclusions as for the IPEC EE-PN were attained. On the other hand, the increase in the *DS* of CAG (from 0.19 in CAG19 to 0.77 in CAG77) decreased IBF release, keeping other conditions constant. For the two CAGs, the molecular weight (M_n) was varied from 134.5 KDa in CAG19 to 196.6 KDa in CAG77. Accordingly, in this case, the influence of the lower *DS* of CAG19 would have been more important than its lower molecular weight, as the cationic component of lower molecular weight allowed for a quicker release. It should be taken into account that unlike PNs, which differ mainly in their molecular weight, CAG19, of lower molecular weight, is actually composed of longer chains of polysaccharide than CAG77, which was further degraded by the more drastic conditions of its substitution reaction, as determined by light scattering measurements. The higher molecular weight of CAG77 is due to the higher number of substituting groups in the polysaccharide backbone. A higher release of IPEC Eudragit L100–chitosan and IPEC Eudragit L100-55–chitosan with the increase in the molecular weight of chitosan has also been reported (Moustafine et al., 2008).

When comparing the swelling of the matrix and drug release profiles for a given IPEC, it was found that the systems showing higher swelling were the ones that released the model drug faster. In this way, IPEC MS-KC reached the higher swelling and drug release. For IPEC EE-PN, the IPEC EE-PN702 presented higher swelling and drug release than IPEC EE-PNRT1. The swelling order for IPEC CAG-PN (IPEC CAG19-PN702 > IPEC CAG19-PNRT1 > IPEC CAG77-PN702 > IPEC CAG77-PNRT1) agreed with that found for the drug release. This trend, of practical utility, is in general satisfied when comparing IPEC systems consisting of the same or similar components. However, some exceptions may be pointed out. Tablets with 50 mg IPEC EE-KC plus 50 mg IBF that presented swelling values of 122% after 8 h released 40.1% of the drug in the same period, whereas tablets with 50 mg IPEC CAG77-PNRT1 plus 50 mg IBF with swelling values of 215% after 8 h released only 30.5% of the drug. Since the drug release process, in addition to matrix swelling, involves other phenomena that can be the rate-limiting step of the global process, care in predicting drug release from swelling data of IPECs composed by polymers of different structure should be taken. Thus, the swelling test should be considered only as a first approach to the dissolution test in the evaluation of new IPECs.

The release from tablets composed of the physical mixtures PM EE-KC, PM EE-PN, and PM CAG-PN plus IBF was slower than that observed from the respective IPECs, despite their higher swelling. Other results for physical mixtures of pectin—chitosan and pectin—arabic gum also showed to release a model drug (chlorpromazine) slower than the corresponding IPECs (Meshali and Gabr, 1993). However, in the case of the physical mixtures PM MS-KC, a faster release in the physical mixture than in the IPEC was found, possibly because the starch in the physical mixture acted as tablet disintegrant exposing IBF to rapid dissolution (Adebayo et al., 2008; Prado et al., 2009). In all cases the physical mixtures presented widely dispersed results among replicates, as reflected in the amplitude of the error bars corresponding to a confidence level of 95% in the figures of the release profiles (Figure 31.7).

Because sink conditions were not attained in the acid stage due to the low solubility of IBF, only experimental release data corresponding to the buffer stage were fitted to a mathematical model (Model I) based on previously reported proposals (Peppas, 1985; Siepmann and Peppas, 2001). Accordingly, experimental data corresponding to fractions of drug released ≤ 60% were employed. Model I equation is as follows:

$$\frac{M_t}{M_\infty} = k(t - t')^n + \alpha \tag{31.6}$$

where

M_t/M_∞ is the fraction of drug released at time t

k is the apparent release constant that takes into account the geometrical and structural characteristics of the drug release system

t is the time elapsed since the beginning of the release test

t' is the duration of the acid stage ($t' = 2$ h)

n is the release exponent

α is a term that considers the amount of drug released in the acid stage (0–2 h) (Huang and Brazel, 2001)

In Figure 31.8, the comparison between experimental data and Model I predictions is presented, for the different IPEC systems. The model characteristic parameters, evaluated

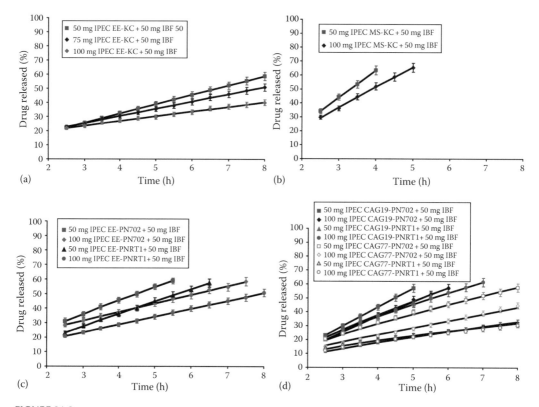

FIGURE 31.8
Comparison between experimental IBF release profiles from the different IPEC formulations for the buffer stage (dots) and those predicted by Model I (solid lines). (a) IPEC EE-KC, (b) IPEC MS-KC, (c) IPECs EE-PN, and (d) IPECs CAG-PN.

TABLE 31.4

Model Characteristic Parameters of Model I (IPECs and Physical Mixtures)

IPEC	IPEC:IBF (mg:mg)[a]	$k\,(h^{-n})$	N	α	R^2
EE-KC	50:50	6.77	0.99	18.85	1.000
	75:50	5.24	0.99	20.80	0.996
	100:50	3.41	0.99	20.14	0.996
MS-KC	50:50	19.98	0.98	24.01	0.996
	100:50	16.01	0.93	20.93	0.999
EE-PNRT1	50:50	9.15	0.96	18.40	0.999
	100:50	5.19	1.02	18.14	1.000
EE-PN702	50:50	10.36	0.93	25.57	0.999
	100:50	5.96	1.00	25.43	0.999
CAG19-PN702	50:50	13.64	1.00	16.29	1.000
	100:50	12.93	0.87	14.27	0.998
CAG19-PNRT1	50:50	13.11	0.89	12.50	0.994
	100:50	12.80	0.81	14.20	0.998
CAG77-PN702	50:50	9.50	0.85	14.19	0.999
	100:50	5.51	0.95	12.94	0.998
CAG77-PNRT1	50:50	5.60	0.81	9.78	0.991
	100:50	5.30	0.86	8.29	0.991
Physical Mixture	**PM:IBF (mg:mg)[a]**	$k\,(h^{-n})$	N	α	R^2
EE-KC	100:50	5.84	0.57	6.66	0.970
MS-KC[b]	100:50	—	—	—	—
EE-PN702	100:50	8.18	0.55	12.81	0.979
CAG19-PN702	100:50	6.79	0.88	13.46	0.969

[a] Weight ratio between IPEC (or physical mixture) and IBF in the tablet.
[b] Model characteristic parameters for both models could not be determined as tablet disintegrated and completely released IBF before the beginning of the buffer stage.

by nonlinear regression analysis of the results corresponding to the buffer stage, are shown in Table 31.4. As can be inferred from R^2 values (≥ 0.991), the model appropriately describes the experimental data. For cylindrical geometry, as is the case of the tablets examined in this chapter, a release exponent (n) of 0.45 points to Fickian diffusion transport, whereas values of n between 0.45 and 0.89 suggest non-Fickian transport. In turn, values of n close to 0.89 indicate that the system releases the drug with zero-order kinetics (Case II transport) independently of the actual release mechanism (Peppas, 1985; Siepmann and Peppas, 2001).

As can be seen in Table 31.4, n values were close to 0.89 for all the IPEC formulations (range $0.81 < n < 1.02$). For all the IPEC systems evaluated, the k parameter for the formulations prepared with 50 mg of a given IPEC was higher than the one for the formulations that contained 100 mg of the same IPEC. It should be noted that for IPEC EE-KC, the k parameter for the formulation containing 50 mg IPEC plus 50 mg IBF is approximately twice the value for the formulation where the double amount of IPEC was used (100 mg IPEC plus 50 mg IBF). An intermediate k parameter was determined for the 75 mg IPEC plus 50 mg IBF formulation. In general, this indicates that the k value could be modified by changing the proportion of the IPEC in the tablets. However, the extent of the variation depends on the specific IPEC system considered. Thus, the 50 mg IPEC CAG77-PNRT1 formulation presented a k value of 5.60 h^{-1}, barely higher than 5.30 h^{-1} for the 100 mg IPEC

CAG77-PNRT1 formulation. Modeling of experimental dissolution data for the physical mixtures led to low R^2 values (0.969–0.979) (Table 31.4).

To further study the mechanisms involved in drug release, experimental data from the buffer stage were fitted to a second model (Model II) based on previous proposals (Peppas, 1985; Siepmann and Peppas, 2001). The equation representing the model used is as follows:

$$\frac{M_t}{M_\infty} = k_1(t-t')^m + k_2(t-t')^{2m} + \alpha' \tag{31.7}$$

The meaning of terms M_t/M_∞, t', is the same as for Model I. The model characteristic parameters k_1, k_2, and m, evaluated by nonlinear regression analysis, are presented in Table 31.5.

It is worth mentioning that in this case, the term α' added is the respective experimental release value at time = 2 h (end of the acid stage) and was included in order to reduce the number of model parameters to be adjusted. Figure 31.9 shows experimental data and Model II predictions. As shown in Table 31.5, R^2 values were equal or greater than 0.992. Accordingly, Model II seems to adequately describe the experimental release data from IPEC matrices. On the contrary, dissolution data for the physical mixtures did not show good fit to Model II. The fact that the release of the model drug from the physical

TABLE 31.5

Model Characteristic Parameters of Model II (IPECs and Physical Mixtures)

IPEC	IPEC:IBF (mg:mg)[a]	k_1 (h^{-n})	k_2 (h^{-2n})	m	R^2
EE-KC	50:50	9.76	3.23	0.52	0.996
	75:50	8.29	3.46	0.46	0.992
	100:50	6.82	2.70	0.38	0.992
MS-KC	50:50	25.40	8.33	0.48	0.996
	100:50	17.35	7.94	0.49	0.996
EE-PNRT1	50:50	8.83	2.76	0.63	0.999
	100:50	6.56	2.10	0.59	0.993
EE-PN702	50:50	11.31	4.68	0.51	0.998
	100:50	9.94	3.58	0.47	0.992
CAG19-PN702	50:50	9.98	5.20	0.65	1.000
	100:50	8.36	5.33	0.56	0.997
CAG19-PNRT1	50:50	9.44	3.53	0.63	0.999
	100:50	9.50	5.68	0.50	0.999
CAG77-PN702	50:50	11.01	1.50	0.60	0.999
	100:50	4.98	0.70	0.80	0.997
CAG77-PNRT1	50:50	0.70	0.40	0.57	1.000
	100:50	6.00	0.60	0.58	0.998
Physical Mixture	**PM:IBF (mg:mg)[a]**	k_1 (h^{-n})	k_2 (h^{-2n})	m	R^2
EE-KC	100:50	4.34	2.20	0.38	0.971
MS-KC[b]	100:50	—	—	—	—
EE-PN702	100:50	8.18	0.57	0.50	0.978
CAG19-PN702	100:50	7.49	2.76	0.52	0.970

[a] Weight ratio between IPEC (or physical mixture) and IBF in the tablet.
[b] Model characteristic parameters for both models could not be determined as tablet disintegrated and completely released IBF before the beginning of the buffer stage.

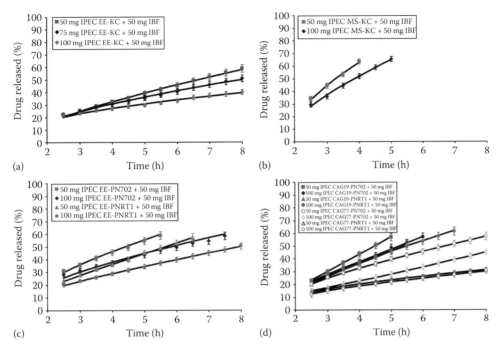

FIGURE 31.9
Comparison between experimental IBF release profiles from the different IPEC formulations for the buffer stage (dots) and those predicted by Model II (solid lines). (a) IPEC EE-KC, (b) IPEC MS-KC, (c) IPECs EE-PN, and (d) IPECs CAG-PN.

mixtures could not be estimated from the swelling tests, and the low R^2 values obtained in the application of Models I and II provide additional support to the observations on the important differences between the behavior of physical mixtures and their corresponding IPECs.

The first term on the right side of Model II (Equation 31.7) represents Fickian diffusional contribution, F, whereas the second term represents the Case II matrix relaxation, R. The ratio of both contributions can be calculated as follows:

$$\frac{R}{F} = \frac{k_2 t^m}{k_1} \tag{31.8}$$

The model characteristic parameters estimated in Table 31.5 and the experimental data from the IPEC systems were used to build Figure 31.10, namely, to represent the R/F ratio versus the drug release percentage.

The results shown in Figure 31.10 indicate that in general, the contribution of Fickian diffusion dominated all formulations, when the percentage of drug released was low (short times). In turn, for a particular drug release percentage, the contribution of matrix relaxation was relatively more important for the formulations containing greater amounts of IPEC. In addition, for each formulation, the relaxation of the matrix also became more important when the percentage of drug released increased, even exceeding diffusion in the cases of 50 mg IPEC EE-KC plus 50 mg IBF, 50 mg IPEC EE-PN702 plus 50 mg IBF, 50 mg IPEC CAG19-PN702 plus 50 mg IBF, 100 mg IPEC CAG19-PN702 plus 50 mg IBF, and 50 mg IPEC CAG19-PNRT1 plus 50 mg IBF tablet formulations.

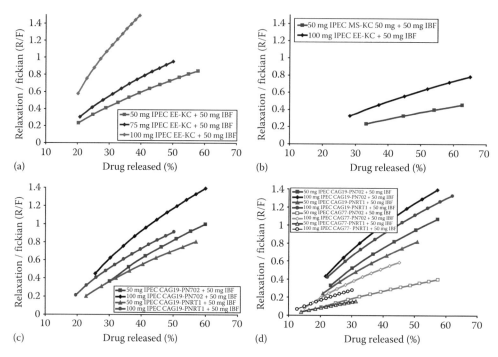

FIGURE 31.10

Ratio between matrix relaxation and Fickian diffusion contributions (R/F), for 50, 75, or 100 mg IPEC (plus 50 mg IBF) formulations. (a) IPEC EE-KC, (b) IPEC MS-KC, (c) IPECs EE-PN, and (d) IPECs CAG-PN.

31.4 Conclusions

Novel IPECs have been prepared employing EE, MS, and CAG as the cationic component and KC and agarans of the red seaweed PN as the anionic ones. The systems were characterized and their potential as controlled drug release matrices was evaluated. Turbidity results indicated that IPEC composition was not affected by the order of addition of the components. Elemental analysis enabled to confirm the formation of stoichiometric complexes (1:1 interaction of the RUs). FTIR spectra of IPECs were different from their starting materials and their physical mixtures, as a result of the ionic interactions between the oppositely charged polyelectrolyte chains. Solid IPEC particles showed characteristic shapes, and IPECs based on EE presented porous structures confirmed by N_2 adsorption measurements. All the IPECs tested exhibited good flowability and compactibility properties allowing their use for full-scale manufacture. Tablets of IPECs and IBF as model drug were prepared by direct compression, which is an advantageous method from both operational and economic viewpoints. No organic solvents were used during the preparation of formulations, nor in the extraction of polysaccharides from PN or in the synthesis of CAGs. Swelling behavior of IPEC tablets was very different from those obtained from physical mixtures. These monolithic matrix systems released the drug with near zero-order kinetics during the buffer stage. The results indicated that release profiles could be controlled by altering the amount of IPEC in the tablets. Also, the change in molecular weight and the *DS* of the components allowed varying release profiles. According to a reported model that allowed an adequate description of the experimental dissolution data in the buffer stage, Fickian diffusion appears to predominate initially over relaxation, with the latter increasing along the release process, to even surpass the first in some systems. These results could be particularly useful to companies interested in controlled drug release technologies but limited to the direct compression technique.

Acknowledgments

This work was supported by grants of the National Research Council of Argentina (CONICET), Agencia Nacional de Promoción Científica y Tecnológica (ANPCyT) and the University of Buenos Aires.

References

Adebayo, S., Brown-Myrie, E., and Itiola, O. 2008. Comparative disintegrant activities of breadfruit starch and official corn starch. *Powder Technol*. 181: 98–103.

Anderson, N. S., Dolan, T. C. S., Penman, A., Rees, D. A., Mueller, G. P., Stancioff, D. J., and Stanley N. F. 1968. Carrageenans. Part IV. Variations in the structure and gel properties of κ-carrageenan, and the characterisation of sulfate esters by infrared spectroscopy. *J. Chem. Soc. C* 602–606.

Annon, 1988. Final report on the safety assessment of polyquaternium-10. *J. Am. Coll. Toxicol*. 7: 335–351.

Arnott, S., Fulmer, A., Scott, W. E., Dea, I. C. M., Moorhouse, R., and Rees, D. A. 1974. The agarose double helix and its function in agarose gel structure. *J. Mol. Biol*. 90: 269–272.

Aspinall, G. O. 1985. *The Polysaccharides*. Academic Press, London, U.K.

Bani-Jaber, A. and Al-Ghazawi, M. 2005. Sustained release characteristics of tablets prepared with mixed matrix of sodium carrageenan and chitosan: Effect of polymer weight ratio, dissolution medium, and drug type. *Drug Dev. Ind. Pharm*. 31: 241–247.

Bhardwaj, T. J., Kanwar, M., Lal, R., and Gupta, A. 2000. Natural gums and modified natural gums as sustained release carriers. *Drug Dev. Ind. Pharm*. 26: 1025–1038.

Bonferoni, M. C., Rossi, S., Ferrari, F., Bertoni, M., Bolhuis, G. K. and Caramella, C. 1998. On the employment of λ carrageenan in a matrix system. III. Optimization of a λ carrageenan–HPMC hydrophilic matrix. *J. Controlled Release* 51: 231–239.

Bonferoni, M. C., Rossi, S., Tamayo, M., Pedraz, J. L., Dominguez-Gil, A., and Caramella, C. 1993. On the employment of λ-carrageenan in a matrix system. I. Sensitivity to dissolution medium and comparison with Na carboxymethylcellulose and xanthan gum. *J. Controlled Release* 26: 119–127.

Bonferoni, M. C., Rossi, S., Tamayo, M., Pedraz, J. L., Dominguez-Gil, A., and Caramella, C. 1994. On the employment of λ-carrageenan in a matrix system. II. λ-Carrageenan and hydroxypropyl-methylcellulose mixtures. *J. Controlled Release* 30: 175–182.

Boraie, N. A. and Naggar V. F. 1984. Sustained release of theophylline and aminophylline from agar tablets. *Acta Pharm. Jugosl*. 34: 247–256.

Capron, I., Yvon, M., and Muller, G. 1996. In-vitro gastric stability of carrageenan. *Food Hydrocolloids* 10: 239–244.

Chiao, C. and Robinson, J. 1998. Sistemas de liberación sostenida de drogas. In: *Remington Farmacia*, Vol. 19, ed. A. Gennaro, Editorial Médica Panamericana, Buenos Aires, Argentina, pp. 2535–2559.

Dautzenberg, H., Kötz, J., Linow, K. J., Philipp, B., and Rother, G. 1994. Static light scattering of polyelectrolyte complex solutions. In: *Macromolecular Complexes in Chemistry and Biology*, eds. P. Dubin, J. Bock, R. Davies, D. Schulz, and C. Thies, Springer, Berlin, Germany, pp. 119–133.

Desai, S. and Bolton, S. 1993. A floating controlled-release drug delivery system: In vitro–in vivo evaluation. *Pharm. Res.* 10: 1321–1325.

Esezobo, S. 1989. Disintegrants: Effects of interacting variables on the tensile strengths and disintegration times of sulfaguanidine tablets. *Int. J. Pharm.* 56: 207–211.

Estévez, J., Ciancia, M., Rodriguez, M., and Cerezo, A. 2003. Ficocoloides de Algas Rojas (Rhodophyta): Carragenanos, Agaranos y DL-Hibridos. Investigaciones en Argentina. *Bol. Soc. Argent. Bot.* 38: 13–28.

Fassihi, A. R. 1989. Characteristics of hydrogel as disintegrant in solid dose technology. *J. Pharm. Pharmacol.* 41: 853–855.

Grant, G. T., Morris, E. R., Rees, D. A., Smith, P. J. C., and Thom, D. 1973. Biological interactions between polysaccharides and divalent cations: The egg-box model. *FEBS Lett.* 32: 195–198.

Gupta, V. K., Hariharan, M., Wheatley, T. A., and Price, J. C. 2001. Controlled-release tablets from carrageenans: Effect of formulation, storage and dissolution factors. *Eur. J. Pharm. Biopharm.* 51: 241–248.

Gursoy, A. and Cevik, S. 2000. Sustained release properties of alginate microspheres and tabletted microspheres of diclofenac sodium. *J. Microencapsul.* 17: 565–575.

Haggett, N. M. W., Hoffmann, R. A., Howlin, B. J., and Webb, G. A. 1997. Molecular modelling of six-ring agarose chains: Effects of explicit and implicit solvent. *J. Mol. Model.* 3: 301–310.

Hariharan, M., Wheatley, T. A., and Price, J. C. 1997. Controlled-release tablet matrices from carrageenans: compression and dissolution studies. *Pharm. Dev. Technol.* 2: 383–393.

Hennink, W. E. and van Nostrum, C. F. 2002. Novel crosslinking methods to design hydrogels. *Adv. Drug Delivery Rev.* 54: 13–36.

Higgins, J. D., Gilmor, T. P., Martelluci, S. A., Bruce, R. D., and Brittain, H. G. 2001. Ibuprofen. In: *Analytical Profiles of Drug Substances*, Vol. 27, ed. H. G. Brittain, Academic Press, San Diego, CA, pp. 265–300.

Hodsdon, A. C., Mitchell, J. R., Davies, M. C., and Melia, C. D. 1995. Structure and behaviour in hydrophilic matrix sustained release dosage forms: 3. The influence of pH on the sustained-release performance and internal gel structure of sodium alginate matrices. *J. Controlled Release* 33: 143–152.

Huang, X. and Brazel, C. S. 2001. On the importance and mechanisms of burst release in matrix-controlled drug delivery systems. *J. Controlled Release* 73: 121–136.

Ito, H., Miyamoto, T., Inagaki, H., Noishiki, Y., Iwata, H., and Matsuda, T. 1986a. In vivo and in vitro blood compatibility of polyelectrolyte complexes formed between cellulose derivatives. *J. Appl. Polym. Sci.* 32: 3413–3421.

Ito, H., Shibata, T., Miyamoto, T., Noishiki, Y., and Inagaki, H. 1986b. Formation of polyelectrolyte complexes between cellulose derivatives and their blood compatibility. *J. Appl. Polym. Sci.* 31: 2491–2500.

Krentz, D. O., Lohmann, C., Schwartz, S., Bratskaya, S., Liebert, T., Laube, J., Heinze, T., and Kulicke, W. M. 2006. Properties and flocculation efficiency of highly cationized starch derivatives. *Starch/Stärke* 58: 161–169.

Larma, I. and Harjula, M. 1999. Stable compositions comprising levosimendan and alginic acid. Patent No WO9955337.

Laurienzo, P. 2010. Review marine polysaccharides in pharmaceutical applications: An overview. *Mar. Drugs* 8: 2435–2465.

Li, L., Fang, Y., Vreeker, R., and Appelqvist, I. 2007. Reexamining the egg-box model in calcium-alginate gels with x-ray diffraction. *Biomacromolecules* 8: 464–468.

Li, J. Y. and Yeh, A. I. 2001. Relationships between thermal, rheological characteristics and swelling power for various starches. *J. Food Eng.* 50: 141–148.

Lieberman, H. A. and Lachman, L. 1980. *Pharmaceutical Dosage Forms: Tablets*. Marcel Dekker, Inc., New York.

Lowman, A. M. 2000. Complexing polymers in drug delivery. In: *Handbook of Pharmaceutical Controlled Release Technology*, ed. D. L. Wise, Marcel Dekker, New York, pp. 89–98.

Meshali, M. M. and Gabr, K. E. 1993. Effect of interpolymer complex formation of chitosan with pectin or acacia on the release behaviour of chlorpromazine HCl. *Int. J. Pharm.* 89: 177–181.

Morris, E. R., Rees, D. A., Thom, D., and Boyd, J. 1978. Chiroptical and stoichiometric evidence of a specific, primary dimerisation process in alginate gelation. *Carbohydr. Res.* 66: 145–154.

Moustafine, R. I., Kabanova, T. V., Kemenova, V. A., and Van den Mooter, G. 2005a. Characteristics of interpolyelectrolyte complexes of Eudragit E100 with Eudragit L100. *J. Controlled Release* 103: 191–198.

Moustafine, R. I., Kemenova, V. A., and Van den Mooter, G. 2005b. Characteristics of interpolyelectrolyte complexes of Eudragit E 100 with sodium alginate. *Int. J. Pharm.* 294: 113–120.

Moustafine, R. I., Margulis, E. B., Sibgatullina, L. F., Kemenova, V. A., and Van den Mooter, G. 2008. Comparative evaluation of interpolyelectrolyte complexes of chitosan with Eudragit® L100 and Eudragit® L100–55 as potential carriers for oral controlled drug delivery. *Eur. J. Pharm. Biopharm.* 70: 215–225.

Moustafine, R. I., Salachova, A. R., Frolova, E. S., Kemenova, V. A., and Van den Mooter, G. 2009. Interpolyelectrolyte complexes of Eudragit® E PO with sodium alginate as potential carriers for colonic drug delivery: Monitoring of structural transformation and composition changes during swellability and release evaluating. *Drug Dev. Ind. Pharm.* 35: 1439–1451.

Moustafine, R. I., Zaharov, I. M., and Kemenova, V. A. 2006. Physicochemical characterization and drug release properties of Eudragit® E PO/Eudragit® L 100-55 interpolyelectrolyte complexes. *Eur. J. Pharm. Biopharm.* 63: 26–36.

Ofner, C. M. III and Klech-Gelotte, C. M. 2007. Gels and jellies. In: *Encyclopedia of Pharmaceutical Technology*, 3rd edn, ed. J. Swarbrick, Informa Healthcare, New York, pp. 1875–1890.

Peppas, N. A. 1985. Analysis of Fickian and Non-Fickian drug release from polymers. *Pharma Acta Helv.* 60: 110–115.

Peppas, N. A., Bures, P., Leobandung, W., and Ichikawa, H. 2000. Hydrogels in pharmaceutical formulations. *Eur. J. Pharm. Biopharm.* 50: 27–46.

Philipp, B., Dautzenberg, H., Linow, K. J., Kötz, J., and Dawydoff, W. 1989. Polyelectrolyte complexes—Recent developments and open problems. *Prog. Polym. Sci.* 14: 91–172.

Picker, K. M. 1999a. Matrix tablets of carrageenans I: A compaction study. *Drug Dev. Ind. Pharm.* 25: 329–337.

Picker, K. M. 1999b. Matrix tablets of carrageenans II: Release behavior and effect of added cations. *Drug Dev. Ind. Pharm.* 25: 339–346.

Prado, H. J., Ciancia, M., and Matulewicz, M. C. 2008a. Agarans from the red seaweed *Polysiphonia nigrescens* (Rhodomelaceae, Ceramiales). *Carbohydr. Res.* 343: 711–718.

Prado, H. J., Matulewicz, M. C., Bonelli, P., and Cukierman, A. L. 2008b. Basic butylated methacrylate copolymer/kappa-carrageenan interpolyelectrolyte complex: Preparation, characterization and drug release behaviour. *Eur. J. Pharm. Biopharm.* 70: 171–178.

Prado, H. J., Matulewicz, M. C., Bonelli, P. R., and Cukierman, A. L. 2009. Preparation and characterization of a novel starch-based interpolyelectrolyte complex as matrix for controlled drug release. *Carbohydr. Res.* 344: 1325–1331.

Prado, H. J., Matulewicz, M. C., Bonelli, P. R., and Cukierman, A. L. 2011. Studies on the cationization of agarose. *Carbohydr. Res.* 346: 311–321.

Prado, H. J., Matulewicz, M. C., Bonelli, P. R., and Cukierman, A. L. 2012. Preparation and characterization of controlled release matrices employing novel seaweed-based interpolyelectrolyte complexes. *Int. J. Pharm* 429: 12–21.

Rodríguez, R., Alvarez-Lorenzo, C., and Concheiro, A. 2003. Cationic cellulose hydrogels: Kinetics of the cross-linking process and characterization as pH-/ion-sensitive drug delivery systems. *J. Controlled Release* 86: 253–265.

Rouquerol, F., Rouquerol, J., and Sing, K. 1999. *Adsorption by Powders and Porous Solids. Principles, Methodology and Applications.* Academic Press, London, U.K.

Rowe, R. C., Sheskey, P. J., and Quinn, M. E. 2009. *Handbook of Pharmaceutical Excipients*, 6th edn. Pharmaceutical Press, London, U.K.

Russo, R., Malinconico, M., and Santagata, G. 2007. Effect on cross-linking with calcium ions on the physical properties of alginate films. *Biomacromolecules* 8: 3193–3197.

Satish, C., Satish, K., and Shiwakumar, H. 2006. Hydrogels as controlled drug delivery systems: Synthesis, crosslinking, water and drug transport mechanism. *Indian J. Pharm. Sci.* 68: 133–140.

Shotton, E. and Leonard, G. S. 1976. Effect of intragranular and extragranular disintegrating agents on particle size of disintegrated tablets. *J. Pharm. Sci.* 65: 1170–1174.

Siepmann, J. and Peppas, N. A. 2001. Modeling of drug release from delivery systems based on hydroxypropyl methylcellulose (HPMC). *Adv. Drug Delivery Rev.* 48: 139–157.

Singh, S. K. and Naini, V. 2007. Dosage forms: Non-parenterals. In *Encyclopedia of Pharmaceutical Technology*, 3rd edn, ed. J. Swarbrick, Informa Healthcare, New York, pp. 988–1000.

Song, Y., Sun, Y., Zhang, X., Zhou, J., and Zhang, L. 2008. Homogeneous quaternization of cellulose in NaOH/urea aqueous solutions as gene carriers. *Biomacromolecules* 9: 2259–2264.

Stanciu, C. and Bennett, J. R. 1974. Alginate/antacid in the reduction of gastro-œsophageal reflux. *Lancet* 303: 109–111.

Stortz, C. and Cerezo, A. 2000. Novel findings in carrageenans, agaroids and "hybrid" red seaweed galactans. *Curr. Top. Phytochemistry* 4: 121–134.

Tapia, C., Costa, E., Moris, M., Sapag-Hagar, J., Valenzuela, F., and Basualto, C. 2002. Study of the influence of the pH media dissolution, degree of polymerization, and degree of swelling of the polymers on the mechanism of release of diltiazem from matrices based on mixtures of chitosan/alginate. *Drug Dev. Ind. Pharm.* 28: 217–224.

Tapia, C., Escobar, Z., Costa, E., Sapag-Hagar, J., Valenzuela, F., Basualto, C., Gau, M. N., and Yasdani-Pedram, M. 2004. Comparative studies on polyelectrolyte complexes and mixtures of chitosan–alginate and chitosan–carrageenan as prolonged diltiazem clorhydrate release systems. *Eur. J. Pharm. Biopharm.* 57: 65–75.

de la Torre, P. M., Enobakhare, Y., Torrado, G., and Torrado, S. 2003. Release of amoxicillin from polyionic complexes of chitosan and poly(acrylic acid) study of polymer/polymer and polymer/drug interactions within the network structure. *Biomaterials* 24: 1499–1506.

Usov, A. 2011. Polysaccharides of the red algae. *Adv. Carbohydr. Chem. Biochem.* 65: 115–217.

USP 30/NF 25, 2007. The United States Pharmacopeia 30/National Formulary 25, United States Pharmacopeial Convention, Inc., Rockville, MD.

Vatier, J., Vallot, T., and Farinotti, R. 1996. Antacid drugs: multiple but too often unknown pharmacological properties. *J. Pharm. Clin.* 15: 41–51.

Zhang, M., Ju, B. Z., Zhang, S. F., Ma, W., and Yang, J. Z. 2007. Synthesis of cationic hydrolyzed starch with high DS by dry process and use in salt-free dyeing. *Carbohydr. Polym.* 69: 123–129.

32

Marine Biomaterials: Role in Drug Delivery and Tissue Engineering toward Biomedical Applications

Devarai Santhosh Kumar and Kota Sobha

CONTENTS

32.1 Introduction: Biomaterials and Drug Delivery Systems

Tissue engineering is the promising therapeutic approach that combines cells, biomaterials, and microenvironmental factors to induce differentiation signals into surgically transplantable formats and promote tissue repair and/or functional restoration. Although several advances have been made in the field of tissue engineering, there are still significant challenges to be addressed in repairing or replacing tissues that serve predominantly biomechanical functions such as articular cartilage. One important obstacle that could be identified is with the scaffolds that play an important role in the extracellular matrix (ECM) but often fail to create the exact/conducive microenvironment during the engineered tissue development to promote the accurate in vitro tissue development. Therefore, the emerging challenge of engineered tissues is to rely on producing scaffolds with an informational function. In other words, informational polymers—the ones containing growth factors facilitating cell attachment, proliferation, and differentiation—are better than noninformational polymers. Growth factors help to manipulate the host healing response at the site of injury facilitating tissue repair and also improve the in vitro tissue growth in order to produce more biofunctional engineered tissues. The strategy is to mimic matrix and provide the necessary information or signaling for cell attachment, proliferation, and differentiation to meet the requirements of dynamic reciprocity for tissue engineering. Thus, proper drug delivery is a prerequisite in tissue-engineering applications. Biopolymers perform a diverse set of functions in their natural environment. To cite an example, proteins function as structural materials and catalysts; carbohydrates function in storage, maintain the functional integrity of membranes, and aid in intracellular communication (Yu et al. 2006). The properties displayed by biological materials and systems are exclusively determined by the physicochemical properties of the monomers and their sequence. In general, a well-defined macromolecular structure can lead to a rich complexity of function, and by virtue of their length and flexibility, they enable a unique control of hierarchical organization and long-range interactions. In many cases, the matrices and scaffolds would ideally be made of biodegradable polymers whose properties closely resemble those of the ECM which is a soft, tough, and elastomeric proteinaceous network that provides mechanical stability and structural integrity to tissues and organs (Guo et al. 2002). Biomaterials should possess mechanical properties capable of withstanding the forces and motions experienced by the normal tissues and have sufficient fatigue strength to ensure a long life of the implant in vivo.

For human and animal health novel delivery systems, common concerns exist in areas of cost-effective treatment, "patient compliance," optimum drug delivery, and bioavailability (Pope 1978). Ideally controlled drug release entails carefully programming the output of a chemical from a physicochemical system such that drug release can be activated on demand. Advanced drug delivery systems possess several advantages over conventional dosage forms. Ideally, they may improve drug potency, control drug release to give a sustained therapeutic effect, provide greater safety, and decrease toxic side effects. Finally, they may target a drug specifically to a desired tissue, organ, or location in the body.

Microencapsulation technology, discovered about five decades ago, is a process whereby small discrete solid particles or small liquid droplets are completely surrounded and enclosed by an intact shell. The structure resembles that of a living cell with a thin membrane or wall surrounding a discrete amount of core material. The method selected to prepare microcapsules depends to a great extent on the core and wall materials used and the ultimate application of the product. Pharmaceutically, the most commonly used membrane materials include cellulose acetate phthalate, gelatin, ethyl cellulose, polyamides, polymethyl methacrylate, polystyrene, rubber, and waxes. Core materials are generally liquids or solids including polymers, waxes, and resins (Mc Ginity et al. 1981). A major advantage of microencapsulated drug products is with drugs which irritate linings in the stomach and intestines. The drug concentration is controlled by slow release characteristics of the microcapsules. Thus, the safety of potential ulcer-producing drugs is increased. Potential pharmaceutical applications of microencapsulation include sustaining or prolonging release of drugs, masking taste and odor of drugs, stabilizing drugs sensitive to atmospheric conditions, preventing vaporization of volatile substances, eliminating incompatibilities via physical separation, overcoming flow problems by formation of free-flowing particles, increasing density of light fluffy powders, overcoming static charge, and turning liquids into solids. Processes for the preparation of biodegradable microspheres containing DL-polylactic acid have been developed. Depending on the physicochemical properties of the drug encapsulated and the drug–polymer ratio, the microspheres will release drug in the body from an intramuscular injection over a period of days to several months. The drug is released by slow diffusion from the particle and by the slow biodegradation of the polymer. By reducing the particle size, it may be possible to target the drug containing microspheres to specific body organs such as the lung, liver, or spleen following intravenous administration. This has been successfully accomplished by other research using liposomes as the targeted drug delivery system. With microparticles, stress conditions like temperature, light, and humidity alter the porosity of the membrane, degrade the drug and polymer, or cause polymorphic or crystalline changes in the encapsulated drug. Scanning electron microscopy, powder x-ray diffraction, and differential staining colorimetry have proven to be invaluable techniques to help explain stability data.

A second specialized delivery system is oral *controlled release tablets* made by one of the three processes, namely, wet granulation, direct compression, and recompression. In addition, there are two more additional advanced drug delivery systems: intravenous fat emulsions and transdermal patch devices. The applications of microemulsions as drug delivery systems for poorly water-soluble drugs show great promise, and the oils in these emulsions include safflower or soybean oil. The intravenous route of administration is valuable when the rapid administration of drugs is required. It is also employed for the long-term infusion of drugs and nutrients via indwelling catheters. However, physical problems may arise with drugs possessing limited aqueous solubility or drugs present in a salt form which can revert to a less soluble form upon IV administration. Drugs with solubility limitations may precipitate at the site of injection leading to severe complications, including thrombophlebitis. Precipitation is a potential problem with poorly soluble drugs because solutions of the drug in mixtures of solvents, such as propylene glycol and ethanol, with water must be employed. Upon injection into the bloodstream, the solvents are rapidly diluted, and this may result in precipitation of the drug at the site of injection. The potential for this to occur with drugs like diazepam and phenytoin has been reported in the literature. The emulsions containing drugs in the oil phase comprise submicron size oil droplets emulsified and stabilized with egg yolk phospholipids.

Transdermal patch devices are applied topically to the skin and contain a reservoir of the drug which slowly diffuses through a rate-controlling membrane prior to absorption through the skin. There are twofold advantages of these devices: one is the controlled release of medication for long periods of time, and the other is the prevention of rapid metabolism of the drug by the liver. The two well-known drugs that are commercially available for human therapy in transdermal systems are scopolamine for the prevention of travel sickness and nitroglycerin for the treatment of angina. Research efforts with these systems are aimed not only to identify candidate drugs for patch devices but to optimize the membrane component of the system that controls the rate of drug release. Many factors related to drug potency, therapeutic index, and site of action must be considered in selection of a drug candidate.

Cell encapsulation is a promising therapeutic approach to deliver cells/drugs to targeted sites to achieve repair. Encapsulation physically isolates a cell mass from an outside environment and aims to maintain normal cellular physiology within a desired permeability barrier. Encapsulation technique involving small spherical vehicles and conformal-coated tissues is called "microencapsulation" while the one that involves larger flat sheet and hollow fiber membranes is called "macroencapsulation." The encapsulated cells can then be cultured in vitro or transplanted in vivo, either to repopulate a defect site or to produce growth factors or other molecules that will have an effect over the targeted cell population. There are several protein-based polymers that find application in research work for drug or cell delivery within the tissue-engineering field. Some of them include collagen, gelatin, silk fibroin, and fibrin/fibrinogen. These protein-based polymers have the advantage of mimicking many features of ECM and hence have the potential to direct migration, growth, and organization of cells during tissue regeneration and wound healing and assist in stabilization of encapsulated and transplanted cells. More than the natural origin polymers which have the drawback of batch variation, recombinant technologies produce proteins with precisely defined properties, predictable placement of cross-linking groups, binding moieties at specific sites along the polypeptide chain, or programmable degradation rates that make them very useful for drug delivery and tissue engineering.

32.2 Biopolymers That Are Widely Investigated for Use in Drug Delivery Systems

32.2.1 Collagen: Properties

Collagen is an ideal scaffold or matrix for tissue engineering as it is the major protein component of the extracellular matrix, providing support to connective tissues such as skin, tendons, bones, cartilage, blood vessels, and ligaments. In its native environment, collagen interacts with cells in connective tissues and transduces essential signals for the regulation of cell anchorage, migration, proliferation, differentiation, and survival (Chunlin et al. 2004). Although 27 types of collagens have been identified to date, collagen type I is the most abundant and most investigated for biomedical applications. Fibril-forming collagen molecules, derived from their precursors after cleavage of C- and N-propeptides, consist of three polypeptide chains of Gly-X-Y amino acid repeats twined around one another to form triple helices. Collagen is defined by high mechanical strength, good biocompatibility, low antigenicity, and ability of being cross-linked and tailored for its mechanical, degradation, and water-uptake properties. Collagen mainly isolated from animal tissues may be a potential antigen owing to viral and prion contamination. However, purification techniques using enzymatic methods may be employed to eliminate the immunogenic telopeptides. Recombinant and nonrecombinant human collagens serve as an alternative for animal-derived collagens but are expensive.

Collagen, appeared very early in evolution in such primitive animals as jellyfish, coral, and sea anemones, is widely applied in tissue-engineering applications and to a less extent in delivery systems.

32.2.2 Collagen in Drug Delivery Systems

The main applications of collagen as drug delivery systems are collagen shields in ophthalmology, sponges for burns/wounds, minipellets, and tablets for protein delivery, gel formulation in combination with liposomes for sustained drug delivery, as controlling material for transdermal drug delivery, and nanoparticles for gene delivery and basic matrices for cell culture systems. Collagen plays an important role in the formation of tissues and organs and is involved in various functional expressions of cells. Collagen is a good surface-active agent and demonstrates its ability to penetrate a lipid-free interface (Fonseca et al. 1996). Collagen exhibits biodegradability, weak antigenecity (Maeda et al. 1999), and superior biocompatibility compared with other natural polymers, such as albumin and gelatin. Collagen finds use in biomedical applications as it can form fibers with extra strength and stability through its self-aggregation and cross-linking. In most of drug delivery systems made of collagen, in vivo absorption of collagen is controlled by the use of cross-linking agents such as glutaraldehyde, chromium tanning, formaldehyde, polyepoxycompounds, acylazide, carbodiimides, and hexamethylenediisocyanate. Physical treatment such as ultraviolet/gamma ray irradiation and dehydrothermal treatment has been efficiently used for the introduction of cross-links to collagen matrix. From the literature, it is evident that under optimized conditions, oxidized and denatured thiolated collagen films are more resistant and rigid than glutaraldehyde-treated ones.

Collagen can be extracted into an aqueous solution and molded into various forms of delivery systems. Besides the major applications of collagen as drug delivery systems, collagen's use as surgical sutures, hemostatic agents, and tissue engineering including basic matrices for cell culture systems and replacement/substitutes for artificial blood vessels and valves is well known. Some disadvantages of collagen-based systems arose from their poor mechanical strength and effectiveness in the management of infected sites. The better collagen delivery systems having an accurate release control can be achieved by adjusting the structure of the collagen matrix or adding other proteins such as elastin, fibronectin, or glycosaminoglycans. A combination of collagen with other polymers, such as collagen/ liposome and collagen/silicone has been proposed to achieve the stability of a system and the controlled release profiles of incorporated compounds.

32.2.3 Types of Collagen-Based Drug Delivery Systems

32.2.3.1 Film/Sheet/Disk

The major application of collagen films is as barrier membrane. Films with a thickness of 0.01–0.5 mm and made of biodegradable materials such as prepared from telopeptide-free reconstituted collagen demonstrated a slow release profile of incorporated drugs. The drugs can be loaded into collagen membranes by hydrogen bonding, covalent bonding, or simple entrapment. They can be sterilized and become pliable upon hydrolyzation, while retaining adequate strength to resist manipulation. Collagen film, when applied to the eye, was found to be completely hydrolyzed after 5–6 h suggesting that collagen-based systems are suitable for resembling current liquid and ointment vehicles. Collagen film/ sheet/disk are used for the treatment of tissue infection such as infected corneal tissue or liver cancer. Soluble ophthalmic insert in the form of a wafer or a film was introduced as a drug delivery system for the treatment of infected corneal tissue using a high dose of antibiotic agents such as gentamicin and tetracycline. The wafer route of administration was found to give the highest tissue concentration of incorporated drugs for sufficiently long duration of about a week. The local application of microfibrous collagen sheets loaded with anticancer agent, etoposide (VP-16), in the liver resulted in a relatively long maintenance of drug concentrations at the target site.

Collagen film and disk as gene delivery systems have many advantages. Systems that isolate transplanted cells from the host immune system might be beneficial and economical as they would allow the use of allogenic or even xenogenic cells in many patients. A combination of collagen and other polymers such as atelocollagen matrix added on the surface of polyurethane films enhanced attachment and proliferation of fibroblasts and supported growth of cells. Thus, studies indicate that collagen-based film/disk systems should contain extra matrices that improve conditions for a long-term cell survival. Matrix films composed of various combinations of collagen and elastin have been developed and evaluated for its uses in tissue calcification and as a controlled delivery device for its uses in tissue calcification and as a controlled delivery device for cardiovascular drugs. Collagen films developed by Lee et al. (2001) were used to simulate the calcification process of implantable biomaterials such as bioprosthetic heart valve (BHV). The differential composition of aortic wall (90% collagen) and leaflet (99% collagen) is found to be responsible for their differences in calcification rates and their response to anticalcification agents, suggesting the elastin concentration effects on the calcification rate of implantable biomaterials. Studies on the total amount of calcium accumulation in a system implanted in the rat subcutaneous model indicated an increase with increase in the concentrations of elastic from 10% to 90% suggesting that elastin has a more critical role in tissue calcification than collagen and that this system can be used as a calcifiable matrix simulating calcification process of implantable tissues such as BHV. This system could also be put to use in local and systemic delivery of various anticalcification agents, cardiovascular drugs, and antibiotics for the treatment of heart diseases.

32.2.3.2 Collagen Shields

These were originally designed for bandage contact lenses which are gradually dissolved in cornea. One of the advantages of the collagen-based drug delivery systems is the ease with which the formulation can be applied to the ocular surface and its potential for self-administration. The collagen corneal shield is fabricated from porcine scleral tissue that closely resembles collagen molecules of the human eye. The mechanical properties of the shield protect the healing corneal epithelium from the blinking action of the eyelids. The collagen corneal shield would promote epithelial healing after corneal transplantation and radial keratomy. Drug delivery by collagen shields depends on loading and a subsequent release of medication by the shield. The collagen matrix acts as a reservoir, and the drugs are entrapped in the interstices of the collagen matrix in a solution for water-soluble drugs or incorporated into the shield for water-insoluble drugs. As tears flush through the shield and the shield dissolves, it provides a layer of biologically compatible collagen solution that seems to lubricate the surface of the eye, minimize rubbing of the lids on the cornea, increase the contact time between the drug and the cornea, and foster epithelial healing. A bolus release of drug from the lenses was attributable to the enhanced drug effect. Thus, this system allows the higher corneal concentration of drug and the more sustained drug delivery into the cornea and the aqueous humor.

Collagen shields were used as delivery devices for the treatment of various local infections, and their therapeutic effects were compared with the conventional formulations. The use of antibiotic collagen shields supplemented by frequent topical applications has been clinically useful for preoperative and postoperative antibiotic prophylaxis, the initial treatment of bacterial keratitis, and the treatment of corneal abrasions. Most studies showed that shields provided equal or better drug delivery of fluorescein, prednisolone acetate, cyclosporine, and ofloxacin to the anterior segment. Delivery of drugs through the impregnated collagen shield was more comfortable and reliable than frequent application of other conventional treatments such as drops, ointment, or daily subconjunctive infection. Delivery of plasmid DNA into the bleb through a collagen shield increased chloramphenicol acetyltransferase, the reporter gene, 30-fold over injection of plasmid DNA through saline vehicle. Gene therapy using naked plasmid DNA and a simple collagen shield delivery was very useful for regulating wound healing after glaucoma surgery.

Modifications of collagen were made to simplify the application, reduce blurring of vision, and enhance the drug concentration and bioavailability of drugs in the cornea and aqueous humor. The cross-linked collagen using glutaraldehyde or chromium tanning can serve as a drug reservoir and provide more desirable drug delivery than non-cross-linked collagen shields by increasing the contact time between the drug and the cornea. Collasomes developed by adding long hydrocarbon side chains to the collagen increase the hydrophobicity of the collagen and the total surface area as well which decreases the diffusion rate of hydrophilic drug molecules from the collagen matrix. Collasomes hydrated in a solution of sodium fluorescein and suspended in a methyl cellulose vehicle as a model for delivery of water-soluble drugs produced fluorescein concentrations much higher in the cornea and aqueous humor compared with fluorescein containing vehicle alone. Collagen shields as a drug carrier for topical agents have several advantages like faster epithelial healing, less stromal edema at the wound sites, protection of keratocytes adjacent to the wound sites, and diminishment of inflammatory reaction. There are also certain disadvantages such as reducing visual activity and causing slight discomfort.

Collagen sponges have been very useful in the treatment of severe burns and as a dressing for many types of wounds such as pressure sores, donor sites, leg ulcers, and decubitus ulcers as well as for in vitro test systems. Collagen sponges have the ability to easily absorb large quantities of tissue exudates, smooth adherence to the wet wound bed with preservation of low-moisture climate as well as its shielding against mechanical harm and secondary bacterial infection. A rapid recovery of skin from burn wounds by an intense infiltration of neutrophils into the sponge was demonstrated with sponge implantation. Coating of a collagen sponge with growth factor further facilitates dermal and epidermal wound healing. To achieve high resilient activity and fluid building capacity, collagen sponges have been combined with other materials like elastin, fibronectin, or glycosaminoglycans. The starting material can be cross-linked with glutaraldehyde and subsequently graft copolymerized with other polymers such as polyhydroxyethyl methacrylate. The grafted PHEMA chains which are hydrophilic keep the membranes wet and increase their tensile strength and thus affect the efficiency in the management of infected wounds and burns.

Collagen sponges were found to be suitable for short-term delivery (3–7 days) of antibiotics such as gentamicin. These collagen sponges were also found to be of use in osteoinduction. When absorbable collagen sponge containing bone morphogenetic protein 2 (rhBMP-2) was tested in the rat model for the evaluation of the efficacy of rhBMP-2 produced in *Escherichia coli* on promoting bone healing, it was found that bacterially expressed rhBMP-2 loaded in collagen sponge was osteogenic in vivo. Similarly, an absorbable collagen sponge containing bone morphogenetic proteins (rhBMP-2) stabilizes endosseous dental implants in bony areas, and normal bone formation was restored without complication. Collagen sponges were also used for delivery of steroids through topical applications such as intravaginal delivery of lipophilic compounds including retinoic acid. Collagen-based sponge was inserted into a cervical cap made of hydrogen hypan which adheres to the wet tissue surfaces by the force of differential osmotic pressure. This novel system is associated with high local concentration of drugs without producing any systemic symptoms and has been very useful for local drug delivery. Collagen sponge as a drug carrier or a vaginal contraceptive barrier showed many advantages, such as the controlled release of spermicidal agents and reducing the tissue irritation activity. The major drawbacks of sponges appear to be the difficulty of assuring adequate supplies and their preservation.

Other problems arose from their poor mechanical strength and ineffectiveness in the management of infected wounds and burns.

32.2.3.3 Gel, Hydrogel, Liposomes: Collagen

Hydrogels containing collagen and polyhydroxy ethyl methacrylate were made to develop a delivery system for anticancer drugs such as 5-FU. Hybrid copolymers of collagen with polyethylene glycol 6000 and polyvinylpyrrolidone were prepared for the controlled delivery of contraceptive steroids. Two synthetic polymers, polyvinyl alcohol (PVA) and polyacrylic acid (PAA), were blended with two biological polymers, collagen and hyaluronic acid, to enhance the mechanical strength of natural polymers and to overcome the biological drawbacks of synthetic polymers. These blends were formulated into hydrogels, films, and sponges and subsequently loaded with growth hormone (GH). The results of this study showed that GH could be released from collagen–PVA hydrogels in a controlled release pattern, and the rate and quantity of GH released were mainly dependent on collagen content in the system. One of the successful applications of collagen for the controlled delivery systems is collagen-based gel as an injectable aqueous formulation. One such example is a combination of collagen and epinephrine for delivery of 5-FU developed for cancer treatment by diffusion after intratumoral injection.

32.2.4 Modifications on Collagen Film/Sheet/Disk

Collagen films cross-linked by chromium tanning, formaldehyde, or a combination of both have been successfully used as implantable delivery systems in achieving the sustained release of medroxy progesterone acetate. A modification by attaching another membrane to collagen-based film/sheet/disk was attempted to achieve the controlled release rate of incorporated drugs. A transdermal delivery device containing nifedipine, whose release rate was well controlled by an attached membrane made of chitosan, showed the highest therapeutic efficacy in the treatment of tissue infection. Collagen film and matrix were used as gene delivery carriers for promoting bone formation. A composite of recombinant human bone morphogenetic protein 2 (rhBMP-2) and collagen was developed to monitor bone development and absorbent change of carrier collagen. The rhBMP-2/collagen only implant resulted in no bone formation. Collagen provides an anchorage for cell differentiation and remains as an artificial matrix in woven bone. Another study indicated that collagen matrix loaded with BMP and placed in a close contact with osteogenic cells achieved direct osteoinduction without causing a cartilage formation.

The marine environment, with its enormous wealth of biological and chemical diversity (Fuhrman et al. 1995; Field et al. 1997; Rossbach and Kniewald 1997), represents a treasure trove of useful materials awaiting discovery. Indeed, a number of clinically useful drugs, investigational drug candidates, and pharmacological tools have already resulted from marine-product discovery programs (Table 32.1). However, a number of key areas for future investigation are anticipated to increase the application and yield of useful marine bioproducts. The broad areas where advances could have substantial impact on drug discovery and development are (1) accessing new sources of marine bioproducts, (2) meeting the supply needs of the drug discovery and development process, (3) improving paradigms for the screening and discovery of useful marine bioproducts, (4) expanding knowledge of the biological mechanisms of action of marine bioproducts and toxins, and (5) streamlining the regulatory process associated with marine bioproduct development.

TABLE 32.1

Some Examples of Commercially Available Marine Bioproducts

S. No.	Products	Application	Original Source	Reference
1	*Pharmaceuticals*			Pomponi (1999)
	Ara-A (acyclovir)	Antiviral drug (herpes infections)	Marine sponge, *Cryptotethya crypta*	
	Ara-C (cytosar-U, cytarabine)	Anticancer drug (leukemia and non-Hodgkin's lymphoma)	Marine sponge, *Cryptotethya crypta*	
2	*Molecular Probes*			
	Okadaic acid	Phosphatase inhibitor	Dinoflagellate	
	Manoalide	Phospholipase A_2 inhibitor	Marine sponge, *Luffariella variabilis*	
	Aequorin	Bioluminescent calcium indicator	Bioluminescent jellyfish, *Aequorea victoria*	
	Green fluorescent protein (GFP)	Reporter gene	Bioluminescent jellyfish, *Aequorea victoria*	
3	*Enzymes*			
	Vent and Deep Vent DNA polymerase (New England BioLabs)	Polymerase chain reaction enzyme	Deep-sea hydrothermal vent bacterium	
4	*Pigment*			
	Phycoerythrin	Conjugated antibodies used in ELISAs and flow cytometry	Red algae	
5	*Cosmetic additives*			
	Resilience® (Estée Lauder)	"Marine extract" additive	Caribbean gorgonian, *Pseudopterogorgia elisabethae*	

32.3 Gelatin

Gelatin is a natural polymer derived by acid and alkaline processing of collagen and is commonly used for pharmaceutical and medical applications because of its biodegradability and biocompatibility in physiological environments. Because of these characteristics, gelatin is used as a safe component in drug formulations or as a sealant for vascular prosthesis. Gelatin with low antigenicity as compared to collagen contains a large number of glycine, proline, and 4-hydroxyproline residues. Two different types of gelatin could be produced depending on the pretreatment type: acidic or alkaline. The alkaline process targets the amide groups of asparagine and glutamine and hydrolyzes them into carboxyl groups, thus producing aspartic and glutamic acids. On the contrary, acidic treatment hardly affects the amide groups, and therefore, gelatin obtained by this treatment will have the isoelectric point similar to that of collagen. Thus, manufacturers produce gelatin with varying isoelectric point values; the most used is the basic gelatin with an isoelectric point of 9.0 and the acidic gelatin with an isoelectric point of 5.0. It is well accepted that a positively or negatively charged polyelectrolyte electrostatically interacts with an oppositely charged molecule to form a polyion complex. Theoretically, gelatin can form polyion complexes with any type of charged molecules: if the biomolecule/drug to be released is acidic, basic gelatin with an isoelectric point of 9.0 is preferable as a matrix, while acidic gelatin with an isoelectric point of 5.0 should be applicable to the control release of a basic protein. As both the gelatins are insoluble in water, a hydrogel (that can form polyion complex with protein) is prepared through chemical cross-linking with water-soluble carbodiimides and glutaraldehyde. The release of the biologically active protein/drug from the hydrogel by its enzymatic degradation with time in the body can be tailored by changing the extent of cross-linking which in turn produces varied water contents. Gelatin-based systems with variations in their electrical and physical properties could be produced by altering the manufacturing methodology and, therefore, find a wide array of applications in the fields of drug delivery, gene therapy, and tissue engineering. Promising properties, safety, and mainly the possibility of polyion complexation make gelatin a polymer of choice in drug delivery for tissue-engineering applications targeting several tissues including bone, cartilage, skin, and adipose tissue. Gelatin, for its easy processability and gelation properties, is manufactured in a range of shapes including sponges and injectable hydrogels. However, the most used carriers are gelatin microspheres which normally are incorporated in a second scaffold such as a hydrogel.

32.4 New Bioproduct Discovery and Supply

The ocean is a rich source of biological and chemical diversity. It covers more than 70% of the earth's surface and contains more than 300,000 described species of plants and animals. A relatively small number of marine plants, animals, and microbes have already yielded more than 12,000 novel chemicals (Faulkner 2001).

Unexamined habitats must be explored to discover new species. Most of the environments explored for organisms with novel chemicals have been accessible by SCUBA (i.e., to 40 m). Although some novel chemicals have been identified at high latitudes, such as the fjords of British Columbia and under the Antarctic ice, the primary focus of marine biodiversity prospecting has been the tropics. Tropical seas are well known to be areas of high biological diversity and, therefore, logical sites of high chemical diversity. Much of the deep sea is yet to be explored, and very little exploration has occurred at higher latitudes. With rare exceptions (e.g., the analysis of deep-sea cores to identify unusual microbes), marine organisms from the deep-sea floor, mid-water habitats, and high-latitude marine environments and most of the sea surface itself have not been studied. The reason for this deficiency is primarily financial: oceanographic expeditions are expensive, and neither federal nor pharmaceutical industry funding has been available to support oceanographic exploration and discovery of novel marine resources. The potential for discovery of novel bioproducts from yet-to-be-discovered species of marine macroorganisms and microorganisms (including symbionts) is high (De Vries and Beart 1995; Cragg and Newman 2000; Mayer and Lehmann 2001).

To optimize identification of marine resources with medicinal potential, the best tools for discovery must be used at all stages of exploration: in new locations, for collection of organisms never before sampled, and for the identification of chemicals with pharmaceutical potential. Increased sophistication in the tools available to explore the deep sea has expanded the habitats that can be sampled and has greatly improved the opportunities for discovery of new species and the chemical compounds that they produce. New and improved vehicles are being developed to take us farther and deeper in the ocean. These platforms need to be equipped with even more sophisticated and sensitive instruments to identify an organism as new, to assess its potential for novel chemical constituents, and if possible, to nondestructively remove a sample of the organism. Tools and sensors that have been developed for space exploration and diagnostic medicine need to be applied to the discovery of new marine resources.

Perhaps the greatest untapped source of novel bioproducts is marine microorganisms (Bentley 1997; Gerwick and Sitachitta 2000; Gerwick et al. 2001). Although new technologies are rapidly expanding our knowledge of the microbial world, research to date suggests that less than 1% of the total marine microbial species diversity can be cultured with commonly used methods. That means chemicals produced by as many as 99% of the microorganisms in the ocean have not yet been studied for potential commercial applications. These organisms constitute an enormous untapped resource and opportunity for discovery of new bioproducts with applications in medicine, industry, and agriculture. Developing creative solutions for the identification, culture, and analysis of uncultured marine microorganisms is a critical need.

With the enormous potential for discovery, development, and marketing of novel marine bioproducts comes the obligation to develop methods for supplying these products without disrupting the ecosystem or depleting the resource. Supply is a major limitation in the development of marine bioproducts (Cragg et al. 1993; Clarke et al. 1996; Turner 1996; Cragg 1998). In general, the natural abundance of the source organisms will not support development based on wild harvest. Unless there is a feasible alternative to harvesting, promising bioproducts will remain undeveloped. Some options for sustainable use of marine resources are chemical synthesis, aquaculture of the source organism, cell culture of the macroorganism or microorganism source, and molecular cloning and biosynthesis in a surrogate organism. Each of these options has advantages and limitations; not all methods will be applicable to supply every marine bioproduct, and most of the methods are still in development. Understanding the fundamental biochemical pathways by which bioproducts are synthesized is key to most of these techniques.

Molecular approaches offer particularly promising alternatives not only to the supply of known natural products (e.g., through the identification, isolation, cloning, and heterologous expression of genes involved in the production of the chemicals) but also to the discovery of novel sources of molecular diversity (e.g., through the identification of genes and biosynthetic pathways from uncultured microorganisms) (Bull et al. 2000). Manipulation of heterologously expressed secondary metabolite biosynthetic genes to produce novel compounds having potential pharmaceutical utility is at the forefront of current scientific achievements and has tremendous potential for creation of novel chemical entities (Khosla et al. 1999; Du and Shen 2001; Floss 2001; Rohlin et al. 2001; Staunton and Wilkinson 2001; Xue and Sherman 2001). In approaches parallel to those used for terrestrial soils, efforts need to be made to clone useful secondary metabolite biosynthetic pathways from natural assemblages of marine microorganisms (e.g., "cloning of the ocean's metagenome"). Use of these approaches to provide solutions to natural product supply and resupply problems should be increased.

Marine organisms have demonstrated their utility as models to understand disease processes in humans. Priority should be given to the identification and development of new model marine organisms to (1) identify novel targets for disease therapy, (2) discover novel chemicals for drug development, and (3) provide alternatives to current animal (and human) testing of drugs. With more complete genome sequences available from novel organisms, it will be more likely that an analogue to human mutations can be found in a convenient test organism. Of critical importance in the development of new models is the availability of genome sequences from marine organisms. Genomic approaches, including whole-genome studies of appropriate model organisms, will accelerate discovery of new targets and new marine-derived drugs.

32.5 Recommendations for Enhancing Drug Discovery with Marine Biotechnology

- Explore new habitats.
- Develop tools to discover new resources.
- Discover and culture new marine microorganisms (including symbionts).
- Provide sufficient supply of bioproducts.
- Develop new screening strategies.
- Pursue strategies to hasten the discovery of new materials.
- Combine resources of academic, governmental, and industrial laboratories to expand access to biological screens in a variety of therapeutic areas.
- Expand research on pharmacological mechanisms.
- Establish new marine model organisms.
- Expand research on marine bioproduct biosynthesis and molecular biology.

32.6 Biomaterials and Bioengineering

Well beyond the obvious providers of food, the world's seas have always been bountiful providers of special materials valued for human health and pleasure. Access to this resource historically has been hindered by the apparent hostility of the seawater environment to manufactured materials and engineering concepts of *terra firma*. In spite of the extraordinary potential of the marine environment for new biomaterials, the environmental risks and exploration costs have been prohibitive.

In the past decade, new tools of biotechnology have been introduced that are producing extraordinary new products and assays based on the new understanding of genetic factors and their expression as complex biological molecules. Applying these tools to the marine environment provides opportunities to unlock similar micromolecular vaults of marine biomedical products so that they can join other macro-biomaterials already harvested from the sea for thousands of years (Tables 32.2 and 32.3).

32.6.1 Novel Characteristics of Macro-Biomaterials from Marine Organisms

Marine biomaterials are a heterogeneous group of organic-, ceramic-, and polysaccharide-based polymers that hold promise for a variety of new approaches to the treatment of disease. The marine environment is home to numerous microporous materials, such as those that provide the framework for coral reefs or those that compose the spines

TABLE 32.2

Some Commercially Available Marine-Derived Biomedical Research Probes

S. No.	Source	Probe	Function	Price
1	Sponge	Manoalide	Phospholipase A_2 inhibitor	$120/mg
		Calyculin A	Protein phosphatase inhibitor	$105/25 μg
		Luffariellolide	Phospholipase A_2 inhibitor	$100/mg
		12-epi-scalaridial	Phospholipase A_2 inhibitor	$136/mg
		Latrunculin B	Actin polymerization inhibitor	$90/mg
		Mycalolide B	Actin polymerization inhibitor	$212/20 μg
		Swinholide A	Actin microfilament disruptor	$100/20 μg
2	Dinoflagellate	Okadic acid	Protein phosphatase inhibitor	$75/25 μg
3	Bryozoan	Bryostatin 1	Protein kinase C activator	$88/10 μg
4	Sea hare	Dolastatin 15	Microtubule assembly inhibitor	$125/mg

TABLE 32.3

Marine-Derived Antitumor Compounds Licensed for Development

S. No.	Marine Source	Drug	Organism	Current Status
1	Sponge	Discodermolide	*Discodermia dissoluta*	To enter Phase I trials in 2002; licensed to Novartis
		Isohomohalichondrin B	*Lissodendoryx* sp.	Licensed to PharmaMar S.A.; in advanced preclinical trials
		Bengamide	*Jaspis* sp.	Synthetic derivative licensed to Novartis; in clinical trials
		Hemiasterlins A and B	*Cymbastella* sp.	Derivatives to enter clinical trials in 2002; licensed to Wyeth-Ayerst
		Girolline	*Pseudaxinyssa cantharella*	Licensed to Rhone Poulenc
2	Bryozoan	Bryostatin 1	*Bugula neritina*	In Phase I/II clinical trials in the United States/Europe; U.S. National Cancer Institute (NCI) sponsored trials

of sea urchins. These macro-biomaterials are characterized by highly interconnected porous networks, with a wide range of porosities (Weber and White 1972). Because of their geometric and material properties, coral structures and urchin spines are used in vascular graft construction and orthopedic surgical repairs. Identification of the natural convoluted geometries and fouling-resistant surface features of coral has been a key factor prompting consideration of other biotechnology approaches to successful biomimicry and biomaterials manufacture. Marine organisms can provide many more novel models for biomolecular materials design.

New biotechnologies have been introduced for biocompatible, self-limiting, implantable biomedical devices based on "storage biopolymers," such as polyhydroxyalkanoates, which are abundant in marine microorganisms (Madison and Huisman 1999). New opportunities also exist for high-value biomedical products, such as drug delivery units, based on chitin from marine crabs and other crustaceans (Felt et al. 1998; Janes et al. 2001; Sato et al. 2001). The enormous supply of chitin and chitosan biopolymers serves as a base for hydrogel-like hosts for various medicinal ingredients, including antibiotics, and provides good wound-dressing qualities for abrasions and ulcers. Work is under way to utilize novel combinations of storage biopolymers, particularly polyhydroxybutyrate, with coral segments to fabricate a scaffold that can be used in bone repair (Laurencin et al. 1996; Madihally and Matthew 1999; Suh and Matthew 2000).

32.6.2 Facilitating Work at Surfaces

Marine surfaces are important planes of research and exploration for biotechnological applications. Of particular interest are the characteristics of submerged natural surfaces that resist corrosion and adhesion and the opposing characteristics of selected organisms that allow them to adhere tightly to wet, slimy surfaces. The oceans' intrinsically nonstick, low-drag plant and animal surfaces and the adaptations of some species to adhere to wet surfaces hold incredible promise for future biomedical applications (Anderson 1996). The most well-known example is perhaps the common blue mussel, *Mytilus edulis*, with its strong byssal threads and adhesion disks which allow it to remain attached in very high-energy environments, including pounding surf. However, to fully commercialize these characteristics, critical issues of cross-link biocatalysis and water displacing posttranslational modifications of secreted adhesive biopolymers must be resolved. In addition to the submerged biological and physical surfaces, the air–sea interface is important as a biomaterial source and model for bioengineering of new artificial lungs and biolubricants. The sea surface is ubiquitously coated with surface-active natural molecules that are the modulators of gas and particle exchange across the liquid–gas interface. Similar analogies exist between sea-surface films and natural biolubricants of human tear films in the blinking human eye.

32.6.3 Applications for Novel Marine Biomaterials

There are many areas in which a better understanding of physiological processes in marine organisms may improve the development of biomedical tools. For example, coral growth and healing may improve the understanding of bone development and healing. A better understanding of the principles of biomimicry of marine surfaces may allow the development of micro- and nanostructured implants for tissue regeneration. Sea-surface explorations should be a routine part of deep-sea and coral examinations for materials with bioengineering and tissue-engineering applications. New photocatalytic materials will likely be found in the uppermost sea-surface zones otherwise neglected in explorations of deep-sea and coral surfaces, as evidenced by the recent discoveries of light-driven photopigment reactions near the sea–air boundary (Béjà et al. 2000, 2001).

Biotechnological tools may reveal how marine biocatalysis promotes secure underwater adhesion, with strength and security yet unmatched by terrestrial sources and synthetic approaches. Underwater self-cleaning and self-lubricating plant and animal surfaces may be better understood with new biotechnology, the results of which could be used for the benefit of dry eye and dry mouth sufferers and lubricant-depleted human tissues.

The sustained productivity and economic successes of collection and bioengineering of kelp and other macroalgal products into agars, alginates, and food products provide models for the future of marine biotechnology as it applies to marine biomaterials. Another goal is to identify and exploit the micro- and nanoscale novel characteristics of marine organisms that can make excellent templates for biomaterials and drug delivery of therapeutic devices with potential application in human medicine and bioengineering.

32.7 Marine Tissue Engineering

According to Global Industry Analysts (GIA), the global market in marine biotechnology is forecast to reach U.S. $4.1 billion by the year 2015. Major potential factors driving market growth include growing interest from medical, pharmaceutical, aquaculture, nutraceutical, and industrial sectors. Further, widening applications in several end-use areas including marine transportation, environmental remediation, cosmetics, research, and food sectors are also contributing to market growth. Marine bioactive substances market is forecast to register the fastest growth rate of more than 4.0% during the period 2009–2015. In terms of end use, health care and biotechnology constitute the largest as well as fastest growing segment in marine biotechnology.

32.8 Bone and Cartilage

Regenerative medicine has shown great potential to address the rapid growing need of treatment of diseases in the twenty-first century (Liu 2007). Special interest has been shown in advanced functional bio-nanomaterial development which holds clues for effective cure of diseases and enhances selectivity as well as sensitivity of detecting biomolecules (Ma 2008). Rapid progress in nanotechnology and its far-reaching technology have triggered the use of nanomaterials to greater potential which mimics biological response in terms of structure, chemical composition, and mechanical properties (Gupta et al. 2009). Several types of materials such as synthetic polymers, metals, composites, and ceramics have been developed and used for different biomedical applications (Ratner and Bryant 2004). Most importantly, biomaterials used in joint replacements and dental implants need to have good biocompatibility; highly corrosive resistance and osteogenicity in response to the biological systems are highly preferred for the development of bone regeneration (Anselme 2000).

Similarly, cartilage (shock absorber) is a connective tissue which is found mainly in between the joints of femur and tibia region. Degenerative cartilage leads to osteoarthritis; it is commonly associated with pain, swelling, inflammation, and no free movement between femur and tibial region of the bone. Cartilage degeneration is one of the major problems to athlete's as well elder orthoclinician patients over 50 years of age. Until the last decade, cartilage repair was performed by drilling, abrasion arthroplasty, microfracture, and transplantation of chondrocytes, perichondrium, meniscal allograft, periosteum, and osteochondral grafts (Steadman et al. 2003; Huade et al. 2009). In another way, cell-based therapies like autologous chondrocyte implantation and matrix-assisted autologous chondrocyte implantation technique were mostly used for osteoarthritic patients (Brittberg et al. 1994). These methods do not have any proper evidence of the capacity of surgery in terms of phenotype biological procedure (Peter et al. 2006; Nakamura et al. 2009). In addition to the earlier mentioned techniques, different biomaterials/scaffolds are also used for the cartilage regeneration (few are listed in Table 32.4). Bioactive glass–ceramic is another type of biomaterials used for the in vitro cartilage regeneration. The rat primary chondrocytes are placed on the biomaterial having the focal contacts containing vinculin and beta1-integrin to facilitate the chondrocyte attachment, cell differentiation, and matrix production. On this biomaterial/scaffold, the round cells formed are separated by a dense ECM with positive collagen II and chondroitin sulfates which are important for cartilage formation (Loty et al. 1997). In this scenario,

TABLE 32.4
Different Biomaterials/Scaffolds Used for Cartilage Regeneration

S. No.	Biomaterials	Type of Cartilage	Mode of Operation	Model	Experimentation	Remarks	Reference
1	Plastics	Articular cartilage	Simple plastic flask	Rabbit	In vitro	Chondrocytes cultured on plastic lose their round shape and dedifferentiate to a fibroblast-like phenotype forming a monolayer of flattened cells	Villar et al. (2004)
2	PLGA	Bovine articular cartilage	Hybrid scaffold entrapped with celline	Mice	In vitro and in vivo	It is important to find that this biomaterial could withstand a longer period with definite shape and structure	Guoping Chen et al. (2004)
3	Bioactive glass–ceramic	Chondrocytes	Focal contacts containing vinculin and beta1-integrin	Rat	In vitro	Improper growth, nonadherent to the membrane, interfacial failure, and loss of implant can occur	Loty et a1. (1997)
4	Alginate, PGA scaffold, monolayer culture	Chondrocytes		Human	In vitro	Alginate contains spherical chondrocytes surrounded by dense ECM leads to diffusion. Increased accumulation of sulfated glycosaminoglycans and biochemical analysis show low level of proliferation than monolayer culture	Mark et al. (2003)
5	PGA	Elastic cartilage	Rotational bioreactors	Adult sheep auricles	In vitro	Biodegradable capacity of the material need for cartilage formation	Shinichi Terada et al. (2005)

in vitro marine scaffold autologous/allogeneic cartilage regenerating implant/transplant is in high demand with cost-effective route. It was observed that primary chondrocytes of rabbit articular cartilage were cultured on the simple plastic in which cells facilitate to dedifferentiation and proliferation with phenotype forming on a monolayer of flattened cells (Villar et al. 2004). Guoping et al. (2004) demonstrated that when bovine articular cartilages of primary chondrocytes were seeded along with the hybrid scaffold, the cartilage formation was observed using mice model. This hybrid sponge facilitated cell seeding along with homogenous cell distribution by secreting extracellular matrices with DL-lactic co-glycolic acid (PLGA) biomaterial, and it showed superior mechanical strength with definite shape (Guoping Chen et al. 2004). Polyglycolic acid (PGA) is another scaffold used for cartilage regeneration in which primary chondrocytes from adult sheep auricles were coated on the PGA hydrogel. It was observed that collagen I and PGA hydrogel coated on the scaffold showed enhanced proliferation and cartilage regeneration (Shinichi et al. 2005). Similarly, in in vitro studies on human chondrocyte, the cells were seeded on the scaffold material where it undergoes redifferentiation process by regaining the spherical shape of fibroblast phenotype with high amount of ECM formation (Schulze-Tanzil et al. 2002; Mark et al. 2003).

32.9 Marine Medical Applications

Basic production of marine drug production toward commercialization was schematically presented in Figure 32.1. Research in this area is at early stages relative to biotechnology research on animal and human. In the case of humans and in the case of some plant species, there have been large-scale research projects going through several phases where, firstly, technology platforms necessary for the research and the development of protein analyses and bioinformatics tools have been developed. Therefore, an advance research of gene-specific study will also address the completed solution to human being to use marine origin. Some of the products already available have been derived from sponges, fish, and other organisms listed in Table 32.5.

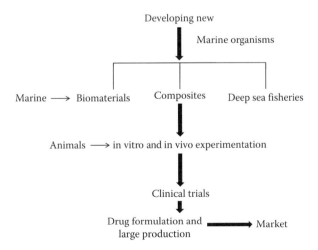

FIGURE 32.1
Marine drug development for commercialization.

TABLE 32.5

Selected Examples of Clinical Trials and Commercial Available Marine Products

S. No.	Drugs	Therapeutic Application	Company	Clinical Status	Marine Organism	Reference
1	Ara-A nucleoside	Herpes simplex virus infections—inhibits viral replication (virostatic agent)	—	Approved	Sponge	Haefner (2003)
	Ara-C nucleoside	Leukemia—inhibits tumor growth (cytostatic agent)	—	Approved	Sponge	
	Ecteinascidin 743 alkaloid	Soft tissue sarcomas, malignant connective tissue tumors—obstructs tumor drug resistance	—	Approved	Tunicate	
	Hydramacin peptide	To fight penicillin-resistant bacteria—antimicrobial effect	—	Not yet approved	Fresh water polyp	
	Ziconotide peptide	Painkiller—obstructs ion channels	—	Approved	Sea snail	
2	Orthopedic implant	Bone grafting	—	Approved	Coral (Family *Isididae*)	Yogesh and Tarun (2010)
	A-Kainic acid	Antiparasitic	—		*Digenia simplex*	
	Okadaic acid	Molecular probe	—		*Prorocentrum belizeanum*	
	Polyketide synthase	Enzyme	—		*Pseudoceratina clavata*	
	Prialt™	Analgesic	—		*Conus magus*	
	Topsentin, Tsistsixenicin A, 3-one	Anti-inflammatory	—		*Spongosporites ruetzleri, Capenella thyrsoidea, Alcyonium valdivae*	
	Sualimine, KRN 7000, Eleutherobin, E7389, Discodermolide	Anticancer	—		Shark, *Agelas mauritianus, Eleutherobia* sp. *Halicondria okadai, Discodermia dissolute*	
	Manzamine A	Antimalarial	—		*Haliclona* sp.	
	Cephalosporins	Antimicrobial	—		*Cephalosporium acremonium*	
	Didemnin B	Antiviral	—		*Tethya crypta*	

No.	Product	Application	Status/Company	Discoverer/Source	Source organism	Reference
3	Biocoral	Bone implant	Available	Inoteb	*Porites, Acropora, Lobophyllia, Montastrea, Dichocoenia*	Clarke et al. (2011)
	ProOsten 200R	Bone implant	Available	Biomet	*Porites*	
	ProOsteon 500R	Bone graft	Available	Biomet	*Goniopora*	
	Algipore	Bone graft	Available	Biomet	*Corallina officinalis*	
4	Conotoxins	Chronic pain	Phase I/II/III	DENTSPLY Friadent	Cone snail	Narsinh et al. (2005)
	GTS21	Alzheimer's disease	Phase I/II	—	Nemertine worm	
	LAF389	Cancer	Phase I	—	Sponge	
	Yondelis™		Phase II/III	—	Sea squirt	
	Dolastatin		Phase II		Sea Slug	
	ILX651		Phase I		Sea slug	
	Cemadotin		Phase II		Sea slug	
	HTI286		Phase I		Sponge	
	Aplidin™		Phase II		Sea squirt	
	Squalamine lactate		Phase II		Shark	
	IPL512602 (steroid)	Inflammation, asthma	Phase II	—	Sponge	
5	Kahalalide F	Antitumor	PharmaMar S.A.	Scheuer, University Illinois	*Elysia rufescens*	Pomponi (2001)
	Isohomohalichondrin B		PharmaMar S.A.	Munro and Blunt, University of Canterbury, New Zealand	*Lissodendoryx* sp.	
	Thiocoraline		PharmaMar S.A.	Canedo, Spain	*Micromonospora marina*	
	Isogranulatimide		Kinetik, Canada	Andersen and Bjerinck, University of British Columbia and Brazil	*Didemnum granulatum*	
	Bengamide		Novartis	California, Santa Cruz	*Jaspis* sp.	

(continued)

TABLE 32.5 (continued)

Selected Examples of Clinical Trials and Commercial Available Marine Products

S. No.	Drugs	Therapeutic Application	Company	Clinical Status	Marine Organism	Reference
6	Vent® DNA polymerase	Polymerase chain reaction			Deep-sea hydrothermal vent bacterium	Pomponi (1999)
	Formulaid®	Fatty acids as additives in infant formula nutrition supplement	Martek Biosciences		Marine microalga	
	Aequorin	Bioluminescent calcium inhibitor			Jellyfish, *Aequorea victoria*	
	GFP	Reporter gene			Jellyfish, *Aequorea victoria*	
	Phycoerythrin	Conjugated antibodies used in ELISAs and flow cytometry			Red algar	
	Resilience® (Estee Lauder)	Marine extracts additive in cosmetics			Caribbean gorgonian, *Pseudopterogorgia elisabethae*	

32.10 Conclusions

As discussed in this chapter, the outmost potential in the area of marine natural products used as drug delivery system which covers a range of pharmaceutical and medical region (leukemia, cancer, anti-infection, inflammation, regeneration, etc.). In this view, ocean and sea has got a huge variety of metabolites and curable medicines for medical application. Therefore, once we develop a proper documentation of these drugs in the aspects of molecular and genetic level, with the available reports, there is a brighter chance that marine generated drugs will entre in the global markets as one of the most important value added products for mankind in health scenario.

References

Anderson, J.M. 1996. Biomaterials and medical implant science: Present and future perspectives: A summary report. *Journal of Biomedical Materials Research* 32: 143–147.

Anselme, K. 2000. Osteoblast adhesion on biomaterials. *Biomaterials* 21(7): 667–681.

Beja, O., L. Aravind, E.V. Koonin et al. 2000. Bacterial bacteriorhodopsin: Evidence for light-driven proton pumping in the sea. *Science* 289: 1902–1906.

Béjà, O., E.N. Spudich, J.L. Spudich, M. Leclere, and E.F. DeLong. 2001. Proteorhodopsin phototrophy in the ocean. *Nature* 411: 786–789.

Bentley, R. 1997. Microbial secondary metabolites play important roles in medicine: Prospects for discovery of new drugs. *Perspectives in Biology and Medicine* 40: 364–394.

Brittberg, M., A. Lindahl, A. Nilsson, C. Ohlsson, O. Isaksson, and L. Peterson. 1994. Treatment of deep cartilage defects in the knee with autologous chondrocyte transplantation. *The New England Journal of Medicine* 331(14): 889–895.

Bull, A.T., A.C. Ward, and M. Goodfellow. 2000. Search and discovery strategies for biotechnology: The paradigm shift. *Microbiology and Molecular Biology Reviews* 64: 573–606.

Chunlin, Y., P.J. Hillas, J.A. Buez et al. 2004. The application of recombinant human collagen in tissue engineering. *BioDrugs* 18: 103–119.

Clarke, K.M., G.C. Lantz, S.K. Salisbury, S.F. Badylak, M.C. Hiles, and S.L. Voytik. 1996. Intestine submucosa and polypropylene mesh for abdominal wall repair in dogs. *Journal of Surgical Research* 60: 107–114.

Clarke, S.A., P. Walsh, C.A. Maggs, and F. Buchanan. 2011. Designs from the deep: Marine organisms for bone tissue engineering. *Biotechnology Advances* 29: 610–617.

Cragg, G.M. 1998. Paclitaxel (Taxol): A success story with valuable lessons for natural product drug discovery and development. *Medical Research Reviews* 18: 315–331.

Cragg, G.M. and D.J. Newman. 2000. Antineoplastic agents from natural sources: Achievements and future directions. *Expert Opinion on Investigational Drugs* 9: 2783–2797.

Cragg, G.M., S.A. Schepaerz, M. Suffness, and M.R. Grever. 1993. The taxol supply crisis. New NCI policies for handling the large-scale production of novel natural product anticancer and anti-HIV agents. *Natural Products* 56: 1657–1668.

De Vries, D.J. and P.M. Beart. 1995. Fishing for drugs from the sea: Status and strategies. *Trends in Pharmacological Science* 16(8): 275–279.

Du, I. and B. Shen. 2001. Biosynthesis of hybrid peptide-polyketide natural products. *Current Opinions in Drug Discovery and Development* 4: 215–228.

Faulkner, D.J. 2001. Marine natural products. *Natural Products Reports* 18: 1–49.

Felt, O., P. Buri, and R. Guthy. 1998. Chitosan: A unique polysaccharide for drug delivery. *Drug Development and Industrial Pharmacy* 24: 979–993.

Field, K.G., D. Gordon, T. Wright et al. 1997. Diversity and depth-specific distribution of SARII cluster rRNA genes from marine planktonic bacteria. *Applied and Environmental Microbiology* 63: 63–70.

Floss, H.G. 2001. Antibiotic biosynthesis: From natural to unnatural compounds. *Journal of Industrial Microbiology and Biotechnology* 27: 183–194.

Fonseca, M.J., M.A. Alsina, and F. Reig. 1996. Coating liposomes with collagen (Mr 50000) increases uptake into liver. *Biochimica et Biophysica Acta* 1279(2): 259–265.

Fuhrman, J.A., K. Mc Callum, and A.A. Davis. 1995. Phylogenetic diversity of subsurface marine microbial communities from the Atlantic and Pacific oceans. *Applied and Environmental Microbiology* 61: 4517.

Gerwick, W.H. and N. Sitachitta. 2000. Nitrogen containing metabolites from marine bacteria. In *The Alkaloids*, G. Cordell (Ed.). Academic Press, San Diego, CA, pp. 239–285.

Gerwick, W.H., L.T. Tan, and N. Sitachitta. 2001. Nitrogen containing metabolites from marine cyanobacteria. In *The Alkaloids*, G. Cordell (Ed.). Academic Press, San Diego, CA, pp. 75–184.

Guo, X.D., Q.X. Zheng, J.Y. Du et al. 2002. Molecular tissue engineering concepts, status and challenge. *Journal of Wuhan University of Technology* 17: 30–34.

Guoping, C., S. Takashi, U. Takashi, O. Naoyuki, and T. Tetsuya. 2004. Tissue engineering of cartilage using a hybrid scaffold of synthetic polymer and collagen. *Tissue Engineering* 10(3–4): 323–330.

Gupta, D., J. Venugopal, S. Mitra, V.R.G. Dev, and S. Ramakrishana. 2009. Nanostructured biocomposite substrates by electrospinning and electrospraying for the mineralization of osteoblasts. *Biomaterial* 30(11): 2085–2094.

Haefner, B. 2003. Drugs from the deep: Marine natural products as drug candidates. *Drug Discovery Today* 8: 536–544.

Huade, L., Z. Qiang, X. Yuxiang, F. Jie, S. Zhongli, and P. Zhijun. 2009. Rat cartilage repair using nanophase PLGA/HA composite and mesenchymal stem cells. *Journal of Bioactive and Compatible Polymers* 24: 83–99.

Janes, K.A., P. Calvo, and M.J. Alonso. 2001. Polysaccharide colloidal particles as delivery systems for macromolecules. *Advanced Drug Delivery Reviews* 47: 83–97.

Khosla, C., R.S. Gokhale, J.R. Jacobsen, and D.E. Cane. 1999. Tolerance and specificity of polyketide synthases. *Annual Reviews of Biochemistry* 68: 219–253.

Laurencin, C.T., M.A. Attawia, H.E. Elgendy, and K.M. Herbert. 1996. Tissue engineered bone-regeneration using degradable polymers: The formation of mineralized matrices. *Bone* 19: 935–995.

Lee, H.C., S. Anuj, and L. Yugyung. 2001. Biomedical applications of collagen. *International Journal of Pharmaceutics* 221: 1–22.

Liu, S.Q. 2007. *Bioregenerative Engineering: Principles and Applications*. Wiley-Interscience, New York.

Loty, C., N. Forest, H. Boulekbache, T. Kokubo, and J.M. Sautier. 1997. Behavior of fetal rat chondrocytes cultured on a bioactive glass ceramic. *Journal of Biomedical Material Research* 37: 137–149.

Ma, P.X. 2008. Biomimetic materials for tissue engineering. *Advanced Drug Delivery Reviews* 60(2):184–198.

Madihally, S.V. and H.W. Matthew. 1999. Porous chitosan scaffolds for tissue engineering. *Biomaterials* 20: 1133–1142.

Madison, L.L. and G.W. Huisman. 1999. Metabolic engineering of poly (3-Hydroxyalkanoates): From DNA to plastic. *Microbiology and Molecular Biology Reviews* 63: 21–53.

Maeda, M., S. Tani, A. Sano, and K. Fujioka. 1999. Microstructure and release characteristics of the minipellet, a collagen based drug delivery system for controlled release of protein drugs. *Journal of Controlled Release* 62: 313–324.

Mark, R.H., H.C. Stanley, L.S. Barbara et al. 2003. Human septal chondrocyte redifferentiation in alginate, polyglycolic acid scaffold, and monolayer culture. *The Laryngoscope* 113(1): 25–32.

Mayer, A. and V.K. Lehmann. 2001. Marine pharmacology in 1999: Antitumor and cytotoxic compounds. *Anticancer Research* 21: 2489–2500.

Mc Ginity, J.W., G.W. Cuff, and A.B. Combs. 1981. Microencapsulation of pharmaceuticals. *Australian Journal of Pharmaceutical Sciences* 10(1): 17–19.

Nakamura, N., T. Miyama, L. Engebretsen, H. Yoshikawa, and K. Shino. 2009. Cell-based therapy in articular cartilage lesions of the knee. *Arthroscopy* 25: 531–552.

Narsinh, L., N.T. Archana, and E.G.M. Werner. 2005. Marine natural products in drug delivery. *Natural Product Radiance* 4(6): 471–477.

Peter, B., B. Thomasr, K. Bodo, and R. Martin. 2006. Matrix-associated autologous chondrocyte transplantation/implantation (MACT/MACI)—5-year follow-up. *The Knee* 13: 194–202.

Pomponi, S.A. 1999. The bioprocess-technological potential of the sea. *Journal of Biotechnology* 70: 5–13.

Pomponi, S.A. 2001. The oceans and human health: The discovery and development of marine-derived drugs. *Oceanography* 14(1): 78–87.

Pope, D.G. 1978. Animal health specialized delivery systems. In *Animal Health Products, Design and Evaluation*, D.C. Monkhouse (Ed.). American Pharmaceutical Association, Washington, DC, pp. 78–114.

Ratner, B.D. and S.J. Bryant. 2004. Biomaterials: Where we have been and where we are going. *Annual Review of Biomedical Engineering* 6: 41–75.

Rohlin, I., M.K. Oh, and J.C. Liao. 2001. Microbial pathway engineering for industrial processes: Evolution, combinatorial biosynthesis and rational design. *Current Opinions in Microbiology* 4: 330.

Rossbach, M. and G. Kniewald. 1977. Concepts of marine specimen banking. *Chemosphere* 34: 1997–2010.

Sato, T., T. Ishil, and Y. Okahata. 2001. In vitro gene delivery mediated by chitosan. Effect of pH, serum and molecular mass of chitosan on the transfection efficiency. *Biomaterials* 22: 2075–2080.

Schulze, T.G., P. de Souza, C.H. Villegas et al. 2002. Redifferentiation of dedifferentiated human chondrocytes in high-density cultures. *Cell Tissue Research* 308: 371–379.

Shinichi, T., Y. Hiroshi, R.F. Julie et al. 2005. Hydrogel optimization for cultured elastic chondrocytes seeded onto a polyglycolic acid scaffold. *Journal of Biomedical Materials Research Part A* 75A(4): 907–916.

Staunton, J. and B. Wilkinson. 2001. Combinatorial biosynthesis of polyketides and nonribosomal peptides. *Current Opinion in Chemical Biology* 5: 159–164.

Steadman, J.R., K.K. Briggs, J.J. Rodrigo, M.S. Kocher, T.J. Gill, and W.G. Rodkey. 2003. Outcomes of microfracture for traumatic chondral defects of the knee: Average 11-year follow-up. *Arthroscopy* 19: 477–484.

Suh, J.K.F. and H.W.T. Matthew. 2000. Application of chitosan-based polysaccharide biomaterials in cartilage tissue engineering: A review. *Biomaterials* 21: 2589–2598.

Turner, D.M. 1996. Natural product source material use in the pharmaceutical industry: The Glaxo experience. *Journal of Ethnopharmacology* 51: 39–43.

Villar-Súarez, V., V.I. Calles, I.G. Bravo et al. 2004. Differential behavior between isolated and aggregated rabbit auricular chondrocytes on plastic surfaces. *Journal of Biomedicine and Biotechnology* 2: 86–92.

Weber, J.,N. and E.W. White. 1972. Carbon-metal graded composites for permanent osseous attachment of non-porous metals. *Materials Research Bulletin* 7: 1005–1016.

Xue, Y. and D.H. Sherman 2001. Biosynthesis and combinatorial biosynthesis of pikromycin-related macrolides in *Streptomyces venezuelae*. *Metabolic Engineering* 3: 15–26.

Yogesh, M. and A. Tarun. 2010. Marine derived pharmaceuticals-development of natural health products from marine biodiversity. *International Journal of ChemTech Research* 2(4): 2198–2217.

Yu, L., K. Dean, and K. Li. 2006. Polymer blends and composites from renewable resources. *Progress in Polymer Science* 31: 576–602.

33

Application of Marine Biomaterials for Gene Delivery

You-Kyoung Kim, Hu-Lin Jiang, Bijay Singh, Yun-Jaie Choi,
Myung-Haing Cho, Toshihiro Akaike, and Chong-Su Cho

CONTENTS

33.1 Introduction

In recent decades, gene therapy is a powerful method in curing a variety of inherited and acquired diseases by replacing defective genes, substituting missing genes, or silencing unwanted gene expression (Kabanov and Kabanov 1995). The lack of effective carriers is a major drawback to progress for clinical applications although most of the gene therapy relies on animal viral vectors because they achieve high efficiency of gene transfer in vivo and in clinical trials. However, use of animal viral vectors has several limitations such as immunogenicity, potential infectivity, inflammation to the human body, and complicated production (Smith 1995). Therefore, nonviral vectors have been rapidly receiving attention as a gene delivery system because of easy production, low immune response against the vector, and high flexibility of size of the delivered gene (Mao et al. 2010). Among nonviral vectors, lipids and polymers are by far the most widely used gene carriers because the lipoplexes are rapidly cleared from the bloodstream and widely distributed in the body (Li and Huang 1997). Cationic synthetic polymers such as polyethylenimine (PEI) (Boussif et al. 1995), poly(L-lysine) (PLL) (Wu and Wu 1987), polyamidoamine dendrimer (Haensler and Szoka1993), and poly(amino ester) (Anderson et al. 2005) have been extensively used due to the several advantages such as selection of appropriate size, conjugation with specific targeting moieties, and chemical modification although a drawback of cationic synthetic polymers as gene carriers is limited knowledge of their biological effects. Natural polymers have been widely used as nonviral vectors because they are biocompatible, less immunogenic, and less toxic. The objective of this chapter is to summarize the use of alginate, chitosan (CHI), and pullulan (PU) among marine biomaterials in delivering DNA and small interference RNA (siRNA) for clinical application in the future.

33.2 Alginate

Alginate as the primary structural component of brown seaweed is the monovalent form of alginic acid and is a linear polysaccharide of β(1→4)-linked D-mannuronic acid and (1→4)-linked L-guluronic acid as shown in Figure 33.1 (Lee and Mooney 2012). The alginate has been widely used for biomedical applications because it is less toxic, is easy to modify chemically, and undergoes gelation in the presence of divalent cations. In this section, we discuss nanoparticles, microspheres, microcapsules, and graft (g) systems using alginate for gene therapy.

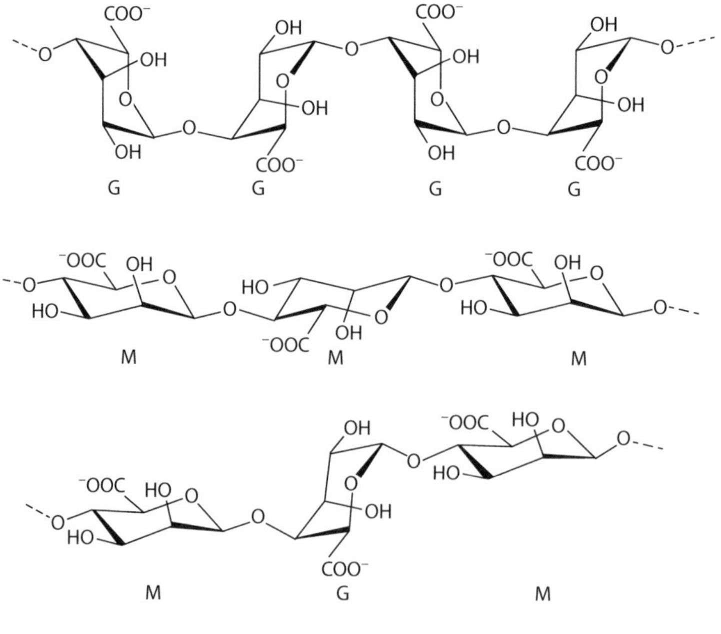

FIGURE 33.1
Chemical structures of G-block, M-block, and alternating block in alginate. (From Lee, K.Y., and Mooney, D.V., *Prog. Polym. Sci.*, 37, 108, 2012. With permission.)

33.2.1 Alginate Nanoparticles

PEI is one of the widely used nonviral carriers because it has an excellent buffering capacity toward endosomal environment. On the other hand, the PEI has high cytotoxicity although cytotoxicity of the PEI is dependent on the molecular weight (MW). Patnaik et al. (2006) prepared PEI/alginate nanoparticles to deliver siRNA into mammalian cells for reducing cytotoxicity by PEI itself. The results indicated that the PEI/alginate nanoparticles showed 80% suppression of GFP expression with lower cytotoxicity although the concentration of alginate is very critical in gene expression.

Douglas and Tabrizian (2005) prepared alginate/CHI nanoparticles as a DNA carrier by adjusting the ratio of alginate to CHI, the MW of the both polymers, and the solution pH, but they did not perform gene transfection. Hong et al. (2008) also made alginate/CHI nanoparticles to deliver smad3 antisense oligonucleotides (ASOs) on the dorsum of C57BL6 mice for accelerated wound healing. It was found that smad3 ASO-loaded alginate/CHI nanoparticles accelerated wound healing faster than other groups. Furthermore, Azizi et al. (2010) used alginate/CHI nanoparticles for release of epidermal growth factor receptor (EGFR) antisense from EGFR-loaded nanoparticles. The results showed that release of EGFR antisense lasted for about 50 h and the freeze-drying of EGFR-loaded nanoparticles did not affect release and degradation of antisense. However, they did not check gene expression.

Recently, Zhao et al. (2012) prepared alginate/$CaCO_3$/DNA nanoparticles to decrease particle sizes and to stabilize $CaCO_3$/DNA nanoparticles. It was found that the gene transfections in 293T and HeLa cells were significantly enhanced by adding alginate to the $CaCO_3$/DNA nanoparticles due to the improved delivery efficiency with the modification of alginate.

33.2.2 Alginate Microspheres

The most common method to prepare alginate microspheres from an aqueous alginate solution is to mix the solution with divalent cations as the cross-linking agents although the divalent cations bind solely to guluronate blocks of the alginate chains as the eggbox model of cross-linking (Grant et al. 1973). Ionically cross-linked alginate microspheres efficiently encapsulate DNA under mild conditions, and the release of DNA from alginate microspheres can be controlled.

Mittal et al. (2001) loaded pMNe-gal-SV40 as a DNA vaccine into alginate microspheres for induction of protective immune responses with DNA on mice. Systemic routes of immunization showed higher β-galactosidase or bovine adenovirus type 3 (BAd3)-specific IgG enzyme-linked immunosorbent assay (ELISA) titers compared to those obtained by mucosal routes of inoculation.

Sone et al. (2002) used alginate microspheres to deliver modified green fluorescent protein gene CaMV35S-sGFP to protoplasts isolated from cultured tobacco cells. About 10-fold higher GFP expression was obtained after 24 h incubation using alginate microspheres compared to naked DNA. However, the transfection efficiency by the alginate microspheres was only 0.22%.

Mierisch et al. (2003) used alginate microspheres to deliver transgenic chondrocytes labeled with enhanced GFP in the rabbit knees for application cartilage of repair. Alginate microspheres promoted expression of cartilage-specific genes and allowed delivery of chondrocytes into osteochondral defects, suggesting the possibility of transgenic chondrocyte delivery by alginate microspheres.

Zachos et al. (2006) studied the potency of adenovirus (Ad) transduction of bone marrow-derived mesenchymal stem cells (BMDMSC) with bone morphogenetic proteins (BMP)-2 and BMP-6 in alginate microspheres. The results indicated that transduction of BMDMSC with Ad-BMP-2 or Ad-BMP-6 accelerated osteogenic differentiation and mineralization of stem cells in alginate microspheres. They also used mesenchymal stem cells (MSC) transduced with BMP-2 in alginate microspheres to promote bone and cartilage repair in nude rats (Zachos et al. 2007). At day 14, only Ad-BMP-2 stem cells in alginate microspheres by direct injection to the rats showed completely healed osteotomies.

de las Heras et al. (2010) encapsulated pDNA-VP2 vaccine for infectious pancreatic necrosis virus (IPNV) in alginate microspheres to avoid the aggressive gastrointestinal conditions experienced after oral administration in fish. The results indicated that the vaccine induced innate immune responses, raising the expression of IFN more than 10-fold by alginate microspheres compared to the empty plasmid.

33.2.3 Alginate Microcapsules

Alginate microspheres prepared by ionic cross-linking between alginate and divalent cations have critical drawback of limited long-term stability in physiological conditions due to exchange reactions with monovalent cations. Moreover, the calcium ions released from the alginate microspheres may promote hemostasis (Lee and Mooney 2012). Therefore, cationic polymers such as CHI and PLL have been used to make alginate microcapsules after coating with cationic polymers.

Xu et al. (2002) entrapped inducible nitride oxide synthase gene (iNOS)-expressing cells within alginate/PLL microcapsules to deliver to tumor sites in a nude mouse model for tumor killing. The results indicated that delivery of these iNOS-expressing cells within these microcapsules to tumors formed from human ovarian cancer SKOV-3 resulted in 100% tumor killing due to the generation of sustainable high concentrations of NO and reactive nitrogen species at tumor sites.

Garcia-Martin et al. (2002) enclosed mouse C_2C_{12} myoblasts and Madin–Darby canine kidney (MDCK) epithelial cells transduced with MFG-FVIII vector into alginate microcapsules and implanted them into mice intraperitoneally to prevent cell immune rejections. It was found that plasma of mice receiving C_2C_{12} and encapsulated MDCK cells had transient therapeutic levels of FVIII in immunocompetent $C_{57}BL/6$ mice.

Zheng et al. (2003) encapsulated NIH3T3 cells modified with murine interleukine-12 (mIL-12) gene into alginate microcapsules and implanted them in tumor-bearing mice to explore the antitumor immunity. The microencapsulated NIH3T3-mIL-12 cells released mIL-12 continuously and stably for a long time. Moreover, mIL-12 released from the microencapsulated NIH3T3-mIL-12 cells resulted in a significant inhibition of tumor proliferation.

Barsoum et al. (2003) encapsulated MDCK cells genetically modified to express either human growth hormone or canine α-iduronidase in alginate/PLL/alginate microcapsules and implanted them into the dog brain to cure neurodegenerative disease. The delivery of both gene products was extremely low and extensive inflammatory reactions were observed.

Cirone et al. (2002) encapsulated non-autologous mouse myoblasts (C_2C_{12}) modified to secrete IL-2 linked to the Fv region of a humanized antibody with affinity to HER-2/*neu* into alginate/PLL/alginate microcapsules and implanted them into a mouse model bearing HER-2/*neu*-positive tumors to suppress tumor. Treatment with these encapsulated cells led to a delay in tumor progression and prolonged survival of the animals.

Madry et al. (2005) encapsulated lapine articular chondrocytes transfected with expression plasmid vectors containing the cDNA for the *Escherichia coli lacZ* gene or the human insulin-like growth factor I (IGF-I) gene into alginate microcapsules and implanted them into osteochondral defects in the trochlear groove of rabbits to repair full-thickness cartilage defects. The transplantation of IGF-I implants improved articular cartilage repair and accelerated the formation of the subchondral bone compared to *lacZ* implants.

Zhang et al. (2006) encapsulated colon carcinoma (CT26) and Lewis lung carcinoma (LL/2c) murine cells transfected with plasmid-borne monokine induced by interferon-γ (pORF-MIG) and cisplatin into alginate microcapsules and implanted them into CT26 colon carcinoma tumor model mice to get thymus-dependent antitumor effects. The results indicated that the combination of pORF-MIG plus cisplatin showed inhibition of angiogenesis and induction of apoptosis or CTL activity.

Ding et al. (2007) encapsulated BMP-2 gene-modified MSCs in alginate/PLL/alginate microcapsules to induce bone formation. It was found that the gene products from the encapsulated BMP-2 cells induced the undifferentiated MSCs to osteoblasts with higher alkaline phosphatase activity compared to control group.

33.2.4 Alginate–Graft–PEI System

Alginate itself cannot be complexed with gene because it does not have any positive charges. Recently, He et al. (2012) prepared alginate-g-PEI by grafting low MW PEI (MW:2000) onto oxidized alginate through Schiff-base reaction and evaluated it as a gene carrier in vitro. The alginate-g-PEI showed higher transfection efficiency than PEI 25 K as a control with lower cytotoxicity. However, they did not check cytotoxicity as the same N/P ratios as gene expression experiment.

33.3 Chitosan

Among natural polymers, CHI and CHI derivatives have been mostly used as gene carriers because they are biocompatible, biodegradable, less immunogenic, and less toxic, carrying positive charges as shown in Figure 33.2 (Onishi and Machida 1999). The CHI obtained by deacetylation of chitin is consisted of repeating β(1→4)-linked D-glucosamine and N-acetyl-D-glucosamine. In this section, only pH-sensitive modification of CHI as the gene carrier will be covered due to the page limitation because one of the critical causes of poor transfection efficiency by CHI across intracellular delivery is inefficient release of gene in CHI/gene complexes from endosomes into the cytoplasm (Park et al. 2003).

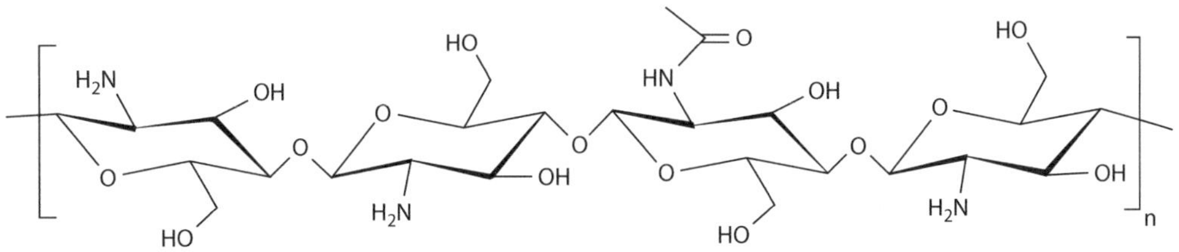

FIGURE 33.2
Chemical structures of CHI. (From Onishi, H. and Machida, Y., *Biomaterials*, 20, 176, 1999. With permission.)

We discuss PEI, imidazole, and spermine (SP) as pH-sensitive groups incorporated into CHI to give buffering capacity.

33.3.1 Chitosan–Graft–PEI

PEI has been used as golden standard among nonviral vectors because it has a high buffering capacity in an endosome and facilitates endosomal escape to the cytoplasm although high MW PEI is very cytotoxic in vitro and in vivo. On the other hand, low MW PEI is less cytotoxic with lower transfection efficiency. Therefore, many researchers have tried to introduce low MW PEI to the CHI through degradable linkages.

Wong et al. (2006) first synthesized PEI-g-CHI through cationic polymerization of aziridine as a monomer by low MW CHI and evaluated it as a gene carrier. The PEI-g-CHI showed higher transfection efficiency than PEI 25 K in vitro and in vivo with lower cytotoxicity due to a synergistic effect of PEI having a buffer capacity and CHI having biocompatibility.

Jiang et al. (2007a) prepared CHI-g-PEI differently through an imine reaction between low MW PEI and oxidized CHI as shown in Figure 33.3. The CHI-g-PEI also showed higher transfection efficiency in three different cell lines than PEI 25 K with lower cytotoxicity.

Lu et al. prepared *N*-maleated CHI (NMC)-g-PEI (Lu et al. 2008) and *N*-succinyl CHI (NSC)-g-PEI (Lu et al. 2009) through grafting of low MW PEI to NMC and NSC, respectively. The NMC-g-PEI showed higher transfection efficiency in 293T and HeLa cells than PEI 25 K although the particle sizes of NMC-g-PEI/DNA complexes were 200–400 nm. The transfection efficiency of NSC-g-PEI was higher than that of PEI 25 K and the transfection was not affected by the presence of serum.

Lou et al. (2009) prepared PEI-g-CHI using ethylene glycol diglycidyl ether as a spacer to increase water solubility and transfection efficiency of CHI. The PEI-g-CHI showed higher transfection efficiency even at high weight ratios of PEI-g-CHI to DNA with lower cytotoxicity.

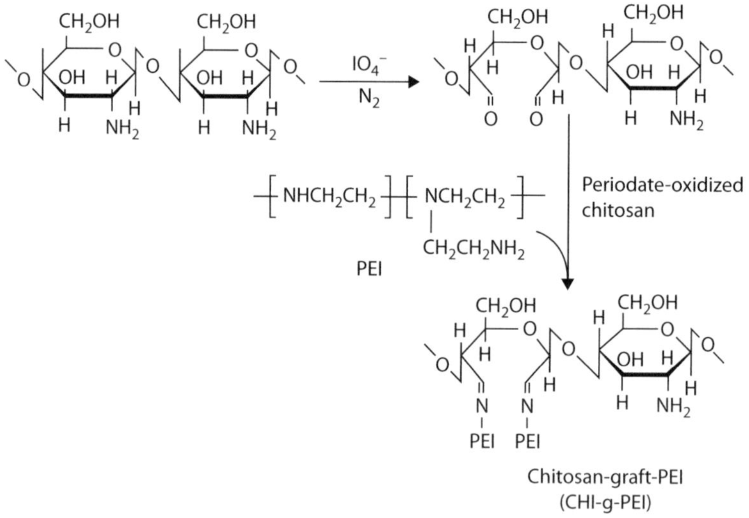

FIGURE 33.3
Proposed reaction scheme for synthesis of CHI-g-PEI. (From Jiang, H.L. et al., *J. Control. Release*, 117, 274, 2007a. With permission.)

Gao et al. (2010) used 1,1′-carbonyldiimidazole as another linking agent between CHI and low MW PEI to prepare CHI-g-PEI. The CHI-g-PEI showed higher transfection efficiency in three different cancer cells than PEI 25 K with lower cytotoxicity and suppressed tumor growth rate when mice was inoculated with the CCL22 gene owing to the rapid escape of the carrier from endosome to the cytoplasm.

Zhang et al. (2010) synthesized poly(ethylene glycol) (PEG)-g-CHI-g-PEI through polymerization of aziridine by PEG-g-CHI prepared by reaction between activated PEG and CHI to increase water solubility and transfection efficiency of CHI. The PEG-g-CHI-g-PEI showed higher transfection efficiency than PEI 25 K with lower cytotoxicity, and the transfection efficiency was not affected by serum due to the PEG in the carrier.

Jere et al. (2009) used CHI-g-PEI for delivery of Akt1 siRNA to A549 cells. The CHI-g-PEI efficiently delivered Akt1 siRNA and silenced oncoprotein Akt1 in A549 cells than PEI 25 K. The silencing of cell survival protein significantly increased apoptosis of A549 cells and decreased lung cancer proliferation malignancy and metastasis of the cells as shown in the schematic representation of Figure 33.4.

Recently, Ping et al. (2011) prepared CHI–g–PEI–β-cyclodextrin (CD) through reductive amination between oxidized CHI and low MW PEI-modified β-CD to deliver siRNA in HEK293 and L929 cell lines. Gene silencing activity mediated by CHI-g-PEI-β-CD showed

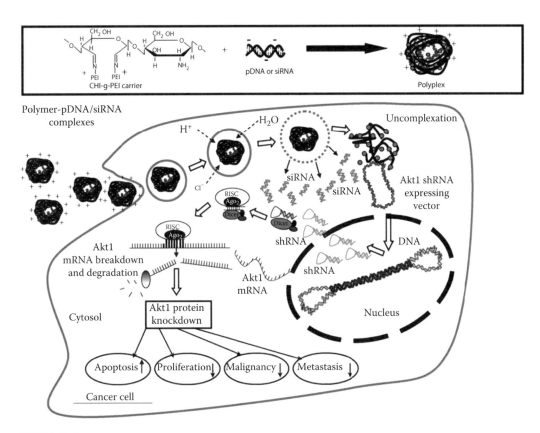

FIGURE 33.4
Schematic representation of oncogene Akt1-targeted shRNA and siRNA delivery to cancer cell using CHI-g-PEI carrier and its consequences on cancer cell survival. (From Jere, D. et al., *Int. J. Pharm.*, 378, 195, 2009. With permission.)

higher knockdown effect in both cells than PEI 25 K with lower cytotoxicity. Moreover, the pendent β-CD in the carrier allowed the supramolecular PEGylation though self-assembly of adamantyl-modified PEG with the β-CD moieties. The supramolecular PEGylation of the polyplexes significantly improved their stability under physiological conditions although there are many steps to prepare the carrier.

33.3.2 Imidazole-Modified Chitosan

Imidazole-containing nonviral vectors have been used as gene carriers because they have buffering capacity and enhance release of complexes into the cytoplasm following adsorptive pinocytosis (Wang et al. 2008).

Kim et al. (2003) coupled urocanic acid (UA) having imidazole group with CHI to have buffering capacity in the modified CHI as shown in Figure 33.5. The UA-modified CHI (UAC) increased about 1000-fold transfection efficiency in 293T cells than CHI itself due to the buffering capacity in the endosomal compartment. They also delivered gene into a K-ras null lung cancer model mouse through nose-only inhalation by UAC (Jin et al. 2006). The UAC/PDCD4 complex suppressed tumor angiogenesis and facilitated apoptosis compared to vector control. Furthermore, they delivered phosphatase and tensin homologue deleted on chromosome 10 (PTEN) into a K-ras lung cancer model mouse through an aerosol route (Jin et al. 2008). The UAC/PTEN complex suppressed lung tumors through Akt-related signal pathways as well as cell cycle arrest.

Wang delivered p53 gene into HepG2 in vitro and into BALB/c nude mice through intra-tumoral injection by UAC (Wang et al. 2008). The UAC/p53 gene complex induced apoptosis by inhibition of HepG2 growth in vitro and suppressed tumor growth in vivo.

Ghosn et al. (2008) coupled imidazole acetic acid (IAA) with CHI to increase water solubility and buffering capacity of CHI. IAA-coupled CHI mediated a 100-fold increase of transfection efficiency compared to CHI itself due to the buffering capacity of imidazole group. Moreira et al. (2009) also prepared IAA-coupled CHI. The transfection efficiency by the IAA-coupled CHI was dependent on the degree of substitution of IAA.

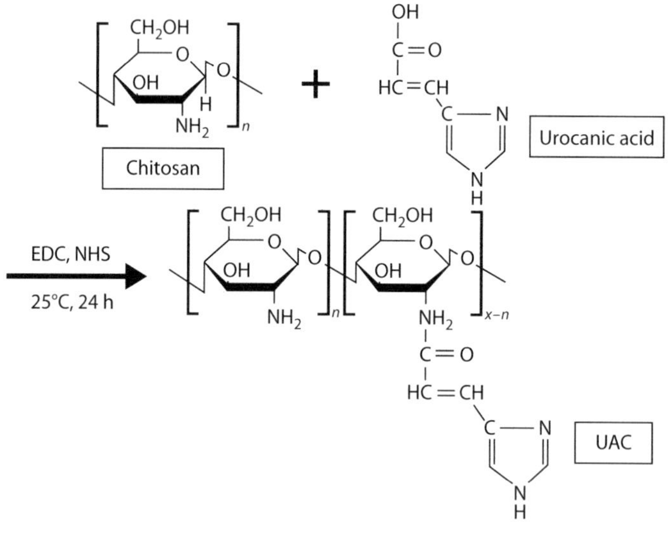

FIGURE 33.5
Synthetic scheme of UAC. (From Kim, T.H. et al., *J. Control. Release*, 93, 393, 2003. With permission.)

IAA-coupled CHI with 22.1% of substitution enhanced β-galactosidase expression in 293T and HepG2 cells.

Chang et al. (2010) introduced histidine into CHI through disulfide bonds between 2-iminothiolane-modified CHI and histidine–cysteine. The histidine-introduced CHI showed enhanced cellular uptake of gene and higher gene expression than CHI due to the buffering capacity of introduced histidine. They also introduced fourth-generation lysine–histidine dendrons to CHI to promote its endosomal escape property (Chang et al. 2011). The gene transfection efficiency of dendron-modified CHI in HEK293 cells was higher than that of CHI due to the high buffering capacity.

Recently, Shi et al. (2012) prepared *N*-imidazolyl-*O*-carboxymethyl CHI to increase water solubility and transfection efficiency of CHI. The polymer was soluble in a wide pH range (4–10) and showed higher transfection efficiency in HEK293 cells than CHI although the transfection efficiency was dependent on the degree of imidazolyl substitution.

Ghosn et al. (2010) delivered glyceraldehyde 3-phosphate dehydrogenase (GAPDH) siRNA to the mouse via either intravenous (IV) or intranasal routes by PEGylated IAA-modified CHI. The PEGylated IAA-modified CHI/GAPDH siRNA complexes significantly knocked down GAPDH enzyme in both lung and liver of mouse after IV delivery.

33.3.3 Chitosan–Graft–Spermine

SP is a tetra-amine with two primary and two secondary amino groups involved in cellular metabolism and is present in all eukaryotic cells (Allen 1983). It reversibly condenses DNA and has a high buffering effect due to the secondary amine in it.

Recently, Jiang et al. (2011) prepared a CHI-g-SP through an imine reaction between periodate-oxidized CHI and SP to improve transfection efficiency of CHI as shown in Figure 33.6. The CHI-g-SP showed higher transfection efficiency than CHI with lower cytotoxicity.

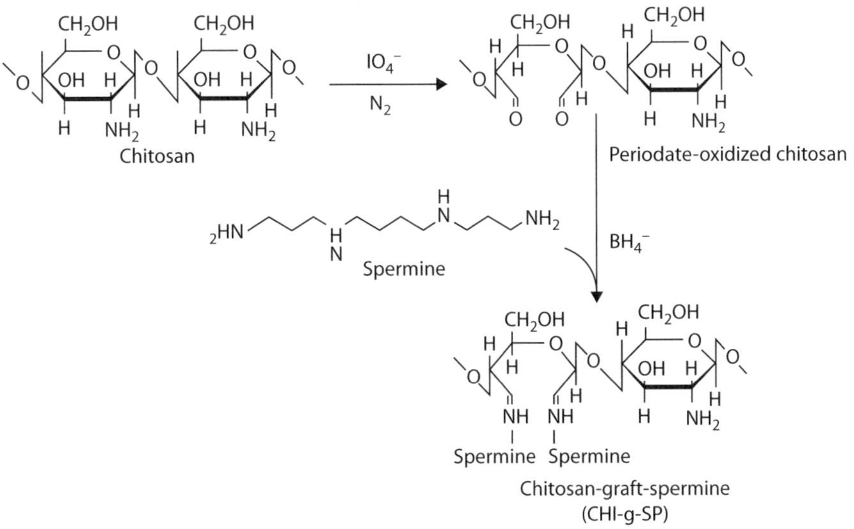

FIGURE 33.6
Proposed reaction scheme for synthesis of CHI-g-SP. (From Jiang, H.L. et al., *Eur. J. Pharm. Biopharm.*, 77, 38, 2011. With permission.)

Alex et al. (2011) introduced SP into galactosylated CHI to increase transfection efficiency and to target in liver as dual purpose because the galactose ligand recognized asialogly-coprotein receptors on the hepatocytes (Jiang et al. 2007b). The galactosylated CHI-g-SP showed higher transfection efficiency in HepG2 cells through receptor-mediated internalization mechanism.

33.4 Pullulan

PU is a water-soluble and neutral linear polysaccharide consisting of maltotriose units connected by an $\alpha(1\rightarrow4)$ glycosidic bond, whereas consecutive maltotriose units are connected to each other by an $\alpha(1\rightarrow6)$ glycosidic bond as shown in Figure 33.7 (Cheng et al. 2011). The PU is purified from the fermentation medium of the *Aureobasidium pullulans* isolated from marine environments (Mishra et al. 2011). The PU has been used as the gene carrier because it is biocompatible, nontoxic, and non-immunogenic.

33.4.1 Pullulan Conjugation Based on Metal Coordination

Hosseinkhani et al. (2002) introduced triethylenetetramine (TE), diethylenetriamine pentaacetic acid (DP), and SP to PU to deliver DNA containing Zn^{2+} ions to obtain conjugate of PU derivatives and DNA with Zn^{2+} coordination and injected them to mice through IV injection. The PU derivatives/DNA conjugates with Zn^{2+} coordination significantly enhanced gene expression in the liver than free DNA because the PU has high affinity to the liver cells (Kaneo et al. 2001).

33.4.2 PU–Graft–SP

Tabata and his coworkers prepared PU-g-SP by reaction of hydroxyl groups of PU and amine ones of SP to deliver p53 gene into T24 cells (Kanatani et al. 2006). The PU-g-SP suppressed in vitro proliferation of T24 cells through clathrin- and raft/caveolae-dependent

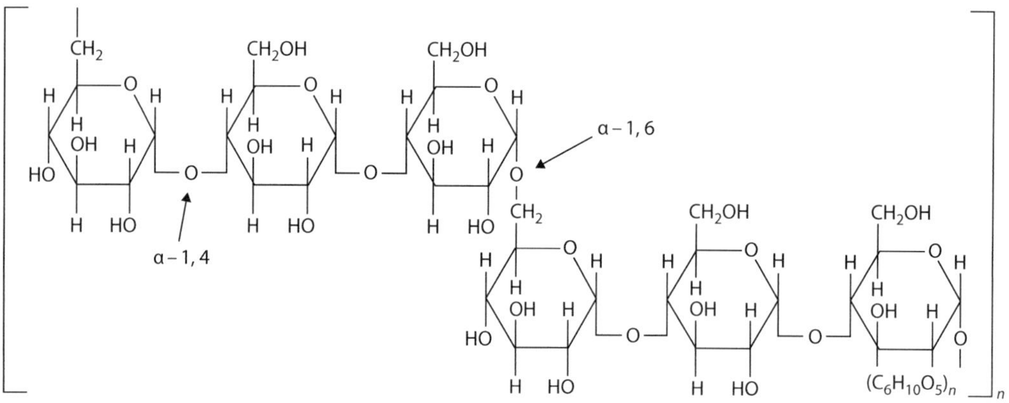

FIGURE 33.7
Structure of PU. (From Cheng, K.C., Demirci, A., and Catchmark, J.M., *Appl. Microbiol. Biotechnol.*, 92, 30, 2011. With permission.)

endocytotic pathways. The gene expression by the PU-g-SP was dependent on the percent SP introduced (Jo et al. 2007a) and MW of PU (Jo et al. 2007b) in the PU-g-SP. They also delivered neuronal gene in rat sensory neuron cell line by PU-g-SP (Thakor et al. 2009). Interestingly, the transfection efficiency by the PU-g-SP was highest for anionic complexes with lower cytotoxicity, which is different from general polycationic vectors although its mechanism is not clear. Furthermore, they delivered the mouse Notch intracellular domain (NICD) gene into bone marrow stromal cells (BMSCs) to induce dopamine-producing neuronal cells using PU-g-SP-mediated reverse transfection method (Nagane et al. 2009). It was found that introduced exogenous plasmid genes were successfully transcribed and expressed as proteins in the cytoplasm of BMSCs with lower cytotoxicity, and finally the differentiation of induced neuronal cells into dopamine-producing cells was promoted. In addition, they delivered gene into rat mesenchymal stromal cells seeded into the gelatin scaffold by the PU-g-SP (Kido et al. 2011). The results indicated that the transfection efficiency depended on the method of complex-containing scaffold preparation, suggesting that cells were transfected with the complexes released from the scaffold.

Recently, Thomsen et al. (2011) delivered plasmid DNA bearing cDNA encoding human growth hormone 1 (hGH1) in brain capillary endothelial cells to secrete protein from brain by the PU-g-SP. The transfection of human brain microvascular endothelial cells with PU-g-SP/DNA complexes led to secretion of hGH1 protein into the growth medium.

33.4.3 PU–Graft–Diethylaminoethyl

San Juan et al. (2007a) prepared PU–graft–diethylaminoethyl (DE) to deliver a plasmid expressing a secreted form of alkaline phosphatase (pSEAP) in smooth muscle cells. The PU-g-DE showed 150-fold SEAP activity than pSEAP alone. The phosphorus oxychloride-cross-linked PU-g-DE 3D matrices protected pSEAP from DNase I degradation and showed high gene transfer without cell toxicity. They also delivered DNA in vascular smooth muscle cells (VSMCs) by the tubular PU-g-DE hydrogel (San Juan et al. 2007b). The transfection in VSMCs was dependent on DE in the PU-g-DE. Furthermore, they used PU-g-DE hydrogel for the coating of stent to deliver siRNA targeted to MMP2 in vascular cells (San Juan et al. 2009). The PU-g-DE hydrogel loaded with siRNA in rabbit balloon-injured carotid arteries induced an uptake of siRNA into the arterial wall and a decrease of pro-MMP2 activity.

33.4.4 PU–Graft–Glycidyl Trimethyl Ammonium

Rekha and Sharma (2009) prepared PU–graft–glycidyl trimethyl ammonium (GT) by reaction of GT and PU to deliver gene in vitro on hepatocytes and in vivo on mice. The PU-g-GT showed high transfection efficiency on HepG2 cells and high liver binding affinity in mice due to the specificity of PU for liver.

33.4.5 PU–Graft–PEI

Recently, Rekha and Sharma (2011) prepared PU-g-PEI by reaction of PU-succinimidyl carbonate and PEI for liver cell gene delivery. The PU-g-PEI showed comparable transfection efficiency to PEI 25 K through ASGPR of the hepatocytes with good hemocompatibility and lower toxicity although they used high MW PEI instead of low MW PEI.

33.5 Summary

As discussed in this chapter, alginate, CHI, and PU among marine biomaterials have been covered as nonviral vectors for gene delivery system. A number of in vitro and in vivo studies on CHI and CHI derivatives as nonviral carriers have been used than alginate and PU. More continued development of structure–gene function relationships and fundamental studies on cellular processes in vitro and in vivo as well as quality control should be necessary for future development of marine biomaterials as gene carriers. Also, most studies performed by far have only been conducted using in vitro and in animal models. Therefore, additional preclinical studies need to be performed for application in clinical trials.

References

Alex, S. M., M. R. Rekha, and C. P. Sharma. 2011. Spermine grafted galactosylated chitosan for improved nanoparticle mediated gene delivery. *International Journal of Pharmaceutics* 410:125–137.

Allen, J. C. 1983. Biochemistry of the polyamines. *Cell Biochemistry and Function* 1:131–140.

Anderson, D. G., A. Akinc, N. Hossain, and R. Langer. 2005. Structure/property studies of polymeric gene delivery using a library of poly(beta-amino esters). *Molecular Therapy* 11:426–434.

Azizi, E., A. Namazi, I. Haririan, S. Fouladdel, M. R. Khoshayand, P. Y. Shotorbani, A. Nomani, and T. Gazori. 2010. Release profile and stability evaluation of optimized chitosan/alginate nanoparticles as EGFR antisense vector. *International Journal of Nanomedicine* 5:455–461.

Barsoum, S. C., W. Milgrram, W. Mackay, C. Coblentz, K. H. Delaney, J. M. Kwiecien, S. A. Kruth, and P. L. Chang. 2003. Delivery of recombinant gene product to canine brain with the use of microencapsulation. *Journal of Laboratory and Clinical Medicine* 142:399–413.

Boussif, O., F. Lezoualc'h, M. A. Zanta, M. D. Mergny, D. Scherman, B. Demeneix, and J. P. Behr. 1995. A versatile vector for gene and oligonucleotide transfer into cells in culture and *in vivo*: polyethylenimine. *Proceedings of the National Academy of Sciences of the United States of America* 92:7297–7301.

Chang, K. L., Y. Higuchi, S. Kawakami, F. Yamashita, and M. Hashida. 2010. Efficient gene transfection by histidine-modified chitosan through enhancement of endosomal escape. *Bioconjugate Chemistry* 21:1087–1095.

Chang, K. L., Y. Higuchi, S. Kawakami, F. Yamashita, and M. Hashida. 2011. Development of lysine-histidine dendron modified chitosan for improving transfection efficiency in HEK293 cells. *Journal of Controlled Release* 156:195–202.

Cheng, K. C., A. Demirci, and J. M. Catchmark. 2011. Pullulan: Biosynthesis, production, and applications. *Applied Microbiology and Biotechnology* 92:29–44.

Cirone, P., J. M. Bourgeois, R. C. Austine, and P. L. Chang. 2002. A novel approach to tumor suppression with microencapsulated recombinant cells. *Human Gene Therapy* 13:1157–1166.

Ding, H. F., R. Liu, B. G. Li, J. R. Lou, K. R. Dai, and T. T. Tang. 2007. Biologic effect and immunoisolating behavior of BMP-2 gene-transfected bone marrow-derived mesenchymal stem cells in APA microcapsules. *Biochemical and Biophysical Research Communications* 362:923–927.

Douglas, K. L. and M. Tabrizian. 2005. Effect of experimental parameters on the formation of alginate-chitosan nanoparticles and evaluation of their potential application as DNA carrier. *Journal of Biomaterials Science, Polymer Edition* 16:43–56.

Gao, J. Q., Q. Q. Zhao, T. F. Lv, W. P. Shuai, J. Zhou, G. P. Tang, W. Q. Liang, Y. Tabata, and Y. L. Hu. 2010. Gene-carried chitosan-linked-PEI induced high gene transfection efficiency with low toxicity and significant tumor-suppressive activity. *International Journal of Pharmaceutics* 387:286–294.

Garcia-Martin, C., M. K. Chuah, A. Van Damme, K. E. Robinson, B. Vanzieleghem, J. M. Saint-Remy, D. Gallardo, F. A. Ofosu, T. Vandendriessche, and G. Hortelano. 2002. Therapeutic levels of human factor VIII in mice implanted with encapsulated cells: Potential for gene therapy of haemophilia A. *The Journal of Gene Medicine* 4:215–223.

Ghosn, B., S. P. Kasturi, and K. Roy. 2008. Enhancing polysaccharide-mediated delivery of nucleic acids through functionalization with secondary and tertiary amines. *Current Topics in Medicinal Chemistry* 8:331–340.

Ghosn, B., A. Singh, M. Li, A. V. Vlassov, C. Burnett, N. Puri, and K. Roy. 2010. Efficient gene silencing in lungs and liver using imidazole-modified chitosan as nanocarrier for small interfering RNA. *Oligonucleotides* 20:163–172.

Grant, G. T., E. R. Morris, D. A. Rees, P. J. C. Smith, and D. Thom. 1973. Biological interactions between polysaccharides and divalent cations: the egg-box model. *FEBS Letters* 32:195–198.

Haensler, J. and F. C. Jr. Szoka. 1993. Polyamidoamine cascade polymers mediate efficient transfection of cells in culture. *Bioconjugate Chemistry* 4:372–379.

He, W., Z. Guo, Y. Wen, Q. Wang, B. Xie, S. Zhu, and Q. Wang. 2012. Alginate-graft-PEI as a gene delivery vector with high efficiency and low cytotoxicity. *Journal of Biomaterials Science, Polymer Edition* 23:315–331.

de las Heras, A. I., S. Rodriguez Saint-Jean, and S. I. Perez-Prieto. 2010. Immunogenic and protective effects of an oral DNA vaccine against infectious pancreatic necrosis virus in fish. *Fish and Shellfish Immunology* 28:562–570.

Hong, H. J., S. E. Jin, J. S. Park, W. S. Ahn, and C. K. Kim. 2008. Accelerated wound healing by smad3 antisense oligonucleotides-impregnated chitosan/alginate polyelectrolyte complex. *Biomaterials* 29:4831–4837.

Hosseinkhani, H., T. Aoyama, O. Ogawa, and Y. Tabata. 2002. Liver targeting of plasmid DNA by pullulan conjugation based on metal coordination. *Journal of Controlled Release* 83:287–302.

Jere, D., H. L. Jiang, Y. K. Kim, R. Arote, Y. J. Choi, C. H. Yun, M. H. Cho, and C. S. Cho. 2009. Chitosan-graft-polyethylenimine for Akt1 siRNA delivery to lung cancer cells. *International Journal of Pharmaceutics* 378:194–200.

Jiang, H. L., Y. K. Kim, R. Arote, J. W. Nah, M. H. Cho, Y. J. Choi, T. Akaike, and C. S. Cho. 2007a. Chitosan-graft-polyethylenimine as a gene carrier. *Journal of Controlled Release* 117:273–280.

Jiang, H. L., J. T. Kwon, Y. K. Kim, E. M. Kim, R. Arote, H. J. Jeong, J. W. Nah et al. 2007b. Galactosylated chitosan-graft-polyethylenimine as a gene carrier for hepatocyte targeting. *Gene Therapy* 14:1389–1398.

Jiang, H. L., H. T. Lim, Y. K. Kim, R. Arote, J. Y. Shin, J. T. Kwon, J. E. Kim et al. 2011. Chitosan-graft-spermine as a gene carrier in vitro and in vivo. *European Journal of Pharmaceutics and Biopharmaceutics* 77:36–42.

Jin, H., T. H. Kim, S. K. Hwang, S. H. Chang, H. W. Kim, H. K. Anderson, H. W. Lee et al. 2006. Aerosol delivery of urocanic acid-modified chitosan/programmed cell death 4 complex regulated apoptosis, cell cycle, and angiogenesis in lungs of K-ras null mice. *Molecular Cancer Therapeutics* 6:1041–1049.

Jin, H., C. X. Xu, H. W. Kim, Y. S. Chung, J. Y. Shin, S. H. Chang, S. J. Park et al. 2008. Urocanic acid- modified chitosan-mediated PTEN delivery via aerosol suppressed lung tumorigenesis in K-ras(LA1) mice. *Cancer Gene Therapy* 15:275–283.

Jo, J., T. Ikai, A. Okazaki, K. Nagane, M. Yamamoto, Y. Hirano, and Y. Tabata. 2007a. Expression profile of plasmid DNA obtained using spermine derivatives of pullulan with different molecular weights. *Journal of Biomaterials Science, Polymer Edition* 18:883–899.

Jo, J., T. Ikai, A. Okazaki, M. Yamamoto, Y. Hirano, and Y. Tabata. 2007b. Expression profile of plasmid DNA by spermine derivatives of pullulan with different extents of spermine introduced. *Journal of Controlled Release* 118:389–398.

Kabanov, A. V. and V. A. Kabanov. 1995. DNA complexes with polycations for the delivery of genetic material into cells. *Bioconjugate Chemistry* 6:7–20.

Kanatani, I., T. Ikai, A. Okazaki, J. Jo, M. Yamamoto, M. Imamura, A. Kanematsu, S. Yamamoto, N. Ito, O. Ogawa, and Y. Tabata. 2006. Efficient gene transfer by pullulan-spermine occurs through both clathrin-and raft/caveolae-dependent mechanisms. *Journal of Controlled Release* 116:75–82.

Kaneo, Y., T. Tanaka, T. Nakano, and Y. Yamaguchi. 2001. Evidence for receptor-mediated hepatic uptake of pullulan in rats. *Journal of Controlled Release* 70:365–373.

Kido, Y., J. I. Jo, and Y. Tabata. 2011. A gene transfection for rat mesenchymal stromal cells in biodegradable gelatin scaffolds containing cationized polysaccharides. *Biomaterials* 32:919–925.

Kim, T. H., J. E. Ihm, Y. J. Choi, J. W. Nah, and C. S. Cho. 2003. Efficient gene delivery by urocanic acid-modified chitosan. *Journal of Controlled Release* 93:389–402.

Lee, K. Y. and D. V. Mooney. 2012. Alginate: properties and biomedical applications. *Progress in Polymer Science* 37:106–126.

Li, S. and L. Huang. 1997. In vivo gene transfer via intravenous administration of cationic lipid-protamine-DNA (LPD) complexes. *Gene Therapy* 4:891–900.

Lou, Y. L., Y. S. Peng, B. H. Chen, L. F. Wang, and K. W. Leong. 2009. Poly(ethylene imine)-g-chitosan using EX-810 as a spacer for nonviral gene delivery vectors. *Journal of Biomedical Materials Research Part A* 88:1058–1068.

Lu, B., Y. X. Sun, Y. Q. Li, X. Z. Zhang, and R. X. Zhuo. 2009. N-succinyl-chitosan-grafted with low molecular weight polyethylenimine as a serum-resistant gene vector. *Molecular BioSystems* 5:629–637.

Lu, B., X. D. Xu, X. Z. Zhang, S. X. Cheng, and R. X. Zhuo. 2008. Low molecular weight polyethylenimine grafted N-maleated chitosan for gene delivery: properties and in vitro transfection studies. *Biomacromolecules* 9:2594–2600.

Madry, H., G. Kaul, M. Cucchiarini, U. Stein, D. Zurakowski, K. Remberger, M. D. Menger, D. Kohn, and S. B. Trippel. 2005. Enhanced repair of articular cartilage defects in vivo by transplanted chondrocytes overexpressing insulin-like growth factor I (IFG-I). *Gene Therapy* 12:1171–1179.

Mao, S., W. Sun, and T. Kissel. 2010. Chitosan-based formulations for delivery of DNA and siRNA. *Advanced Drug Delivery Reviews* 62:12–27.

Mierisch, C. M., H. A. Wilson, M. A. Turner, T. A. Milbrandt, L. Berthoux, M. L. Hammarskjöld, D. Rekosh, G. Balian, and D. R. Diduch. 2003. Chondrocyte transplantation into articular cartilage defects with use of calcium alginate: the fate of the cells. *The Journal of Bone and Joint Surgery* 85-A:1757–1767.

Mishra, B., S. Vuppu, and K. Rath. 2011. The role of microbial pullulan, a biopolymer in pharmaceutical approaches: A review. *Journal of Applied Pharmaceutical Science* 1:45–50.

Mittal, S. K., N. Aggarwal, G. Sailaja, A. van Olphen, H. HogenEsch, A. North, J. Hays, and S. Moffatt. 2001. Immunization with DNA, adenovirus or both in biodegradable alginate microspheres: Effect of route of inoculation on immune response. *Vaccine* 19:253–263.

Moreira, C., H. Oliveira, L. R. Pires, S. Simoes, M. A. Barbosa, and A. P. Pego. 2009. Improving chitosan-mediated gene transfer by the introduction of intracellular buffering moieties into the chitosan backbone. *Acta Biomaterialia* 5:2995–3006.

Nagane, K., M. Kitada, S. Wakao, M. Dezawa, and Y. Tabata. 2009. Practical induction system for dopamine-producing cells from bone marrow stromal cells using spermine-pullulan-mediated reverse transfection method. *Tissue Engineering Part A* 15:1655–1665.

Onishi, H. and Y. Machida. 1999. Biodegradation and distribution of water-soluble chitosan in mice. *Biomaterials* 20:175–182.

Park, I. K., T. H. Kim, S. I. Kim, Y. H. Park, W. J. Kim, T. Akaike, and C. S. Cho. 2003. Visualization of transfection of hepatocytes by galactosylated chitosan-graft-poly(ethylene glycol)/DNA complexes by confocal laser scanning microscopy. *International Journal of Pharmaceutics* 257:103–110.

Patnaik, S., A. Aggarwal, S. Nimesh, A. Goel, M. Ganguli, N. Saini, Y. Singh, and K. C. Gupta. 2006. PEI-alginate nanocomposites as efficient in vitro gene transfection agents. *Journal of Controlled Release* 114:398–409.

Ping, Y., C. Liu, Z. Zhang, K. L. Liu, J. Chen, and J. Li. 2011. Chitosan-graft-(PEI-β-cyclodextrin) copolymers and their supramolecular PEGylation for DNA and siRNA delivery. *Biomaterials* 32:8328–8341.

Rekha, M. R. and C. P. Sharma. 2009. Blood compatibility and in vitro transfection studies on cationically modified pullulan for liver cell targeted gene delivery. *Biomaterials* 30:6655–6664.

Rekha, M. R. and C. P. Sharma. 2011. Hemocompatible pullulan-polyethyleneimine conjugates for liver cell gene delivery: in vitro evaluation of cellular uptake, intracellular trafficking and transfection efficiency. *Acta Biomaterialia* 7:370–379.

San Juan, A., M. Bala, H. Hlawaty, P. Portes, R. Vranckx, L. J. Feldman, and D. Letourneur. 2009. Development of a functionalized polymer for stent coating in the arterial delivery of small interfering RNA. *Biomacromolecules* 10:3074–3080.

San Juan, A., G. Ducrocq, H. Hlawaty, I. Bataille, E. Guénin, D. Letourneur, and L. J. Feldman. 2007a. Tubular cationized pullulan hydrogels as local reservoirs for plasmid DNA. *Journal of Biomedical Materials Research Part A* 83:819–827.

San Juan, A., H. Hlawaty, F. Chaubet, D. Letourneur, and L. J. Feldman. 2007b. Cationized pullulan 3D matrices as new materials for gene transfer. *Journal of Biomedical Materials Research Part A* 82:354–362.

Shi, B., Z. Shen, H. Zhang, J. Bi, and S. Dai. 2012. Exploring *N*-imidazolyl-*O*-carboxymethyl chitosan for high performance gene delivery. *Biomacromolecules* 13:146–153.

Smith, A. E. 1995. Viral vectors in gene therapy. *Annual Review of Microbiology* 49:807–838.

Sone, T., E. Nagamori, T. Ikeuchi, A. Mizukami, Y. Takakura, S. Kajiyama, E. Fukusaki, S. Harashima, A. Kobayashi, and K. Fukui. 2002. A novel gene delivery system in plants with calcium alginate micro-beads. *Journal of Bioscience and Bioengineering* 94:87–91.

Thakor, D. K., Y. D. Teng, and Y. Tabata. 2009. Neuronal gene delivery by negatively charged pullulan-spermine/DNA anioplexes. *Biomaterials* 30:1815–1826.

Thomsen, L. B., J. Lichota, K. S. Kim, and T. Moos. 2011. Gene delivery by pullulan derivatives in brain capillary endothelial cells for protein secretion. *Journal of Controlled Release* 151:45–50.

Wang, W., J. Yao, J. P. Zhou, Y. Lu, Y. Wang, L. Tao, and Y. P. Li. 2008. Urocanic acid-modified chitosan-mediated p53 gene delivery inducing apoptosis of human hepatocellular carcinoma cell line HepG2 is involved in its antitumor effect in vitro and in vivo. *Biochemical and Biophysical Research Communications* 377:567–572.

Wong, K., G. Sun, X. Zhang, H. Dai, Y. Liu, C. He, and K. W. Leong. 2006. PEI-g-chitosan, a novel gene delivery system with transfection efficiency comparable to polyethylenimine in vitro and after liver administration *in vivo*. *Bioconjugate Chemistry* 17:152–158.

Wu, G. Y. and C. H. Wu. 1987. Receptor-mediated in vitro gene transformation by a soluble DNA carrier system. *Journal of Biological Chemistry* 262:4429–4432.

Xu, W., L. Liu, and I. G. Charles. 2002. Microencapsulated iNOS-expressing cells cause tumor suppression in mice. *FASEB Journal* 16:213–215.

Zachos, T., A. Diggs, S. Weisbrode, J. Bartlett, and A. Bertone. 2007. Mesenchymal stem cell-mediated gene delivery of bone morphogenetic protein-2 in an articular fracture model. *Molecular Therapy* 15:1543–1550.

Zachos, T. A., K. M. Shields, and A. L. Bertone. 2006. Gene-mediated osteogenic differentiation of stem cells by bone morphogenetic proteins-2 or –6. *Journal of Orthopaedic Research* 24:1279–1291.

Zhang, W., S. Pan, Y. Wen, X. Luo, and X. Zhang. 2010. Synthesis of poly(ethylene glycol)-g-chitosan-g-poly(ethylene imine) co-polymer and in vitro study of its suitability as a gene-delivery vector. *Journal of Biomaterials Science, Polymer Edition* 21:741–758.

Zhang, R., L. Tian, L. J. Chen, F. Xiao, J. M. Hou, X. Zhao, G. Li et al. 2006. Combination of MIG (CXCL9) chemokine gene therapy with low-dose cisplatin improves therapeutic efficacy against murine carcinoma. *Gene Therapy* 13:1263–1271.

Zhao, D., R. X. Zhuo, and S. X. Cheng. 2012. Alginate modified nanostructured calcium carbonate with enhanced delivery efficiency for gene and drug delivery. *Molecular BioSystems* 8:753–759.

Zheng, S., Z. X. Xiao, Y. L. Pan, M. Y. Han, and Q. Dong. 2003. Continuous release of interleukin 12 from microencapsulated engineered cells for colon cancer therapy. *World Journal of Gastroenterology* 9:951–955.

34

Advantages of Chitin-Based Nanobiomaterials in Nanomedicine

S. Sowmya, Shantikumar V. Nair, and R. Jayakumar

CONTENTS

34.1 Introduction

Chitin, the second most abundant natural biomaterial composed of $\beta(1\rightarrow4)$-linked 2-acetamido-2-deoxy-β-D-glucose units (or N-acetylglucosamine units), is well recognized as a substance providing many valuable biological properties, namely, biocompatibility, hemostasis, and antibacterial/anti-infectious property (Jayakumar et al., 2011). It is a fairly cytocompatible material that promotes the attachment and spreading of diverse cells such as normal human keratinocytes, fibroblasts, osteoblasts, and many more. Chitin is highly biodegradable in nature due to the activity of lysozymes present in the human body (Kurita et al., 2000; Noh et al., 2006). It is being used in the fabrication of a variety of medical devices and regenerative medical components due to its high crystallinity, biochemical significance, and biocompatibility (Yimin et al., 2008). The excellent and unique properties of chitin offer a large and active surface area, making it suitable for different applications, and hence, these properties are being explored in the fields of engineering, technology, and medicine (Muzzarelli, 2011). The main disadvantage of chitin is its insolubility in organic solvents and acids. However, chitin is soluble in saturated $CaCl_2$–methanol solvent system (Tamura et al., 2011). Using this solvent system, chitin solution was prepared (Tamura et al., 2011). This chitin solution can be easily regenerated into gel or nanogel by the addition of water/methanol (Sanoj Rejinold et al., 2011, 2012; Tamura et al., 2011). Chitin hydrogel is subjected to lyophilization to obtain chitin scaffolds (Madhumathi et al., 2010; Jayakumar et al., 2011;

Sowmya et al., 2011; Tamura et al., 2011). This chapter will focus on the advantages of chitin nanofibers, nanogels, and nanocomposite scaffolds in drug delivery, tissue engineering, and wound healing in detail.

34.2 Chitin Nanofibers in Tissue Engineering and Wound Dressing

Electrospinning process is a versatile technique because it can produce fibers with diameter ranging from tens of nanometers to several micrometers. The various parameters that determine the diameter of the fibers are molecular weight, molecular-weight distribution and architecture (branched, linear, etc.) of the polymer, solution properties (viscosity, conductivity, and surface tension), electric potential, flow rate and concentration, distance between the capillary and collection screen, ambient parameters (temperature, humidity, and air velocity in the chamber), motion of target screen (collector), and needle gauge (Jayakumar et al., 2010b). Chitin nanofibers in comparison to microfibers offer various advantages such as high surface area to volume ratio, enhanced cellular properties such as attachment and proliferation. Biocompatible chitin nanofibers have been used for tissue engineering and wound healing applications (Jayakumar et al., 2010a,c, 2011a,b). Chitin has an accelerating effect on the wound healing process. The main biochemical activities of chitin-based materials in wound healing are polymorphonuclear cell activation, fibroblast activation, cytokine production, giant cell migration, and stimulation of type IV collagen synthesis (Mezzana, 2008). The cytocompatibility of chitin nanofibrous scaffold was studied for wound healing applications (Noh et al., 2006). Chitin nanofibrous scaffolds were developed using different polymeric materials or combination of polymers, which were found to promote cell attachment and spreading of normal human keratinocytes and fibroblasts compared to chitin microfibers. This may be a consequence of the high surface area available for cell attachment due to their 3D features and high surface area to volume ratio, which are favorable parameters for cell attachment, growth, and proliferation. Chitin/poly(glycolic acid) (PGA) (Park et al., 2006b) and chitin/silk fibroin (SF) (Park et al., 2006a) fibrous scaffolds proved to be cytocompatible wherein the matrix consisting of 25% PGA or SF and 75% chitin had the best results. Bovine serum albumin (BSA) coating was given to the chitin/PGA fibrous scaffold, which was considered as a good candidate for tissue engineering applications (Park et al., 2006b). Normal human epidermal fibroblast (NHEF) and normal human epidermal keratinocyte (NHEK) cells spread uniformly throughout the chitin/SF fibrous scaffold. Therefore, these scaffolds could be suitable for wound healing applications (Park et al., 2006a). Similarly electrospun water-soluble carboxymethyl chitin (CMC)/poly(vinyl alcohol) (PVA) blend nanofibrous scaffolds for tissue engineering applications were developed (Shalumon et al., 2009). The nanofibers prepared were bioactive and biocompatible. Cytotoxicity and cell attachment studies of the nanofibrous scaffold were evaluated using human mesenchymal stem cells (hMSCs) by the 3-(4,5-dimethylthiazol-2-yl)-2,5-diphenyltetrazolium bromide (MTT) assay. Cell attachment studies revealed that cells were able to attach and spread uniformly throughout the nanofibrous scaffolds. These results confirmed that the cytocompatible nature of nanofibrous CMC/PVA scaffold supports cell adhesion/attachment and proliferation, and hence, this scaffold can be a useful candidate for applications in tissue engineering (Shalumon et al., 2009).

34.3 Chitin Nanocomposite Scaffolds in Tissue Engineering and Wound Healing

Scaffolds are 3D porous structures made of ceramic or polymer or metals or a combination of all these together (Sachlos and Czernuszka, 2003). They play an important role in various fields such as tissue engineering and wound healing. The scaffold provides the necessary support for cells to attach, proliferate, and maintain their differentiated function. Nano-hydroxyapatite (nHA) with the chemical formula $Ca_{10}(PO_4)_6(OH)_2$ is commonly used for biomedical applications owing to its unique functional properties of high surface area to volume ratio, and it also mimics the apatite-like structure and composition of hard tissues such as enamel, dentin, and bone (Ge et al., 2004; Farzadi et al., 2011). It is stable in body fluids, bioactive, osteoconductive, nontoxic, noninflammatory, non-immunogenic, and nonbiodegradable (Murugan and Ramakrishna, 2004; Peter et al., 2010). It has the ability to form a direct chemical bond with the surrounding hard tissues (Chen et al., 2002). In addition, it offers other advantages such as ease of fabrication, handling, and close surface contact with the surrounding tissues (Jiang et al., 2008). β-chitin/nHA nanocomposite scaffolds were synthesized from a mixture of β-chitin hydrogel and nHA by freeze-drying technique (Sudheesh Kumar et al., 2011b). The cytocompatibility of the nanocomposite scaffolds was studied using MG-63, Vero, NIH 3T3, and HDF cells. The results indicated that the cells were viable and showed enhanced attachment and proliferation onto the nanocomposite scaffolds. Similar results were observed with α-chitin/nHA nanocomposite scaffolds synthesized from α-chitin hydrogel and nHA by freeze-drying approach (Sudheesh Kumar et al., 2011a). These results essentially signify that the synthesized nanocomposite scaffolds can serve as potential candidates for bone tissue engineering and wound healing (Sudheesh Kumar et al., 2011a,b).

Another important bioceramic is bioactive glasses that are silicate-based materials used for bone repair and are widely used in orthopedics and dentistry (Hench, 1991; Wheeler et al., 2000). They can bond to both soft and hard tissues and are superior to HA in their ability for osseointegration, osteoblast and marrow stromal cell proliferation, and differentiation (Kokubo, 1991; Xynos et al., 2000; Valerio et al., 2004; Verrier et al., 2004; Bosetti and Cannas, 2005; Foppiano et al., 2007; Hench, 2009). In comparison to other bioactive ceramics, bioactive glass bonds to bone at faster rate due to the formation of carbonated apatite on their surface in the presence of physiological fluid. In addition, the bioactive glass ceramics influence osteoblastic cell differentiation with an increase in the level of differentiation markers like ALP, osteocalcin, and osteopontin (Xynos et al., 2000; Valerio et al., 2004). Bioactive glass ceramic nanoparticles (nBGC) were prepared using solgel technique that offers certain advantages in comparison to fusion method such as homogeneity, higher purity, and surface area (Peter et al., 2009; Sowmya et al., 2011). The α-chitin/nBGC and β-chitin/nBGC composite scaffolds were prepared using α-chitin/β-chitin hydrogel with nBGC by lyophilization technique (Peter et al., 2009; Sowmya et al., 2011). The biocompatibility of the composite scaffolds was studied using MTT assay and cell attachment studies on MG63 and POB cells. Results confirmed the cytocompatible nature of the scaffolds with no signs of toxicity, and the MG63 and POB cells were well adhered onto the scaffolds. These results suggested that the developed composite scaffolds have promising applications in alveolar bone tissue engineering (Peter et al., 2009; Sowmya et al., 2011).

Addition of silica nanoparticles (NPs) enhances the bioactivity and biocompatibility of chitin. Silica serves as active filler in various polymeric systems. Stabilization of these NPs is essential to prevent aggregation/agglomeration (Jerzy and Ludomir, 2003). Recently, α-chitin composite scaffold containing nanosilica was developed using α-chitin hydrogel (Madhumathi et al., 2009). Bioactivity, swelling ability, and cytotoxicity of α-chitin composite scaffolds were analyzed in vitro. These scaffolds were found to be bioactive in SBF and biocompatible with MG63 cell line. The α-chitin/nanosilica composite scaffolds showed higher biocompatibility. These results suggest that α-chitin/nanosilica composite scaffolds can be useful for bone tissue engineering (Madhumathi et al., 2009).

In a similar way, β-chitin/nanosilver composite scaffolds were prepared for wound tissue engineering applications using β-chitin hydrogel with silver NPs (Sudheesh Kumar et al., 2010). The antibacterial, blood clotting, swelling, cell attachment, and cytotoxicity studies of the prepared composite scaffolds were evaluated. The prepared β-chitin/nanosilver composite scaffolds had bactericidal effect against *Escherichia coli* and *Staphylococcus aureus* and showed good blood clotting ability as well. The scaffolds were cytocompatible wherein Vero (epithelial cells) were well adhered on the scaffolds. Similarly, α-chitin/nanosilver composite scaffolds showing similar results were developed for wound tissue engineering applications using α-chitin hydrogel with silver NPs (Madhumathi et al., 2010). These results essentially signify that chitin/nanosilver composite scaffolds could be potential candidates for wound tissue engineering NPs (Madhumathi et al., 2010; Sudheesh Kumar et al., 2010).

34.4 Chitin Nanoparticles in Drug Delivery

CMC is a water-soluble derivative of chitin and used for drug delivery and tissue engineering applications (Jayakumar et al., 2010a,c). Ashish Dev et al. (2010) prepared CMC nanoparticles (CMC NPs) by cross-linking CMC with $CaCl_2$ and $FeCl_3$. MTT assay was applied to evaluate the cytocompatibility of the CMC NPs. These NPs were nontoxic to L929 mouse fibroblast cells. The antibacterial and magnetic properties of the CMC NPs were also studied. The major magnetic component was paramagnetic in nature. In this study, the model hydrophobic anticancer drug, 5-fluorouracil (5-Fu), was loaded into CMC NPs via emulsion cross-linking method. The drug-loaded CMC NPs reduced the viability with increasing concentration of 5-Fu in oral epithelial carcinoma (KB) cells. Drug release studies showed that the CMC NPs showed controlled and sustained drug release at pH 6.8. These results indicated that CMC NPs are a promising carrier system for controlled drug delivery (Ashish Dev et al., 2010).

34.5 Chitin Nanogels in Drug Delivery and Imaging

Nanogels are hydrogels confined to nanoscopic dimensions with many attractive properties such as size tunability, large surface area useful for multivalent bioconjugation, excellent drug-loading capacity, controlled release, and their responsiveness to environmental stimuli. These properties make them very attractive to be an ideal drug delivery system

(Jung et al., 2007). Sanoj Rejinold et al. (2012) developed biodegradable chitin nanogels (CNGs) of size 65 nm by controlled regeneration method followed by characterization. These CNGs having reduced particle size will improve the blood circulation time and extravasation rate into tumors. The CNGs showed higher swelling and degradation in acidic pH compared to other pH. This is attributed to the swelling ability of CNG at a pH below its pKa value (6.1). The in vitro cytocompatibility, cellular uptake, cell trafficking, and hemolysis assay were analyzed on an array of cell lines. Cell uptake studies were done by conjugating CNGs with the rhodamine-123 dye (rhodamine-123–CNGs), which showed retention of nanogels inside the cells. The hemolytic ratio was <5%, the critical safe level according to ISO/TR 7406. These studies confirmed that the CNGs could be useful for the delivery of drugs, growth factors for drug delivery, and tissue engineering (Sanoj Rejinold et al., 2012). For multifunctionalization, CNGs was conjugated with mercaptopropionic acid (MPA)-capped cadmium telluride quantum dots (CdTe-QDs) (QD-CNGs) for the in vitro cellular localization studies (Sanoj Rejinold et al., 2011). In addition, the BSA was loaded on to QD-CNGs (BSA-QD-CNGs). The CNGs, QD-CNGs, and BSA-QD-CNGs were characterized by scanning electron microscope (SEM) and atomic force microscope (AFM). The size of the nanogels was in the range of <100 nm. The nanogels were cytocompatible to L929, NIH-3T3, KB, MCF-7, PC3, and Vero cells. The cell uptake studies of the QD-CNGs were analyzed, which showed retention of these nanogels inside the cells (L929, PC3, and Vero). The hemolytic ratio was <5% as stated in the previous study. In addition, the protein-loading efficiency of the nanogels has also been analyzed. The study revealed that these multifunctionalized nanogels could be useful for drug delivery with simultaneous imaging (Sanoj Rejinold et al., 2011).

Jayakumar et al. (2012) prepared doxorubicin-loaded CNGs and were characterized by SEM, dynamic light scattering (DLS), and Fourier transform infrared spectroscopy (FTIR) for cancer drug delivery. The size distribution was in the range of 130–160 nm for the doxorubicin-loaded CNGs. The in vitro cytotoxicity studies of doxorubicin-loaded CNGs were studied using L929, PC3, MCF-7, A549, and HEPG2 cell lines that reduced the viability of cancer cells when compared to normal L929 cells. The loading efficiency was increased with the increase in incubation time. Release studies indicated enhanced drug release at acidic pH. The internalization studies showed a significant uptake of doxorubicin-loaded CNGs in all the tested cell lines. All these results indicated that doxorubicin-loaded CNGs can be used for prostate, breast, lung, and liver cancer (Jayakumar et al., 2012).

Curcumin-loaded CNGs (CCNGs) were developed using biocompatible and biodegradable chitin with curcumin, an anticancer drug for skin cancer via the transdermal route (Sabitha et al., 2012). The developed CCNGs form a very good and stable dispersion in water. The CCNGs were characterized using DLS, SEM, and FTIR. Spherical particles in a size range of 70–80 nm were observed. The CCNGs showed controlled release and higher release at acidic pH compared to neutral pH. The cytotoxicity of the nanogels was analyzed on human dermal fibroblast cells (HDF) and A375 (human melanoma) cell lines. The results showed specific toxicity of the CCNGs on melanoma but less toxicity toward HDF cells. The confocal analysis confirmed the uptake of CCNGs by A375. Control CNG exhibited no significant apoptosis, whereas apoptosis was observed at a higher concentration of cytotoxic range of CCNGs. The histopathology studies of the porcine skin samples treated with the prepared materials showed normal epidermis and dermis morphology facilitating penetration with no observed signs of inflammation. The CCNGs offer specific advantage wherein these CCNGs showed specific toxicity toward melanoma cells thus suitable for the treatment of melanoma, the most common and serious type of skin cancer, by effective transdermal penetration (Sabitha et al., 2012).

34.6 Conclusions

This chapter essentially describes the applications of chitin in tissue engineering, wound healing, and drug delivery. Chitin nanofibers were compared with chitin microfibers that enhanced its compatibility with different cell types suitable for tissue engineering and wound healing applications. The presence of HA, bioactive glass, silica NPs, etc. enhanced the properties and functions of nanocomposite scaffolds. Also the presence of silver NPs imparted antibacterial ability to the nanocomposite scaffolds. Chitin NPs and CNGs found their application in drug delivery and imaging. Different combinations of drugs loaded into chitin NPs and nanogels could be applicable for prostrate, breast, lung, liver, and skin cancer therapy. Overall chitin is a truly remarkable natural polymer useful for biomedical applications due to its unique biological functions and physical properties.

Acknowledgments

The authors are grateful to the Nanomission, Department of Science and Technology, and Department of Biotechnology, Government of India, for supporting the research fund under Nanoscience and Nanotechnology Initiative Program. One of the authors, Sowmya Srinivasan, is thankful to the Council of Scientific and Industrial Research (CSIR) for the financial support through Senior Research Fellowship Award (SRF).

References

Ashish, D., N. S. Binulal, A. Anitha, S. V. Nair, T. Furuike, H. Tamura, and R. Jayakumar. 2010. Preparation of novel poly(lactic acid)/chitosan nanoparticles for anti-HIV drug delivery applications. *Carbohydrate Polymers* 80: 833–838.

Bosetti, M. and M. Cannas. 2005. The effect of bioactive glasses on bone marrow stromal cells differentiation. *Biomaterials* 26: 3873–3879.

Chen, F., Z. C. Wang, and C. J. Lin. 2002. Preparation and characterization of nano-sized hydroxyapatite particles and hydroxyapatite/chitosan nano-composite for use in biomedical materials. *Materials Letters* 57: 858–861.

Farzadi, A., M. Solati-Hashjin, F. Bakhshi, and A. Aminian. 2011. A synthesis and characterization of hydroxyapatite/β-tricalcium phosphate nanocomposites using microwave irradiation. *Ceramic International* 37: 65–71.

Foppiano, S., S. J. Marshall, G. W. Marshall, E. Saiz, and A. P. Tomsia. 2007. Bioactive glass coatings affect the behavior of osteoblast-like cells. *Acta Biomaterialia* 3: 765–771.

Ge, Z., S. Baguenard, L. Y. Lim, A. Weec, and E. Khor. 2004. Hydroxyapatite-chitin tissue engineered bone substitutes. *Biomaterials* 25: 1049–1058.

Hench, L. L. 1991. Bioceramics: From concept to clinic. *Journal of American Ceramic Society* 74: 1487–1510.

Hench, L. L. 2009. Genetic design of bioactive glass. 2009. *Journal of the European Ceramic Society* 29: 1257–1265.

Jayakumar, R., Amrita Nair, N. Sanoj Rejinold, S. Maya, and S. V. Nair. 2012. Doxorubicin loaded pH responsive chitin nanogels for drug delivery to cancer cells. *Carbohydrate Polymers* 87: 2352–2356.

Jayakumar, R., K. P. Chennazhi, S. Sowmya, S. V. Nair, T. Furuike, and H. Tamura. 2011b. Chitin scaffolds in tissue engineering. *International Journal of Molecular Sciences* 12: 1876–1887.

Jayakumar, R., Deepthy Menon, K. Manzoor, S. V. Nair, and H. Tamura. 2010a. Biomedical applications of chitin and chitosan based nanomaterials-A short review. *Carbohydrate Polymers* 82: 227–232.

Jayakumar, R., S. V. Nair, N. Selvamurugan, M. Prabaharan, S. Tokura, and H. Tamura. 2010c. Novel carboxymethyl derivatives of chitin and chitosan materials and their biomedical applications. *Progress in Materials Science* 55: 675–709.

Jayakumar, R., M. Prabaharan, S. V. Nair, and H. Tamura. 2010b. Novel chitin and chitosan nanofibers in biomedical applications. *Biotechnology Advances* 28: 142–150.

Jayakumar, R., M. Prabaharan, P. T. Sudheesh Kumar, S. V. Nair, and H. Tamura. 2011a. Biomaterials based on chitin and chitosan in wound dressing applications. *Biotechnology Advances* 29: 322–337.

Jerzy, C. and S. Ludomir. 2003. Synthesis of nanosilica by the sol-gel method and its activity toward polymers. *Materials Science* 21: 461–469.

Jiang, L., Y. Li, X. Wang, L. Zhang, J. Wen, and M. Gong. 2008. Preparation and properties of nano-hydroxyapatite/chitosan/carboxymethyl cellulose composite scaffold. *Carbohydrate Polymers* 74: 680–684.

Jung, K. O., J. S. Daniel, and M. Krzysztof. 2007. Synthesis and biodegradation of nanogels as delivery carriers for carbohydrate drugs. *Biomacromolecules* 8: 3326–3331.

Kokubo, T. 1991. Bioactive glass ceramics: Properties and applications. *Biomaterials* 12: 155–163.

Kurita, K., Y. Kaji, T. Mori, and Y. Nishiyama. 2000. Enzymatic degradation of β-chitin: Susceptibility and the influence of deacetylation. *Carbohydrate Polymers* 42: 19–21.

Madhumathi, K., K. C. Kavya, P. T. Sudheesh Kumar, T. Furuike, H. Tamura, S. V. Nair, and R. Jayakumar. 2009. Novel chitin/nanosilica composite scaffolds for bone tissue engineering applications. *International Journal of Biological Macromolecules* 45: 289–292.

Madhumathi, K., P. T. Sudhessh Kumar, S. Abhilash, V. Sreeja, H. Tamura, K. Manzoor, S. V. Nair, and R. Jayakumar. 2010. Development of novel chitin/nanosilver composite scaffolds for wound dressing applications. *Journal of Materials Science: Materials in Medicine* 21: 807–813.

Mezzana, P. 2008. Clinical efficacy of a new chitin nanofibrils-based gel in wound healing. *ActaChirurgiaePlasticae* 50: 81–84.

Murugan, R. and S. Ramakrishna. 2004. Bioresorbable composite bone paste using polysaccharide based nano hydroxyapatite. *Biomaterials* 25: 3829–3835.

Muzzarelli, R. A. A. 2011. New techniques for optimization of surface area and porosity in nanochitins and nanochitosans. *Advances in Polymer Science* 244: 167–186.

Noh, H. K., S. W. Lee, J. M. Kim, J. E. Oh, K. H. Kim, C. P. Chung et al. 2006. Electrospinning of chitin nanofibers: Degradation behavior and cellular response to normal human keratinocytes and fibroblasts. *Biomaterials* 27: 3934–3944.

Park, K.E., S. Y. Jung, S. J. Lee, B. M. Min, and W. H. Park. 2006a. Biomimetic nanofibrous scaffolds: Preparation and characterization of chitin/silk fibroin blend nanofibers. *International Journal of Biological Macromolecules* 38: 165–173.

Park, K.E., H. K. Kang, S. J. Lee, B. M. Min, and W. H. Park. 2006b. Biomimetic nanofibrous scaffolds: preparation and characterization of PGA/chitin blend nanofibers. *Biomacromolecules* 7: 635–643.

Peter, M., G. Nitya, N. Selvamurugan, S. V. Nair, T. Furuike, H. Tamura, and R. Jayakumar. 2010. Preparation and characterization of chitosan-gelatin/nanohydroxyapatite composite scaffolds for tissue engineering applications. *Carbohydrate Polymers* 80: 687–694.

Peter, M., P. T. Sudheesh Kumar, N. S. Binulal, S. V. Nair, H. Tamura, and R. Jayakumar. 2009. Development of novel chitin/nanobioactive glass ceramic nanocomposite scaffolds for tissue engineering applications. *Carbohydrate Polymers* 78: 926–931.

Sabitha, M., N. Sanoj Rejinold, Amrita Nair, Vinoth-Kumar Lakshmanan, S. V. Nair, and R. Jayakumar. 2012. Curcumin loaded chitin nanogels for skin cancer treatment via the transdermal route. *Nanoscale* 4: 239–250.

Sachlos, E. and J. T. Czernuszka. 2003. Making tissue engineering scaffolds work. Review on the application of solid freeform fabrication technology to the production of tissue engineering scaffolds. *European Cells and Materials* 5: 29–40.

Sanoj Rejinold, N., Amrita Nair, M. Sabitha, K. P. Chennazhi, H. Tamura, S.V. Nair, and R. Jayakumar. 2012. Synthesis, characterization and in vitro cytocompatibility studies of chitin nanogels for biomedical applications. *Carbohydrate Polymers* 87: 936–942.

Sanoj Rejinold, N., K. P. Chennazhi, H. Tamura, S. V. Nair, and R. Jayakumar. 2011. Multifunctional chitin nanogels for simultaneous drug delivery, bioimaging and biosensing. *ACS Applied Materials and Interfaces* 3: 3654–3665.

Shalumon, K. T., N. S. Binulal, N. Selvamurugan, S. V. Nair, D. Menon, T. Furuike, H. Tamura, and R. Jayakumar. 2009. Electrospinning of carboxymethyl chitin/poly(vinyl alcohol) nanofibrous scaffolds for tissue engineering applications. *Carbohydrate Polymers* 77: 863–869.

Sowmya, S., P. T. S. Sudheesh Kumar, K. P. Chennazhi, S. V. Nair, H. Tamura, and R. Jayakumar. 2011. Biocompatible β-chitin hydrogel/nanobioactive glass ceramic nanocomposite scaffolds for periodontal bone regeneration. *Trends in Biomaterials and Artificial Organs* 25: 1–11.

Sudheesh Kumar, P. T., S. Abhilash, K. Manzoor, S. V. Nair, H. Tamura, and R. Jayakumar. 2010. Preparation and characterization of novel β-chitin/nano silver composite scaffolds for wound dressing applications. *Carbohydrate Polymers* 80: 761–767.

Sudheesh Kumar, P. T., S. Sowmya, K. L. Vinoth, H. Tamura, S. V. Nair, and R. Jayakumar. 2011a. Synthesis, characterization and cytocompatibility studies of α-chitin hydrogel/nano hydroxy-apatite composite scaffolds. *International Journal of Biological Macromolecules* 49: 20–31.

Sudheesh Kumar, P. T., S. Sowmya, K. L. Vinoth, H. Tamura, S. V. Nair, and R. Jayakumar. 2011b. β-Chitin hydrogel/nano hydroxyapatite composite scaffolds for tissue engineering applications. *Carbohydrate Polymers* 85: 584–591.

Tamura, H., T. Furuike, S. V. Nair, and R. Jayakumar. 2011. Biomedical applications of chitin hydrogel membranes and scaffolds. *Carbohydrate Polymers* 84: 820–824.

Valerio, P., M. M. Pereira, A. M. Goes, and F. Leite. 2004. The effect of ionic products from bioactive glass dissolution on osteoblast proliferation and collagen production. *Biomaterials* 25: 2941–2948.

Verrier, S., J. J. Blaker, M. Maquet, L. L. Hench, and R. A. A. Boccaccinia. 2004. PDLLA/bioglass composites for soft-tissue and hard-tissue engineering: An in vitro cell biology assessment. *Biomaterials* 25: 3013–3021.

Wheeler, D. L., M. J. Montfort, and S. W. McLoughlin. 2000. Differential healing response of bone adjacent to porous implant coated with hydroxyapatite and bioactive glass. *Journal of Biomedical Materials Research* 55: 603–612.

Xynos, I. D., A. J. Edgar, L. D. K. Buttery, L. L. Hench, and J. M. Polak. 2000. Ionic products of bioactive glass dissolution increase proliferation of human osteoblasts and induce insulin-like growth factor II mRNA expression and protein synthesis. *Biochemical Biophysics Research Communication* 276: 461–465.

Yimin, F., S. Tsuguyuki, and I. Akira. 2008. Preparation of chitin nanofibers from squid pen β-chitin by simple mechanical treatment under acid conditions. *Biomacromolecules* 9: 1919–1923.

35

Chitin Nanofibrils for Biomimetic Products: Nanoparticles and Nanocomposite Chitosan Films in Health Care

P. Morganti, G. Tishchenko, M. Palombo, I. Kelnar, L. Brozova,
M. Spirkova, E. Pavlova, L. Kobera, and F. Carezzi

CONTENTS

35.1 Recent Advances in Application of Chitin-Based Micro- and Nanoparticles in Cosmetics

35.1.1 Introduction

35.1.1.1 Polymeric Nanoparticles

Polymeric nanoparticles (PNs) are extensively studied as attractive particulate carriers for drug and cosmetic delivery systems, because of their controlled and sustained-release properties, subcellular size, and biocompatibility with tissue and cells (Grund et al., 2011). For these purposes, PNs are defined as solid colloidal particles ranging in size from 10 to 400 nm. They consist of macromolecular materials, in which the biological active agent is dissolved, entrapped, encapsulated, or absorbed, or to which the active agent is attached (Muthu and Singh, 2009; Dinarvand et al., 2011).

The term "nanoparticle" is a collective name for both nanospheres and nanocapsules (Figure 35.1).

In a *nanosphere*, the active agent can be surface-absorbed or particle-encapsulated owing to its matrix-type structure (Pinto et al., 2006). Differently, a *nanocapsule* is a vesicular system, in which an active agent is confined into a cavity and forms an inner liquid core surrounded by a polymeric membrane (Couvreur et al., 1995; Vinetsky and Madgassi, 1999). The submicron size of PNs over microparticles offers many recognized advantages, for example, their relatively high intraparticle uptake of active ingredients (Benoit et al., 1986; McClean et al., 1998; Sopprimath et al., 2001; Binks, 2002).

When PNs are dispersed into multiple nanoemulsions (NEs) for application in personal care and cosmetics, their biological efficacy increases in many times, mainly, because of easier penetrability through the skin layers owing to their small size in the emulsion droplets. However, NEs consisting of oil in water (O/W) or water in oil (W/O) droplets' phases with fine dispersions of 20–50 nm droplet sizes possess a higher kinetic stability.

It is important to underline that in PNs preparation, the optimization of phases of NEs represents important step for achieving stable emulsification and production processes,

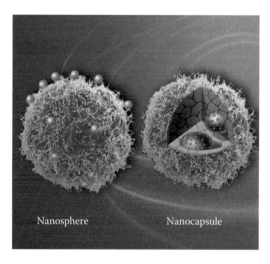

FIGURE 35.1
Imagination of the spatial structure of a nanosphere and a nanocapsule.

which depend, mainly, on the interfacial tension and bulk viscosity, phase transition region, structure, and concentration of a surfactant (Davies and Haydon, 1957; Davies and Rideal, 1961; Aveyard et al., 1986; Millers and Raney, 1993; Miller, 1996; Lopes-Montilla et al., 2002; Bouchemal et al., 2004a,b).

There are two types of NEs: thermodynamically stable and metastable ones, both depending on the preparation method (Sarker, 2005; Tirnaksiz et al., 2010). The Brownian motion of PNs prevents their sedimentation or creaming. Owing to very small sizes of the droplets, the physical stability of NEs increases but, however it requires stabilization with specific emulsifying agents, which must not form the lyotropic liquid crystalline phases. The right selection of an appropriate composition, the control of the addition order of all ingredients, the use of right surfactants, the application of high-energy technique, and the high-pressure homogenization are all together absolutely necessary for obtaining stable emulsions with very small sizes of droplets. In any way, the coalescence rates of NEs are closely related to the molecular weight of the surfactant absorbed on the O/W or W/O interface: the longer a surfactant molecule is, the more stable emulsion is formed (Sing et al., 1999; Tirnaksiz and Kalsin, 2005).

The number of homogenization cycles, the homogenization pressure, and the temperature affecting the droplet sizes of each NE represent other important parameters for maintaining the physical stability of the system as a whole (Yuan et al., 2008).

35.1.2 Production and Release of Nanoparticles

In nanocapsule and nanosphere production, the primary step is the preparation of NE by the nanoprecipitation method (Fessi et al., 1992) or, alternatively, by the interfacial polycondensation method accompanied with the spontaneous emulsification process (Bouchemal et al., 2004a).

35.1.2.1 Preparation of Micro- and Nanoparticles

A *nanosphere* is a spherical nanoparticle prepared from a definite polymer while that of a *nanocapsule* is a nanoparticle, which has a core surrounded by a material distinctly different from its composition (Samd et al., 2010). For preparing these particulate systems, the following 10 prerequisites referring to the utilized material and to the final formulation should be fulfilled: (1) *longer duration of action*, (2) *control of content release*, (3) *increase in activity with a biological efficacy*, (4) *protection of the active ingredients and* (5) *absence of toxicity*, (6) *bio- and ecocompatibility for all selected ingredients and final formulation*, (7) *sterilizability*, (8) *relative stability in both short and long period of the emulsion storage*, (9) *water solubility or dispersibility, and* (10) *easy targetability*.

Different methods may be used in preparation of chitin and chitosan (CS) particulate systems by using chitin nanofibrils (CNs). Selection of any method depends upon the desired particle size, thermal and chemical stability of the entrapped active ingredient, reproducibility of the released kinetic profiles, stability, and low toxicity of the final product. The nature of the active ingredients and type of the designed delivery process should be taken into consideration as well.

Chitin and/or CS nanoparticles may be formed as a spontaneous block-polymer complex when the aqueous suspensions of polycationic CN and/or CN-CS are added under stirring to polyanions such as hyaluronic acid (HA) or tripolyphosphate (STP) according to the ionic gelation technique (Calvo et al., 1997; De Campos et al., 2001; Xu and Du, 2003). The obtained CN-HA nanoparticles with diameters between 200 and 500 nm are usually separated by centrifugation or spray drying. As usual, their shape is quasispherical under transmission electron microscopy (TEM). Depending on the preparation method, it is possible to obtain CN-HA nanoparticles or HA-CN ones positively or negatively charged on their surface, respectively, and containing one or more hydro- or liposoluble active ingredients in the core, if they are previously solubilized or dispersed into CN and/or HA aqueous suspensions.

The polycationic CN has the ability to link the oppositely charged polyanionic HA forming a new block-*co*-polymer called *complex coacervate*. If it has to be present in the particle core together with some active ingredient(s), the nanocapsules' wall (coating layer) should be formed. Since the active groups of the anionic polymer and ingredients used for interacting with CN may vary significantly depending on their nature and quantity, the physicochemical properties of a coacervate will be also varied because of the difference in quantity and electrical charges of raw materials used (polyanionic HA or polycationic CN, etc.). Therefore, for a definite combination of a polycationic CN, with a polyanionic polymer, and an active ingredient, the successful microencapsulation will depend on many factors such as CN/anionic polymer/active ingredient ratio, pH, presence of electrolytes in solution, interfacial tension, and homogenization equipment.

35.1.2.2 Preparation of Emulsions and Nanoemulsions

To obtain the best efficiency and compatibility of the final cosmetic formulation, it should be better to use double emulsions, where the droplets of the dispersed phases contain even smaller dispersed droplets. These double emulsions may be W/O/W (water/oil/water) or O/W/O (oil/water/oil) ones, in which the external continuous phase is water or oil, respectively. They may be organized as *microemulsion* (ME) or as *nanoemulsion* (NE) systems. Differently from NEs, where nanoparticles cover the size range of 20–500 nm, the particles in MEs have sizes between 5 and 500 nm (Figure 35.2).

The considerably smaller dimensions of PNs over microparticles offer the number of distinct advantages. Therefore, PNs have to be adequately prepared to control and stabilize their droplet sizes and distribution. Sometimes, they may lose their transparency with time as a result of an increase in droplet size. In any way, PNs have to ensure complete protection of entrapped material and dissolved incompatible substances in the internal and external phase of the same product, to modulate the entrapped substances release (Bonina et al., 1992; Ozer and Aydin, 2009). Many comparative studies of PNs and MPs both in vitro and in vivo have shown that the former improve both transepidermal and transdermal delivery properties including the skin intercorneocytal uptake (Kreilgaard et al., 2000; Alvarez Figueroa and Blanco-Menden, 2001; Kreilgaard, 2001). Therefore, it is possible to obtain innovative cosmetic products by the combination of PNs with different sizes (*containing different active ingredients at their core*) and multiple MEs and NEs.

The formation of NEs requires energy input from conventional mechanical devices refined often on high-pressure two-stage homogenizers and microfluidizers or from the chemical potential of the components used (Hasrani et al., 1983; Washington and Davis, 1988; Lidgate et al., 1990). The long-term physical stability of NEs without apparent flocculation or coalescence makes them unique. In this case, they are sometimes considered as thermodynamically stable (Shrinivas et al., 2009).

Thus, it is possible to formulate new *cosmeceuticals* by using CN characterized by different superficial electrical charges, absorbing, incorporating, or selecting biologically active molecules. The MEs or NEs dispersed in the right way possess also much higher surface for contact with the skin structures. For all these reasons, these new products, ensuring

	Lipocapsules® (Gelatin)	Lipocapsules® (PMU/MMM)	Lipospheres®	Lipobead™	Lipoparticle™
Form	Soft/pliable	Hard/brittle	Soft and pliable spheres	Water swellable dry bead	Dry particles
Size (micron)	15–3000	5–100	500–4000	700 and 1500	5 and 500
Internal phase	60%–97%	50%–80%	25% maximum	5% maximum	30% maximum
Structure	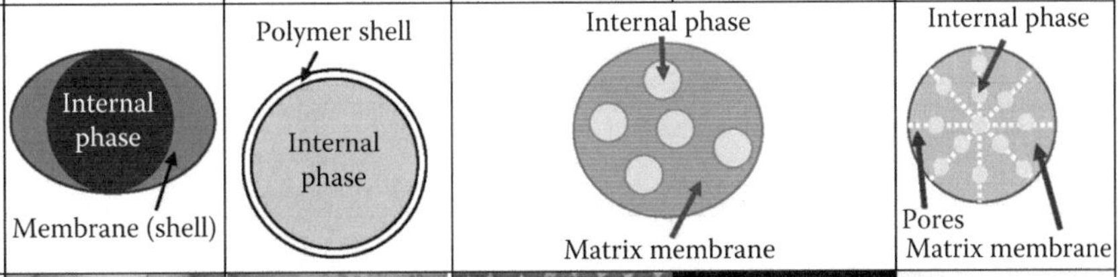 Internal phase / Membrane (shell)	Polymer shell / Internal phase	Internal phase / Matrix membrane		Internal phase / Pores / Matrix membrane
Appearance	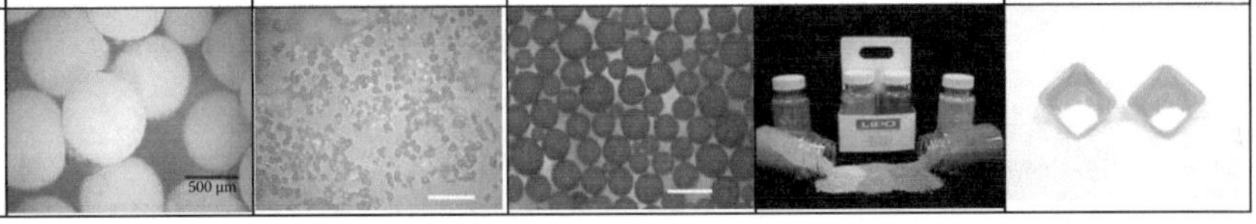				

FIGURE 35.2
Physicochemical parameters and appearance of the commercial ME and microparticle delivery systems. (From Mayer, P., Microencapsulation Technologies, 2008.)

higher penetration of the active ingredients with a better distribution and elimination, will give as result a higher efficient activity at level of both the skin layers and the entire human body. Thus, the final NEs constitute a new extremely fruitful cosmetic form for the release of many active ingredients at different rates (Lee et al., 2003).

35.1.2.3 Release of Active Ingredients

The most important parameter of PNs, containing encapsulated or entrapped active ingredients is the capacity for their release during storage and after skin application. The active ingredients, may be released by two ways: (1) mechanically by squeezing or rubbing under the applied pressure or (2) by diffusion through the coating layers of PNs (Kawashima et al., 1985a,b; Bodmeier et al., 1989; Liu et al., 1997). The efficiency of an active ingredient depends on its bioavailability, that is the way in which the ingredient is distributed and delivered to the skin (Figure 35.3). It is, therefore, essential to know how an active ingredient reaches its estimated site of action being released for a prolonged period of time at the same site of action. It is possible to obtain a *long-lasting* or *slow-releasing* cosmetic activity (Polk et al., 1994; Morganti, 2009a,b, 2010, 2011). Thus, the bioavailability of the selected ingredients depends not only on the type and form of used PNs but also on their physicochemical characteristics and the final emulsion designed. For obtaining the best results and the global efficiency of the cosmetic formula, it is necessary to choose the best preparation method and the best polymer(s) for achieving more efficient entrapment of the active ingredient(s).

The charge of a nanoparticle surface is also a very important variable in targeting delivery of an active ingredient. Once applied on the negatively charged skin or hair, the positively charged PNs of chitin/CS can easily and rapidly adhere on these human surfaces, allowing the control of the active ingredient(s) penetration. A great attention should be

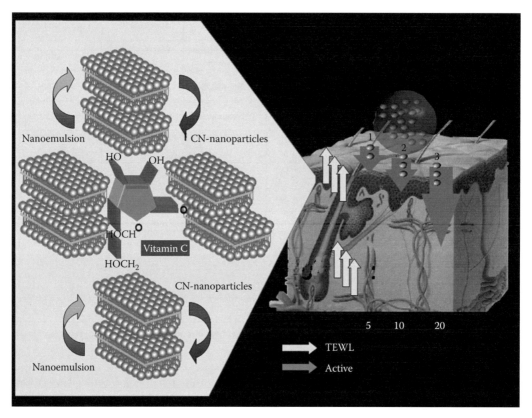

FIGURE 35.3
NE containing chitin nanoparticles with entrapped vitamin C (left). (right) ⇨ penetration of vitamin C into skin layers: 1 (stratum corneum), 2 (stratum spinosum), and 3 (dermis) after 5, 10, and 20 days of skin treatment with NE. ➡ TEWL is the transdermal water loss.

paid to the product design since the final formulation composed of the emulsified micro/ nanoparticles, the selected vehicles and the active ingredients encapsulated and/or entrapped into the nanospheres may regulate the corneocyte turnover, modulating the skin barrier function or repairing the damaged parts on the surface of the hair's cuticular structure, protecting its inner root sheath and cortex also (Biagini et al., 2008; Morganti, 2011).

It should be emphasized that the activity of the final cosmetic formulation depends not only on the micro- and nanodimensions of both the vehicles and active compounds, but also on the biological efficacy of the selected ingredients and, of course, on their release at the right targeted sites.

35.1.2.4 Release of Lutein

The release of ingredients entrapped in CN nanoparticles will be reported in detail elsewhere (Morganti et al., 2012a,b), while the lutein release from CS nanoparticles from both amorphous and crystal CN ones has shown (Figure 35.4) that lutein was in accordance with the composition and size of the nanoparticles used.

For nanoparticles based on CS and amorphous CN, the maximum release of lutein achieved 80%–98% during 20 h after dissolution, while for nanoparticles prepared

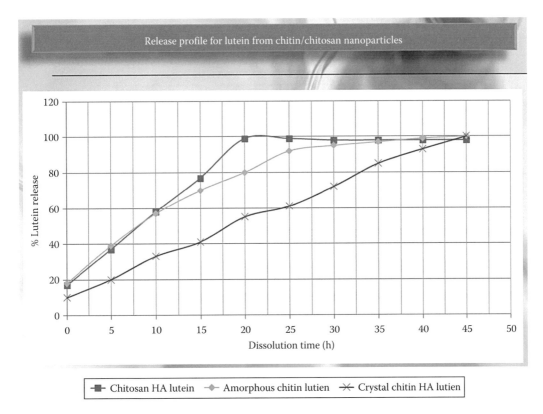

FIGURE 35.4
Kinetics of the release of lutein entrapped in nanoparticles based on CS, amorphous or crystal CN, and HA. ■, CS-HA-lutein; ◆, amorphous CN-HA-lutein; ×, crystal CN-HA-lutein.

from crystal CN, the release has shown a more regular and constant dissolution rate during 48 h. The different dissolution rates of these PNs seem to be attributed to the difference in their size, lutein entrapment capacity, and binding affinity to both water and lutein. The nanoparticles from crystal CN had the higher nanoparticle yield (42%), lutein loading content (35%), and entrapment efficiency (66%) (Table 35.1). Their mean size was the smallest (185 nm) compared with that of nanoparticles based on CS and amorphous chitin.

It should be concluded that all nanoparticles based on the studied chitin derivatives have shown high bioavailability together with very low toxicity. Owing to considerably higher crystallinity of CN in comparison to amorphous chitin, the former induced more continuous and constant release of lutein during about 48 h. This result reveals that the physicochemical structure of the studied polysaccharides influenced not only the loading capacity, which is higher for nanoparticles with smaller sizes, but also the more complete binding of the active ingredients such as lutein. The stable nanoparticles based on different chitin derivatives can be easily produced. However, for obtaining the best biorelease of the entrapped active ingredients and for their good bioavailability at the human skin application, the physicochemical structure of the chitin derivatives, the molecular size of the selected active ingredients, and the method used for its entrapment together with the design of the final emulsion should be chosen correctly.

TABLE 35.1

Characteristics of Nanoparticles Based on Chitin Derivatives
(CS, Amorphous and Crystal Chitin) Complexed with HA and Containing
the Entrapped Lutein

Polymer	Nanoparticle Yield (%)	Lutein Loading Content (%)	Entrapment Efficacy (%)	Particle Mean Size (nm)
Chitoson-HA-lutein	33 ± 9	10 ± 3	32 ± 5	458 ± 14
Amorphous chitin-HA-lutein	31 ± 10	18 ± 3	40 ± 5	355 ± 13
Crystal-chitin HA(CN) lutein	42 ± 9	35 ± 3	66 ± 6	185 ± 13

Note: All measurements were performed in triplicate.
Abbreviations: CN, Chitin Nanofibrils; HA, Hyaluronic acid.

35.1.3 Stability and Characterization of Chitin Micro- and Nanoparticles

Unlike MEs stable at high surfactant content, NEs keep their long-term physical stability at lower surfactant concentration attracting a great attention for application in personal cosmetics and healthcare products. Particularly, CN-based NEs are preferred by consumers and patients owing to the nature of their fluidity and admissible low toxicological profile and because of their aesthetic character and high skin feel (Gopal, 1968).

One of the most important physical characteristics of any NE is the size distribution of its droplets depending on the, so-called, spontaneity of the emulsification process (Gopal, 1968; Shahizdadeh et al., 1999). The spontaneity of both the emulsification process and the obtained droplets with small sizes is controlled by different mechanisms and affected by physicochemical characteristics of all the used ingredients. The sizes of NE droplets are widely varied and depend on the surfactant system and nature of the oil used. The higher the viscosity of oil and the values of the relative hydrophilic/lipophilic balance (HLB), the smaller the sizes of drops obtained.

Taking into account the experience of other authors (Seijo et al., 1990; Niwa et al., 1993; Guinebretière et al., 2002), our group has obtained the NEs based on CN with the smallest size of drops, when the balanced combination of hydrophilic (Pluronic®F68) and lipophilic (Lipoid®S75) surfactants was used. The synergistic interactions between these two surfactants with different HLB ensured the long-term stability of NEs owing to their, probably, very low interfacial tension at the oil–water interface (Tirnaksiz and Kalsin, 2005; Farahmad et al., 2006).

Another important aspect of the emulsification process is the miscibility of nanoparticles with the used water-solvent system. This is extremely important for producing the stable nanoparticles to be inserted into a designed cosmetic emulsion. The selection of organic solvents, if they are used, is the routine requirement in production of nanoparticles containing the entrapped active ingredients. The solvent(s) selected for the spontaneous emulsification has to be quasi-totally miscible with the continuous aqueous phase, and their toxicity must be low. The optimization of the spontaneous emulsification consists in the right choice of the balanced composition of the organic phase (oils), the used lipophilic surfactant(s), and the water-miscible solvent(s) used in the aqueous phase together with hydrophilic surfactant(s) and water. The final size of nanoparticles and their size distribution in NEs depend on the kinetics of the emulsification process, which, in its turn, is mainly controlled by the solubility of the selected organic solvent in water (Wehrle et al., 1995). After the complete removal of the water-miscible solvent by evaporation, the spontaneous emulsification is going on faster, when the miscibility of the organic phase and aqueous one is better. Selection of the right solvent is, therefore, another important requirement characterizing the structure of final NEs and, consequently, the size distribution of nanoparticles.

Naturally, the choice of both the suitable polymer and the emulsification/evaporation processes is another fundamental rule for obtaining the stabilized nanoparticles dispersed in stable NEs. The first step on preparation of HA-CN nanoparticles is carried out by the ionic gelation method using a dispersing agent (emulsifier compound) and high-energy stirring under vacuum. The polycationic CN is suspended in aqueous solution containing the active ingredient(s), while the polyanionic HA is dispersed in water forming the suspension of nanodroplets and containing or not other active ingredients (Morganti et al., 2012a,b). Due to the complexation between species bearing the opposite charges, CN undergoes ionic gelation and precipitates forming lamellar particles, which may be transformed in spherical nanoparticles by the homogenization process. It is possible to obtain a block-*co*-polymer in the form of nanospheres by this method; the active ingredient(s) is finely dispersed in the polymer network successively. In a second step, this aqueous suspension of nanospheres is dispersed into a multiple emulsion.

Water can be evaporated by increasing temperature under pressure and continuous stirring. Alternatively, it can be removed by applying the stream of hot air. For activation of polymer precipitation and the consequent formation of nanoparticles, it is necessary to promote the right diffusion of the dispersed phase being water or solvent.

Other important factors are, of course, the high oil(s), the combination of the selected surfactants, and the solvent/water miscibility. All are the key factors for promoting the self-emulsification of NEs with small sizes of droplets. Nanoparticle surface and its physicochemical character are very important parameters in targeting cosmetic delivery as well (Tice and Gillex, 1985; Wehrle et al., 1995; Grossiord and Seiller, 1998; Farahmand et al., 2006; Meyer et al., 2009; Morganti et al., 2012a,b).

The HLB in the polymeric composition, the surface charge, the biodegradation profile of the nanoparticles, the type of adjuvant substances, the associated active ingredient(s), and their molecular weight, charge, and localization in nanospheres controlled by absorption or incorporation process have all a great influence on penetration of the active ingredients through the skin and on their biodistribution and elimination (Quintanar-Guerrero et al., 1998). Thus, nanoparticles from hydrophilic positively charged polymers such as CN and CS have shown the binding affinity to follicle-associated epithelia and good bioadhesive properties to mucous membranes as well (Biagini et al., 2008).

The design of any preparation method of micro- and nanoparticles depends upon the nature of active ingredients and the type of the delivery device. Organic solvents with low toxicity (class III according to the EU Pharmacopeia) have to be used for the safety reasons. In some cases, other methods such as the ionic gelation should be preferred because of toxicological problems and technical difficulties to use the solvent method.

35.1.3.1 Nanoparticle Characterization and Stability

As will be published elsewhere (Morganti et al., 2012a,b), our group has reported about the possibility to produce the stable nanoparticles by the spontaneous formation of complexes at the simple mixing of polycations such as CS and CN with different polyanions (HA, collagen, alginate, carrageen, or pectin). Compared with the solvent method, this technique has the advantage since only water is utilized as the continuous phase of emulsion. In this case, there is no additional step—the removal of used organic solvents. The obtained block-*co*-polymer–nanoparticles may be easily dispersed into multiple NEs by this solvent-free method, in which the nanoparticle size is governed by the rate of stirring, the type and amount of dispersing agent(s), the viscosity of aqueous phase, and temperature. The dependence of nanoparticle sizes, their yield, the lutein loading content, and its entrapment efficiency on the type of chitin derivative (CS, amorphous or crystal CN), forming block-*co*-polymers with HA, have shown (Table 35.1) that the smallest average diameters of nanoparticles can be obtained if the crystal CN instead of amorphous chitin or CS is used (Morganti et al., 2012a,b). It has been confirmed by monthly control that the droplets of emulsion remain stable without sedimentation or creaming during 1 year at different temperatures.

It is interesting to underline that the production of CN-HA nanoparticles, by the ionic gelation method, eliminating the washing steps, improves the economical system reducing energy consumption. The conventional mechanical equipment and/or high-power ultrasound device are the main advantages of the spontaneous emulsification process ensuring the easy preparation of nanodroplets. This low-energy and time-saving method is a mild process suitable for encapsulating the unstable biological substances such as vitamins and unsaturated fatty acids. As concerns the release of a drug or any active cosmetic ingredient, it is affected by many factors such as polymer degradation, its molecular weight and crystallinity (i.e., if amorphous or crystal chitin is used), binding affinity of an active ingredient, its hydrophilicity or hydrophobicity, and its capability to be incorporated into the polymeric matrix with high loading content (Gref et al., 1994; Sain et al., 1998; Yeong et al., 2003).

The determination of the release behavior of an ingredient from each kind of polymer nanoparticles is a rather complicated process. The aspects regarding the nanometric dimensions, final stability of emulsions, and the release of active ingredients remain still unclear and require further investigations. In any way, the use of CN for entrapment of various active cosmetic or medical ingredients has opened a new avenue for creation of eco- and biocompatible nanoparticles with very low toxicity and improved consumer compliance (Morganti et al., 2012a,b). CN, being an easily biodegradable polymer with low toxicity and good biocompatibility (Morganti, 2009a,b; Morganti and Li, 2011; Morganti et al., 2011a,c) is finally degraded forming oligomers and individual monomers, which may be metabolized in the body via Krebs cycle and eliminated as carbon dioxide and water (Morganti, 2009a,b). Among the natural polymers utilized nowadays, CN is a very promising ingredient for the preparation of novel cosmetic delivery systems since the method of its manufacturing does not cause environmental problems and the raw source of chitin being produced from the fish waste is easy of access at low cost. The applications of this clarified natural polymer are not limited by cosmetic use described earlier. It is used in biomedicine for preparation of biomembranes and human implants, in pharmacy, in food packaging, and in production of biotextiles (Morganti, 2009b).

35.1.4 Safety and Biocompatibility of Chitin Micro- and Nanoparticles

CN derivatives and their block-*co*-polymers were evaluated in this paragraph from the point of view of their safety as potential drug and cosmetic ingredients and/or active carriers.

The cytotoxicity of CN and block CN-*co*-HA nanoparticles was determined by the MTT method (Musmann, 1983; Natthan et al., 2010) using ex vivo cultures of keratinocytes

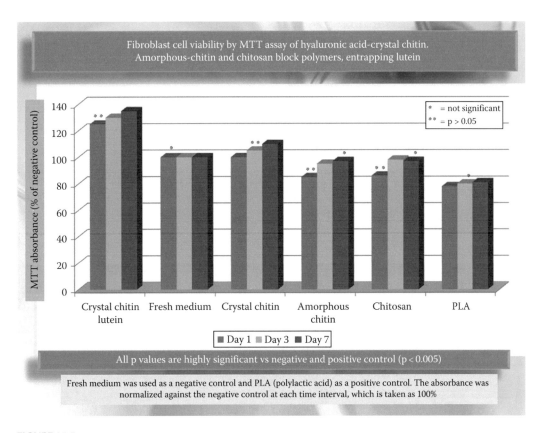

FIGURE 35.5
Dependence of the viability of fibroblast cells on the lutein release from □ CS-HA, ■ amorphous chitin–HA, and ⊠ crystal chitin–HA nanoparticles. Fresh medium and PLA are the negative and positive controls, respectively. The relative absorbance was determined by MTT assay (in % from negative control accepted as 100%) at first, third, and seventh day of the fibroblast cells contact with the tested nanoparticles.

and fibroblasts; comparing their viability in the presence of both the tested nanoparticles and polylactic acid (PLA), known as safe compound in drug delivery (Morganti et al., 2012a,b) was compared. CN and block CN-*co*-HA polymer nanoparticles (Figures 35.5 and 35.6) have shown a very low toxicity and high relative safety and may be considered as safe components for drug or cosmetic delivery. The ex vivo results obtained have been confirmed by the in vivo tape and scrub methods. These techniques made it possible to control the skin penetration of different NEs containing CN and block CN-*co*-HA polymer nanoparticles with entrapped lutein as active ingredient. It was possible to obtain nanoparticles positively or negatively charged on their surface by changing the producing process. Lutein was detected in all stratum corneum layers at different concentrations in dependence on the method used and the obtained electrical charge. Lutein was much more concentrated at the first five SC stripped layers (second strip) for the positively charged nanoparticles (Figures 35.7 and 35.8). In contrast, the negatively charged nanoparticles were practically recovered only on the outermost SC surface (about 90% on first strip) with overall negative net charge (of about 18% on second strip and 0% on the others).

Increasing in the number of scrubs at different times of treatment, the recovery of lutein in the corneocytes' layers is higher in dependence on (1) the *days of treatment* with the NE and (2) the *electrical charges* of the designed nanoparticles. The more forced scrubs gave rise

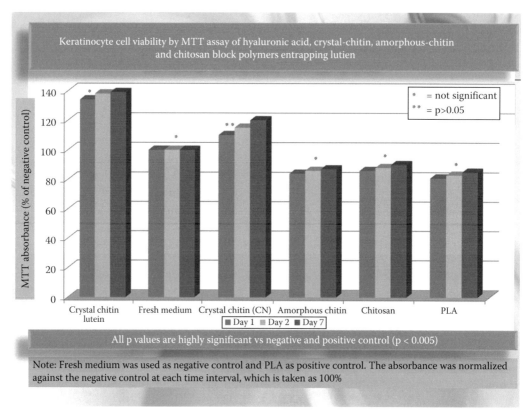

FIGURE 35.6
Dependence of the viability of keratinocyte cells on the lutein release from □ CS-HA, ■ amorphous chitin–HA, and ⊠ crystal chitin–HA nanoparticles. For details, see the caption to Figure 35.5. The relative absorbance was determined by MTT assay (in % from negative control accepted as 100%) at first, second, and seventh day of the keratinocyte cells contact with the tested nanoparticles.

to verify the last corneocytes, living near the dermis. Increasing the days of treatment with positively charged nanoparticles, lutein penetrated deeper through the corneocytes layers. This phenomenon is clear at using the positively charged CN-HA nanoparticles. On the contrary, the negatively charged HA-*co*-CN nanoparticles were recovered only in the first corneocytes' layers. However, 100% lutein was recovered in the outermost (deeper) SC layers depending on the number of stripping or scrubs, days of treatment, and nanoparticle charge. Lutein did never penetrate into the inner metabolically active skin strata. This difference in the recovered activity implies that nanoparticles are capable to disturb the assembled lipid lamellae in dependence on their electrical charge, thus favoring the diffusion of active molecules entrapped into the nanoparticles in different corneocytes' layers.

It should be noted in conclusion that it seems to be possible to produce the safe nanocarriers bearing biologically active ingredients, which are selectively released in the superficial epidermis layers. These innovative nanoparticles based on CN have good skin tolerability. They are capable to change the physical properties of SC without provoking evident side effects and improve the diffusivity of active compounds without using the invasive technologies.

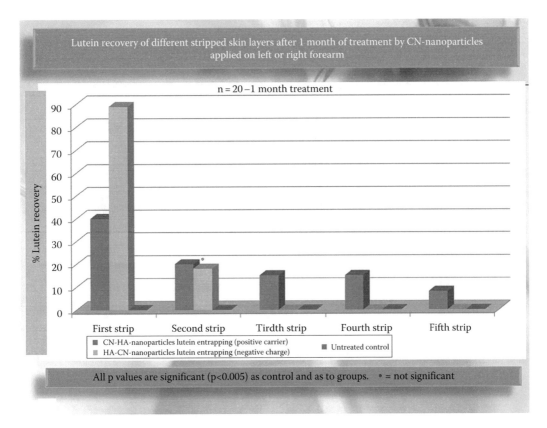

Lutein recovery of different stripped skin layers after 1 month of treatment by CN-nanoparticles applied on left or right forearm

n = 20 – 1 month treatment

All p values are significant (p<0.005) as control and as to groups. * = not significant

FIGURE 35.7
Dependence of the lutein recovery in different skin layers on the charge of nanoparticles: ≤ CN-HA-lutein (positive charge), ■ HA-CN-lutein (negative charge), ⊠ untreated control. Corneocytes from first to fifth strips were obtained after 1-month treatment of left or right forearms with the tested nanoparticles.

35.1.5 Biodegradability

35.1.5.1 Cell Metabolism and Enzymes

It is well known that many natural human and environmental processes such as the natural skin turnover and cell sloughing are controlled by enzymes (Brooks et al., 2002). The chemical reactions, which are carried out inside the plant or human cells, will occur at much higher temperatures outside the cells. For this reason, each reaction requires a specific boost for controlling the chemical reactivity (Brooks et al., 2002). This control is exerted through specialized proteins called *enzymes*, each of which accelerates or catalyzes many possible reactions. There are two opposing streams of chemical reactions occurring in cells: (1) the *catabolic* pathways, which breakdown foodstuffs into small molecules necessary for cells as building blocks and also generating energy, and (2) the *anabolic* or biosynthetic pathways, which use the energy obtained by catabolism to drive the synthesis of many other molecules that form the cells. For example, specific enzymes secreted by the keratinocytes are the effective cellular catalysts dissolving the desmosomes, which release the dead surface skin cells. Their active sites are sulfhydryl groups, which cleave

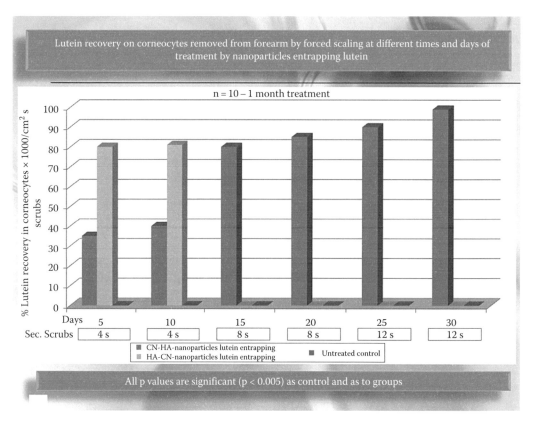

FIGURE 35.8
Illustration of the vibration modes in an acetylated glucosamine group. Amide I is referred to the stretching vibrations of C=O group, amide II implies N–H bending and C–N stretching vibrations, and amide III is a very complex vibration mode resulting from in-phase combination of C–N stretching and N–H in-plane bending, with some contribution from C–C stretching and C=O bending vibrations.

the peptide bonds by the same way as the thioglycolic acid and cysteine do breaking down the peptide bonds in hairs at permanent wave (Johnson et al., 2008).

Enzymes are highly specific and complex protein catalysts acting in both the human body and environment and controlling thousands of catabolic and anabolic reactions on degradation and elimination of waste materials. They help to carry out most chemical reactions, which are necessary to the cells to maintain their viability (Brooks et al., 2002; Johnson et al., 2008). Enzymes are extremely efficient compounds and work by reducing entropy between the products and reactants so that the activation energy decreases and reaction can occur rapidly. When this happens, the substrate's ground-state energy level increases. Then, the activated substrate binds with the enzyme's reactive site. For controlling the possibility to degrade the chitin/CS nanoparticles without interfering with the skin cell's activity, the different enzymes were used. After the enzymatic hydrolysis, the more or less degradability of different nanoparticles was assessed (Table 35.2) by measuring their weight variation resulting from the activity of different enzymes such as cellulase, lysozyme, pectinase, amylase, and collagenase (Morganti et al., 2012a,b). The nanoparticles were indifferent or prone particularly to the enzymatic degradation without

TABLE 35.2

Efficiency of the Enzymatic Degradation of Nanoparticles Based on Chitin Derivatives Complexed with HA and Containing the Entrapped Lutein after 48 Day Hydrolysis at 25°C

Enzyme	Relative Weight Loss [(Wi − Wf)/Wi] × 100 (%)[a]		
	Crystal CN-HA-Lutein	Amorphous CN-HA-Lutein	Amorphous CS-HA-Lutein
Cellulose	99.47	99.67	0.2
Pectinase	99.7	99.8	0.25
Amylase	99.9	99.9	0.4
Lysozyme	99.95	99.85	0.4
Collagenase	99.7	99.76	0.3

[a] Wi and Wf are the weight of nanoparticles (g) before and after enzymatic degradation. All measurements were performed in triplicate.

visible differences between all chitin derivatives (amorphous or crystal CN and CS) and the tested enzymes. These results demonstrate that all synthesized nanoparticles being totally and readily degraded by the enzymes, which are normally present in humans and environment, have to be considered as healthy and eco-compatible active carriers for noninvasive transepidermal drug and cosmetic delivery.

35.2 Skin Wound Healing and Repair

The repairing of normal wounds as the consequence of an injury gives rise to an innate immune response involving inflammation activated by enzymes with different activities. Wound healing is an orchestrated cascade of events that lead to repair of the skin, when the underlying dermis is also compromised, but lead also to an anatomic regeneration, when the epidermis is injured. The majority of wounds are polymicrobial ones with both aerobes and anaerobes present and with the prevalence of aerobic pathogens, such as *Staphylococcus aureus*, *Pseudomonas aeruginosa*, and *beta-hemolytic streptococci*.

Inflammation, as a beneficial host response, contributes to the pathogenesis of a large number of diseases. Proper balance between the levels of proteinase and inhibitors of keratinocytes' enzymatic activity is crucial for resolving the inflammation and wound reepithelialization. For example, the metalloproteinases degrade all components of the extracellular matrix. It seems that *fibrin* accelerates keratinocyte activation and reduces the time of wound closure. Skin's integrity and its normal functioning depend on keratinocytes' position in the epidermal structure. They *recognize and translate* the epidermal continuous intercellular signals and perform their functions at any particular time. Keratinocytes not only communicate with each other but also communicate with dermis and the local immune system creating a constant flow of information (Freeberg et al., 2001; Tomic-Canic et al., 2003).

Many sophisticated dressings are available for wound care, which can be used without or in combination with the absorbers of exudates, and combat odors and infections, relieve the pain, and provide and maintain moist environment at the wound surface, necessary for facilitation of the production of granulation tissue and epithelialization process (Thomas, 2003). There is a broad spectrum of occlusive or semiocclusive dressings such as woven and nonwoven tissue and nanocomposite films used in healing the acute and chronic wounds. These dressings have to be kept moist to heal the wounds and increase their superficial epithelialization. Simultaneously, the dressings can also increase the population of microorganisms and, hence, induce wound infections. For controlling the antiseptic activity and moisture in wounds, the special CS and CN films releasing nanocrystallite silver have been developed. The increase in stability and cytocompatibility of silver nanoparticles and their antiseptic efficacy at simultaneous reduce in their potential toxicity are achieved by some low quantity of Ag ions entrapped and slowly released from these innovative semiocclusive films (Morganti et al., 2012a,b).

35.2.1 Nanocomposite Films from Chitosan and Chitin Nanoparticles

The considered, in this chapter, nanocomposite films from CS and CN exhibit excellent biocompatibility with skin at application in cosmetics and dermatology (Morganti, 2010). In comparison with CS films cross-linked through covalent bonds by natural (genipin) or synthetic (glutaraldehyde, STP, ethylene glycol, diglycidyl ether, and diisocyanate) cross-linkers (Muzzarelli, 2009b), the CN-CS films are considerably more biodegradable since both components are strengthened by only a developed system of relatively weak hydrogen (H) bonds and hydrophobic interactions. In applying to the skin, the humidity inside a CN-CS film grows, followed by increase in water content and decrease in the interchains binding in CS matrix. As a result, the distance between the chains increases, and easier biodegradation of a nanocomposite film occurs.

The intensive investigations on preparation and application of nanocomposite CS films, especially, in the health care (Muzzarelli et al., 2007; Muzzarelli, 2009a) are carried out by the scientific groups headed by Muzzarelli and Morganti, although some attempts have been already made by other researches in preparing edible and packing films by reinforcing some natural and synthetic polymers with CN (Muzzarelli et al., 2007).

Analysis of the published results on preparation and characterization of CS films reinforced with CN has shown that the thermal stability and the apparent degree of crystallinity of the CS matrix did not practically change after introducing CN. The tensile strength of CN-reinforced CS films increased from that of the pure CS films with initial increase in the CN content to reach a maximum at their content of about 3 wt% and decreased gradually with further increase in the CN content, while the percentage of elongation at break decreased from that of the pure CS with initial increase in the CN content and leveled off when their content was greater than or equal to about 3 wt% (Sriupayo et al., 2005). The heat treatment helped improve water resistance of the CN-CS films, leading to decreased values of their relative weight loss and degree of swelling. As evidenced by atomic force microscopy (AFM), the CNs were homogeneously dispersed in the CS matrix in the nanocomposites. The water uptake studies showed that cross-linking and chitin incorporation in the CS matrix both decreased the equilibrium water uptake although cross-linking had a more pronounced impact on permselectivity and stability toward pH variations. It was also found that incorporation of CN in CS matrix did not affect its inherent characteristics like biodegradability, transparency, and antibacterial properties (Mathew et al., 2009).

35.2.2 Preparation of Nanocomposite Chitin–Chitosan Films

The solution casting, having been invented shortly after World War II by Glen Howatt for producing the ceramic capacitors (Twiname and Mistler, 1999), is nowadays a leading method in nanotechnology for preparation of composite films with very homogeneous distribution of nanoparticles, uniform properties, and thickness, for example, therapeutic films for drug delivery. One of the obvious advantages of the solution casting consists in that the viscous solutions of biopolymers are processed at ambient condition. Therefore, this method seems to be the most suitable (Thayer, 2003) for production of the composite films from polysaccharides such as CN and CS, which are not thermoplastics.

At the lab scale, the solution casting is usually carried out as follows: a homogeneous mixture consisting of, for example, an aqueous CS solution, desired quantities of CN, and a plasticizer is degassed, cast on a support using a knife to ensure the desired thickness of a film, and dried under ambient conditions. The dried films are removed from the supports and ready for in vitro testing and further in vivo biological applications.

In practice, it is sometimes required to enhance the antimicrobial activity by preparing the therapeutically oriented films. For these purposes, various physiologically active substances such as antibiotics or Ag nanoparticles (Vimala et al., 2010) are incorporated to the nanocomposite films. In this case, the preparation procedure differed from that described earlier by the fact that the therapeutic ingredient is introduced by spraying the surface of the cast CN-CS films before they are dried. It is also possible to entrap the active ingredient previously into CN before producing the films. The latter method resulted in higher activity of Ag-CN-CS films.

35.2.3 Physicochemical Characteristics

For successful preparation of new composite materials and optimization of their properties, the knowledge of the physicochemical properties (chemical structure, physical state, and functionality) of the components is the sine qua non. The functionality of the components defines their compatibility at mixing and homogeneity of the composites and, hence, their mechanical properties, which help to evaluate the durability of a composite material and to give instructions at its practical applications.

The chemical structure of CN and CS is practically the same. Both these components consist of glucosamine ($GlcNH_2$) and *N*-acetylglucosamine ($GlcNH-COCH_3$) moieties bound with each other through 1,4-β-glycosidic bonds in linear chains. CN and CS differed in the values of DA* that, in its turn, defines the difference in their physical state: CNs are nanofibrils insoluble in water even acidified to pH 2 and form a stable aqueous suspension, whereas CS is water soluble at pH about 5 and forms transparent viscous honey-like solutions.

More detailed information about difference in functionality of CS and CN is usually obtained by Fourier transform infrared (FTIR) spectroscopy, which is the most powerful tool for identifying types of chemical bonds (functional groups) since each of them absorbs light of the definite wavelength.[†]

---

* The contents of $GlcNH-COCH_3$ moieties in the used CN and chitosan were about 90 and 20 mol%, respectively.
† An FTIR spectrum of a pure compound is generally so unique that it is like a molecular "fingerprint." By interpreting the infrared absorption spectrum, the chemical bonds in a molecule can be determined.

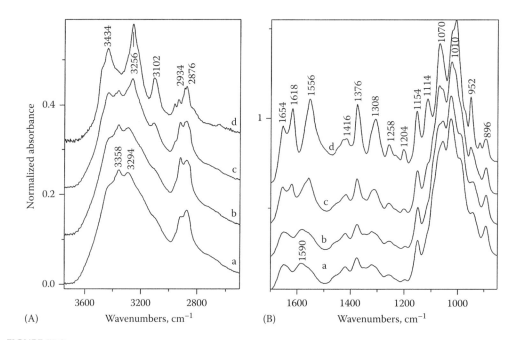

FIGURE 35.9

FTIR spectra (16 scans with 4 cm⁻¹-resolution) of CS and nanocomposite CN-CS films with CN content, wt%: a, 0 (CS); b, 6; c, 36; d, 100 (CN). Spectra were recorded using a spectrophotometer PerkinElmer Paragon 1000PC and attenuated total reflection technique Specac MKII Golden Gate Single Reflection ATR system with a diamond crystal; the incidence angle was 45° and evaluated using Spectrum 2.00 software. The range of wavenumbers, cm⁻¹: (A) 3750–2500 and (B) 1700–850.

The difference in normalized* FTIR spectra of CN and CS (Figure 35.9) is mainly defined by the difference in their DA. The absorption intensity of all vibration modes in the spectrum of CN (curves d) is considerably higher than that in CS one (curve a). The reason of this phenomenon is very likely higher packing density of the chains in CN than in CS. This supposition is fulfilled if the molecular orientation of chitin chains in CN is the same as in CS (Zhang et al., 1998). This is especially true of both CS and α-CN used since their chains are arranged in an antiparallel fashion. The FTIR spectra of CN and CS show that the most essential distinctions are observed in the interval of wave numbers 3500–3000 and 1700–1500 cm⁻¹. In the latter interval, the appearance of the characteristic bands in the FTIR spectrum of CN is explained by the high content of *N*-acetylated amine groups, giving the bands assigned to the vibrations of amides I, II, and III (Figure 35.10) (Paulino et al., 2006; Kumirska et al., 2010).

Amide I is referred to the stretching vibrations of C=O group, amide II implies N–H bending and C–N stretching vibrations, and amide III is a very complex vibration mode resulting from in-phase combination of C–N stretching and N–H in-plane-bending, with some contribution from C–C stretching and C=O bending vibrations.

In the FTIR spectrum of CN, the amide I band is split into two components at 1654 and 1618 cm⁻¹ due to the influence of H-bonds; the amide II band is observed at 1556 cm⁻¹

---

* Normalization of FTIR spectra was carried out by dividing all absorbance values at a spectrum to maximum absorbance value (max A_X) in this spectrum. The wave number X corresponding to the max A_X was 1028 cm⁻¹, 1010 cm⁻¹, 1028 cm⁻¹, or 1026 cm⁻¹ for chitosan; CN; composite CN-CS films with 6 and 36 wt% CN content, respectively.

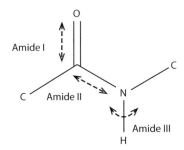

FIGURE 35.10
Illustration of the vibration modes in the acetylated glucosamine group.

(Kumirska et al., 2010). The presence of amide III in CN spectrum is confirmed by the bands at 3100 and 3256 cm^{-1} assigned to NH bending and stretching, respectively.

A progressive weakening of all these bands is usually observed during *N*-deacetylation of chitin. The changes in absorption intensity of these bands in CS spectrum are considered as a confirmation of the really occurred *N*-deacetylation reaction. In contrast to CN spectrum, in the CS one, the intensification of the peak at 1590 cm^{-1} and a decrease at 1652 cm^{-1} are observed. This reveals the prevalence of NH$_2$ groups, which appeared in CS after deacetylation of *N*-acetylglucosamine moieties. The bands at 3434 and 3358 cm^{-1} are assigned to the stretching vibration of hydroxyl groups (Paulino et al., 2006). Their absorption intensity is higher in CN spectrum than in CS one, where these bands are shifted to 3358 and 3294 cm^{-1} due to H-bonding. Some changes in the wave numbers of the rest bands corresponding to the vibration intensity of other functional groups such as –CH, –OH, C–O–C, glucose ring, –CH$_3$, and –CH$_2$ presenting in both CN and CS are less pronounced between the spectra. Very likely, less sharpness of the peaks in CS spectrum than in CN one is mainly affected by H-bonds involved in intra- and interchain interactions, which have been recently analyzed in detail by molecular dynamics (MD) simulations (Franca et al., 2008, 2011). The analysis of 3D structures of chitin and CS has shown that, namely, intra- and interchain H-bonds* stabilize the tridimensional structure of both chitin and CS in the solid state resulting in their ordered fibrillar structure with rather high degree of crystallinity (Mogilevskaya et al., 2006), which is considerably higher for chitin than for CS. The developed system of H-bonds affecting the spatial packing of CS chains manifests itself the more the higher is DA. In the ^{13}C CP/MAS NMR spectra of CS, CN, and their composites (Figure 35.11), the peaks corresponding to the resonance of ring carbons C1-C6, carbonyl C7 carbon, and methyl C8 carbon (i.e., CO and CH$_3$ groups in GlcNH-CO-CH$_3$ moieties, respectively) in CN spectrum (curve b) are noticeably sharper, and their resolution is considerably better than in CS one (curve a). In CS, the chains have greater rotation and more degrees of freedom because of lower amount of acetyl groups participating in H-bonding and restricting the motion of chains around the glycosidic linkage (Errington et al., 1993). That is why the cross-polarization efficiency is the highest

---

* It was shown that one intrachain H-bond is formed between OH group at C3 and bridge oxygen of the same chain of chitin in the solid state. In the interchain H-bond, CH$_2$OH group at C6 of one chain and the NHCOCH$_3$ group at C2 of a glucosamine unit of another chain are involved (Franca, 2011). These H-bonds force the chains to adopt mainly one conformation (a twofold helix) in chitin that results in its low conformational changes, that is, low flexibility of chains. In chitosan, the chains exist in four main helical conformations (extended twofold helix, relaxed twofold helix, 4/1 helix, and 5/3 helix) that ensure their considerably higher flexibility and, hence, lower crystallinity than that of CN.

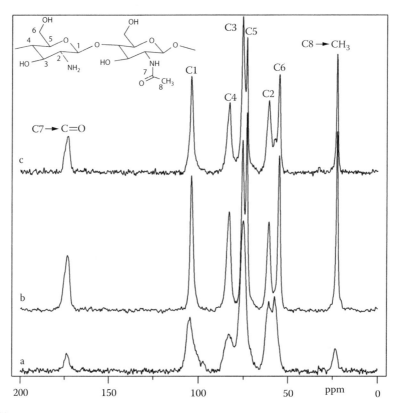

FIGURE 35.11

1D solid-state NMR spectra of CS film (a); CN (b) and a nanocomposite CN-CS film (c) with 36 wt% content of CN. The spectra were measured using a Bruker Avance 500 NMR spectrometer at magic angle spinning frequency of the sample 10 kH and amplitude modulated cross-polarization with duration 1 ms to for obtaining ^{13}C CP/MAS NMR spectra with 5s recycle delay. The ^{13}C scale was calibrated with glycine as external standard (176.03 ppm—low-field carbonyl signal).

for highly crystalline CN consisting of chains, the spatial conformation of which is fixed by multiple H-bonds and hydrophobic interactions. The spectra of composites, in which the relative content of more amorphous CS decreases, occupy some intermediate posts; they become more similar to that of CN when higher content of nanofibrils is incorporated to CS matrix (curve c). Although CN-CS films are the nanocomposites of practically a "single" polymer,* nevertheless, the reinforcing nanofillers (slender "nanorods" with high rigidity) influence on spatial packing of CS chains in composites considerably.

For visualizing the morphological changes in composite materials on the micro- and nanolevels, the scanning electron microscopy (SEM), TEM, and AFM are the most popular methods. In SEM micrographs, the fracture of CN-CS films (Figure 35.12c) looks more relief (rougher) than that of CS one (Figure 35.12a). When higher magnified (Figure 35.12d), the distribution of nanofibrils in CS matrix seems to be homogeneous, confirming the

---

* It is generally accepted that chitin is considered and named as chitosan if it is *N*-deacetylated to such a degree that it becomes soluble in dilute acidic medium. It is typical for chitosan that its DA values are ranged in the interval 40–60 mol % (Paulino, 2006).

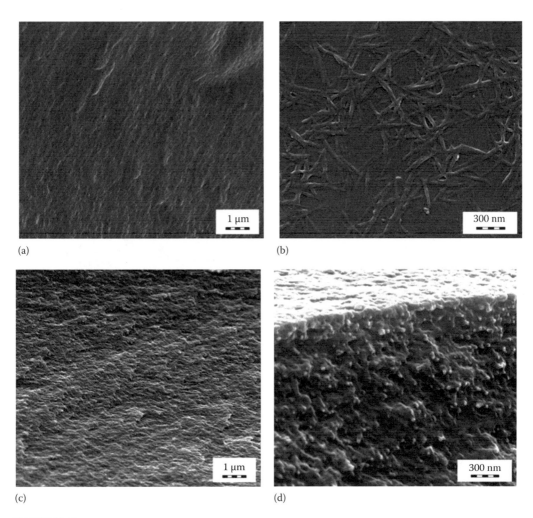

(a)   (b)

(c)   (d)

FIGURE 35.12
Field emission gun scanning electron microscopy (FEGSEM) micrographs of a CS film fracture (a); a drop of CN aqueous emulsion air dried on a microscopic glass (b); fractures (c, d) of a nanocomposite CN-CS films with 36 wt% CN content at low and high magnifications. All samples were covered with a thin platinum layer (~4 nm) in order to limit sample damage and increase resolution (Vacuum sputter coater SCD 050, Balzers). The micrographs were obtained in high-vacuum mode, at high acceleration voltage (30 kV, small spot size 2 nm), and secondary electrons detector using a microscope Quanta 200 FEG (FEI, Czech Republic).

good compatibility of both components. The nanocomposite films do not lost their macroscopic homogeneity and transparency even at high content of CN* (Figure 35.12b).

At the nanoscale level in the AFM 3D height images (10 × 10 μm²) (Figure 35.13a), a CS film and a nanocomposite CN-CS one look heterogeneous, but the surface of the former film seems to be more ordered than that of the latter one (Figure 35.13b). CS chains interacting with each other through multiple H-bonds formed elongated clusters packed rather regularly as can be seen in the phase image of a CS film (Figure 35.13c). In contrast,

* The CNs evaluated by SEM have the average diameter ~30 nm, length ~300 nm, and average aspect ratio about 10.

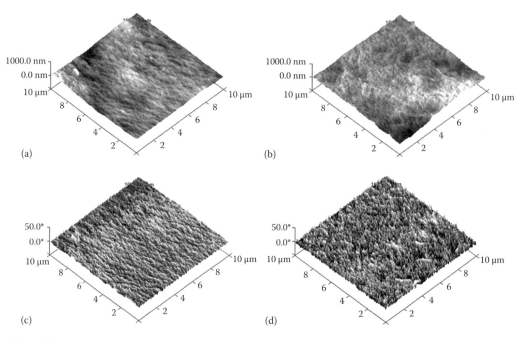

FIGURE 35.13

AFM 3D height (a, b) and phase (c, d) images of a CS film (a, c) and a nanocomposite CN-CS (b, d) one with 36 wt% CN content. Tested area: 10×10 μm². The images were obtained using an atomic force microscope (MultiMode Digital Instruments NanoScopeTM Dimension IIIa) equipped with the SSS-NCL probe, Super Sharp Silicon™-SPM-Sensor (NanoSensors™ Switzerland) at spring constant 35 nm⁻¹ and resonant frequency ~170 kHz using the tapping mode AFM technique.

the aggregates of CS chains look disordered in the phase image of a nanocomposite CN-CS film (Figure 35.13d). This happens because CS chains being more mobile more easily interact with functional groups exposed on the surface of rigid nanofibrils. The latter being considerably larger in dimensions force highly flexible CS chains to immobilize on their surface. The interchain bindings, which have existed in CS phase, are demolished when it is filled with rigid CN. This disturbance of the packing order of CS chains on the surface of composite CN-CS films is qualified with the phase images.

The water uptake is very important characteristics of each new material to be assumed for skin application in both cosmetics and dermatology. Solubility and swelling of CS are known to be influenced by crystallinity, which is correlated to the percentage and distribution of acetyl groups along the biopolymer chain (Sannan et al., 1976). The water uptake within the composite CN-CS films (Figure 35.14) increases continuously with growing pressure of water vapors (Figure 35.14A) from 0 to 3 kPa. Simultaneously, the water absorption decreases with increasing the CN content. It is obviously because CNs with remarkably higher DA are more hydrophobic than CS in spite of the fact that CNs have hydrated water molecules participating in H-bonds (Franca et al., 2008, 2011). Therefore, the relative water uptake* within composite CN-CS films (Figure 35.14B) decreases progressively with increase in CN content and achieves its constant value at 36 wt% CN content.

---

* The relative water uptake was calculated as the ratios of the water absorption capacities of a composite plaster and a CS film.

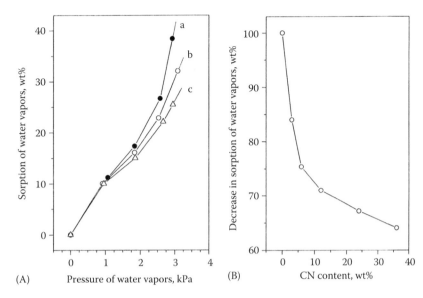

FIGURE 35.14
Water absorption from vapor phase (A) with CS (a) and nanocomposite CN-CS (b, c) films with 6 and 36 wt% content measured at $25 \pm 0.1°C$ using a Sartorius balance at the water vapor pressures 1, 2, 2.5, and 3 kPa. Zero point: the constant weight of a film into evacuated balance chamber. (B) Decrease in absorption of water vapors with increasing CN content.

The water absorption from the vapor phase within the dried nanocomposite films is also accompanied by some rearrangement of CS chains due to their hydration. When the pressure rises from 0 to 1 kPa, the water absorption grows sharply due to easy hydration of the surface-exposed amine and hydroxyl groups. In the interval 1–2 kPa, the water uptake increases somewhat slower because of insufficient permeability of CS network, which keeps its structural stability owing to multiple intra- and interchain H-bonds and hydrophobic interactions. Further increase in pressure of water vapors results in disruption of some H-bonds inside CS matrix, and the water absorption achieves higher values because of an increase in the distance between the CS chains (Ferreira et al., 2008).

The structural rearrangement of CS network with pressure is more pronounced for a non-cross-linked CS film. Compared with CS, the structural stability of the composite CN-CS films is higher because of the presence of highly hydrophobic CN.

The permeability (in Barrers*) of nanocomposite CS films with 36 wt% CN content in relation to some gases is low, 0.83 (N_2), 2.16 (O_2), 2.63 (CH_4), 4.34 (H_2), and 42.56 (CO_2), and comparable with that of soft hydrogels used in production of contact lenses. This is explained by the absence of real transport pores in nanocomposite films; the penetration of gas molecules occurs through them by diffusion owing to fluctuation of CS chains. Nevertheless, in spite of negligible gas permeability, CN-CS films cannot be considered as barrier materials. The highest permeability is observed in relation to more polar molecules of carbon dioxide. This finding can be useful at application of the nanocomposite films as skin plasters.

---

* A Barrer is a non-SI unit of gas permeability used in the contact lens industry, especifically for oxygen permeability (Effron, 2002). For example, the oxygen permeability of contact lenses prepared from soft hydrogels is equal to 7 Barrers and increases up to 40 Barrers at 36% and 80% water content, respectively.

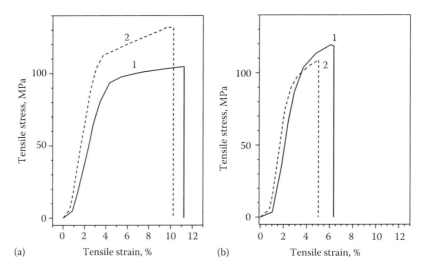

FIGURE 35.15
Tensile stress as a function of the tensile strain of CS (a) and nanocomposite CN-CS (b) films determined at a crosshead speed of 1 mm/min at reciprocally perpendicular stretching directions (1) and (2) using an Instron 5800 apparatus equipped with Bluehill 2 software. (a) CS film; (b) nanocomposite CS film with 36 wt% content of CN.

The mechanical properties (the ultimate tensile strength and Young's module)* give information about how a polymer material actually behaves on a macroscopic scale. From practical point of view, the determination of mechanical characteristics of any new material allows to compare them with those of known materials of the same type and to choose the best operation conditions in dependence on practical application.

As documented (Figure 35.15), CNs impart rather significant reinforcement to CS phase mainly by increase in Young's modulus and decrease in elongation at break. This is most probably caused by synergistic effects originating from interactions between components resulting in both immobilization of CS chains on the CN surface and changes induced by CN in packing of CS chains in composites. The effect of incorporated CN increases with their content in nanocomposite films.

The difference between the values of the ultimate tensile strength for films from pure CS and from composites with 36 wt% relative content of CN is not so high, 100–130 and 107–120 MPa, respectively. It means that the newly formed system of H-bonds and hydrophobic interactions does not yield in efficiency to that in pure CS matrix although they both differ from each other.

Quite unexpected feature is the difference in mechanical characteristics of the nanocomposite CN-CS films when the test specimens were cut perpendicular to each other's directions (Table 35.3). It is obvious that the relatively low (corresponding to the scatter of measurements) but systematic difference in properties (namely, the tensile strength and Young's modulus) measured in both directions is not accidental.

The therapeutic effect of nanocomposite CN-CS films not only depends on their behavior in contact with skin, as consequence of injury, but also gives rise to an innate response involving inflammation, activated especially on swelling and permeability to enzymes but

---

* For similar nanocomposite CN-CS films, the ultimate tensile strength, which quantifies how much stress a tested material will endure before suffering permanent deformation, changed from 85 to 75 MPa at 3 wt% CN content, whereas Young's modulus, which quantifies the elasticity of a material, decreased from 12 to 7 wt% (Sriupayo, 2005). The Young's modulus defined for small strains as the ratio of rate of change of stress to strain.

TABLE 35.3

Mechanical Characteristics of the Nanocomposite CN-CS Films

CN Content wt%	A			B		
	MPa		%	MPa		%
	Young's Modulus	Break Stress	Break Strain	Young's Modulus	Break Stress	Break Strain
0	4922 ± 1227	108 ± 8	9 ± 2	5719 ± 765	120 ± 11	11 ± 3
1.5	5437 ± 779	118 ± 13	10 ± 2	5657 ± 1363	109 ± 13	9 ± 3
3	5779 ± 669	109 ± 9	8 ± 3	6347 ± 933	114 ± 11	7 ± 2
6	5682 ± 654	113 ± 9	8 ± 1	6006 ± 793	113 ± 6	8 ± 1
12	6192 ± 350	106 ± 9	7 ± 2	6304 ± 633	111 ± 13	8 ± 2
24	5869 ± 982	104 ± 8	6 ± 1	5880 ± 1146	107 ± 13	8 ± 2
36	6041 ± 962	119 ± 7	6 ± 2	7352 ± 711	113 ± 16	5 ± 1
36[a]	6727 ± 454	116 ± 12	6 ± 1	7531 ± 1329	123 ± 11	5 ± 1

Note: The directions of stretching A and B were perpendicular to each other.

[a] The composite films dried under the applied electric field (6 kV).

also on the type of the incorporated active ingredient and its distribution in the films. The difference in the therapeutic effect of nanocomposite CN-CS films themselves and with phase-incorporated Ag-CN is analyzed in Section 35.2.4.

35.2.4 Activity, Biocompatibility, and Antibacterial Properties of Nanocomposite Ag–CN–CS Films in Medical Applications

The special active dressings such as nanocomposite CN-CS films and NEs, which maintain controlled release of the entrapped active ingredients during the treatment period without deactivation by the skin enzymes (Yang et al., 2001; Vuniak-Novadovic, 2003; Morganti and Hong-Duo Chen, 2011a), are extremely desirable in medical applications. The controlled tissue repair and regeneration require such dressings or emulsions, which ensure the sustained effect of wound healing, especially, when it goes on regular and continuous. In this case, the dressing and/or the NE acts for a longer time. Notable efforts are made to provide longer-term release of the entrapped active ingredients, so that they may ensure their therapeutic efficacy. A wide range of engineered tissue dressings have been applied for accommodation of different active molecules participating in repair and regeneration of skin tissue in normal and chronic wounds (Mathew et al., 2009; Plotner and Mostov, 2010).

The new nanocomposite CN-CS films have been designed by us to repair, regenerate, and/or replace the damaged skin; to maintain its own moisture; and to suppress the growth of pathogenic microorganisms. Owing to the excellent film-forming properties of CS, these film dressings have the tridimensional structure similar to skin and are biologically active due to the entrapped multiple NEs based on the block-*co*-polymer–nanoparticles. The physicochemical properties of the nanocomposite CN-CS films produced at the laboratory scale were described in Sections 35.2.1 through 35.2.3. Their activity and biocompatibility will be reported in detail elsewhere (Morganti et al., 2012a,b).

Here, we report about the regenerative–rejuvenation activity, which was found by a double-blind study on the skin type IV of 40 women with the photo-aged skin treated by a pulsed-dye laser (nonablative technique) for three sessions. The nonablative laser and light source techniques are known as treatments inducing a wound healing response in

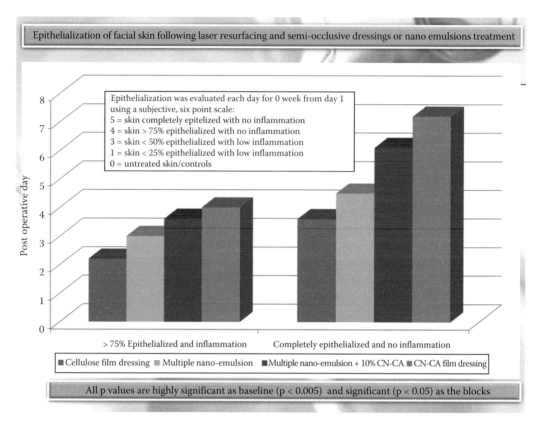

FIGURE 35.16

Effect of the dressing type on the epithelialization of the skin of face following laser resurfacing. The epithelialization was evaluated daily during a week beginning from the first post-operative day. The appearance of the facial skin was as follows: >25% of the epithelialized skin with low inflammation (first post-operative day), <50% of the epithelialized skin with low inflammation (third), 75% of the epithelialized skin with no inflammation (fourth), completely epithelialized skin with no inflammation (fifth). ■ cellulose film semiocclusive dressing, ☐ multiple NE, ⊠ multiple NE + 10% (CN-CS), ☐ CN-CS film dressing.

the papillary and upper reticular dermis without epidermal ablation (Menaker et al., 1999). The cellulosic film or CN-CS one (5 × 5 cm), a multiple NE or multiple NE containing additionally 10% of CN-CS nanoparticle–block-*co*-polymers, was applied in double blind on the treated area of the face (left or right). Everyone can see (Figure 35.16), when comparing the effect of CN-CS film with that of cellulosic one, that the use of an effective moisture-retentive dressing enhances more or less wound healing and modulates the inflammatory process by creating the cellular environment necessary for wound healing at the best rate, temperature, humidity, and pH during the repair (Vitto and Perejda, 1987). The dressing with entrapped antimicrobial compound, such as the nanosized silver particles used, is useful for maintaining the normal level of free-floating bacteria and for eliminating the formation of the pathogenic bacterial biofilms. These biofilms are also referred as *bioburden* ones comparable with the metabolic load imposed by bacteria. They are implicated in chronic infections, which are often resistant to antimicrobial agents (Costerton et al., 1995; Bello et al., 2001).

It is interesting to underline that the nanocomposite CN-CS films with entrapped nanosized silver particles at a very low final concentration (20 ppm) were noncytotoxic and also

TABLE 35.4

Assessment of the Antibacterial Activity of the Nanocomposite CN-CS
and CN-CS-Ag Films after 18 h Incubation at 36°C on Agar Containing the
Culture of Bacteria Taken from Bioburden Skin Tissue

Sample	Bacterial Growth (CFU/g)
Agar + culture of bacteria from bioburden skin tissue (CB)	10^7
Agar + CB + CS-CN nanocomposite film	10^5
Agar + CB + CS-CN-Ag nanocomposite film	10^3

modulate the presence of free-floating bacteria without encouraging the relative micro-bial proliferation of the pathogenic bacteria or delaying the wound healing process. The obtained significant delay in proliferation of *bioburden bacteria* from 10^7 CFU/g (Table 35.4) to 10^3CFU/g was observed at application of the CS-CN-Ag films. The growth of *bioburden bacteria* decreased from 10^7 to 10^5 CFU/g at using the CS-CN films. The antimicrobial effect of the latter was lower because of lower germicidal activity of both CN and CS than that of silver particles (data in progress).

Nevertheless, the results obtained confirmed the positive effect of the polyaminogly-coside (CN-CS) carrier itself, which, being degraded by the skin enzymes, gives rise to nutrients and energy to the cells modulating all their catabolic and anabolic reactions and stimulating the immune response that suppresses the growth of the *bioburden bacteria*. It should be noted that among many factors, the abnormal microbiologic environment of a wound is considered as a causal one in retarding the healing.

Bacteria presenting in wound consume glucose and oxygen leading to the temporary anoxia. This is the main rationale for preferable using the CS-CN films with entrapped nanosized silver particles in treatment of the open wounds to prevent infection and increase the rate of healing process. In the environment with high moisture, the nanocom-posite CS-CN-Ag films help to keep in equilibrium the keratinocytes' biochemical signal-ing, ameliorating the global cellular responsiveness. These innovative films are capable to modulate the water content and the level of the reactive oxygen species (ROS) in the wound bed as well. In this case, the molecular communication is activated; the injured keratinocytes are sent out to regulate the activities of proteases, which reequilibrate the inflammatory process also (data not shown). Wounds with adequate tissue hydration and the right production of ROS demonstrate fast and more direct course of epithelialization (Fisher and Maibach, 1972; Hebda and Sandulache, 2004). During the inflammatory pro-cess, ROS are generated, blood flow increases (proteases are activated), and immune cells are attracted by chemical signals to the site of injury (Pillai et al., 2005; Ha et al., 2006; Briganti and Picardo, 2009). For these reasons, the proper balance between proteases, the level of inhibitors, and ROS production are crucial to resolve the inflammatory process and reepithelialize the wound subsequently.

The biological safety of the nanocomposite CS-CN and CS-CN-Ag films was controlled in accordance with EN ISO 10993 used for the biological evaluation of medical devices and will be reported elsewhere (Morganti et al., 2012a,b). The obtained results on the biocompatibility of the tested nanocomposite films in relation to keratinocytes and fibro-blasts and their proliferation (ex vivo cultures) (Figures 35.17 and 35.18) have shown that both nanocomposite CS-CN and CS-CN-Ag films did not interfere in the regular growth of these skin cells. The cytotoxicity and the irritation potential tests, which were carried out on the same cells using these polyaminoglucoside compounds, have demonstrated high effectiveness and safety of both these films in the wound healing. None of the

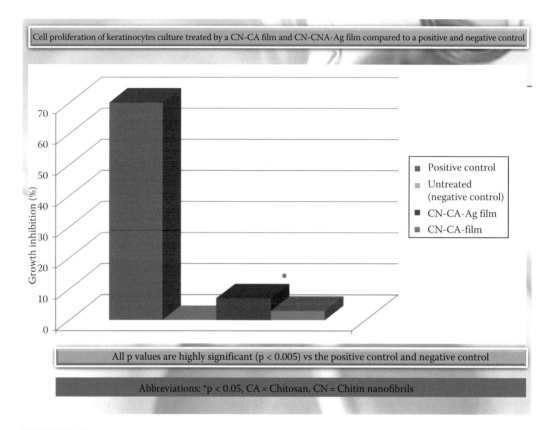

FIGURE 35.17
Cell proliferation of the keratinocytes culture treated with ⊠ a CN-CS film and □ Ag-CN-CS film in comparison with □ untreated (negative control) and ■ treated keratinocytes with PLA (positive control).

tested nanocomposite films have shown any toxic and/or irritation effects on the cells (data not shown).

35.3 Conclusive Remarks

CN nanoparticles and the nanocomposite CN-CS films (Mezzana, 2008; Morganti et al., 2008; Morganti et al., 2010, 2011a–c) were prepared and characterized with the aim to determine their physicochemical and biological properties and to evaluate the safety of these products to be used as potential carrier of active ingredients in cosmetics and skin care and in wound healing, respectively.

The clinical antiaging (Morganti et al., 2010) or anti-acne (Morganti et al., 2011b) effects of some CN nanostructured block-*co*-polymer complexes (Morganti et al., 2012a–c) were excellent as well as their good possibility in repairing the disrupted skin barrier in wound healing (Mezzana, 2008; Morganti et al., 2011a–c, 2012a–c). All these studies were carried out successfully in both in vitro and in vivo. Nevertheless, for large-scale applications of these innovative CN-CS films without and with entrapped active ingredients, further

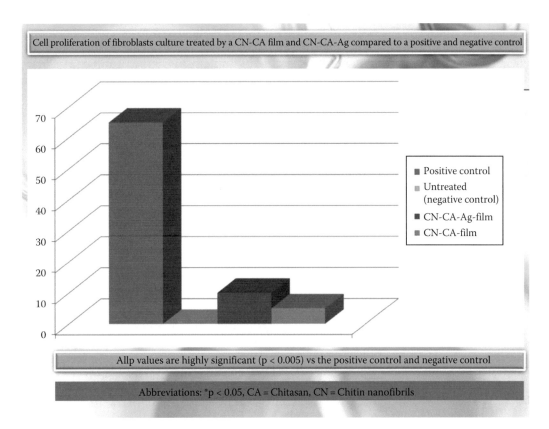

Cell proliferation of fibroblasts culture treated by a CN-CA film and CN-CA-Ag compared to a positive and negative control

Legend:
- Positive control
- Untreated (negative control)
- CN-CA-Ag-film
- CN-CA-film

Allp values are highly significant (p < 0.005) vs the positive control and negative control

Abbreviations: *p < 0.05, CA = Chitasan, CN = Chitin nanofibrils

FIGURE 35.18
Cell proliferation of fibroblasts culture treated with T CN-CS film and □ Ag-CN-CS film in comparison with □ untreated (negative control) and ■ treated fibroblasts with PLA (positive control).

in vivo confirmation of their efficacy is needed. The steps regarding to the production of CN nanocapsules and nanocomposite films should be studied deeper to achieve more economic scale-up optimization, to improve the yield and entrapment efficiency of the active ingredients for better industrial applicability of the process.

The development and practical application of the innovative products for enhancing the healing of wounds, especially chronic ones, the wound treatment, and the management must be optimized. In connection with this, it is necessary to remember that all the cells presenting in the environment of wound bed have the potential to "cross talk" with each other in order to synchronize the overall response to injury. Therefore, attention must be paid to all cellular components and, of course, to the used ingredients in order to obtain a generalized, integrated picture of the wound healing response regarding also to the continuous intercellular signaling (Hebda and Sandulache, 2004). Thus, these natural moist-retaining and slow-releasing antiseptic nanocomposite CN-CS films with the specific performance parameters, such as permeability to gases, absorbency, and the physical form similar to skin, may be considered as useful innovative surgical product for bettering the wound care management.

On the basis of the obtained results, it should be concluded that both the CN-based nanoparticles and nanoparticulate systems are the promising candidates with luminous future and an important place in the global cosmetic and medical market since they increase the efficacy of the active ingredients used normally. The CN-based nanocomposite products are involved in the catabolic and anabolic reactions and act by the innovative NICE (nervous, immune, cutaneous, and endocrine systems) way (Morganti et al., 2011d; Morganti and Hong-Duo Chen, 2011a,b) activating the immune system and increasing the efficacy of active ingredients. They help to transmit the activated signals from outside to inside the cell as well (Morganti et al., 2012c).

It should be emphasized that CN/CS-based nanoparticles can be considered as unique carries because they can be successfully eliminated being degraded by the chitinolytic enzymes working in humans, such as the highly conserved chitotriosidase expressed by activated phagocytes in plasma and acid mammalian chitinase (AMCase) found in the gastrointestinal tract and lungs (Eide et al., 2011). In connection with this, the application of CN/CS-based nanoparticles could be really the great breakthrough in the treatment of various chronic diseases associated as with external as internal surfaces of human body.

References

Alvarez-Figueroa MJ and Blanco-Menden C. 2001. Transdermal delivery of methotrexate: Iontophoretic delivery from hydrogels and passive delivery from emulsions. *Int. J. Pharm.* 215: 57–65.

Aveyard R, Binks BP, and Mead J. 1986. Interfacial tension minima in oil-water-surfactant systems. *J. Chem. Soc. Faraday Trans. I* 82: 1755.

Bello YM, Falabella AF, Decarlho H, Nayyar G, and Kirsner RS. 2001. Infection and wound healing. *Wounds* 13(4): 127–131.

Benoit JP, Couvreur R, Devissaguet JP, Fessi H, Puisieux F, and Roblot-Treupel L. 1986. Les fromes vectorisées ou distribution modulée, nuveaux sistèmes d'administration medicaments. *J. Pharm. Belg.* 41: 319–329.

Biagini G, Zizzi A, Giantomassi F, Orlando F, Lucarini G, Mattioli Belmonte M, Tucci MG, and Morganti P. 2008. Cutaneous absorption of nanostructured chitin associated with natural synergistic molecules (lutein). *J. Appl. Cosmetol.* 26: 69–80.

Binks BP. 2002. Particles as surfactants: Similarities and differences. *Curr. Opin. Colloid Interface Sci.* 7(1–2): 21–41.

Bodmeier R, Oh KH, and Pramar Y. 1989. Preparation and evaluation of drug–containing chitosan leads. *Drug. Dov. Ind. Pharm.* 15: 1475–1494.

Bonina F, Bader S, Montenegro L, Scrofani C, and Visca M. 1992. Three phase emulsions for controlled delivery in the cosmetic field. *Int. J. Cosmet. Sci.* 14: 65–74.

Bouchemal K, Briancon S, Perrier E, Fessi H, Bonnet I, and Zidowicz N. 2004a. Synthesis and characterization of polyurethane and poly (ether urethane) nanocapsules using a new technique of interfacial polycondensation combined to spontaneous emulsification. *Int. J. Pharm.* 269(1): 89–100.

Bouchemal K, Briancon S, Perrier E, and Fessi H. 2004b. Nano-emulsion formulation using spontaneous emulsification: Solvent, oil and surfactant optimisation. *Int. J. Pharm.* 280: 241–251.

Briganti S and Picardo M. 2009. Antioxidant activity, lipid peroxidation and skin diseases. *J. Eur. Acad. Dermatol. Venereol.* 17(6): 663–669.

Brooks G, Scholz DB, Parish D, and Bennet J. 2002. Aging and the future of enzymes in cosmetics. In: AC Kozlowski (Ed), *Cosmeceuticals: Active Skin Treatment*, Allured Publishing Corporation, Carol Stream, IL, pp. 206–218.

Calvo P, Remunan-Lopez C, Vila-Jato JL, and Alonso MJ. 1997. Chitosan and chitosan/ethylene oxide block copolymer nanoparticles as novel carriers for protein and vaccines. *Pharm. Res.* 14: 1431–1436.

Costerton JW, Lewandowski Z, Caldwell DE, Korber DR, and Lappin-Scott HM. 1995. Microbial biofilms. *Annu. Rev. Microbiol.* 49: 711–745.

Couvreur R, Dubernet C, and Puisieux F. 1995. Controlled drug delivery with nanoparticles: Current possibilities and future trends. *Eur. J. Pharm. Biopharm.* 41: 2–13.

Davies JT and Haydon DA. 1957. Spontaneous emulsification. *Int. Congr. Surf. Act 2nd* 1: 417–425.

Davies JT and Rideal KK. 1961. Diffusion through interfaces. In: H Willmer (Ed.) *Interfacial Phenomena*, 1st edn. Academic Press, New York, pp. 417–425.

De Campos M, Sanchez A, and Alonso MJ. 2001. Chitosan nanoparticles: A new vehicle for the improvement of the delivery of drugs to the ocular surface. *Int. J. Pharm.* 224(1/2): 159–168.

Dinarvand R, Sepehri N, Manoochehri S, Roohani H, and Atyabi F. 2011. Polylactide-co-glycolide nanoparticles for controlled delivery of anticancer agents. *Int. J. Nanomed.* 6: 877–895.

Eide KB, Norberg AL, Heggset EB, Lindbom AR, Vårum KM, Eijsink VG, and Sørlie M. 2012. Human chitotriosidase-catalyzed hydrolysis of chitosan. *Biochemistry* 51: 487–495.

Errington, N, Harding SE, Varum KM, and Illum L. 1993. Dynamic characterization of chitosans varying in degree of acetylation. *Int. J. Biol. Macromol.* 15: 113–117.

Farahmand S, Tajerzadeh H, and Farboud ES. 2006. Formulation, and evaluation of vitamin C multiple emulsion. *Pharm. Dev. Technol.* 11: 255–261.

Ferreira ML, Pedroni VI, Alimenti GA, Gschaider ME, and Schulz PC. 2008. The interaction between water vapor and chitosan II: Computational study. *Colloids Surf. A: Physicochem. Eng. Aspects* 315: 241–249.

Fessi H, Devissaguet JP, and Puisieux F. 1992. Procede de preparation de systemes colloidaux dispersibles d'une susbstance, sous forme de nanoparticulates EP 0275 796 B1.

Fisher LD and Maibach HI. 1972. The effect of occlusive and semipermeable dressings on the mitotic activity of normal and wounded human epidermis. *Br. J. Dermatol.* 86: 593–600.

Franca EF, Freitas LCG, and Lins RD. 2011. Chitosan molecular structure as a function of N-acetylation. *Biopolymers* 95(7): 448–460.

Franca EF, Lins RD, Freitas LCG, and Straatsma TP. 2008. Characterization of chitin and chitosan molecular structure in aqueous solution. *J. Chem. Theory Comput.* 4(12): 2141–2149.

Freeberg M, Tomic-Canic M, Komine M, and Blumberg M. 2001. Keratins and the keratinocytes activation cycle. *J. Invest. Dermatol.* 116: 633–640.

Gopal RES. 1968. Principles of emulsion formation. In: P Shermqn (Ed.) *Emulsion Science*. Academic Press, London, U.K., pp. 1–75.

Gref R, Minamitake Y, Peracchia MT, Trubetskoy V, Torchilin V, and Langer R. 1994. Biodegradable long-circulating polymer nanospheres. *Science* 263: 1600–1603.

Grossiord JL and Seiller M. 1998. *Multiple Emulsions: Structure, Properties and Applications*. Editions de Santé, Paris, France.

Grund S, Bauer M, and Fischer D. 2011. Polymers in drug delivery-state of the art and future trends. *Adv. Eng. Mater.* 13(3): B61–B87.

Guinebretière S, Briançon S, Fessi H, Teodorescu VS, and Blanchin MG. 2002. Nanocapsules of biodegradable polymers: Preparation and characterization by direct high resolution electron microscopy. *Mater. Sci. Eng.* C21: 137–142.

Ha HJ, Kim J, Ryoo ZJ, and Kim TJ. 2006. Inhibition of the TPA-induced cutaneous inflammation and hyperplasice by EC-SOD. *Biochem. Biophys. Res. Commun.* 348: 450–458.

Hasrani PK, Davis SS, and Grove MJ. 1983. The preparation and properties of injectable emulsions by a spontaneous emulsification process. *Int. J. Pharm.* 89: 139–146.

Hebda PA and Sandulache VC. 2004. The biochemistry of epidermal healing. In: DT Rovee and HI Maibach (Eds.) *The Epidermis in Wound Healing*. CRC Press, New York, pp. 59–86.

Johnson A, Lewes J, Roberts K, and Walter P. 2008. *Molecular Biology of the Cell*, 5th edn. Garland Science, New York.

Kawashima K, Handa T, Kabai H, Takenada H, and Lin SY. 1985a. The effect of thickness and hardness of the coating film on the drug release of theophylline granules. *Chem. Pharm. Bull.* 33: 2469–2474.

Kawashima K, Handa T, Takenada H, Lin SY, and Ando Y. 1985b. Novel method for the preparation of controlled–release theophylline granules coated with a polyelectrolyte complex of sodium polyphosphate chitosan. *J. Pharm. Sci.* 74: 264–268.

Kothekar SC, Waghmare JT, and Momin SA. 2009. Rationalizing and producing nanoemulsions for personal care. In A Kuzlowski (Ed.) *Formulating Strategies in Cosmetic Science.* Allured Books, New York, pp. 165–176.

Kreilgaard M. 2001. Dermal pharmacokinetics of microemulsion formulations determined by in vitro microdialysis. *Pharm. Res.* 18: 367–373.

Kreilgaard M, Pedersen EJ, and Jaroszewski JW. 2000. NMR characterization and transdermal drug delivery potentials of microemulsion systems. *J. Controlled Release* 69: 421–433.

Kumirska J, Czerwicka M, Kaczyñski Z, Bychowska A, Brzozowski K, Thöming J, and Stepnowski P. 2010. Application of spectroscopic methods for structural analysis of chitin and chitosan. *Mar. Drugs* 8: 1567–1636.

Lee PJ, Langer R, and Ghastri VP. 2003. Novel microemulsions enhancer formulation for simultaneous transdermal delivery of hydrophilic and hydrophobic drugs. *Pharm. Res.* 20: 264–269.

Lidgate DM, Fu RC, and Fleitman JS. 1990. Using a microfluidizer to manufacture parental emulsions. *Pharm. Technol.* 14: 30–33.

Liu LS, Liu SQ, Ng SY, Froix M, Ohno T, and Heller S. 1997. Controlled release of interleukin-2 for tumor immunotherapy using alginate: Chitosan porous microspheres. *J. Controlled Release* 43: 65–74.

Lopes-Montilla JC, Herrera-Morales PE, and Pandey DO. 2002. Spontaneous emulsification: Mechanisms, physicochemical aspects, modelling, and applications. *J. Dispers. Sci. Technol.* 23(1/3): 219–268.

Mathew AP, Laborie MPG, and Oksman K. 2009. Cross-linked chitosan/chitin crystal nanocomposites with improved permeation selectivity and pH stability. *Biomacromolecules* 10: 1627–1632.

Mc Clean S, Prosser E, Meehan E, Malley D, Clarke N, Ramtoola Z et al. 1998. Binding and uptake of biodegradable poly-lactide micro and nanoparticles in intestinal epithelia. *Eur. J. Pharm. Pharm. Sci.* 6: 153–163.

Menaker GM, Wrone DA, Williams RM, and Moy R. 1999. Treatment of facial rhytides with a nonablative laser: A clinical and histological study. *Dermatol. Surg.* 25: 440–444.

Meyer J, Polak G, and Schuermann R. 2009. Preparing PIC emulsions with a very fine particle size. In: A Kozlowski (Ed.) *Formulating Strategies in Cosmetic Science.* Allured Books, New York, pp. 192–208.

Mezzana P. 2008. Clinical efficacy of a new nanofibrils-based gel in wound healing. *Acta Chirurgiae Plasticae* 50: 81–84.

Miller CA. 1996. Solubilisation and intermediate phase formation in oil-water-surfactant systems. *Tenside Surf. Det.* 33: 191–196.

Millers CA and Raney KH. 1993. Solubilisation-emulsification mechanisms of detergency. *Colloids Surf. A* 74: 169–215.

Mogilevskaya EL, Akopova TA, Zelenetskii AN, and Ozerin AN. 2006. The crystal structure of chitin and chitosan. *Polym. Sci. Ser. A* 48: 116–123.

Morganti P. 2009a. Beauty from inside and outside. Natural products works in multiple ways. In: A Tabor and R Blair (Eds.) *Nutritional Cosmetics. Beauty from Within.* Elsevier, New York, pp. 95–111.

Morganti P. 2009b. Chitin nanofibrils in skin treatment. *J. Appl. Cosmetol.* 27: 251–270.

Morganti P. 2010. Use and potential of nanotechnology in cosmetic dermatology. *Clin. Cosmet. Invest. Dermatol.* 3: 5–13.

Morganti P. 2011. Chitin nanofibrils and their derivatives as cosmeceuticals. In: S-K Kim (Ed.) *Chitin, Chitosan, Oligosaccharides and their Derivatives.* CRC Press, New York, pp. 531–542.

Morganti P, Berardesca E, Guarneri B, Guarneri F, Fabrizi G, Palombo P, and Palombo M. 2010b. Topical clindamycin 1% vs phosphatidylcholine linoleic acid-rich and nicotinamide 4% in the treatment of acne: A multicenter—Randomized trial. *Int. J. Cosmet. Sci.* 33: 1–10.

Morganti P and Chen H-D. 2011a. Skin cell management: More than a cosmetic approach. *Biomed. Sci.* 55(7): 400–464.

Morganti P and Chen H-D. 2011b. Skin life and cell management: The NICE approach. *Pers. Care* 4(n1): 29–36.

Morganti P and Li YH. 2011b. From waste material skin-friendly nanostructured products to save humans and environment. *J. Cosmet. Dermatol. Sci. Appl.* 3: 99–105. http://www.SciRP.org/journal/jcdsa

Morganti P and Palombo M. 2012a. Topical chitosan-chitin nanofibrils film-assisted pulsed-dye laser treatment for facial rejuvenation. *J. Appl. Cosmetol.*, In print.

Morganti P, Del Ciotto P, and Carezzi F. 2012c. Unpublished data.

Morganti P, Del Ciotto P, and Gao XH. 2012a. Skin delivery and controlled release of active ingredients nanoencapsulated by chitin nanofibrils: A new approach. *Cosmetic Science and Technology.* In print.

Morganti P, Del Ciotto P, Fabrizi G, Guarneri F, Cardillo A, Palombo M, and Morganti G. 2012b. Safety and tolerability of chitin nanofibrils-hyaluronic acid nanoparticles entrapping lutein. Note I nanoparticles characterization and bioavailability. *Dermatology Research and Practice.* In print.

Morganti P, Del Ciotto P, Morganti G, and Fabien-Soulè V. 2011a. Application of chitin nanofibrils and collagen of marine origin as bioactive ingredients. In: SK Kim (Ed.) *Marine Cosmeceuticals: Latest Trends and Perspectives.* CRC-Press, New York, pp. 267–290.

Morganti P, Fabrizi G, Guarneri F, Palombo M, Palombo P, Cardillo A, Ruocco E, Del Ciotto P, and Morganti G. 2011c. Repair activity of skin barrier by chitin-nanofibrils complexes. *SÖFW. J.* 5: 10–23.

Morganti P, Fabrizi G, Palombo M, Guarneri F, Cardillo A, and Morganti G. 2011b. New chitin complexes and their anti-aging activity from inside out. *J. Nutr. Health Aging,* In press.

Morganti P, Li YH, and Chen HD. 2011d. NICE *melody* for innovative mind-body skin care. *Cosmet. Sci. Technol.* 1: 49–59.

Morganti P, Morganti G, Fabrizi G, and Cardillo A. 2008. A new sun to rejuvenate the skin. *J. Appl. Cosmetol.* 26: 159–168.

Morganti P, Morganti G, and Morganti A. 2011e. Transforming nanostructured chitin from crustacean waste into beneficial health products: A must for our society. *Nanotechnol. Sci. Appl.* 4: 1–7.

Morganti P, Palombo M, Palombo P, Fabrizi G, Cardillo A, Carezzi F, Morganti G, Ruocco E, and Dziergowski S. 2010a. Cosmetic science in skin aging: Achieving the efficacy by the chitin nanostructured crystallites. *SOFW J.* 136(3): 14–24.

Musmann T. 1983. Rapid colorimetric assay for cellular growth and survival: Application to proliferation and cytotoxicity assays. *J. Immunol. Methods* 65(2–2): 55–63.

Muthu MS and Singh SS. 2009. Targeted nanomedicines: Effective treatment modalities for cancer, AIDS and brain disorders. *Nanomedicine* 4(11): 105–118.

Muzzarelli RAA. 2009a. Chitins and chitosans for the repair of wounded skin, nerve, cartilage and bone. *Carbohydr. Polym.* 76: 167–182.

Muzzarelli RAA. 2009b. Genipin-crosslinked chitosan hydrogels as biomedical and pharmaceutical aids. *Carbohydr. Polym.* 77: 1–9.

Muzzarelli RAA, Morganti P, Morganti G, Palombo P, Palombo M, Biagini G, Belmonte MM, Giantomassi F, Orlandi F, and Muzzarelli C. 2007. Chitin nanofibrils/chitosan glycolate composites as wound medicaments. *Carbohydr. Polym.* 70: 274–284.

Natthan C, Praneet O, Theerasak R, Tanasait N, and Pitt S. 2010. Preparation and characterization of chitosan-hydroxybenzotriazole/polyvinylchool blend nanofibers by the electrospinning technique. *Carbohydr. Polym.* 81: 675–680.

Niwa T, Takeuchi H, Hino T, Kunou N, and Kawashima Y. 1993. Preparations of biodegradable nanospheres of water-soluble and insoluble drugs with D, L–lactic/glycolide copolymer by a novel spontaneous emulsification solvent diffusion method, and drug release behaviour. *J. Controlled Release* 25: 89–98.

Ozer O and Aydin B. 2009. Effect of oil type on stability of W/O/W emulsions. In: A Kuzlowski (Ed.) *Formulating Strategies in Cosmetic Science.* Allured Books, New York, pp. 179–190.

Paulino AT, Simionato JI, Garcia JC, and Notami J. 2006. Characterization of chitosan and chitin produced from silkworm chrysalides. *Carbohydr. Polym.* 64: 98–103.

Pillai S, Oresajo C, and Hayward J. 2005. Ultraviolet radiation and skin aging: Roles of reactive oxygen species, inflammation and protease activation, and strategies for prevention of inflammation-induced matrix degradation. A review. *Int. J. Cosmet. Sci.* 27(1): 17–34.

Pinto Reis C, Nenfeld RJ, Ribeiro AJ, and Veiga F. 2006. Nanoencapsulation I method for preparation of drug-loaded polymeric nanoparticles. *Nanomed. Nanotechnol. Biol. Med.* 2: 8–21.

Plotner AN and Mostow EN. 2010. A review of bioactive materials and chronic wounds. *Cutis* 85: 259–266.

Polk A, Amsden B, Yao KD, Peng T, and Goosen MF. 1994. Controlled release of albumin from chitosan-alginate microcapsules. *J. Pharm. Sci.* 83: 178–185.

Quintanar-Guerrero D, Allemann E, Fessi H, and Doelker E. 1998. Preparation techniques and mechanism of formation of biodegradable nanoparticles from preformed polymers. *Drug Dev. Ind. Pharm.* 24: 1113–1128.

Sain IG, Kim SY, Lee YM, Cho CS, and Sung YK. 1998. Methoxypoly(ethylene glycol)/ε-caprolactone amphiphilic block copolymeric micelle containing indomethacin I. Preparation and characterization. *J. Controlled Release* 51: 1–19.

Samd A, Tariq M, Intakhab Alam M, and Akher Ms. 2010. Microsphere: A novel drug delivery system. In: F Monzer (Ed.) *Colloids in Drug Delivery*. CRC Press, New York, pp. 455–478.

Sannan T, Kurita K, and Iwakura Y. 1976. Studies on chitin. 2. Effect of deacetylation on solubility. *Macromol. Chem.* 177: 3589–3600.

Sarker DK. 2005. Engineering of nanoemulsions for drug delivery. *Curr. Drug Delivery* 2: 297–310.

Seijo B, Fattal E, Roblot-Treupel L, and Couvreur P. 1990. Design of nanoparticles of less than 50 nm diameter: Preparation and characterization. *Int. J. Pharm.* 62: 1–7.

Shahizdadeh N, Bonn D, Aguerre-Chariol O, and Meunier J. 1999. Spontaneous emulsification: Relation to microemulsion phase behaviour. *Colloids Surf. A Physiochem. Eng. Aspects* 147: 375–380.

Shrinivas CK, Jyotsna TW, and Shamim AM 2009. Rationalizing and producing nanoemulsions for personal care. In: A Kuzlowski (Ed), *Formulating Strategies in Cosmetic Science*, Allured Books, New York, pp. 165–176.

Sing AJF, Graciaa A, Lachaise J, Brochette P, and Salarger JL. 1999. Interactions and coalescence of nanodroplets in translucent O/W emulsions. *Colloids Surf. A Physicochem. Eng. Aspects* 152: 31–39.

Sopprimath KS, Aminabhavi TM, Kulkarni E, Xiao JX, and Kissel T. 2001. Biodegradable polymeric nanoparticles as drug delivery devices. *J. Controlled Release* 70: 1–20.

Sriupayo J, Supaphol P, Blackwell J, and Rujiravanit R. 2005. Preparation and characterization of α-chitin whisker-reinforced chitosan nanocomposite films with or without heat treatment. *Carbohydr. Polym.* 62: 130–136.

Thayer AM. 2003. Nanomaterials. *Chem. Eng. News* 81: 15–22.

Thomas S. 2003. Wound dressings. In DT Rovee and H Maibach (Eds.) *The Epidermis in Wound Healing*. CRC Press, New York, pp. 215–241.

Tice TR and Gillex RM. 1985. Preparation of injectable controlled- release microcapsules by solved–evaporation process. *J. Controlled Release* 2: 243–252.

Tirnaksiz F and Kalsin O. 2005. A topical W/O/W multiple emulsion prepared with Tetronic 908 as a hydrophilic surfactants: Formulation, characterization and release study. *J. Pharm. Pharmaceut. Sci.* 8: 299–315.

Tirnaksiz F, Akkus S, and Celebi N. 2010. Nanoemulsions as drug delivery systems. In F Monzer (Ed.) *Colloids in Drug Delivery*. CRC Press, New York, pp. 221–244.

Tomic-Canic M, Agren MS, and Alvarez OM. 2003. Epidermal repair and the chronic wound. In DT Rovee and H Maibach (Eds.) *The Epidermis in Wound Healing*. CRC Press, New York, pp. 25–57.

Twiname ER and Mistler RE. 1999. In J Wachtman Jr. (Ed.) *"Tape Casting," Ceramic Innovations in the 20th Century*. The American Ceramic Society, Westerville, OH, p. 54.

Vimala K, Mohana YM, Sivudu KS, Varaprasad K, Ravindra S, Reddya NN, Padma Y, Sreedhar B, and Raju KM. 2010. Fabrication of porous chitosan films impregnated with silver nanoparticles: A facile approach for superior antibacterial application. *Colloids Surf. B Biointerf.* 76: 248–258.

Vinetsky Y and Magdassi S. 1999. Microcapsules in cosmetics. In: S Magdassi and E Touitou (Ed.) *Novel Cosmetic Delivery Systems*. Marcel Dekker Inc, New York, pp. 295–313.

Vitto J and Perejda AJ. 1987. *Connective Tissue Disease, Molecular Pathology of the Extracellular Matrix*. Marcel Dekker, New York.

Vuniak-Novadovic G. 2003. The fundamentals of tissue engineering: Scaffolds and bioreactors. In *Tissue Engineering of Cartilage and Bone*. Novadis Fundation, John Wiley & Sons, New York, pp. 34–51.

Washington C and Davis SS. 1988. The production of parental feeding emulsions by microfluidizer. *Int. J. Pharm*. 94: 169–176.

Wehrle P, Magenheim B, and Benita S. 1995. The influence of process parameters on the PLA nanoparticles size distribution, evaluated by means of factorial design. *Eur. J. Pharm. Biopharmacol*. 41: 19–26.

Xu Y and Du Y. 2003. Effect of molecular structure of chitosan on protein delivery properties of chitosan nanoparticles. *Int. J. Pharm*. 250(1): 215–226.

Yang S, Leong KF, Du Z, and Chua CK. 2001. The design of scaffolds for use in tissue engineering. Part I traditional factors. *Tissue Eng*. 7: 679–689.

Yeong JC, Lee J, and Cho K. 2003. Effects of crystalline microstructure on drug release behaviour of poly (ε-caprolactone) microspheres. *J. Controlled Release* 92: 249–258.

Yuan Y, Gao Y, Zhao J, and Mao L. 2008. Characterization and stability evaluation of β-carotene nanoemulsions prepared by high pressure homogenization under various emulsifying conditions. *Food Res. Int*. 41: 61–68.

Zhang J, Zhao J, Zhang HL, Li HL, and Liu ZF. 1998. Effect of the molecular interaction on molecular packing and orientation in azobenzene-functionalized self-assembled monolayers on gold. *Thin Solid Films* 327–329: 195–198.

36

Role of Nanocomposites and Nanostructured Biomaterials in Biomedical and Nanobiotechnology

Abdul Bakrudeen Ali Ahmed, R. Arun Kumar, and Rosna Mat Taha

CONTENTS

36.1 Introduction

The Food and Agriculture Organization (FAO) of the United Nations and the World Health Organization (WHO, 2008) have recognized a need for scientific advice on any food safety implications that may arise from the use of nanotechnologies in the food and agriculture sectors through its horizon-scanning activities. With the advent of nanotechnology, the prospects for using medical imaging, disease diagnoses, drug delivery, cancer treatment, gene therapy, and other areas have progressed rapidly. The worldwide market for products produced using nanotechnology is estimated to reach US$1 trillion by 2015 (Roco, 2005).

Nanobiotechnology represents the convergence of nanotechnology and biotechnology, yielding materials and products that use biological molecules in their construction or are designed to affect biological systems. Several applications of nanotechnology include engineering biomolecules for nonbiological use such as DNA-based computer circuits, using nanotechnology tools such as medical diagnostic devices and medical imaging to study biology and combining nanomaterials with biological systems for outcomes such as targeted drug therapies. Nanobiotechnology often studies existing elements of nature in order to fabricate new device (Brooks et al., 1983). Therefore, the unbridled growth and uses of nanobiotechnology in medical and human health evaluations open society, and it could become the asbestos of the twenty-first century.

36.2 Nanoparticle for Medical Application

Scientists have taken to naming their particles after the real-world shapes that they might represent. Nanospheres (Agam and Guo, 2007), nanoreefs (Choy et al., 2004), nanoboxes, and more have appeared in the literature. Biological processes that contribute to both health and disease occur at the nanoscale, the size scale of proteins, nucleic acids, pores, cellular membranes, and other biomolecules. In addition, the benefits and uses of nanoparticles (NPs) in drug delivery, cancer treatment, and gene therapy may cause unintentional human exposure. Present-day nanomedicine exploits carefully structured NP such as dendrimers (Borges and Schengrund, 2005), carbon fullerenes buckyballs (Mashino et al., 2005), and nanoshells to target specific tissues and organs. These NPs may serve as diagnostic and therapeutic antiviral, antitumor, or anticancer agents, and their efforts are given next.

36.2.1 Alzheimer's Disease

Alzheimer's disease (AD) is a progressive and ultimately fatal neurodegenerative disorder, afflicting approximately 40% of the population over 80 years of age. There are around 30 million people worldwide. By 2010, it is estimated that there will be half a million AD sufferers in the United Kingdom. Currently, there are approximately 600 million persons aged 60 years and older, and this number will reach close to 2 billion in 2050. The latest 2008 data for the United States alone estimate that 5 million Americans have the disease, with an estimated increase to 11–16 million by 2050. One of the most promising applications of nanoscience is in AD. As patients can be definitely diagnosed after they pass away and their brain is examined for the telltale damage, scientists are hunting for test that would help make a diagnosis in living patients.

One possible biomarker for AD is a protein called amyloid beta–derived diffusible ligands (ADDLs). Support for the role of ADDLs comes from their neurotoxicity and presence at elevated levels in the brains of AD patients as compared with the age-matched controls (Gong et al., 2003). The correlation of cerebrospinal fluid (CSF) ADDL levels with the disease state offers promise for improved AD diagnosis and early treatment. This finding was made possible by combining ADDL-specific monoclonal antibodies (Lambert et al., 2001; Chang et al., 2003) with an ultrasensitive, NP-based protein detection strategy termed biobarcode amplification (BCA) (Nam et al., 2003). The BCA strategy used by Klein, Mirkin, and coworkers (Georganpoulou et al., 2005) makes clever use of NPs as DNA carrier to enable million-fold improvements over ELISA sensitivity. CSF is first exposed to monoclonal anti-ADDL antibodies bound to magnetic microparticles. After ADDL binding, the microparticles are separated with a magnetic field and washed before addition of secondary antibodies bound to DNA–Au NP conjugates. These conjugated to contain covalently bound DNA as well as complementary barcode DNA that is attached via hybridization. Unreacted antibody DNA: Au: NP conjugates are removed during a second magnetic separation, after which elevated temperature and low-salt conditions release the barcode DNA for analysis (Keating, 2005). Because the pathology of AD is thought to begin decades before the first symptoms, it would be very interesting to learn at what stage of disease progression ADDL levels in the CSF rise above those in healthy individuals.

36.2.2 Anticancer

Cancer is an enormous socioeconomic problem. According to the National Cancer Institute (NCI), it is estimated that in 2007, there will be over 1.4 million new cases of cancer (of any type) and over 550,000 deaths from cancer in the United States from the American Cancer Society. This makes cancer the second deadliest disease category, after heart diseases. The conventional anticancer treatments are nonspecific to target killing of tumor cells, may induce severe systemic toxicity, and produce drug-resistant phenotypic growth. An exciting potential use of nanotechnology in cancer treatments is the exploration of tumor-specific thermal scalpels to heat and burn tumors (O'Neal et al., 2004). It was observed in mice that selective photothermal ablation of tumor using near-infrared (NIR)-absorbing polyethylene-coated gold nanoshells of 130 nm inhibited tumor growth and enhanced survival of animals for up to 90 days compared with controls (Perkel, 2004). Furthermore, it was reported that antibody-coated magnetic iron NPs were effective to heat and literally cook the tumors. Similar work performed in athymic mice using an antibody-coated iron NP (DeNardo et al., 2005) showed specific targeted binding to tumors and tumor necrosis within 24 h after therapy with better response. The efficacy of different antibodies conjugated to NPs, including transferring epidermal growth factor receptor, was examined in animal studies (El-Sayed et al., 2006). In cancer therapy, enzyme-mediated liposome destabilization and specific phospholipase A2 activation with synergistic membrane perturbing and permeability were reported to be more effective (Andresen et al., 2004). Nanoshells can be used for photothermal ablation of tumor (Loo et al., 2004) tissue as demonstrated both in human breast carcinoma cells in vitro and in a murine model in vivo (Hirsch et al., 2003). However, electromagnetic interactions between the gold NPs change the property of the metal, making it absorb light from the NIR, which can easily penetrate several centimeters of (human) tissue without harming it.

In the murine model, poly (ethylene glycol)-passivated gold-coated silica nanoshells were injected interstitially ~5 mm into the tumor volume (tumor size 3–5.5 mm). Poly (ethylene glycol) is used to increase circulation time (Gref et al., 1994) as well as to reduce nonspecific attachment or uptake (Agam and Guo, 2007). The blood vessels inside tumors develop poorly, allowing the nanoshells to leak out and accumulate inside tumors. Six hours after the injections, an external laser source of NIR light (power density approx. 4–35 W/cm^2) is applied through the skin for 3–7 min. The gold NPs readily absorb the energy and turn it into heat resulting in an average temperature increase of ~37°C, which induced irreversible cancerous tissue damage. The heating is localized and does not affect healthy tissue adjacent to the tumor. The mice remain cancer-free after the treatment, whereas growth of tumors in the control group, i.e., no treatment and sham group, continues rapidly. It is also possible to attach biological markers, such as antibodies and proteins, to the nanoshells, in order to direct them to their target tissues (Loo et al., 2005). The advantage of using smaller particles is that they can be inserted into any part of the human body to treat cancer cells in their infancy.

Hyperthermia can be produced by NIR laser irradiation of gold NPs present in tumors and thus induces tumor cell killing via a bystander effect. To be clinically relevant, however, several problems still need to be resolved. In particular, selective delivery and physical targeting of gold NPs to tumor cells are necessary to improve therapeutic selectively. Considerable progress has been made with respect to retargeting adenoviral vectors for cancer gene therapy. Therefore, it was hypothesized that covalent coupling of gold NPs to retargeted adenoviral vectors would allow selective delivery of the NPs to tumor cells, thus feasibilizing hyperthermia and gene therapy as a combinatorial therapeutic approach. For this, sulfo-*N*-hydroxysuccinimide-labeled gold NPs were reacted to adenoviral vectors encoding a luciferase reporter gene driven by the cytomegalovirus promoter. Covalent coupling could be achieved, while retaining virus infectivity and ability to retarget tumor-associated antigens. These results indicate the possibility of using adenoviral vectors as carriers for gold NPs (Events et al., 2006). Development of these new medicines will be a fantastic voyage that we are literally betting our lives on.

36.2.3 Gene Therapy

NP-based gene therapy to be effective in systemic gene treatment of lung cancer has to use a novel tumor suppressor gene, FUS1 (Gopalan et al., 2004). Chitosan, a polymer long used in gene therapy, was reported to have increased transfection efficiency and decreased cytotoxicity (Mansouri et al., 2006). Oral gene delivery in BALB/c mice using poly-ʟ-lysine-modified silica NPs has shown success with the distribution of particle throughout the intestinal mucous cell with limited cytotoxicity (Li et al., 2005). Recent in vitro work in breast cancer cells has shown the potential efficiency of NP-mediated gene delivery of the wild-type p53. Cancer cell exposed to this NP-based gene delivery showed an increased and sustained antiproliferative activity not seen in cell exposed to vector alone (Prabha and Labhasetwar, 2004). A nonviral vector for in vivo gene delivery and fluorescent visualization of transfection using organically modified silica NPs has promising success for targeted brain therapy (Bharali et al., 2005). Recent gene therapy studies are work against Parkinson's disease; results have chronic progressive disorder of the central nervous system and loss of cells in the brain (substantia nigra).

Those cells produce dopamine, a chemical messenger responsible for transmitting signals within the brain. Loss of dopamine causes critical nerve cells in the brain, or neurons, to fire out of control, leaving patients unable to direct or control their movement in a normal manner. They plan to use this technology to transduce brain cells so that they express proteins beneficial to the cells' survival and test the feasibility of delivering condensed DNA NPs that encode for a neurotrophic factor to the brain as a means to halt or prevent the neurodegenerative process in an animal model of Parkinson's disease. Neurotrophic factors are capable of protecting neurons from dying, thereby rescuing essential neurons in the brain. In animal studies, neurotrophic factors have revived dormant brain cells, caused them to produce dopamine, and prompted dramatic improvement of symptoms. The MJFF Rapid Response Innovation Awards support projects that may have little to no existing preliminary data but that hold potential to significantly impact understanding or treatment of Parkinson's disease.

36.3 Magnetic Nanoparticles

Magnetic NPs such as superparamagnetic iron oxide NPs (~15 nm in diameter) (Jordan et al., 1999, 2001), paramagnetic copper–nickel alloy NPs (Bettge et al., 2004), or magnetite (Fe_3O_4) cationic liposomes (Shinkai et al., 1996) are becoming more and more important for many applications in medical science and data storage technique. In medical applications, the magnetic NPs are used for diagnostics and therapy (Albrecht et al., 2005). For example, they can serve as a contrast medium in magnetic resonance imaging. The magnetisms were deposited on a substrate and magnetized vertically before measuring and the stray field of four single particles with a diameter of about 40 nm each. The picture correlates with the vertically magnetized magnetic dipoles. This investigation pointed out that magnetisms are single-domain particles showing a remanent magnetization. The saturation magnetization m and the anisotropy constant k_{eff} of MNP ensembles were measured using a SQUID susceptometer. The data achieved will serve as input parameters for the analysis and the validation of the MRX data and the demonstrator. The validation is needed to ensure the quality of the data measured using the new equipment in clinical applications and production.

36.3.1 Nanorobots

The engineering of molecular products needs to be carried out by robotic devices, which have been termed as nanorobots. Hence, the nanorobots are essentially a controllable machine at the nanometer or molecular scale that is composed of nanoscale components. Development of microelectronics in the 1980s has led to new tools for biomedical instrumentation, the manufacturing of nanoelectronics (Das et al., 2007), and will similarly permit further miniaturization toward integrated medical systems, providing efficient methodologies for pathological prognosis (Narayan et al., 2004; Hede and Huilgol, 2006). The use of microdevices in surgery and medical treatments is a reality that has brought many improvements in clinical procedures in recent years. More complex molecular machines, or nanorobots, having embedded nanoscopic features represent new tools for medical procedures (Freitas, 2005; Patel et al., 2006).

36.3.2 Surgical Nanorobotics

Surgical nanorobots are introduced into the body through the vascular system (or) at the ends of catheters into various vessels and other cavities of the human body. A surgical nanorobot, programmed or guided by a human surgeon, could act as a semiautonomous on-site surgeon inside the human body. Axotomy of the roundworm neurons was performed by femtosecond laser surgery, after which the axons functionally regenerated (Yanik et al., 2004). A femtolaser acts like a pair of nanoscissor by vaporizing tissue locally while leaving adjacent tissue unharmed. Femtolaser surgery was performed for localized nanosurgical ablation of focal adhesions adjoining live mammalian epithelial cells (Kohli et al., 2005), microtubule dissection inside yeast cells (Sacconi et al., 2005), noninvasive intratissue nanodissection of plant cell walls, selective destruction of intracellular single plastids or selected parts of them (Tirlapur and Konig, 2002), and even the nanosurgery of individual chromosomes (selectively knocking out genomic nanometer-sized regions within the nucleus of living Chinese hamster ovary cells).

36.3.3 Intracranial Therapy

Considering the properties of nanorobots to navigate as blood-borne devices, they can help on important treatment processes of complex diseases in early diagnosis and smart drug delivery. Their application of different tasks can be performed through embedded nanosensors to identify medical targets inside the human body. Numerical analysis and advanced computational simulation techniques are used to investigate nanorobot interaction and activation for sensing gradient changes of relevant chemical pattern for brain aneurysm. Thus, a detained approach is described serving as a test bed to support the fast development of molecular machines toward new therapies and treatments. An important and interesting aspect in the current development is the fact that the similar hardware architecture and sensing methodology presented for nanorobots to identify intracranial harmful vessel growth can also be used for a broad range of problems in medicine, including specialized brain therapies, neurodegenerative problems, and surgery (Gao et al., 2004). A key factor to increase the changes for patients in having a satisfactory treatment from cerebral aneurysm relies on detection of vessels deformation in early stages of bulbs development.

36.4 Carbon Nanotubes

Carbon nanotubes are among the astonishing objects that science sometimes discovers and that will likely revolutionize technological developments of the twenty-first century. Since the carbon nanotube discovery in 1991 by Iijima, it has been investigated by many researchers all over the world. It can be seen as the nearly 1D form of fullerenes. Carbon nanotubes are 100 times stronger than steel, impervious to temperatures up to 6500°F, and only one to a few nanometers in width. Carbon nanotube arrays can play a key role in the artificial cochlea development. It has been established that growing of the carbon nanotubes requires use of small metal catalyst particles (5–100 nm). Recent discoveries of various forms of carbon nanostructures have stimulated research on their applications of diverse fields. They hold promise for applications in medicine, drug, and gene delivery area (Rao and Cheetham, 2001).

36.4.1 Cancer Treatment

Single-walled carbon nanotubes having noncovalent attachment of various functional groups such as proteins, peptides, enzymes, polysaccharides, porphyrin, DNA, and sodium dodecyl sulfonate have been synthesized. Owing to their semiconducting properties, single-walled carbon nanotubes have been proposed as chemical sensor for gaseous molecule, such as NO_2 or NH_3 (Kong et al., 2000). Main application of these carbon nanotubes in the therapeutic field is photothermal therapy for cancer. Indeed, although biological systems are transparent to 700–110 nm NIR light, the intrinsic strong absorbance of single-walled carbon nanotubes in this window can be used for optical stimulation of carbon nanotubes inside living cells to afford various useful functions. Kam and his coworkers have shown that this singular property of single-walled carbon nanotubes can be used to destroy cancer cells selectively upon irradiation with NIR light (Kam et al., 2005). This selective cancer cell destruction by appropriately functionalized single-walled carbon nanotubes provides new opportunities in the area of cancer therapy. Researchers today have started conducting studies where they use carbon nanotubes as sensors that can locate harmful toxins that damage DNA, as a drug delivery system, and as tools to destroy cancerous cells.

36.4.2 Bone Fixations

Multiwalled carbon nanotubes are flexible and resilient tubular structure with diameter of 10–40 nm, length is 10–150 μm, and strength 50–100 times greater than steel at fraction of weight. For the first time, catalytic growth of multiwalled carbon nanotubes by CVD was proposed by Soltesz et al. (2005). Witzmann and Monteiro analyzed human epidermal keratinocytes (HEKs) exposed to multiwalled carbon nanotubes in cell culture using large format of 2D gel electrophoresis and mass spectrometry (MS). Compared with controls, 24 h of multi-walled carbon nanotubes exposure altered the expression of 36 proteins (P < .01), whereas 106 were altered at 48 hours. Peptide mass fingerprinting identified most of the differentially expressed proteins, and the various proteins identities reflected a complex cellular response to multiwalled carbon nanotube exposure. In addition, the proteins are associated with metabolism, cell signaling, and stress; they observed a consistent effect on the expression of cytoskeletal elements and vesicular trafficking components. These data clearly showed that multiwalled carbon nanotubes are capable of altering protein expression in a target epithelial cell that constitutes a primary route of occupational exposure in target epithelial cells for manufactured nanotubes (Witzmann and Monteiro-Riviere, 2006). The addition of multiwalled carbon nanotubes improved the fatigue performance of acrylic bone cement by as much as seven times. As the bone cement was loaded, the multiwalled carbon nanotubes resisted the separation of the crack faces. Although, it is unlikely that one carbon nanotube could provide enough resistance to slow the growth of the crack, it is likely that thousands of carbon nanotubes, working in parallel, can greatly slow the rate of crack growth. The cumulative effects of crack bridging, therefore, were slower crack growth and increased fatigue life. These findings suggest that the addition of multiwalled carbon nanotubes is a promising solution to the problem of fatigue failure.

For the third issue, in new bone formation, the scientists used bone morphogenetic proteins (BMPs), a group of proteins known for their ability to induce the formation of bone and cartilage. They made a composite consisting of BMP, multiwalled carbon nanotubes, and collagen and implanted it in the dorsal musculature of mice. Again, they found that multiwalled carbon nanotube particles were integrated entirely into new bone and bone marrow but also that, in comparison to a control group using only BMP/collagen, the multiwalled carbon nanotubes seemed to accelerate new bone formation in response to BMP. Furthermore, it is finally confirmed that hydroxyapatite was formed and crystallized on the multiwalled carbon nanotube surface in simulated body fluid remarkably quickly and that the multiwalled carbon nanotubes acted as the core for the initial hydroxyapatite crystallization. The results of these experiments demonstrate that multiwalled carbon nanotubes possess good bone compatibility, as indicated by minimal inflammatory reaction. Their results thus indicate the compatibility of multiwalled carbon nanotubes with biomaterial positioned in contact with bone and their suitability for use in regions of bone healing such as fracture sites, and this finding should facilitate development of new drug delivery systems or scaffold materials for bone regeneration using multiwalled carbon nanotubes. Furthermore, multiwalled carbon nanotubes included in implants for the treatment of fractures, such as plates and screws, may promote bone repair and thus facilitate rapid fracture healing. As is true generally, safety-related testing involving carcinogenesis and other toxicity is necessary prior to carbon nanotube use in humans.

36.4.3 Monitoring Blood Glucose

Carbon nanotubes are promising to sense candidates to monitor glucose in blood and urine. Multiwalled carbon nanotubes as well as single-walled carbon nanotubes have been used to develop enzymatic amperometric biosensors (Wang et al., 2003; Joshi et al., 2005) or fluorimetric biosensors (Barone et al., 2004). The enzyme glucose oxidase is either immobilized inside multiwalled carbon nanotubes or noncovalently attached to the surface of single-walled carbon nanotubes or noncovalently attached to the surface of single-walled carbon nanotubes enabling the catalysis of glucose with hydrogen peroxide as coproduct. For the amperometric biosensor, the enzyme immobilization allows for the direct electron transfer from enzyme to a gold or platinum transducer producing the response current. The fluorescence biosensor could be used in a new type of implantable biological sensor such as NIR nanoscale sensor. This sensor could be inserted into tissue, excited with a laser pointer, and provide real-time, continuous monitoring of blood glucose levels. It consists of protein-encapsulated single-walled carbon nanotubes functionalized with potassium ferrocyanide, a substance that is sensitive to hydrogen peroxide. The ferrocyanide ion adsorbs on the surface through the porous monolayer. When present, hydrogen peroxide will form a complex with the ion, which changes the electron density of the carbon nanotube and, consequently, its optical properties. The more glucose that is present, the brighter the carbon nanotube will fluoresce. The sensor can be loaded into a porous capillary and inserted into tissue. As carbon nanotubes do not degrade like organic molecules that fluoresce, these NP optical sensors would be suitable for long-term monitoring applications. Proof-of-concept studies to detect glucose levels have been performed in vitro, i.e., in blood samples. Practical use is 5–10 years ahead, according to the researchers. Self-assembled peptide nanotube can be used in an electrochemical biosensor (Yemini et al., 2005). The presence of the peptide nanotubes improves the sensitivity of the device severalfold. Peptide nanotube offers several advantages over carbon nanotubes, since they are biocompatible, water soluble, inexpensive, easy to manufacture, and can be chemically modified by targeting their amino or carboxyl groups. The sensing technique can be used as a platform for ultrasensitive detection of biological and chemical agents.

36.5 Capnography

Carbon nanotube–based chemical gas sensors have great potential in medical applications. Currently, Nanomix Inc. is developing a medical capnography sensor using polyethyleneimine-coated carbon nanotubes. Capnography is the measurement of carbon dioxide concentration in human respiration and is an indication of patient status during administration of anesthesia. The tiny, low-power sensor will be the first disposable electronic capnography sensor and has the potential to extend the reach of quantitative respiratory monitoring beyond the operating room and into ambulatory and emergency settings, as well as doctor's offices. Various applications have been reported illustrating the broad potential of carbon nanotube–based biosensors, such as biosensing platforms for the simultaneous detection of dopamine and ascorbic acid for the diagnosis of Parkinson's disease (Wang et al., 2002), and dopamine and serotonin (Wu et al., 2003), and a nitric oxide radical biosensor (Wang et al., 2005). Recently, a more generalized approach for enzyme-based biosensors has been demonstrated by immobilizing enzymes in redox hydrogels incorporating single-walled carbon nanotubes (Joshi et al., 2005).

36.5.1 Protein Transporters

Many therapeutic agents may turn out to be proteins, but proteins can be difficult to get across the cell membrane and into the cytoplasm while still retaining their biological function. Single-walled carbon nanotubes could become a new class of a generic tool of delivering small peptides (Pantarotto et al., 2004) and proteins (Kam and Dai, 2005) into cells in vitro as well as in vivo. Acid-oxidized single-walled carbon nanotubes bind various types of protein and transport them through the cell membrane. These acid-treated carbon nanotubes are stable in water and do not aggregate, as do untreated carbon nanotubes. The uptake mechanism is not fully understood, and proposed mechanisms are endocytosis (Kam et al., 2004), phagocytosis (Cherukuri et al., 2004), and insertion and diffusion through the lipid bilayer of the cell membrane (Bianco et al., 2005). In many instances, a cell breaks down proteins transported via endocytosis, but the single-walled carbon nanotube–bound proteins avoid this fate if concurrently a small amount of the antimalarial drug chloroquine is delivered leading to swelling of the endosomal compartments and eventual rupture (Ogris et al., 1998). For reasons that are still unclear, acid-treated carbon nanotubes are able to bind a large protein, human immunoglobulin, but are not able to transport that protein across the cell membrane. To test if carbon nanotubes can deliver small proteins that then retain their biological activity once inside the cell, single-walled carbon nanotubes were used to deliver the protein cytochrome C (Cyt-c) that triggers apoptosis. Cell line experiments showed that single-walled carbon nanotube–bound Cyt-c retained its biological activity and did cause significantly higher rates of apoptosis than did either Cyt-c or the nanotubes into the cytoplasm have to be elucidated, and these were unambiguous help to medical fields.

36.5.2 Nanowires

Nanowires can be synthesized using a large variety of materials such as metals, e.g., Ag (Braun et al., 1998), semimetals, e.g., Bi (Zhang et al., 1998), semiconductors, e.g., Cds (Routkevitch et al., 1996), and superconductors, e.g., Zn (Li et al., 2000). Silicon nanowire field-effect transistor devices have been used as pH sensors (Cui and Lieber, 2001). Photocurrent response to UV light irradiation suggests that ZnO nanowires could be a good candidate for optoelectronic switches (Kind et al., 2002). Nanowires have also been proposed for use in inorganic–organic solar cells (Huynh et al., 2002). The multifunctional nanowire is the presence of bioscaffolds with titanium (Dong et al., 2007). In addition, nanoscale light-emitting diodes with colors ranging from the ultraviolet to NIR region could be combined with microfluidics in lab-on-a-chip systems to produce highly integrated analytic systems that might enable applications ranging from high-throughput screening to medical diagnostics to be developed (Huang et al., 2005).

36.5.3 Viruses Detection

Semiconducting silicon nanowires can be configured as field-effect transistors for the electrical detection of viruses in solutions (Patolsky et al., 2004). When a single charged virus binds to receptors (e.g., antibodies) linked to the nanodevice, the conductance of a semiconducting nanowire changes from the baseline value, and when the virus unbinds, the conductance returns to the baseline value. The conductance of a second nanowire device without receptors should show no change during the same time period and can serve as an internal control. Nanowires are confined to a central region that is coupled to a microfluidic channel for sample delivery, and the conductance response can be recorded while solutions with viruses flow at a constant rate. Modification of different nanowires within an array with receptors specific for different viruses provides a means for simultaneous detection of multiple viruses at the single particle level. The potential of nanowire-based electrical detection of viruses exceeds the capabilities of other methods such as polymerase chain reaction–based assays (Gardner et al., 2003) and micromechanical devices (Gupta et al., 2004).

36.5.4 Cancer Detection

Investigators at the University of California have developed a simple and cost-effective method of building conducting polymer nanowires that can detect a wide range of levels of a cancer biomarker (Bangar et al., 2009). Ashok Mulchandani's research team developed a new device. At its heart lies polypyrole nanowires connected to a pair of gold electrode spaced a mere 3 μm apart and also use an applied electric field to move individual nanowires into proper alignment on the gold electrodes. They coat the nanowires with material known as EDC that can serve as an attachment point for antibodies and other molecules that bind to specific cancer biomarkers. The investigators attached an antibody that binds to the cancer biomarker CA 125. When solutions with known concentrations of CA 125 were applied to the biosensor, the device accurately measured concentration as low as 1 enzymatic unit per milliliter (U/mL) of solution to as high as 1000 U/mL. The maximal normal blood level of CA 125 is considered to be 35 U/mL. The researchers obtained identical results when they tested human blood plasma for CA 125 levels. The researchers noted that their next step would be to create a device capable of measuring a panel of disease markers simultaneously. They also planned to incorporate their biosensor into a microfluidic device that would be suitable for use in portable disease detection system.

36.6 Spectrum Application

36.6.1 Antidiabetic Effect

Permanent solution for diabetic patients could be artificial pancreas. The original idea was first described in 1974. The concept of its work is simple, a sensor electrode repeatedly measures the level of blood glucose; this information feeds into a small computer that energizes an infusion pump, and the needed units of insulin enter the bloodstream from a small reservoir (Hanazaki et al., 2006). However, the main problem and the reason why most patients refused to have such an artificial organ was its size. Today, it is logical to assume that nanotechnology can solve the problem.

An American company, Medtronic MiniMed, has been working on a device called long-term sensor system (LTSS), which links an implantable long-term glucose mini sensor with an implantable insulin mini pump. The main problem is how to develop and refine a sophisticated algorithm to translate glucose levels determined by the sensor into appropriate insulin dosages. Testing of the LTSS to date is promising, and MiniMed scientists predict they can bring an artificial pancreas to marker by the year 2008. It is not hard to imagine what the artificial pancreas might bring to diabetes patients. Ideally, it would mean nearly normal glycemic, no checking of blood glucose levels, no risk of hyper/hypoglycemia, no chronic diabetic complications, no chronic immunosuppression as in islet transplantation, etc. There is no doubt that with its small size, artificial pancreas would be an acceptable solution for every diabetic patient. Another one great alternative for pancreatic tissue transplantation could be the so-called artificial beta cell. The cells can be genetically altered so that they could not only produce insulin but could also respond to the rise and fall of blood glucose, just as normal pancreatic beta cells do (Dinsmoor, 2006). Dr. Illani Atwater from Sansum Medical Research Institute, Santa Barbara, CA, was working on inserting the proinsulin gene into a keratinocyte cell line attached to a glucose-sensitive promoter gene, as well as the genes for GLUT2 glucose transporters and glucokinase phosphorylation enzymes. No matter which way leads toward the solution, the result will be the same, i.e., artificial beta cell will produce insulin in response to the rise of blood glucose, and no target for immune system. Medical applications of cantilever-based sensors have been proposed for early diagnosis of diabetes mellitus (Lang et al., 2002) and can improve blood glucose monitoring using small and ultrasensitive analytical platforms (Yan et al., 2004). In patients with diabetes mellitus, ketones are produced due to the deterioration of blood insulin concentrations. Acetone is one of these ketones that is excreted in urine or expired as vapor in exhaled air. Disposable test kits are used to detect acetone in urine. Acetone in exhaled air can only be detected by the physician as a putrid smell without any quantification. Small amounts of acetone in a patient's breath can be detected by cantilever array sensor technique, which may attribute to early diagnosis of diabetes mellitus.

36.7 Quantum Dots Applications

Quantum dots are spherical nanosized crystals. They can be made of nearly every semiconductor metal (e.g., Cds, CdSe, CdTe, ZnS, PbS), but alloys and other metals (e.g., Au) can also be used (Zheng et al., 2004). The prototypical quantum dot is cadmium selenite (CdSe). Quantum dots range between 2 and 10 nm in diameter. In the early 1990s, quantum dots were mainly prepared in aqueous solution with added stabilizing agents. This procedure yielded low-quality quantum dots with poor fluorescence efficiencies and large size variations. Biomedical monitoring applications have taken considerable advantage of using quantum dots for sensitive optical imaging in fixed cells and tissues, living cells, and animal models. In addition, quantum dots can be conjugated to biological molecules such as proteins, oligonucleotides, and small molecules, which are used to direct binding of the quantum dot to area of interest for biolabeling and biosensing (Bruchez et al., 1998). Quantum dots are now used extensively for labeling in biomedical research (Chan and Nie, 1998), and this use is predicted to grow because of their many advantages over alternative labeling methods. Moreover, quantum dots have brighter emission and good photostability.

36.7.1 Treatment for Tumor

Targeted molecular imaging of tumors was first demonstrated in nude mice using quantum dots (Gao et al., 2004b). Nude mice lack a thymus and a functional immune system. Therefore, a human xenograft of tumor cells will be accepted and grow in nude mice. This xenograft tumor model is therefore an excellent model to study in vivo targeting of therapeutics to human cancer cells. Moreover, the vasculature of most cancer tissue is highly disordered, causing exposed interstitial tissue, so that tumor antigens are in direct contact with blood. Nude mice with human prostate tumors were injected intravenously with poly (ethylene glycol)-conjugated quantum dots functionalized with antibodies against the prostate-specific membrane antigen. The permeability and retention effect is due to the inherent vasculature permeability of the microenvironment of cancerous tissue, combined with the lack of lymphatic drainage. Due to the permeability and retention effect alone, it was found that nonconjugated poly (ethylene glycol) quantum dots accumulated in induced mouse tumors, demonstrating tumor contrast, but much less efficiently than actively targeted probes. Recently, an intraoperative highly sensitive technique for pulmonary sentinel lymph node mapping using NIR fluorescent quantum dots has been developed (Soltesz et al., 2005). The study showed the feasibility of the techniques for mapping pulmonary lymphatic drainage and guiding excision of the sentinel lymph node in a porcine model. In addition, the application of quantum dots in multiphoton intravital microscopy shows great versatility for studying tumor pathophysiology (Stroh et al., 2005). Intravital microscopy is a powerful imaging technique that allows continuous noninvasive monitoring of molecular and cellular processes in intact living tissue with 1–10 μm resolution (Jain et al., 2002). Quantum dots can be customized to concurrently image and differentiate tumor vessels from both perivascular cells and matrix and to monitor the trafficking of bone marrow–derived precursor cells to the tumor vasculature allowing to investigate the degree to which the vascular and perivascular structures are formed or remodeled in response to cell homing.

36.7.2 Treatment for Blindness

Emerging nanotechnologies have a great potential to uncover the cause of cataract and may provide a good solution for its treatment. The lens is comprised of tightly packed epithelial cells and lens fibers, enclosed in a thin capsule, although the lens fibers have few organelles and their protein content is very high. The lens consists of 35% protein and 65% water. In addition, there are three classes of proteins in the human lens. The researchers used intact porcine lenses from 5 month- old pigs, intact human lenses obtained from three donors aged 41, 42, and 45 years, and section of human lens cortex obtained from four donors aged 11, 19, and 32 years, and these were incubated for 72 h at 7°C in aqueous solution of green (566 nm) and red (652 nm) fluorescent water-soluble cadmium tellurium NPs. Future studies are required to determine the critical variables necessary for the diffusion of NPs through the lens capsule, and these researchers reveal that fluorescent NPs are used to enhance visualization of the lens capsule during cataract surgery (Schachar et al., 2008).

36.7.3 Detection of Immunity

Antibodies linked to quantum dots, in combination with a technique known as multispectral imaging, to detect 11 clusters of differentiation markers in fixed human lymphoid tissue samples are used. The researchers attached quantum dots with unique emission spectra, the color of light they emit when irradiated with light to each of 11 commercially available antibodies that target these differentiation markers. Mainly streptavidin-conjugated quantum dots with distinct emission spectra were tested for their utility in indentifying a variety of differentially expressed antigens. Slides were analyzed using confocal laser scanning microscopy, which enabled with a single excitation wavelength

(488 argon laser) the detection of up to seven signals (streptavidin-conjugated quantum dots 525, 565, 585, 605, 655, 705, and 805 nm) plus the detection of 4′,6-diamidino-2-phenylindole with an infrared laser turned to 760 nm for two photon excitation. Each of these signals was specific for the intended morphologic immunohistochemical target. In addition, five of the seven streptavidin-conjugated quantum dots tested were used on the same tissue section and could be analyzed simultaneously on routinely processed formalin-fixed, paraffin-embedded sections. Applications of this multiplexing method will enable investigators to explore the clinically relevant multidimensional cellular interactions that underlie diseases, simultaneously, and the development of multitarget quantum dot–based diagnostic systems; there are still many factors that need to be examined to optimize the use of these nanoscale beacons (Fountaine et al., 2006).

36.7.4 Detection of Cell Death

Researchers have developed an NP that can spot apoptosis, using both MRI and fluorescence imaging. Animals test showed that this NP can provide anatomical information using MRI and cellular level information using fluorescence imaging. Imaging-programmed cell death in the body could provide an early indication that an antitumor therapy is indeed killing cancer cells. Importantly, biocompatible molecular structure is capable of binding strongly to eight gadolinium atoms and then linked multiple carriers to each fluorescent quantum dot and also attached one molecule of annexing A5 (Prabha and Labhasetwar, 2004). The resulting NP contained enough gadolinium atoms to produce a strong MRI signal that would be detectable even if only a few of the NPs were able to bind an apoptotic cell. To test the imaging ability of this NP, the investigators added it to cells triggered to start apoptosis. During the initial stages of apoptosis, the researchers were able to detect small patches of green fluorescence on the cell membrane. As apoptosis continued, these green patches spread across the entire cell membrane. MRI experiments showed that the NP produced an imaging signal that was approximately 40 times stronger than that produced by the gadolinium carrier alone. Subsequent imaging experiments were able to detect injury-induced apoptosis in mice.

36.8 Conclusion

Nanotechnology offers important new tools expected to have a great impact on many areas in medical technology. It provides extraordinary opportunities to improve materials and medical devices, and they contain several chemical, physical, engineering, and biological sciences. The nanometer scale is helpful to determine the molecular components within the living cells and gives enormous spectrum with emergent properties; the convergence scale has been applied for to improve the human health development. In particular, relevant applications are reported in surgery, cancer diagnosis and therapy, biodetection of disease markers, molecular imaging, implant technology, tissue engineering, and devices for drug, protein, gene, and radionuclide delivery. The future that can be envisioned for improvements in public health through the application of nanotechnologies, including nanomedicine and nanobiotechnology, seems bright, and these discoveries already are revolutionizing manufacturing processes of many materials and devices that find broad application in society.

References

Agam, M.A. and Guo, Q. (2007), Electron beam modification of polymer nanospheres, *J. Nanosci. Nanotechnol.*, 7, 3615–3619.

Albrecht, M. et al. (2005), Scanning force microscopy study of biogenic nanoparticles for medical applications, *J. Magn. Magn. Mat.*, 290, 269–271.

Andresen, T.L., Davidsen, J., Begtrup, M., Mouritsen, O.G., and Jorgensen, K. (2004), Enzymatic release of antitumor ether lipids by specific phospholipase A2 activation of liposome forming prodrugs, *J. Med. Chem.*, 47, 1694–1703.

Bangar, M.A., Shirale, D.J., Chen, W., Myung, N.V., and Mulchandani, A. (2009), Single conducting polymer nanowire chemiresistive label-free immunosensor for cancer biomarker, *Anal. Chem.*, 8, 2168–2175.

Barone, P.W., Baik, S., Heller, D.A., and Strano, M.S. (2004), Near-infrared optical sensors based on single-walled carbon nanotubes, *Nat. Mater.*, 4, 86–92.

Bettge, M., Chatterjee, J., and Haik, Y. (2004), Physically synthesized Ni-Cu nanoparticles for magnetic hyperthermia, *Biomagn. Res. Technol.*, 2, 4–9.

Bharali, D.J. et al. (2005), Organically modified silica nanoparticles: A non-viral vector for in vivo gene delivery and expression in the brain, *Proc. Natl. Acad. Sci. USA*, 102, 11539–11544.

Bianco, A. et al. (2005), Cationic carbon nanotubes bind to CpG oligo deoxynucleotides and enhance their immune-stimulatory properties, *J. Am. Chem. Soc.*, 127, 58–59.

Borges, A.R. and Schengrund, C.L. (2005), Dendrimers and antivirals: A review, *Curr. Drug Targets Infect. Disord.*, 5, 247–254.

Braun, E., Eichen, Y., Sivan, U., and Ben-Yoseph, G. (1998), DNA-templated assembly and electrode attachment of a conducting silver wire, *Nature*, 391, 775–778.

Brooks, B.R. et al. (1983), Program for macromolecular energy, minimization, and dynamics calculations, *J. Comp. Chem.*, 4, 187–217.

Bruchez, M., Moronne, M., Gin, P., Weiss, S., and Alivisatos, A.P. (1998), Semiconductor nanocrystals as fluorescent biological labels, *Science*, 281, 2013–2016.

Chan, W.C. and Nie, S. (1998), Quantum dot bio-conjugates for ultrasensitive non-isotopic detection, *Science*, 281, 2016–2018.

Chang, L., Bakhos, L., Wang, Z., Venton, D.L., and Klein, W.L. (2003), Femtomole immunodetection of synthetic and endogenous amyloid-beta oligomers and its application to Alzheimer's disease drug candidate screening, *J. Mol. Neurosci.*, 20, 305–313.

Cherukuri, P., Bachilo, S.M., Litovsky, S.H., and Weisman, R.B. (2004), Near-infrared fluorescence microscopy of single-walled carbon nanotubes in phagocytic cells. *J. Am. Chem. Soc.*, 126, 15638–15639.

Choy, J.H., Jang, E.S., Won, J.H., Chung, J.H., Jang, D.J., and Kim, Y.W. (2004), Hydrothermal route to ZnO nanocoral reefs and nanofibers, *Appl. Phys. Lett.*, 84, 287.

Cui, Y. and Lieber, C.M. (2001), Functional nanoscale electronic devices assembled using silicon nanowire building blocks, *Science*, 291, 851–853.

Das, S. et al. (2007), Designs for ultra-tiny, special-purpose nanoelectronic circuits, *IEEE Trans. Circuits Syst. I*, 54, 2528–2540.

DeNardo, S.J. et al. (2005), Development of tumor targeting bio-probes (111In-chimeric L6 monoclonal antibody nanoparticles) for alternating magnetic field cancer therapy, *Clin. Cancer Res.*, 11, 7087–7092.

Dinsmoor, R.S. (2006), Islet cell transplantation. http://www.childrenwithdiabetes.com/_on_701.htm

Dong, W. et al. (2007), Multifunctional nanowire bio-scaffolds on titanium. *Chem. Mater.*, 19, 4454–4459.

El-Sayed, I.H., Huang, X., and El-Sayed, M.A. (2006), Selective laser photo-thermal therapy of epithelial carcinoma using anti-EGFR antibody conjugated gold nanoparticles, *Cancer Lett.*, 239, 129–135.

Everts, M. et al. (2006), Covalently linked Au nanoparticles to a viral vector: Potential for combined photothermal and gene cancer therapy, *Nano Lett.*, 6, 587–591.

Fountaine, T.J., Wincovitch, S.M., Geho, D.H., Garfield, S.H., and Pittalunga, S. (2006), Multispectral imaging of clinically relevant cellular targets in tonsil and lymphoid tissue using semiconductor quantum dots, *Mod. Pathol.*, 19, 1181–1191.

Freitas, R.A. (2005), Nanotechnology, nanomedicine and nanosurgery, *Int. J. Surg.*, 3, 1–4.

Gao, Q. et al. (2004a), Disruption of neural signal transducer and activator of transcription 3 causes obesity, diabetes, infertility, and thermal dys-regulation, *Proc. Natl. Acad. Sci. USA*, 101, 4661–4666.

Gao, X., Cui, Y., Levenson, R.M., Chung, L.W., and Nie, S. (2004b), In vivo cancer targeting and imaging with semiconductor quantum dots, *Nat. Biotechnol.*, 22, 969–976.

Gardner, S.N., Kuczmarski, T.A., Vitalis, E.A., and Slezak, T.R. (2003), Limitations of TaqMan PCR for detecting divergent viral pathogens illustrated by hepatitis A, B, C, and E viruses and human immunodeficiency virus, *J. Clin. Microbiol.*, 41, 2417–2427.

Georganopoulou, D.G. et al. (2005), Assessment of CSF levels of tau protein in mildly demented patients with Alzheimer's disease, *Proc. Natl. Acad. Sci. USA*, 102, 2273–2276.

Gong, Y. et al. (2003), Alzheimer's disease-affected brain: Presence of oligomeric A β ligands (ADDLs) suggests a molecular basis for reversible memory loss, *Proc. Natl. Acad. Sci. USA*, 100, 10417–10422.

Gopalan, B. et al. (2004), Nanoparticle based systemic gene therapy for lung cancer: Molecular mechanisms and strategies to suppress nano-particle-mediated inflammatory response, *Technol. Cancer Res. Treat.*, 3, 647–657.

Gref, R. et al. (1994), Biodegradable long circulating polymeric nanospheres. *Science*, 263, 1600–1603.

Gupta, A., Akin, D., and Bashir, R. (2004), Single virus particle mass detection using microresonators with nanoscale thickness, *Appl. Phys. Lett.*, 84, 1976–1978.

Hanazaki, K., Nose, Y., and Brunicardi, F.C.H. (2006), Artificial endocrine pancreas, *J. Am. Coll. Surg.*, 193, 310–322.

Hede, S. and Huilgol, N. (2006), Nano: The new nemesis of cancer, *J. Cancer Res. Ther.*, 2, 186–195.

Hirsch, L.R. et al. (2003), Nanoshell-mediated near-infrared thermal therapy of tumors under magnetic resonance guidance, *Proc. Natl. Acad. Sci. USA*, 100, 13549–13554.

Huang, Y., Duan, X., and Lieber, C.M. (2005), Nanowires for integrated multicolor nanophotonics, *Small*, 1, 142–147.

Huynh, W.U., Dittmer, J.J., and Alivisatos, A.P. (2002), Hybrid nanorod-polymer solar cells, *Science*, 295, 2425–2427.

Jain, R.K., Munn, L.L., and Fukumura, D. (2002), Dissecting tumour pathophysiology using intravital microscopy, *Nat. Rev. Cancer*, 2, 266–276.

Jordan, A. et al. (2001), Presentation of a new magnetic field therapy system for the treatment of human solid tumors with magnetic fluid hyperthermia, *J. Magn. Magn. Mater.*, 225, 118–126.

Jordan, A., Scholz, R., Wust, P., Fahling, H., and Roland, F. (1999), Magnetic fluid hyperthermia (MFH): Cancer treatment with AC magnetic field induced excitation of biocompatible superparamagnetic nanoparticles, *J. Magn. Magn. Mater.*, 201, 413–419.

Joshi, P.P., Merchant, S.A., Wang, Y., and Schmidtke, D.W. (2005), Amperometric biosensors based on redox polymer-carbon nanotube-enzyme composites, *Anal. Chem.*, 77, 3183–3188.

Kam, N.W.S. and Dai, H. (2005), Carbon nanotubes as intracellular protein transporters: Generality and biological functionality, *J. Am. Chem. Soc. USA*, 127, 6021–6026.

Kam, N.W.S., Jessop, T.C., Wender, P.A., and Dai, H. (2004), Nanotube molecular transporters: Internalization of carbon nanotube-protein conjugates into mammalian cells, *J. Am. Chem. Soc. USA*, 126, 6850–6851.

Kam, N.W., O'Connell, M., Wisdom, J.A., and Dai, H. (2005), Carbon nanotube as multifunctional biological transporters and near infrared agent for selective cancer cell destruction, *Proc. Natl. Acad. Sci. USA*, 102, 11600–11605.

Keating, C.D. (2005), Nanoscience enables ultrasensitive detection of Alzheimer's biomarker, *PNAS*, 7, 2263–2264.

Kind, H., Yan, H., Messer, B., Law, M., and Yang, P. (2002), Nanowire ultraviolet photodetectors and optical switches, *Adv. Mater.*, 14, 158–160.

Kohli, V., Elezzabi, A.Y., and Acker, J.P. (2005), Cell nanosurgery using ultra-short (femtosecond) laser pulses: Applications to membrane surgery and cell isolation, *Lasers Surg. Med.*, 37, 227–230.

Kong, J., Franklin, N.R., and Zhou, C. (2000), Nanotube molecular wires as chemical sensors, *Science*, 287, 622–625.

Lambert, M.P. et al. (2001), Vaccination with soluble A-beta oligomers generates toxicity neutralizing antibodies, *J. Neurochem.*, 79, 595–605.

Lang, H.P., Hegner, M., Meyer, E., and Gerber, C.H. (2002), Nanomechanics from atomic resolution to molecular recognition based on atomic force microscopy technology, *Nanotechnology*, 13, 29–36.

Li, Y., Cheng, G.S., and Zhang, L.D. (2000), Fabrication of highly ordered ZnO nanowire arrays in anodic alumina membranes, *J. Mater. Res.*, 15, 2305–2308.

Li, Z., Zhu, S., Gan, K., Zhang, Q., Zeng, Z., and Zhou, Y. (2005), Poly-l-lysine-modified silica nanoparticles: A potential oral gene delivery system, *J. Nanosci. Nanotechnol.*, 5, 1199–1203.

Loo, C. et al. (2004), Nanoshell-enabled photonics-based imaging and therapy of cancer, *Technol. Cancer Res. Treat.*, 3, 33–40.

Loo, C., Lowery, A., Halas, N., West, J., and Drezek, R. (2005), Immunotargeted nanoshells for integrated cancer imaging and therapy, *Nano Lett.*, 5, 709–711.

Mansouri, S. et al. (2006), Characterization of folate-chitosan-DNA nano-particles for gene therapy, *Biomaterials*, 27, 2060–2065.

Mashino, T. et al. (2005), Human immunodeficiency virus-reverse transcriptase inhibition and hepatitis C virus RNA-dependent RNA polymerase inhibition activities of fullerene derivatives, *Bioorg. Med. Chem. Lett.*, 15, 1107–1109.

Nam, J.M., Thaxton, C.S., and Mirkin, C.A. (2003), Nanoparticle based bio-bar codes for the ultra sensitive detection of proteins, *Science*, 301, 1884–1886.

Narayan, R.J. et al. (2004), Nanostructured ceramics in medical devices: Applications and prospects, *JOM*, 56, 38–43.

Ogris, M. et al. (1998), The size of DNA/transferrin-PEI complexes is an important factor for gene expression in cultured cells, *Gene Ther.*, 5, 1425–1433.

O'Neal, D.P., Hirsch, L.R., Halas, N.J., Payne, J.D., and West, J.L. (2004), Photo thermal tumor ablation in mice using near infrared-absorbing nanoparticles, *Cancer Lett.*, 209, 171–176.

Pantarotto, D., Briand, J.P., Prato, M., and Bianco, A. (2004), Translocation of bioactive peptides across cell membranes by carbon nanotubes, *Chem. Commun. Camb.*, 1, 16–17.

Patel, G.M., Patel, G.C., Patel, R.B., Patel, J.K., and Patel, M. (2006), Nano-robot: A versatile tool in nanomedicine, *J. Drug Target*, 14, 63–67.

Patolsky, F. et al. (2004), Electrical detection of single viruses, *Proc. Natl. Acad. Sci. USA*, 101, 14017–14022.

Perkel, J.M. (2004), The ups and downs of nano-biotech, *Scientist*, 18, 14–18.

Prabha, S. and Labhasetwar, V. (2004), Nanoparticle-mediated wild-type p53 gene delivery results in sustained antiproliferative activity in breast cancer cells, *Mol. Pharmacol.*, 1, 211–219.

Rao, C.N.R. and Cheetham, A.K. (2001), Science and technology of nanomaterials: Current status and future prospects, *J. Mater. Chem.*, 11, 2887–2894.

Roco, M.C. (2005), Environmentally responsible development of nanotechnology, *Environ. Sci. Technol.*, 39, 106–112.

Routkevitch, D., Bigioni, T., Moskovits, M., and Xu, J.M. (1996), Electrochemical fabrication of CdS nanowire arrays in porous anodic aluminum oxide templates, *J. Phys. Chem.*, 100, 14037–14047.

Sacconi, L., Tolic Norrelykke, I.M., Antolini, R., and Pavone, F.S. (2005), Combined intracellular three dimensional imaging and selective nanosurgery by a nonlinear microscope, *J. Biomed.*, 10, 14002.

Schachar, R.A. et al. (2008), Diffusion of nanoparticles into the capsule and cortex of a crystalline lens, *Nanotechnology*, 19, 25102.

Shinkai, M. et al. (1996), Intracellular hyperthermia for cancer using magnetite cationic liposomes: In vitro study, *Jpn. J. Cancer Res.*, 87, 1179–1183.

Soltesz, E.G. et al. (2005), Intraoperative sentinel lymph node mapping of the lung using near-infrared fluorescent quantum dots, *Ann. Thorac. Surg.*, 79, 269–277.

Stroh, M. et al. (2005), Quantum dots spectrally distinguish multiple species within the tumor milieu *in vivo, Nature Med.,* 11, 678–682.

Tirlapur, U.K. and Konig, K. (2002), Femtosecond near infrared laser pulses as a versatile non invasive tool for intra tissue nanoprocessing in plants without compromising viability, *Plant J.,* 31, 365–374.

Wang, Y., Li, Q., and Hu, S. (2005), A multiwall carbon nanotubes film-modified carbon fiber ultramicroelectrode for the determination of nitric oxide radical in liver mitochondria, *Bioelectrochemistry,* 65, 135–142.

Wang, Z., Liu, J., Liang, Q., Wang, Y., and Luo, G. (2002), Carbon nanotube-modified electrodes for the simultaneous determination of dopamine and ascorbic acid, *Analyst,* 127, 653–658.

Wang, S.G., Zhang, Q., Wang, R., and Yoon, S.F. (2003), A novel multi-walled carbon nanotube-based biosensor for glucose detection, *Biochem. Biophys. Res. Commun.,* 311, 572–576.

Witzmann, F.A. and Monteiro-Riviere, N.A. (2006), Multi walled carbon nanotube exposure alters protein expression in human keratinocytes, *Nanomed. Nanotechnol.,* 2, 158–168.

Wu, K., Fei, J., and Hu, S. (2003), Simultaneous determination of dopamine and serotonin on a glassy carbon electrode coated with a film of carbon nanotubes, *Anal. Biochem.,* 318, 100–106.

Yan, X., Ji, H.F., and Lvov, Y. (2004), Modification of microcantilevers using layer-by-layer nanoassembly film for glucose measurement, *Chem. Phys. Lett.,* 396, 34–37.

Yanik, M.F. et al. (2004), Neurosurgery: Functional regeneration after laser axotomy, *Nature,* 432, 822.

Yemini, M., Reches, M., Rishpon, J., and Gazit, E. (2005), Novel electrochemical biosensing platform using self-assembled peptide nanotubes, *Nano Lett.,* 5, 183–186.

Zhang, Z., Ying, J.Y., and Dresselhaus, M.S. (1998), Bismuth quantum-wire arrays fabricated by a vacuum melting and pressure injection process, *J. Mater. Res.,* 13, 1748.

Zheng, J., Zhang, C., and Dickson, R.M. (2004), Highly fluorescent, water-soluble, size-tunable gold quantum dots, *Phys. Rev. Lett.,* 93, 77402.

Part IV

Industrial Applications of Marine-Derived Biomaterials

37

Industry Perspectives of Marine-Derived Proteins as Biomaterials

Se-Kwon Kim, Dai-Hung Ngo, Thanh-Sang Vo, and BoMi Ryu

CONTENTS

37.1 Introduction

In recent years, consumer's demand for products with functional ingredients has increased, and this situation has underlined the need to guarantee the safety, traceability, authenticity, and health benefits of such products. According to recent knowledge, foods derived from marine seem to be by far the greatest sources of bioactive protein. Hence, commercially available marine food protein products have also prompted newer challenges. Marine bioactive food proteins have been isolated from fish, algae, mollusk, crustacean, and marine by-products including substandard muscles, viscera, skins, trimmings, and shellfish. Bioactive proteins derived from marine organisms as well as from marine fish processing by-products have greater potential for the development of functional foods for new commercial trends by industries. Marine food proteins have long been recognized for their nutritional and functional properties (Larsen et al. 2011). They have been used as essential raw materials in most industries. They have potential in novel commercial trends, as they are widely commercialized in food, beverage, pharmaceutical, and cosmetic industries, in addition to other fields such as medicine, biotechnology, photography, textiles, leather, and electronic. The industrialists are eager to embrace a novel product if it can deliver what consumers want and, at the same time, industry needs to balance its involvement against the perceived market potential for a new trend. This chapter presents an overview of the current status, future industrial perspectives, and commercial trends of marine bioactive food proteins.

37.2 Industry Perspectives of Marine Proteins

37.2.1 Food Industry

The improvement of solubility and foaming properties of marine food proteins perceives novel trends for consumer appealing. To improve a protein's solubility and foaming properties, mild hydrolysis can be first used to remove the amide nitrogen group, which increases the number of negatively charged groups. Further hydrolysis then reduces the protein's average molecular weight. Chemical modification techniques have been the subject of much research. Besides chemical and enzymatic modifications, genetically modified proteins are available, but global acceptance of these has limited their use. The perspective of improving functional characteristics of marine food proteins could be the way to novel food products. The antifreeze proteins of polar fishes' proteins that act as nucleating agents could have useful applications in frozen food systems. The former could be used to lower temperature and retard crystallization during frozen storage and the latter to give the desirable crystal size and texture when added to ice-cream formulations.

Furthermore, marine capture fisheries contribute over 50% of total world fish production, and more than 70% of this production has been utilized for processing. As a result, every year, a considerable amount of total catch is discarded as processing leftovers and that includes trimmings, fins, frames, skin, and viscera (Kim and Mendis 2006). Among the by-products from fish processing plants are fish frames, which include head, bone, and tail, which are very important protein sources. Therefore, there is a great potential in marine bioprocess industry to convert and utilize more of fish processing waste as valuable products. One of the approaches for the effective protein recovery from these by-products is enzymatic hydrolysis, which is widely applied to improve and upgrade the functional and nutritional properties of proteins.

Lipid oxidation by reactive oxygen species such as superoxide, hydroxyl radicals, and H_2O_2 causes a decrease in nutritional value of lipid foods and affects their safety and appearance. Therefore, in food and pharmaceutical industries, many synthetic commercial antioxidants such as hydroxytoluene (BHT), butylated hydroxyanisole (BHA), tert-butylhydroquinone (TBHQ), and propyl gallate (PG) have been used to retard the oxidation and peroxidation processes. However, the use of these synthetic antioxidants is under strict regulation due to their potential health risk. Hence, the search for natural antioxidants as safe alternatives is important to the food industry. Furthermore, natural bioactive food proteins such as phycobiliproteins can be derived from marine blue–green and red algae, which also have potential as natural food colorants. Therefore, marine bioactive food proteins have important functional properties that could be scaled up and economically favorable as nutraceutical ingredients for the food industry (Hettiarachchy et al. 1996; Park et al. 2001).

37.2.2 Pharmaceutical Industry

Marine food-derived proteins are important ingredients in pharmaceutical products. Some of them are currently used as drugs, for example, insulin, while others are used to provide filler for other drugs and therapeutic agents in the pharmaceutical industry. Thus, novel marine food proteins have the potential to be used as novel drugs. Components of proteins in marine foods are containing sequences of bioactive peptides, which could exert a physiological effect in the body (Jung et al. 2006). Recently, marine bioactive peptides have been shown to possess numerous biological functions such as antioxidative, antihypertensive, antimicrobial, anticancer, antithrombotic, antihypercholesterol, opioid agonistic, immunomodulatory, prebiotic, and mineral-binding activities (Clare and Swaisgood 2000; Elias et al. 2008; Betoret et al 2011; Rajanbabu and Chen 2011). Therefore, new applications are appearing for them as novel natural pharmaceuticals. Recently, it has been observed that most synthetic drugs have several side effects. For instance, synthetic antihypertensive drugs have shown several side effects (Atkinson and Robertson 1979). Furthermore, the use of heparin may be accompanied by side effects such as thrombocytopenia, hemorrhagic effect, ineffectiveness in congenital or acquired antithrombin deficiencies, and incapacity to inhibit thrombin bound to fibrin (Costa et al. 2010). Therefore, marine bioactive peptides have potential as novel drugs in the pharmaceutical industry without the undesirable side effects. In addition, the need to discover new antimicrobial substances is important due to progressive development of resistance by pathogenic microorganisms against conventional antibiotics. Marine-derived antibacterial peptides play a significant role as antimicrobial agents and have shown potencies that make them useful in the pharmaceutical industry.

37.2.3 Cosmetic Industry

Marine proteins have been well recognized for their biologically active substances with a great potential to be used as cosmetics. Novel perspectives in cosmetic industry have been arisen by the young generation toward beauty as well as maintaining a young appearance with novel cosmetics containing natural bioactive ingredients. Hence, the search for safe and inexpensive natural bioactive ingredients from marine proteins as cosmetic ingredients is promising (Kim et al. 2008). Phycoerythrin pigment protein in red algae can be used as a pigment in cosmetics. Incorporating marine proteoglycans as a nutricosmetic in skin capsules is said to boost collagen, help strengthen cell cohesion, and improve skin density, creating firmer skin. In addition, marine food proteins have potential as functional ingredients in cosmetics such as sunscreen lotions, shampoo, conditioners, hair gel, nail polish, and lipstick.

Recently, the cosmetic application of collagen and gelatin, derived from terrestrial animals like cow and pig, is declining because of animal diseases and some ethnic or religious barriers. New trends are pushing to use other food sources such as marine fish–derived collagen and gelatin. They are excellent functional ingredients for the cosmetic industry. Collagen and gelatin have a high moisturizing property and can be produced as novel cosmetic creams and gels. Collagen for skin care has been produced mainly from cold water fish skins such as cod, haddock, and salmon. Collagen is being commercially produced from fish scale, such as tilapia, by decalcification and enzymatic hydrolysis. The uniqueness of scale collagen is its molecular weight, which is lower (~1000 Da) than skin collagen.

With the invention of UV radiation protection compounds, antiwrinkling agents, and antiaging compounds in the cosmetic industry, new trends have focused on the manufacture of sunscreen lotions, creams, and other cosmetics. In this case, marine-derived bioactive food proteins are promising functional ingredients for these new cosmeceuticals with pharmaceutical benefits.

37.2.4 Other Industries

The perspective for use of marine bioactive food proteins is promising in other industries such as printing and photography, electronic, textiles, and leather.

37.3 Marine-Derived Proteins with Commercial Trends

37.3.1 Gelatin

Gelatin, one of the most popular biopolymers, is widely used in food, pharmaceutical, cosmetic, and photographic industries because of its unique functional and technological properties. For industrial purposes, gelatin is extracted mainly from skins and bones of cattle and pigs. However, due to highly infectious and contagious animal diseases and some religious barriers, industrial use of gelatin from these sources is becoming limited. Therefore, marine-derived gelatin is an alternative with safe and economical advantages.

In the food industry, gelatin is utilized in confections (mainly for providing chewiness, texture, and foam stabilization), low-fat spreads (to provide creaminess, fat reduction, and mouth feel), dairy (to provide stabilization and texturization), baked goods (to provide emulsification, gelling, and stabilization), and meat products (to provide water binding). Gelatin has a tendency to form complexes with other proteins and hydrocolloids. This property makes gelatin useful for precipitating materials that cause haze or cloudiness in wines, beer, cider juice, and vinegar. Hence, gelatin can be used in the food industry as a clarification agent. In addition, the use of gelatin in the nutraceutical industry is widespread. It not only serves as an excipient but also is an excellent and economical source of multiple amino acids. Therefore, gelatin can serve as a functional ingredient in medicinal food formulas. It is also widely utilized in nutritional bars, sports drinks, and energy drinks and reduces carbohydrate content in foods formulated for diabetic patients. Gelatin, being low in calories, is normally recommended for use in foodstuffs to enhance protein levels and is especially useful in body-building foods.

In the pharmaceutical and medical fields, gelatin is used as a matrix for implants, in injectable drug delivery microspheres, and in intravenous infusions. There are also reports in which live attenuated viral vaccines used for immunization against measles, mumps, rubella, rabies, and tetanus toxin contain gelatin as stabilizer. Moreover, gelatin is widely used in the pharmaceutical industry for the manufacture of hard and soft capsules, plasma expanders, and in wound care. As a protein, gelatin is low in calories and melts in the mouth to give excellent sensory properties resembling fat, making it ideal for use in low-fat products. Low gelling temperature of gelatin offers new potential applications such as use in dry products (for microencapsulation), and in fact, one of the major application is in the encapsulation of vitamins and other pharmaceutical additives such as azoxanthine. Moreover, gelatin can be used to microencapsulate food flavors.

Gelatin could be utilized as the base for light-sensitive coatings that are important to the electronics trade due its low-temperature gelling property. In addition, it is a good medium for precipitating silver halide emulsions since this process can be carried out at a lower temperature. The photography industry uses large quantities of gelatin in several applications due to this phenomenon. In the cosmetic industry, gelatin has been used for many years as hydrolyzed animal protein in shampoos, conditioners, lipsticks, and nail formulas. Recently, additional uses of gelatin have been found as a collagen source in topical creams and other value-added cosmetic products (Gómez-Guillén et al. 2002).

37.3.2 Collagen

Collagen is the protein that is found in the highest concentration, about 30%, in the living body. It is the main structural element of bones, cartilage, skin, tendons, ligaments, blood vessels, teeth, cornea, and all other organs of vertebrates. The molecular structure of collagen contains three polypeptide α chains wound together in a tight triple helix. Each polypeptide called α chain consists of repeated sequence of triplet $(Gly-X-Y)_n$, where X and Y are often proline (Pro) and hydroxyproline (Hyp). Nowadays, consumer demand has arisen for marine-derived collagens due to animal disease and religious issues as discussed for collagen (Senaratne et al. 2006).

On the industrial front, most of the applications for collagen are direct result that collagen can be synthesized into gelatin, which turns out to be a highly useful raw material in the food industry. It is now well known and scientifically proven that hydrolyzed collagen significantly contributes to maintaining bone and joint health and prevents osteoporosis and osteoarthritis. Additionally, collagen improves the elasticity of skin by stimulating the production of collagen by the skin cells themselves thus maintaining youthful and vibrant skin and neutralizing the skin's continuous aging deterioration by redensifying the dermis. To take advantage of all these healthy claims, a number of functional foods or nutraceuticals have been introduced in the market (Mendis et al. 2005).

Collagen has also found application in the manufacture of photography aids, as well as in the production of cosmetic and pharmaceutical products. In addition, polythene–collagen hydrolysate blends have been shown to be a successful alternative to thermoplastic industry as environmentally friendly biodegradable plastics. Blends of collagen hydrolysate and low-density polyethylene up to a 20%–30% content of collagen hydrolysate produce transparent, cohesive, and flexible films that are characterized by satisfactory thermal and mechanical responses and can be applied in packaging and agriculture fields.

In the medical field, collagen can be intended to promote healing of skin that has been damaged or removed as a result of skin grafting, ulceration, burns, cancer, excision, or mechanical trauma. This type of artificial skin prevents moisture and heat loss from the wounded skin and also prevents microbial infiltration to the body. Artificial skin is used not only to limit entrance of foreign matter into the body and prevent mass and heat transfer out of the body but also to provide a continuous cellular layer over the skin. Moreover, collagen can be applied to restructure dental damage and for manufacturing of artificial bones in the medicine. Collagen has high potential in the search for manufacturing artificial bones in medicine because of its high biocompatibility; it is the main protein component in human bones (Karim and Bhat 2009).

37.3.3 Bioactive Peptides

Marine bioactive peptides have been identified to possess nutraceutical potentials that are beneficial in human health promotion. They can be produced by either one of three methods such as solvent extraction, enzymatic hydrolysis, and microbial fermentation of marine food proteins. They usually contain 3–20 amino acid residues, and their activities are based on their amino acid composition and sequence. These short chains of amino acids are inactive within the sequence of the parent protein, but can be released during gastrointestinal digestion, food processing, or fermentation. Depending on the amino acid sequence, marine bioactive peptides have been shown to display a wide range of biological functions that benefit health including antihypertensive, antagonists, immunomodulatory, anticoagulant, antioxidant, anticancer, antimicrobial, antiobesity, and calcium-binding activities in addition to nutrient utilization (Byun and Kim 2001; Rajapakse et al. 2005; Kim et al. 2007; Jo et al. 2008; Liu et al. 2008; Sheih et al. 2009). Some marine bioactive peptides have shown multifunctional effects based on their structure and other factors including hydrophobicity, charge, or microelement binding properties.

Recently, bioactive peptides have been isolated widely by enzymatic hydrolysis of marine organisms. However, in fermented marine food sauces, enzymatic hydrolysis has already been done by microorganisms, and bioactive peptides can be purified without further hydrolysis. In addition, several bioactive peptides have been isolated from marine processing by-products or wastes. Furthermore, some of these bioactive peptides have been identified to possess nutraceutical activities that are beneficial in human health promotion, and it has been shown that marine bioactive peptides can decrease the risk of cardiovascular diseases. Moreover, increasing consumer knowledge of the link between diet and health has raised the awareness and demand for functional food ingredients and nutraceuticals. This is leading to the avoidance and undesirable side effects associated with organically synthesized chemical drugs and also avoidance of the high cost of drug therapies. Bioactive peptides derived from marine organisms as well as fish processing by-products have potential in the development of functional foods, and they can act as potential physiological modulators of metabolism after absorption. Therefore, marine bioactive peptides can be used as versatile raw materials to produce nutraceuticals and pharmaceuticals for human beings.

Recent researches have provided evidence that marine-derived bioactive peptides play a vital role in human health and nutrition. The possibilities of designing new pharmaceuticals and functional foods that support reduced diet-related chronic malfunctions are promising. According to the recent studies, the anticancer activity of marine peptides has been evident due to induction of apoptosis and inhibition of cell proliferation in vitro. These peptides were obtained from anchovy sauce, sea slug, sea hare, squid (Alemán et al. 2011), cod, plaice, salmon, tuna dark muscle (Hsu et al. 2011), fish backbone (Naqash and Nazeer 2011), and shrimp shell (Kannan et al. 2011). Moreover, Wergedahl and colleagues have revealed that protein hydrolysate of salmon was able to reduce the risk of cardiovascular diseases via lowering plasma cholesterol level and inhibiting the activity of Acyl-CoA/cholesterol acyltransferase in Zucker rats (Wergedahl et al. 2004).

Although the anticoagulant marine peptides have rarely been reported, they have been found from marine organisms such as marine starfish, blue mussel, and echiuroid worm (Jo et al. 2008). Moreover, marine anticoagulant proteins have also been purified from yellowfin sole and ark shell. These marine-derived anticoagulant peptides are noncytotoxic and have the potential to be used as functional ingredients in nutraceuticals or pharmaceuticals.

Several lines of studies have been provided by finding the efficient agents and potential targets for antiobesity therapeutics. Herein, cholecystokinin, a biomarker associated with satiety, is identified as a promising target to reduce obesity.

Meanwhile, low-molecular-weight peptides (1–1.5 kDa) from shrimp head protein hydrolysates have been found to be an effective agent for stimulation of cholecystokinin release in STC-1 cells (Cudennec et al. 2008). Thus, these peptides are suggested as a promising functional food against obesity via regulation of cholecystokinin release. Hence, novel pharmaceuticals developed from marine bioactive peptides can be applied as oral administration instead of intravenous administration. For that reason, marine bioactive peptides have the potential to be used in the formulation of health-enhancing nutraceuticals, cosmetics, and as potent drugs with well-defined pharmacological effects.

Components that bind and solubilize minerals such as calcium can be considered to be beneficial in the prevention of dental caries, osteoporosis, hypertension, and anemia. Notably, some peptides derived from hoki and Alaska pollack frame proteins have been known due to their calcium-binding capability (Jung and Kim 2007). Moreover, the improved calcium retention with hoki phosphopeptide intake was observed in osteoporosis model rats to the same level as a commercially prepared casein oligophosphopeptide preparation. Calcium-binding peptides derived from marine may have applications as dairy-free functional food or beverage ingredients for people with lactose intolerance, anticarcinogenic ingredients, or as agents for reducing the risk of osteoporosis.

37.3.4 Algal Proteins

In recent years, algae have gained much attention due to interest in their nutraceutical potential and development of algae-based functional foods and nutraceuticals worldwide. Because of their low content of energy but high concentration of dietary fibers, minerals, and vitamins, they seem to be a good source of healthy food. Algae provide a significant amount of nitrogen compounds, namely, amino acids and proteins as well. The protein content of marine algae varies greatly with species. In general, red seaweeds contain high levels of protein (maximum 47% of the dry weight), green seaweeds contain moderate contents (9%–26% of the dry weight), while brown seaweeds contain much lower protein amounts (3%–15% of the dry weight). A few studies are available on the nutritional value of algal proteins, and some perspectives on the potential applications and commercialization trends of algal proteins for the development of new foods or additives for human consumption are promising (Fleurence 1999). With respect to their high-protein content and amino acid composition, the red seaweeds appear to be an interesting potential source of food proteins and in the development novel functional foods. In addition, the red seaweeds contain a particular protein called phycoerythrin, which is already used in biotechnology applications as a dye in immunofluorescence reactions.

Besides, the high-protein content of various microalgal species and their amino acid pattern, which compares favorably with that of other food proteins, is a good endorsement of microalgae as an alternative protein source. For instance, *Chlorella* (*Chlorella vulgaris* and *Chlorella pyrenoidosa*) is rich in protein (40%–60%), chlorophyll, and carotenoids. It exhibits putative anticarcinogenic, immunomodulatory, hypolipidemic, gastric mucosal–protective, and detoxification activities. *Spirulina platensis* provides immune enhancement and protein supplementation (65%–71% by weight) and has putative health benefits including anemia prevention, hypocholesterolemic, antioxidant, hepatoprotective, and antiallergic activities. Furthermore, the industrial scale growth of the microalga *Dunaliella* can turn out protein extract at about 100 times greater productivity than that reported in agriculture and 50-fold greater than in fish farming (Lordan et al. 2011).

37.3.5 Enzymes

Enzymes are widely used in the food industry, food-grade enzymes. New enzyme trends have arisen in the fat and oil industries, for processing margarine, and the removal of phospholipids in vegetable oils (degumming), using a highly selective microbial phospholipase. Furthermore, enzymes are potential candidates in the textile industry, beverage industry, animal feed industry, detergent industry, and organic chemical synthesis industry. Due to advances in modern biotechnology, enzymes can be developed today for processes where no one would have expected an enzyme to be applicable just a decade ago. Common to most applications, the trends for enzymes due to cost-effective catalysts working under mild conditions result in significant savings in resources such as energy and water for the benefit of both the industry in question and the environment (Kirk et al. 2002). New commercial trends show promise in using underutilized marine food or fish waste to extract enzymes, which can be applicable in industrial purposes (Kim et al. 2003).

37.3.6 Lectins

Lectins (agglutinins) are multivalent carbohydrate-binding proteins or glycoproteins that are finding valuable commercialization trends in the biomedical industry. Thus, lectins derivatized with fluorescent dyes, gold particles, or enzymes are employed as histochemical and cytochemical reagents for detection of glycoconjugates in tissue sections, on cells and subcellular organelles, and in investigations of intracellular pathways of protein glycosylation. Lectin binding has been used to demonstrate that membrane receptors for hormones, growth factors, neurotransmitters, and toxins are glycoconjugates. Another trend in clinical application is that lectins can be used for blood typing. A large amount of lectins have been isolated and characterized from sponges, tunicates, crustaceans, and mollusks. Molchanova et al. (2007) described the purification, characterization, carbohydrate specificity, and anti-HIV-l activity of the new Ca^{2+}-independent GlcNAc-specific lectin from the sea worm *Serpula vermicularis*. In addition, Wang et al. (2006) reported that a 30 kDa beta-galactose-specific lectin isolated from the marine worm *Chaetopterus variopedatus* possesses anti-HIV-1 activity in vitro. Furthermore, some marine algal lectins can be developed as antibiotics against marine vibrios. In the food industry, calcium-binding lectins can be incorporated in neutraceutical or functional food to prevent calcium deficiency (Jung et al. 2003).

37.4 Conclusions

Marine organisms are rich sources of structurally novel and bioactive materials with valuable industrial potentials. Recently, marine bioactive proteins appear to fit the criteria for development as functional ingredients. They are naturally occurring compounds, and their isolation/extraction is relatively cost-effective. They are widely available, with a guaranteed supply. Most importantly, they are functional—their biological activities affect the pathogenesis of several diseases. Hence, marine-derived food proteins are excellent alternative sources of novel functional foods and pharmaceuticals that can contribute to consumer's well-being by replacing synthetic ingredients and cosmetics. The possibilities of designing new functional foods and pharmaceuticals that support reduced the prevalence and severity of chronic diseases are promising.

References

Alemán, A., E. Pérez-Santín, S. Bordenave-Juchereau, I. Arnaudin, M. C. Gómez-Guillén, and P. Montero. 2011. Squid gelatin hydrolysates with antihypertensive, anticancer and antioxidant activity. *Food Research International* 44:1044–1051.

Atkinson, A. B. and J. I. S. Robertson. 1979. Captopril in the treatment of clinical hypertension and cardiac failure. *Lancet* 2:836–839.

Betoret, E., N. Betoret, D. Vidal, and P. Fito. 2011. Functional foods development: trends and technologies. *Trends in Food Science and Technology* 22:498–508.

Byun, H. G. and S. K. Kim. 2001. Purification and characterization of angiotensin I converting enzyme (ACE) inhibitory peptides from Alaska Pollack (*Theragra chalcogramma*) skin. *Process Biochemistry* 36:1155–1162.

Clare, D. A. and H. E. Swaisgood. 2000. Bioactive milk peptides: A prospectus. *Journal of Dairy Science* 83:1187–1195.

Costa, L. S., G. P. Fidelis, S. L. Cordeiro, R. M. Oliveira, D. A. Sabry, R. B. G. Câmara, L. T. D. B. Nobre et al. 2010. Biological activities of sulfated polysaccharides from tropical seaweeds. *Biomedicine Pharmacotherapy* 64:21–28.

Cudennec, B., R. Ravallec-Plé, E. Courois, and M. Fouchereau-Peron. 2008. Peptides from fish and crustacean by-products hydrolysates stimulate cholecystokinin release in STC-1 cells. *Food Chemistry* 111:970–975.

Elias, R. J., S. S. Kellerby, and E. A. Decker. 2008. Antioxidant activity of proteins and peptides. *Critical Reviews in Food Science and Nutrition* 48:430–441.

Fleurence, J. 1999. Seaweed proteins: biochemical, nutritional aspects and potential uses. *Trends in Food Science and Technology* 10:25–28.

Gómez-Guillén, M. C., J. Turnay, M. D. Fernández-Díaz, N. Ulmo, M. A. Lizarbe, and P. Montero. 2002. Structural and physical properties of gelatin extracted from different marine species: A comparative study. *Food Hydrocolloids* 16:25–34.

Hettiarachchy, N. S., K. C. Glenn, R. Gnanasambandan, and M. G. Johnson. 1996. Natural antioxidant extract from fenugreek (*Trigonella foenumgraecum*) for ground beef patties. *Journal of Food Science* 61:516–519.

Hsu, K. C., E. C. Y. Li-Chan, and C. L. Jao. 2011. Antiproliferative activity of peptides prepared from enzymatic hydrolysates of tuna dark muscle on human breast cancer cell line MCF-7. *Food Chemistry* 126:617–622.

Jo, H. Y., W. K. Jung, and S. K. Kim. 2008. Purification and characterization of a novel anticoagulant peptide from marine echiuroid worm, *Urechis unicinctus*. *Process Biochemistry* 43:179–184.

Jung, W. K., R. Karawita, S. J. Heo, B. J. Lee, S. K. Kim, and Y. J. Jeon. 2006. Recovery of a novel Ca-binding peptide from Alaska pollack (*Theragra chalcogramma*) backbone by pepsinolytic hydrolysis. *Process Biochemistry* 41:2097–2100.

Jung, W. K. and S. K. Kim. 2007. Calcium-binding peptide derived from pepsinolytic hydrolysates of hoki (*Johnius belengerii*) frame. *European Food Research and Technology* 224:763–767.

Jung, W. K., P. J. Park, and S. K. Kim. 2003. Purification and characterization of a new lectin from the hard roe of skipjack tuna, *Katsuwonus pelamis*. *International Journal of Biochemistry and Cell Biology* 35:255–265.

Kannan, A., N. S Hettiarachchy, M. Marshall, S. Raghavan, and H. Kristinsson. 2011. Shrimp shell peptide hydrolysates inhibit human cancer cell proliferation. *Journal of the Science of Food and Agriculture* 91:1920–1924.

Karim, A. A. and R. Bhat. 2009. Fish gelatin: properties, challenges, and prospects as an alternative to mammalian gelatins. *Food Hydrocolloids* 23:563–576.

Kim, S. Y., J. Y. Je, and S. K. Kim. 2007. Purification and characterization of antioxidant peptide from hoki (*Johnius belengeri*) frame protein by gastrointestinal digestion. *Journal of Nutritional Biochemistry* 18:31–38.

Kim, S. K. and E. Mendis. 2006. Bioactive compounds from marine processing byproducts—A review. *Food Research International* 39:383–393.

Kim, S. K., P. J. Park, H. G. Byun, J. Y. Je, S. H. Moon, and S. H. Kim. 2003. Recovery of fish bone from hoki (*Johnius belengeri*) frame using a proteolytic enzyme isolated from mackerel intestine. *Journal of Food Biochemistry* 27:255–266.

Kim, S. K., Y. D. Ravichandran, S. B. Khan, and Y. T. Kim. 2008. Prospective of the cosmeceuticals derived from marine organisms. *Biotechnology and Bioprocess Engineering* 13:511–523.

Kirk, O., T. V. Borchert, and C. C. Fuglsang. 2002. Industrial enzyme applications. *Current Opinion in Biotechnology* 13:345–351.

Larsen, R., K. E. Eilertsen, and E. O. Elvevoll. 2011. Health benefits of marine foods and ingredients. *Biotechnology Advances* 29:508–518.

Liu, Z., S. Dong, J. Xu, M. Zeng, H. Song, and Y. Zhao. 2008. Production of cysteine-rich antimicrobial peptide by digestion of oyster (*Crassostrea gigas*) with alcalase and bromelain. *Food Control* 19:231–235.

Lordan, S., R. P. Ross, and C. Stanton. 2011. Marine bioactives as functional food ingredients: potential to reduce the incidence of chronic diseases. *Marine Drugs* 9:1056–1100.

Mendis, E., N. Rajapakse, H. G. Byun, and S. K. Kim. 2005. Investigation of jumbo squid (*Dosidicus gigas*) skin gelatin peptides for their in vitro antioxidant effects. *Life Sciences* 77:2166–2178.

Molchanova, V., I. Chikalovets, O. Chernikov, N. Belogortseva, W. Li, J. H. Wang, D. Y. O. Yang, Y. T. Zheng, and P. Lukyanov. 2007. A new lectin from the sea worm *Serpula vermicularis*: Isolation, characterization and anti-HIV activity. *Comparative Biochemistry and Physiology, Part C* 145:184–193.

Naqash, S. Y. and R. A. Nazeer. 2011. In vitro antioxidant and antiproliferative activities of bioactive peptide isolated from *Nemipterus japonicus* backbone. *International Journal of Food Properties* 15(6):1200–1211.

Park, P. J., W. K. Jung, K. D. Nam, F. Shahidi, and S. K. Kim. 2001. Purification and characterization of antioxidative peptides from protein hydrolysate of lecithin-free egg yolk. *Journal of American Oil Chemists Society* 78:651–656.

Rajanbabu, V. and J. Y. Chen. 2011. Antiviral function of tilapia hepcidin 1–5 and its modulation of immune-related gene expressions against infectious pancreatic necrosis virus (IPNV) in Chinook salmon embryo (CHSE)-214 cells. *Fish and Shellfish Immunology* 30:39–44.

Rajapakse, N., W. K. Jung, E. Mendis, S. H. Moon, and S. K. Kim. 2005. A novel anticoagulant purified from fish protein hydrolysate inhibits factor XIIa and platelet aggregation. *Life Sciences* 76:2607–2619.

Senaratne, L. S., P. J. Park, and S. K. Kim. 2006. Isolation and characterization of collagen from brown backed toadfish (*Lagocephalus gloveri*) skin. *Bioresource Technology* 97:191–197.

Sheih, I. C., T. J. Fang, and T. K. Wu. 2009. Isolation and characterization of a novel angiotensin I-converting enzyme (ACE) inhibitory peptide from the algae protein waste. *Food Chemistry* 115:279–284.

Wang, J. H., J. Kong, W. Li, V. Molchanova, I. Chikalovets, N. Belogortseva, P. Luck'yanov, and Y. T. Zeng. 2006. A β-galactose-specific lectin isolated from the marine worm *Chaetopterus variopedatus* possesses anti-HIV-1 activity. *Comparative Biochemistry and Physiology C* 142:111–117.

Wergedahl, H., B. Liaset, O. A. Gudbrandsen, E. Lied, M. Espe, Z. Muna, S. Mork, and R. F. Berge. 2004. Fish protein hydrolysate reduces plasma total cholesterol, increases the proportion of HDL cholesterol, and lowers Acyl-CoA:cholesterol acyltransferase activity in liver of Zucker rats. *Journal of Nutrition* 134:1320–1327.

38

Marine Polysaccharide (Chitosan) and Its Derivatives as Water Purifier

Y. Dominic Ravichandran and R. Rajesh

CONTENTS

38.1 Introduction

Water is one of the essential components of nature, frequently polluted by agricultural, industrial, and man-made activities. The exponential growth of population and industrial development has made potable water a rare commodity (Szygu et al. 2009). Chitosan, a biopolymer, is an aminopolysaccharide composed of glucosamine, 2-amino-2-deoxy-β-D-glucose. It is prepared by alkaline deacetylation of chitin, a biopolymer extracted from shell fish sources. Chitosan exhibits a variety of physicochemical and biological properties, which could be used in the fields of biotechnology, agriculture, textile, biomedical engineering, food processing, pharmaceuticals, and ophthalmology. It is a weak cationic base insoluble in water and organic solvent but soluble in aqueous acidic solution with many amine ($-NH_2$) and hydroxyl ($-OH$) groups and acts as a chelate to form complex with metal ion (Zeng et al. 2008, Bina et al. 2009, Renault et al. 2009). The nature of the pollutants present in the water and wastewater depends on the source generation that varies from place to place (Bhatnagar and Sillanpa 2009). Chitosan has been widely used for water treatment to remove the pollutants. It is a well-known biosorbent for metal cations; the reactive amino group binds with metal ion to remove the metal present in the water by ion exchange. Several methods have been used to modify the natural chitosan in order to improve the adsorption capacity (Miretzky and Cirelli 2009). Water treatment plants face many problems when removing turbidity from raw untreated water to produce drinking water. Inorganic coagulants such as aluminum sulfate (alum) and polyaluminum chloride have been widely used for the removal of raw water turbidity because it is cost-effective and easy to handle. However, the sludge obtained from those treatment leads to disposal problems and contains higher aluminum in treated water. Cationic polyelectrolytes have been used as effective coagulants or flocculants in which chitosan, a biodegradable, nontoxic, and high-molecular-weight polymer, has also been used as an eco-friendly coagulant and flocculant (Chatterjee et al. 2009).

Dye used in textile, food, plastic, and pharmaceutical industry generates the colored impurities in water. Moreover, synthetic dyes are toxic and carcinogenic and decrease the photosynthesis, which in turn disturbs the aquatic ecosystem. Chitosan-based composite biosorbent is found to remove the dyes in an effective manner (Copello et al. 2011). Fluoride is another important parameter in water for dental health; the higher concentration of fluoride causes dental and skeletal fluorosis. Removal of fluorine can be done by various methods including ion exchange, electrochemical, and coagulation, but all these processes are expensive. Chitosan prepared in several shapes, gel beads, microspheres, and nanoparticles is also used to remove the fluorine (Miretzky and Cirelli 2011). Higher concentration of nitrate present in ground and surface water leads to blue baby diseases, which can be avoided by using treated water by sorption on protonated cross-linked chitosan gel beads (Jaafari et al. 2004).

38.2 Physicochemical Characteristics of Chitosan

Chitosan is obtained by partial or total deacetylation of chitin, which in turn depends upon the isolation of chitin from raw material and experimental procedure. The degree of deacetylation makes chitosan different from chitin and their solubility in dilute acidic solution. Forty percent deacetylation makes chitosan soluble in dilute acidic solution. Even though the polymer backbone of chitosan consists of hydrophilic functional group, it is insoluble in water at near-neutral pH and most of the organic solvent. The crystalline nature of chitosan is due to the intermolecular and intramolecular hydrogen bonding between the chains and sheets, respectively. The mechanical and chemical properties of chitosan can be modified by physical or chemical process. The efficiency of the adsorbent mainly depends upon the physicochemical properties including porosity, particle size of adsorbents, and surface area. The adsorption of heavy metal ions by chitosan is due to the presence of the following properties:

- High hydrophilicity due to presence of large number of hydroxyl groups of glucose units
- Presence of a large number of functional groups including hydroxyl group, primary amino group, and acetamido group, which have high chemical reactivity
- Flexible structure of polymer chains

The chemical modification of chitosan does not change the skeleton of chitosan but shows new or improved properties (Miretzky and Cirelli 2009, 2011).

38.2.1 Chitosan as Natural Flocculants or Coagulant

Alum is one of the widely used coagulants in water and wastewater treatment. The sludge produced by this method is difficult to dehydrate; its efficiency depends upon the pH. The other disadvantages of using higher concentration of aluminum are the health hazards. Chitosan possesses characteristics of both coagulant and flocculant nature, i.e., high cationic charge density, long polymer chains, bridging of aggregates, and precipitation. The major advantages of using chitosan as coagulant/flocculant include its nontoxic nature biodegradability, high settling speed of flocs, and chelating behavior. The physicochemical properties to interact with various contaminants including inorganic, organic suspensions, and dissolved organic substances make it unique. The sludge produced by chitosan as coagulant is of high density and can facilitate its drying compared to sludge produced with metal salts and is degradable by microorganisms, which make them environment friendly. The organic matter released during coagulation step increases the disinfection property (Rizzo et al. 2008). The modified water-soluble chitosan has been prepared and used for coagulation and flocculation process, which shows more effectiveness than commercial one (Reyna et al. 2010). It has been used for coagulation of bentonite suspension in which maximum coagulation was achieved at 5 mg/L chitosan concentration. Coagulation of bentonite by chitosan was pH sensitive, and at acidic pH, coagulation takes place effectively (Chatterjee et al. 2009). The disadvantages are its pH-dependent and heterogeneous properties (Renault et al. 2009).

38.2.2 Separation of Water from Alcohol Mixture

Pervaporation is an attractive conventional method for the separation of water from aqueous alcohol mixture. This technique works on the selective permeation of membrane producing permeate stream enriched in the preferentially permeating species (Feng and Huang 1996). The modified chitosan membrane has also been used to separate water from alcohol mixture. Some of them are carboxymethyl chitosan, acetic acid complex chitosan, sulfonated chitosan, amidoxime chitosan, polyacronitrile chitosan, and phosphorylated chitosan membrane (Lee et al. 1997).The advantages of modified chitosan are that it is easy to separate chitosan from the azeotropic mixtures and it is less costly (Wang et al. 1996). Currently, there are several membranes to separate water, and one of them is chitosan N-methylol nylon six blend membrane for the separation of water–ethanol mixture. The permselectivity of this blend membrane was improved by acid treatment. The salting-out effect of ionized group in the chitosan matrix excludes organic solvents and decreased the permeability of ethanol while retaining the total permeability of water (Shieh and Huang 1998).

38.2.3 Recoveries of Protein from Surimi Wash Water

Protein flocculation is one of the techniques used for the removal of surimi from the wash water. Complexation of chitosan with pectin, carrageenan, or alginate yielded coagulating agent with improved protein adsorption and reduction of turbidity compared to free chitosan Chitosan–alginate complex is used to recover soluble proteins from surimi wash water at slightly acidic pH of 6. The electrostatic interaction between amino group and anionic group of chitosan was found to be the reason for this behavior (Wibowo et al. 2005). This process not only resulted in the decreased turbidity in the surimi wash water but effectively recovered the soluble protein that would otherwise be discarded in the environment as waste (Wibowo et al. 2007).

38.2.4 Removal of Dyes

Water pollution due to dyes present in the effluents of textile, leather, paper, and dye manufacturing industry is one of the major environmental concerns. The dyes used not only pollute the water but also reduce the productivity of the soil by their toxic nature. This colored dye effluents are considered to be toxic to the aquatic biota and affect the symbiotic process by disturbing the natural equilibrium through reduced photosynthetic activity. Some of the dyes also cause allergy, skin irritation, and cancer in humans. Thus the removal of dyes from water has become inevitable, and use of chitosan-based biosorbent is one of the methods of removal (Bhatnagar and Sillanpa 2009).

The removal of dyes including acid yellow 73 (Iqbal et al. 2011), acid green 25 (Wong et al. 2003, Mahmoodi et al. 2011), acid orange 10 and 12 (Wong et al. 2003, Zhou et al. 2011), acid red 18, 37, and 73, (Wong et al. 2003, Kamari et al. 2009, Shen et al. 2010), acid blue 25 (Kamari et al. 2009), food dye acid blue 9, food yellow 3 (Dotto and Pinto 2011), methylene blue (Wang et al. 2010, Chatterjee et al. 2011a), and disodium 6-hydroxy-5-((2-methoxy-5-methyl-4-sulfophenyl)azo)-2-naphthalenesulfonate (Piccin et al. 2011) using chitosan as powder, flakes, beads, and hydrogels has already been reported and summarized in the Tables 38.1 and 38.2.

38.2.5 Removal of Phenol

Phenol is one of the environmental water pollutants generated mainly from industries such as paper, plastic, metals, pharmaceuticals, and resin. Because of their toxicity, it has to be removed from water in order to maintain the ecological balance. Many synthetic resin, low-cost natural adsorbents, and microbiological water treatment are used for the removal of phenol. However, the water-soluble phenol is not satisfactorily removed from water by the aforesaid methods. The chitosan-conjugated thermoresponsive polymers have also been used to remove the phenol in water. One of the examples is the polymer prepared by condensation of chitosan with poly(*N*-isopropylacrylamide-co-acrylic acid) [PNIPPAm-AA] mediated through water-soluble imide 1-ethyl-3-(3-dimethylaminopropyl) carbodimide hydrochloride. Phenol is removed from water by tyrosine-induced oxidation in which phenol is converted to catechol and subsequently oxidized to o-quinone. The o-quinone molecules react with themselves to form dark brown oligomers, which can bind with amino moiety of chitosan to form Schiff bases or Michael-type adducts and thus get separated from water on filtration (Saitoh et al. 2009, 2011).

38.2.6 Removal of Fluoride

Fluoride is an essential element in water for dental health. The concentration of fluoride in drinking water should not exceed 1.5 mg/L. There are several methods to remove excessive fluoride from drinking water. Among them, absorption using chitosan derivatives seems to be effective, economical, and environment friendly. Fluoride ion is more electronegative and small in ionic size; because of these properties, it can possess strong affinity toward transition and rare earth metals. It is also well known that N in the NH_2 group of chitosan can act as electron donor and form chelates with metal ions. The N in the NH_2 group of chitosan can act as electron donor and form chelated complexes with metal ions, and the OH^- group can complete the coordination shells of the metals. Depending upon the pH, the OH^- groups can be protonated and adsorb F^- ions through exchange mechanism (Miretzky et al. 2011).

TABLE 38.1

Removal of Dyes Using Chitosan

Adsorbent	Adsorbate	Adsorption Capacity (mg/g)	pH	Isotherm	References
Chitosan	Acid green 25	645.1	—	Langmuir	Wong et al. (2003)
Chitosan	Acid green 25	178.0	2.0	Tempkin	Mahmoodi et al. (2011)
Chitosan	Acid orange 10	922.9	—	Langmuir	Wong et al. (2003)
Chitosan	Acid orange 12	973.3	—	Langmuir	Wong et al. (2003)
Chitosan	Acid red 18	693.2	—	Langmuir	Wong et al. (2003)
Chitosan	Acid red 73	728.2	—	Langmuir	Wong et al. (2003)
Chitosan	Direct red 23	155.0	2.0	Tempkin	Mahmoodi et al. (2011)
Chitosan	Food dye acid blue 9	226.0	3.0	Elovich	Dotto and Pinto (2011)
Chitosan	Food yellow 3	352.6	3.0	Elovich	Dotto and Pinto (2011)
Chitosan	Disodium 6-hydroxy-5-((2-methoxy-5-methyl-4-sulfophenyl) azo)-2-naphthalenesulfonate	300.0	5.7	Elovich	Piccin et al. (2011)
Chitosan beads	Acid red 37	128.2	6.0	Langmuir	Kamari et al. (2009)
Chitosan beads	Acid red 37	357.1	6.0	Langmuir	Kamari et al. (2009a)
Chitosan beads	Acid blue 25	263.1	4.0	Langmuir	Kamari et al. (2009)
Chitosan beads	Acid blue 25	178.5	4.0	Langmuir	Kamari et al. (2009a)
Chitosan hydrogel beads	Methylene blue	226.2	—	Sips	Chatterjee et al. (2011)
Chitosan flakes	Acid yellow 73	—	3.0	Langmuir and Freundlich	Iqbal et al. (2011)

Magnesia (MgO) is a well-known absorbent against fluoride. The adsorption of MgO can be improved by the preparation of composite with chitosan. The chitosan-modified MgO acts as efficient defluorinating agent when compared with MgO alone (Sundaram et al. 2009). Like chitosan-modified MgO, some of the metals bind with chitosan such as titanium–aluminum binary metal oxide supported beads of chitosan (Thakre et al. 2010), lanthanum-incorporated chitosan (Kamble et al. 2007, Thakre et al. 2010a, Jagtap et al. 2011), and neodymium-modified chitosan (Yao et al. 2009) and were used for defluoridation. From the brackish underground water, fluoride can be removed by chitosan. However, the efficiency of this support in salt water is very weak. Electrodialysis method for salt water to remove fluoride is more effective but is costly. The combination

TABLE 38.2

Removal of Dyes Using Chitosan Derivatives

Adsorbent	Adsorbate	Adsorption Capacity (mg/g)	pH	Isotherm	References
Chitosan grafted acrylamide	Remazol yellow gelb 3RS	1211.0	2.0	Langmuir–Freundlich	Kyzas and Lazaridis (2009)
Chitosan grafted acrylic acid	Basic yellow 37	595.0	10.0	Langmuir–Freundlich	Kyzas and Lazaridis (2009)
Chitosan grafted poly(methyl methacrylate)	Procion yellow MX	250.0	7.0	Langmuir and Freundlich	Singh et al. (2009)
Chitosan grafted poly(methyl methacrylate)	Remazol brilliant violet	357.0	7.0	Langmuir and Freundlich	Singh et al. (2009)
Chitosan grafted poly(methyl methacrylate)	Reactive blue H5G	178.0	7.0	Langmuir and Freundlich	Singh et al. (2009)
Chitosan hydrogel beads (by alkali) grafted polyethyleneimine	Reactive black 5	709.3	6.0	Langmuir	Chatterjee et al. (2011b)
Chitosan hydrogel beads (by sodium dodecyl sulfate) grafted polyethyleneimine	Reactive black 5	413.2	6.0	Langmuir	Chatterjee et al. (2011b)
Chitosan–glutaraldehyde beads	Acid blue 25	127.0	4.0	Langmuir	Kamari et al. (2009)
Chitosan–glutaraldehyde beads	Acid red 37	166.7	6.0	Langmuir	Kamari et al. (2009)
Chitosan–sulfuric acid beads	Acid blue 25	102.5	4.0	Langmuir	Kamari et al. (2009)
Chitosan–sulfuric acid beads	Acid red 37	139.3	6.0	Langmuir	Kamari et al. (2009)
Chitosan cross-linked with ethylenediamine	Eosin Y	294.1	5.0	Langmuir	Huang et al. (2011)
Tetraethylenepentamine-modified chitosan	Eosin Y	292.4	5.0	Langmuir	Huang et al. (2011a)
Chitosan–ethylene glycol diglycidyl ether beads	Acid red 37	59.5	6.0	Langmuir	Kamari et al. (2009)
Chitosan–ethylene glycol diglycidyl ether beads	Acid blue 25	142.8	4.0	Langmuir	Kamari et al. (2009)
Ethylenediamine-modified magnetic chitosan nanoparticles	Acid orange 7	1215.0	4.0	Langmuir	Zhou et al. (2011)
Ethylenediamine-modified magnetic chitosan nanoparticles	Acid orange 10	1017.0	3.0	Langmuir	Zhou et al. (2011)
Chitosan with 4-formyl-1,3-benzene sodium disulfonate	Basic blue 3	166.5	3.0	Langmuir	Crini et al. (2008)

TABLE 38.2 (continued)

Removal of Dyes Using Chitosan Derivatives

Adsorbent	Adsorbate	Adsorption Capacity (mg/g)	pH	Isotherm	References
N-benzyl disulfonate derivatives of chitosan	Basic blue 9	121.9	3.0	—	Crini et al. (2008a)
N,O-carboxymethyl-chitosan	Methylene blue	349.0	8.0	Langmuir	Wang et al. (2010)
γ-Fe_2O_3-SiO_2-chitosan composite	Methyl orange	34.3	2.9	Freundlich	Zhu et al. (2011)
β-cyclodextrin–chitosan modified Fe_3O_4 nanoparticles	Methyl blue	2780.0	5.0	Langmuir	Fan et al. (2012)
Chitosan coated on magnetite (Fe_3O_4)	Alizarin red	40.12	3.0	Langmuir	Fan et al. (2012a)

of both these methods removes fluoride from brackish groundwater effectively and economically (Sahlia et al. 2007). Chemically modified and protonated chitosan beads for the removal of fluoride from water are reviewed and given in Table 38.3 (Viswanathan et al. 2009).

38.2.7 Removal of Metal Ions

Activated carbon has been used as a sorbent to remove the metal ions from water. However, the use of activated carbon is expensive, so there is an increasing interest to prepare other adsorbent material with low cost. Chitosan is an excellent biosorbent to remove metal cation from water at neutral pH. Several methods are used to modify the natural biopolymer chitosan either by physical or chemical methods to improve the adsorption capacity of chitosan (Miretzky and Cirelli 2009). Some of the metal ions removed by chitosan and chitosan derivates are shown in Tables 38.4 through 38.10.

38.2.8 Removal of Nitrate

Groundwater or surface water resource all over the globe is heavily contaminated by nitrate ion. The high concentration of nitrate in drinking water is undesirable and causes blue baby syndrome due to the conversions of hemoglobin in to methemoglobin, inhibiting the oxygen transport. The conventional methods used for denitrification are biological denitrification and ion exchange process. In biological denitrification process, the use of carbonaceous substrate makes it cumbersome and expensive. Moreover, it is effective only at low temperature, i.e., below 7°C. In ion exchange resin process, the chloride ion concentration in water is increased. Electrodialysis or reverse osmosis to remove the nitrate is not a usual method because of the cost involved. Protonated gel beads of chitosan effectively remove the nitrate from groundwater and are cheaper. The sorption capacity of the chitosan beads depend upon the pH, and in the pH range of 3–5, it is more efficient, whereas the efficiency is reduced as the pH is 2 or less. This may be due to the breakage of chitosan beads (Jaafari et al. 2004).

TABLE 38.3

Removal of Fluoride Using Chitosan and Its Derivatives

Adsorbent	Adsorption Capacity (mg/g)	pH	Isotherm	References
Chitosan-based mesoporous Ti–Al binary metal oxide beads	2.22	3.0–9.0	Langmuir	Thakre et al. (2010)
Neodymium-modified chitosan	22.38	7.0	Langmuir	Yao et al. (2009)
Lanthanum-incorporated chitosan beads	4.70	5.0	Langmuir	Bansiwal et al. (2009)
Lanthanum-impregnated chitosan beads	1.27	6.7	Freundlich	Jagtap et al. (2011)
La(III)-incorporated carboxylated chitosan beads	11.95	7.0	Langmuir, Freundlich	Viswanathan and Meenakshi (2008a)
Magnetic chitosan	22.49	7.0	Langmuir and Bradley's	Ma et al. (2007)
Fe(III)-loaded carboxylated chitosan beads	15.38	7.0	Langmuir, Freundlich	Viswanathan and Meenakshi (2008b)
Glutaraldehyde-cross-linked protonated chitosan beads	7.32	7.0	Langmuir, Freundlich	Viswanathan et al. (2009a)
Carboxylated cross-linked chitosan beads	11.11	7.0	Langmuir, Freundlich	Viswanathan et al. (2009b)
MgO–chitosan composite	11.23	3.0–11.0	Langmuir, Freundlich	Sundaram et al. (2009)
Nanohydroxyapatite–chitosan	2.04	3.0	Langmuir, Freundlich	Sundaram et al. (2008)
Aluminum–chitosan composite	10.42	7.0	Langmuir, Freundlich	Viswanathan and Meenakshi (2010a)
Zr(IV)-entrapped carboxylated chitosan beads	13.69	7.0	Freundlich, Langmuir and Dubinin–Radushkevich	Viswanathan and Meenakshi (2009a)
Chitosan-supported zirconium(IV) tungstophosphate composite	7.63	3.0	Langmuir, Freundlich	Viswanathan and Meenakshi (2010b)
Neodymium-modified chitosan	22.38	7.0	Langmuir	Yao et al. (2009)
Cerium (III)-encapsulated carboxylated chitosan beads	9.00	7.0	Langmuir, Freundlich	Viswanathan and Meenakshi (2009b)

TABLE 38.4

Removal of Cadmium (II)

Adsorbent	Adsorption Capacity (mg/g)	pH	Isotherm	References
Xanthated chitosan	357.14	8.0	Langmuir	Sankararamakrishnan et al. (2007)
Thiocarbamoyl chitosan flakes	666.70	7.5	Langmuir	Chauhan et al. (2012)
Chitosan–graft-γ-cyclodextrin	833.33	8.5	Langmuir	Mishra and Sharma (2011)
Chitosan–cellulose acetate blend membrane	17.88	8.0	Langmuir	Zhang et al. (2011)
5,10,15,20-Tetrakis (1-methyl-4-pyridinio) porphyrin tetra (p-toluenesulfonate) immobilized chitosan–cellulose acetate blend membrane	43.77	8.0	Langmuir	Zhang et al. (2011)
Procion Brown MX 5BR immobilized poly(hydroxyethylmethacrylate–chitosan) composite membranes	18.50	5.0	—	Genc et al. (2002)
Chitosan hydrogel beads	61.35	6.3	Freundlich	Beigi et al. (2009)

TABLE 38.5

Removal of Nickel (II)

Adsorbent	Adsorption Capacity (mg/g)	pH	Isotherm	References
Reactive blue 2 dye immobilized chitosan	11.20	8.5	Langmuir	Vasconcelos et al. (2007)
Chitosan-grafted acrylonitrile	358.54	5.5	Langmuir	Ramya et al. (2011)
Chitosan-grafted-poly(2-amino-4,5-pentamethylene-thiophene-3-carboxylic acid N′-acryloyl-hydrazide) chelating resin	49.40	6.0	Langmuir	Bekheit et al. (2011)
Chitosan/magnetite nanocomposite beads	52.55	6.0	Langmuir	Tran et al. (2010)
Chitosan-coated polyvinyl chloride beads	120.50	5.0	Langmuir and Freundlich	Popuri et al. (2009)

TABLE 38.6

Removal of Chromium (VI)

Adsorbent	Adsorption Capacity (mg/g)	pH	Isotherm	References
Chitosan	166.00	4.0	Langmuir-Freundlich	Kyzas et al. (2009a)
Fe-cross-linked chitosan	295.00	4.8	Langmuir–Freundlich	Zimmermann et al. (2010)
Chitosan-grafted poly(acrylamide)	935.00	4.0	Langmuir-Freundlich	Kyzas et al. (2009a)
Chitosan-grafted poly(acrylic acid)	518.00	4.0	Langmuir-Freundlich	Kyzas et al. (2009a)
Chitosan-grafted polyacrylonitrile	218.82	5.5	Langmuir	Shanmugapriya et al. (2011)
Glutaraldehyde-cross-linked grafted chitosan beads	4057.00	4.0	Langmuir	Kousalya et al. (2010)
Glutaraldehyde-cross-linked protonated chitosan beads	3239.00	4.0	Langmuir	Kousalya et al. (2010)
Glutaraldehyde-cross-linked carboxylated chitosan beads	3647.00	4.0	Langmuir	Kousalya et al. (2010)
Glutaraldehyde-cross-linked chitosan-xanthated beads	256.40	3.3	Langmuir	Sankararamakrishnan et al. (2006)
Glutaraldehyde-cross-linked chitosan-xanthated flakes	625.00	3.0	Langmuir	Sankararamakrishnan et al. (2006)
Xanthated chitosan column	202.25	3.0	—	Chauhan and Sankararamakrishnan (2011)
Thiocarbamoyl chitosan flakes	434.80	2.0	Langmuir	Chauhan et al. (2012)
Chitosan coated with poly 3-methylthiophene	127.62	2.0	Langmuir	Hena (2010)
Alumina–chitosan composite	8.62	4.0	Dubinin–Radushkevich	Gandhi et al. (2010)

TABLE 38.7

Removal of Copper (II)

Adsorbent	Adsorption Capacity (mg/g)	pH	Isotherm	References
Chitosan beads	80.71	6.0	Langmuir	Ngah et al. (2002)
Chitosan cross-linked with glutaraldehyde beads	59.67	6.0	Langmuir	Ngah et al. (2002)
Chitosan cross-linked with epichlorohydrin beads	62.47	6.0	Langmuir	Ngah et al. (2002)
Chitosan-grafted acrylonitrile	230.79	5.0	Langmuir	Ramya et al. (2011)
Epichlorohydrin-cross-linked chitosan	35.46	6.0	Langmuir	Chen et al. (2008a)
Epichlorohydrin-cross-linked xanthate chitosan	43.47	5.0	Langmuir	Kannamba et al. (2010)
Chitosan cross-linked with ethylene glycol diglycidyl ether beads	45.94	6.0	Langmuir	Ngah et al. (2002)
Carboxylated chitosan-bound Fe3O4 magnetic nanoparticles	21.50	5.0	Langmuir	Chang and Chen (2005)
Chitosan-grafted poly(2-amino-4,5-pentamethylene-thiophene-3-carboxylic acid N′-acryloyl-hydrazide) chelating resin	137.64	6.0	Langmuir	Bekheit et al. (2011)
Chitosan-grafted polyacrylonitrile	239.31	7.0	Langmuir	Shanmugapriya et al. (2011)
Reactive blue 2 dye immobilized chitosan	57.00	7.0	Langmuir	Vasconcelos et al. (2007)
Chitosan-grafted polyacrylonitrile	239.31	7.0	Langmuir	Shanmugapriya et al. (2011)
Chitosan-grafted poly(acrylamide)	166.00	6.0	Langmuir-Freundlich	Kyzas et al. (2009a)
Chitosan-grafted poly(acrylic acid)	318.00	6.0	Langmuir-Freundlich	Kyzas et al. (2009a)
Chitosan	208.00	6.0	Langmuir-Freundlich	Kyzas et al. (2009a)
Chitosan-coated polyvinyl chloride beads	87.90	4.0	Langmuir and Freundlich	Popuri et al. (2009)

TABLE 38.8

Removal of Lead (II)

Adsorbent	Adsorption Capacity (mg/g)	pH	Isotherm	References
Chitosan	47.39	6.0	Langmuir	Asandei et al. (2009)
Chitosan–alginate beads	60.27	4.5	Langmuir	Ngah and Fatinathan (2010)
Glutaraldehyde-cross-linked chitosan-xanthated beads	322.60	4.0	Langmuir	Chauhan and Sankararamakrishnan (2008)
Epichlorohydrin-cross-linked chitosan	34.13	6.0	Langmuir	Chen et al. (2008a)
Chitosan/magnetite nanocomposite beads	63.33	6.0	Langmuir	Tran et al. (2010)
Pb(II)-imprinted chitosan biosorbent using diatomite as core material	139.60	7.0	Langmuir	Jiang et al. (2010)
Chitosan/TiO2 hybrid film	36.80	3.0	Freundlich	Tao et al. (2009)
Chitosan beads	34.98	4.5	Langmuir and Freundlich	Ngah and Fatinathan (2010)
Chitosan–glutaraldehyde beads	14.24	4.5	Langmuir and Freundlich	Ngah and Fatinathan (2010)
Procion Brown MX 5BR immobilized poly(hydroxyethylmethacrylate–chitosan) composite membranes	22.70	5.0	—	Genc et al. (2002)

TABLE 38.9

Removal of Arsenic

Adsorbent	Adsorbate	Adsorption Capacity (mg/g)	pH	Isotherm	References
Chitosan nanospheres	As (V)	270	5.2	Langmuir	Singh et al. (2011)
As(III)-loaded α-Fe$_2$O$_3$-chitosan composite	As (III)	6.18	5.0	Langmuir	Liu et al. (2011)
Iron-impregnated chitosan beads	As (III)	6.48	8.0	Freundlich	Gang et al. (2010)
Molybdate-impregnated chitosan beads column	As (III)	1.98	5.0	—	Chen et al. (2008)
Molybdate-impregnated chitosan beads column	As (V)	2.00	5.0	—	Chen et al. (2008)
3,4-Diamino benzoic acid functionalized chitosan	As (V)	82.00	3.0	—	Sabarudin et al. (2005)

38.3 Conclusion

In recent times, there is an increasing interest in the development of marine polysaccharides for various applications including water treatment because of its availability and low cost. The high reactivity against water pollutants has made them a potential candidate for

TABLE 38.10

Removal of Other Metal Ions

Adsorbent	Adsorbate	Adsorption Capacity (mg/g)	pH	Isotherm	References
Procion Brown MX 5BR immobilized poly(hydroxyethylmethacrylate–chitosan) composite membranes	Hg(II)	68.80	5.0	—	Genc et al. (2002)
Chitosan–montmorillonite composites	Se(VI)	18.40	—	Langmuir	Bleiman and Mishael (2010)
3,4-Diamino benzoic acid functionalized chitosan	Se(IV)	64.00	3.0	—	Sabarudin et al. (2005)
3,4-Diamino benzoic acid functionalized chitosan	Se(VI)	88.00	2.0 and 3.0	—	Sabarudin et al. (2005)
Chitosan-grafted poly(2-amino-4,5-pentamethylene-thiophene-3-carboxylic acid N′-acryloyl-hydrazide) chelating resin	Co(II)	102.51	6.0	Langmuir	Bekheit et al. (2011)
Epichlorohydrin-cross-linked chitosan	Zn(II)	10.21	6.0	Langmuir	Chen et al. (2008)

the water treatment. The modification of chitosan to its derivatives has shown that the marine polysaccharide chitosan can be tailor-made to any requirement. The multidimensional usage of chitosan and its derivative as water purifier has been well established and reviewed in this chapter.

References

Asandei, D., L. Bulgariu, and E. Bobu. 2009. Lead (II) removal from aqueous solutions by adsorption onto chitosan. *Cellulose Chemistry and Technology* 43:211–216.

Bansiwal, A., D. Thakre, N. Labhshetwar, S. Meshram, and S. Rayalu. 2009. Fluoride removal using lanthanum incorporated chitosan beads. *Colloids and Surfaces B: Biointerfaces* 74:216–224.

Beigi, M. S., V. Maghsoodi, S. M. Mousavi, and N. Rajabi. 2009. Batch equilibrium and kinetics studies of Cd (ii) ion removal from aqueous solution using porous chitosan hydrogel beads. *Iranian Journal of Chemistry and Chemical Engineering* 28:81–89.

Bekheit, M. M., N. Nawar, A. W. Addison, D. A. A. Latif, and M. Monier. 2011. Preparation and characterization of chitosan-grafted-poly(2-amino-4,5-pentamethylene-thiophene-3-carboxylic acid N′-acryloyl-hydrazide) chelating resin for removal of Cu(II), Co(II) and Ni(II) metal ions from aqueous solutions. *International Journal of Biological Macromolecules* 48:558–565.

Bhatnagar, A. and M. Sillanpa. 2009. Applications of chitin- and chitosan-derivatives for the detoxification of water and wastewater—A short review. *Advances in Colloid and Interface Science* 152:26–38.

Bina, B., M. H. Mehdinejad, M. Nikaeen, and H. M. Attar. 2009. Effectiveness of chitosan as natural coagulant aid in treating turbid waters. *Iranian Journal of Environmental Health, Science and Engineering* 6:247–252.

Bleiman, N. and Y. G. Mishael. 2010. Selenium removal from drinking water by adsorption to chitosan-clay composites and oxides: Batch and column tests. *Journal of Hazardous Materials* 183:590–595.

Chang, Y. C. and D. H. Chen, 2005. Preparation and adsorption properties of monodisperse chitosan-bound Fe_3O_4 magnetic nanoparticles for removal of Cu(II) ions. *Journal of Colloid and Interface Science* 283:446–451.

Chatterjee, S., T. Chatterjee, and S. R. Lim. 2011a. Adsorption of a cationic dye, methylene blue, on to chitosan hydrogel beads generated by anionic surfactant gelation. *Environmental Technology* 32:1503–1514.

Chatterjee, T., S. Chatterjee, and S. H. Woo. 2009. Enhanced coagulation of bentonite particles in water by a modified chitosan biopolymer. *Chemical Engineering Journal* 148:414–419.

Chatterjee, S., T. Chatterjee, and S. H. Woo. 2011b. Influence of the polyethyleneimine grafting on the adsorption capacity of chitosan beads for reactive black 5 from aqueous solutions. *Chemical Engineering Journal* 166:168–175.

Chauhan, D., M. Jaiswal, and N. Sankararamakrishnan. 2012. Removal of cadmium and hexavalent chromium from electroplating waste water using thiocarbamoyl chitosan. *Carbohydrate Polymers* 88:670–675.

Chauhan, D. and N. Sankararamakrishnan. 2008. Highly enhanced adsorption for decontamination of lead ions from battery wastewaters using chitosan functionalized with xanthate. *Bioresource Technology* 99:9021–9024.

Chauhan, D. and N. Sankararamakrishnan. 2011. Modeling and evaluation on removal of hexavalent chromium from aqueous systems using fixed bed column. *Journal of Hazardous Materials* 185:55–62.

Chen, C. Y., T. H. Chang, J. T. Kuo, Y. F. Chen, and Y.C. Chung. 2008. Characteristics of molybdate-impregnated chitosan beads (MICB) in terms of arsenic removal from water and the application of a MICB-packed column to remove arsenic from wastewater. *Bioresource Technology* 99:7487–7494.

Chen, A. H., S. C. Liu, C. Y. Chen, and C. Y. Chen. 2008a. Comparative adsorption of Cu(II), Zn(II), and Pb(II) ions in aqueous solution on the crosslinked chitosan with epichlorohydrin. *Journal of Hazardous Materials* 154:184–191.

Copello, G. J., A. M. Mebert, M. Raineri, M. P. Pesenti, and L. E. Diaza. 2011. Removal of dyes from water using chitosan hydrogel/SiO_2 and chitin hydrogel/SiO_2 hybrid materials obtained by the sol–gel method. *Journal of Hazardous Materials* 186:932–939.

Crini, G., F. Gimbert, C. Robert, B. Martel, O. Adam, N. M. Crini, F. D. Giorgi, and P. M. Badot. 2008. The removal of Basic Blue 3 from aqueous solutions by chitosan-based adsorbent: Batch studies. *Journal of Hazardous Materials* 153:96–100.

Crini, G., B. Martel, and G. Torri. 2008a. Adsorption of C.I. Basic Blue 9 on chitosan-based materials. *International Journal of Environment and Pollution* 34:451–465.

Dotto, G. L. and L. A. A. Pinto. 2011. Adsorption of food dyes acid blue 9 and food yellow 3 onto chitosan: Stirring rate effect in kinetics and mechanism. *Journal of Hazardous Materials* 187:164–170.

Fan, L., Y. Zhang, X. Li, C. Luo, F. Lu, and H. Qiu. 2012a. Removal of alizarin red from water environment using magnetic chitosan with Alizarin Red as imprinted molecules. *Colloids and Surfaces B: Biointerfaces* 91:250–257.

Fan, L., Y. Zhang, C. Luo, F. Lu, H. Qiu, and M. Sun. 2012. Synthesis and characterization of magnetic β-cyclodextrin–chitosan nanoparticles as nano-adsorbents for removal of methyl blue. *International Journal of Biological Macromolecules* 50:444–450.

Feng, X. and R. Y. M. Huang. 1996. Pervaporation with chitosan membranes. I. Separation of water from ethylene glycol by a chitosan/polysulfone composite membrane. *Journal of Membrane Science* 116:67–76.

Gandhi, M. R., N. Viswanathan, and S. Meenakshi. 2010. Preparation and application of alumina/chitosan biocomposite. *International Journal of Biological Macromolecules* 47:146–154.

Gang, D.D., B. Deng, and L. S. Lin. 2010. As(III) removal using an iron-impregnated chitosan sorbent. *Journal of Hazardous Materials* 182:156–161.

Genc, O., C. Arpa, G. Bayramoglu, M. Y. Arica, and S. Bektas. 2002. Selective recovery of mercury by Procion Brown MX 5BR immobilized poly(hydroxyethylmethacrylate/chitosan) composite membranes. *Hydrometallurgy* 67:53–62.

Hena, S. 2010. Removal of chromium hexavalent ion from aqueous solutions using biopolymer chitosan coated with poly 3-methyl thiophene polymer. *Journal of Hazardous Materials* 181:474–479.

Huang, X.Y., J. P. Bin, H. T. Bu, G. B. Jiang, and M. H. Zeng. 2011. Removal of anionic dye eosin Y from aqueous solution using ethylenediamine modified chitosan. *Carbohydrate Polymers* 84:1350–1356.

Huang, X. Y., X. Y. Mao, H. T. Bu, X. Y. Yu, G. B. Jiang, and M. H. Zeng. 2011a. Chemical modification of chitosan by tetraethylenepentamine and adsorption study for anionic dye removal. *Carbohydrate Research* 346:1232–1240.

Iqbal, J., F. H. Wattoo, M. H. S. Wattoo, R. Malik, S. A. Tirmizi, M. Imran, and A. B. Ghangro. 2011. Adsorption of acid yellow dye on flakes of chitosan prepared from fishery wastes. *Arabian Journal of Chemistry* 4:389–395.

Jaafari, K., T. Ruiz, S. Elmaleh, J. Coma, and K. Benkhouja. 2004. Simulation of a fixed bed adsorber packed with protonated cross-linked chitosan gel beads to remove nitrate from contaminated water. *Chemical Engineering Journal* 99:153–160.

Jagtap, S., M. K. Yenkie, S. Das, and S. Rayalu. 2011. Synthesis and characterization of lanthanum impregnated chitosan flakes for fluoride removal in water. *Desalination* 273:267–275.

Jiang, W., H. Su, H. Huo, and T. Tan. 2010. Synthesis and properties of surface molecular imprinting adsorbent for removal of pb^{2+}. *Applied Biochemistry and Biotechnology*, 160:467–476.

Kamari, A., W. S. W. Ngah, M. Y. Chong, and M. L. Cheah. 2009a. Sorption of acid dyes onto GLA and H_2SO_4 cross-linked chitosan beads. *Desalination* 249:1180–1189.

Kamari, A., W. S. W. Ngah, and L. K. Liew. 2009. Chitosan and chemically modified chitosan beads for acid dyes sorption. *Journal of Environmental Sciences* 21:296–302.

Kamble, S. P., S. Jagtap, N. K. Labhsetwar, D. Thakare, S. Godfrey, S. Devotta, and S. S. Rayalu. 2007. Defluoridation of drinking water using chitin, chitosan and lanthanum-modified chitosan. *Chemical Engineering Journal* 129:173–180.

Kannamba, B., K. L. Reddy, and B. V. AppaRao. 2010. Removal of Cu(II) from aqueous solutions using chemically modified chitosan. *Journal of Hazardous Materials* 175:939–948.

Kousalya, G. N., M. R. Gandhi, and S. Meenakshi. 2010. Sorption of chromium(VI) using modified forms of chitosan beads. *International Journal of Biological Macromolecules* 47:308–315.

Kyzas, G. Z., M. Kostoglou, and N. K. Lazaridis. 2009a. Copper and chromium(VI) removal by chitosan derivatives-equilibrium and kinetic studies. *Chemical Engineering Journal* 152:440–448.

Kyzas, G. Z. and N. K. Lazaridis. 2009. Reactive and basic dyes removal by sorption onto chitosan derivatives. *Journal of Colloid and Interface Science* 331:32–39.

Lee, Y. M., S. Y. Nam, and D. J. Woo. 1997. Pervaporation of ionically surface crosslinked chitosan composite membranes for water-alcohol mixtures. *Journal of Membrane Science* 133:103–110.

Liu, B., D. Wang, H. Li, Y. Xu, and L. Zhang. 2011. As(III) removal from aqueous solution using α-Fe_2O_3 impregnated chitosan beads with As(III) as imprinted ions. *Desalination* 272:286–292.

Ma, W., F. Q. Ya, M. Han, and R.Wang. 2007. Characteristics of equilibrium, kinetics studies for adsorption of fluoride on magnetic-chitosan particle. *Journal of Hazardous Materials* 143:296–302.

Mahmoodi, N. M., R. Salehi, M. Arami, and H. Bahrami. 2011. Dye removal from colored textile wastewater using chitosan in binary systems. *Desalination* 267:64–72.

Miretzky, P. and A. F. Cirelli. 2009. Hg (II) removal from water by chitosan and chitosan derivatives: A review. *Journal of Hazardous Materials* 167:10–23.

Miretzky, P. and A. F. Cirelli. 2011. Fluoride removal from water by chitosan derivatives and composites: A review. *Journal of Fluorine Chemistry* 132:231–240.

Mishra, A. K. and A. K. Sharma. 2011. Synthesis of γ-cyclodextrin/chitosan composites for the efficient removal of Cd(II) from aqueous solution. *International Journal of Biological Macromolecules* 49:504–512.

Ngah, W. S. W., C. S. Endud, and R. Mayanar. 2002. Removal of copper(II) ions from aqueous solution onto chitosan and cross-linked chitosan beads. *Reactive and Functional Polymers* 50:181–190.

Ngah, W. S. W. and S. Fatinathan. 2010. Pb(II) biosorption using chitosan and chitosan derivatives beads: Equilibrium, ion exchange and mechanism studies. *Journal of Environmental Sciences* 22(3):338–346.

Piccin, J. S., G. L. Dotto, M. L. G. Vieira, and L. A. A. Pinto. 2011. Kinetics and mechanism of the food dye fd&c red 40 adsorption onto chitosan. *Journal of Chemical and Engineering Data* 56:3759–3765.

Popuri, S. R., Y. Vijaya, V. M. Boddu, and K. Abburi. 2009. Adsorptive removal of copper and nickel ions from water using chitosan coated PVC beads. *Bioresource Technology* 100:194–199.

Ramya, R., P. Sankar, S. Anbalagan, and P. N. Sudha. 2011. Adsorption of Cu(II) and Ni(II) ions from metal solution using crosslinked chitosan-g-acrylonitrile copolymer. *International Journal of Environmental Sciences* 1:1323–1338.

Renault, F., B. Sancey, P. M. Badot, and G. Crini. 2009. Chitosan for coagulation/flocculation processes—An eco-friendly approach. *European Polymer Journal* 45:1337–1348.

Reyna, R. R., S. Schwarz, G. Heinrich, G. Petzold, S. Schütze, and J. Bohrisch. 2010. Flocculation efficiency of modified water soluble chitosan versus commonly used commercial polyelectrolytes. *Carbohydrate Polymers* 81:317–322.

Rizzo, L., A. D. Gennaro, M. Gallo, and V. Belgiorno. 2008. Coagulation/chlorination of surface water: A comparison between chitosan and metal salts. *Separation and Purification Technology* 62:79–85.

Sabarudin, A., K. Oshita, M. Oshima, and S. Motomizu. 2005. Synthesis of chitosan resin possessing 3,4-diamino benzoic acid moiety for the collection/concentration of arsenic and selenium in water samples and their measurement by inductively coupled plasma-mass spectrometry. *Analytica Chimica Acta* 542:207–215.

Sahlia, M. A. M., S. Annouar, M. Tahaikt, M. Mountadar, A. Soufiane, and A. Elmidaoui. 2007. Fluoride removal for underground brackish water by adsorption on the natural chitosan and by electrodialysis. *Desalination* 212:37–45.

Saitoh, T., K. Asano, and M. Hiraide. 2011. Removal of phenols in water using chitosan—Conjugated thermo-responsive polymers. *Journal of Hazardous Materials* 185:1369–1373.

Saitoh, T., Y. Sugiura, K. Asano, and M. Hiraide. 2009. Chitosan-conjugated thermo-responsive polymer for the rapid removal of phenol in water. *Reactive and Functional Polymers* 69:792–796.

Sankararamakrishnan, N., A. Dixit, L. Iyengar, and R. Sanghi. 2006. Removal of hexavalent chromium using a novel cross linked xanthated chitosan. *Bioresource Technology* 97:2377–2382.

Sankararamakrishnan, N., A. K. Sharma, and R. Sanghi. 2007. Novel chitosan derivative for the removal of cadmium in the presence of cyanide from electroplating wastewater. *Journal of Hazardous Materials* 148:353–359.

Shanmugapriya, A., R. Ramya, S. Ramasubramaniam, and P. N. Sudha. 2011. Studies on removal of Cr(VI) and Cu(II) ions using chitosan grafted-polyacrylonitrile. *Archives of Applied Science Research* 3(3):424–435.

Shen, C., S. Song, L. Zang, X. Kang, Y. Wen, W. Liu, and L. Fu. 2010. Efficient removal of dyes in water using chitosan microsphere supported cobalt (II) tetrasulfophthalocyanine with H_2O_2. *Journal of Hazardous Materials* 177:560–566.

Shieh, J. J. and R. Y. M. Huang. 1998. Chitosan/N-methylol nylon 6 blend membranes for the pervaporation separation of ethanol-water mixtures. *Journal of Membrane Science* 148:243–255.

Singh, P., J. Bajpai, A. K. Bajpai, and R. B. Shrivastava. 2011. Removal of arsenic ions and bacteriological contamination from aqueous solutions using chitosan nanospheres. *Indian Journal of Chemical Technology* 18:403–413.

Singh, V., A. K. Sharma, D. N. Tripathi, and R. Sanghi. 2009. Poly(methylmethacrylate) grafted chitosan: An efficient adsorbent for anionic azo dyes. *Journal of Hazardous Materials* 161:955–966.

Sundaram, C. S., N. Viswanathan, and S. Meenakshi. 2008. Uptake of fluoride by nano-hydroxyapatite/chitosan, a bioinorganic composite. *Bioresource Technology* 99:8226–8230.

Sundaram, C. S., N. Viswanathan, and S. Meenakshi. 2009. Defluoridation of water using magnesia/chitosan composite. *Journal of Hazardous Materials* 163:618–624.

Szygu, A., E. Guibal, M. A. Palacin, M. Ruiz, and A. M. Sastre. 2009. Removal of an anionic dye (Acid Blue 92) by coagulation–flocculation using chitosan. *Journal of Environmental Management* 90:2979–2986.

Tao, Y., L. Ye, J. Pan, Y. Wang, and B. Tang. 2009. Removal of Pb(II) from aqueous solution on chitosan/ TiO_2 hybrid film. *Journal of Hazardous Materials* 161:718–722.

Thakre, D., S. Jagtap, A. Bansiwal, N. Labhsetwar, and S. Rayalu. 2010a. Synthesis of La- incorporated chitosan beads for fluoride removal from water. *Journal of Fluorine Chemistry* 131:373–377.

Thakre, D., S. Jagtap, N. Sakhare, N. Labhsetwar, S. Meshram, and S. Rayalu. 2010. Chitosan based mesoporous Ti–Al binary metal oxide supported beads for defluoridation of water. *Chemical Engineering Journal* 158:315–324.

Tran, H. V., L. D. Tran, and T. N. Nguyen. 2010. Preparation of chitosan/magnetite composite beads and their application for removal of Pb(II) and Ni(II) from aqueous solution. *Materials Science and Engineering C* 30:304–310.

Vasconcelos, H. L., V. T. Favere, N. S. Goncalves, and M. C. M. Laranjeira. 2007. Chitosan modified with Reactive Blue 2 dye on adsorption equilibrium of Cu(II) and Ni(II) ions. *Reactive and Functional Polymers* 67:1052–1060.

Viswanathan, N. and S. Meenakshi. 2008a. Enhanced fluoride sorption using La(III) incorporated carboxylated chitosan beads. *Journal of Colloid and Interface Science* 322:375–383.

Viswanathan, N. and S. Meenakshi. 2008b. Selective sorption of fluoride using Fe(III) loaded carboxylated chitosan beads. *Journal of Fluorine Chemistry* 129:503–509.

Viswanathan, N. and S. Meenakshi. 2009a. Synthesis of Zr(IV) entrapped chitosan polymeric matrix for selective fluoride sorption. *Colloids and Surfaces B: Biointerfaces* 72:88–93.

Viswanathan, N. and S. Meenakshi. 2009b. Enhanced and selective fluoride sorption on Ce(III) encapsulated chitosan polymeric matrix. *Journal of Applied Polymer Science* 112:1114–1121.

Viswanathan, N. and S. Meenakshi. 2010a. Enriched fluoride sorption using alumina/chitosan composite. *Journal of Hazardous Materials* 178:226–232.

Viswanathan, N. and S. Meenakshi. 2010b. Development of chitosan supported zirconium(IV) tungstophosphate composite for fluoride removal. *Journal of Hazardous Materials* 176:459–465.

Viswanathan, N., C. S. Sundaram, and S. Meenakshi. 2009a. Removal of fluoride from aqueous solution using protonated chitosan beads. *Journal of Hazardous Materials* 161:423–430.

Viswanathan, N., C. S. Sundaram, and S. Meenakshi. 2009b. Sorption behaviour of fluoride on carboxylated cross-linked chitosan beads. *Colloids and Surfaces B: Biointerfaces* 68:48–54.

Wang, L., Q. Li, and A. Wang. 2010 Adsorption of cationic dye on N,O-carboxymethyl chitosan from aqueous solutions: Equilibrium, kinetics, and adsorption mechanism. *Polymer Bulletin* 65:961–975.

Wang, X. P., Z. Q. Shen, F. Y. Zhang, and Y. F. Zhang. 1996. A novel composite chitosan membrane for the separation of alcohol-water mixtures. *Journal of Membrane Science* 119:191–198.

Wibowo, S., G. Velazquez, V. Savant, and J. A. Torres. 2005. Surimi wash water treatment for protein recovery: Effect of chitosan–alginate complex concentration and treatment time on protein adsorption. *Bioresource Technology* 96:665–671.

Wibowo, S., G. Velazquez, V. Savant, and J. A. Torres. 2007. Effect of chitosan type on protein and water recovery efficiency from surimi wash water treated with chitosan–alginate complexes. *Bioresource Technology* 98:539–545.

Wong, Y. C., Y. S. Szeto, W. H. Cheung, and G. McKay. 2003. Equilibrium studies for acid dye adsorption onto chitosan. *Langmuir* 19:7888–7894.

Yao, R., F. Meng, L. Zhang, D. Ma, and M. Wang. 2009. Defluoridation of water using neodymium-modified chitosan. *Journal of Hazardous Materials* 165:454–460.

Zeng, D., J. Wu, and J. F. Kennedy. 2008. Application of a chitosan flocculant to water treatment. *Carbohydrate Polymers* 71:135–139.

Zhang, L., Y. H. Zhao, and R. Bai. 2011. Development of a multifunctional membrane for chromatic warning and enhanced adsorptive removal of heavy metal ions: Application to cadmium. *Journal of Membrane Science* 379:69–79.

Zhou, L., J. Jin, Z. Liu, X. Liang, and C. Shang. 2011. Adsorption of acid dyes from aqueous solutions by the ethylenediamine-modified magnetic chitosan nanoparticles. *Journal of Hazardous Materials* 185:1045–1052.

Zhu, H. Y., R. Jiang, Y. Q. Fu, J. H. Jiang, L. Xiao, and G.M. Zeng. 2011. Preparation, characterization and dye adsorption properties of γ-Fe_2O_3/SiO_2/chitosan composite. *Applied Surface Science* 258:1337–1344.

Zimmermann, A. C., A. Mecabo, T. Fagundes, and C. A. Rodrigues. 2010. Adsorption of Cr(VI) using Fe-crosslinked chitosan complex (Ch-Fe). *Journal of Hazardous Materials* 179:192–196.

39

Industrial Applications of Marine Polysaccharides

S.N. Joshi, A.N. Bedekar, and P.N. Sudha

CONTENTS

39.1 Introduction

Marine poly-oligosaccharides have been found to have significant commercial importance to various industrial applications. These have been developed over the years with demand for improvements in material or process or performance of final desired product. Presently, many industrial applications of natural polymers and their derivatives are most fascinating and they are most investigated. For this purpose, biodegradable natural polymers such as polysaccharides and proteins find way into industries. The very nature of these oligosaccharides has been understood over the years, and applications are developed to reduce cost and better performance with the use of biodegradable material. The field of natural polysaccharides of marine origin is already large and however expanding rapidly. Seaweed is the most abundant source of polysaccharides such as *alginates, agar, and agarose as well as carrageenan,* while *chitin and chitosan* are extracted from exoskeleton of marine crustaceans. Such a wide variety of poly-oligosaccharides can be derived from plant or animal origin using chemical or biological methods. Advances in biotechnology have led the way to produce a couple of these polysaccharides in vitro using microorganisms controlling growth mechanism. Alginic acid, chitin, chitosan, agar, and carrageen are naturally occurring abundant and cheap marine polysaccharides. Paola (2010) and Steinbuckel and Rahee (2010) have recently reviewed applications of marine polysaccharides to pharmaceutical and food industry.

Production figures across the world are estimated to be increasing over the years. Table 39.1 gives approximate quantities of such industrially produced poly-oligosaccharides. Biopolymers have an advantage of being biodegradable, and these materials contain certain similar structural groups to natural extracellular components. The present review focuses on progress in discovering commercial applications of marine polysaccharides.

39.2 Chitin/Chitosan Polysaccharides

Chitin is the second most abundant polysaccharide in the world, dominated only by cellulose (Nishimura et al. 1991). Although chitin is found naturally in large amounts through many sources, chitosan is only found in some fungi with limited quantities. The chitosan used in industrial applications is typically derived from chitin through the use of chemical or enzymatic treatments of the shells of shrimp or crab secured from the waste products of the crabbing and shrimping industries (Duck et al. 2009). Structure of chitin and chitosan is shown in Figures 39.1 and 39.2, respectively.

TABLE 39.1

Worldwide Production Figures

Name	MT/Year
Chitin	>200,000
Agar	~9,000
Alginate	~26,500
Carrageenan	~50,000

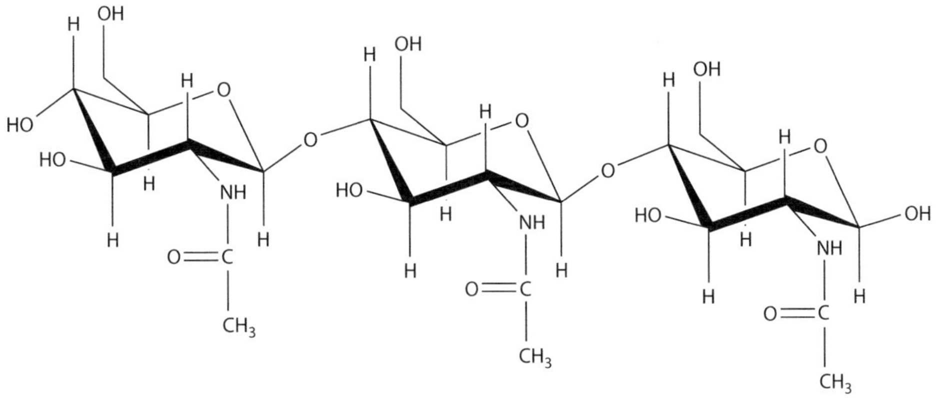

FIGURE 39.1
Structure of chitin.

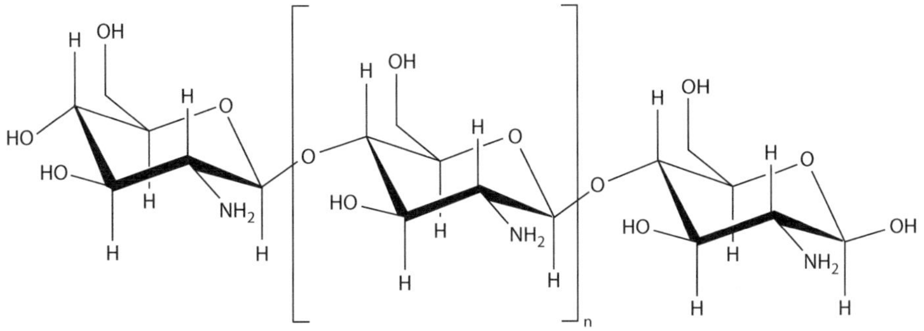

FIGURE 39.2
Structure of chitosan.

39.2.1 Water Treatment

Application of chitinous products in wastewater treatment has received considerable attention in recent years in the literature. In particular, the development of chitin- and chitosan-based materials as useful adsorbent polymeric matrices is an expanding field in the area of adsorption science. Groundwater/bore well water or even swimming pool water can be treated with oligosaccharides to reduce hardness and active/suspended particles. Today, there is growing interest in developing natural low-cost alternatives to synthetic polymers (Crini 2006). *The properties of chitin and chitosan enable them to attach to a variety of organic contaminants (bacteria, algae, urea, sweat), minerals, metals, and oil. Chitosan therefore dramatically increases the effectiveness of filtration systems, being sand or cartridges, which normally cannot capture fine particles and solved pollutant.* If these waste products are used for wastewater treatment, it not only increases the potential of applications but also reduces the environmental pollution caused by the disposal of these underutilized by-products (Sudha 2010).

Chitosan possesses interesting characteristics that also make it an effective biosorbent for the removal of color with outstanding adsorption capacities. Compared with conventional commercial adsorbents such as commercial activated carbons for removing dyes from solution, adsorption using chitosan-based materials as biosorbent offers several advantages.

The sorption of heavy metals from gold mining wastewater using chitosan was studied by Benavente et al. (2011). The results showed that the solution pH strongly affects the adsorption capacity of chitosan. It was observed that the greatest adsorption of Cu(II), Hg(II), Pb(II), and Zn(II) occurs at high pH, with an optimum adsorption pH of between 4 and 6. The Redlich–Peterson isotherm fits the experimental data well for Hg and Zn, while the Cu and Pb equilibrium data are best fitted by the Langmuir and Sips isotherms, respectively. The adsorption of the metals on chitosan follows the sequence Hg > Cu > Pb > Zn. Biolog-HEPPE AG, Germany, commercially produces such poly-oligosaccharides. Other companies producing chitin and chitosan along with their derivatives are Primex, Kreber, India Sea Foods, Mathani Exports, Quindou, Bannwach bioline, etc. It has been found that low molecular weight chitosan (CS) compounds do react much faster than high molecular weight ones.

39.2.2 Wastewater Engineering

Flocculating or coagulation agent for various industrial effluents wastewater is being commercially exploited. For example, electroplating, metalizing, dyes, biotechnology companies, food processing, and pharmaceutical industry let out large amounts of wastewater, which needs to be treated effectively. Oligosaccharides play an important role in treatment of such wastewaters from a wide variety of industry. It is eco-friendly as the complexes are generally biodegradable and does not leave any chemical substance behind as such. Sacco and Msotti (2010) and No et al. (2000) have shown such a wide range of industrial wastewater treatment applications.

The biopolymers have generally reactive group or groups at regular intervals due to their high molecular weight. This molecule generally scavenges various types of negatively charged ions to form a complex and either precipitates or remains in solution or even forms a film type structure. This material can be easily filtered off, and wastewater can be easily recycled for reuse. There are numerous companies in China, Thailand, India, and Vietnam which produce large quantities of chitin and chitosan products apart from Japan, the United States, Canada, Iceland, and parts of European countries.

Chitosan is well known also for its excellent biosorption for metal cation removal in near-neutral solutions because of the large number of NH_2 groups. The excellent adsorption characteristics of chitosan for heavy metals can be attributed to (1) high hydrophilicity due to large number of hydroxyl groups of glucose units, (2) presence of a large number of functional groups (acetamido, primary amino, and/or hydroxyl groups), (3) high chemical reactivity of these groups, and (4) flexible structure of the polymer chain (Crini 2005). The reactive amino group selectively binds to virtually all group III transition metal ions but does not bind to groups I and II (alkali and alkaline earth metal ions) (Muzzarelli 1985). Also, due to its cationic behavior, in acidic media, the protonation of amine groups leads to adsorption of metal anions by ion exchange (Guibal 2004). Hence, chitin, chitosan, and their grafted and cross-linked derivatives of the same are found to be highly efficient for dye removal, COD removal, and heavy metal removal thereby making it as an excellent material for treating industrial wastewater.

The removal of Cr (VI) ions from aqueous solutions has been investigated using nanochitosan (NC)/carboxymethyl cellulose (CMC) blend (Govindarajan et al. 2011). Chitosan-coated carbon was used for the removal of heavy metal chromium and found as a favorable adsorbent due to the synergistic action of both carbon and chitosan

(Souundarrajan et al. 2011). Kenaf dust-filled chitosan biocomposite was prepared for the adsorption of Cu (II) metal ion, and the maximum adsorption capacity of the composite was found to be around 232 mg/g (Annie Kamala Florence et al. 2011). The adsorption capacity of chromium (VI) metal ion onto the chitosan/starch binary blend in the presence of cross-linker glutaraldehyde was investigated and found very effective by Ramasubramanian et al. (2012). The functional groups on the biosorbent surface were found to play a role in the entrapment of the target chromium ions. Biosorbent used in this work is freely, abundantly, locally available, and expected to be viable for removal of chromium ion from aqueous solution. Chitosan with nylon 6 membrane was evaluated as adsorbent to remove copper and cadmium ions from synthetic wastewater. The results show that the process can be easily scaled up for the recovery of copper and cadmium from industrial wastewater without resorting to rotation to overcome mass transfer limitations (Prakash et al. 2012). The maximum adsorption of the heavy metals was favorable at acidic pH of the medium in all the abovementioned cases.

Oligosaccharides have been shown to be effective even in the treatment of radioactive waste (Moattanr and Haveripour 2004) and in the removal of low levels of radioactive substances with chitin + alginate combination. Particularly, it is suggested for cancer treatment of hospital sanitary wastewater, which may contain some traces of radioactive waste. Treatment of such wastewater with oligosaccharides is suggested to be effective in reducing concentration of radioactive substances, and there is no need to hold such wastewater for a long time until decay occurs. Due to its complex formation with biopolymers, the radioactivity can be immediately reduced in wastewater, which may be released as sewage water (Moattanr and Hayeripour 2004).

Food processing industrial wastewater has variety of substances from suspended particles, natural dyes, and even bioactive ingredients. These molecules can be made to react with biopolymers/chitosan at pH 5–7 to be removed by complexation followed by filtration. Such water may be recycled for reprocessing or gardening. The food processing industry needs large amount of water, and hence, it is imperative to conserve and reuse process water. German company BIOLOG-HEPPE producer of chitosan oligomers commercially supplies for such applications under trade name (HEPPIX).

39.2.3 Preservative and Biotechnology

Biopolymers have been shown to have specific application to preserve certain natural dyes. It is very specific and hence required to use with caution. Giri Dev (2000) has studied application to preserve natural Henna in its original color. At least 100 dyes, mainly anionic dyes, have been so far studied. Chitosan has an extremely high affinity for many classes of dyes. In particular, it has demonstrated outstanding removal capacities for anionic dyes such as acid, reactive, and direct dyes. This is due to its unique polycationic structure (Crini and Badot 2010).

Chitosan is used as a stationary phase for chromatography of various biomolecules, for example, proteins and saccharides. Porous beads are manufactured from chitosan by cross-linking and are available commercially in Japan—Chitoperl*—with a range of specifications, including chemically modified material. Other applications include chiral recognition, ion exchange, gel permeation, and affinity chromatography as well as immobilization of cells, enzymes, antibodies, or other polypeptides. Microbial and mammalian cells are also immobilized by encapsulation, often alginates as the negatively charged polymer component.

39.2.4 Biomedical Applications

Biomedical applications include a wide variety from *wound healing* to sustained drug release for special treatment of diseases and even for skin burn. Wound healing bandages have been developed and commercialized during the last 10 years or so. It is mainly using chitosan with medium to low molecular weight compounds. Films that are formed using this molecule have shown good oxygen permeability, moisture retention, and wound healing properties. These films are made in the form of bandage to form cuts/injuries. HemCon, a company in the United States, produces these wound healing bandages commercially. Marina Burkatovskaya et al. (2008) studied the effect of using HemCon® bandage in wound healing in mice. HemCon bandage is an engineered chitosan acetate preparation designed as a hemostatic dressing and is under investigation as a topical antimicrobial dressing. The effect of the bandage application on excision wounds that were or were not infected with *Staphylococcus aureus*, in normal mice or mice previously pretreated with cyclophosphamide (CY). Chitosan acetate bandage reduced the number of inflammatory cells in the wound at days 2 and 4 and had an overall beneficial effect on wound healing especially during the early period where its antimicrobial effect is most important. Chitosan film was used as a wound dressing in male Wister rats (Khan and Peh 2003). The results suggested that chitosan film treatment might have beneficial influence on various phases of wound healing such as fibroplasias, collagen synthesis, and contraction resulting in faster healing. It was possible that the enhanced healing of wounds in rats by chitosan film was a result of its stimulating activity and/or its capacity to stimulate fibroblast proliferation resulting in the progression of wound healing. It was also suggested that chitosan might induce fibroblasts to release interleukin-8, which is involved in migration and proliferation of fibroblasts and vascular endothelial cells (Mori et al. 1997).

New technique of *controlled drug release* agent have been tested and found to be effective using biopolymers or oligosaccharides. These are used as specific drug carriers for certain drugs, which need to be released for direct absorption into the blood and reach target organ. Many clinical trials are underway to make it effective, and it has been found to give positive results.

Blood cholesterol levels have been shown to be controlled by intake of chitosan in small dosages. It scavenges the cholesterol molecule, which gets excreted through the system. Chitosan as such is very inert and doesn't react with mild acidic conditions in stomach. It is therefore suggested to be safe to use; however, there are some scientific reports contradicting this argument (Dodane and Vilvalam 1998). Many supplements can help in the fat reduction process, including pyruvate and chitosan. Pyruvate, found in red apples, some types of cheese, and red wine, stimulates fat loss and boosts exercise performance. Chitosan attaches itself to fat in the stomach before it is digested, thus trapping the fat and preventing its absorption by the digestive tract (Sun et al. 2003). Hypercholesterolemia is an important risk factor for cardiovascular disease. Orally administered chitosan binds lipids in the small intestine and reduces their absorption. Chitosan has been shown to decrease serum cholesterol in animal and human studies (Bokura1 and Kobayashi 2003). When animals were fed for 20 weeks on a diet containing 5% chitosan or on a control diet, the blood cholesterol levels were significantly lower in the chitosan-fed animals throughout the study and at 20 weeks were 64% of control levels (Douglas et al. 1998). This study was the first to show a direct correlation between lowering of serum cholesterol with chitosan and inhibition of atherogenesis and suggests that the agent could be used to inhibit the development of atherosclerosis in individuals with hypercholesterolemia.

Biopolymers or the oligosaccharides have shown film-forming capability. It is this property that has been exploited to either alone or in composite form for *skin burn patients*. Such film or composite film can cover the skin till it is recovered; it even stops water oozing out from skin or loss of liquid from body. This kind of film can also prevent external contamination. This film can help tissue building faster and hence healing recovery process itself (Nicekraszewicz 2005). Polish company Tricomed on commercial scale produces various medical application devices. Wound closure requires a material that restores the epidermal barrier function and becomes incorporated into the healing wound (Tompkins and Burke 1996). Integra artificial skin is currently the most widely accepted synthetic skin substitute to be developed for use in burn patients. It was described originally by Yannas et al. (1980). Integra has a bilaminar structure, consisting of cross-linked bovine collagen and glycosaminoglycan, coated on one side with a silicone membrane that provides epidermal function. Chitosan SRT used is also shown to have similar inflammatory, angiogenesis, and tissue in-growth responses to Integra and could serve as an alternative to Integra and HSA as a skin substitute (Shah et al. 2011). Chitin is used as a dental filling, and the chewing gum and mouthwash containing chitosan are used as good candidate for oral hygiene.

To date, several immobilized enzyme-based processes have proved to be economic and have been implemented on a larger scale, mainly in the food industry, and in the manufacture of fine specialty chemicals and pharmaceuticals, particularly where asymmetric synthesis or resolution of enantiomers to produce optically pure products is involved (Wiseman 1993). The properties of immobilized enzymes are governed by the properties of both the enzyme and the support material (Tischer and Wedekind 1999). As enzyme immobilization supports chitin- and chitosan-based materials that are used in the form of powders, flakes, and gels of different geometrical configurations. Chitin/chitosan powders and flakes are available as commercial products among others from Sigma-Aldrich and chitosan gel beads (Chitopearl) from Fuji Spinning Co. Ltd. (Tokyo, Japan) (Barbara 2004).

Active immobilization of cells on inert supports enables facilitation of segregation of cells from the aqueous phase, and recovery of cells after a bioreaction is completed. To achieve cell immobilization, entrapment of cells within porous matrices appears to be the most desirable method. The polymers commonly used in such a preparation include agar, alginate, κ-carrageenan, polyacrylamide, and chitosan (Bickerstaff 1997).

39.2.5 Antimicrobial Applications

Face mask with antimicrobial coating is recommended in operation theaters, to support staff at hospitals or epidemic outbreak, or for biological control for the staff working on eventualities. Commercially, M/s Crosstex, a U.S. company, produces BIOSAFE facemasks for H1N1-type infection protection. Chitin and chitosan have excellent properties such as biodegradability, biocompatibility, and nontoxicity and have been shown to enhanced wound healing in animals and humans (Jayakumar et al. 2011).

Photo cross-linked electrospun mats containing quaternary chitosan (QCS) were efficient in inhibiting growth of Gram-positive bacteria and Gram-negative bacteria (Ignatova et al. 2007). These results suggested that the cross-linked QCS/PVP electrospun mats are promising materials for wound-dressing applications. A polyelectrolyte complex (PEC), which consists of chitosan as a cationic and γ-poly (glutamic acid) (γ-PGA) as an anionic polyelectrolyte, was developed as a wound-dressing material (Tsao et al. 2011). Chitosan/alginate composite membrane incorporated with ciprofloxacin HCl had the potential for wound-dressing application (Dong et al. 2010). Biocompatible carboxyethyl chitosan/poly(vinyl alcohol) (CECS/PVA) nano-fibers were prepared by electrospinning of aqueous CECS/PVA solution (Zhou et al. 2008) as wound-dressing material. Medical gear for doctors and paramedical staff who work very close to patients can wear this antimicrobial-coated fabric clothing while on duty/at workplace. Biological epidemic outbreak: Preventive measure for biosafety application for field staff who on their jobs.

Textile fabric coating applications have been developed mainly for medical applications. Swiss company SWICOFIL produces fabrics with chitosan fibers for various applications, such as sportswear and undergarments.

Optical instrument storages like microscopes, variety of analytical instruments, binoculars, etc., get affected by ingress of moisture and deposition on lenses, which makes the expensive instrument nonfunctional. When the instruments are preserved with biopolymer-coated fabric, moisture gets arrested and hence life of the instrument can be extended. It acts similar to silica gel bag application. Cameras and lens are expensive, and to increase life of such, it has been found to prevent moisture ingress and life and functional improvements. Hearing aid instruments can get wet due to body moisture and possible malfunction. When preserved with coated fabric, the instrument remains dry and life of small battery can be extended (Everest Biotech).

39.2.6 Agricultural Applications

Both chitin and chitosan have shown antiviral, antibacterial, and antifungal properties and are explored for agricultural applications. They have been used to control diseases or reduce their spread and to chelate nutrients and minerals preventing pathogens to access them or innate plant defense. Plant protection is a great concern all over the world due to infestation from pathogens. Recent review published by El Hadrami (2010) recapitulates properties and uses of chitin/chitosan and their derivatives on mechanism and plant–pathogen interaction. Fragments from chitin/chitosan have known eliciting activities leading to defense response in host plant in response to microbial infection including accumulation of phytoalexins, pathogen-related proteins, proteinase inhibitors, lignin synthesis, and callus formation. Other practical agricultural applications include antifungal treatment, spraying on the plants, additives to groundwater for water retention, seed coating, fruits preservation, and ripening again by coating on them.

Chitosan is often used for plant disease control as powerful elicitor rather than direct antimicrobial or toxic agent. Its direct toxicity remains dependent on properties such as the concentration applied, molecular weight, degree of deacetylation, solvent, pH, and viscosity. The degree of deacetylation defines number of active sites with which nucleophilic groups react, and viscosity provides environment that could extend duration and intensity of reaction.

Biopolymer-coated fabric application to agricultural products: Everest Biotech (2010) has patented such application for agriculture including postharvest management and industry (Everest Biotech). Sugar storage for a long time (>1 year) is a challenge due to hygroscopic nature. When packed with inner layer of coated fabric, storage life gets extended without lump formation. Flours of various grains do contain moisture that leads to microbial activity within a short time. Wheat, rice, and pulse flours are extensively used, transported, and stored for a long time. To extend life of such material is extremely important, and when packed with inner layer coated fabric, moisture is removed by the fabric and hence microbial activity gets reduced, thereby life of packed substance gets extended.

Postharvest management of essential oil herbage before oil extraction can be done very economically without loss of oil contents and production of good quality of oil, for example, patchouli, rosemary, and stevia. All such essential oils have significant industrial demand. Other types of spices such as ginger and cut onions can be dried without energy usage (drying tunnel/ovens). Grain storage for long duration without any microbial activity has been shown to be effective in very hot or humid climatic conditions. The fabric forms an inner layer for packing of 25/50 kg with outer cover of woven polypropylene sack.

39.2.7 Cosmetics Applications

Chitosan is found in wide variety in cosmetic items from creams and lotions to hair care products. Few companies however have developed and commercialized such products. Various molecular weights and concentrations have been used in combination to develop applications for skin care and hair care products (COGNIS Deutschland GmbH). The company produces various types of creams for both face and body including sunblock, aftershaves, and facial cleansers. Film-forming capability of chitosan has been utilized to make moisturizing creams or preventive sunblock lotion. The positive electrical charge and high molecular weight of chitosan make it act as a good moisturizer as it cannot penetrate the skin. The formulations containing chitosan are already in the market as skin care products in different brand names. Chitosan and hair are complementary to each other as chitosan is positively charged and hair negative. A clear solution of chitosan can increase the strength and smoothness of hair. Hence, chitosan can be used in shampoos, hair colorants, and rinses (Dutta et al. 2004).

Contact lens: These have to be biocompatible and should be capable of handling over a period of time. Attempts have been made to develop contact lenses using modified forms of oligosaccharides. Contact lens made from partially depolymerized chitosan are clear and tough and possess the required mechanical properties (Dutta et al. 2004). Meron Biopolymers and Chinese researchers have developed chitosan + gelatin composite as contact lens material (Xin-Yuan and Wei 2004).

39.2.8 Paper Technology

Cellulosic paper pulp and chitosan have resembling structure and are compatible with each other. Cellulose and chitosan monomers have very close structural properties except that the reactive –NH2 group is attached to chitosan molecule. Composites with cellulose/paper have been developed. Chitosan has been used as composite material to produce paper sheets for packaging applications. Hosokawa et al. (1990) have shown composite properties of paper are far more superior like tensile strength. Its high oxygen gas barrier capacity makes such paper suitable for packaging. Another packaging-related work has been done by Gaellstedt et al. (2005) by coating chitosan on packaging paper applications to improve quality and printability of paper. The ink gets fixed permanently, and quality of print is good and long lasting. Kuusipalo et al. (2005) have shown antimicrobial properties of chitosan-coated paper that can be best used for packaging fruits, vegetables, and other agro products.

Handmade paper: By incorporating small amounts of biopolymers in the paper pulp, it has been shown to improve tensile strength of the paper particularly for handmade/recycled paper.

39.2.9 Current Problems and Limitations

Chitin is a typical naturally derived biopolymer. Production of chitin on large is limited to availability of crabs and shrimps, which are potential resources with seasonal variations. These are either sweet water cultivated or directly obtained from open sea fishing activity. The natural material has to be processed in short time. There is variation in quality of chitin produced from different geographical location across the world. Value-added products derived from chitin can vary from batch to batch. It has been discussed in international forums, and standardization is being done to ascertain quality aspect. There are other issues related to environmental pollution due to usage of high alkali levels and its disposal; unless it is recycled however, cost of neutralization is high. There are also soluble calcium salts unutilized or discarded during the processing. Current production estimates are placed in Table 39.1.

39.3 Applications of Carrageenan

Carrageenan is a generic name for a family of polysaccharide. It is a sulfated linear polysaccharide extracted with water or alkali from certain red seaweeds of the *Rhodophyceae* class. They have been extensively used in food industry as thickening, gelling, and protein-suspending agents. All carrageenan fractions are water soluble, being insoluble in organic solvents, oils, and fats. It is a hydrocolloid that mainly consists of salts of sodium, potassium, and calcium or magnesium sulfate esters of galactose and 3,6-anhydro galactose copolymers (Therkelsen 2003). Carrageenan has a wide variety of applications. Chemical structure of carrageenan is shown in Figure 39.3.

39.3.1 Food Industry

In the food industry, carrageenans are widely utilized due to their excellent physical functional properties, such as thickening, gelling, and stabilizing abilities, and have been used to improve the texture of cottage cheese, to control the viscosity and texture of puddings and dairy desserts, and as binders and stabilizers in the meat-processing industry for the manufacture of patties, sausages, and low-fat hamburgers. The food industry accounts for 70%–80% of the total world production, estimated at about 45,000 MT/year, of which about 45% goes to dairy products and 30% to meat and meat derivatives.

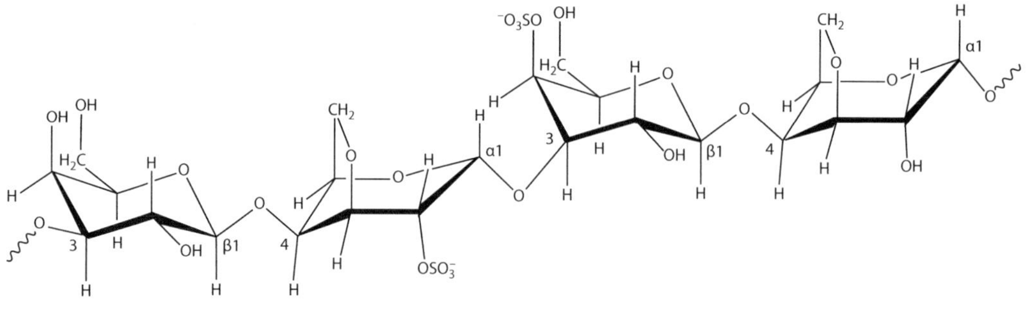

FIGURE 39.3
Structure of carregneenan.

39.3.2 Pharmaceutical Applications

In pharmaceutical industry applications, carrageenan is recommended as excipient in pills and tablets. It is used as emulsifiers for mineral oil and insoluble drugs (Urukpa et al. 2006). It is also recommended in medical applications for many anti-inflammatory drugs. Due to higher degree of sulfation, it is considered for drugs. They are also known for biological activities related to inflammatory and immune responses. Carrageenans are potent inhibitors of herbs and HPV viruses, and there are indications that these polysaccharides may suffer some protection against HIV infections. He et al. (1997) demonstrated that synthetic j-selenocarrageenans may inhibit the proliferation of breast cancer cells.

Hu et al. (2006) used kappa-carrageenases extracted from the marine bacterium Cytophaga MCA-2 to produce low molecular weight j-carrageenans. These derivatives showed much higher in vivo tumor inhibition than the parent compounds, and the observed weight increase of immune organs such as the thymus suggested that the antitumor mechanism of the carrageenan oligosaccharides may be initiated via organ-mediated defense reactions. These findings are complementary to the studies of Mou et al. (2003) in which depolymerized j-carrageenans were sulfate by the use of chlorosulfonic acid in formamide and the resulting oligosaccharides showed in vitro antitumor activity.

They are also suggested for sustained drug delivery for pharmaceuticals drugs that has been demonstrated by Bharadwaj et al. (2000) and Lazazarini et al. (2006). Grafting of j-carrageenan with methyl methacrylate was carried out by Prasad et al. (2006) employing microwave irradiation. The resultant crystalline product could be obtained rapidly (2 min). The copolymerization of j-carrageenan with acrylic acid and 2-acrylamido-2-methylpropanesulfonic acid led to the development of biodegradable hydrogels with potential use for novel drug delivery systems (Pourjavadi et al. 2007).

Since carrageenan was active against HIV only at concentrations about 1000 times higher than those required to inhibit papillomaviruses (Buck et al. 2006). However, carrageenans may serve as models for designing novel anti-HIV agents, improving their therapeutic properties through chemical modifications.

Porous nanocomposites were prepared by coprecipitation of calcium phosphates into a j-carrageenan matrix (Daniel-da-Silva et al. 2007), whose resulting porosity and morphology were suitable for application in bone tissue engineering. The association between carrageenan, nanohydroxyapatite, and collagen resulted in an injectable bone substitute biomaterial, suitable for bone reconstruction surgery (Gan and Feng 2006).

39.3.3 Enzyme Immobilization

The carrageenan hydrogels (grafting of kappa-carrageenan with methyl methacrylate) are very promising for industrial immobilization of enzymes since the immobilization procedures result in increases of the storage and thermal stability of the enzymes necessary for use in continuous systems (Tumturk et al. 2007). It is also considered for electrophoresis experiments.

39.3.4 Cosmetic Applications

Carrageenans are also extensively used in nonfood industry products such as cosmetics, printing, and textile formulations (Imeson 2000). They make toothpaste more stable, absorb body fluids, when formulated in wound dressing and interact with human carotene to give soft skin. They made hand lotion preparations smooth and are also recommended for shampoo formulations.

39.3.5 Water Treatment

By grafting of poly(*N*-vinyl formamide) onto j-carrageenan, efficient flocculants have been obtained, and they could be used for the treatment of coal wastewater. By incorporation of poly(*N*-vinyl formamide) graft onto j-carrageenan through graft copolymerization, the drag reduction effectiveness can be enhanced, and biodegradation can be minimized. All types of carrageenan have been extensively used for beverage clarification. It is added to beer or wine, which serves as fining agent by complexation with proteins. Filtration or centrifugation removes insoluble particles (Ruiter and Rudolph 1997).

In oil well drilling, carrageenan and other polysaccharides are used to increase the viscosity of drilling fluid. Increased viscosity enhances the carrying capacity of the fluid. Water-based paints and ink carry 0.15%–0.25% of carrageenan to increase thickness (viscosity), and for obtaining uniform flow properties, it is even used up to 0.8%. It is also used to suspend and stabilize insolubles in abrasive suspensions and ceramic glaze.

39.3.6 Current Problems and Limitations

Industry is at high competition over the years with price war, and further development has not progressed due to limitation of funding for R&D. It is competing today with pectin, and one finds that patents on pectin-related products/processes are at least 10 times higher than carrageenan applications.

39.4 Applications of Alginate

Alginate is a natural occurring polymer of guluronic acid and mannuronic acid, quite abundant in nature as structural component in marine brown algae and as capsular polysaccharide in soil bacteria. Brown algae biomass generally consists of mineral or inorganic/organic compound. The isolating process of alginate from brown algae biomass is simple, including stages of pre-extraction with HCl followed by washing, filtration, and neutralization with alkali. Sodium alginate is precipitated from solution by alcohol (isopropyl or ethanol) and usually re-precipitated (for high purity) in the same way. However, commercial scale production process is much complicated with large number of unit processes (Rowley et al. 1990). Chemical structure of basic alginate molecule is shown in Figure 39.4.

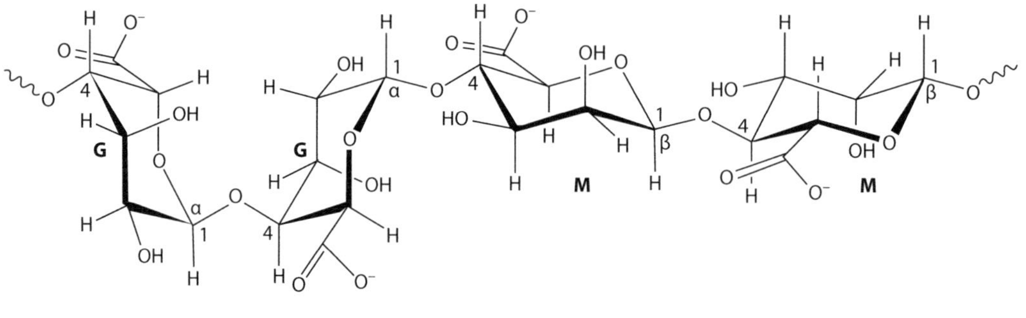

FIGURE 39.4
Structure of alginate

An interesting property of alginate is instantaneous formation of gel spheres at pH > 6 by ionotropic gelation with divalent cations such as Ca, Ba, and Zn, and for this, it is widely used for microencapsulation of drugs. On the other hand, at low pH, hydration of alginic acid leads to the formation of a high-viscosity "acid gel." The ability of alginate to form two types of gel dependant on pH, that is, an acid gel and an ionotropic gel, gives the polymer unique properties compared to natural macromolecules, and it can be tailor-made for a wide range of applications. Typical applications include the following.

39.4.1 Food Applications

Alginate with high guluronic acid contents contributes to some modification of appetite sensation but not food intake in healthy adults. As alginates are viscous dietary fibers, they would be expected to reduce intestinal uptake and potentially lower the glycemic response and/or cardiovascular disease risk. A number of previous studies have reported that alginates may reduce the activity of certain digestive enzymes within the upper GI tract. In vitro determination of protease activity under physiological conditions has suggested that low concentrations (<0.1%) of alginate reduce pepsin activity by up to 80% (Sunderland et al. 2000); they also have a small inhibitory effect on trypsin activity.

39.4.2 Pharmaceutical Applications

The conventional role of alginate in pharmaceutics includes serving as thickening, gel-forming, and stabilizing agents, as alginate can play a significant role in controlled release drug products.

Great attention has also been focused on biopolymer-based hydrogels for use as potential carriers in controlled drug delivery. Recently, much research efforts have been concentrated to develop calcium alginate beads loaded with various low molecular weight therapeutic agents. In various studies, alginate beads have been used as excellent vehicles. Polymethylmethacrylate (PMMA)-coated microcapsules of diclofenac sodium (DFS) were prepared by a modified water-in-oil-in-water (W1/O/W2) emulsion solvent evaporation method using sodium alginate as a matrix material in the internal aqueous phase. Their performance with respect to controlled release of the drug in simulated gastric fluid and simulated intestinal fluid was evaluated and compared with non-matrix microcapsules prepared by the conventional W1/O/W2 emulsion solvent evaporation method. The matrix microcapsules appeared to be suitable for releasing lesser amounts of DFS in simulated gastric fluid and providing extended release in simulated intestinal fluid (Pal et al. 2011).

Sustained release microparticles were successfully prepared by Chakraverty (2012) by employing ionotropic gelation technique where the natural water-soluble polymer, namely, sodium alginate prolongs the release of the drug norfloxacin. Chitosan-coated alginate microcapsules were developed as oral sustained delivery carriers for antitubercular drugs in order to improve patient compliance and to reduce dose/dosing frequency in the management of tuberculosis (TB), which otherwise demands prolonged chemotherapy. The microcapsules exhibited a slow and sustained release over a period of 72 h (Sabitha et al. 2010).

39.4.3 Protein Delivery

The protein drug market is rapidly growing, and various protein drugs are now available owing to the development of recombinant DNA technology. Alginate is an excellent candidate for delivery of protein drugs, since proteins can be incorporated into alginate-based formulations under relatively mild conditions that minimize their denaturation, and the gels can protect them from degradation until their release.

39.4.4 Wound Dressings

Alginate-based wound dressings offer many advantageous features. Traditional wound dressings (e.g., gauze) have provided mainly a barrier function—keeping the wound dry by allowing evaporation of wound exudates while preventing entry of pathogen into the wound (Boateng et al. 2008). In contrast, modern dressings (e.g., alginate dressings) provide a moist wound.

Blends of alginate, chitin/chitosan, and fucoidan gels have been reported to provide a moist healing environment in rats, with an ease of application and removal (Murakami et al. 2010). The addition of silver into alginate dressings also enhanced the antioxidant capacity (Wiegand et al. 2009). Alginate fibers cross-linked with zinc ions have also been proposed for wound dressings, as zinc ions may generate immunomodulatory and antimicrobial effects, as well as enhanced keratinocyte migration and increased levels of endogenous growth factors (Ågren and Wilkinson 1999).

39.4.5 Tissue Engineering

One of the first applications of alginate gels in tissue engineering involved the transplantation of encapsulated pancreatic islet allografts and xenografts in an effort to cure type I diabetes. Tissue engineering is a potential approach to provide hepatic tissues for replacement of a failing liver, and alginate gels encapsulating hepatocytes may offer a suitable platform for developing a bioartificial liver as they are easily manipulated and can be cryopreserved (Selden and Hodgson 2004; Koizumi et al. 2007).

39.4.6 Bone Tissue Engineering

Alginate has also been combined with inorganic materials to enhance bone tissue formation. Alginate/hydroxyapatite (HAP) composite scaffolds with interconnected porous structures were prepared by a phase separation method, which enhanced the adhesion of osteosarcoma cells (Lin and Yeh 2004).

39.4.7 Cell Culture

Alginate gels are increasingly being utilized as a model system for mammalian cell culture in biomedical studies. These gels can be readily adapted to serve as either 2-D or more physiologically relevant 3-D culture systems.

39.4.8 Nerve Repair

Alginate gels have also been investigated for the repair of the central and peripheral nerve systems. Alginate-based highly anisotropic capillary gels, introduced into acute cervical spinal cord lesions in adult rats, were integrated into the spinal cord parenchyma without major inflammatory responses and directed axonal regrowth (Prang et al. 2006).

39.4.9 Paper and Adhesive Industry

The main use for alginate in the paper industry is in surface sizing. Alginate added to the normal starch sizing gives a smooth continuous film and a surface with less fluffing. The oil resistance of alginate films gives a size with better oil resistance and enhances grease-proof properties. An improved gloss is obtained with high gloss inks.

39.5 Applications of Agar

Agar-agar is a phycolloid, which is constructed from complex polysaccharide molecules extracted from certain species of red algae. Agar and its variant contain also variable amounts of pyruvate and urinate substances. Agar as such is insoluble in cold water but readily dissolves in boiling water. Agar when dissolved in hot water and permitted to cool forms thermally reversible gel, without need of acidic condition or oxidizing agent. This characteristic gives agars the ability to perform a reversible gelling process without losing their mechanical and thermal properties. Agar forms a super gel with glutaraldehyde. Used as in enzymological studies in various applications like protein receptors, nitrogenous material fixation, and cross-linking with agarose to immobilize enzymes (Gupta 2000).

Chemical structure of agar is presented in Figure 39.5.

39.5.1 Food Applications

In the human food industry, agar is used mainly as a gelling agent and in a secondary way as a stabilizing agent and for controlling viscosity. It is used as an additive, not as a nutrient. In confectionery, it is used to prepare jellies, marshmallows, and candies or candy fillers. In bakery, agar is used to cover cakes and in icing doughnuts, and when it is applied to chocolate, it allows a good adherence to the base without cracking. Agar is also important in fruit jelly preparations. When compared with pectin, agar has the advantage of not needing high sugar concentrations to form a gel. In marmalade production, agar is used as a thickening and gelling agent.

39.5.2 Pharmaceutical Applications

In microbiology, agar is the medium of choice for culturing bacteria on solid substrate. Agar is also used in some molecular microbiological culture medium. Agar is typically

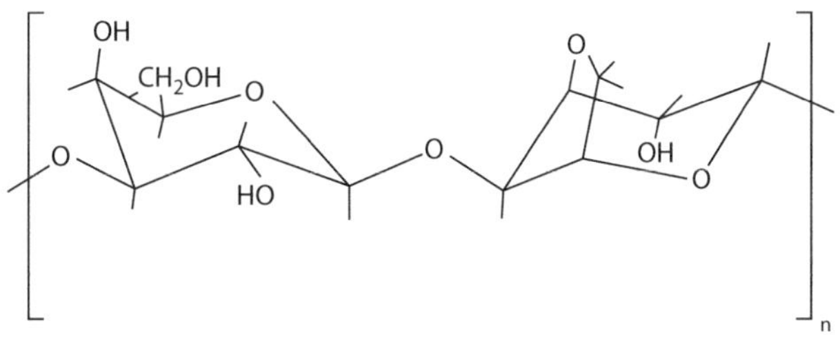

FIGURE 39.5
Structure of agar.

used in a final concentration of 1%–2% for solidifying culture media. Smaller quantities (0.05%–0.5%) are used in media for motility studies (0.5% w/v) and for growth of anaerobes (0.1%) and microaerophiles. Microbiology techniques to obtain DNA information (Dumitriu 1988). More recently, agar was used in a newly developed medium, that is, combined deactivators-supplemented agar medium (CDSAM), to evaluate the viability of dermatophytes in skin scales (Adachi and Watanabe 2007).

Agar beads instantaneously are formed by gelification. The results of dissolution and release studies indicated that agar beads could be useful for the preparation of sustained release dosage forms, although no many further studies have been developed (Bao et al. 2008).

Dental impression materials: Agar was first introduced into dentistry for recording crown impressions in 1937 by Sears. The commercial agar dental impression material can be managed by changing the gel into a sol with heat.

39.5.3 Biomedical Applications

Agar is used as an ingredient in the preparation of capsules and suppositories, in surgical lubricants, in the preparation of emulsions, and as suspending agent for barium sulfate in radiology.

Electrophoresis: Agar gel is the good medium for immunodiffusion and immunoelectrophoresis. As a substance for simple zone electrophoresis, that is, for separating a mixture into its components, agar gel is not quite so well known, though it has been used for this purpose for a long time. It has a number of special features; being a gel, zones will tend to be sharper and better separated than in powdery or fibrous media, though it has less resolving power than other gels like starch and acrylamide, which have more marked sieve-like properties. For certain purposes, agar gel is the medium of choice, for instance, the separation of hemoglobin F from A and for the separation of certain constituents of the immunoglobulin complex. Its transparency and ease of drying to thin film make agar gel suitable for storage, photography, and photometric scanning (Wiener 1965).

39.5.4 Enzyme Immobilization

Agar is an easily available and inexpensive matrix with easy immobilization procedure was used. Both the agarose and agar matrix proved to be a good support for the enzyme showing more or less about 75% immobilization by Prakash and Jaiswal (2011). The optimum pH of the immobilized enzyme was observed to be 7.0 showing its potential for use in detergent industries.

39.5.5 Other Industrial Applications

Agar is also used for clarifying beer, wine, or Japanese "sake." It finds applications in photographic stripping films and paper. It is used in solidified alcohol fuel, in dyed coatings for paper, textiles, and metals, in pressure-sensitive tapes, as flash inhibitor in sulfur mining explosives, as an ingredient in cosmetic creams and lotions, as corrosion inhibitor for aluminum, and for the action of nicotine as insecticide in plant sprays. Agar is mixed with shellac and wax for shoe and leather polishes.

References

Adachi M. and Watanabe S. 2007. Evaluation of combined deactivators-supplemented agar medium (CDSAM) for recovery of dermatophytes from patients with tinea pedis. *Med Mycol.* 45(4):347–349.

Ågren M.S. and Wilkinson E. 1999. Zinc in wound repair. *Arch. Dermatol.* 135:1273–1274.

Annie Kamala Florence J., Gomathi T., and Sudha P.N. 2011. Equilibrium adsorption and kinetics study of chitosan-dust kenaf fiber composite. *Arch. Appl. Sci. Res.* 3(4):366–376.

Araki C.1966. Some recent studies on the polysaccharides of agarophytes. *Proc. Seaweeds Symp.* 3:3–19.

Bao L., Yang W., Mao X., Muo S., and Tang S. 2008. Agar/collagen membrane as skin dressing for wound. *Biomed. Mater.* 3:044108.

Barbara K. 2004. Application of chitin- and chitosan-based materials for enzyme immobilizations: A review. *Enzyme Microb. Technol.* 35:126–139.

Benavente M., Moreno L., and Joaquin M. 2011. Sorption of heavy metals from gold mining wastewater using chitosan. *J. Taiwan Inst. Chem. Eng.* 339:1–13.

Bharadwaj T.R., Kanwar M., Lad R., and Gupta A. 2000. Natural gums and modified natural gums, as sustained drug release carriers. *Drug Dev. Ind. Pharm.* 26:1025–1038.

Bickerstaff G.F. (Ed.). 1997. Methods in biotechnology. In *Immobilization of Enzymes and Cells*, Vol. 1, pp. 1–11. Humana Press Inc., Totowa, NJ.

Bixler H.J. and Porse H. 2010. A decade of change in the Seaweed hydrocolloids industry, *J. Appl. Phycol.* 23:321–335.

Boateng J.S., Matthews K.H., Stevens H.N., and Eccleston G.M. 2008. Wound healing dressings and drug delivery systems: a review. *J. Pharm. Sci.* 97:2892–2923.

Bokura1 H. and Kobayashi S. 2003. Chitosan decreases total cholesterol in women: a randomized, double-blind, placebo-controlled trial. *Eur. J. Clin. Nutr.* 57:721–725.

Buck C.B., Thompson C.D., Roberts J.N., Muller M., Lowy D.R., and Schiller J.T. 2006. Carrageenan is a potent inhibitor of papillomavirus infection. *PLoS Pathog.* 2:671–680.

Burkatovskaya M., Castano A.P., Demidova-Rice T.N., Tegos G.P., and Hamblin M.R. 2008. Effect of chitosan acetate bandage on wound healing in infected and noninfected wounds in mice. *Wound Repair Regen.* 16(3):425–431.

Chakraverty R. 2012. Preparation and evaluation of sustained release microsphere of norfloxacin using sodium alginate. *Int. J. Pharm. Sci. Res.* 3(1):293–299.

Crini G. 2005. Recent developments in polysaccharide-based materials used as adsorbents in wastewater treatment. *Prog. Polym. Sci.* 30:38–70.

Crini, G. 2006. Non-conventional low-cost adsorbents for dye removal; a review. *Bioresour. Technol.* 97:1061–1085.

Crini G. and Badot P.-M. 2010. Starch-based biosorbents for dyes in textile wastewater treatment. *Int. J. Environ. Technol. Manag.* 12(2–4):129–150.

Daniel-da-Silva A.L., Lopes A.B., Gil A.M., and Correia R.N. 2007. Synthesis and characterization of porous kappa-carrageenan/calcium phosphate nanocomposite scaffolds. *J. Mater. Sci.* 42:8581–8591.

Dodane V. and Vilvalam V.D. 1998. Pharmaceutical applications of Chitosan. *Pharm. Sci. Technol.* 1:246–253.

Dong Y., Liu H.Z., Xu L., Li G., Ma Z.N., Han F., Yao H.M., Sun Y.H., and Li S.M. 2010. A novel CHS/ALG bilayer composite membrane with sustained antimicrobial efficacy used as wound dressing. *Chin. Chem. Lett.* 21:1011–1014.

Douglas J.O., Affiliations.

Duck W.L., Lim H., Chong H.N., and Shim W.S. 2009. Advances in chitosan material and its hybrid derivatives: A review. *Open Biomater. J.* 1:10–20.

Dumitriu S. 1988. *Polysaccharide: A Structural Diversity and Functional Versatility*, Marcel Dekker Publisher, New York.

Dutta P.K., Dutta J., and Tripathi V.S. 2004. Chitin, chitosan: Chemistry, properties and applications. *J. Sci. Ind. Res.* 63:20–31.

El Hadrami A., Adam L.R., El Hadrami I., and Daayf F. 2010. Chitosan in plant protection (review). *Mar. Drugs* 8:968–987.

Everest Biotech. Indian Patent 2938/CHE/2010.

Gaellstedt M., Brottman A., and Hedenqvist M.S. 2005. Packaging related properties of protein and chitosan coated paper. *Packag. Technol. Sci.* 18:160–170.

Gan S. and Feng Q. 2006. Preparation and characterization of a new injectable bone substitute-carrageenan/nano-hydroxyapatite/collagen. *Zhongguo Yixue Kexueyuan Xuebao* 28:710–713.

Giri Dev V.R., Venugopal J., Sudha S., Deepika, G., and Ramakrishna. S. 2009. Dyeing and anti-microbial characteristics of chitosan treated wool fabrics with henna dye. *Carbohydr. Polym.* 75(4):646–650.

Govindarajan C., Ramasubramaniam S., Gomathi T., Narmadha D.A., and Sudha P.N. 2011. Sorption studies of Cr (VI) from aqueous solution using nanochitosan-carboxymethyl cellulose blend. *Arch. Appl. Sci. Res.* 3(4):127–138.

Guibal E. 2004. Interactions of metal ions with chitosan—Based sorbents: A review. *Sep. Purif. Technol.* 38:43.

Gupta M.N. (Ed.) 2000. *Methods & Tool in Biosciences & Medicine*, Birkhauser Verlag, Basel, Switzerland. Non aqueous enzymology, pp. 37–50.

Holmes C.C. and Miller T.E. 1998. Dietary chitosan inhibits hypercholesterolaemia and athero-genesis in the apolipoprotein E-deficient mouse model of atherosclerosis. *Atherosclerosis.* 138(2):329–334.

He G., Cheng C., and Lu R. 1997. Studies on biological effects of kappaselenocarrageenan on human breast cancer cell line BCaP-37. *Zhonghua Yufang Yixue Zazhi.* 31:103–106.

Hosokawa J., Nishiyama M., Yoshihara K., and Kubo T. 1990. Biodegradable film derived from chitosan & homogenized cellulose. *Ind. Eng. Chem. Res.* 29:800–805.

Hu X., Jiang X., Aubree E., Boulenguer P., and Critchley A.T. 2006. Preparation and in vivo antitumor activity of k-carrageenan oligosaccharides. *Pharm. Biol.* 44:646–650.

Ignatova M., Manolova N., and Rashkov I. 2007. Novel antibacterial fibers of quaternized chitosan and poly(vinyl pyrrolidine) prepared by electrospinning. *Eur. Polym. J.* 43:1112–1122.

Imeson A.P. 2000. Carrageenans. In *Handbook of Hydrocolloids*, pp. 87–102, Philips G.O. and Williams P.A. Eds., Woodhead Pub. Ltd., Cambridge, U.K..

Jayakuman R., Prabaharan M., Sudheesh Kumar P.T., Nair S.V., Furuike T., and Tamura H. 2011. *Novel Chitin and Chitosan Materials in Wound Dressing, Biomedical Engineering, Trends in Materials Science*, Laskovski A.N. Ed., ISBN: 978–953–307–513–6, InTech, Available from: http://www.intechopen.com/articles/show/title/novel-chitin-and-chitosan-materials-in-wound-dressingdrug release agents

Khan T.A. and Peh K.K. 2003. A preliminary investigation of chitosan film as dressing for punch biopsy wounds in rats. *J. Pharm. Pharmaceut. Sci.* 60(1):20–26.

Koizumi T., Aoki T., Kobayashi Y., Yasuda D., Izumida Y., Jin Z.H., Nishino N. et al. 2007. Long-term maintenance of the drug transport activity in cryopreservation of microencapsulated rat hepa-tocytes. *Cell Transplant.* 16:67–73.

Kuusipalo J., Kaunisto M., Laine A., and Kellomäki M. 2005. Chitosan as a coating additive in paper and paperboard. *Tappi J.* 4:17–21.

Laurienzo P. 2010. Marine polysaccharides in pharmaceutical application: An overview. *Mar. Drugs* 8:2435–2465.

Lazazarini R., Maiorka P.C., Liu J., Papadopoulos V., and Palermo-Neto J. 2006. Diazepam effects on carrageenan induced inflammatory paw edema in rats. Role of nitric oxide. *Life Sci.* 78(26):3027–3034.

Lin H.R. and Yeh Y.J. 2004. Porous alginate/hydroxyapatite composite scaffolds for bone tissue engi-neering: Preparation, characterization, and in vitro studies. *J. Biomed. Mater. Res. Part B.* 71:52–65.

Miyazaki S., Nakayam A.M., Oda M., and Takada D. 2004. Chitosan & sodium alginate based bio-adhesives for intraoral drug delivery *Artwood. Biol. Pharma. Bull.* 17:745–747.

Moattanr F. and Haveripour S. 2004. Applications of Chitin & zeolite absorbents for low level radioactive liquid wastes. *Int. J. Sci. Tech.* 1(1):45–50.

Mori T., Okumura M., Matsura M., Ueno K., Tokura S., Okamoto Y., Minami S., and Fujinaga T. 1997. Effect of chitin and its derivatives on the proliferation and cytokine production of fibroblasts *in vitro. Biomaterials* 18:947–995.

Mou H., Jiang X., and Guan H. 2003. A kappa-carrageenan derived oligosaccharide prepared by enzymatic degradation containing anti-tumor activity. *J. Appl. Phycol.* 15:297–303.

Murakami K., Aoki H., Nakamura S., Nakamura S.I., Takikawa M., Hanzawa M., Kishimoto S. et al. 2010. Hydrogel blends of chitin/chitosan, fucoidan and alginate as healing-impaired wound dressings. *Biomaterials.* 31:83–90.

Muzzarelli R.A.A. 1985. Chitin. In *The Polysaccharides*, Vol. 3, pp. 417–447, Aspinall G.O. Ed., Academic Press, London, U.K.

Muzzarelli R.A.A 1998. Some modified chitosans and their niche applications. In *Chitin Handbook*, pp. 47–51, Muzzarelli R.A.A. and Peter M.G. Eds., European Chitin Society, Italy.

Nicekraszewicz A. 2005. Chitosan medical dressings. *Fibres Text. East. Eur.* 13(6) (54):16–18.

Nishimura S., Kohgo O., Kurita K., and Kuzuhara H. 1991. Chemospecific manipulations of a rigid polysaccharide synthesis of novel chitosan derivatives with excellent solubility in common organic solvents by regioselective chemical modifications. *Macromolecules* 24:4745–4748.

No H.K. and Meyers S.P. 2000. Review of environmental contamination of waste water. *Rev. Environ. Contam. Toxicol.* 563:1–28.

Pal T., Paul S., and Sa B. 2011. Polymethylmethacrylate coated alginate matrix microcapsules for controlled release of diclofenac sodium. *Pharmacol. Pharm.* 2(2):56–66.

Paola L. 2010. Marine polysaccharides in pharmaceutical applications—An overview. *Mar. Drugs* 8, 2435–2465.

Paul W. and Sharma, C.P. 2004. Chitosan & alginate wound dressing: A short review. *Trends Biomater. Artif. Organs* 18(1):18–24.

Perez-Perez C., Regalado-González C., Rodríguez-Rodríguez C.A., Barbosa-Rodríguez J.R., and Villaseñor-Ortega F. 2006. Incorporation of antimicrobial agents in food packaging films and coatings. In *Advances Agriculture & Food Biotechnology*, pp. 194–216, Gerardo R., Gonzalez G., and Torres-Pacheco I. Eds., Research Signpost Publication.

Prakash O. and Jaiswal N. 2011. Immobilization of a thermostable-amylase on agarose and agar matrices and its application in starch stain removal. *World Appl. Sci. J.* 13(3):572–577.

Prakash N., Sudha P.N., and Renganathan, N.G. 2012. Copper and cadmium removal from synthetic industrial wastewater using chitosan and nylon 6. Environmental Science and Pollution Research. Published online February 2012.

Prang P., Muller R., Eljaouhari A., Heckmann K., Kunz W., Weber T., Faber C., Vroemen M., Bogdahn U., and Weidner N. 2006. The promotion of oriented axonal regrowth in the injured spinal cord by alginate-based anisotropic capillary hydrogels. *Biomaterials.* 27:3560–3569.

Prasad K., Meena R., and Siddhanta A.K. 2006. Microwave-induced rapid one-pot synthesis of kappa-carrageenan-g-PMMA copolymer by potassium persulphate initiating system. *J. Appl. Polym. Sci.* 101:161–166.

Raheem, El Helw, El Said El A.Y. 1988. Preparation and characterization of alginate beads containing phenobarbitone sodium. *J. Microencapsul.* 5:159–163.

Ramasubramaniam S., Govindarajan C., Gomathi T., and Sudha P.N. 2012. Removal of Chromium (VI) from aqueous solution using chitosan—Starch blend. *Der Pharmacia Lettre* 4(1):240–248.

Rowley J.A., Madlambayan G., and Mooney D.J. 1990. Alginate hydrogels as synthetic extracellular matrix. *Biomaterials* 20:45–53.

Ruiter C.A. and Rudolph B. 1997. Carrageenan biotechnology. *Trends food Sci. Technol.* 8:389–405.

Sabitha P., Vijaya Ratna J., and Ravindra Reddy K. 2010. Design and evaluation of controlled release chitosan-calcium alginate microcapsules of anti tubercular drugs for oral use. *Int. J. Chem. Tech. Res.* 2(1):88–98.

Sacco D. and Msotti L.A. 2010. Application of chitosan flocculants to ground water treatment. *Mar. Drugs* 8:1518–1525.

Sears A.W. 1937. Hydrocolloid impression technique for inlays and fixed bridges. *Dent. Digest.* 43:230–234.

Selden C. and Hodgson H. 2004. Cellular therapies for liver replacement. *Transpl. Immunol.* 12:273–288.

Shah Jumaat M.Y., Ahmad S.H., Arman Zaharil M.S., and Hasnan J. 2011. Evaluation of the biocompatibility of a bilayer chitosan skin regenerating template, human skin allograft, and integra implants in rats. *ISRN Mater. Sci.* Article ID 857483,1–7.

Sharma D.N. Chapter 8.7, In *Chemical Science & Engineering*, BARC Highlights 71, in Water Chemistry for Nuclear Fuel cycle. "Nuclear effluent polishing by chitosan".

Souundarrajan M., Gomathi T., and Sudha P.N. 2012. Adsorptive removal of chromium (VI) from aqueous solutions and its kinetics study. *Arch. Appl. Sci. Res.* 4(1):225–235.

Steinbuckel A. and Rahee S.K. Eds. 2010. *Polysaccharides and Polyamides in Food Industry*, Wiley-VCH Publication, Weinheim, Germany.

Sudha P.N. 2010. Chitin/chitosan and derivatives for waste water treatment. In *Chitin, Chitosan, Oligosaccharides and Their Derivatives Biological Activities and Applications*, Kim S.-K. Eds., Pub. CRC publishers, Boca Raton, FL, ISBN 978–1–4398–1603–5.

Sun T., Xu P., Liu Q., Xue J., and Xie W. 2003. Graft copolymerization of methacrylic acid onto carboxymethyl chitosan. *Eur. Polym. J.* 39(1):189–192.

Sunderland A.M., Dettmar P.W., and Pearson J.P. 2000. Alginates inhibit pepsin activity in vitro; A justification for their use in gastro-oesophageal reflux disease (GORD). *Gastroenterology* 118:347.

Therkelsen G.H. 2003. *Carragenan in Industrial Polysaccharides & Their Derivatives*, pp. 145–180, Whistler R.L. and BeMiller J.N. Eds., Academic Press, San Diego, CA.

Tischer W. and Wedekind F. 1999. Immobilized enzymes: Methods and applications. *Top Curr. Chem.* 200:95–126.

Tompkins R.G. and Burke J.E. 1996. Alternative wound coverings. In *Total Burn Care*, 1st edn., pp. 164–172, Herndon D. Ed., WB Saunders, Philadelphia, PA.

Tsao C.T., Chang C.H., Lin Y.Y., Wu M.F., Wang J.L., Young T.H., Han J.L., and Hsieh K.H. 2011. Evaluation of chitosan/γ-poly(glutamic acid) polyelectrolyte complex for wound dressing materials. *Carbohydr. Polym.* 84(2):812–819.

Tumturk H., Karaca N., Demirel G., and Sahin F. 2007. Preparation and application of poly(N,N-dimethylacrylamide-co-acrylamide) and poly(N-isopropylacrylamide-co-acrylamide)/kappa-carrageenan hydrogels for immobilization of lipase. *Int. J. Biol. Macromol.* 40:281–285.

Urukpa F.O., Arntfield S.D., and L W T 2006. Network formulation of canola proteins k-carrageenan mixture as affected by salt, urea & lithouortol. *Food Sci. Technol.* 39:939–945.

Wiegand C., Heinze T. and Hipler U.-C. 2009. Comparative in vitro study on cytotoxicity, antimicrobial activity, and binding capacity for pathophysiological factors in chronic wounds of alginate and silver-containing alginate. *Wound Repair Regen.* 17(4):511–521.

Wiener R.J. 1965. *Agar Gel Electrophoresis*, p. 425, Elsevier, Amsterdam, the Netherlands.

Wiseman A. 1993. Designer enzyme and cell applications in industry and in environmental monitoring. *J. Chem. Tech. Biotechnol.* 56:3–13.

Xin-Yuan S. and Wei T.T. 2004. New contact lens based on chitosan + gelatin composites. *J. Bioact. Compat. Polym.* 19:467–475.

Yannas I.V., Burke J.F., Gordon P.L., Huang C., and Rubenstein R.H. 1980. Design of an artificial skin. II. Control of chemical composition. *J. Biomed. Mater. Res.* 14(2):107–131.

Zhou Y., Yang D., Chen X., Xu Q., Lu F., and Nie J. 2008. Electrospun Water-soluble carboxyethyl chitosan/poly(vinyl alcohol) nanofibrous membrane as potential wound dressing for skin regeneration. *Biomacromolecules* 9:349–354.

Commercial Organizations websites:

Bannwach Bioline (Bioline.co.th)

Biologe-Heppe.com

Cognis.com

Crosstex.com

Everestbio.com

Hemcon.com
Indiaseafood.co.in
Ivancic.com
Kreber.com.de
Mathanichitosan.co.in
Meronbiopolyers.com
Primex.com.is
Swicofil.com

40

Application of Enzymes from Marine Microorganisms

Xiujuan Shi, E. Song, and Chen Zhang

CONTENTS

40.1 Introduction

Marine microorganisms represent the most common source of enzymes because of their broad biochemical diversity, feasibility of mass culture, and ease of genetic manipulation (Niehaus et al. 1999). The world's oceans cover more than 70% of our planet surface; countless marine microorganisms contain biochemical secrets that can provide new insights and understanding of enzymes. Because the microbial enzymes are relatively more stable and active than the corresponding enzymes derived from plants or animals, marine microorganisms have been attracting more and more attention as a resource for new enzymes (Kin 2006).

With the recent advent of biotechnology, there has been a growing interest and demand for enzymes with novel properties. The diversity and complexity of marine environment might make the enzymes generated by marine microorganisms significantly different with homologous enzymes from terrestrial microorganisms. In recent years, researchers have isolated a variety of enzymes with special activities from marine bacteria, actinomycetes, fungi, and other marine microorganisms, and some products have already been used in industrial applications. Especially, some marine microbial enzymes have yielded a considerable number of drug candidates. A review of the enzymes in marine environment is presented.

40.2 Polysaccharide-Degrading Enzymes

40.2.1 Alginate Lyases

The brown alga is one of the largest marine biomass resources. Alginate has a wide range of applications; further, the degraded low-molecular fragment shows more potential. Alginate lyases, characterized as either mannuronate or guluronate lyases, a complex copolymer of α-L-guluronate and its C5 epimer β-D-mannuronate. They have been isolated from a wide range of organisms, including algae, marine invertebrates, and marine and terrestrial microorganisms. In recent years, the marine microbial alginate lyases have been greatly developed. Discovery and characterization of alginate lyases will enhance and expand the use of these enzymes to engineer novel alginate polymers for applications in various industrial, agricultural, and medical fields (Gacesa 1992).

40.2.2 Chitinase and Chitosanase

Chitin is widely distributed in nature as a biopolymer with nontoxic properties. It is the second most abundant natural biopolymer after cellulose in the nature and is the major structural component of most fungi cell wall and also quite abundant in the crust of insects and crustaceans. Chitin and chitosan have the similar chemical structure. Chitin is made up of a linear chain of acetylglucosamine groups. And chitosan is the deacetylated form of chitin. After hydrolysis, chitin and chitosan could enhance immune function, promote digestive function, and eliminate toxins from the body, even inhibit tumor cell growth and involve in other important physiological functions (Ngo et al. 2008). Therefore, hydrolysis of chitin and chitosan becomes a hot topic recently.

As the marine zooplankton is regularly supposed to shed, there is a large number of abandoned chitin, which could be a rich source of carbon and energy for growth and reproduction of chitin-degrading microorganisms. The total production of chitin in the whole marine biocycle is at least of 2.3 million metric tons per year (Charles et al. 1991). Until now, researchers have found a wide range of microorganisms, which can produce chitinase or chitosanase, including *Aspergillus, Penicillium, Rhizopus, Myxobacteria, Sporocytophaga, Bacillus, Enterobacter, Klebsiella, Pseudomonas, Serratia, Chromobacterium, Clostridium, Flavobacterium, Arthrobacter,* and *Streptomyces* (Fukamizo 2000).

40.2.3 Agarases

Agar is a highly heterogeneous polysaccharide. Neutral agarose is an alternating polymer of D-galactose and 3,6-anhydro-L-galactose linked by alternating β1 → 4 and α1 → 3 bonds. Agar oligosaccharides have a wide range of applications in food industry; it can be used for beverages, bread, and some low-calorie food production. Japanese use agar oligosaccharide as a moisturizing cosmetic additive that also has good hair conditioning effects (Yaphe and Duckworth 1972).

Nowadays, the acid degradation of agar is replacing by enzymatic degradation with the advantages of easy control and mild reaction. Agarase-producing bacteria were isolated from bacteria associated with seawater; agar-degrading microorganisms can be divided into two groups: bacteria soften the agar; the other violently liquefies the agar. Marine bacterial agarase has a high level of activity for the degradation of complex polysaccharides such as agar and agarose. In 1902, Gran isolated agar-degrading *Pseudomonas galactica* from seawater. Until now, from species within the genus *Cytophaga, Bacillus, Vibrio, Alteromonas, Pseudoalteromonas, Streptomyces*, researchers have found the presence of agarase (Parro et al. 1998).

40.2.4 Cellulose and Hemicellulose Hydrolase

Cellulose is an organic compound with the formula $(C_6H_{10}O_5)_n$, a polysaccharide consisting of a linear chain of several hundred to over ten thousand $\beta(1 \rightarrow 4)$-linked D-glucose units. Hemicellulose is a polysaccharide related to cellulose, and in contrast to cellulose, it can be derived from several sugars including glucose, xylose, mannose, galactose, rhamnose, and arabinose. Hemicellulose consists of shorter chains of around 200 sugar units. Cellulose is the maximum available saccharide in nature and is about 50% of all plant matter, and hemicellulose is about 20%–30%, while the remainder is mainly lignin (Klemm et al. 2005).

Cellulolysis is the process of breaking down cellulose through hydrolysis reaction into smaller polysaccharides called cellodextrin. Because cellulose molecules strongly bind to each other, cellulolysis is relatively difficult when compared to the breakdown of other polysaccharides (Brás et al. 2008). Until now, it was found that bacteria can produce cellulase, including *Cytophaga, Cellulomonas, Vibrio, Clostridium, Nocardia*, and *Streptomyces*, and for certain fungi, it was found that *Trichoderma, Aspergillus, Fusarium, Chaetomium, Phoma, Sporotrichum, Penicillium*, etc., are also able to produce cellulase. Hemicellulase generally refers to the hydrolase, which can hydrolyze polysaccharides, for example, xylanase, galactanase, and arabanase, among which xylanase has particular economic value (Tong et al. 1980).

Cellulase can be used for biotextile auxiliaries, cotton and linen product processing, and biofertilizer processing. With the rapid development of seaweed industry, a mass of waste release into the environment leads to very serious pollution problems. Cellulases degrade seaweed processing waste to low molecular fragments, which can be easily absorbed by plants as biofertilizer.

Xylanases are hydrolases depolymerizing the plant cell component xylan, the second most abundant polysaccharide. Xylanases could be produced by fungi, bacteria, yeast, marine algae, etc., but the principal commercial source is filamentous fungi. Xylanase could be used on semicellulose to produce products with high economic value, such as xylitol. In paper and pulp industry, using xylanase can improve the lignin dissolution rate and reduce the usage of Cl_2 and ClO_2, thereby reducing pollution and improving pulp properties. Xylanase also can degrade some polysaccharides in juice or beer; thus, it could contribute to beverage clarification (Brás et al. 1980; Doi 2008).

40.2.5 Carrageenases

Carrageenan or carrageenin is a family of linear sulfated polysaccharides, which are extracted from red seaweeds. 80% of the carrageenan is used in food and food-related industry, and it can be used as coagulant, adhesives, stabilizer, and emulsifier.

In addition, it also has been widely applied in pharmaceutical and cosmetic industries. The oligosaccharides obtained from carrageenan degradation showed a variety of specific physiological activities, such as antivirus, antitumor, anticoagulation, and so on (Roberts et al. 2007). As early as 1943, Mori extracted carrageenase from marine mollusk. Right now, *Pseudomonas*, *Cytophaga*, *Alteromonas atlantica*, *Alteromonas carrageeno vora*, and some unidentified strains have been found to possess the carrageenan-degrading enzymes. Sarwar et al., using carrageenan-containing medium, cultured *Cytophaga* lk-C783 and obtained extracellular κ-carrageenase with a molecular weight of 10 kD (Sarwar et al. 1987). In 2004, Mou et al. isolated an extracellular κ-carrageenase with a molecular weight of 30 kD from marine *Cytophaga* MCA-2 (Renner and Breznak 1998). A distinct λ-carrageenan-degrading *Pseudoalteromonas* bacterium (CL19) was isolated from a deep-sea sediment sample in 2006 by Yukari and Yuji; the molecular mass of this purified enzyme was approximately 100 kD (Ohta and Hatada 2006).

40.2.6 Other Polysaccharide Hydrolases

Amylases were found in bread making, and they can break down complex sugars such as starch into simple sugars such as glucose, maltose, and dextrin. They can be classified into α-amylase, β-amylase, and γ-amylase. Unlike the other forms of amylase, γ-amylase is most efficient in acidic environments. To date, researchers have found some terrestrial microorganisms, which can produce extracellular amylase, such as *Arxula adeninivorans*, *Lipomyces*, *Saccharomycopsis*, *Schwanniomyces*, *Candida japonica*, and *Filobasidium capsuligenum* (Gupta et al. 2003). With the development of marine science and technology, researchers reported more and more microorganisms from marine habitats capable of producing amylase. The marine yeast strain *Aureobasidium pullulans* N13d, producing an extracellular amylase, was isolated from the deep-sea sediments of Pacific Ocean (Li et al. 2007).

Fucoidan is a complex sulfated polysaccharide, constituted by fucose, galactose, xylose, mannose, arabinose, and uronic acid. The fucoidan oligosaccharide with molecular weight <1000 Da can be used as human epidermal keratinocyte activator, Furukawa purified fucoidanase, generated from marine *Vibrio*, and obtained three kinds of enzymes, which can hydrolyze substrate to small-molecule oligosaccharides (Furukawa et al. 1992). Yaphe and Morgan reported that marine bacteria *Pseudomonas atlantica* and *Pseudoalteromonas carrageenovora* were cultured in medium for 3 days by using fucoidan as the sole carbon source, with the substrate utilization as 31.5% and 29.9%, respectively (Yaphe and Morgan 1959).

Japanese researcher isolated *Bacillus circulans* from Tokyo Bay sea mud, which do not grow in conventional culture medium, but when the medium was properly diluted, it may grow and produce a new glucanase. This glucanase can act on α-1,3 bond and α-1,6 bond in glucan. From the marine *Bacillus*, a new glucanase has been isolated, which showed the optimum activity at 37°C, and this property is suitable for oral and other health care (Yahata et al. 1990).

40.3 Extremozymes

The marine environment is extremely complex, including the low-temperature, high-temperature, high hydrostatic pressure, strong acid, strong alkali, and a very poor nutritional conditions. An extremophilic microorganism is a microorganism that thrives in and may even require physically or geochemically extreme conditions that are detrimental to the majority of life on Earth. Extremophilic microorganisms are adapted to survive in ecological niches; they must adaptively change their physiological structure and metabolism in order to get adapted to the extreme environmental conditions.

Therefore, extremophilic microorganisms screened from these environments may have some specific physiological principle, which can produce unique biocatalysts that function under extreme conditions comparable to those prevailing in various industrial enzymes. Because of this reason, in recent years, research program about extremophilic microorganisms is very popular and became a new area of interest in microbial research (Niehaus et al. 1999).

There are some regions in the ocean. Microorganisms from these locales are commonly highly acidophilic or alkalophilic, and they can live in pH 5, even below pH 1 or over pH 9 conditions. Extracellular enzymes secreted these microorganisms that are commonly acidophilic enzyme (optimum pH < 3.0) or alkalophilic enzyme (optimum pH > 9.0). Compared with the neutral enzymes, the extreme pH enzymes show a good stability in environment; it is due to the particular enzyme molecule containing high proportion of acidic amino acids or basic amino acids. The enzymes produced by acidophilic or alkalophilic microorganisms could have wide application for compound synthesis in extreme pH conditions. In ocean, the average seawater salinity is about 3.5%, but in some regions it could be higher. A large number of salt-tolerant or halophilic microorganisms will survive in these high-salinity areas, and enzymes from halophilic microorganisms can maintain the stability at high salt concentrations (David and Michael 1999).

Near the deep-sea volcanoes, some microorganisms can survive in extreme conditions, even like the over 100°C temperature. Therefore, these microorganisms are supposed to have unique enzyme system, which can work in this high-temperature condition. For example, the nucleic acid enzymes, such as DNA polymerase, ligase and restriction endonuclease, have a significant application value in molecular biology research. Iundberg's group purified a thermostable DNA polymerase from thermophilic archaea (*Pyrococcus furiosus*), which has polymerizing and proofreading double functions, and it still has high activity even at 100°C. Hence, this polymerase can be applied in high-fidelity PCR experiments (Cowan et al. 1987). In 2008, a novel thermostable nonspecific nuclease from thermophilic bacteriophage GBSV1 was isolated by Song's group, and this nonspecific nuclease can degrade various nucleic acids, including RNA, single-stranded DNA, and double-stranded DNA (Song and Zhang 2008).

Algoriphagus, Psychrotrophs, and other low-temperature microorganisms have obvious advantages in the ecology. The low-temperature microorganisms cannot readily be involved in contamination. Their culture condition is simple, and the enzymes from these microorganisms have high enzyme activity and high-catalytic-efficiency advantages. Hence, with the assistance of low-temperature microbial enzymes, it can greatly shorten the processing time and save the expensive heating/cooling system, thus saving considerable energy. Cold-adapted enzymes from marine microorganisms, especially the lipase and protease, have considerable potential, particularly in cleaning industry. Many studies have shown that Antarctic marine bacteria about 77% are resistant to cold environment and 23% are addicted to cold environment. Because of unique geography and climate characteristics in Antarctica, it forms a dry, bitterly cold, strong radiation environment, in which microorganisms have to survive with the corresponding unique molecular mechanism, physiological and biochemical characteristics. For these reasons, the Antarctic marine bacteria are thought to produce new bioactive substances with significant potential (Kano et al. 1997). In 1994, Feller screened α-amylase-generating bacteria *Alteromonas haloplanktis* from Antarctic, which can grow well at 4°C; however, cell proliferation and enzyme secretion would be suppressed at 18°C; meanwhile, at 0°C–30°C, the activity of this α-amylase is seven times higher than α-amylases from homeothermic animals (Feller et al. 1994). Kolenc transferred TOL plasmid pWWO of mesophilie *Psychrotrophs putida* PaW1 to the psychrotroph *Psychrotrophs putida* Q5. Expression of the genes was shown that the transconjugant had the capacity to degrade and utilize toluate (1000 mg/L) as a sole source of carbon at temperatures as low as 0°C (Kolenc et al. 1988). Transferring the useful gene from mesophilic microorganisms to psychrophilic ones was established to promote low-temperature microbial biological feature, which may have enormous potential in removing pollution in cold environment.

Studies have shown hydrostatic pressure can obviously promote the enzyme thermal stability. Generally, enzymes have a good 3D specificity under hydrostatic pressure, but when pressure exceeds to a certain range, the enzyme's weak bond could be easily destroyed, thereby leading to the disintegration of the enzyme conformation. The deep sea is regarded as an extreme environment with conditions of high hydrostatic pressure. Enzymes from deep-sea microorganisms are thought to have characteristic pressure-adaptation mechanisms in structure and function, and they can be utilized in high-hydrostatic-pressure environment without disintegration. Microorganisms obtained from deep-sea environment appear to be an important source of modern enzyme industries. The first barophilic bacteria has been isolated from a deep-sea sample and has been found to grow optimally at about 500 bars and 2°C–4°C in 1979. Japanese scientists isolated multiple strains of bacteria addicted to pressure from the marine environment and found that the in vivo genes, proteins, and enzymes in the deep sea still have a high ability. The discovery and research of the marine barophilic microorganisms provide a good foundation for further development on extreme enzymes.

40.4 Protease

Total protease sales represent more than 60% of all industrial enzyme sales in the world. In modern society, the protease share widely applications in detergent industry, leather industry, and also proteases could be used for pharmaceutical applications, such as digestive drugs, anti-inflammatory drugs (Ilona and Zdzislaw 2007). In 1960, Dane first got alkaline protease from *Bacillus licheniformis*. So far, it still has been found that microorganisms are the most suitable resources for protease production. In 1972, Nobou Kato got a new type of alkaline protease from marine *Psychrobacter*, after quite a few proteases continually are obtained from marine microorganisms. Qiu et al., from the seawater, mud, fish, and other samples, selected 30 kinds of marine bacteria; after UV mutagenesis, they got N1-35 strain, and this strain produced protease compared with the terrestrial ones that have significant advantages (Graham et al. 1980). A yeast strain (*Aureobasidium pullulans*) with high yield of alkaline protease was isolated from sea saltern of China Yellow Sea by Chi et al. in 2007, and the maximum production of enzyme was 623.1 U/mg protein (7.2 U/mL) (Chi et al. 2007). In 2009, *Bacillus mojavensis* A21 producing alkaline proteases was isolated from seawater by Haddar et al., and they purified two detergent stable alkaline serine proteases (BM1 and BM2) from this strain. Both proteases showed high stability toward nonionic surfactants. In addition, both of them showed excellent stability and compatibility with a wide range of commercial liquid and solid detergents (Haddar et al. 2009).

40.5 Lipase

Lipases are ubiquitous enzymes that catalyze the breakdown of fats and oils with subsequent release of free fatty acids, diacylglycerols, monoglycerols, and glycerol (Babu et al. 2008). Lipases have received considerable attention in recent years, as evidenced by the increasing amount of information about lipases in the current literature. The majority of microbial lipases are used in detergents, paper production, cosmetic production, food flavoring, organic synthesis, and some other industrial applications. With marine resource exploitation, the pelagic fishes have become the primary target of fishery. However, human have to face the certain difficulties for fish preservation, processing, and marketing. Compared with traditional methods, using lipases has incomparable advantages. Therefore, applications of lipases in the fish-processing field are causing growing concern (Kojima and Shimizu 2003).

40.6 Prospects

The twenty-first century is the century of ocean, and the ocean is a vast treasure of human life. Recently, most countries face similar problems such as high population, resource consumption, and pollution. Meanwhile, the marine biological progress and development would give another option to human. Marine microbial enzymes, especially marine extreme microbial enzyme applications, have become more and more important.

Because enzymes have unequaled advantages, many industries are keenly interested in adapting enzymatic methods to the requirements of their processes. Clinical application of enzymes has been developing also. For example, surgeons used proteolytic enzymes for debridement of wounds, and promising clinical results have been reported by injection of certain enzymes such as streptokinase, crystalline trypsin, and chymotrypsin. Since increased therapeutic use of enzymes, presently unpredictable, rapid advances in this field may be expected (Underkofler et al. 1958). Uses of enzymes have increased greatly during the past few years. Prospects are excellent for continuing increased usage of presently available enzymes in present applications and in new uses and of new enzymes for many purposes. And also some new field, like metagenomics, offers a powerful lens for viewing the microbial world that may have the potential to revolutionize understanding of the marine microbial enzymes. Japan constantly increases its support to marine microbial enzyme research, and from 1992, the Japanese government made a series of marine microorganisms and planned to discover and clone proteins or enzymes with some special activity. In addition, Canada, Spain, Finland, and Russia and other countries have also stepped up on marine bioenzyme research.

Collectively, due to marine biological diversity and specificity of biological metabolism, the study of a global scale is still just beginning, but it has a huge potential for development and applications with industrial benefits.

Acknowledgments

This study was supported by a grant from National Natural Science Foundation of China (grant number 81100673) and a grant from Marine Bioprocess Research Center of the Marine Biotechnology program funded by the Ministry of Land, Transport and Maritime, Republic of Korea.

References

Babu, J., Pramod, W.R., George, T. 2008. Cold active microbial lipases: Some hot issues and recent developments. *Biotechnology Advances* 26: 457–470.

Brás, N.F., Cerqueira, N.M.F.S.A., Fernandes, P.A., Ramos, M.J. 2008. Carbohydrate binding modules from family 11: Understanding the binding mode of polysaccharides. *International Journal of Quantum Chemistry* 108: 2030–2040.

Charles, J., Marie F. Voss-Foucart. 1991. Chitin biomass and production in the marine environment. *Biochemical Systematics and Ecology* 19: 347–356.

Chi, Z.M., Ma, C., Wang, P., Li, H.F. 2007. Optimization of medium and cultivation conditions for alkaline protease production by the marine yeast *Aureobasidium pullulans*. *Bioresource Technology* 98: 534–538.

Cowan, D.A., Smolenski, K.A., Daniel, R.M., Morgan, H.W. 1987. An extremely thermostable extracellular proteinase from a strain of the archaebacterium Desulfurococcus growing at 88°C. *Biochemical Journal* 247: 121–133.

David, W.H., Michael, J.D. 1999. Extremozymes. *Current Opinion in Chemical Biology* 3: 39–46.

Doi, R.H. 2008. Cellulases of mesophilic microorganisms: Cellulosome and noncellulosome producers. *Annals of the New York Academy of Sciences* 1125: 267–279.

Feller, G., Payan, F., Theys, M. 1994. Stability and structural analysis of α-amylase from the antarctic psychrophile Alteromonas haloplanctis A23. *European Journal of Biochemistry* 222: 441–447.

Fukamizo, T. 2000. Chitinolytic enzymes: Catalysis, substrate binding, and their application. *Current Protein and Peptide Science* 1: 105–124.

Furukawa, S.I., Fujikawa, T., Koga, D. 1992. Purification and some properties of exo-type fucoidanases from *Vibrio* sp. N-5. *Bioscience, Biotechnology, and Biochemistry* 56: 1829–1834.

Gacesa, P. 1992. Enzymatic degradation of alginates. *International Journal of Biochemistry* 24: 545–552.

Graham, C.R., David, R.W., Frank, T.R. 1980. Peptone induction and rifampin-insensitive collagenase production by *Vibrio alginolyticus*. *Journal of Bacteriology* 142: 447–454.

Gupta, R., Gigras, P., Mohapatra, H., Goswami, V.K., Chauhan, B. 2003. Microbial α-amylases: A biotechnological perspective. *Process Biochemistry* 38: 1599–1616.

Haddar, A., Agrebi, R., Bougatef, A., Hmidet, N., Sellami-Kamoun, A., Nasri, M. 2009. Two detergent stable alkaline serine-proteases from *Bacillus mojavensis*A21: Purification, characterization and potential application as a laundry detergent additive. *Bioresource Technology* 100: 3366–3373.

Ilona, K., Zdzislaw, E.S. 2007. Neutral and alkaline muscle proteases of marine fish and invertebrates a review. *Journal of Food Biochemistry* 20: 349–364.

Kano, H., Taguchi, S., Momose, H. 1997. Cold adaptation of a mesophilic serine protease, subtilisin, by in vitro random mutagenesis. *Applied Microbiology and Biotechnology* 47: 46–51.

Kin, S.L. 2006. Discovery of novel metabolites from marine actinomycetes. *Current Opinion in Microbiology* 9: 245–251.

Klemm, D., Heublein, B., Fink, H.P., Bohn, A. 2005. Cellulose: Fascinating biopolymer and sustainable raw material. *ChemInform* 22: 3358–3393.

Kojima, Y., Shimizu, S. 2003. Purification and characterization of the lipase from *Pseudomonas fluorescens* HU380. *Journal of Bioscience and Bioengineering* 96: 219–226.

Kolenc, R.J., Inniss, W.E., Glick, B.R. 1988. Transfer and expression of mesophilic plasmid-mediated degradative capacity in a psychrotrophic bacterium. *Environmental Microbiology* 54: 638–641.

Li, H.F., Chi, Z.M., Wang, X.H., Ma, C.L. 2007. Amylase production by the marine yeast *Aureobasidium pullulans* N13d. *Journal of Ocean University of China* 6: 61–66.

Ngo, D.N., Qian, Z.J., Je, J.Y., Kim, M.M., Kim, S.K. 2008. Aminoethyl chitooligosaccharides inhibit the activity of angiotensin converting enzyme. *Process Biochemistry* 43: 119–123.

Niehaus, F., Bertoldo, C., Kähler, M., Antranikian, G. 1999. Extremophiles as a source of novel enzymes for industrial application. *Applied Microbiology and Biotechnology* 51: 711–729.

Ohta, Y., Hatada, Y. 2006. A novel enzyme, lambda-carrageenase, isolated from a deep-sea bacterium. *Journal of Biochemistry* 140: 475–481.

Parro, V., Mellado, R.P., Harwood, C.R. 1998. Effects of phosphate limitation on agarase production by *Streptomyces lividans* TK21. *FEMS Microbiology Letters* 158: 107–113.

Renner, M.J., Breznak, J.A. 1998. Purification and properties of ArfI, an α-L-arabinofuranosidase from *Cytophaga xylanolytica*. *Applied and Environmental Microbiology* 64: 43–52.

Roberts, J.N., Christopher, B.B., Cynthia, D.T., Rhonda, K., Marcelino, B., Peter, L.C., Douglas, R.L., John, T.S. 2007. Genital transmission of HPV in a mouse model is potentiated by nonoxynol-9 and inhibited by carrageenan. *Nature Medicine* 13: 857–861.

Sarwar, G., Matoyoshi, S., Oda, H. 1987. Purification of a α-carrageenan from marine Cytophaga species. *Microbiology and Immunology* 31: 869–877.

Song, Q., Zhang, X.B. 2008. Characterization of a novel non-specific nuclease from thermophilic bacteriophage GBSV1. *BMC Biotechnology* 8: 43.

Tong, C.C., Cole, A.L., Shepherd M.G. 1980. Purification and properties of the cellulases from the thermophilic fungus *Thermoascus aurantiacus*. *Biochemical Journal* 191: 83–94.

Underkofler, L.A., Barton, R.R., Rennert, S.S. 1958. Production of microbial enzymes and their applications. *Applied Microbiology* 6: 212–221.

Yahata, N., Watanabe, T., Nakamura, Y., Yamamoto, Y., Kamimiya, S., Tanaka, H. 1990. Structure of the gene encoding beta-1,3-glucanase A1 of *Bacillus circulans* WL-12. *Gene* 86: 113–117.

Yaphe, W., Duckworth, M. 1972. The relationship between structures and biological properties of agars. In *Proceedings of the 7th International Seaweed Symposium*, Sappora, Japan, pp. 15–22.

Yaphe, W., Morgan, K. 1959. Enzymatic hydrolysis of fucoidan by Pseudomonas atlantica and Pseudomonas carrageenovora. *Nature* 183: 761–762.

Index

For Product Safety Concerns and Information please contact our
EU representative GPSR@taylorandfrancis.com Taylor & Francis
Verlag GmbH, Kaufingerstraße 24, 80331 München, Germany